The Science and Treatment of Psychological Disorders

Sixteenth Edition

ANN M. KRING
University of California, Berkeley

SHERI L. JOHNSON
University of California, Berkeley

Vice President: Amanda Miller
Editorial Director: Justin Jeffryes
Executive Editor: Glenn Wilson
Senior Managing Editor: Judy Howarth
Senior Editorial Assistant: Kelly Gomez

Creative Product Design Lead: Jon Boylan
Senior Creative Product Designer: Thomas Nery
Senior Manager, Content Enablement & Operations: Simon Eckley
Cover Photo: © imaginima/Getty Images

This book was typeset in 9.5/12 STIX Two Text at Lumina Datamatics.

Wiley is a global leader in research and education, unlocking human potential by enabling discovery, powering education, and shaping workforces. For over 200 years, Wiley has fueled the world's knowledge ecosystem. Today, our high-impact content, platforms, and services help researchers, learners, institutions, and corporations achieve their goals in an ever-changing world. Visit us at Wiley.com.

Readers should be aware that websites listed in this work may have changed or disappeared between when this work was written and when it is read. Neither the publisher nor authors shall be liable for any loss of profit or any other commercial damages, including but not limited to special, incidental, consequential, or other damages.

Evaluation copies are provided to qualified academics and professionals for review purposes only, for use in their courses during the next academic year. These copies are licensed and may not be sold or transferred to a third party. Upon completion of the review period, please return the evaluation copy to Wiley. Return instructions and a free of charge return shipping label are available at www.wiley.com/go/returnlabel. If you have chosen to adopt this textbook for use in your course, please accept this book as your complimentary desk copy. Outside of the United States, please contact your local representative.

EPUB ISBN: 978-1-394-22170-7

The inside back cover will contain printing identification and country of origin if omitted from this page. In addition, if the ISBN on the cover differs from the ISBN on this page, the one on the cover is correct.

Library of Congress Cataloging-in-Publication Data

Names: Kring, Ann M., author. | Johnson, Sheri L., author.
Title: The science and treatment of psychological disorders / Ann M. Kring, University of California, Berkeley, Sheri L. Johnson, University of California, Berkeley.
Other titles: Abnormal psychology
Description: Sixteenth edition. | [Hoboken, NJ] : Wiley, [2024] | Preceded by: Abnormal psychology / Ann M. Kring and Sheri L. Johnson. DSM-5-TR update, fifteenth edition. [2022]. | Includes bibliographical references and index.
Identifiers: LCCN 2024008995 (print) | LCCN 2024008996 (ebook) | ISBN 9781394221752 (paperback) | ISBN 9781394221714 (adobe pdf) | ISBN 9781394221707 (epub)
Subjects: LCSH: Psychology, Pathological.
Classification: LCC RC454 .A244 2024 (print) | LCC RC454 (ebook) | DDC 616.89—dc23/eng/20240327
LC record available at https://lccn.loc.gov/2024008995
LC ebook record available at https://lccn.loc.gov/2024008996

Printed in the United States of America.

SKY10082219_081724

To

Angela Hawk

Daniel Rose, Robert Sangster, and Vickie Davis

About the Authors

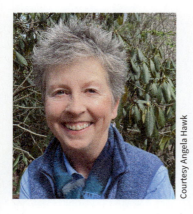

Courtesy Angela Hawk

ANN M. KRING is Professor of Psychology at the University of California at Berkeley. She received her B.S. from Ball State University and her M.A. and Ph.D. from the State University of New York at Stony Brook. Her internship in clinical psychology was completed at Bellevue Hospital and Kirby Forensic Psychiatric Center, both in New York. From 1991 to 1998, she taught at Vanderbilt University. She joined the faculty at UC Berkeley in 1999, served two terms as Director of the Clinical Science Program and Psychology Clinic, and was Chair of the Psychology Department from 2015 to 2020. She received a Distinguished Teaching Award from UC Berkeley in 2008. She was elected President of the Society for Research in Psychopathology and President of the Society for Affective Science. She is a past member of the Board of Directors of the Association for Psychological Science.

She was given a Young Investigator Award by the National Alliance for Research on Schizophrenia and Depression (NARSAD) and the Joseph Zubin Memorial Fund Award in recognition of her research on schizophrenia. She is a fellow of the American Association for the Advancement of Science, the Association for Psychological Science, the Society for Experimental Psychologists, and the Society for Personality and Social Psychology. Her research has been supported by grants from the Scottish Rite Schizophrenia Research Program, NARSAD, and the National Institute of Mental Health. She is co-editor (with Denise Sloan) of *Emotion Regulation and Psychopathology* (Guilford Press) and co-author (with Janelle Caponigro, Erica Lee, and Sheri Johnson) of *Bipolar Disorder for the Newly Diagnosed* (New Harbinger Press). She is also the author of more than 130 articles and book chapters. Her current research focuses on emotion and psychopathology, with a specific interest in the emotional features, negative symptoms, and social factors of schizophrenia. As part of a follow-up study of children whose mothers were enrolled in a study in the early 1960s, she is also studying how early development might influence clinical, cognitive, social, and neural outcomes in late middle age.

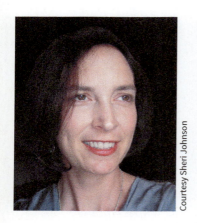

Courtesy Sheri Johnson

SHERI L. JOHNSON is Distinguished Professor of Psychology at the University of California at Berkeley. She received her B.A. from Salem College and her Ph.D. from the University of Pittsburgh. She completed an internship and postdoctoral fellowship at Brown University, and she was a clinical assistant professor at Brown from 1993 to 1995. From 1995 to 2008, she taught in the Department of Psychology at the University of Miami, where she was recognized three times with the Excellence in Graduate Teaching Award. In 1993, she received a Young Investigator Award from the National Alliance for Research in Schizophrenia and Depression (NARSAD). She is an associate editor for *Psychological Bulletin* and a consulting editor for *Clinical Psychological Science* and *Journal of Psychopathology and Clinical Science*. She has served as President of the Society for Research in Psychopathology and is a fellow of the Academy of Behavioral Medicine Research, the Association for Behavioral and Cognitive Therapies, and the Association for Psychological Science.

Her work has been funded by NARSAD, the National Cancer Institute, the National Science Foundation, the National Institute of Mental Health, and the Wellcome Trust. She has authored over 300 publications, and her findings have been published in leading journals such as *Biological Psychiatry, Journal of Abnormal Psychology, Psychological Bulletin*, and *American Journal of Psychiatry*. She is co-editor or co-author of six books, including *Psychological Treatment of Bipolar Disorder* (Guilford Press), *Bipolar Disorder for the Newly Diagnosed* (New Harbinger Press), *Bipolar Disorder: Advances in Psychotherapy Evidence-Based Practice* (Hogrefe Publishing), and *Emotion and Psychopathology* (American Psychological Association). Her work focuses on bipolar disorder, emotion, emotion-related disorders, and impulsivity.

The focus of this book has always been on the balancing and blending of research and clinical application and on the effort to involve the learner in the problem solving engaged in by clinicians and scientists. We continue to emphasize an integrated approach, showing how psychopathology is best understood by considering multiple perspectives and how these varying perspectives can provide us with the clearest accounting of the causes of these disorders as well as the best possible treatments. With the sixteenth edition, we have once again emphasized the recent and comprehensive research coverage that has been the hallmark of the book.

We have removed "Abnormal Psychology" from the title of the book because the term "abnormal" is out-of-date, inaccurate, and stigma-promoting in the field of clinical psychological science. We are not alone in making this change. One of the oldest academic journals, formerly called *Journal of Abnormal Psychology* changed its name in 2022 to *Journal of Psychopathology and Clinical Science.* Many college courses in Abnormal Psychology have changed their names as well. We agree with the editors at the *Journal of Psychopathology and Clinical Science* that "… human diversity is too broad to be contained—or constrained—by the metaphor of abnormality." Our contention is that people with psychological disorders are first and foremost people and that the term *abnormal* is overly broad and can be misconstrued to the detriment of people who have psychological disorders.

The cover image represents a neural network model. Just as in a complex network, there are myriad influences that contribute to psychological disorders. People are shaped by the interaction of their neurobiology and environment, which is what the study of psychological disorders is all about: different influences (genetic, neuroscience, personality, cognitive, behavioral, and social) coming together to shape the development and course of different psychological disorders. This is also how science works. New discoveries help to reshape the domains of scientific inquiry, shifting the connecting points in the network of our current understanding of psychological disorders.

Goals of the Book

With each new edition, we update, make changes, and streamline features to enhance both the scholarly and the pedagogical characteristics of the book. We also work to couch complex concepts in prose that is sharp, clear, and vivid. The domains of psychopathology and intervention continue to become more multifaceted and technical. Therefore, good coverage of psychological disorders must engage students in order to foster the focused attention necessary to acquire a deep, critical understanding of the material. Some of the most exciting breakthroughs in psychopathology research and treatment that we present in the book have come in complex areas such

as molecular genetics, neuroscience, and cognitive science. Rather than oversimplify these knotty issues, we have instead worked to make the explanations clear and accessible.

We strive to present up-to-date theories and research on the causes of and treatments for psychological disorders and to convey some of the intellectual excitement of the search for answers to some of the most puzzling questions facing us today. We encourage students to participate with us in a process of discovery as we sift through the evidence on the origins of psychological disorders and the effectiveness of specific interventions.

As always, we emphasize ways in which we can help to erase the stigma unfortunately still associated with psychological disorders. That was one of our motivations for changing the title of the book. Despite the ubiquity of psychological disorders, such stigma can keep some individuals from seeking treatment, keep our legislatures from providing adequate funding for treatment and research, and keep myths about psychological disorders alive and well. A major goal for this book is to combat the stigma and present a positive and hopeful view on the causes and treatments of these disorders.

Organization of the Sixteenth Edition

In Chapters 1 through 4, we place the field in historical context, introduce the major approaches to understanding psychological disorders, describe the *Diagnostic and Statistical Manual of Mental Disorders,* Fifth Edition Text Revision (DSM-5-TR) and critically discuss its validity and reliability, provide an overview of major approaches and techniques in clinical assessment, and then look at the major research methods of the field. These chapters provide the foundation for interpreting and understanding the later chapters. Specific psychological disorders and their treatment are discussed in Chapters 5 through 15. Chapter 16 covers legal and ethical issues in the science and treatment of psychological disorders.

Throughout the book, we discuss several influences relevant to understanding the causes and treatments of psychological disorders, including genetic, neuroscience, cognitive behavioral, personality, and socioemotional influences. We also emphasize the importance of adopting an integrative approach, which recognizes that these domains interweave to contribute to psychological disorders. For instance, genetic influences are important in attention-deficit/hyperactivity disorder, but genes do their work via the environment. In the anxiety disorders, conditioning models are prominent, and the neurobiological studies help enrich our understanding of how conditioning works. In disorders such as depression, social influences such as trauma can drive neurobiological shifts. For still other disorders—for example, dissociative disorders—cognitive factors involving consciousness are believed to be central, and researchers are considering how neural profiles might relate to gaps in consciousness.

We continue to include considerable material on the role of culture, race, and ethnicity in the study of causes and treatment of psychological disorders, as well as the role of trauma, childhood maltreatment, and interpersonal issues. Throughout all the chapters, we point to specific examples of the important role of these influences. For example, in Chapter 3, "Diagnosis and Assessment," we discuss cultural bias in assessment and ways to guard against this selectivity in perception. In Chapter 4, we discuss a growing body of work on the efficacy of psychotherapy across racial and ethnic groups. We also include new information on the role of race and culture in anxiety, depression, PTSD, OCD, schizophrenia, eating disorders, sexual disorders, childhood disorders, and substance use disorders.

New to This Edition

The sixteenth edition contains many exciting changes. First, as the research on each disorder has burgeoned, we continue to focus on only the most exciting, replicable, and accepted theories, research, and treatments. This edition, like past ones, contains hundreds of updated references. Second, we have simplified the writing throughout the book to increase the clarity of presentation and to highlight the key issues in the field. We have updated or added new figures and tables to carefully illustrate various concepts.

We have continued to add pedagogy based on feedback from students and professors. We continue to include a feature introduced in the last edition called Read More About It, in which we highlight recent important books about different disorders. We also include Focus on Discovery boxes to showcase cutting-edge research on selected topics or important historical highlights. In addition, we have modified and added Check Your Knowledge questions so that students can do a quick check to see if they are learning and integrating the material. Drawing on evidence supporting the importance of generative thinking for learning, we include open-ended questions. There are many photos providing illustrations of real-world applications of psychopathology, including photos of some of the highly successful and well-known people who have come forward in the past several years to discuss their own psychological disorders. The end-of-chapter summaries continue to be consistent across the chapters, using a bulleted format to summarize the descriptions, causes, and treatments of the disorders covered.

New and Expanded Coverage

We are excited about the new features of this edition. The major new material in this edition is outlined by chapter here.

Chapter 1: Introduction and Historical Overview

- Streamlined discussion of defining psychological disorder
- Expanded historical information to include the Islamic world
- New information in the section on mental health professionals

Chapter 2: Current Approaches in Psychopathology

- Expanded discussion of multiple influences on psychological disorders and how they are important individually and collectively
- Updated information on genetics, including GWAS
- Updated information on brain connectivity and networks
- New information on cognitive behavioral approaches to psychopathology
- New information on discrimination, race, ethnicity, and gender
- New information on trauma and childhood maltreatment

Chapter 3: Diagnosis and Assessment

- New section covering childhood adverse experiences and stress associated with discrimination and minority status
- New information on brain stimulation methods
- New coverage of the personality inventory MMPI-3
- New information on avoiding racial and cultural bias in assessment
- Removed dhat syndrome and uppgivenhets syndrome
- Edited the number of diagnoses in DSM-5TR as previous work had conflated specifiers and diagnoses in these counts

Chapter 4: Research Methods in Psychopathology

- Noted availability of large-scale longitudinal studies, such as the ABCD study
- Added information about diversity in experimental studies
- Summarized that more than 20 meta-analyses have concluded that the effects of psychotherapy are as powerful for racial and ethnic minorities as they are for whites
- Updated table of empirically supported treatments
- Updated information on the science of placebo effects

Chapter 5: Mood Disorders

- Updated information about the diminishing age of onset for depression over time
- Updated GWAS and neuroimaging findings
- More specificity about cytokines as predictors of depression
- New section on sleep and circadian problems in depression and bipolar disorder
- New section on integrating biological, psychological, and social influences, focused on reward sensitivity rather than cortisol and inflammation
- Cultural adaptations for CBT noted
- Updates on mindfulness-based cognitive therapy, now supported for a broader range of depression profiles
- More concise and updated section on adjunctive therapy for bipolar disorder
- New analyses of the efficacy of antidepressants based on datasets filed with the FDA
- More information on approaches to treatment-resistant depression, including esketamine and a new form of rTMS
- Information on antipsychotics for the treatment of bipolar depression.
- Removed DBS given the broader range of fully FDA approved treatments for depression
- Updated epidemiology of suicide section
- Updated information on the genetic vulnerability to death by suicide
- Noted that rapid effects of ketamine in lowering suicidal ideation
- Included information on the U.S. national suicide hotline
- Removed sections on neurotransmitters, seasonal affective disorder, and cortisol dysregulation due to nonreplications

Chapter 6: Anxiety Disorders

- Reorganized and updated material on age of onset to cover anxiety disorders generally rather than separately for each anxiety disorder
- Updated information on disability related to anxiety disorders
- Noted that phobias were first recognized as a discrete syndrome by an Islamic writer in the ninth century
- Added note about increases in anxiety during COVID-19 in countries with higher rates of infection
- Updated section on neuroimaging
- Given the limited empirical work available, removed the section on the specific etiology of agoraphobia
- Updated evidence for the contrast avoidance theory of GAD

- New paragraphs on treatment availability and cultural adaptations of treatment
- Updated material on the efficacy of psychological and medication treatments
- Removed material on cortisol awakening response, on acquisition of classically conditioned fears, and on classical conditioning of prepared stimuli in humans due to nonreplications

Chapter 7: Obsessive-Compulsive-Related and Trauma-Related Disorders

- New data shows that ASD symptoms do predict the severity of PTSD symptoms
- Added information about suicidality in OCD and BDD
- Added findings that clutter is a key predictor of impairment in hoarding disorder
- Added information about the influence of COVID on OCD symptoms
- Retitled the cortico-striatal networks as the cortico-striatal-thalamic-cortical (CSTC) loop, and added a figure to show the thalamic part of this circuitry, and noted that support for this loop is provided by brain stimulation studies
- Updated behavioral model of OCD to focus on slowed extinction to conditioned fear
- Added new computational model of OCD, focused on difficulties trusting evidence
- Highlighted the importance of addressing family accommodation strategies as part of ERP for OCD
- Updated findings regarding efficacy of cognitive therapy and ERP in OCD and hoarding
- Added information about case management for hoarding disorder
- New information about the epidemiology of trauma exposure
- Added information about refugee risk for PTSD in the section on culture
- Added information about intimate partner violence as one key type of trauma
- Added information about the low rates of receipt of adequate PTSD treatment
- Updated information about efficacy of psychological treatments
- Removed material on habit in OCD, due to nonreplication
- Removed material on cognitive deficits other than categorization in hoarding disorder
- Removed information about emotion regulation training in PTSD, as little research is available

Chapter 8: Dissociative Disorders and Somatic Symptom and Related Disorders

- New information about sleep and dissociation
- Added information that the Dissociative Experiences Scale has been shown to have poor reliability
- Added findings that those with DID appear to be more suggestible
- Noted that safety behaviors may intensify distress in somatic symptom and related disorders
- Added findings that conversion disorder appears linked to aberrant connectivity of the amygdala with regions involved in motor control and motor processing
- Added findings supporting benefits of CBT for health anxiety and conversion disorder

Chapter 9: Schizophrenia

- New information on racial disparities in schizophrenia
- Removed of nonreplicated and outdated material on candidate gene approach
- Addition of latest GWAS and discussion of nonspecificity of findings
- New information on rTMS in schizophrenia
- New and updated neuroscience information
- Critical evaluation of the evidence for neurotransmitters in the cause of schizophrenia
- New information on urbanicity
- New information on medication and tDCS treatments for schizophrenia
- New section on community care needs

Chapter 10: Substance Use Disorders

- New information on opioids, including updates on fentanyl overdoses and treatment
- New research on the nonbenefits of moderate drinking
- Updated information on prevalence rates of substance use and disorders in all tables and figures
- New Read More About It feature on Beth Macy's *Raising Lazarus: Hope, Justice, and the Future of America's Opioid Crisis*
- New information on e-cigarettes and vaping
- Updated genetics information
- Information on legalization and potential benefits of hallucinogens
- Information on how the COVID-19 pandemic influenced drug and alcohol use

- New information on treatments for nicotine use disorder
- New information on cannabis and the long-term impact on cognition and the effects of higher concentrations of THC
- Reorganized and streamlined section on psychosocial influences
- New information on treatments for alcohol and drug use disorders

Chapter 11: Eating Disorders

- New information on obesity in Focus on Discovery 11.1
- New discussion of atypical anorexia nervosa
- New information on genetic influences
- New information on media influences
- New information on eating disorders in men, including sexual minoritized men
- New information on culture, race, and ethnicity and eating disorders
- New information on the brain's reward system, dopamine, and eating disorders
- New information on treatment effectiveness

Chapter 12: Sexual Disorders

- Updated information about LGQBT rates
- Reduced content on the history of Master's and Johnson's work
- Noted the import of sensitivity to cultural factors in treatment of sexual dysfunction
- Added mindfulness to treatments of sexual dysfunction
- Updated biological treatments for female sexual interest/arousal disorder

Chapter 13: Disorders of Childhood

- New information on girls and attention-deficit/hyperactivity disorder (ADHD) and longitudinal outcomes
- New information on parenting and conduct disorder
- New information on callous and unemotional traits in conduct disorder
- Removal of older and poorly replicated molecular genetics research
- New information on depression in youth, including discussion of the influence of screen time
- New information on the prevalence of anxiety and depression in youth
- New information on treatment for anxiety, including general and specific treatments

- New information on the causes and treatment of depression in children and adolescents
- Updated information on the genetics of autism spectrum disorder
- Updated information on the brain and autism
- Updated information on treatment of autism spectrum disorder

Chapter 14: Late Life and Neurocognitive Disorders

- Updated statistics about centenarians
- Added findings that older Americans sustained higher levels of happiness than younger Americans even during the pandemic.
- Updated information about the Baltimore study of aging
- Added findings that telecare and internet delivery of psychotherapy have been empirically supported in late life samples
- Updated prevalence estimates and projections for dementia, including estimates of the higher rates of disease among Back and Hispanic Americans
- Added information that blood tests can identify biomarkers of plaques and tangles
- Added new material on biological and lifestyle risk factors, and on health disparities
- Updated statistics on Huntington's disease
- New section on medications designed to reduce amyloid plaques and other basic mechanisms
- New evidence that antidepressants are not effective in reducing agitation for patients with dementia
- New data on the modest effects of caregiver interventions
- Included information on the FINGER trial, a major multimodal intervention designed to address modifiable lifestyle factors in individuals at-risk for dementia.
- Updated delirium to note the high rates among those with dementia and those with COVID-19, and that prevention programs are estimated to reduce risk by 40%
- Removed information about stereotype priming in older adults, cognitive training programs, and full cognitive recovery after delirium given mixed evidence

Chapter 15: Personality Disorders

- Reworked section on trauma and personality disorder, to integrate findings from representative community samples and twin studies
- Updated findings showing a much higher rate of conversion to schizophrenia among those initially diagnosed with schizotypal personality disorder

- Updated information showing very high correlation of the number of psychopathic traits with the number of antisocial personality disorder symptoms.
- New section on the psychological risk factors for psychopathy
- New content on over-diagnosis, on interpersonal sensitivity and emotion regulation, and on findings from repetitive transcranial magnetic stimulation in borderline personality disorder
- Removed focus on trauma in borderline personality disorder given coverage earlier in the chapter
- More succinct coverage of fragile self-esteem in narcissistic personality disorder
- New material on overlap between OCPD and OCD
- Reorganized treatment section, and placed larger focus on the two most well-validated treatments for borderline personality disorder: dialectical behavior therapy and mentalization-based therapy
- Removed content on MAO-A gene × environment interaction due to nonreplications
- Removed studies of threat insensitivity and inattention during reward pursuit from the antisocial personality disorder section due to the small effect sizes

Chapter 16: Legal and Ethical Issues

- New information on violence and mental illness
- New information on jail diversion programs and the crisis intervention team approach
- Streamlined chapter overall

Special Features for Students

Several features of this book are designed to help students to master and enjoy the material.

Clinical Cases   We include Clinical Cases throughout the book. These cases provide a clinical context for the theories and research that occupy most of our attention in the chapters, and they help make vivid the real-life implications of the empirical work of psychopathologists and clinicians.

Focus on Discovery   In-depth discussions of selected topics appear throughout the book as stand-alone Focus on Discovery boxes, allowing us to involve readers in specialized topics without detracting from the flow of the main chapter text. Sometimes a Focus on Discovery expands on a point discussed in the chapter; sometimes it deals with an entirely separate but relevant issue—often a controversial one.

Read More About It   Read More About It features discuss selected books on the topics covered in the chapters. Included are first-person accounts of experiencing a psychological disorder and works detailing the origins of disorders and their consequences or discussing psychological disorders in a broader community context.

Quick Summaries   We include short summaries of sections throughout the chapters to give students an opportunity to pause and assimilate the material. These can help students keep track of the multifaceted and complex issues that surround the study of psychopathology.

End-of-Chapter Summaries   At the end of each chapter we review the chapter material in a bulleted summary. In Chapters 5–15, we organize these summaries into sections on clinical descriptions, causes,, and treatment—the major sections of every chapter covering the disorders. We believe that this format makes it easier for readers to review and remember the material. In fact, we suggest that students read the summary before beginning the chapter itself to get a good sense of what lies ahead. Reading the summary again after completing the chapter will enhance students' understanding and provide an immediate sense of the knowledge acquired in just one reading of the chapter.

Check Your Knowledge Questions   Throughout each chapter, we provide three to seven sets of review questions covering the material discussed. These questions are intended to help students assess their understanding and retention of the material, as well as to provide them with samples of the types of questions that often are found in course exams. We believe that these review questions will be useful aids for students as they make their way through the chapters.

Glossary   When an important term is introduced, it is boldfaced and defined or discussed immediately. Most such terms appear again later in the book, where they are not highlighted in this way. All these terms are listed again at the end of each chapter in an alphabetical list of key terms, and definitions appear at the end of the book in a glossary.

Defining Symptoms Boxes   We include a box with the defining symptoms of each of the disorders we cover in the book. The symptoms in these lists represent the fifth edition of the *Diagnostic and Statistical Manual of Mental Disorders*, known as DSM-5-TR, as well as the eleventh edition of the *International Classification of Disease*, known as ICD-11. We discuss both of these works in Chapter 3. We make considerable use of DSM-5-TR, though in a selective and occasionally critical manner. Sometimes we find it more effective to discuss theory and research on a problem in a way that is different from DSM conceptualization.

To Learn More

This 16th edition *of The Science and Treatment of Psychological Disorders* is available in two formats: as a print text and as an enhanced e-text. The enhanced e-text and practical printed text options offer the flexibility to suit multiple course formats, whether they be face-to-face, a hybrid/blended learning environment, or an online class.

Students who opt for the enhanced e-text have Case Study Videos and other interactive study tools integrated with the text. The collection of 7- to 10-minute Case Study Videos presents an encompassing view of 16 psychological disorders. Produced by documentary filmmaker Nathan Friedkin in collaboration with Ann Kring and Sheri Johnson, each case study features people with psychological disorders and their families, describing symptoms from their own perspective. In addition, each video also provides concise information about the available treatment options and commentary from a mental health professional. Along with the Case Study Videos, the enhanced e-text includes a variety of Interactivities that promote engagement and Flashcards that give students the opportunity to easily test their knowledge of key terms and vocabulary.

All instructors have access to a Book Companion Website that provides access to the Case Study Videos and a variety of Instructor Resources including a complete Test Bank, Lecture Presentation Slides, and an Instructor's Manual with Lecture Launchers, Discussion Stimulators, Handouts, suggestions for a variety of demonstrations and activities, and an annotated list of Web Resources for each chapter that puts useful online resources into the context of your course.

Acknowledgments

We are grateful for the contributions of our colleagues and staff, for it was with their assistance that this edition was able to become the book that it is. We have benefited from the skills and dedication of the folks at Wiley. For this update, we have many people to thank. Specifically, we thank Executive Editor Glenn Wilson; working with you on this edition has been a pleasure. In addition, we would like to thank Dan'el Nighting for the copy editing. And finally, we would like to thank Rajeev Kumar for guiding us through the production process.

From time to time, students and faculty colleagues have sent us their comments; these communications are always welcome. Readers can e-mail us at kring@berkeley.edu, sljohnson@berkeley.edu.

Finally, and most important, our heartfelt thanks go to people in our lives who gave their continued support and encouragement along the way. A great big thanks to Angela Hawk (AMK) and Daniel Rose, Robert Sangster and Vickie Davis (SLJ), to whom this book is dedicated with love and gratitude.

March 2024

ANN M. KRING

SHERI L. JOHNSON

Brief Contents

Contents

Introduction and Historical Overview

LEARNING GOALS

1. Explain the meaning of stigma as it applies to people with psychological disorders.

2. Understand the characteristics that define psychological disorder.

3. Understand how the causes and treatments of psychological disorders have changed over the course of history.

4. Describe the historical forces that have helped to shape our current view of psychological disorders, including biological and psychological views.

5. Understand what we have (and have not) learned from history.

6. Describe the different mental health professions, including the training involved and the expertise developed.

Clinical Case

Jack

Jack dreaded family gatherings. His parents' house would be filled with his brothers and their families, and all the little kids would run around making a lot of noise. His parents would urge him to "be social" and spend time with the family, even though Jack preferred to be alone. He knew that the kids called him "crazy Uncle Jack." In fact, he had even heard his younger brother Kevin call him "crazy Jack" when Kevin stopped by to see their mother the other day. Jack's mother admonished Kevin, reminding him that Jack had been doing very well on his new medication. "Schizophrenia is an illness," his mother had said.

Jack had not been hospitalized with an acute episode of schizophrenia for over 2 years. Even though Jack still heard voices, he had learned not to talk about them in front of his mother because she would then start hassling him about taking his medication or ask him all sorts of questions about whether he needed to go back to the hospital. He hoped he would soon be able to move out of his parents' house and into his own apartment. The landlord at the last apartment he had tried to rent rejected his application once he learned that Jack had schizophrenia. His mother and father needed to cosign the lease, and they had inadvertently said that Jack was doing very well with his illness. The landlord asked about the illness, and once his parents mentioned schizophrenia, the landlord became visibly uncomfortable. The landlord called later that night and said the apartment had already been rented. When Jack's father pressed him, the landlord admitted he "didn't want any trouble" and that he was worried that people like Jack were violent.

Clinical Case

Felicia

Felicia didn't like to think back to her early school years. Elementary school was not a very fun time. She couldn't sit still or follow directions very well. She often blurted out answers when it wasn't her turn to talk, and she never seemed to be able to finish her class papers without many mistakes. As if that wasn't bad enough, the other girls often laughed at her and called her names. She still remembers the time she tried to join in with a group of girls during recess. They kept running away, whispering to each other, and giggling. When Felicia asked what was so funny, one of the girls laughed and said, "You are hyper, girl! You fidget so much in class, you must have ants in your pants!"

When Felicia started fourth grade, her parents took her to a psychologist. She took several tests and answered all sorts of questions. At the end of these testing sessions, the psychologist diagnosed Felicia with attention-deficit/hyperactivity disorder (ADHD). Felicia began seeing a different psychologist, and her pediatrician prescribed the medication Ritalin. She enjoyed seeing the psychologist because she helped her learn how to deal with the other kids' teasing and how to do a better job of paying attention. The medication helped, too—she could concentrate better and didn't seem to blurt out things as much anymore.

Now in high school, Felicia is much happier. She has a good group of close friends, and her grades are better than they have ever been. Though it is still hard to focus sometimes, she has learned several ways to deal with her distractibility. She is looking forward to college, hoping she can get into the top state school. Her guidance counselor has encouraged her, thinking her grades and extracurricular activities will make for a strong application.

We all try to understand other people. Determining why another person does or feels something is not easy to do. In fact, we do not always understand our own feelings and behavior. Figuring out why people behave in normal, expected ways is difficult enough; understanding seemingly abnormal behavior, such as the behavior of Jack and Felicia, can be even more difficult.

Psychological Disorders and Stigma

In this book, we will consider the description, causes, and treatments of several different **psychological disorders**. We will also demonstrate the numerous challenges professionals in this field face. As you approach the study of **psychopathology**, the field concerned with the nature, development, and treatment of psychological disorders, keep in mind that the field is continually developing and adding new findings. As we proceed, you will see that the field's interest and importance are ever-growing.

The focus of the book, human behavior, is personal and powerfully affecting. Who has not experienced irrational thoughts or feelings? Most of us have known someone, a friend or a relative, whose behavior was upsetting or difficult to understand, and we realize how frustrating it can be to try to understand and help a person with psychological difficulties.

College courses in clinical psychology are among the most popular in the entire curriculum, not just in psychology departments. Our feeling of familiarity with the topic draws us to the study of psychopathology, but it also has a distinct disadvantage: We bring to the study our preconceived notions of the subject matter. Each of us has developed certain ways of thinking and talking about psychological disorders, certain words and concepts that somehow seem to fit. As you read this book and try to understand the psychological disorders it discusses, we may be asking you to adopt different ways of thinking about psychological disorders from those to which you are accustomed.

Perhaps most challenging of all, we must not only recognize our own preconceived notions of psychological disorders, but also confront and work to change the **stigma** we often associate with these conditions. Stigma refers to the destructive beliefs and attitudes held by a society that are ascribed to groups considered different in some manner, such as people with psychological disorders. More specifically, stigma has four characteristics (see **Figure 1.1**):

1. A label is applied to a group of people that distinguishes them from others (e.g., "crazy").
2. The label is linked to deviant or undesirable attributes by society (e.g., crazy people are dangerous).
3. People with the label are seen as essentially different from those without the label, contributing to an "us" versus "them" mentality (e.g., we are not like those crazy people).
4. People with the label are discriminated against unfairly (e.g., a clinic for crazy people can't be built in our neighborhood).

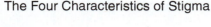

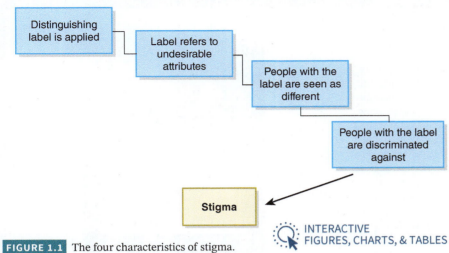

The Four Characteristics of Stigma

INTERACTIVE
FIGURES, CHARTS, & TABLES

FIGURE 1.1 The four characteristics of stigma.

The case of Jack illustrates how stigma can lead to discrimination. Jack was denied an apartment because of his schizophrenia. The landlord believed Jack's schizophrenia meant he would be violent. However, a person with a psychological disorder is more likely to be a victim of violence than a perpetrator of it (Desmarais, Van Dorn, et al., 2014), even though people with psychological disorders can be violent if they do not receive treatment (Torrey, 2014).

As we will see, the treatment of people with psychological disorders throughout recorded history has not generally been good, and this has contributed to their stigmatization, to the extent that they have often been brutalized and shunned by society. In the past, torturous treatments were held up to the public as miracle cures, and even today, terms such as *crazy*, *insane*, *retard*, and *schizo* are tossed about without thought of the people who have psychological disorders and for whom these insults and the intensely distressing feelings and behaviors they refer to are a reality of daily life. The cases of Jack and Felicia illustrate how hurtful using such careless and mean-spirited names can be.

Psychological disorders remain the most stigmatized of conditions in the 21st century, despite advances in the public's knowledge about the origins of psychological disorders (Hinshaw, 2018). Throughout this book, we hope to fight this stigma by showing you the latest evidence about the nature and causes of these disorders, together with treatments, dispelling myths and other misconceptions as we proceed. As part of this effort, we will try to put a human face on psychological disorders by including descriptions of actual people with these disorders. Additional ways to fight stigma are presented in **Read More About It 1.1**.

But you will have to help in this fight, for the mere acquisition of knowledge does not ensure the end of stigma (Corrigan, 2015). Many mental health practitioners and advocates had hoped that the more people learned about the many causes of psychological disorders, the less stigmatized these disorders would be. Although people's knowledge has increased, unfortunately stigma has not decreased, at least not for all disorders (Pescosolido, Halpern-Manners, et al., 2021). In one study, researchers surveyed people's attitudes and knowledge about psychological disorders at two points in time: 1996 and 2006 (Pescosolido, Martin, et al., 2010). Compared with people in 1996, people in 2006 were more likely to believe that psychological disorders such as schizophrenia, depression, and alcohol addiction had a neurobiological cause, but stigma toward these disorders did not decrease. In fact, in some cases it increased. For example, people in 2006 were less likely than people in 1996 to want to have a person with schizophrenia as their neighbor. Sadly, evidence from other studies backs up the findings from this study: Knowing more about the causes or available treatments of psychological disorders like schizophrenia or depression does not decrease stigma, according to studies in 13 different countries around the world (Pescosolido, Medina, et al., 2013). Knowing more is linked to a *greater* desire for more social distance from people with some psychological disorders (Kvaale, Haslam, & Gottdiener, 2013; Loughman & Haslam, 2018). One bit of positive news: Data from a 2018 survey found that between 2006 and 2018, people were less like

Read More About It 1.1

The Mark of Shame and Another Kind of Madness

The psychologist Stephen Hinshaw published two important books about stigma and mental illness. In 2007, he published *The Mark of Shame: The Stigma of Mental Illness and an Agenda for Change*. In this important book, Hinshaw discusses several steps that can be taken to end stigma surrounding psychological disorders. In 2017, he published a second book, entitled *Another Kind of Madness: A Journey Through the Stigma and Hope of Mental Illness*, which is a deeply personal story about the toll that stigma can take on families. Hinshaw works to humanize mental illness by telling his own personal story about his father, who had bipolar disorder. In both of these books, Hinshaw makes a strong case for why stigma is a "final frontier for human rights" (see also Hinshaw, 2018).

Here, we briefly discuss some of the key suggestions for fighting stigma in many arenas, including community, mental health professions, and individual/family behaviors and attitudes.

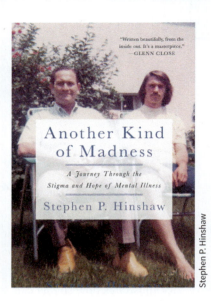

Stephen P. Hinshaw

Community Strategies

Housing Options   Rates of homelessness in people with psychological disorders are too high, and more programs to provide community residences and group homes are needed. However, many neighborhoods are reluctant to embrace the idea of people with a psychological disorder living among them. Lobbying legislatures and community leaders about the importance of adequate housing is a critically important step toward providing housing for people with psychological disorders and reducing stigma.

Personal Contact   Providing greater housing opportunities for people with psychological disorders will likely mean that people with

these disorders will shop and eat in local establishments alongside people without these disorders. Research suggests that this type of contact—where status is relatively equal—can reduce stigma. In fact, personal contact can be more effective than education in reducing stigma (Corrigan, Morris, et al., 2012). Informal settings, such as local parks and churches, can also help bridge the personal contact gap between people with and without psychological disorders.

Mental Health and Health Profession Strategies

Mental Health Evaluations   Many children see their pediatricians for well-baby or well-child exams. The goal of these visits is to prevent illness before it occurs. Hinshaw (2007) makes a strong case for including similar efforts to prevent psychological disorders among children and adolescents by, for example, using rating scale assessments from parents and teachers to help identify problems before they become more serious.

Education, Training, and Support   Mental health professionals should receive training in stigma issues (Hinshaw, 2018). This type of training would undoubtedly help professionals recognize the pernicious signs of stigma, even within the very profession that is charged with helping people with psychological disorders. In addition, mental health professionals need to keep current on the descriptions, causes, and empirically supported treatments for psychological disorders. This would certainly lead to better interactions with people and might also help educate the public about the important work being done by mental health professionals. Indeed, some evidence suggests that mental health professionals can exhibit stigma even though they have devoted their professional lives to helping others with psychological disorders (Corrigan & Nieweglowski, 2019). Mental health professionals should also seek support as they do this important work to help others, to guard against burnout and the development of stigma.

Individual and Family Strategies

Education for Individuals and Families   It can be frightening and disorienting for families to learn that a loved one has been

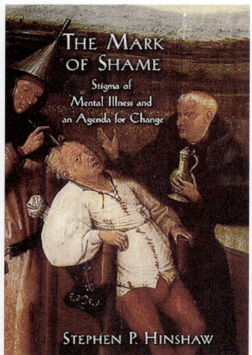

Stephen P. Hinshaw

diagnosed with an illness, and this may be particularly true for psychological disorders. Receiving current information about the causes and treatments of psychological disorders is crucial because it helps to alleviate blame and remove stereotypes families might hold about psychological disorders. Educating people with a psychological disorder is also extremely important. Sometimes termed *psychoeducation*, this type of information is built into many types of treatments, whether pharmacological or psychosocial. For people to understand why they should adhere to certain treatment regimens, it is important for them to know the nature of their illness and the treatment alternatives available.

Support and Advocacy Groups Participating in support or advocacy groups can be a helpful adjunct to treatment for people with psychological disorders and their families. Websites such as Mind Freedom International (http://www.mindfreedom.org) are designed to provide a forum for people with psychological disorders to find support. These sites, developed and run by people with psychological disorders, contain useful links, videos, and other helpful resources. In-person support groups are also helpful, and many communities have groups supported by the National Alliance on Mental Illness (http://www.nami.org). Finding peers in the context of support groups can be beneficial, especially for emotional support and empowerment.

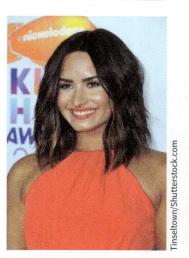

The singer Demi Lovato has talked about her struggles with bipolar disorder and substance use.

likely to desire more social distance from people with depression (Pescosolido, et al., 2021). We hope that this trend continues for other psychological disorders.

Two factors that can reduce stigma are contact and familiarity. A recent meta-analysis (see Chapter 4) of studies around the world found that coming into contact with someone with a psychological disorder can reduce stigma, and this reduction persists a year later (Maunder & White, 2019). Familiarity refers to whether a person knows someone with a severe mental illness. In general, familiarity is associated with less stigma (Corrigan & Nieweglowski, 2019). That is, if you work or live with someone who has a psychological disorder, you are less likely to exhibit stigma. Unfortunately, though, there is some evidence that greater familiarity, as in being a caretaker or mental health professional, is associated with more stigma (Corrigan & Nieweglowski, 2019). How can this be? Researchers have suggested that family burden and job burnout can foster stigma, which points to the importance of providing support for family members and mental health professionals. Clearly, there is work to be done.

Other efforts to reduce stigma have been quite creative in their use of social media and other means to get the message out that psychological disorders are common and affect us all in one way or another. Indeed, over 57 million people in the United States (i.e., about 1 in 5 people) had some type of psychological disorder in 2021, according to the National Survey on Drug Use and Health conducted by the Substance Abuse and Mental Health Services Administration (SAMHSA, 2022). For example, the website Bring Change to Mind (http://bringchange2mind.org) is a platform for personal stories that seeks to end stigma associated with psychological disorders; it was co-founded by the actress Glenn Close and her sister Jessie, who has bipolar disorder (see Chapter 5), and her nephew Calen, who has schizophrenia (see Chapter 9). Many podcasts feature people talking poignantly about their lives with different psychological disorders, and these accounts help to demystify and therefore destigmatize the disorders. For example, podcasts such as "The Mental Illness Happy Hour," "All in the Mind," and "Inside Mental Health" include discussions of psychological disorders and psychology topics more broadly. Strong365 (http://strong365.org) features stories of people living with different psychological disorders. Patients Like Me (http://www.patientslikeme.com) is a social networking site for people with all sorts of illnesses.

Celebrities or public figures with psychological disorders can also help reduce stigma. For example, the singer and songwriter Demi Lovato and the actor Chyler Leigh openly discuss their lives with bipolar disorder and have worked to help reduce stigma.

In this chapter, we first discuss what we mean by the term *psychological disorder*. Then we look briefly at how our views of psychological disorders have evolved through history to the more scientific perspectives of today. We conclude with a discussion of the current mental health professions.

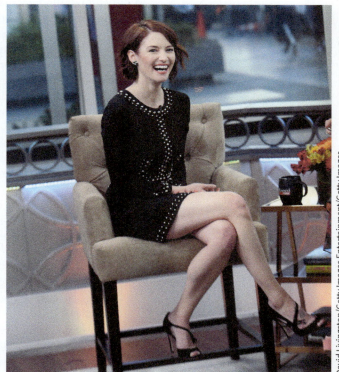

Actor Chyler Leigh co-starred in *SuperGirl*, and she has also talked about her life with bipolar disorder.

Quick Summary

This book focuses on the description, causes, and treatments of several different psychological disorders. It is important to note at the outset that the personal impact of our focus on psychological disorders requires us to make a conscious, determined effort to remain open-minded as we learn more. Stigma remains a central problem in the field of psychopathology. Stigma has four components that involve the labels for psychological disorders and their uses. Even the use of everyday terms such as *crazy* or *schizo* can contribute to the stigmatization of people with psychological disorders.

1.1 Check Your Knowledge

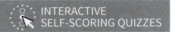
INTERACTIVE
SELF-SCORING QUIZZES

(Answers are at the end of the chapter.)

1. Characteristics of stigma include all the following *except*:
    a. a label reflecting desirable characteristics
    b. discrimination against those with the label
    c. focus on differences between those with and without the label
    d. labeling a group of people who are different

2. *True or false?*

Psychological disorders remain the most stigmatized of conditions in the 21st century.

3. *True or false?*

Close to 20 million people in the United States had some type of psychological disorder in 2022, according to the National Survey on Drug Use and Health conducted by SAMHSA.

Defining Psychological Disorder

A difficult but fundamental task facing those in the field of psychopathology is to define psychological disorder. The best current definition of psychological disorder is one that contains several characteristics. The definition of *mental disorder* presented in the current edition of the American diagnostic manual, the *Diagnostic and Statistical Manual of Mental Disorders, Fifth Edition, Text Revision* (DSM-5-TR), includes several characteristics essential to the concept of psychological disorder (Stein, Phillips, et al., 2010), as shown in **Table 1.1**.

In the following sections, we consider three key characteristics that should be part of any comprehensive psychological disorder definition: personal distress, disability and dysfunction (see **Figure 1.2**). We will see that no single characteristic can fully define the concept, although each has merit and each captures some part of what might be a full definition. Consequently, psychological disorder is usually determined based on the presence of several characteristics at one time.

TABLE 1.1 The DSM-5-TR Definition of Mental Disorder

The DSM-5-TR definition of *mental disorder* includes the following:
- The disorder occurs within the individual.
- It involves clinically significant difficulties in thinking, feeling, or behaving.
- It usually involves personal distress of some sort, such as in social relationships or occupational functioning.
- It involves dysfunction in psychological, developmental, and/or neurobiological processes that support mental functioning.
- It is not a culturally specific reaction to an event (e.g., death of a loved one).
- It is not primarily a result of social deviance or conflict with society.

Personal Distress

One characteristic used to define psychological disorder is personal distress—that is, a person's behavior may be classified as disordered if it causes him or her great distress. Felicia felt distress about her difficulty in paying attention and the social consequences of this difficulty—that is, being called names by other schoolgirls. Jose was distressed about falling to the floor after hearing the sound of popping balloons. Personal distress also characterizes many of the forms of psychological disorder considered in this book—people experiencing anxiety disorders and depression suffer greatly. But not all psychological disorders cause distress. For example, an individual with antisocial personality disorder may treat others coldheartedly and violate the law without experiencing any guilt, remorse, anxiety, or other type of distress. And not all behavior that causes distress is disordered—for example, the grief after the loss of a loved one.

Disability

Disability—that is, impairment in some important area of life (e.g., work or personal relationships)—can also characterize psychological disorder. For example, substance use disorders are defined in part by the social or occupational disability (e.g., serious arguments with one's spouse or poor work performance) created by substance abuse. Being rejected by peers, as Felicia was, is also an example of this characteristic. Phobias can produce both distress and disability—for example, if a severe fear of flying prevents someone living in California from taking a job in New York. Like distress, however, disability alone cannot be used to define psychological disorder because some, but not all, disorders involve disability. For example, the disorder bulimia nervosa involves binge eating and compensatory purging (e.g., vomiting) to control weight, but it does not necessarily involve disability. Many people with bulimia lead lives without impairment, while bingeing and purging in private.

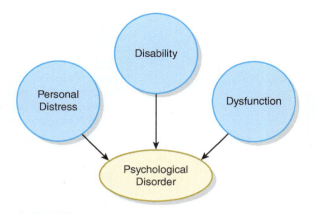

FIGURE 1.2 **Three characteristics of a comprehensive definition of psychological disorder.**

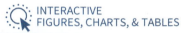
INTERACTIVE FIGURES, CHARTS, & TABLES

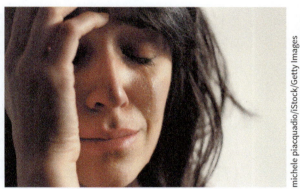

Personal distress can be part of the definition of psychological disorder.

michele piacquadio/iStock/Getty Images

Clinical Case

José

José didn't know what to think about his nightmares. Ever since he returned from the war, he couldn't get the bloody images out of his head. He woke up nearly every night with nightmares about the carnage he had witnessed as a soldier stationed in Fallujah. Even during the day, he would have flashbacks to the moment his Humvee was nearly sliced in half by a rocket-propelled grenade. Watching his friend die sitting next to him was the worst part; even the occasional pain from shrapnel still embedded in his shoulder was not as bad as the recurring dreams and flashbacks. He seemed to be sweating all the time now, and whenever he heard a loud noise, he jumped out of his chair. Just the other day, his grandmother stepped on a balloon left over from his "welcome home" party. To José, it sounded like a gunshot, and he immediately dropped to the ground.

His grandmother was worried about him. She thought he must have *ataque de nervios*, just as her father had back home in Puerto Rico. She said her father had been afraid all the time and felt like he was going crazy. She kept going to Mass and praying for José, which he appreciated. The army doctor said he had post-traumatic stress disorder (PTSD). José was supposed to go to the Veterans Administration (VA) hospital for an evaluation, but he didn't really think there was anything wrong with him. Yet his buddy Jorge had been to a group session at the VA, and he said it made him feel better. Maybe he would check it out. He wanted these images to get out of his head.

Dysfunction

Dysfunction refers to something that has gone wrong and is not working as it should. The DSM-5-TR definition, shown in Table 1.1, provides a broad concept of dysfunction, which is supported by the current body of evidence. Specifically, the DSM definition of dysfunction refers to the fact that developmental, psychological, and biological dysfunctions are all interrelated. That is, the brain impacts behavior, and behavior impacts the brain; thus, dysfunction in these areas is interrelated.

Quick Summary

Defining psychological disorder remains difficult. Several different definitions have been offered, but none can entirely account for the full range of disorders. A behavior causing personal distress can be a characteristic of psychological disorder. Behaviors that cause a disability or are unexpected can be considered part of a psychological disorder. Taken together, each definition of psychological disorder has something helpful to offer in the study of psychopathology.

1.2 Check Your Knowledge

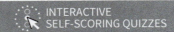
INTERACTIVE
SELF-SCORING QUIZZES

(Answers are at the end of the chapter.)

1. *True or false?*

Phobias can produce both distress and disability.

2. Which of the following definitions of psychological disorder is currently thought best?
    a. personal distress
    b. disability and dysfunction
    c. norm violation
    d. none of the above

3. What is an advantage of the DSM-5-TR definition of psychological disorder?
    a. It includes information about the brain.
    b. It includes many components, none of which alone can account for psychological disorder.
    c. It is part of the current diagnostic system.
    d. It recognizes the limits of our current understanding.

Early History of Psychological Disorders

Many textbooks begin with a chapter on the history of the field. Why? It is important to consider how concepts and approaches have changed (or not) over time, because we can learn from mistakes made in the past and because we can see that our current concepts and approaches are likely to change in the future. As we consider the history of psychological disorders, we will see that many new approaches to their treatment throughout time have appeared to go well at first and been heralded with much excitement and fanfare, only to eventually fall into disrepute. These are lessons that should not be forgotten as we consider more contemporary approaches to treatment and their attendant enthusiasm.

Supernatural Explanations

Before the age of scientific inquiry, all good and bad manifestations of power beyond human control—eclipses, earthquakes, storms, fire, diseases, the changing seasons—were regarded as supernatural. Behavior seemingly out of individual control was also ascribed to supernatural causes. Many early philosophers, theologians, and physicians who studied the troubled mind believed that disturbed behavior reflected the displeasure of the gods or possession by demons.

Examples of supernatural explanations are found in the records of the early Chinese, Egyptians, Babylonians, Arabs, and Greeks. Among the Hebrews, odd behavior was attributed to possession of the person by bad spirits, after God in his wrath had withdrawn protection. The New Testament includes the story of Christ curing a man with an unclean spirit by casting out the devils from within him and hurling them onto a herd of swine (Mark 5:8–13).

The belief that odd behavior was caused by possession led to treating it by **exorcism**, the ritualistic casting out of evil spirits. Exorcism typically took the form of elaborate rites of prayer, noisemaking, forcing the afflicted to drink terrible-tasting brews, and on occasion more extreme measures, such as flogging and starvation, to render the body uninhabitable to devils.

Early Biological Explanations

In the fifth century BCE, Hippocrates (460?–377? BCE), often called the father of modern medicine, separated medicine from religion, magic, and superstition. He rejected the prevailing Greek belief that the gods sent mental disturbances as punishment and insisted instead that such illnesses had natural causes and hence should be treated like other, more common maladies, such as colds and constipation. Hippocrates regarded the brain as the organ of consciousness, intellectual life, and emotion; thus, he thought that disordered thinking and behavior were indications of some kind of brain pathology. Hippocrates is often considered one of the earliest proponents of the notion that something wrong with the brain contributes to psychological disorders.

Hippocrates classified psychological disorders into three categories: mania, melancholia, and phrenitis, or brain fever. Hippocrates believed that healthy brain functioning, and therefore mental health, depended on a delicate balance among four humors, or fluids of the body—namely, blood, black bile, yellow bile, and phlegm. An imbalance of these humors produced disorders. For example, if a person had a preponderance of black bile, the explanation was melancholia; too much yellow bile explained irritability and anxiousness; and too much blood, changeable temperament.

Through Hippocrates' teachings, the phenomena associated with psychological disorders became more clearly the province of physicians rather than religious figures. The treatments he suggested were quite different from exorcism. For melancholia, for example, he prescribed tranquility, sobriety, care in choosing food and drink, and abstinence from sexual activity. Hippocrates left behind remarkably detailed records clearly describing many of the symptoms now recognized in seizure disorders, alcohol use disorder, stroke, and paranoia.

Hippocrates' ideas, of course, did not withstand later scientific scrutiny. However, his basic premise—that human behavior is markedly affected by bodily structures or substances and that odd behavior is produced by physical imbalance or even damage—did foreshadow aspects of contemporary thought.

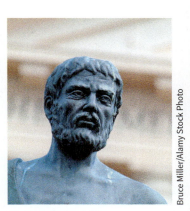

The Greek physician Hippocrates held a biological view of psychological disorders, considering psychological disorders to be diseases of the brain.

The Dark Ages: Back to the Supernatural

Historians have often pointed to the death of Galen (CE 130–200), the second-century Greek who is regarded as the last great physician of the classical era, as the beginning of the so-called Dark Ages in Western European medicine and in the treatment and investigation of psychological disorders. In Europe, the Church had gained influence, and the papacy was declared independent of the state. Christian monasteries, through their missionary and educational work, replaced physicians as healers and as authorities on psychological disorders.

The monks in the monasteries cared for and nursed the sick, including people with psychological disorders, by praying over them and touching them with relics; they also concocted fantastic potions for them to drink in the waning phase of the moon. Many people with psychological disorders roamed the countryside, destitute and progressively becoming worse. During this period, there was a return to a belief in supernatural causes of psychological disorders.

Although the Dark Ages represented a period during which supernatural explanations reemerged, this was not true in all parts of the world. Indeed, the teachings of Galen continued to be influential in the Islamic world. For example, the Persian physician alAl-Bh-Razi (865–925) established a facility for the treatment of people with psychological disorders in Baghdad and was an early practitioner of psychotherapy. Another Islamic scholar, Ibn Sina (980–1037) wrote about phobias and panic, noting that a person's pulse might speed up when someone was in a panic state (Awaad & Ali, 2016). This period in the Islamic world was referred to as the Golden Era, and writings from this period contain descriptions of psychological disorders that are remarkably similar to our descriptions today. For example, Al-Balkhi (849–934) described obsessional disorders that are very similar to the DSM-5-TR criteria for obsessive compulsive disorder, which we discuss in Chapter 7 (Awaad & Ali, 2015).

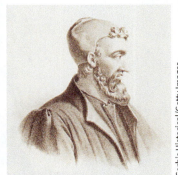

Galen was a Greek physician who followed Hippocrates' ideas and is regarded as the last great physician of the classical era.

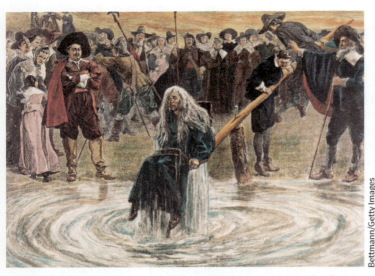

In the dunking test, if the woman did not drown, she was considered to be in league with the devil (and punished accordingly); this is the ultimate no-win situation.

Lunacy Trials From the 13th century on, as the cities of Europe grew larger, hospitals began to come under secular jurisdiction. Municipal authorities, gaining in power, tended to supplement or take over some of the activities of the Church, one of these being the care of people with psychological disorders. The foundation deed for the Holy Trinity Hospital in Salisbury, England, dating from the mid-14th century, specified the purposes of the hospital, one of which was that the "mad are kept safe until they are restored of reason." English laws during this period allowed people with psychological disorders to be hospitalized. Notably, the people who were hospitalized were not described as being possessed (Allderidge, 1979).

Beginning in the 13th century, lunacy trials to determine a person's mental health were held in England. As explained by Neugebauer (1979), the trials were conducted under the Crown's right to protect people with psychological disorders, and a judgment of insanity allowed the Crown to become guardian of the person's estate. The defendant's orientation, memory, intellect, daily life, and habits were at issue in the trial. Usually, strange behavior was attributed to physical illness or injury or to some emotional shock. Interestingly, the term *lunacy* comes from a theory espoused by the Swiss physician Paracelsus (1493–1541), who attributed odd behavior to a misalignment of the moon and stars (the Latin word for "moon" is *luna*). Even today, many people believe that a full moon is linked to odd behavior; however, there is little scientific evidence to support this belief.

Development of Asylums

Until the 15th century, there were very few hospitals in Europe for people with psychological disorders. Old, unused leprosy hospitals were converted to **asylums**, refuges for the housing and care of people with psychological disorders.

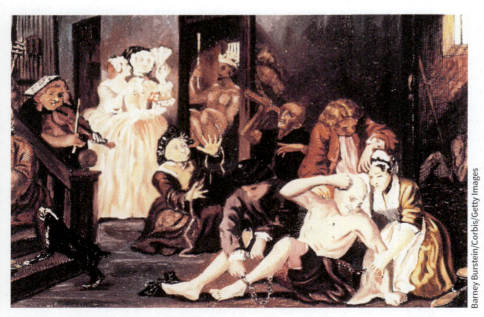

In this 18th-century painting by Hogarth, two upper-class women find amusement in touring St. Mary's of Bethlehem (Bedlam).

Bethlehem and Other Early Asylums The Priory of St. Mary of Bethlehem was founded in 1243. Records indicate that in 1403 it housed six men with psychological disorders. In 1547, Henry VIII handed it over to the city of London, thereafter to be a hospital devoted solely to the housing of people with psychological disorders. The conditions in Bethlehem were deplorable. Over the years, the word *bedlam*, the popular name for this hospital, came to mean a place or scene of wild uproar and confusion (Jay, 2016). Bethlehem eventually became one of London's great tourist attractions by the 18th century, rivaling both Westminster Abbey and the Tower of London. Even as late as the 19th century, viewing the people housed in Bethlehem was considered entertainment, and people bought tickets to see them. Similarly, in the Lunatics Tower, which was constructed in Vienna in 1784, people were confined in the spaces between inner square rooms and the outer walls, where they could be viewed by passersby.

Unfortunately, housing people with psychological disorders in hospitals and placing their care in the domain of medicine did not necessarily lead to more effective treatment. In fact, the medical treatments were often crude and painful. Benjamin Rush (1745–1813), for example, began practicing medicine in Philadelphia in 1769 and is considered the father of American psychiatry. Yet he believed that psychological disorder was caused by an excess of blood in the brain, for which his favored treatment was to draw great quantities of blood from people with psychological disorders (Farina, 1976). Rush also believed that many people with psychological disorders could be cured by being frightened. Thus, one of his recommended procedures was for the physician to convince the patient that death was near!

Pinel's Reforms

Philippe Pinel (1745–1826) has often been considered a primary figure in the movement for more humane treatment of people with psychological disorders in asylums. In 1793, while the French Revolution raged, he was put in charge of a large asylum in Paris known as La Bicêtre, where many of the people were kept locked up in chains.

Many texts assert that Pinel removed the chains of the people in La Bicêtre. Historical research, however, indicates that it was not Pinel who released the people from their chains. Rather, it was a former patient, Jean-Baptiste Pussin, who had become an orderly at the hospital. In fact, Pinel was not even present when the people were released (Weiner, 1994). Several years later, though, Pinel praised Pussin's efforts and began to follow the same practices.

Pinel came to believe that people in his care were first and foremost human beings, and thus these people should be approached with compassion and understanding and treated with dignity. He surmised that if their reason had left them because of severe personal and social problems, it might be restored to them through comforting counsel and purposeful activity. Thus, light and airy rooms replaced dungeons. People formerly considered dangerous now strolled through the hospital and grounds without creating disturbances or harming anyone.

Although Pinel did much good for people with psychological disorders, he was no paragon of enlightenment and egalitarianism. He reserved the more humanitarian treatment for the upper classes; people of the lower classes were still subjected to terror and coercion as a means of control, with straitjackets replacing chains.

Moral Treatment

For a time, asylums established in Europe and the United States were relatively small, privately supported, and operated along the lines of the humanitarian changes at La Bicêtre. In the United States, the Friends' Asylum, founded in 1817 in Pennsylvania, and the Hartford Retreat, established in 1824 in Connecticut, were set up to provide humane treatment. In accordance with this approach, which became known as **moral treatment**, people had close contact with attendants, who talked and read to them and encouraged them to engage in purposeful activity; residents led lives as close to normal as possible and in general took responsibility for themselves within the constraints of their disorders. Further, there were to be no more than 250 people in any given hospital (Whitaker, 2002).

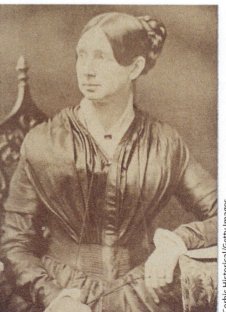

Moral treatment was largely abandoned in the latter part of the 19th century. Ironically, the efforts of Dorothea Dix (1802–1887), who was a crusader for improved conditions for people with psychological disorders and fought to have hospitals created for their care, helped effect this change. Dix, a Boston school teacher, taught a Sunday school class at the local prison and was shocked at the deplorable conditions in which the inmates lived. Her interest spread to the conditions at mental hospitals and to people with psychological disorders who had nowhere to go for treatment. She campaigned vigorously to improve the lives of people with psychological disorders and personally helped see that 32 hospitals were built. These large public hospitals took in many of the people whom the private hospitals could not accommodate. Unfortunately, the small staffs of these new hospitals were unable to provide the individual attention that was a hallmark of moral treatment (Powers, 2017; Scull, 2022). (See **Focus on Discovery 1.1** for an examination of whether the conditions have improved in today's mental hospitals.)

In the 19th century, Dorothea Dix played a major role in the establishment of more mental hospitals in the United States.

Focus on Discovery 1.1

The Mental Hospital Today

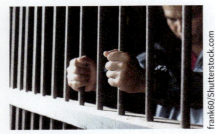

frank60/Shutterstock.com

In the United States, more people with psychological disorders are found in jails and prisons than in mental hospitals—a national disgrace.

In the late 1960s and early 1970s, concerns about the restrictive nature of confinement in a mental hospital, along with unrealistic enthusiasm about community-based treatments (Torrey, 2014), led to the so-called deinstitutionalization (i.e., release from the hospital) of many people with psychological disorders. Budget cuts beginning in 1980 and ongoing today have caused this trend to continue. But sometimes people with a psychological disorder do need treatment in a hospital setting, and, unfortunately, we still do not do a good job of this, even in the 21st century (as we will discuss in more detail in Chapter 16). Treatment in public mental hospitals today is often "just enough" to provide some protection, food, shelter, and, in most cases, medication. Indeed, people with psychological disorders in a public hospital may receive little treatment beyond medication.

Public mental hospitals in the United States are funded either by the federal government or, more often, by the state in which they are located. Many Veterans Administration hospitals and general medical hospitals also contain units for people with psychological disorders. Since the mid-1950s, the number of public mental hospitals has decreased substantially. In 1955, there were 340 beds in public hospitals for people with psychological disorders for every 100,000 people; by 2016, there were just 11.7 beds for every 100,000 people (Fuller, Sinclair, et al., 2016). States differ in the number of mental hospitals they have and, importantly, in the laws that determine whether a person can be involuntarily committed to such a hospital, a topic we return to in Chapter 16 (Berger, Dailey, et al., 2018).

One of the many unfortunate consequences of having fewer mental hospitals today is that people with severe psychological disorders go to hospital emergency departments in search of care. A 2019 report from the Treatment Advocacy Center reported that over 2.2 million people with a severe disorder such as schizophrenia or bipolar disorder went to emergency departments (EDs) in 2014. The stays in EDs (up to 24 hours or more) are much longer for people with these disorders than for people who arrive for other reasons, such as a heart attack (Treatment Advocacy Center, 2019).

Another very unfortunate consequence of having fewer mental hospitals is the fact that jails have become the de facto mental hospitals in many cities in the United States (Baillargeon, Binswanger, et al., 2009; Rosenberg, 2019; Roth, 2018; Torrey, 2014). Sadly, jails in Los Angeles County and Cook County (in Chicago) are now the largest "mental hospitals" in the United States, housing 10 times more people with psychological disorders than any actual mental hospital (Steinberg, Mills, & Romano, 2015). Moreover, a report from the Treatment Advocacy Center and the National Sheriffs' Association that drew from 2004–2005 data in the United States indicated that there are more people with psychological disorders in jails or prisons than in mental hospitals (Torrey, Kennard, et al., 2010). Furthermore, of the people currently in prison or jail, over half have a psychological disorder (James & Glaze, 2006).

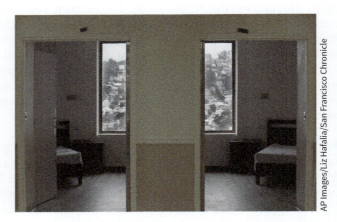

AP Images/Liz Hafalia/San Francisco Chronicle

Most rooms at public mental hospitals are bleak and unstimulating.

Quick Summary

Early explanations of psychological disorders included not only supernatural but also biological approaches, as evidenced by the ideas of Hippocrates. During the Dark Ages, some people with psychological disorders were cared for in monasteries, but many simply roamed the countryside. Treatments for people with psychological disorders have changed over time, though not always for the better. Exorcisms did not help. Treatments in asylums could also be cruel and unhelpful, but pioneering work by Dix and others made asylums more humane places for treatment. Unfortunately, their good ideas did not last, as the mental hospitals became overcrowded and understaffed.

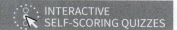
(Answers are at the end of the chapter.)

True or false?

1. Benjamin Rush is credited with beginning moral treatment in the United States.
2. Exorcism was an early biological treatment.
3. Hippocrates was one of the first to propose that psychological disorders had a biological cause.
4. The term *lunatic* is derived from the ideas of Paracelsus.

Historical Antecedents of Contemporary Views

As horrific as the conditions were in Bethlehem Hospital (and in many ways, continue to be in mental hospitals today; see Focus on Discovery 1.1), the physicians at the time were nonetheless interested in what caused the maladies of their patients. Table 1.2 lists the hypothesized causes of the illnesses exhibited by people in 1810 that were recorded by William Black, a physician working at Bethlehem at the time (Appignanesi, 2008). It is interesting to observe that about half of the presumed causes were biological (e.g., fever, hereditary, venereal) and half were psychological (e.g., grief, love, jealousy). Only about 10% of the causes were supernatural (Hunter & MacAlpine, 1963).

TABLE 1.2   Causes of Maladies Observed Among People in Bethlehem in 1810

Cause	Number of People
Childbed*	79
Contusions/fractures of skull	12
Drink/intoxication	58
Family/hereditary	115
Fevers	110
Fright	31
Grief	206
Jealousy	9
Love	90
Obstruction	10
Pride	8
Religion/Methodism	90
Smallpox	7
Study	15
Venereal	14
Ulcers/scabs dried up	5

Source: Adapted from Appignanesi (2008), Hunter and MacAlpine (1963).

*Childbed refers to childbirth—perhaps this malady is akin to what we now call postpartum depression.

Contemporary developments in biological and psychological approaches to the causes and treatments of psychological disorders were heavily influenced by theorists and scientists working in the late 19th and early 20th centuries. In this section, we review the historical antecedents of these more contemporary approaches.

Biological Approaches

Discovering Brain and Behavior Relationships

The anatomy and workings of the nervous system were partially understood by the mid-1800s, and several discoveries linking areas of the brain to specific behaviors were made. For example, the French surgeon Paul Broca (1824–1880) identified an area of the brain in the left frontal lobe that was linked to the ability to speak out loud. The German neurologist Carl Wernicke (1848–1905) identified an area of the brain in temporal lobe that was linked to the ability to comprehend speech. By the early 1900s, researchers had determined that the microorganism that caused syphilis could infect the brain and that this infection was causing the steady deterioration of both mental and physical abilities and progressive paralysis called *general paresis.*

Exciting as these discoveries were, not enough was known to allow investigators to conclude whether the structural brain abnormalities presumed to cause various psychological disorders were present. Nevertheless, causal links had been established between infection, damage to certain areas of the brain, and behavior associated with psychological disorders. If one type of psychological disorder had a biological cause, so could others. Biological approaches gained credibility, and searches for more biological causes were off and running.

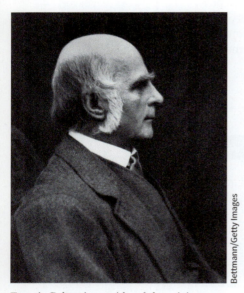

Francis Galton is considered the originator of genetics research.

Bettmann/Getty Images

Genetics

Francis Galton (1822–1911), often considered the originator of genetic research because of his study of twins in the late 1800s in England, attributed many behavioral characteristics to heredity. He is credited with coining the terms *nature* and *nurture* to talk about differences in genetics (nature) and environment (nurture). In the early 20th century, investigators became intrigued by the idea that psychological disorders might run in families, and beginning at that time, many studies documented the heritability of psychological disorders such as schizophrenia, bipolar disorder, and depression. These studies would set the stage for later theories about the genetic influences on psychological disorders.

Unfortunately, Galton is also credited with creating the eugenics movement in 1883 (Brooks, 2004). Advocates of this movement sought to eliminate what the movement deemed as undesirable characteristics from the population by restricting the ability of certain people to have children (e.g., by enforced sterilization). Many of the early efforts in the United States to determine whether psychological disorders could be inherited were associated with the eugenics movement, and this stalled research progress. Indeed, in a sad page from U.S. history, state laws in the late 1800s and early 1900s prohibited people with psychological disorders from marrying and forced them to be sterilized to prevent them from "passing on" their illness. Such laws were upheld by the U.S. Supreme Court in 1927 (Stern, 2015), and it wasn't until much later that these abhorrent practices were halted. For example, the eugenics law in California was not repealed until 1979. Some states have now provided compensation to people who experienced this horrible practice (Stern, Novak, et al., 2017).

Biological Treatments

The general warehousing of people in mental hospitals in the early part of the 20th century, coupled with the shortage of professional staff, created a climate that allowed, perhaps even subtly encouraged, experimentation with radical interventions. In the early 1930s, the practice of inducing a coma with large dosages of insulin was introduced by Sakel (1938), who claimed that up to three-quarters of the people with schizophrenia whom he treated showed significant improvement. Later findings by other researchers were less encouraging, and insulin-coma therapy—which presented serious risks to health, including irreversible coma and death—was gradually abandoned.

Early in the 20th century, **electroconvulsive therapy (ECT)** was originated by two Italian physicians, Ugo Cerletti and Lucino Bini. Cerletti was interested in epilepsy and was seeking a way to induce seizures experimentally. He found that by applying electric shocks to the sides of the human head he could produce full epileptic seizures. Then, in Rome in 1938, he used the technique on a person with schizophrenia.

In the decades that followed, ECT was administered to people with schizophrenia and severe depression, usually in hospital settings. As we will discuss in Chapter 5, it is still used today for people with severe depression. Fortunately, important refinements in the ECT procedures have made it less problematic, and it can be an effective treatment for some people.

In 1935, Egas Moniz, a Portuguese psychiatrist, introduced the *prefrontal lobotomy*, a surgical procedure that destroys the tracts connecting the frontal lobes to other areas of the brain. His initial reports claimed high rates of success (Moniz, 1936), and over the next 20 years thousands of people with psychological disorders underwent variations of this psychosurgery. The procedure was used especially for those whose behavior was violent. Many people did indeed quiet down and could even be discharged from hospitals, but largely because their brains were damaged. During the 1950s, this intervention fell into disrepute for several reasons. After surgery, many people became dull and listless and suffered serious losses in their emotional experience and cognitive capacities—for example, becoming unable to carry on a coherent conversation with another person—which is not surprising given the destruction of parts of their brains that support emotion, thought, and language.

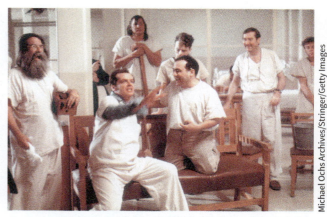

Scene from *One Flew Over the Cuckoo's Nest*. The character portrayed by Jack Nicholson was lobotomized in the film.

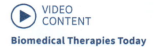

▶ VIDEO CONTENT
Biomedical Therapies Today

Psychological Approaches

The search for biological causes of psychological disorders dominated until well into the 20th century, no doubt partly because of the discoveries made about the brain and genetics. But beginning in the late 18th century, various psychological points of view emerged that attributed psychological disorders to psychological malfunctions. These theories were fashionable first in France and Austria and later in the United States, leading to the development of psychotherapeutic interventions based on the tenets of the individual theories.

Mesmer and Charcot
During the 18th century in Western Europe, many people were observed to be subject to *hysteria*, which referred to physical incapacities, such as blindness or paralysis, for which no physical cause could be found. Franz Anton Mesmer (1734–1815), an Austrian physician practicing in Vienna and Paris in the late 18th century, believed that hysteria was caused by a distribution of a universal magnetic fluid in the body. Moreover, he thought that one person could influence the fluid of another to bring about a change in the other's behavior.

Mesmer conducted meetings cloaked in mystery and mysticism, and he originally developed a technique that used rods to influence a person's alleged magnetic fields. Later, Mesmer perfected his routines so that he would simply look at people rather than using rods.

Although Mesmer regarded hysteria as having strictly biological causes, we discuss his work here because he is generally considered one of the earlier practitioners of modern-day hypnosis. (The word *mesmerism* is a synonym for *hypnotism*; the phenomenon itself was known to the ancients of many cultures, where it was part of the sorcery and magic of conjurers and faith healers.) Mesmer came to be regarded as a quack by his contemporaries, which is ironic, since he had earlier helped discredit an exorcist, Father Johann Joseph Gassner, who was performing similar rituals (Harrington, 2008). Nevertheless, hypnosis gradually became respectable.

The great Parisian neurologist Jean-Martin Charcot (1825–1893) also studied hysterical states. Although Charcot believed that hysteria was a problem with the nervous system and had a biological cause, he was also persuaded by psychological explanations. One day, some of his enterprising students hypnotized a healthy woman and, through suggestion, induced her to display certain hysterical symptoms. Charcot was deceived into believing that she was an actual patient with hysteria. When the students showed him how readily they could remove

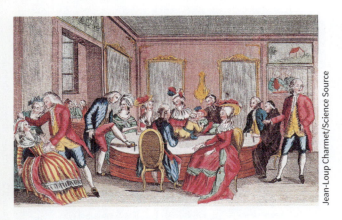

Mesmer's procedure for manipulating magnetism was generally considered a form of hypnosis.

the symptoms by waking the woman, Charcot became interested in psychological interpretations of these very puzzling phenomena. Given Charcot's prominence in Parisian society, his support of hypnosis as a worthy treatment for hysteria helped to legitimize this form of treatment among medical professionals of the time (Harrington, 2008; Hustvedt, 2011).

Breuer and Freud   In the late 19th century, Viennese physician Josef Breuer (1842–1925) treated a young woman with a number of hysterical symptoms, including partial paralysis, impairment of sight and hearing, and often difficulty speaking. This young woman, whose identity was disguised under the pseudonym Anna O., sometimes went into a dreamlike state, or "absence," during which she mumbled to herself, seemingly preoccupied with troubling thoughts. Breuer hypnotized her, and while hypnotized, she began talking more freely and, ultimately, with considerable emotion about upsetting events from her past. Frequently, on awakening from a hypnotic session, she felt much better. Breuer found that the relief of a particular symptom seemed to last longer if, under hypnosis, she was able to recall the event associated with the first appearance of that symptom and if she was able to express the emotion she had felt at the time. Reliving an earlier emotional trauma and releasing emotional tension by expressing previously forgotten thoughts about the event was called *catharsis*, and Breuer's method became known as the *cathartic method*. In 1895, Breuer and a younger colleague, Sigmund Freud (1856–1939), jointly published *Studies in Hysteria*, partly based on the case of Anna O.

Ironically, a later investigation revealed that Breuer and Freud reported the case of Anna O. incorrectly. Historical study by Ellenberger (1972) indicates that Breuer's talking cure helped the young woman only temporarily. Hospital records discovered by Ellenberger confirmed that Anna O. continued to rely on morphine to ease the "hysterical" problems that Breuer is reputed to have cured by catharsis.

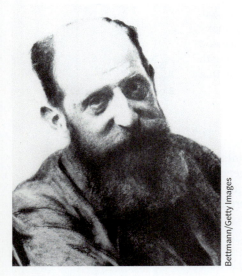

Josef Breuer, an Austrian physician and physiologist, collaborated with Freud in the early development of psychoanalysis.

Freud and Psychoanalysis   The apparently powerful role played by factors of which people seemed unaware led Freud to postulate that much of human behavior is determined by forces that are inaccessible to awareness. Although he was very much influenced by the ideas of Charcot, he believed that symptoms of hysteria could be explained more often by psychological causes than by neurological causes (Harrington, 2019). The central assumption of Freud's theorizing was that psychopathology results from **unconscious** conflicts in the individual. In the next sections, we take a brief look at Freud's theory.

Structure of the Mind   Freud divided the mind into three principal parts: id, ego, and superego. According to Freud, the id is present at birth and is the repository of all the energy needed to run the mind, including the basic urges for food, water, elimination, warmth, affection, and sex. Trained as a neurologist, Freud saw the source of the id's energy as biological and unconscious. That is, a person cannot consciously perceive this energy—it is below the level of awareness.

The **id** seeks immediate gratification of its urges. When the id is not satisfied, tension is produced, and the id drives a person to get rid of this tension as quickly as possible. For example, a baby feels hunger and is impelled to move about, sucking, in an attempt to reduce the tension arising from the hunger urge.

According to Freud, the **ego** begins to develop from the id during the second 6 months of life. Unlike the contents of the id, those of the ego are primarily conscious. The task of the ego is to deal with reality, and it mediates between the demands of reality and the id's demands for immediate gratification.

The **superego**—the third part of the mind in Freud's theory—can be roughly conceived of as a person's conscience. Freud believed that the superego develops throughout childhood, arising from the ego much as the ego arises from the id. As children discover that many of their impulses—for example, biting—are not acceptable to their parents, they begin to incorporate parental values as their own to receive the pleasure of parental approval and avoid the pain of disapproval.

Defense Mechanisms

According to Freud, and as elaborated by his daughter Anna (Freud, 1946/1966), herself an influential psychoanalyst, discomforts experienced by the ego as it attempts to resolve conflicts and satisfy the demands of the id and superego can be reduced in several ways. A **defense mechanism** is a strategy used by the ego to protect itself from anxiety. Examples of defense mechanisms are presented in **Table 1.3**.

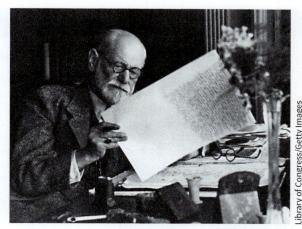

Sigmund Freud developed a theory of the structure and functions of the mind (including explanations of the causes of psychological disorders) and psychoanalysis, a method of therapy based on it.

Psychoanalytic Therapy

Psychotherapy based on Freud's theory is called **psychoanalysis**, or psychoanalytic therapy. It is still practiced today, although not as commonly as it once was.

In psychoanalytic and newer psychodynamic treatments, the goal of the therapist is to understand the person's early childhood experiences, the nature of key relationships, and the patterns in current relationships. The therapist is listening for core emotional and relationship themes that surface again and again.

One component of psychoanalytic therapy is the analysis of **transference**. Transference refers to the person's responses to his or her analyst that seem to reflect attitudes and ways of behaving toward important people in the person's past. For example, a person might feel that the analyst is generally bored by what he or she is saying and as a result might struggle to be entertaining; this pattern of response might reflect the person's childhood relationship with a parent rather than what's going on between the person and the analyst. The analyst might suggest that the person was made to feel boring and unimportant as a child and could gain parental attention only through humor.

Continuing Influences of Freud and His Followers

Freud's ideas and methods have been heavily criticized over the years. One of the main criticisms has to do with the lack of research to support them. In **Focus on Discovery 1.2**, we discuss two other historical figures who began as followers of Freud but then developed their own theories.

TABLE 1.3   **Selected Defense Mechanisms**

Defense Mechanism	Definition	Example
Repression	Keeping unacceptable impulses or wishes from conscious awareness	A professor starting a lecture she dreaded giving says, "In conclusion."
Denial	Not accepting a painful reality into conscious awareness	A victim of childhood abuse does not acknowledge it as an adult.
Projection	Attributing to someone else one's own unacceptable thoughts or feelings	A man who hates members of a racial group believes that it is they who dislike him.
Displacement	Redirecting emotional responses from their real target to someone else	A child gets mad at her brother but instead acts angrily toward her friend.
Rationalization	Offering acceptable reasons for an unacceptable action or attitude	A parent berates a child out of impatience, then indicates that she did so to "build character."

Focus on Discovery 1.2

Extensions and Variations on Freud's Theories

Several of Freud's contemporaries met with him periodically to discuss his theory. As often happens when a brilliant leader attracts brilliant followers and colleagues, disagreements arose about many general issues, such as the relative importance of id versus ego, of biological versus sociocultural forces on psychological development, of unconscious versus conscious processes, and of childhood versus adult experiences. We discuss two influential historical figures here: Carl Jung and Alfred Adler.

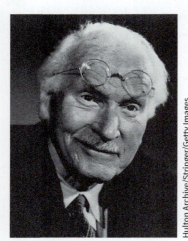

Carl Jung was the founder of analytical psychology.

Hulton Archive/Stringer/Getty Images

Jung and Analytical Psychology

Carl Gustav Jung (1875–1961), originally considered Freud's heir apparent, broke with Freud in 1914 over many issues. Jung proposed ideas radically different from Freud's, ultimately establishing *analytical psychology*. Jung hypothesized that, in addition to the personal unconscious postulated by Freud, there is a *collective unconscious*, a part of the unconscious that is common to all human beings and that consists primarily of what Jung called *archetypes*, or basic categories that all human beings use in conceptualizing about the world.

Adler and Individual Psychology

Alfred Adler (1870–1937) also broke with Freud's views, and Freud remained quite bitter toward Adler after their relationship ended. Adler's theory, which came to be known as *individual psychology*, regarded people as inextricably tied to their society because he believed that fulfillment was found in doing things for the social good (Adler, 1930).

A central element in Adler's work was his focus on helping people change their illogical and mistaken ideas and expectations. He believed that feeling better and behaving better depend on thinking more rationally, an approach that anticipated contemporary developments in cognitive behavior therapy (discussed in Chapter 2).

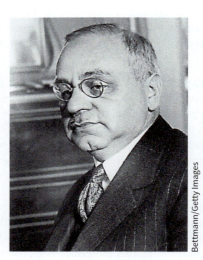

Alfred Adler was the founder of individual psychology.

Bettmann/Getty Images

Though perhaps not as influential as it once was, the work of Freud and his followers continues to have an impact on the field of psychopathology (Westen, 1998). This influence is most evident in the following three commonly held assumptions:

1. *Childhood experiences help shape adult personality.* Contemporary clinicians and researchers still view childhood experiences and other environmental events as crucial. They seldom focus on the psychosexual stages about which Freud wrote, but some emphasize problematic parent–child relationships in general and how they can influence later adult relationships in negative ways.

2. *There are unconscious influences on behavior.* As we will discuss in Chapter 2, the unconscious is a focus of contemporary research in cognitive neuroscience and psychopathology. This research shows that people can be unaware of the causes of their behavior. However, most current researchers and clinicians do not think of the unconscious as a repository of id instincts.

3. *The causes and purposes of human behavior are not always obvious.* Freud and his followers sensitized generations of clinicians and researchers to the nonobviousness of the causes and purposes of human behavior. Contemporary psychodynamic theorists continue to caution us against taking everything at face value. A person expressing disdain for another, for example, may actually like the other person very much, yet be fearful of admitting positive feelings. This tendency to look under the surface, to find hidden meanings in behavior, is perhaps Freud's best-known legacy.

The Rise of Behaviorism

After some years, many in the field began to lose faith in Freud's approach. Instead, the experimental procedures of the psychologists who were investigating learning in animals assumed a more dominant role in psychology. **Behaviorism** focuses on observable behavior rather than on consciousness or mental functioning. We will look at three types of learning that influenced the behaviorist approach in the early and middle parts of the 20th century and that continue to be influential today: **classical conditioning**, **operant conditioning**, and **modeling**.

Classical Conditioning   Around the turn of the 20th century, the Russian physiologist and Nobel laureate Ivan Pavlov (1849–1936) discovered classical conditioning, quite by accident. As part of his study of the digestive system, Pavlov gave a dog meat powder to make it salivate. Before long, Pavlov's laboratory assistants became aware that the dog began salivating when it saw the person who fed it. As the experiment continued, the dog began to salivate even earlier, when it heard the footsteps of its feeder. Pavlov was intrigued by these findings and decided to study the dog's reactions systematically. In the first of many experiments, a bell was rung behind the dog and then the meat powder was placed in its mouth. After this procedure had been repeated several times, the dog began salivating as soon as it heard the bell and before it received the meat powder.

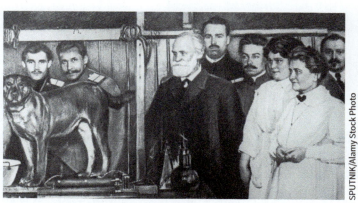

Ivan Pavlov, a Russian physiologist and Nobel laureate, made important contributions to the research and theory of classical conditioning.

In this experiment, because the meat powder automatically elicits salivation with no prior learning, the powder is termed an **unconditioned stimulus (UCS)** and the response of salivation an **unconditioned response (UCR)**. When the offering of meat powder is preceded several times by a neutral stimulus, the ringing of a bell, the sound of the bell alone (the **conditioned stimulus**, or CS) can elicit the salivary response (the **conditioned response**, or CR) (see **Figure 1.3**). As the number of paired presentations of the bell and the meat powder increases, the number of salivations elicited by the bell alone increases. What happens to an established CR if the CS is no longer followed by the UCS—for example, if repeated soundings of the bell are not followed by meat powder? The answer is that fewer and fewer CRs (salivations) are elicited, and the CR gradually disappears. This is termed **extinction**.

Classical conditioning can even instill fear. A famous but ethically questionable experiment conducted by John Watson (1878–1958) and Rosalie Rayner (Watson & Rayner, 1920) involved introducing a white rat to an 11-month-old boy, Little Albert. The boy showed no fear of the animal and appeared to want to play with it. But whenever the boy reached for the rat, the experimenter made a loud noise (the UCS) by striking a steel bar behind Albert's head. This caused Little Albert great fright (the UCR). After five such experiences, Albert became very frightened (the CR) by the sight of the white rat, even when the steel bar was not struck.

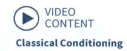

VIDEO CONTENT

Classical Conditioning

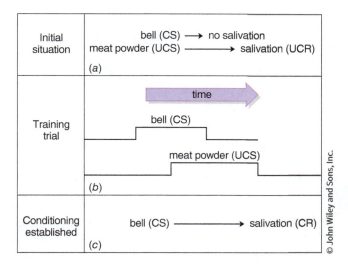

FIGURE 1.3   **The process of classical conditioning. (a)** Before learning, the meat powder (UCS) elicits salivation (UCR), but the bell (CS) does not. **(b)** A training or learning trial consists of presentations of the CS, followed closely by the UCS. **(c)** Classical conditioning has been accomplished when the previously neutral bell elicits salivation (CR).

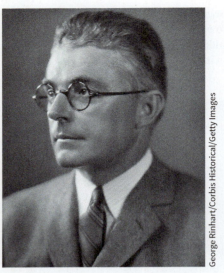

John B. Watson, an American psychologist, was a major figure in establishing behaviorism.

The fear initially associated with the loud noise had come to be elicited by the previously neutral stimulus, the white rat (now the CS). This study suggests a possible relationship between classical conditioning and the development of certain disorders, in this instance a phobia.

Operant Conditioning   In the 1890s, Edward Thorndike (1874–1949) began work that led to the discovery of another type of learning. Rather than investigate the association between stimuli, as Pavlov did, Thorndike studied the effects of consequences on behavior. Thorndike formulated what was to become an extremely important principle, the **law of effect**: Behavior that is followed by consequences satisfying to the organism will be repeated, and behavior that is followed by unpleasant consequences will be discouraged.

B. F. Skinner (1904–1990) introduced the concept of operant conditioning, so called because it applies to behavior that operates on the environment. Renaming Thorndike's "law of effect" the "principle of reinforcement," Skinner distinguished two types of reinforcement. **Positive reinforcement** refers to the strengthening of a tendency to respond by virtue of the presentation of a pleasant event, called a positive reinforcer. For example, a puppy will be more likely to sit if it is given a treat after doing so. **Negative reinforcement** also strengthens a response, but it does so via the removal of an aversive event, such as when the beeping noise in your car stops once you fasten your seatbelt. One other important reinforcement principle is *intermittent reinforcement*— rewarding a response only a portion of the times it appears. Intermittent reinforcement makes new behavior more enduring. It is the principle at work in maintaining some problem behaviors, such as gambling (see Chapter 10).

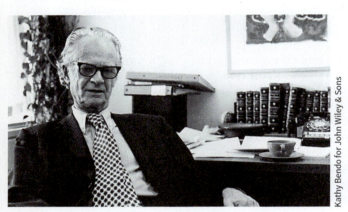

B. F. Skinner originated the study of operant conditioning and promoted the extension of this approach to education, psychotherapy, and society as a whole.

Modeling   Learning often goes on even in the absence of reinforcers. We all learn by watching and imitating others, a process called *modeling*. In the 1960s, experimental work demonstrated that witnessing someone perform certain activities can increase or decrease diverse kinds of behavior, such as sharing, aggression, and fear. For example, Bandura and Menlove (1968) used a modeling treatment to reduce fear of dogs in children. After witnessing a fearless model engage in various activities with a dog, initially fearful children showed an increased willingness to approach and touch a dog. Children of parents with phobias or substance use problems may acquire similar behavior patterns in part by observing their parents' behavior.

The Importance of Cognition   Beginning in the 1960s, the study of cognition began to become prominent. Researchers and clinicians realized that the ways in which people think about, or *appraise*, situations can influence behavior in dramatic ways. For example, walking into a room of strangers can elicit thoughts such as "Great! I am so

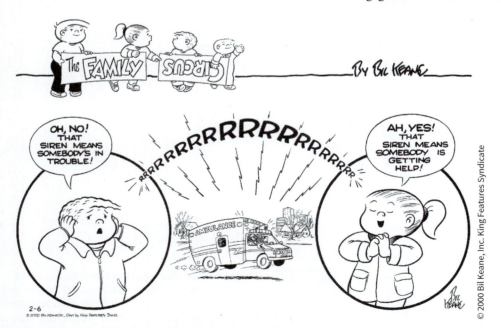

Appraisals are an important part of cognitive therapy. As illustrated, appraisals can change the meaning of a situation.

excited to meet all sorts of new and interesting people" or "I do not know any of these people, and I am going to look and sound ridiculous!" A person who has the first thought is likely to approach a group of people enthusiastically and join in the conversation. A person who has the second thought, however, is likely to turn right around and leave the room. The study of cognition greatly informed the development of cognitive behavioral therapy (CBT), which we discuss throughout the book. In CBT, therapists typically begin by helping clients become more aware of their thoughts. Therapists hope that by changing cognition, people can change their feelings, behaviors, and symptoms.

VIDEO CONTENT

Comparing and Contrasting Classical and Operant Conditioning

Quick Summary

The 19th and 20th centuries saw a return to biological explanations for psychological disorders. Developments outside the field of psychopathology, such as the positing of the germ theory of disease and the discovery of the cause of syphilis, illustrated how the brain and behavior are linked. Early investigations into the genetics of psychological disorders led to a tragic emphasis on eugenics and the enforced sterilization of many thousands of people with psychological disorders. Biological approaches to treatment, such as induced insulin coma and lobotomy, eventually gave way to drug treatments. Psychological approaches to psychopathology began with Mesmer's manipulation of "magnetism" to treat hysteria (late 18th century), proceeded through Breuer's conceptualization of the cathartic method in his treatment of Anna O. (late 19th century), and culminated in Freud's theory of the mind and psychoanalysis (early 20th century). The theories of Freud and other psychodynamic theorists do not lend themselves to systematic study, which has limited their acceptance in the field. Although Freud's early work is often criticized, his theorizing has been influential in the study of psychopathology in that it has made clear the importance of early experiences, the notion that we can do things without conscious awareness, and the insight that the causes of behavior are not always obvious.

Behaviorism began its ascendancy in the 1920s and continues to be an important part of various psychotherapies. John Watson built on the work of Ivan Pavlov in showing how some behaviors can be conditioned. B. F. Skinner, building on the work of Edward Thorndike, emphasized the contingencies associated with behavior, showing how positive and negative reinforcement could shape behavior. Research on modeling helped to explain how people can learn even when no obvious reinforcers are present. Early behavior therapy techniques that are still used today include intermittent reinforcement and modeling. The study of cognition became popular beginning in the 1960s.

1.4 Check Your Knowledge

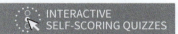

INTERACTIVE SELF-SCORING QUIZZES

(Answers are at the end of the chapter.)

1. Who was a French neurologist whose work was influenced by Mesmer?
2. Who developed the cathartic method, which Freud later built on in the development of psychoanalysis?
3. The _____ is driven by the pleasure principle.
4. In psychoanalysis, _____ refers to interpreting the relationship between therapist and client as indicative of the client's relationship to others.
5. What refers to increasing a desired behavior?
6. A cat comes running at the sound of a treat jar rattling, and his human friend then gives him a treat. The conditioned stimulus in this example is _____.

Have We Learned from History?

Many students of psychopathology grumble about having to read about the history of our field; they are excited to get right into learning about the clinical descriptions, causes, and treatments for psychological disorders. After all, many students of psychopathology aspire to a career as a mental health professional, not a historian. As we began our tour of history, however, we noted that it is important for us to consider the history of our field so that we can see how things have and have not changed over time. Ideally, we will learn from our historical mistakes.

Certainly, we have made many advancements over the centuries. We've learned that many people will experience a psychological disorder in their lifetime, and major models are available that integrate biology, psychology, and social influences for almost every psychological disorder we will cover in this book. Many psychological treatments have been developed, and thousands of publications each year focus on the genetic, neurobiological, and psychosocial causes of psychological disorders.

Despite these advances, we still have much to learn from history when it comes to reducing stigma and treating people with psychological disorders with respect, compassion, and dignity. Consider, for example, recent popular "reality" television shows such as *Hoarders*, *Many Sides of Jane*, *Obsessed*, *Addiction Unplugged*, and *Intervention*, which, respectively, showcase the lives of people with hoarding disorder (see Chapter 7), dissociative identity disorder (see Chapter 8), obsessive-compulsive disorder (see Chapter 7), and substance use disorder (see Chapter 10). Perhaps these shows help to educate people about psychological disorders, but perhaps also they perpetuate stigma by serving as the 21st-century version of the 18th-century practice of viewing people in asylums for entertainment. On the other hand, other television shows present realistic and compassionate portrayals of psychological disorders—for example, *Homeland* (bipolar disorder; see Chapter 5) and *Mr. Robot* (dissociative identity disorder; see Chapter 8). Yet even these shows can simplify or magnify some of the rarer aspects of psychological disorders, perhaps to amplify their entertainment value.

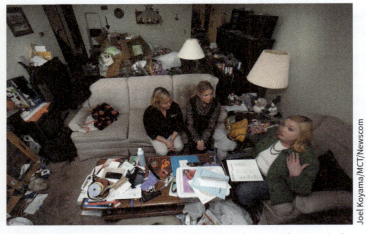

Are contemporary television shows such as *Hoarders* a modern equivalent of aristocrats viewing people in St. Mary's of Bethlehem (aka Bedlam) for entertainment?

Joel Koyama/MCT/Newscom

What about the living conditions for people with psychological disorders? People with serious disorders, such as schizophrenia, bipolar disorder, or severe depression, are often in need of short stays in hospitals. Unfortunately, many such hospitals have closed since the 1950s, making it extremely difficult to stay in a hospital when needed. As we will discuss in more detail in Chapter 16, conditions inside many of the hospitals were deplorable. Yet, instead of improving these conditions, many hospitals simply closed, leaving a large gap in treatment services for people with particularly severe disorders. With nowhere else to go, at least a third of unhoused people in the United States have a severe psychological disorder (Scull, 2022). Today, the new "hospital" for psychological disorders is jail. That is, people with severe psychological disorders are more likely to be housed in a jail than in a hospital (Rosenberg, 2019; Roth, 2018; Scull, 2022). Many people with psychological disorders are not able to work and thus have very little income. These economic realities increase the likelihood of living in low-income housing, such as a single-room occupancy hotel, or SRO, to avoid homelessness. A recent study of such living accommodations found that nearly 75% of the residents of an SRO in Vancouver, Canada, had some type of psychological disorder and that 95% of the residents had a substance use disorder (Vila-Rodriguez, Panenka, et al., 2013).

As we will see in the following chapters, we still have some way to go when it comes to finding effective treatments with a tolerable set of side effects. Many people take medications to help with the symptoms of psychological disorders: In 2020, nearly 16.5% of adults in the United States had at least one prescription for such a medication (Terlizzi & Norris, 2021). However, these medications can have some very unpleasant side effects. For example, medications commonly used to treat schizophrenia can cause weight gain, dry mouth, blurred vision, and extreme fatigue. Imagine your life as a student if you had blurred vision nearly all the time! Some of these side effects contribute to the development of other health problems (e.g., weight gain increases the risk of developing type 2 diabetes). It is perhaps not surprising, then, that some people with schizophrenia opt not to take these medications to avoid the side effects. Of course, current medications may not be as horrid as treatments of old, like bleeding or prefrontal lobotomy. In addition, there are effective psychotherapy treatments for some psychological disorders that do not involve medication at all. However, as we will see in the coming chapters, even though cognitive behavior therapy is an effective treatment for several psychological disorders, it does not help all people.

Have we learned from history? It seems that the answer is both yes and no. The lessons of history are therefore important for those who are headed toward careers as clinical scientists and mental health professionals. And we hope that readers of this book, regardless of their current or future careers, will recognize that we can all do something to reduce stigma, first and foremost by understanding that our current approaches to psychological disorders can and must continue to improve.

Quick Summary

Studying history can help us identify mistakes from the past that can ideally be avoided in the future. And although much progress has been made, we still have a ways to go when it comes to reducing stigma. For example, television shows that feature people with different psychological disorders could perpetuate the stigma and serve as entertainment, much as did strolls through hospitals like Bethlehem in the 18th and 19th centuries. In addition, hospitals and living conditions more generally for some people with psychological disorders is still substandard. Although biological treatments such as medication or ECT have improved, they still have significant side effects.

1.5 Check Your Knowledge

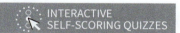
INTERACTIVE
SELF-SCORING QUIZZES

(Answers are at the end of the chapter.)

True or False

1. History has helped us to eradicate stigma surrounding psychological disorders.
2. Television shows depicting people with psychological disorders may be entertaining, but they can also depict realistic portrayals of these conditions.
3. The answer to whether or not we have learned from history regarding psychological disorders is a resounding yes. _____

The Mental Health Professions

As views of psychological disorders have evolved, so too have the professions associated with the field. Professionals authorized to provide psychological services include clinical psychologists, psychiatrists, psychiatric nurses, and social workers. The need for such professionals has never been greater. In this section, we discuss the different types of mental health professionals who treat people with psychological disorders and the different types of training they receive.

Clinical psychologists (such as the authors of this textbook) must have a Ph.D. (or Psy.D.) degree, which entails 4 to 8 years of graduate study. Training for the Ph.D. in clinical psychology or clinical science is similar to the training in other psychological specialties, such as developmental or cognitive neuroscience. It requires a heavy emphasis on research, statistics, and the empirically based study of human behavior. As in other fields of psychology, the Ph.D. is basically a research degree, and candidates are required to produce independent research. But what distinguishes candidates in clinical psychology from other Ph.D. candidates in psychology is that they learn skills in two additional areas. First, they learn techniques of assessment and diagnosis of psychopathology; that is, they acquire the skills necessary to determine whether a person's symptoms or problems indicate a particular disorder. Second, they learn how to practice psychotherapy, a primarily verbal means of helping people change their thoughts, feelings, and behavior to reduce distress and to achieve greater life satisfaction. Students take courses in which they master specific techniques and treat people under close

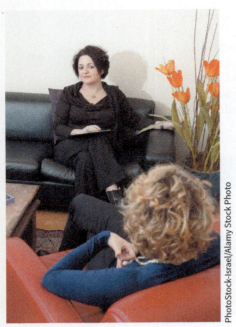

PhotoStock-Israel/Alamy Stock Photo

Clinical psychologists are trained to deliver psychotherapy.

professional supervision; then, during an intensive internship, they refine and bolster these skills.

Other graduate programs are more focused on clinical practice. For example, another degree option for clinical psychologists is the Psy.D. (doctor of psychology), for which the curriculum is similar to that required of Ph.D. students, but with less emphasis on research and more on clinical training. The thinking behind this approach is that clinical psychology has advanced to a level of knowledge and certainty that justifies intensive training in specific techniques of assessment and therapeutic intervention rather than combining practice with research. **Counseling psychologists** also obtain a Ph.D. degree and typically work in a practice setting to helping people handle difficult life circumstances and challenges. The focus of a counseling psychologist is less on psychological disorders and more on well-being, prevention, and education. There are other counseling degree programs not in psychology that focus on mental health, careers, school, or rehabilitation counseling.

Psychiatrists hold an M.D. degree and have had postgraduate training, called a *residency*, in which they have received supervision in the practice of diagnosis and pharmacotherapy (administering medications). By virtue of the medical degree, and in contrast to psychologists, psychiatrists can function as physicians—giving physical examinations, diagnosing medical problems, and the like. Most often, however, the only aspect of medical practice in which psychiatrists engage is prescribing medications, that can influence how people feel and think. Psychiatrists may receive some training in psychotherapy as well, though this is not a strong focus of their training.

A **psychiatric nurse** typically receives training at the bachelor's or master's level. Nurses can also receive more specialized training to become an advanced practice psychiatric nurse, which allows them to prescribe medications. There are nearly 16,000 psychiatric nurses in the United States, and the demand is growing, particularly for advanced practice psychiatric nurses (Delaney, Drew, & Rushton, 2018).

Social workers have an M.S.W. (master of social work) degree. Training programs are shorter than Ph.D. programs, typically requiring 2 years of graduate study. The focus of training is on psychotherapy. Those in social work graduate programs do not receive training in psychological assessment. Some M.S.W. programs offer specialized training and certification in marriage and family therapy.

Summary

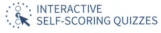

INTERACTIVE SELF-SCORING QUIZZES
Chapter 1 Practice Quiz

- The study of psychopathology is a search to explain why people behave, think, and feel in unexpected, sometimes odd, and possibly self-defeating ways. Unfortunately, people who have a psychological disorder are often stigmatized. Reducing the stigma associated with psychological disorders remains a great challenge for the field.

- In evaluating whether a behavior is part of a psychological disorder, psychologists consider several different characteristics—notably, personal distress, disability, and dysfunction. Each characteristic tells us something about what can be considered a psychological disorder, but no one by itself provides a fully satisfactory definition.

- Since the beginning of scientific inquiry into psychological disorders, supernatural, biological, and psychological points of view have vied for attention. Supernatural viewpoints posited that people with psychological disorders are possessed by demons or evil spirits, leading to treatments such as exorcism. Early

biological viewpoints originated in the writings of Hippocrates. In the Dark Ages, the biological perspective became less prominent in Western Europe, and supernatural thinking regained ascendancy. However, biological and psychological perspectives were strong in the Islamic world. Beginning in the 15th century, people with psychological disorders were often confined in asylums, such as London's Bethlehem. Treatment in asylums was generally poor or nonexistent until various humanitarian reforms were instituted in the 18th century. In the 20th century, genetics and psychological disorders became an important area of inquiry, though the findings from genetic studies were used to the detriment of people with psychological disorders as a result of the eugenics movement.

- In the 19th century, psychological viewpoints emerged from the work of Charcot and the writings of Breuer and Freud. Freud's theory emphasized the importance of unconscious processes and defense mechanisms. Psychoanalysis, which is based on

Freud's theory, makes use of techniques such as the analysis of transference to allow people to confront and understand their conflicts and find healthier ways of dealing with them.

- Behaviorism suggested that behavior develops through classical conditioning, operant conditioning, or modeling. B. F. Skinner introduced the ideas of positive and negative reinforcement and showed that operant conditioning can influence behavior.

- The study of cognition became widespread in the 1960s. Appraisals and evaluating thoughts are part of cognitive behavioral therapy.

- There are several different mental health professions, including clinical psychologist, counseling psychologist, psychiatrist, psychiatric nurse, and social worker. Each involves a training program of different length and with different emphases on research, psychological assessment, psychotherapy, and psychopharmacology.

Answers to Check Your Knowledge Questions

1.1 1. a; 2. True; 3. False

1.2 1. True; 2. d; 3. b

1.3 1. False; 2. False; 3. True; 4. True

1.4 1. Charcot; 2. Breuer; 3. id; 4. transference; 5. positive reinforcement; 6. sound of the jar rattling

1.5 1. False; 2. True; 3. False

Key Terms

asylums   10
behaviorism   19
classical conditioning   19
clinical psychologist   23
conditioned response (CR)   19
conditioned stimulus (CS)   19
defense mechanism   17
ego   16
electroconvulsive therapy (ECT)   14
exorcism   8
extinction   19

id   16
law of effect   20
modeling   19
moral treatment   11
negative reinforcement   20
operant conditioning   19
positive reinforcement   20
psychiatric nurse   24
psychiatrists   24
psychoanalysis   17
psychological disorders   2

psychopathology   2
psychotherapy   17
social workers   24
stigma   2
superego   17
transference   17
unconditioned response (UCR)   19
unconditioned stimulus (UCS)   19
unconscious   16

Current Approaches in Psychological Disorders

LEARNING GOALS

1. Describe the essentials of genetic, neuroscience, and cognitive behavioral influences on psychological disorders.

2. Describe the essentials of socioemotional influences, including emotion, culture, ethnicity, stress, trauma, and interpersonal influences, on the study and treatment of psychological disorders.

3. Recognize the importance of integration across many influences to understanding the causes and treatments for psychological disorders.

In this chapter, we present several types of influences that guide the study and treatment of psychological disorders: genetic, neuroscience, cognitive behavioral, and socioemotional. These influences are important for our understanding of the description, causes, and treatments of all the disorders we will discuss in this book.

Current thinking about psychological disorders is integrative and multifaceted. The work of clinicians and researchers is informed by an awareness of several influences on psychological disorders. For this reason, current approaches to psychological disorders and their treatment typically integrate several influences. That is, no one influence offers the "best" conceptualization of psychological disorders. Rather, for most disorders, each offers some important information about causes and treatment, but only part of the picture.

Genetic Influences

Genes do not, on their own, make us smart, dumb, sassy, polite, depressed, joyful, musical, tone-deaf, athletic, clumsy, literary or incurious. Those characteristics come from a complex interplay within a dynamic system. Every day in every way you are helping to shape which genes become active. Your life is interacting with your genes.

(Shenk, 2010, p. 27)

It has been more than two decades since researchers decoded the human genome; in 2023, researchers reported on progress on the pangenome, which is a decoding of a more diverse group of people from around the world (Liao, Asri, et al., 2023). These exciting milestones have been augmented with the virtual explosion of information regarding human genetics. One of the most important insights from this research is that we no longer must wonder, "Is nature or nurture responsible for human behavior?" We now know that (1) almost all behavior is heritable to some degree (i.e., it involves genes) and (2) despite this, genes do not operate in isolation from the environment. Instead, throughout the life span, the environment shapes how our genes are expressed, and our genes also shape our environments (Plomin, DeFries, et al., 2003; Rutter & Silberg, 2002; Turkheimer, 2000).

The current way to think about genes and the environment is cast as "nature via nurture" (Ridley, 2003). In other words, researchers are learning how environmental influences, such as stress, relationships, and culture (the nurture part), shape which of our genes are turned on or off and how our genes (the nature part) influence our bodies and brain. We know that without genes, a behavior might not be possible. But without the environment, genes could not express themselves and thus contribute to the behavior.

People have 23 pairs of chromosomes, or 46 total. Each chromosome is made up of many **genes**, the carriers of the genetic information (DNA) passed from parents to child. People have between 20,000 and 25,000 genes; the absolute number is hard to fully estimate (Human Genome Project, 2008).

Surprisingly, people don't have many more genes than insects; the mere fruit fly has around 14,000 genes! How can this be? Surely human beings are several times more complex than a fly! As it turns out, however, one of the exciting discoveries about genes was the revelation from dozens of genetic labs that the number of genes was not all that important. Instead, it is the sequencing, or ordering, of these genes, as well as what the genes actually *do*, that makes us unique. What genes do is make proteins that in turn make the body and brain work. Some of these proteins switch other genes on and off, a process called **gene expression**. Learning about the flexibility of genes and how they turn on or off has closed the door on beliefs about the inevitability of the effects of genes, good or bad. And with respect to most psychological disorders, there is not one gene that contributes vulnerability. Instead, psychological disorders are **polygenic**, meaning that the influence of several genes, perhaps operating at different times during development, turning themselves on and off as they interact with a person's environment, is the essence of genetic vulnerability (Sullivan & Geschwind, 2019; Visscher, Wray, et al., 2017).

We now know that we do not inherit psychological disorders from our genes alone; we develop them through the interaction of our genes with our environments (Mukherjee, 2016; Shenk, 2010). This is a subtle but very important point. It is easy to fall into the trap of thinking a person inherits a disorder like schizophrenia from their genes. What genetics research today is telling us, however, is that a person *develops* schizophrenia from the interaction between genes and the environment [as well as the body (e.g., hormones) and brain].

An important term that will be used throughout this book is **heritability**. Unfortunately, it is a term that is easily misunderstood and often misused. Heritability refers to the extent to which variability in a particular behavior (or disorder) in a population can be accounted for by genetic influences. There are two important points about heritability to keep in mind:

1. Heritability estimates range from 0.0 to 1.0: the higher the number, the greater the heritability.

2. Heritability is relevant *only* for a large population of people, not a particular individual. Thus, it is incorrect to talk about any one person's heritability for a particular behavior or disorder. Knowing that the heritability of attention-deficit/hyperactivity disorder (ADHD) is around 0.70 does not mean that 70% of Jane's ADHD is the product of her genes and 30% other influences. Rather, it means that in a population (e.g., a large sample in a study), the variation in ADHD is understood as being attributed to 70% genetic influences and 30% environmental influences. There is no heritability of ADHD (or any disorder) for a particular individual.

Other factors that are just as important as genes in genetic research are environmental influences. **Shared environment** factors include those things that members of a family have in common, such as family income level, child-rearing practices, and parents' marital status and quality. **Nonshared environment** (sometimes referred to as *unique environment*) factors are those things believed to be distinct among members of a family, such

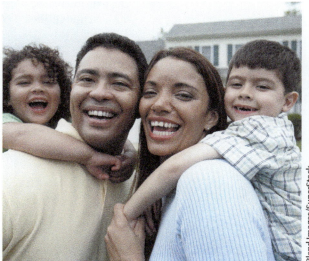

Blend Images/SuperStock

Shared environment refers to things families have in common, like marital quality.

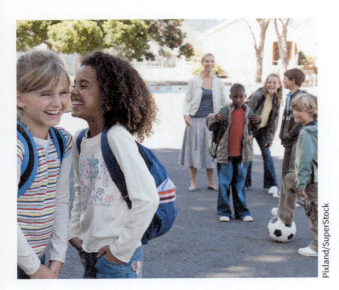

Nonshared environment refers to factors that are distinct among family members, such as having different groups of friends.

as relationships with friends or specific events unique to a person (e.g., being in a car accident or on the swim team), and these are believed to be important in understanding why two siblings from the same family can be so different. Consider an example. Jason is a 34-year-old man who has alcohol use disorder and is struggling to keep his job. His sister, Joan, is a 32-year-old executive in a computer company in San Jose and has no alcohol or drug problems. Jason did not have many friends as a child; Joan was one of the most popular girls in high school. Jason and Joan shared several influences, including their family atmosphere growing up. They also had unique, nonshared experiences, such as differences in peer relationships. Behavior genetics research suggests that shared environmental factors are important for the development of child psychopathology (Burt, 2009, 2014). The nonshared, or unique, environmental experiences can also play a role, although these can be difficult to measure and change a great deal, at least during childhood and adolescence (Burt, Klahr, & Klump, 2015).

We now turn to a review of two broad approaches to understanding genetic influences on psychological disorders: behavior genetics and molecular genetics. We then discuss the exciting evidence on the ways in which genes and environments interact.

Behavior Genetics

Behavior genetics is the study of the degree to which genes and environmental factors influence behavior. Note that behavior genetics is not the study of *how* genes or the environment determines behavior. Many behavior genetics studies estimate the heritability of a psychological disorder without providing any information about how the genes might work. The total genetic makeup of an individual, consisting of inherited genes, is referred to as the genotype (the physical sequence of DNA); the genotype cannot be observed outwardly. In contrast, the totality of observable behavioral characteristics, such as level of anxiety, is referred to as the phenotype.

The phenotype is the product of an interaction between the genotype and the environment. For example, a person may be born with the capacity for high intellectual achievement, but whether he or she develops this genetically given potential depends on environmental influences such as upbringing and education. Hence, intelligence is an index of the phenotype.

A study by Turkheimer, Haley, et al. (2003) shows how genes and environment may interact to influence IQ. Research has demonstrated high heritability for IQ (e.g., Plomin, 1999) and has even identified a constellation of over 50 genes that may be involved (Sniekers, Stringer, et al., 2017). What Turkheimer and colleagues found, though, was that heritability depends on environment. The study included 319 pairs of 7-year-old twins (114 identical, 205 fraternal). Many of the children were living in families either below the poverty line or with a low family income. Among the families of lower socioeconomic status (SES), 60% of the variability in children's IQ was attributable to the environment. Among the higher SES families, the opposite was found. That is, variability in IQ was more attributable to genes than to environment. Thus, being in an impoverished environment may have deleterious effects on IQ, whereas being in a more affluent environment may not help out all that much. It is important to point out that these interesting findings deal with IQ scores, a measure of what psychologists consider to be intelligence, not achievement (we discuss this issue in more detail in Chapter 3). In Chapter 4, we will discuss the major research designs used in behavior genetics research—including family, twin, and adoption studies—to estimate the heritability of different disorders.

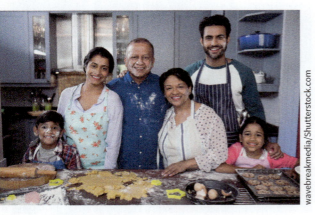

Behavior genetics studies the degree to which characteristics, such as physical resemblance or psychopathology, are shared by family members with shared genes.

Molecular Genetics

Molecular genetics studies seek to identify genes and their functions. A human being has 46 chromosomes (23 chromosome pairs) and each chromosome is made up of hundreds or thousands of genes that contain DNA (see **Figure 2.1**). Different forms of the same gene are called **alleles**. The alleles of a gene are found at the same location, or locus, of a chromosome pair. A genetic **polymorphism** refers to a difference in DNA sequence on a gene that has occurred in a population.

The DNA in genes is transcribed to RNA. In some cases, the RNA is then translated into amino acids, which then form proteins, and proteins make cells (see **Figure 2.2**). All of this is a remarkably complex system, and variations along the way, such as different combinations or sequences of events, lead to different outcomes.

A current focus in molecular genetics research is on identifying differences between people in the *sequence* of their genes and in the *structure* of their genes. One area of interest in the study of gene sequence involves identifying what are called **single nucleotide polymorphisms**, or SNPs (pronounced *snips*). A SNP refers to a difference between people in a single nucleotide (A, T, G, or C; see **Figure 2.3**) in the DNA sequence of a particular gene. Figure 2.3 illustrates what a SNP looks like in a strand of DNA.

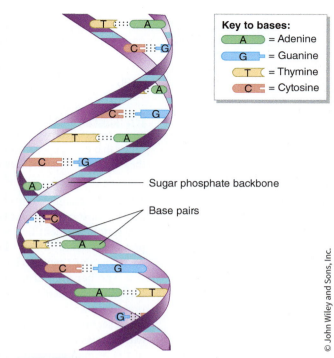

Key to bases:
A = Adenine
G = Guanine
T = Thymine
C = Cytosine

Sugar phosphate backbone

Base pairs

© John Wiley and Sons, Inc.

FIGURE 2.1 This figure shows a strand of DNA with four chemical bases: A (adenine), T (thymine), G (guanine), and C (cytosine).

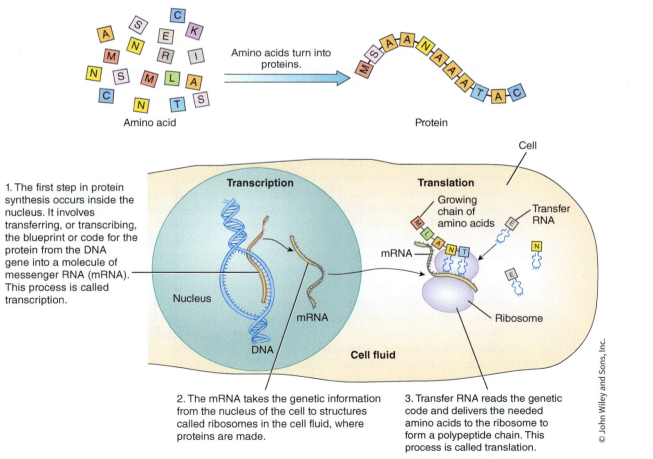

Amino acids turn into proteins.

Amino acid

Protein

Cell

Transcription

Translation

1. The first step in protein synthesis occurs inside the nucleus. It involves transferring, or transcribing, the blueprint or code for the protein from the DNA gene into a molecule of messenger RNA (mRNA). This process is called transcription.

Growing chain of amino acids

Transfer RNA

mRNA

Nucleus

mRNA

DNA

Cell fluid

Ribosome

2. The mRNA takes the genetic information from the nucleus of the cell to structures called ribosomes in the cell fluid, where proteins are made.

3. Transfer RNA reads the genetic code and delivers the needed amino acids to the ribosome to form a polypeptide chain. This process is called translation.

© John Wiley and Sons, Inc.

FIGURE 2.2 This figure shows gene transcription, the process by which DNA is transcribed to RNA. In some cases, the RNA is then translated into amino acids, which then form proteins, and proteins make cells.

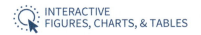
INTERACTIVE
FIGURES, CHARTS, & TABLES

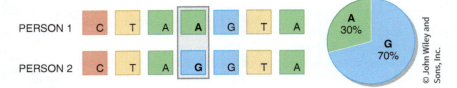

© John Wiley and Sons, Inc.

FIGURE 2.3 Illustration of what a single nucleotide polymorphism, or SNP, looks like in a comparison of two people. The two strands are the same except for a single nucleotide. The illustration to the right shows that the position of G in the sequence is far more common in a large population of people than the position of A in the sequence.

The gray rectangle points out the single nucleotide difference between the two strands. SNPs are the most common types of polymorphisms in the human genome, with nearly 10 million different SNPs identified so far. SNPs have been studied in several disorders, including schizophrenia, autism, anxiety disorders, eating disorders, and mood disorders. Heritability estimates based on SNPs can also be calculated and are referred to as h^2_{SNP} or SNP-based heritability.

Another area of interest is the study of differences between people in gene structure, including the identification of so-called **copy number variations (CNVs)**. A CNV can be present in a single gene or multiple genes. The name refers to an abnormal copy of one or more sections of DNA within the gene(s). These abnormal copies can be *additions*, where extra copies are abnormally present, or *deletions*, where copies are missing. As much as 5% of the human genome contains CNVs, which can be inherited from parents or can be what are called spontaneous (*de novo*) mutations—appearing for the first time in an individual. A method called genome-wide CNV analysis identifies CNVs using very large samples. Later, we will discuss studies that have identified CNVs in different disorders, particularly schizophrenia (Chapter 9), autism spectrum disorder, and ADHD (Chapter 13).

Genome-wide association studies (GWAS, pronounced *gee-waas*) are a key method for identifying SNPs. Using powerful computers, researchers look at all the thousands of genes to isolate differences in the sequence of genes between people who have a psychological disorder and people who do not. Remarkably, a person's entire genome can be obtained from a simple swab on the inside of the cheek! The saliva is then analyzed to reveal millions of sequences across the thousands of genes for each person. Because millions of sequences are analyzed, GWAS require very large samples. To date, GWAS with thousands of participants are available for schizophrenia, bipolar disorder, autism spectrum disorder, ADHD, anorexia, PTSD, anxiety disorders, depression, and Alzheimer's disease (Smoller, Andreassen, et al., 2019; Giangrande, Weber, & Turkheimer, 2022). If certain SNPs are found more often in the group of people with a certain diagnosis, such as schizophrenia, they are said to be associated with schizophrenia. Results from GWAS are often then translated into estimates of individual genetic risk by computing what is called a **polygenic risk score**. These scores have been in predicting the risk of developing Alzheimer's disease (Bellenguez, Küçükali, et al., 2022), a topic we discuss in Chapter 14.

Results from GWAS have led to two key insights about the role of genetics in psychological disorders. First, these studies have confirmed that many genes are involved in disorders. That is, the disorders are polygenic. Second, these studies have identified striking genetic similarities across disorders. That is, rather than identifying genes or genetic mutations such as SNPs that are specific to particular disorders, many studies are finding that diverse disorders share common genetic risk (Baselmans, Yengo, et al., 2021; Caspi & Moffitt, 2018; Giangrande, Weber, & Turkheimer, 2022). In one study of over a million people, a collaborative research group from around the world called the Brainstorm Consortium found evidence for common genetic risk for schizophrenia, bipolar disorder, major depressive disorder, ADHD, and the anxiety disorders (Anttila, Bulik-Sullivan, et al., 2018; Smoller et al., 2019).

Gene–Environment Interactions

As we noted earlier, we know now that genes and environments work together. Life experience shapes how our genes are expressed, and our genes guide us in behaviors that lead to the selection of different experiences. A **gene–environment interaction** means that a given person's sensitivity to an environmental event is influenced by genes.

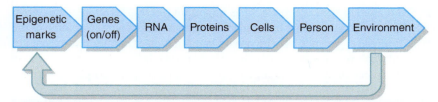

FIGURE 2.4 The dynamic process by which epigenetics influences whether genes are switched on or off. Importantly, the environment influences epigenetics.

Take a simple (and made-up) example. If a person has gene XYZ, he or she might respond to a snakebite by developing a fear of snakes. A person without the XYZ gene would not develop a fear of snakes after being bitten. This simple relationship involves both genes (the XYZ gene) and an environmental event (snakebite).

The study of how the environment can alter gene expression or function is called **epigenetics**. The term *epigenetic* means "above or outside the gene" and refers to the chemical "marks," such as DNA methyl tags or histones, that are attached to and protect the DNA in each gene. These epigenetic marks are what control gene expression, and the environment can directly influence the work of these marks, as shown in **Figure 2.4** (Champagne, 2016; Zhang & Meaney, 2010). In studies with animals, research has shown that epigenetic effects can be passed down across multiple generations—from parents (mothers *and* fathers; Braun & Champagne, 2014) to children and even from grandparents to grandchildren (Champagne, 2016).

Evaluating the Role of Genetic Influences in Psychological Disorders

Genetics is an important part of the study of psychological disorders, and there are many ways in which genes might be involved. The models that will help us understand how genes are implicated in psychological disorders are the ones that take the contemporary view that genes do their work through the environment.

There are three huge challenges facing scientists working to understand the role of genetics in psychological disorders (Giangrande, Weber, & Turkheimer, 2022). The first is to specify exactly how genes and environments reciprocally influence one another. Making the leap to understanding how genes interact with complex human environments throughout the course of development is a great challenge. The second challenge is to recognize the complexity of the task, knowing that several genes (not just one) will contribute to a specific disorder and that there is a long pathway between the genes and the complex behaviors that make up psychological disorders, with several biological processes unfolding along the way. Consider how short the pathway between genes and eye color is: Genes give instructions for production of the chemicals that produce pigment. Indeed, just one SNP accounts for blue eye color (Sturm, Duffy, et al., 2008). By contrast, the pathway between genes and the behavioral phenotypes of psychological disorders is a long and winding road, filled with many biological and psychosocial processes, each of which is influenced by multiple genes. Thus, each individual SNP, CNV, or other polymorphism may reveal a very small effect. Putting all the small genetic pieces together to tell the gene-via-environment story for psychological disorders remains an enormous challenge. For example, polygenic risk scores will be even more helpful in predicting risk for developing psychological disorders by showing how these scores interact with environmental factors (Murray, Lin, et al., 2021).

Third, most of the genetic vulnerability appears to increase risk for many psychological disorders more than risk for specific disorders. Some genetic vulnerability is related to "internalizing disorders" such as depression and anxiety; some genetic vulnerability is related to "externalizing disorders" such as substance use disorders, alcohol use disorders, and disorders that involve rule breaking (such as antisocial personality disorders); and some genetic vulnerability is related to disorders involving psychosis, such as bipolar disorder and schizophrenia. A growing body of work suggests that genetic vulnerability may also operate to increase the very general tendency toward mental health problems, without regard to the type of symptoms (Caspi & Moffit, 2018). Other variables then likely influence how the genetic vulnerability is shaped.

This is an exciting time for genetics research, as important discoveries about genes, environments, and psychological disorders are being made at a rapid rate. In addition, some of the most exciting breakthroughs in genetics have involved a combination of methods from genetics and neuroscience. Although we present genetic and neuroscience influences separately, they go hand in hand when it comes to understanding the possible causes of psychological disorders.

Quick Summary

The study of genetics in psychological disorders focuses on questions such as whether certain disorders are heritable and, if so, what is actually inherited. Heritability is a population statistic, not a metric of the likelihood that a person will inherit a disorder. Environmental effects can be classified as shared or not shared (sometimes called *unique*). Molecular genetics studies seek to identify differences in the sequence (SNPs) and structure of genes (CNVs) that may be involved in psychological disorders. GWAS has identified SNPs common across psychological disorders as well as those specific to certain disorders. Research has emphasized the importance of gene–environment interactions because genes do their work via the environment. Examples in which genetic influence is manifested only under certain environmental conditions (e.g., poverty and IQ) make it clear that we must look not just for the genes associated with psychological disorders but also for the conditions under which these genes may be expressed.

2.1 Check Your Knowledge

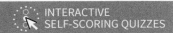
INTERACTIVE
SELF-SCORING QUIZZES

(Answers are at the end of the chapter.)

1. The process by which genes are turned on or off is referred to as:
   a. heritability.
   b. gene expression.
   c. polygenic.
   d. gene switching.

2. Sam and Sally are twins raised by their biological parents. Sam excelled in music and was in the high school band; Sally was the star player on the basketball team. They both received top-notch grades, and they both had part-time jobs at the bagel store. An example of a shared environment variable would be _____.
   a. school activities
   b. band for Sam
   c. basketball for Sally
   d. their parents' relationship

3. What refers to different forms of the same gene?
   a. allele
   b. polygenic
   c. polymorphism
   d. RNA

4. SNPs tell us about the _____ of genes.
   a. DNA
   b. RNA
   c. sequence
   d. polymorphism

5. GWAS involve:
   a. examining the entire genomes of people.
   b. large samples of participants.
   c. analysis of millions of gene sequences to look for SNPs.
   d. all of the above.

Neuroscience Influences

In this section, we look at three domains of neuroscience research in which the data are particularly interesting for understanding influences in psychological disorders: neurons and neurotransmitters, brain structure and function, and the neuroendocrine system.

Neurons and Neurotransmitters

The cells in the nervous system are called neurons, and the nervous system is composed of billions of neurons. Although neurons differ in some respects, each **neuron** has four major parts: (1) the cell body; (2) several dendrites, the short and thick extensions; (3) one or more axons of varying lengths, but usually only one long, thin axon that extends a considerable distance from the cell body; and (4) terminal buttons on the many end branches of the axon (**Figure 2.5**). When a neuron is appropriately stimulated at its cell body or through its dendrites, a nerve impulse travels down the axon to the terminal endings. Between the terminal endings of the sending axon and the cell membrane of the receiving neuron there is a small gap, called the **synapse** (**Figure 2.6**).

For neurons to send a signal to the next neuron so that communication can occur, the nerve impulse must have a way of bridging the synaptic space. The terminal buttons of each axon contain synaptic vesicles, small structures that are filled with **neurotransmitters**. Neurotransmitters are chemicals that allow neurons to send a signal across the synapse to another neuron. As the neurotransmitter flows into the synapse, some of the molecules reach the receiving, or postsynaptic, neuron. The cell membrane of the postsynaptic neuron contains receptors. Receptors are configured so that only specific neurotransmitters can fit into them. When a neurotransmitter fits into a receptor site, a message can be sent to the postsynaptic cell. What actually happens to the postsynaptic neuron depends on the integration of thousands of similar messages. Sometimes these messages are excitatory, leading to the creation of a nerve impulse in the postsynaptic cell; at other times, the messages are inhibitory, making the postsynaptic cell less likely to create a nerve impulse.

Once a presynaptic neuron (the sending neuron) has released its neurotransmitter, the last step is for the synapse to return to its normal state. Not all of the released neurotransmitter has found its way to postsynaptic receptors. Some of what remains in the synapse is broken down by enzymes, and some is taken back into the presynaptic cell through a process called **reuptake**.

Several key neurotransmitters have been implicated in psychological disorders, including **dopamine**, **serotonin**, **norepinephrine**, and **gamma-aminobutyric acid (GABA)**. Serotonin and dopamine may be involved in depression, mania, and schizophrenia. Norepinephrine is a neurotransmitter that communicates with the sympathetic nervous system, where it is involved in producing states of high arousal and may be involved in the anxiety disorders and other stress-related conditions (see **Focus on Discovery 2.1** for more on the sympathetic nervous system). GABA inhibits nerve impulses throughout most areas of the brain and may be involved in the anxiety disorders.

There are several ways in which neurotransmitters may contribute to psychological disorders though the mechanisms by which this happens are not currently well understood. Neurotransmitters are synthesized in the neuron through a series of metabolic steps, beginning with an amino acid. Each reaction along the way to producing an actual neurotransmitter is catalyzed by an enzyme. Neurotransmitter activity can be influenced by errors in these metabolic

VIDEO CONTENT

Neurons and Neuronal Communication

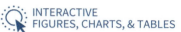
INTERACTIVE FIGURES, CHARTS, & TABLES

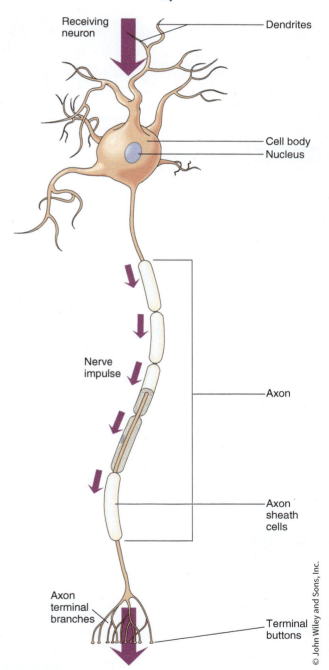

Receiving neuron — Dendrites — Cell body — Nucleus — Nerve impulse — Axon — Axon sheath cells — Axon terminal branches — Terminal buttons

© John Wiley and Sons, Inc.

FIGURE 2.5 The neuron is the basic unit of the nervous system.

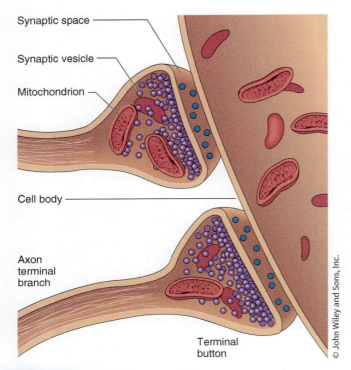

Synaptic space
Synaptic vesicle
Mitochondrion
Cell body
Axon terminal branch
Terminal button

© John Wiley and Sons, Inc.

FIGURE 2.6 A synapse, showing the terminal buttons of two axon branches in close contact with a very small portion of the cell body of another neuron.

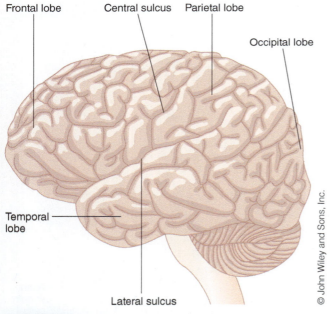

Frontal lobe   Central sulcus   Parietal lobe
Occipital lobe
Temporal lobe
Lateral sulcus

© John Wiley and Sons, Inc.

FIGURE 2.7 Surface of the left cerebral hemisphere, showing the four lobes and the central and lateral sulci.

steps. Other problems with neurotransmitters might result from alterations in the usual processes by which transmitters are deactivated after being released into the synapse. For example, a failure to pump leftover neurotransmitter back into the presynaptic cell (reuptake) would leave excess neurotransmitters in the synapse. Some research has focused on the possibility that the neurotransmitter receptors are at fault in some disorders. This reasoning comes largely from our understanding of how medications used to treat psychological disorders have an impact on receptors.

Structure and Function of the Human Brain

The cortex of the human brain is composed of the neurons that form the thin outer covering of the brain, the so-called **gray matter** of the brain. **Figure 2.7** shows the surface of the cortex on one side of the brain. The cortex consists of six layers of tightly packed neurons, estimated to number close to 16 billion. The cortex is vastly convoluted; the ridges are called *gyri*, and the depressions between them, *sulci*. The sulci are used to define different regions of the brain, much like guide points on a map. The frontal lobe lies in front of the central sulcus, the parietal lobe is behind it and above the lateral sulcus, the temporal lobe is located below the lateral sulcus, and the occipital lobe lies behind the parietal and temporal lobes (see Figure 2.7). The very front of the cortex is called the **prefrontal cortex**.

If the brain is sliced in half, separating the two cerebral hemispheres, additional important structures can be seen. The gray matter of the cerebral cortex does not extend throughout the interior of the brain. Much of the interior is **white matter**, made up of large tracts of myelinated (sheathed) fibers that connect cell bodies in the cortex with those in the spinal cord and in other areas of the brain.

Deep within the brain are cavities called **ventricles**. These ventricles are filled with cerebrospinal fluid. Cerebrospinal fluid circulates through the brain through these ventricles, which are connected with the spinal cord.

A set of deeper, mostly subcortical, structures are implicated in different psychological disorders. Some of these structures are shown in **Figure 2.8**. Important structures are the **anterior cingulate**; the **hippocampus**, which is associated with memory; the **hypothalamus**, which regulates metabolism, temperature, perspiration, blood pressure, sleeping, and appetite; and the **amygdala**, which is an important area for attention to emotionally salient stimuli.

The development of the human brain is a complex process that begins early in the first trimester of pregnancy and continues into early adulthood. It has been estimated that about a third of our genes are expressed in the brain, and many of these genes are responsible for laying out the structure of the brain. The development of the cells and the migration of these cells to the appropriate layers of cortex comprise an intricate dance. Unfortunately, missteps can happen, and current thinking about several disorders, such as schizophrenia, places the beginnings of the problem in these early developmental stages. Brain development continues throughout childhood, adolescence, and even into adulthood. What is happening during this time is cell development and a honing of the connections between cells and brain areas. The gray matter of the brain continues to develop, filling with cells, until early adolescence. Then, somewhat surprisingly, a number of synaptic connections begin to be eliminated—a process called **pruning**. Throughout early adulthood, the connections in the brain may become fewer, but they also become faster. The areas that develop the quickest are areas linked to sensory processes, like the cerebellum and occipital lobe. The area that develops last is the frontal lobe.

Most current research on the brain and psychological disorders examines not just areas or regions of the brain, but rather the **connectivity** between different areas of the brain. This type of inquiry aims to identify how different areas of the brain are connected with one another. Broadly speaking, there are three types of connectivity. *Structural (or anatomical) connectivity* refers to how different structures of the brain are connected via white matter. Problems in structural connectivity have been found in several psychological disorders, particularly for schizophrenia (Koshiyama, Fukunaga, et al., 2020). *Functional connectivity* refers to the connectivity between brain regions based on correlations between their blood oxygen level dependent (BOLD) signals measured with a brain imaging method called fMRI (see Chapter 3). For example, several studies have found reduced functional connectivity in people diagnosed with schizophrenia (Dong, Wang, et al., 2018) and at high risk for developing schizophrenia (Del Fabro, Schmidt, et al., 2021).

Effective connectivity combines both types of connectivity. It reveals not only correlations between BOLD activations in different brain regions but also the direction and timing of those activations, showing, for example, that when someone is viewing pictures of objects, activation in the occipital cortex comes first, followed by activation on the frontal cortex (Friston, 1994).

These connectivity methods have revealed several **brain networks**. Networks are clusters of brain regions that are connected to one another in that activation in these regions is reliably correlated when people perform certain types of tasks or are at rest (see **Figure 2.9**). For example, the frontoparietal network involves activation of the frontal and parietal cortices, and this network is activated when people are doing cognitive tasks. The default-mode network involves areas of the prefrontal cortex and temporal cortex and is activated when people are daydreaming or thinking about the future and recalling memories.

We will discuss several of these brain areas and networks throughout the book. For example, people with schizophrenia have been found to have diminished connectivity between the

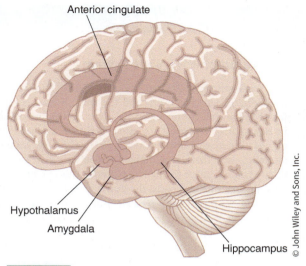

FIGURE 2.8 Subcortical structures of the brain.

© John Wiley and Sons, Inc.

:cursor: INTERACTIVE
FIGURES, CHARTS, & TABLES

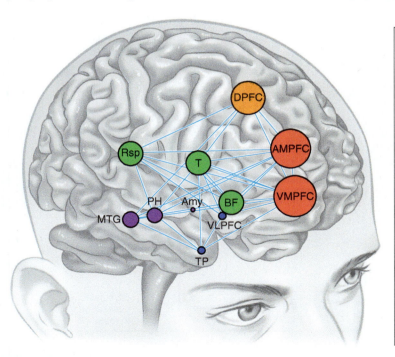

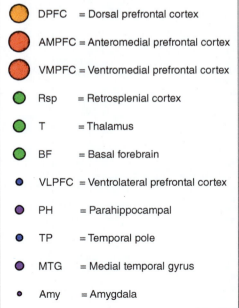

🟠	DPFC	= Dorsal prefrontal cortex
🔴	AMPFC	= Anteromedial prefrontal cortex
🔴	VMPFC	= Ventromedial prefrontal cortex
🟢	Rsp	= Retrosplenial cortex
🟢	T	= Thalamus
🟢	BF	= Basal forebrain
🔵	VLPFC	= Ventrolateral prefrontal cortex
🟣	PH	= Parahippocampal
🔵	TP	= Temporal pole
🟣	MTG	= Medial temporal gyrus
•	Amy	= Amygdala

Adapted from Alves, P.N., Foulon, C., Karolis, V. et al. An improved neuroanatomical model of the default-mode network reconciles previous neuroimaging and neuropathological findings. Commun Biol 2, 370 (2019). https://doi.org/10.1038/s42003-019-0611-3

FIGURE 2.9 This figure shows some of the brain areas that are part of the default mode network. The different sizes of the circles represent how much a region is in the network; the different colors represent the relationships between areas.

Focus on Discovery 2.1

The Autonomic Nervous System

The **autonomic nervous system (ANS)** innervates the endocrine glands, the heart, and the smooth muscles that are found in the walls of the blood vessels, stomach, intestines, kidneys, and other organs. Much of our behavior is dependent on a nervous system that operates very quickly, generally without our awareness, and that has traditionally been viewed as beyond voluntary control, hence the term *autonomic*. This nervous system is itself divided into two parts: the **sympathetic nervous system** and the **parasympathetic nervous system** (**Figure 2.10**). A simple way to think about these two components of the ANS is that the sympathetic nervous system prepares the body for "fight or flight" and the parasympathetic nervous system helps "calm down" the body.

The autonomic nervous system figures prominently in anxiety disorders. For example, people with panic disorder tend to misinterpret normal changes in their nervous system, such as shortness of breath after running up a flight of stairs. Instead of attributing this to being out of shape, people with panic disorder may think they are about to have another panic attack. In essence, they come to fear the sensations of their own autonomic nervous system.

Clinicians and researchers measure sympathetic and parasympathetic nervous system activity, including heart rate, tension in the muscles, breathing rate, and electrodermal activity (or how much the skin perspires). These measures can be helpful in using exposure to treat a person with an anxiety disorder, as it would be useful to know the extent to which the person shows nervous system reactivity when exposed to the stimuli that create anxiety.

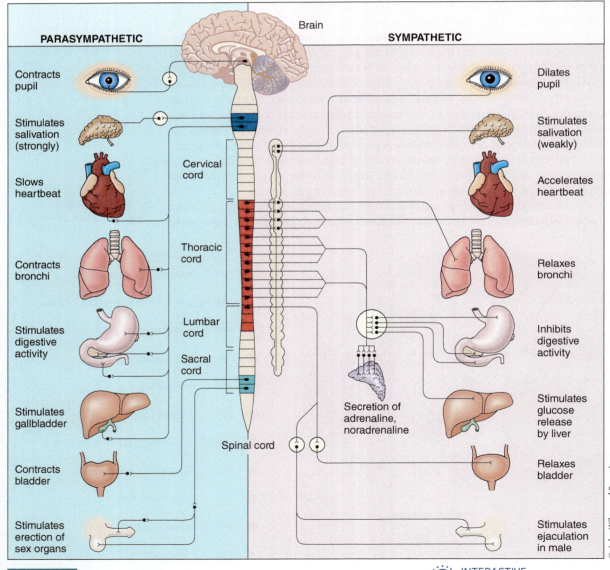

© John Wiley and Sons, Inc.

FIGURE 2.10 The autonomic nervous system.

INTERACTIVE
FIGURES, CHARTS, & TABLES

frontoparietal and default-mode networks (Chapter 9); the size of the hippocampus is reduced among some people with posttraumatic stress disorder, depression, and schizophrenia, perhaps due to overactivity of their stress response systems (Chapters 5, 7, and 9); brain size among some children with autism expands at a much greater rate than it does in typical development (Chapter 13).

The Neuroendocrine System

The neuroendocrine system has been implicated in psychological disorders as well, and we will consider the evidence throughout this book. One of the systems we will return to again and again is the hypothalamic-pituitary-adrenal (HPA) axis (shown in **Figure 2.11**). The **HPA axis** is central to the body's response to stress, and stress figures prominently in many of the disorders we discuss in this book.

When people are faced with a threat, the hypothalamus releases corticotropin-releasing factor (CRF), which then communicates with the *pituitary gland*. The pituitary then releases adrenocorticotropic hormone, which travels via the blood to the adrenal glands. The outer layers of the adrenal glands are referred to as the *adrenal cortex*; this area promotes the release of the hormone **cortisol**. For most people, cortisol is at its highest level first thing in the morning after awakening. It then gradually decreases over the day, with a slight increase around the middle of the afternoon. Cortisol is often referred to as the "stress hormone" because its release and pattern are influenced by stress. The HPA axis is not a fast-moving system, like the autonomic nervous system, reviewed in Focus on Discovery 2.1. Rather, it takes about 20 to 40 minutes for cortisol release to peak. After the stress or threat has remitted, it can take up to an hour for cortisol to return to baseline (i.e., prior to stress) levels (Dickerson & Kemeny, 2004). Chronic stress can lead to long-lasting changes in cortisol release. For some, the pattern of release throughout the day can be flattened, such that it does not decline as much over the course of a day, either because it starts off at a lower level in the morning or because it does not decline as much as the day goes on. As we will see, chronic stress and its effects on the HPA axis are linked to disorders as diverse as schizophrenia, depression, and posttraumatic stress disorder.

Studies of stress and the HPA axis are uniquely integrative. That is, they begin with a psychological concept (stress) and examine how stress is manifested in the body (the HPA axis). As in our discussion of genetic influences earlier, it is hard to consider biology and environment separately—biology may create increased reactivity to the environment, and early experiences may influence biology. One interesting longitudinal study (see Chapter 4) examined how stress impacts the HPA axis over time (Young, Farrell, et al., 2019). The researchers studied a sample of 90 people who had participated in stress assessments 19 times between the ages of 1 and 37. Parents completed a stress interview on behalf of the children until age 17; participants completed their own stress interview from age 23 to 37. (We discuss the assessment of stress using interviews in Chapter 3.) The research team assessed cortisol at the age-37 interview. They found that those people who had experienced a good deal of stress early in life exhibited a flatter pattern of cortisol release at age 37, but only if they were also experiencing a good deal of stress at age 37. This suggests that exposure to stress early in life may "sensitize" the HPA axis to respond in a certain way when faced with stress even into adulthood. Later, we will discuss the role of childhood stress and psychological disorders.

The Immune System

Stress also has effects on the immune system. Reviews of nearly 300 studies confirmed that a wide range of stressors produce problematic changes in the immune system, including medical school examinations, depression and bereavement, marital discord and divorce, job loss, and caring for a relative with Alzheimer's disease, among others (Kiecolt-Glaser & Glaser, 2002; Segerstrom & Miller, 2004). Given that stress is important in psychological disorders, it is perhaps not surprising that the immune system is involved as well.

The immune system involves a broad array of cells and proteins that respond when the body is infected or invaded. The body's first

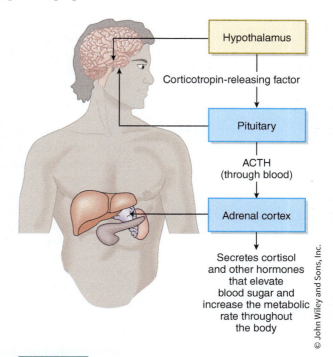

FIGURE 2.11   The HPA axis.

© John Wiley and Sons, Inc.

and quickest line of defense against infectious microorganisms is to unleash cells, such as macrophages, natural killer cells, and T-cells, to destroy these invaders. Inflammation or swelling is a sign of these immunity cells at work. Activation of macrophages in turn stimulates the release of proteins called **cytokines**, which help initiate such bodily responses to infection as fatigue, inflammation, and activation of the HPA axis. Cytokines that produce helpful inflammation are called pro-inflammatory cytokines. Pro-inflammatory cytokines such as interleukins (IL-1, IL-6, IL-8), and tumor necrosis factor alpha (TNF-alpha) have been implicated in depression, anxiety disorders, bipolar disorder, PTSD, and schizophrenia (Fineberg & Ellman, 2013; Goldsmith, Bekhbat, et al., 2023).

Neuroscience Approaches to Treatment

The use of psychiatric drugs continues to increase. For example, in 2019, 15.8% of people in the United States took some type of psychiatric medication (Terlizzi & Zablotsky, 2020). Prescriptions for depression and anxiety medications rose in 46 U.S. states during the COVID-19 pandemic and remained at these high levels in 2023. In 2016, antidepressants were the most commonly prescribed medication for adults between the ages of 40 and 59 in the United States and Canada (Hales, Servais, et al., 2019).

Antidepressants, such as Prozac, increase neural transmission in neurons that use serotonin as a neurotransmitter by inhibiting the reuptake of serotonin. Benzodiazepines, such as Xanax, can be effective in reducing the tension associated with some anxiety disorders, perhaps by stimulating GABA neurons to inhibit other neural systems that create the symptoms of anxiety. Antipsychotic drugs, such as Olanzapine, used in the treatment of schizophrenia, work on dopamine and serotonin. Stimulants, such as Adderall, are often used to treat children with attention-deficit/hyperactivity disorder; they operate on several neurotransmitters that help children focus.

It should be noted that a person could hold a neuroscience view about the nature of a disorder and yet recommend psychological intervention. We have known for over two decades that psychosocial interventions can also influence brain functioning. For example, psychotherapy that teaches a person how to stop performing compulsive rituals, which is an effective and widely used behavioral treatment for obsessive-compulsive disorder, has measurable effects on brain activity (Baxter, Ackermann, et al., 2000).

Evaluating the Role of Neuroscience Influences in Psychological Disorders

Over the past several decades, neuroscientists have made great progress in elucidating brain–behavior relationships. Although we view these developments in a positive light, we also want to caution against reductionism.

Reductionism refers to the view that whatever is being studied can and should be reduced to its most basic elements or constituents. In the case of psychological disorders, reductionism happens when scientists try to reduce complex mental and emotional responses to only what happens in the brain.

Basic elements, such as individual neurons, are organized into more complex brain networks. The properties of these networks cannot be deduced from the properties of the individual neurons. The whole is greater than the sum of its parts. A good example is provided by computers. Students writing papers for their courses use programs like Google Docs. These programs consist of many levels of code that communicate with the computer. The program necessarily relies on low-level communication with the computer, involving a series of 0's and 1's and electronic signals. Yet we don't conceptualize the program in terms of binary digits or electrical impulses. If the spell-checker stopped working, the first place to begin repairs would not be with the computer chips. Instead, we would want the programmer to fix the bug in the code. To be sure, the program could not run without the computer, but the program is more than just the impulses sent by the chips. In the same way, although a complex behavior like a hallucination necessarily involves the brain and neurons firing, it is not likely that we can fully capture the process by knowing about specific neurons.

Although you might assume that we have learned which neurotransmitters are involved in a disorder and then used that information to determine pharmacological treatments, this is often not the case. Rather, the reverse has often happened: A drug is found that influences symptoms, and then researchers are inspired to study the neurotransmitters influenced by that drug. As we will see, the evidence suggesting that neurotransmitters are causal in psychological disorders is not very strong.

Finally, as more and more research has been done using brain imaging (see Chapter 3), key insights about the brain and psychological disorders have emerged. First, there is not just one area of the brain that is linked to specific psychological disorders. Instead, networks of regions have been implicated. Second, as we discussed in the section on genetic influences, recent neuroscience research has underscored the commonality of brain network dysfunction across disorders. In other words, many of the same brain regions and networks have been found to be disrupted across many different disorders, ranging from schizophrenia to ADHD to obsessive-compulsive disorder to major depressive disorder (Etkin, 2019; Sprooten, Rasgon, et al., 2017).

Quick Summary

Neurotransmitters such as serotonin, norepinephrine, dopamine, and GABA have been implicated in many disorders. Several different brain areas and connectivity between them and brain networks are also a focus of research. The HPA axis is responsible for the body's response to stress and thus is relevant for several stress-related disorders. Stress can also produce problematic changes in the immune system, and this can have an impact on psychological disorders such as major depressive disorder. Cytokines help initiate such bodily responses to infection as fatigue, inflammation, and activation of the HPA axis. Pro-inflammatory cytokines have been linked to different psychological disorders. Treatments derived from neuroscience, primarily medications, are effective for some disorders, but they are not necessarily treating the cause of the disorders. Although the brain plays an important role in our understanding of the causes of psychological disorders, we must be careful to avoid reductionism.

2.2 Check Your Knowledge

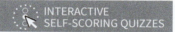 INTERACTIVE SELF-SCORING QUIZZES

(Answers are at the end of the chapter.)

Answer the following questions.

1. List four subcortical areas of the brain.

2. The _____ matter of the brain consists of the tracts of myelinated fibers that connect cells.

3. Neurotransmitters that are studied in psychological disorders include _____, which can produce states of high arousal, and GABA, which inhibits nerve impulses.

4. What does the HPA axis consist of?

5. What part of the immune system are associated with depression?

Cognitive Behavioral Influences

Cognitive behavioral influences include learning principles and cognitive science concepts, such as attention, memory, schema, and appraisal. As we will see, the basic principles from classical and operant conditioning (see Chapter 1) as well as cognitive science have shaped the development of many cognitive behavioral therapies.

Influences from Behaviorism

As discussed in Chapter 1, one key influence from behaviorism is the notion that problem behavior is likely to continue if it is reinforced. In one type of behavior therapy for depression called **behavioral activation (BA) therapy** (Dimidjian, Barrera, et al., 2011), a therapist helps a person identify and engage in tasks and behaviors that provide an opportunity for positive reinforcement.

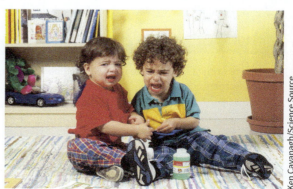

Aggressive responses in children are often rewarded, which makes them more likely to occur in the future. In this photo, the more aggressive child gets to keep the toy.

Ken Cavanagh/Science Source

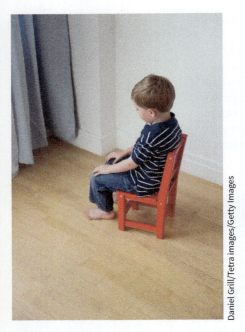

Time-out is a behavioral therapy technique based on operant conditioning; the consequence for misbehavior is removal to an environment with no positive reinforcers.

Reinforcement principles also help explain the persistence of unwanted behavior, such as aggressive behavior, which is a key feature of conduct disorder (see Chapter 13). Aggression is often reinforced (rewarded), as when one child hits another to secure the possession of a toy (getting the toy is the reinforcer). Parents may also unwittingly reinforce aggression by giving in when their child becomes angry or threatens violence to achieve some goal, such as staying up late to watch Netflix or play video games.

Once the source of reinforcement has been identified, behavior therapy may be employed to alter the consequences of the problem behavior. For example, if it was established that getting attention reinforced the problem behavior, the treatment might be to ignore the behavior. This can help to extinguish the undesirable behavior. Another way to extinguish the problem behavior is with a **time-out**, where the person is sent for a period of time to a location where positive reinforcers are not available. Today, time-out is a commonly used parenting technique for children who exhibit a problematic behavior of some sort.

In Chapter 1, we introduced the idea that certain disorders, such as a specific phobia, might develop based on classical conditioning principles. Modeling may also play a role, as we discuss in Chapter 6. One behavior therapy technique that is based on classical conditioning principles and used to treat phobias and anxiety is called **exposure**. The basic idea is that the anxiety will extinguish if the person can face the object or situation long enough with no actual harm occurring. Sometimes this exposure can be conducted in real-life situations. For example, if someone has a fear of flying, you might have them take an actual flight. Or if a person fears a dog, you may gradually expose the person to the dog. To address fears such as rape, trauma, or contamination, where exposure cannot be conducted in real life, *imaginal exposure* will be used. In other situations, both types of exposure are used. We discuss this treatment in more detail in Chapters 6 and 7.

As influential as these behavior therapy techniques were (and still are), behaviorism and behavior therapy were often criticized for minimizing the importance of two factors: thinking and feeling. And the way we think and feel about things undoubtedly influences our behavior. These limitations of behavioral points of view led some behavioral researchers and clinicians to include cognitive and emotion variables in their conceptualizations of psychopathology and therapy.

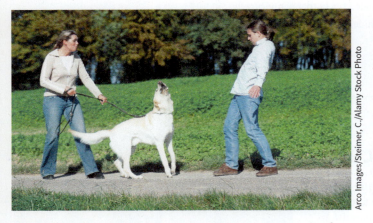

Exposure treatment is one of the most well-supported approaches for anxiety disorders.

Cognitive Science

Cognition is a term that groups together the mental processes of perceiving, recognizing, conceiving, judging, and reasoning. Cognitive science focuses on how people structure their experiences, how they make sense of them, and how they relate their current experiences to past ones that have been stored in memory.

At any given moment, we are bombarded by far more stimuli than we can possibly respond to. How do we filter this overwhelming input, put it into words or images, form hypotheses, and arrive at a perception of what is out there?

Cognitive scientists regard people as active interpreters of a situation, with people's past knowledge imposing a perceptual funnel on the experience. A person fits new information into an organized network of already accumulated knowledge, often referred to as a **schema**, or cognitive set (Neisser, 1976). New information may fit the schema; if not, the person reorganizes the schema to fit the information or construes the information in such a way as to fit the schema. The following scenario, inspired by the pioneering work of Bransford and Johnson (1973), illustrates how a schema may alter the way in which information is processed and remembered:

The woman worked all night finalizing the code for the new dating app. She rushed home to take a quick shower and grab some breakfast before the presentation to the VC firm. She picked out an outfit that was professional yet casual. While eating breakfast, she quickly scanned several apps on her phone and sent a few text messages. As she was leaving, she ran into the landlord, who asked about the rent again. She rushed past, realizing she had left her car keys in the apartment. Not wanting to return for her keys and pass the landlord, she requested Uber even though she was going to be charged premium pricing given the time of day, which soured her mood. And having to wait might make her late.

Now read the excerpt again but add the word *unemployed* before the word *woman*. Now read it a third time, substituting *Google employee* for *woman*. Notice how differently you understand the passage. Ask yourself what apps these women might have checked. If you were asked on a questionnaire to recall this information and you no longer had access to the excerpt, you might answer "Craigslist jobs" for the unemployed woman and "a technology site like ReCode" for the Google employee. Since the passage does not specify what apps or sites were checked, these answers are wrong, but in each instance the error would have been a meaningful, predictable one.

Other important contributions from cognitive science include the study of attention. As we will see, people with disorders as diverse as anxiety disorders, mood disorders, and schizophrenia have problems with attention. For example, individuals with anxiety disorders tend to focus their attention on threatening or anxiety-producing events or situations in the environment, as we discuss in more detail in Chapter 6. People with schizophrenia have a hard time concentrating their attention.

Of course, the concepts of schema and attention are related to each other. If a person has a particular set or schema about the world (e.g., the world is dangerous), that person may be more likely to pay attention to threatening or dangerous things in the environment. Furthermore, this person may be more likely to interpret ambiguous things in the environment as threatening. For example, seeing a stranger standing on a front porch may be interpreted as a sign of danger to someone with such a "danger" schema. For someone without such a schema, this person may be viewed simply as the person who lives in that house.

One of the exciting advances in cognitive science in the past 20 years is the access to and analysis of "big data." Traditional cognitive science experiments involve bringing a sample (say, of 50 to 100 people) into a laboratory to do a set of tasks. Big data approaches, by contrast, can include thousands of participants completing experiments online. Griffiths (2015) describes several exciting new ways in which cognitive scientists are testing theories and hypotheses about cognitive and behavioral processes like decision making, memory, preference learning, and categorization using many participants or huge online databases. Understanding why people make the choices they do can be enormously useful for psychopathology research to determine, for example, why certain people may be more prone to gambling problems than others (Chapter 10) or which people might benefit most from online interventions for various problems.

The Role of the Unconscious

As far back as Freud (see Chapter 1), much of human behavior was presumed to be unconscious, or outside the awareness of the individual. The unconscious has been a hot topic of study among cognitive psychologists for over 50 years. For example, in one classic study, participants were presented with different shapes for 1 millisecond (one-thousandth of a second) (Kunst-Wilson & Zajonc, 1980). Later, they showed virtually no ability to recognize the shapes they had seen, but when they rated how much they liked the various shapes, they preferred the ones they had been shown to other ones. We know that familiarity affects judgments of stimuli; people tend to like familiar stimuli more than unfamiliar ones. This study indicates that some aspects of the stimuli must have been absorbed, even though participants said that they did not recognize the shapes.

Cognitive neuroscientists have more recently explored how the brain supports behavior that is outside conscious awareness. For example, the concept of *implicit memory* refers to the idea that a person can, without being aware of it, be influenced by prior learning. If a person is shown a list of words so quickly that he or she cannot identify the words, the person will be able to recall those words later even though the words were not consciously perceived during the rapid initial presentation. Thus, a memory is formed implicitly (i.e., without conscious awareness). Implicit memory has been studied by psychopathology researchers, who have found, for example, that people with social anxiety and depression have trouble with these tasks (Amir, Foa, & Coles, 1998; Watkins, 2002).

Contemporary studies of the unconscious, such as studies of implicit memory, are a long way from Freud's original theorizing about the unconscious. For cognitive neuroscientists, the unconscious reflects the incredible efficiency and automaticity of the brain. That is, there are simply too many things going on around us all the time for us to be aware of everything. Thus, our brains have developed the capacity to register information for later use even if we are not aware of it.

Cognitive Behavior Therapy

Cognitive behavior therapy (CBT) incorporates theory and research on cognitive processes. Cognitive behavior therapists pay attention to private events—thoughts, perceptions, judgments, self-statements, and even tacit (unconscious) assumptions—and have studied and manipulated these processes in their attempts to understand and modify overt and covert disturbed behavior. **Cognitive restructuring** is a general term for changing a pattern of thought. People with depression may not realize how often they think self-critically, and those with anxiety disorders may not realize that they tend to be overly sensitive to possible threats in the world. Therapists hope that people can change their feelings, behaviors, and symptoms by changing their cognition. The therapist begins by tracking the daily thoughts a person experiences but then moves to understanding more about core cognitive biases and schemas that might shape those daily negative thoughts.

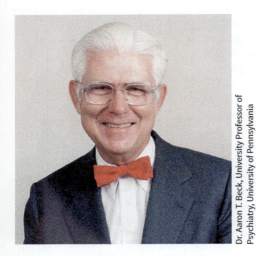

Aaron Beck developed a cognitive theory of depression and a cognitive behavioral therapy for people with depression.

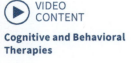

VIDEO CONTENT

Cognitive and Behavioral Therapies

Dr. Aaron T. Beck, University Professor of Psychiatry, University of Pennsylvania

Beck's Cognitive Therapy
Psychiatrist Aaron Beck (1921–2021) developed a cognitive therapy for depression based on the idea that depressed mood is caused by distortions in the way people perceive life experiences (Beck, 1976; Salkovskis, 1996). For example, a person with depression may focus exclusively on negative happenings and ignore positive ones. Imagine that a woman's romantic partner both praises and criticizes her. If the woman attends to the praise and remembers it the next day, she is likely to feel happy. But if she focuses on the criticism and continues to dwell on it the next day, she is likely to feel unhappy. Beck's therapy, which has now been adapted for many other disorders in addition to depression, is a collaborative treatment between a therapist and the person seeking treatment. When a person with depression expresses feeling that nothing ever goes right, for example, the therapist offers counterexamples, pointing out how the person has overlooked favorable happenings. The general goal of Beck's therapy is to provide people with experiences, both inside and outside the therapy room, that will alter their negative schemas, enabling them to have hope rather than despair.

There have also been many extensions of behavior therapy and CBT. The so-called "third wave" behavioral treatments include dialectical behavior therapy (see Chapter 15), mindfulness-based cognitive therapy (see Chapter 5), and acceptance and commitment therapy. The newer treatments differ from traditional CBT by incorporating a focus on spirituality, values, emotion, and acceptance. Another theme is strategies to minimize emotional avoidance. For example, in acceptance and commitment therapy (Hayes, 2005), a person might be taught that much of the destructive power of emotions lies in the way we respond to them cognitively and behaviorally. An overarching goal of these therapies is to help a person learn to be more aware of emotions but to avoid immediate, impulsive reactions to those emotions. In the case of mindfulness-based cognitive therapy, this is facilitated through the use of meditation (Segal, Williams, & Teasdale, 2003). Overall, a rich array of cognitive behavioral approaches have been developed.

Evaluating the Role of Cognitive Behavioral Influences in Psychological Disorders

Cognitive behavioral explanations of psychological disorders have generated a great deal of research over the past several decades. Yet some cognitive explanations do not appear to explain much. That a person with depression has negative schemas tells us that the person thinks gloomy thoughts. But such a pattern of thinking is actually part of the diagnosis of depression. What is distinctive in cognitive behavioral approaches is that the thoughts are given causal status; that is, the thoughts are regarded as causing the other features of the disorder, such as sadness. Research suggests that negative cognitive tendencies can predict the onset of depressive disorders, anxiety disorders, and PTSD. For example, cognition measured before a military recruit goes into the war zone can predict whether the person will develop PTSD. Left unanswered is the question of where the negative thoughts came from in the first place. Much of the current research is focused on understanding what types of mechanisms sustain the negative thoughts typical of many different psychological disorders.

Clinical Case

An Example of Beck's Cognitive Therapy

The following examples illustrate ways of beginning to help a person change negative cognitions.

Therapist: You said that you feel like a failure since Bill left you. How would you define "failure"?

Patient: *Well, the marriage didn't work out.*

Therapist: So, you believe that the marriage didn't work out because you, as a person, are a failure?

Patient: *If I had been successful, then he would still be with me.*

Therapist: So, would we conclude that we can say, "People whose marriages don't work out are failures"?

Patient: *No, I guess I wouldn't go that far.*

Therapist: Why not? Should we have one definition of failure for you and another for everyone else?

People who define *failure* as less than "extraordinarily successful" can see that their definitions are polarized in all-or-nothing terms—that is, "complete success" versus "complete failure." A variation on this technique is to ask the patient how others would define "success" or "failure."

Therapist: You can see that your definition of "failure" is quite different from the way other people might see it. Few people would say that a person who is divorced is a failure. Let's focus on the positive end right now. How would most people define "success" in a person?

Patient: *Well, they might say that someone has success when they accomplish some of their goals.*

Therapist: OK. So, would we say that if someone accomplishes some goals they have success?

Patient: *Right.*

Therapist: Would we also say that people can have different degrees of success? Some people accomplish more goals than others?

Patient: *That sounds right.*

Therapist: So, if we applied this to you, would we say that you have accomplished some of your goals in life?

Patient: *Yes, I did graduate from college and I have been working for the past six years. I've been busy raising Ted—he had some medical problems a couple of years ago, but I got the right doctors for him.*

Therapist: So, would we call these some successful behaviors on your part?

Patient: *Right, I've had some successes.*

Therapist: Is there a contradiction, then, in your thinking—calling yourself a "failure" but saying that you have had several successes?

Patient: *Yes, that doesn't make sense, does it?*

Source: From Leahy, R. L. (2017). *Cognitive Therapy Techniques: A Practitioner's Guide*, pp. 52–53. Guilford Press.

Quick Summary

Cognitive behavioral influences include research from behaviorism and cognitive science. Treatment techniques designed to alter the consequences or reinforcers of a behavior include behavior activation therapy, time-out, and exposure. Cognitive science focuses on concepts such as schema (a network of accumulated knowledge or a cognitive set), attention, memory, and the unconscious, and these concepts are part of cognitive behavioral theories and treatments of psychological disorders. For example, research on implicit memory promoted acceptance of the ideas of unconscious influences on behavior. Cognitive behavior therapy uses behavior therapy techniques and cognitive restructuring. Aaron Beck is an influential cognitive behavior therapist.

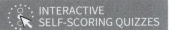

2.3 Check Your Knowledge

INTERACTIVE
SELF-SCORING QUIZZES

(Answers are at the end of the chapter.)

Fill in the blank.

1. _____ is based on the idea that anxiety will extinguish if a bad outcome or harm does not occur.

2. A treatment that focuses on increasing positively reinforcing activities is called _____.

3. One technique that seeks to remove positive reinforces is called _____.

True or false?

4. A schema refers to an organized network of cognitive knowledge.

5. Beck's theory suggests that people have distortions in the way they perceive life's experiences.

6. Current research on the unconscious is conducted in much the same way as it was when Freud talked about the unconscious.

Socioemotional Influences

Additional sets of influences that we will consider throughout this book are emotional, sociocultural, and interpersonal influences. Some type of disturbance in emotion can be found in nearly all psychological disorders. In addition, we will see that sex, race, culture, ethnicity, and social relationships bear importance on the descriptions, causes, and treatments of different disorders. Stress, whether in the form of early life adversity, discrimination, trauma, or difficult life experiences, also influences nearly all psychological disorders. In the next sections, we introduce these concepts and give some examples of why they are so important in psychological disorders.

The Importance of Emotion

Emotions influence how we respond to problems and challenges in our environment. They help us organize our thoughts and actions, both explicitly and implicitly, and they guide our behavior. Perhaps because our emotions exert such widespread influence, we spend a good deal of time trying to regulate how we feel and how we present our emotions to others. Given their centrality, it is not surprising that disturbances in emotions figure prominently in psychological disorders. By one analysis, as many as 85% of psychological disorders include disturbances in emotional processing of some kind (Thoits, 1985).

What is emotion? The answer to that question could fill an entire textbook on its own. Emotions are believed to be fairly short-lived states, lasting for a few seconds, minutes, or at most hours. Sometimes the word *affect* is used to describe short-lasting emotional feelings. Moods, on the other hand, are emotional experiences that endure for a longer period of time. Current theories on emotion suggest that we use information from our bodies, memories, and environment to make sense of and report on how we feel (Barrett, 2017).

To understand emotion in psychological disorders, it is helpful to use several different measures of emotions. The *expressive*, or *behavioral*, *measure* of emotion typically refers to facial expressions of emotion. The *experience*, or *subjective feeling*, measure of emotion refers to how someone reports they feel at any given moment or in response to some event. For example, learning that you received an A on your midterm might elicit feelings of happiness, pride, and relief. Learning you received a C might elicit feelings of anger, anxiety, or embarrassment. The *physiological measure* of emotion involves changes in the body, such as those due to the autonomic nervous system activity that accompanies emotion. For example, if a car almost runs you down as you are crossing the street, you may show a frightened look on your face, feel fear, and experience an increase in your heart rate and breathing rate.

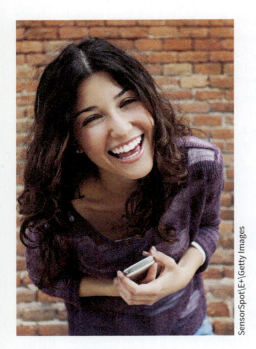

SensorSpot\(E+\)Getty Images

Emotion consists of many components, including expression (shown here), experience, and physiology.

When we consider emotional disturbances in psychological disorders, it is important to consider which emotion measures are affected. For example, people with schizophrenia do not readily express their emotions outwardly, but they report feeling emotions very strongly. People with panic disorder experience excessive fear when no actual danger is present. People with depression may experience prolonged sadness and other negative feelings. A person with antisocial personality disorder may not feel empathy.

Another important consideration in the study of emotion and psychological disorders is the concept of *ideal affect*, which simply refers to the kinds of emotional states that a person ideally wants to feel. At first glance, you might presume that happiness is the ideal affect for everyone. After all, who doesn't want to feel happy? However, research shows that ideal affects vary depending on cultural factors (Tsai, 2017). Thus, people from Western cultures, such as that of the United States, do indeed value happiness as their ideal state. However, people from East Asian cultures, like China, value less arousing positive emotions, such as calmness, more than happiness (Tsai, Knutson, & Fung, 2006). Cross-nationally, more people in the United States seek treatment for cocaine and amphetamines, drugs that are stimulating and associated with feelings of excitement and happiness; more people in China seek treatment for heroin, a drug that has calming effects (for more on the effects of these drugs, see Chapter 10).

Sociocultural Influences

A good deal of research has focused on the ways in which sociocultural influences, such as sex assigned at birth, gender, race, culture, ethnicity, and income inequality and poverty, can influence different psychological disorders. The range of variables considered and the ways of studying those variables cover a lot of ground.

Several studies consider the role of sex assigned at birth in different disorders. These studies have shown that some disorders affect men and women differently. For example, depression is nearly twice as common among women as among men. On the other hand, antisocial personality disorder and alcohol use disorder are more common among men than women. Childhood disorders, such as attention-deficit/hyperactivity disorder, affect boys more than girls, but some researchers question whether this reflects a true difference between boys and girls or a bias in the diagnostic criteria. Current research is looking beyond whether men and women differ in the prevalence rates of certain disorders to ask questions about risk factors that may differently impact men and women in the development of these disorders. For example, father-to-son genetic transmission appears to be an important risk factor in the development of alcohol use disorder for men, whereas sociocultural standards of thinness may be a risk factor in the development of eating disorders for women. Research has also begun to consider gender identify and psychological disorders, for example examining psychological disorders among nonbinary individuals—that is, among people who do not identify as male or female. Research has also focused on studying psychological disorders in sexual minoritized individuals (e.g., gay, lesbian, or bisexual) as well as gender minoritized individuals (e.g., transgender). For example, eating disorders, particularly anorexia nervous, are more common among sexual or gender minoritized men than cisgender, heterosexual men (Brown & Keel, 2023; Calzo, Blashill, et al., 2017).

Other studies show that poverty is a major influence on psychological disorders. For example, poverty is related to antisocial personality disorder, anxiety disorders, and depression. Income inequality is associated with mental health outcomes—in areas where income inequality is greater, people experience more psychological disorders, including depression and psychosis (Ribeiro, Bauer, et al., 2017). What remains to be more clearly sorted out is the causal direction: Does income inequality predict the onset of disorders or do disorders interfere with earning power and thus exacerbate income inequality?

Cultural, racial, and ethnic differences in psychological disorders have also been examined. Some questions, such as whether the disorders we diagnose and treat in the United States are observed in other parts of the world, have been fairly well studied. This research has demonstrated that several disorders are observed in diverse parts of the world. Indeed, no country or culture is without psychological disorders of some sort. For example, schizophrenia is observed in diverse cultures, but the conceptualization and meaning of the symptoms may vary. For example, *nuthkavihak* in the Inuit culture and *were* in the Yoruba culture include talking to oneself, refusing to talk, delusional beliefs, and bizarre behavior (Murphy, 1976). People with schizophrenia in the

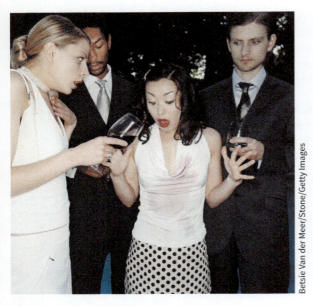

Betsie Van der Meer/Stone/Getty Images

Culture, race, and ethnicity play an important role in the descriptions, causes, and treatments of psychological disorders.

United States consider their auditory hallucinations (hearing voices) to be part of their illness, but people with schizophrenia in India and Ghana are less likely to consider these hallucinations as part of their illness (Luhrmann, Padmavati, et al., 2015). In Chapter 6, we discuss a few anxiety conditions around the world that look very similar to the symptoms of panic disorder. Other disorders are apparently specific to particular cultures. In Chapter 11, we consider the evidence that eating disorders are specific to Western culture. As we discuss in Chapter 3, the current diagnostic system includes cultural influences in the discussion of every category of disorder, and this may be an important step toward increasing research in this area.

Even though there are some similarities in psychological disorders across cultures, there are also many profound cultural influences on the symptoms expressed in different disorders, the availability of treatment, and the willingness to seek treatment. We consider these issues throughout this book.

We must also consider the role of race in psychological disorders. As Anglin and colleagues have pointed out, being a particular race is not a causal factor, but experiencing discrimination and racism can create a social environment that adversely impacts the development and maintenance of psychological disorders (Anglin, Ereshefsky, et al., 2021). Some disorders, such as schizophrenia, are diagnosed more often among Blacks than Whites. Does schizophrenia occurs more often in this group, or does it mean that some type of racial bias might be operating in diagnostic assessments? Black Americans are much less likely to receive an appropriate diagnosis or recommended care for their bipolar disorder, which in turn is tied to greater risk of hospitalization for their symptoms (McMaster & Johnson, 2014). The use of drugs and their effects also vary by race. White Americans are more likely to use or abuse many drugs, such as nicotine, hallucinogens, methamphetamine, prescription painkillers, and, depending on the age group, alcohol. Yet Black American smokers are more likely to die from lung cancer. Eating disturbances and body dissatisfaction are greater among White women than Black women, particularly in college, but differences in actual eating disorders, particularly bulimia, do not appear to be as great. The reasons for these differences are not yet well understood and are the focus of current research. Table 2.1 shows data on sex, ethnic, and racial differences in the number of people reporting certain psychological disorders in 2019 out of a total of 6,945,521 (SAMHSA, 2022).

TABLE 2.1	Number of People in the United States with a Psychological Disorder Among Different Sex, Ethnic, and Racial Groups in 2020							
	Sex Assigned at Birth		**Ethnicity**		**Race**			
Disorder	**Male**	**Female**	**Not of Hispanic or Latino Origin**	**Hispanic or Latino Origin**	**Asian**	**Black**	**White**	**Other**
Trauma-related disorders	530,123	761,230	944,583	235,861	14,546	209,379	783,816	137,128
Anxiety disorders	527,839	874,137	1,053,876	240,877	15,418	150,861	966,447	128,138
ADHD	439,432	212,894	490,524	114,465	4,199	129,730	390,624	70,284
Bipolar disorders	281,146	431,079	573,885	89,965	5,937	116,699	492,718	50,810
Depression disorders	686,701	1,143,469	1,367,174	320,270	26,378	293,485	1,151,672	187,781
Schizophrenia and other psychotic disorders	476,145	288,121	587,311	92,660	17,642	241,020	372,795	72,550

Table values are percentages.

Source: From SAMHSA (2022). Mental Health Annual Report 2015-2020: Use of Mental Health Services: National Client Level Data (https://www.samhsa.gov/data/data-we-collect/mh-cld-mental-health-client-level-data). Public Domain.

Interpersonal Influences and the Role of Stress

Many researchers have published articles on how the quality of relationships influences different disorders. Other researchers are interested in understanding the role of trauma, or serious life events, and stress in psychological disorders. Researchers who study such influences all share the premise that environmental influences can trigger, exacerbate, or maintain the symptoms that make up the different disorders. We will describe some of the ways people measure life events in the next chapter. But the influence of stress within the context of social relationships plays a role in just about all the disorders we will consider.

Family and marital relationships, social support, and even the amount of casual social contact all play a role in influencing the course of disorders. In **Focus on Discovery 2.2**, we discuss couples and family approaches to psychotherapy. Within relationships, researchers have looked for ways to measure not only the relative closeness and support offered but also the degree of hostility displayed.

Interpersonal Therapy   **Interpersonal therapy (IPT)** emphasizes the importance of current relationships in a person's life and how problems in these relationships can contribute to psychological symptoms. The therapist first encourages the patient to identify feelings about their relationships and to express these feelings and then helps the patient generate solutions to interpersonal problems. IPT has been shown to be an effective treatment for depression (a topic we turn to in more detail in Chapter 5). IPT has also been used to treat eating disorders, anxiety disorders, and personality disorders.

Focus on Discovery 2.2

Couples and Family Therapies

Given that interpersonal influences are important in nearly all disorders we discuss in this book, it is not surprising that therapies have been developed to focus on these relationships. In addition to interpersonal therapy, discussed in the text, we consider here two other types of therapies: couples therapy and family therapy.

Couples Therapy

Conflict is inevitable in any long-term partner relationship. Between 40% and 50% of marriages in the United States end in divorce, and most of these divorces happen within the first 7 years of marriage (Bradbury & Bodenmann, 2020; Karney & Bradbury, 2020). People in a distressed marriage are two to three times as likely to experience a psychological disorder (Whisman &

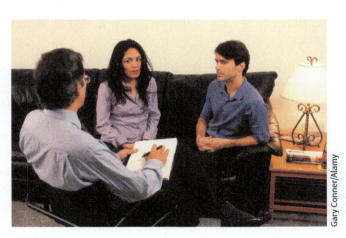

When a problem involves a couple, treatment is most effective if the couple is seen together.

Gary Conner/Alamy

Uebelacker, 2006). In some couples, distress may be a consequence of the psychological disorder, but it is also clear that distress can contribute to psychological disorders (South, 2021). Couples therapy is often used in the treatment of psychological disorders, particularly when they occur in the context of major relationship distress. When one partner is experiencing depression, couples therapy can be just as effective for reducing the depression as individual therapy (Barbato, D'Avanzo, & Parabiaghi, 2018).

In couples therapy, the therapist works with both partners together to reduce relationship distress. Treatments for most couples focus on improving communication, problem solving, satisfaction, trust, and positive feelings (Bradbury & Bodenmann, 2020).

Family Therapy

Family therapy is based on the idea that the problems of the family influence each member and that the problems of each member influence the family. As such, family therapy is used to address specific symptoms of a given family member, particularly for the treatment of childhood problems.

Family therapy is often tailored to the specific disorder. In family approaches for conduct disorder, the therapist may focus on improving parental monitoring and discipline. For adolescents with other externalizing problems, the goal of family therapy may be to improve communication, to change roles, or to address a range of family problems. With disorders like schizophrenia and bipolar disorder, family therapy often includes psychoeducation as a supplement for the medication treatment provided to the individual. Psychoeducation focuses on improving understanding of the disorder, reducing expressed family criticism and hostility, and helping families learn skills for managing symptoms, as in the Clinical Case of Clare (Miklowitz, George, et al., 2003). In anorexia nervosa, family members are used strategically to help the adolescent gain weight. In sum, the goals and strategies of family therapy will be adjusted to meet the needs of different clients.

Clinical Case

Clare

Clare, a 17-year-old girl who lived with her parents and her 15-year-old brother, was referred for family-focused treatment (FFT) of bipolar disorder as an adjunct to medication treatment. She had received a diagnosis of bipolar I disorder in early adolescence and was treated with lithium carbonate and quetiapine but had never fully responded to medications.

During an individual assessment session, Clare explained that she thought about suicide almost daily and had made two prior attempts, both by overdosing on her parents' medications. Clare had kept both attempts secret from her parents. Ethically, clinicians need to take steps to keep a client safe, and in this case, one measure would be to let Clare's parents know about her suicidality. The clinician explained this to Clare.

The first goal in FFT is to provide psychoeducation about bipolar disorder. As the symptoms of bipolar disorder were being reviewed, the clinician asked Clare to discuss her suicide attempts with her parents. When Clare did so, her parents were surprised. Her father, who had experienced his own father's suicide, was particularly concerned.

After psychoeducation, a goal in FFT is to choose one problem for the family to address and to help them learn new problem-solving skills in the process. In this family, the focus of problem solving was how to keep Clare safe from her suicidal impulses. To begin problem solving, the therapist worked with the family to define the problem and its context. The therapist asked the family to discuss situations that seemed to place Clare at most risk for suicide. The family was able to pinpoint that both previous attempts had followed interpersonal losses.

The next phase of problem solving is to generate potential solutions. To help with this process, the clinician framed questions in the problem-solving process for the family, including whether Clare could share her suicidal thoughts with her parents, how to establish whether she was safe, what responses would be helpful from them, and what other protective actions should be taken. Using this structure, the family was able to agree on the plan that Clare would phone or text her parents when she was feeling self-destructive. Clare and her parents generated a plan in which her parents would help Clare engage in positive and calming activities until her suicidal thoughts were less intrusive. Clare and her parents reported feeling closer and more optimistic.

The therapist then began to conduct the next phase of therapy, which focused directly on symptom management. This phase consisted of training Clare to monitor her moods, to identify triggers for mood changes, and to help her cope with those triggers.

As is typical in FFT, the clinician introduced the communication enhancement module during the eighth session. A goal of this module is to role-play new communication skills. Family members practice skills such as "active listening" by paraphrasing and labeling the others' statements and by asking clarifying questions. At first, Clare and her brother protested against the role-play exercises.

Clare experienced another loss during this period when her one and only close, long-term friend announced that she was going to be moving out of state. Clare took an overdose of Tylenol in a suicide attempt. Soon after overdosing, she became afraid and induced vomiting, and later she told her parents about the attempt.

The next session focused on the suicide attempt. Her parents, particularly her father, were hurt and angry. Clare in turn reacted angrily and defensively. The therapist asked the family to practice active listening skills regarding Clare's suicidality. Clare explained that she had acted without even thinking about the family agreement because she had been so distressed about the idea of losing her friend. Clare's parents were able to validate her feelings using active listening skills. The therapist reminded the parents that suicidal actions are common in bipolar disorder and noted that Clare's ability to be honest about her suicide attempt was an indicator of better family connectedness. The therapist also recommended that Clare see her psychiatrist, who increased her dosage of lithium.

By the end of treatment after 9 months, Clare had not made any more suicide attempts, had become more willing to take her medications, and felt closer to her parents. Like many people with bipolar disorder, though, she remained mildly depressed. Clare and her family continued to see the therapist once every 3 months for ongoing support. [Adapted from Miklowitz and Taylor (2005) with permission of the authors.]

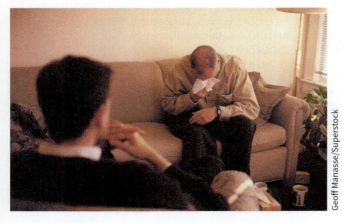

Geoff Manasse/Superstock

Unresolved grief is one of the issues discussed in interpersonal therapy.

In IPT, four interpersonal issues are assessed to examine whether one or more of them might be having an impact on symptoms:

- *Unresolved grief*—for example, experiencing delayed or incomplete grieving following a loss
- *Role transitions*—for example, transitioning from child to parent or from worker to retired person
- *Role disputes*—for example, resolving different relationship expectations between romantic partners
- *Interpersonal or social deficits*—for example, not being able to begin a conversation with an unfamiliar person or finding it difficult to negotiate with a boss at work

In sum, the therapist helps the patient understand that a psychological disorder occurs in a social or relationship context and that getting a better handle on relationship patterns is necessary to reduce symptoms of the disorder.

Challenging interpersonal relationships can be quite stressful. Domestic violence by a partner or ex-partner is the most common type of violence against women, with over a third of women around the world reporting such abuse, and the perpetrators are most often men (World Health Organization, 2013). Domestic violence against women is associated with a greater risk of several psychological disorders, including depression, posttraumatic stress disorder (PTSD), anxiety disorders, eating disorders, and substance use disorders (Trevillion, Oram, et al., 2012). As we discuss in Chapter 4, cross-sectional studies that report correlations between two things such as domestic violence and psychological disorder cannot determine causality. Nevertheless, there is evidence that domestic violence increases the chance of becoming depressed, and that experiencing depression increases the chance of experiencing domestic abuse (Devries, Mak, et al., 2013). Given the unfortunate frequency with which domestic violence occurs and its association with psychological disorders, mental health professionals ought to assess for the occurrence of domestic violence (Oram, Khalifeh, & Howard, 2017).

More generally, many different types of life stressors besides interpersonal stress can influence the onset and course of psychological disorders. Broadly, **stress** can be defined as the subjective experience of distress in response to perceived environmental problems. Severe stress, such as experiencing or witnessing someone else experience exposure to death (actual or threatened), sexual violence, or serious injury, is considered to be a traumatic event in the current diagnostic system (see Chapter 3; American Psychiatric Association, 2013). As many as 70% of people around the world have experienced such a traumatic event, the most common being the unexpected death of a loved one (Benjet, Bromet, et al., 2016). Exposure to a traumatic event is one of the diagnostic criteria for PTSD, but exposure to such events is also associated with many other psychological disorders (Scott, Koenen, et al., 2013).

Other types of stress are also implicated in psychological disorders, as we will discuss throughout the rest of the book. Stress during childhood, sometimes referred to as trauma or maltreatment, is associated with a higher chance of developing a psychological disorder in adulthood (Bjorkenstam, Burstrom, et al., 2016), pointing to the importance of implementing prevention programs to help prevent psychological disorders from occurring (Caspi & Moffitt, 2018). Maltreatment or trauma during childhood or adolescence, no matter what shape it takes (physical abuse, sexual abuse, or neglect), is a risk factor for nearly all disorders we will discuss in this book (Caspi & Moffitt, 2018).

Evaluating the Role of Socioemotional Influences in Psychological Disorders

One of the challenges in studying the role of any influences, including environment and socioemotional influences, is discerning whether these factors are causal. As we discuss in Chapter 4, the best way to identify causal factors is by doing experiments and randomly assigning participants to different conditions. Alas, we cannot randomly assign people to experience trauma or not to see which people are more likely to develop a psychological disorder. We must therefore use other methods to determine causality, such as longitudinal studies (also discussed in Chapter 4). Another challenge to studying the role of socioemotional influences is that many of these factors are strongly related to one another. For example, living in poverty can be very stressful: Determining the role of poverty separately from that of stress is nearly impossible. Interpersonal difficulties are associated with many emotions, such as sadness, anger, despair, or disgust. Yet, these emotions can be experienced and expressed differently based on sex, gender identity, genetics, and stress.

In **Focus on Discovery 2.3**, we illustrate how adopting a single perspective to the exclusion of others can bias your perspective of the critical targets for treatment.

Focus on Discovery 2.3

Multiple Perspectives on a Clinical Problem

To provide a concrete example of how it is possible to conceptualize a clinical case by considering multiple influences, we present a case and discuss how the information provided is open to several interpretations.

Your conceptualization of this case likely will depend on the types of influences you choose to focus on. If you recognize the importance of genetic influences, you are attentive to the family history, noting that Arthur's father had similar difficulties with alcohol. You are probably aware of the research (to be reviewed in Chapter 10) that suggests a genetic contribution to alcohol use disorder. You understand, though, that genes do their work via the environment, and you hypothesize about the ways in which genetic influences interact with different environmental influences (e.g., stress at work and in his relationships), in turn possibly increasing the likelihood that Arthur will turn to alcohol to cope.

Now suppose that you focus on the importance of cognitive behavioral influences, which encourages you to approach psychological disorders in terms of reinforcement patterns as well as cognitive variables. You may focus on Arthur's self-consciousness at college, which seems related to the fact that, compared with his fellow students, he grew up with few advantages. Economic insecurity and hardship may have made him unduly sensitive to criticism and rejection. Alcohol has been his escape from such tensions. But heavy drinking, coupled with persistent doubt about his own worth as a human being, has worsened an already deteriorating marital relationship, further undermining his confidence. As a cognitive behavior therapist, you may decide on cognitive behavior therapy to convince Arthur that he need not obtain universal approval for every undertaking.

If you adopted an integrative perspective, you would recognize that multiple influences contribute to Arthur's difficulties. You would acknowledge the likely genetic contribution to Arthur's alcohol use disorder, but you would also identify key triggers (e.g., job stress) that might lead to greater bouts of drinking. You would likely employ many of the therapeutic techniques noted in this chapter.

Clinical Case

Arthur

Arthur's childhood had not been a particularly happy one. His mother died suddenly when he was 6, and for the next 10 years he lived either with his father or with a maternal aunt. His father drank heavily, seldom managing to get through a day without some alcohol. His father's income was so irregular that he could rarely pay bills on time or afford to live in any but the most run-down neighborhoods. At times, Arthur's father was totally incapable of caring for himself, let alone his son. Arthur would then spend weeks, sometimes months, with his aunt in a nearby suburb.

Despite these early life circumstances, Arthur completed high school and entered college. He qualified for student loans and other financial aid, but he also needed to wait tables and tend bar to make ends meet. During these college years, he felt an acute self-consciousness with people he felt had authority over him—his boss, his professors, and even some of his classmates, with whom he compared himself unfavorably.

Like many people in college, Arthur attended his fair share of parties. He pledged a fraternity at the end of his first year, and this was the source of most of his socializing. It was also the source of a lot of alcohol. He drank heavily at the weekend parties. By his senior year, however, he was drinking daily, often to deal with the stress of being in school and working at the same time.

Two years after college, Arthur married his college girlfriend. He could never quite believe that his wife, as intelligent as she was beautiful, really cared for him. As the years wore on, his doubts about himself and about her feelings toward him would continue to grow.

After college, Arthur began a job at a publishing company, serving as an assistant editor. This job proved to be even more stressful than college. The deadlines and demands of the senior editors were difficult. He constantly questioned whether he had what it took to be an editor. Like his father, he often drank to deal with this stress.

Several years later, when it seemed that life should be getting easier, he found himself in even greater turmoil. Now 35 years old, with a fairly secure job that paid reasonably well, he was arguing more often with his wife. She continually complained about his drinking; he denied that there was a problem. After all, he was only drinking four beers a night. His wife wanted to start a family, but he was not sure if he wanted to have this additional stress in his life. His brooding over his marriage led him to drink even more heavily until finally, one day, he realized he was drinking too much and needed to seek help.

Quick Summary

Disturbances in emotion figure prominently in psychological disorders, but the ways in which emotions can be disrupted vary quite a bit. It is important to distinguish between measures of emotion, including expression, experience, and physiology. In addition, mood can be distinguished from emotion. The concept of ideal affect illustrates how people from different cultures may have different ideal feeling states. Psychological disorders have different types of emotion disturbances, and thus it is important to consider which of the emotion components are affected. In some disorders, all emotion components may be disrupted, whereas in others just one might be problematic.

Sociocultural influences, such as culture, race, ethnicity, sex, gender identity, and socioeconomic status, are important influences in the study of psychological disorders. Some disorders, like schizophrenia and anxiety, appear to be universal across cultures, yet their manifestations may differ somewhat and the ways in which society regards them may also differ. Other disorders, like eating disorders, may be specific to particular cultures. Some disorders are more frequently diagnosed in some racial groups than in others. It is not clear whether this reflects a true difference in the presence of disorder, however; it seems likely that bias is influencing clinical decisions in some cases.

Current research is examining whether risk factors associated with various disorders differ for men and women. Interpersonal relationships can be important buffers against stress and have benefits for physical and mental health.

2.4 Check Your Knowledge

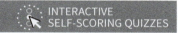
INTERACTIVE SELF-SCORING QUIZZES

(Answers are at the end of the chapter.)

True or false?

1. Emotion can be measured in at least three domains: expression, experience, and physiology.
2. Childhood maltreatment is a risk factor for just a few psychological disorders.
3. Examining the problem-solving interactions of family members is useful for understanding key dimensions in relationships.
4. Domestic violence against women is associated with a greater risk of several psychological disorders.
5. Interpersonal therapy may focus on four types of interpersonal problems: unresolved grief, role transitions, role disputes, and social deficits.

Summary

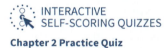
INTERACTIVE SELF-SCORING QUIZZES

Chapter 2 Practice Quiz

- Current thinking about psychological disorders is integrative and multifaceted. The work of clinicians and researchers is informed by an awareness of the many influences on psychological disorders.

- The study of genetic influences in psychological disorders considers genes and environments. Molecular genetics research is identifying differences in gene sequence and structure that may be associated with vulnerability to psychological disorders. Epigenetics refers to the ways in which environments influence the expression of genes. An additional focus of study is how genes and the environment interact in complex ways.

- Neuroscience influences in psychological disorders include brain structure, function, and connectivity; brain networks; neurotransmitters, and other systems, such as the immune system

and the HPA axis. Neuroscience treatments, including medications, are widely used.

- Studies of cognitive behavioral influences emphasize schemas, attention, and cognitive distortions about life experiences and their influence on behavior. Reinforcement principles, modeling, and classical conditioning are learning models that influence our understanding of the cause of some disorders and also inform treatment. Cognitive neuroscience research follows from the early work of Freud, highlighting the importance of childhood experiences, the unconscious, and the fact that the causes of behavior are not always obvious. Cognitive scientists are testing theories and hypotheses about decision making, memory, preference learning, or categorization that inform our understanding of psychological disorders. Cognitive behavior therapy focuses on cognitive restructuring.

- Emotion plays a prominent role in many disorders. It is important to distinguish among measures of emotion that may be disrupted, including expression, experience, and physiology.

- Sociocultural factors, including culture, ethnicity, race, sex assigned at birth, and poverty, are also important to consider in the study and treatment of psychological disorders. The prevalence and meaning of disorders may vary by culture, race, and ethnicity; men and women may have different risk factors for different disorders.

- Interpersonal factors, including social support and relationships, are also important influences in psychological disorders. Social relationships can be an important buffer against stress, and stress in relationships is associated with psychological disorders. Trauma, whether in childhood or in adulthood, is also a risk factor for nearly all psychological disorders.

- Because multiple influences have something to offer in enhancing our understanding of psychological disorders, an integrative approach is the most comprehensive and useful.

Answers to Check Your Knowledge Questions

2.1 1. b; 2. d; 3. a; 4. c; 5.d.

2.2 1. hypothalamus, anterior cingulate, hippocampus, amygdala; 2. white; 3. norepinephrine; 4. hypothalamus, pituitary gland, adrenal cortex; 5. pro-inflammatory cytokines

2.3 1. Exposure; 2. behavioral activation therapy; 3. time-out; 4. True; 5. True; 6. False

2.4 1. True; 2. False; 3. True; 4. True; 5. True

Key Terms

allele   29
amygdala   34
anterior cingulate   34
autonomic nervous system (ANS)   36
behavior genetics   28
behavioral activation (BA) therapy   39
brain networks   35
cognition   40
cognitive behavior therapy (CBT)   42
cognitive restructuring   42
connectivity   35
copy number variation (CNV)   30
cortisol   37
cytokines   38
dopamine   33
emotion   44
epigenetics   31
exposure   40

gamma-aminobutyric acid (GABA)   33
gene   27
gene–environment interaction   30
gene expression   27
genome-wide association studies (GWAS)   30
genotype   28
gray matter   34
heritability   27
hippocampus   34
HPA axis   37
hypothalamus   34
interpersonal therapy (IPT)   47
molecular genetics   29
neuron   33
neurotransmitters   33
nonshared environment   27
norepinephrine   33
parasympathetic nervous system   36

phenotype   28
polygenic   27
polygenic risk score   30
polymorphism   29
prefrontal cortex   34
pruning   35
reuptake   33
schema   40
serotonin   33
shared environment   27
single nucleotide polymorphism (SNP)   29
stress   49
sympathetic nervous system   36
synapse   33
time-out   40
ventricles   34
white matter   34

Diagnosis and Assessment

LEARNING GOALS

1. Describe the purposes of diagnosis and assessment.
2. Distinguish the different types of reliability and validity.
3. Identify the basic features, strengths, and weaknesses of the DSM and broader concerns about diagnosis.
4. Describe the goals, strengths, and weaknesses of psychological approaches to assessment.
5. Understand key approaches to neurobiological assessment.
6. Understand the ways in which culture and ethnicity impact diagnosis and assessment.

Clinical Case

Aaron

Hearing the sirens in the distance, Aaron realized someone must have called the police. He didn't mean to get upset with the people sitting next to him at the bar, but he just knew they were talking about him and plotting to have his special status with the CIA revoked. He could not let this happen again. The last time people conspired against him, he wound up in the hospital. He did not want to go to the hospital again and endure all the evaluations. Different doctors would ask him all sorts of questions about his work with the CIA, which he simply was not at liberty to discuss. They asked other odd questions, such as whether he heard voices or believed others were putting thoughts into his head. He was never sure how they knew that he had those experiences, but he suspected there were electronic bugging devices in his room at his parents' house, perhaps in the electrical outlets.

Just yesterday, Aaron began to suspect that someone was watching and listening to him through the electrical outlets. He decided that the safest thing to do was to stop speaking to his parents. Besides, they were constantly hounding him to take his medication. But when he took this medication, his vision got blurry and he had trouble sitting still. He reasoned that his parents must somehow be part of the group of people trying to remove him from the CIA. If he took this medication, he would lose his special powers that allowed him to spot terrorists in any setting, and the CIA would stop leaving messages for him in phone booths or in the commercials on Channel 2. Just the other day, he had found a tattered paperback book in a phone booth, which he interpreted to mean that a new assignment was imminent. The voices in his head were giving him new clues about terrorist activity. They were currently telling him that he should be wary of people wearing the color purple, as this was a sign of a terrorist. If his parents were trying to sabotage his career with the CIA, he needed to keep out of the house at all costs. That was what had led him to the bar in the first place. If only the people next to him hadn't laughed and looked toward the door. He knew this meant that they were about to expose him as a CIA operative. If he hadn't yelled at them to stop, his cover would have been blown.

Diagnosis and assessment are the critically important first steps in the study and treatment of psychological disorders. In the case of Aaron, a clinician might begin treatment by determining whether he meets the diagnostic criteria for a mood disorder, schizophrenia, or perhaps a substance use disorder. To help them make the correct diagnosis, clinicians and researchers use a variety of assessment procedures, beginning with a clinical interview. Broadly speaking, all clinical assessment procedures are more or less formal ways of finding out what is wrong with a person, what may have caused problems, and what can be done to improve the person's condition. Assessment procedures can help in making a diagnosis, and they can also provide information beyond a diagnosis. Indeed, a diagnosis is only a starting point. In the case of

Aaron, for example, many other questions remain unanswered. Why does Aaron behave as he does? Why does he believe he is working for the CIA? What can be done to resolve his conflicts with his parents? What intellectual and other strengths can be used in helping Aaron in his career? What obstacles might interfere with treatment? These are the types of questions that mental health professionals address in their assessments.

In this chapter, we will describe the official diagnostic system used by many mental health professionals, as well as the strengths and weaknesses of this system. We will then turn to a discussion of the most widely used assessment techniques, including interviews, psychological assessment, and neurobiological assessment. We will then conclude the chapter with an examination of a sometimes neglected aspect of assessment, the role of cultural bias. Before considering diagnosis and assessment in detail, however, we begin with a discussion of two concepts that play a key role in diagnosis and assessment: reliability and validity.

Cornerstones of Diagnosis and Assessment: Reliability and Validity

The concepts of reliability and validity are the cornerstones of any diagnostic or assessment procedure. Without them, the usefulness of our methods would be seriously limited. That said, these two concepts are quite complex. Here we provide a general overview.

Reliability

Reliability refers to consistency of measurement. An example of a reliable measure would be a wooden ruler, which produces the same value every time it is used to measure an object. In contrast, an unreliable measure would be a flexible, elastic-like ruler whose length changes every time it is used. Several types of reliability exist, and here we will discuss the types that are most central to assessment and diagnosis.

Inter-rater reliability refers to the degree to which two independent observers agree on what they have observed. To take an example from baseball, two umpires may or may not agree as to whether the ball is fair or foul. Inter-rater reliability is relevant with interviews but not with self-rated questionnaires.

Test–retest reliability measures the extent to which people being observed twice or taking the same test twice, perhaps several weeks or months apart, receive similar scores. This kind of reliability makes sense only when we can assume that the people will not change appreciably between test sessions on the underlying variable being measured; intelligence tests are a prime example of a measure for which this type of reliability is typically high. On the other hand, we cannot expect people to be in the same mood at a baseline assessment and at a follow-up assessment 4 weeks later, and thus the test–retest reliability of a mood measure would likely be low.

Sometimes psychologists use two forms of a test rather than giving the same test twice, particularly when they are concerned that test takers might remember their answers from the first round of taking the test and aim merely to be consistent. This approach enables the tester to determine **alternate-form reliability**, the extent to which scores on the two forms of the test are consistent.

Finally, **internal consistency reliability** assesses whether the items on a test are related to one another. For example, one would expect the items on an anxiety questionnaire to correlate with one another if they truly tap anxiety. A person who reports a dry mouth in a threatening situation would be expected to report increases in muscle tension as well, since both are common characteristics of anxiety.

Reliability is typically measured on a scale from 0 to 1.0. For all types of reliability, the closer the number is to 1.0, the better the

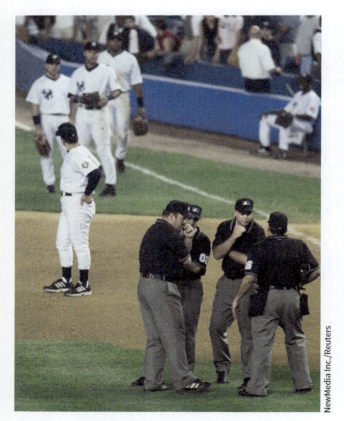

NewMedia Inc./Reuters

Reliability is an essential property of all assessment procedures. One means of establishing reliability is to determine whether different judges agree, as happens when two umpires witness the same event in a baseball game.

reliability. For example, a test with an internal consistency reliability of .65 is only moderately reliable; a different test with an internal consistency reliability of .91 is very reliable.

Validity

Validity is a complex concept, generally related to whether a measure measures what it is supposed to measure. For example, if a questionnaire is supposed to measure a person's hostility, does it do so? Before we describe types of validity, it is important to note that validity is related to reliability—unreliable measures will not have good validity. Because an unreliable measure does not yield consistent results (recall our example of a ruler whose length changes every time it is used), it will not relate very strongly to other measures. For example, an unreliable measure of coping is not likely to show how a person adjusts to stressful life experiences. Reliability, however, does not guarantee validity. For example, height can be measured very reliably, but height would not be a valid measure of anxiety.

Perhaps the most common form of validity in developing tests is **criterion validity**, which assesses whether test scores are correlated with scores on other tests designed to assess the same dimension. For example, scores on a new test designed to assess social anxiety ought to correlate with scores on other tests designed to measure social anxiety. Here we also focus on two types of validity that are often used in considering diagnosis and symptoms.

Content validity refers to whether a measure adequately samples the domain of interest. For example, a test to assess social anxiety ought to include items that cover feelings of anxiety in different social situations. It would have excellent content validity if it contained questions about all the symptoms associated with social anxiety (see Chapter 6). For other uses, though, the same test might have poor content validity. The test doesn't cover questions about anxiety in nonsocial situations, so it would have poor content validity if one were trying to assess specific phobias about heights or snakes.

Construct validity is a more complex concept. It is relevant when we want to interpret a test as a measure of some characteristic or construct that is not observed directly or overtly (Cronbach & Meehl, 1955). A construct is an inferred attribute, such as distorted cognition. Content validity does not ensure high construct validity.

As shown in **Figure 3.1**, construct validity is evaluated by looking at a wide variety of data. For example, suppose people diagnosed as having an anxiety disorder and people without such a diagnosis were compared using their scores on our self-report measure of anxiety proneness. The self-report measure would achieve some construct validity if the people with anxiety disorders scored higher than the people without anxiety disorders. Whereas criterion validity is demonstrated when an anxiety scale is highly correlated with other anxiety scales, greater construct validity would be achieved by showing that the self-report measure was related to other measures thought to reflect anxiety, such as observations of fidgeting and trembling, and physiological indicators, such as increased heart rate and rapid breathing. When the self-report measure is closely associated with these multiple other measures of related concepts (diagnosis, observational indicators, physiological measures), its construct validity is high.

More broadly, construct validity is related to theory. For example, we might hypothesize that being prone to anxiety is in part caused by a family history of anxiety. We

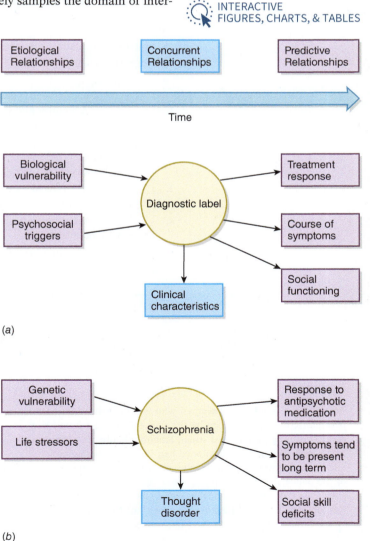

INTERACTIVE FIGURES, CHARTS, & TABLES

FIGURE 3.1 Construct validity. An example of the types of information a diagnosis with high construct validity might help predict.

could then obtain further evidence for the construct validity of our questionnaire by showing that it relates to a family history of anxiety. At the same time, we would also have gathered support for our theory of anxiety proneness. Thus, construct validity provides an important way to test theory.

Quick Summary

With all assessment measures, reliability (consistency of measurement) and validity (whether an assessment measures what it is designed to measure) should be evaluated. Reliability can be estimated by examining how well raters agree, how consistent test scores are over time, how scores from alternate forms of a test compare, or how well items correlate with each other.

Although criterion validity is commonly considered in developing a test, content and construct validity are critically important in test development.

3.1 Check Your Knowledge

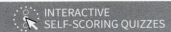
INTERACTIVE
SELF-SCORING QUIZZES

(Answers are at the end of the chapter.)

Determine which type of reliability or validity is tested with each of the following procedures:

a. inter-rater reliability

b. test–retest reliability

c. construct validity

d. criterion validity

1. _____ A group of high school students is given the same IQ test 2 years in a row. Researchers examine whether students obtain similar scores at both time points.

2. _____ A measure of the tendency to blame oneself is developed, and researchers then test whether it predicts depression, whether it is related to childhood abuse, and whether it is related to less assertiveness in the workplace.

3. _____ A self-rated measure of depression is developed, and researchers then test whether it predicts other interview-based and self-rated measures of depression.

4. _____ People are interviewed by two different doctors. Researchers examine whether the doctors agree about the diagnosis.

5. Which type of reliability cannot be tested with self-report measures?

6. Which type of validity is most helping in testing a broad theory?

Clinical Case

Roxanne

Roxanne is a middle-aged woman who was brought to the local psychiatric emergency room by the police. They had found her running through a crowded street, laughing loudly and running into people. When they questioned her, she was speaking rapidly, and her thoughts were hard to follow. At the ER, she wrestled free of the police and began running down the hallway. She knocked over two staff members during her flight, while bellowing at the top of her lungs, "I am the resurrection! Come follow me!" Police brought her back to the exam room, and the staff began to form hypotheses. Clearly, she was full of energy. Had she been through some trauma? She believed she had special religious powers—could this be a delusion? Unfortunately, the staff was unable to gain much information from an interview due to her rapid and incoherent speech. Treatment could not proceed without an understanding of the reason for her unusual behavior. When efforts to calm Roxanne failed, police helped the staff to contact family members, who were relieved to hear that Roxanne was safe. She had disappeared from home the day before. Family members described a long history of bipolar disorder, and they reported having been concerned for the past couple weeks because Roxanne had stopped taking medications for both her bipolar disorder and her high blood pressure. Treatment was able to proceed based on the idea that Roxanne was experiencing a new manic episode of her long-standing bipolar disorder.

The DSM-5-TR diagnosis for Roxanne might look as follows.

Diagnoses: bipolar I disorder, current or most recent episode manic; high blood pressure

Diagnosis

Diagnosis can be the first major step in good clinical care. Having a correct **diagnosis** will allow the clinician to describe base rates, causes, and treatment for Aaron and his family, all of which are important aspects of good clinical care. More broadly, imagine that your doctor told you, "There is no diagnosis for what you have." Rather than experiencing this alarming scenario, receiving a diagnosis can provide relief in several different ways. Many disorders, such as depression and anxiety, are extremely common; knowing that their diagnosis is common can help a person feel less unusual. A diagnosis also can help a person begin to understand why certain symptoms are occurring, which can be a huge relief. Diagnosis enables clinicians and scientists to communicate accurately with one another about cases or research. Indeed, establishing a new diagnosis often fosters research on the topic. For example, autism spectrum disorder (ASD) was only recognized in the *Diagnostic and Statistical Manual* in 1980. Since that time, research on the causes and treatments of ASD has grown exponentially.

The Diagnostic System of the American Psychiatric Association: DSM-5-TR

In this section, we focus on the diagnostic system used by many mental health professionals, **DSM-5-TR**, or the Diagnostic and Statistical Manual of Mental Disorders, 5th edition, Text Revision. In 1952, the American Psychiatric Association published its first *Diagnostic and Statistical Manual* (DSM). The DSM has been revised many times since 1952 (see **Focus on Discovery 3.1** for more on the history of the DSM). The fifth edition of the DSM, referred to as DSM-5, was released in 2013, and a text revision, referred to as DSM-5-TR, was released in 2022 (www.dsm5.org). We will review the major features of DSM-5-TR, and then we will outline some strengths and criticisms of the DSM as well as of diagnosis in general.

The DSM-5-TR provides information about each disorder. To begin, the DSM-5-TR provides specific diagnostic criteria—symptoms for a given diagnosis. These criteria have become more detailed over time. **Table 3.1** compares the descriptions of a manic episode given in DSM-II to those given in DSM-5-TR. Notice how DSM-5-TR is much more detailed and concrete. For each disorder, the DSM-5-TR also describes diagnostic features as well as associated features, such as

TABLE 3.1   **Mania in DSM-II Versus DSM-5-TR**

DSM-II (1968)
Mania was described in DSM-II in just a short paragraph. The paragraph described mania with five symptoms (elevated mood, irritable mood, racing thoughts, rapid talking, and rapid movement). There was no mention of how many symptoms were needed to meet the criteria for a manic episode.

DSM-5-TR (2022)
DSM-5-TR provides a list of symptoms with descriptive detail for each symptom. The symptom description is divided into four parts, which we briefly summarize here. The actual DSM-5-TR offers more detail for all four parts.

1. The first part describes the mood and energy symptoms for mania. A person must show an elevated or irritable mood as well as unusual levels of activity and energy. These mood and energy symptoms must last for at least 1 week unless symptoms are severe enough to require hospitalization.

2. In addition to the mood and energy symptoms, a person also must have three or more of the following symptoms (or four if the mood was irritable and not elated): racing thoughts, rapid talking, very little need for sleep, very high self-esteem or grandiose ideas about the self, distractibility, participation in behaviors that could cause trouble (e.g., excessive spending or sexual encounters), and excessive activity.

3. The symptoms include psychosis, or interfere with work, social interactions, or safety.

4. The last part of the diagnosis is a "rule out" section to clarify whether the symptoms cannot be better accounted for by something else, such as another disorder or the effects of a drug (legal or not).

Focus on Discovery 3.1

A History of Classification and Diagnosis

Emil Kraepelin (1856–1926) authored an influential early classification system, which he included in his textbook of psychiatry published in 1883. Kraepelin noted that certain symptoms clustered together as a *syndrome*. He labeled a set of syndromes and hypothesized that each had its own biological cause, course, and outcome. Even though effective treatments had not been identified, at least the course of the disease could be predicted.

Kraepelin proposed two major groups of severe psychological disorders: dementia praecox (an early term for schizophrenia) and manic-depressive psychosis (an early term for bipolar disorder). He postulated a chemical imbalance as the cause of dementia praecox and an irregularity in metabolism as the explanation of manic-depressive psychosis. Though his theories about causes were not quite correct, Kraepelin's classification scheme influenced the current diagnostic categories.

Development of the WHO and DSM Systems

In 1939 the World Health Organization (WHO) added psychological disorders to its *International List of Causes of Death*. In 1948 the list was expanded to become *the International Statistical Classification of Diseases, Injuries, and Causes of Death*. Unfortunately, the psychological disorders section was not widely accepted. Even though American psychiatrists had played a prominent role in the WHO effort, the American Psychiatric Association published its own *Diagnostic and Statistical Manual* (DSM) in 1952.

In 1969 the WHO published a new version, referred to as the *International Classification of Disease* (ICD), which was more widely accepted. In the United Kingdom, a glossary of definitions was produced to accompany the WHO system. A second version of the American Psychiatric Association's DSM, DSM-II, published in 1968, was similar to the WHO system. But true consensus still eluded the field. Even though DSM-II and the British *Glossary of Mental Disorders* specified some symptoms of diagnoses, the two systems defined different symptoms for a given disorder! Thus diagnostic practices still varied widely. With each revision, greater consensus has been achieved

between the DSM and the ICD. The 11th edition of the ICD was released in 2022.

In 1980 the American Psychiatric Association published an extensively revised diagnostic manual, DSM-III, and a somewhat revised version, DSM-III-R, followed in 1987. One of the big changes in DSM-III that remained in place for 33 years was the introduction of the multiaxial system. Diagnoses were listed on separate dimensions, or axes, as shown in **Figure 3.2**. This multiaxial classification system, by requiring judgments on each of the five axes, forced the diagnostician to consider a broad range of information. DSM-5 no longer uses these distinct axes.

In 1994 the American Psychiatric Association published DSM-IV. For the first time, the committees shaping the new DSM were tasked with explicitly reviewing research data and describing the data guiding any changes in diagnoses. A revision to the supporting text of the DSM-IV, not the actual diagnostic criteria, was published in 2000 and named DSM-IV-TR, with "TR" standing for "text revision."

The development of DSM-5 began in 1999. As with the process for DSM-IV, work groups reviewed each set of diagnoses. Study groups were also formed to consider issues that cut across diagnostic categories, such as life-span developmental approaches, gender and cross-cultural issues, medical issues, impairment and disability, and diagnostic assessment instruments. To protect the process from commercial interests, all work group members signed conflict-of-interest agreements stating that they would accept no more than $10,000 per year from pharmaceutical and industry groups while working on the DSM-5 revision. As was done with DSM-IV, field trials were conducted to assess how the DSM-5 criteria performed in mental health settings. Additional revisions were made based on these data. In the final stages of DSM-5 development, the leaders made changes that were not always consistent with the data and recommendations of the work groups (see Chapter 15 on personality disorders for a stark example of this problem).

The DSM-5 includes many changes from the DSM-IV-TR. Indeed, even conventions for labeling the edition shifted—the Roman numeral used to denote the edition (e.g., DSM-IV) was replaced with

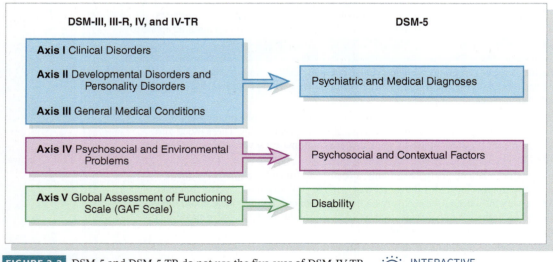

FIGURE 3.2 DSM-5 and DSM-5-TR do not use the five axes of DSM-IV-TR.

INTERACTIVE
FIGURES, CHARTS, & TABLES

an Arabic number (i.e., DSM-5) to facilitate electronic printing. As has happened with each new edition of the DSM, several new diagnoses were added to DSM-5. For example, disruptive mood dysregulation disorder, hoarding disorder, binge-eating disorder, premenstrual dysphoric disorder, and gambling disorder were added. Some of the DSM-IV-TR diagnoses were combined in the DSM-5 because there was not enough evidence for differential causes, course, or treatment response to justify separate diagnostic categories. For example, the DSM-IV-TR diagnoses of substance abuse and dependence were replaced with the DSM-5 diagnosis of substance use disorder. The DSM-IV-TR diagnoses of autism and Asperger's disorder were replaced with the DSM-5 diagnosis of autism spectrum disorder.

The crafters of the DSM-5 aimed to create a living document that will change as new research evidence emerges. Several supplements to the DSM-5 have been published.

A text revision to the DSM-5 was published in 2022. The changes were broader than the DSM-IV-TR revisions were, in that the DSM-5-TR included revisions to clarify that diagnostic criteria for a few disorders and added a new disorder, prolonged grief disorder.

laboratory findings (e.g., enlarged ventricles in schizophrenia) and results from physical exams (e.g., electrolyte imbalances in people who have eating disorders). Next, the DSM-5-TR provides information about age of onset, course, prevalence, risk, prognosis, cultural factors, gender ratios, and differential diagnosis (i.e., how to distinguish similar diagnoses from each other).

Organizing Diagnoses by Symptoms Versus Causes

DSM-5-TR defines diagnoses based on symptoms. Some have argued that advances in our understanding of causes could help us rethink this approach. For example, should symptoms that emerge in the context of serious life adversity be treated in the same way as symptoms that emerge out of the blue? Perhaps the social context could be weighted more heavily in considering whether to diagnose a set of symptoms (Lewis-Fernandez & Aggarwal, 2013; Wakefield, 2013). Others have proposed organizing diagnoses based on parallels in neurotransmitter activity, temperament, or emotion dysregulation. Unfortunately, our knowledge base is not yet strong enough to organize diagnoses around causes (Hyman, 2010). With the exception of dementia, we have no neurobiological markers or genetic indicators to use in making diagnoses. The DSM-5-TR uses symptoms as the basis for diagnosis.

Although DSM-5-TR relies on symptoms as the criteria for diagnoses, overlap in the causes of disorders is considered in a different way—DSM-5-TR chapters are organized to reflect patterns of comorbidity and shared causes (see **Figure 3.3**). For example, DSM-5-TR includes a chapter on obsessive-compulsive and other related disorders. This chapter includes disorders that often co-occur and share some risk factors, including obsessive-compulsive disorder, hoarding disorder, and body dysmorphic disorder.

Ethnic and Cultural Considerations in Diagnosis

Psychological disorders are universal. There is not a single culture in which people are free of psychological disorders. But culture influences the risk factors for psychological disorders (e.g., social cohesion, access to drugs of abuse, and stress), the types of symptoms experienced, stigma, the willingness to seek help, and the treatments available. Sometimes the differences across cultures are profound. For example, although mental health care is widely available in the United States, it is estimated that there is less than one psychiatrist for every million people living in sub-Saharan Africa (World Health Organization, 2015).

Cultural differences do not always play out in the way one might expect. For example, even though they are only half as likely to receive mental health treatment as people in the United States, people with serious psychological disorders in Nigeria remain much more engaged in key roles than do those in other countries (Demyttenaere, Bruffaerts, et al., 2004). This fits with previous findings that outcomes for schizophrenia were more favorable in Nigeria, India, and Colombia than in more industrialized

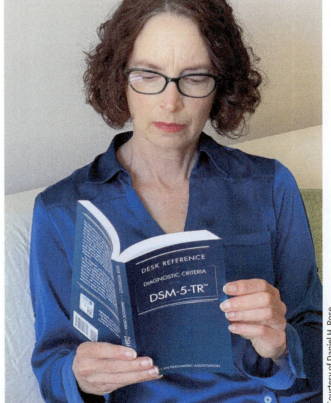

DSM-5-TR is the current diagnostic system of the American Psychiatric Association. It was published in 2022.

Courtesy of Daniel H. Rose

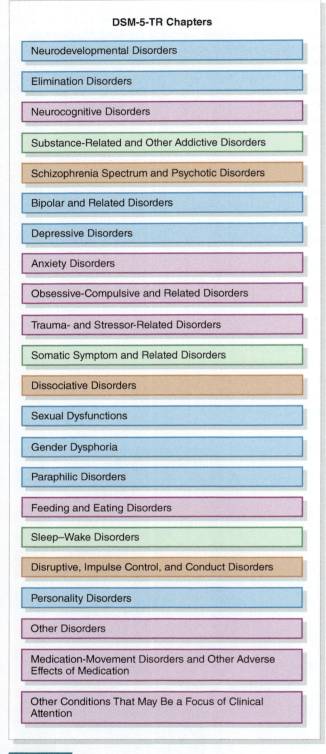

FIGURE 3.3 Chapters in DSM-5-TR.

countries, including the United States (Sartorius, Jablensky, et al., 1986). As shown in **Table 3.2**, rates of psychological disorders tend to be higher in the United States than in many other countries. People who immigrate from Mexico to the United States are initially about half as likely to meet the criteria for a psychological disorder as native-born citizens in the United States, but over time, they and their children begin to show an increase in certain disorders, such as substance use disorder, such that their risk for disorder begins to approximate that of people born in the United States (Alegria, Canino, et al., 2008). A similar profile has been shown among Asian Americans; those who immigrate to the United States have a markedly lower prevalence of psychological diagnoses than Asian Americans who were born in the United States (Hong, Walton, et al., 2014). If we hope to understand how culture influences risk, symptom expression, and outcomes, we need a diagnostic system that can be applied reliably and validly in different countries and cultures (Kessler, Aguilar-Gaxiola, et al., 2009).

Previous editions of the DSM were criticized for their lack of attention to cultural and ethnic variations in psychological disorders. DSM-5 added several features to enhance cultural sensitivity:

- Culture-related issues are discussed in the text for almost all disorders.
- A cultural formulation interview provides 16 questions clinicians can use to help understand how culture may be shaping the clinical presentation.
- An appendix describes syndromes that appear in particular cultures, culturally specific ways of expressing distress, and cultural explanations about the causes of symptoms, illness, and distress.

DSM-5-TR cautions clinicians not to diagnose symptoms unless they are atypical and problematic within a person's culture. Extremely quiet behavior and reticence to speak may seem like social anxiety in one culture but could be a sign of respect in another culture (Lewis-Fernandez & Aggarwal, 2013).

DSM-5-TR provides information about ways in which culture can shape the symptoms and expression of a given disorder. For example, it is more likely in Japan than in the United States for anxiety to be focused around fears of offending others (Kirmayer, 2001). In evaluating symptoms, clinicians also need to be aware that cultures may shape the language used to describe distress. In many cultures, for example, it is common to describe grief or anxiety in physical terms—"I am sick in my heart" or "My heart is heavy"—rather than in psychological terms. In general, clinicians are advised to be constantly mindful of how culture and ethnicity influence diagnosis and treatment.

The DSM-5-TR appendix includes nine **cultural concepts of distress** used to describe syndromes that are observed within specific regions of the world or cultural groups. The following are some examples of these cultural concepts of distress:

- *Shenjing shuairuo.* A syndrome commonly diagnosed in China, characterized by weakness, mental fatigue, negative emotions, and sleep problems. People describing these symptoms often report concerns about work or family stressors, loss of face, or failure.
- *Taijin kyofusho* (interpersonal fear disorder). The fear that one could offend others through inappropriate eye contact, blushing, a perceived body deformation, or body odor. This disorder is most common in Japan, but similar syndromes are observed in cultures that place a strong emphasis on social appropriateness and hierarchy (Lim, 2015).

TABLE 3.2	Twelve-Month Prevalence Rates of the Most Common DSM-IV-TR Diagnoses by Country			
Country	**Anxiety Disorders**	**Mood Disorders**	**Substance Disorders**	**Any Psychological Disorder**
Americas				
Colombia	14.4	7.0	2.8	21.0
Mexico	8.4	4.7	2.3	13.4
United States	19.0	9.7	3.8	27.0
Europe				
Belgium	8.4	5.4	1.8	13.2
France	13.7	6.5	1.3	18.9
Germany	8.3	3.3	1.2	11.0
Italy	6.5	3.4	0.2	8.8
Netherlands	8.9	5.1	1.9	13.6
Spain	6.6	4.4	0.7	9.7
Middle East and Africa				
Lebanon	12.2	6.8	1.3	17.9
Nigeria	4.2	1.1	0.9	6.0
Asia				
Japan	4.2	2.5	1.2	7.4
China	3.0	1.9	1.6	7.1

Source: From Kessler, Aguilar-Gaxiola, et al. (2009).

Diagnoses were assessed with the Composite International Diagnostic Interview. Values are percentages.

Note: In the European countries, bipolar disorder (a form of mood disorder) and non–alcohol-related substance use disorders were not assessed. Obsessive-compulsive disorder (which was considered an anxiety disorder in this survey) was not assessed in Asian countries.

- *Khyâl cap* (wind attacks). A syndrome observed in Cambodian, Thai, and Vietnamese cultural groups. Symptoms overlap with those of panic attacks, including dizziness, rapid heart rate, shortness of breath, and other indicators of intense anxiety and autonomic arousal. This syndrome is often accompanied by the belief that *khyâl* (a windlike substance) is rising in the body and may cause serious physical harm (Hinton, Pich, et al., 2010).

- *Ataque de nervios*. Intense anxiety, anger, fear, or grief; screaming and shouting uncontrollably; crying; trembling; sensations of heat rising from the chest into the head; and verbal or physical aggression. These symptoms are most common among people from Latino cultures and are usually preceded by an acute life stressor (Lim, 2015).

- *Ghost sickness*. An extreme preoccupation with death and those who have died, found among certain Native American tribes.

- *Hikikomori* (withdrawal). A syndrome observed in Japan, Taiwan, and South Korea in which a person, most often an adolescent boy or young adult man, shows profound withdrawal from school, work, family, friendships, and other social roles. Most typically, he shuts himself in his bedroom for 6 months or more and does not socialize with anyone outside the room.

Some have argued that we should try to identify broad syndromes that can be identified across cultures and, to this end, have argued against differentiating cultural concepts of distress from other diagnostic syndromes (Lopez-Ibor, 2003). In support of this position, these researchers point to several cultural concepts of distress that are not so different from the main DSM diagnoses. For example, many Chinese people who have been diagnosed with *shenjing*

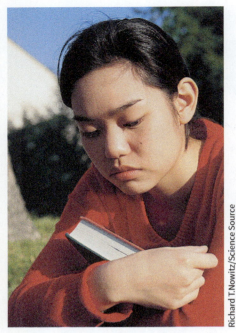

The core symptoms of depression appear to be similar cross-culturally.

shuairuo meet the criteria for a major depressive disorder and will respond to antidepressant medication (Kleinman, 1986). The symptoms of *taijin kyofusho* overlap with those of social anxiety disorder (excessive fear of social interaction and evaluation) and body dysmorphic disorder (the mistaken belief that one is deformed or ugly), which are more commonly diagnosed in the United States. In one study, 100% of the attacks of *khyâl cap* met diagnostic criteria for panic disorder (Hinton et al., 2010). Hence, some researchers believe we should focus on the commonalities in psychological syndromes across cultures.

In contrast, others believe that cultural concepts of distress are central. Surveys that estimate prevalence of psychiatric disorders may vastly underestimate prevalence if cultural concepts of distress are not assessed (Steel, Silove, et al., 2009). For example, almost half of people diagnosed with *hikikomori* or *shenjing shuairuo* do not meet diagnostic criteria for another DSM-5-TR psychiatric disorder (Koyama, Miyake, et al., 2010; Lim, 2015). Moreover, the local beliefs that shape cultural concepts of distress are a key issue in understanding and treating psychological disorders (Hinton & Jalal, 2019). Whether one advocates for a cross-cultural or culture-specific approach to diagnosis, all mental health professionals ought to, at the very least, be aware of the cultural influences that can and do influence the expression of symptoms as well as attitudes toward treatment (Hinton & Patel, 2017).

Specific Criticisms of the DSM

Some specific questions and concerns have been raised about the DSM. We review some of these concerns in the following sections.

Too Many Diagnoses? In the past, up to half of the people seeking treatment described mild symptoms that fell just below the threshold for a diagnosis (Helmuth, 2003). To make it easier to assign a diagnosis to these minor symptoms, DSM-5-TR includes more diagnoses, requires fewer months that symptoms must persist for some diagnoses, and requires fewer symptoms for other diagnoses. DSM-5-TR even includes the category "unspecified," which is to be used when a person meets many but not all of the criteria for a diagnosis.

Some have criticized the large number and scope of diagnostic categories. The DSM-5-TR contains more than 150 diagnoses, and some have questioned whether all of those diagnoses should exist. For example, DSM-5-TR includes a diagnosis for caffeine intoxication—should a person who drinks too much caffeine in one day be considered to have a psychological disorder? DSM-5-TR also includes a category for acute stress disorder to capture symptoms in the first month after a severe trauma. Should these relatively common reactions to trauma be pathologized by being diagnosed as a psychological disorder (Harvey & Bryant, 2002)? By expanding its coverage, the authors of the DSM seem to have made too many problems into psychological disorders without good justification for doing so (Wakefield, 2015).

Others argue that the DSM system includes too many minute distinctions based on small differences in symptoms. One side effect of the huge number of diagnostic categories is a phenomenon called **comorbidity**, which refers to the presence of a second diagnosis. Comorbidity is the norm rather than the exception. Among people who met criteria for at least one DSM-IV psychological diagnosis, 45% met criteria for at least one more psychological diagnosis (Kessler, Berglund, et al., 2005). Some argue that this overlap is a sign that we are dividing syndromes too finely (Hyman, 2010).

One of the reasons for comorbidity is that some symptoms appear in more than one diagnostic category. For example, although delusions and hallucinations are often considered the quintessential symptoms of schizophrenia, they are not specific to schizophrenia and can occur in other psychological disorders, including bipolar disorder, major depressive disorder, and substance use disorders, to name just a few. Someone presenting with these symptoms may be incorrectly given a diagnosis of schizophrenia. In **Read More About It 3.1**, we discuss the case of a

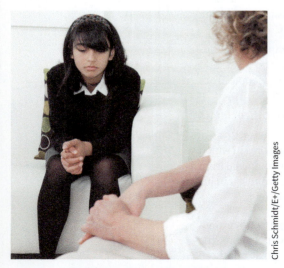

A therapist must be mindful of the role of culture in shaping how people describe their problems.

Read More About It 3.1

Brain on Fire: My Month of Madness

A successful young woman who is a reporter for a major city newspaper begins to feel inklings of paranoia. At first, it doesn't seem like paranoia but more like jealousy. She looks through her boyfriend's drawers for evidence he is cheating on her—something not atypical for new relationships.

But later, she begins to think people are taking special notice of her, that she is receiving special messages from TV, that her family is plotting against her. People are talking about her, whispering her name. People are spying on her and trying to hurt her. When others don't take her concerns seriously, she erupts into rages and becomes very agitated and then, without warning, begins sobbing uncontrollably.

She reports that she sees bright colors; then she reports having visions and seeing things that are most definitely not observed by others. In short, she begins to have visual hallucinations.

She begins to feel like she is having an out-of-body experience, like she is looking down on herself from above, watching her every move. She writes down random musings in a journal, but the thoughts are not connected and are very disorganized. Then, she has a seizure.

What can account for these symptoms, including hallucinations, paranoid delusions, disorganized thinking and behavior, and rapidly changing moods? Is it schizophrenia? Bipolar disorder with psychotic features? A substance use disorder? A seizure disorder? All of these are plausible diagnoses for the symptoms this young woman presented with. Yet none of them was correct.

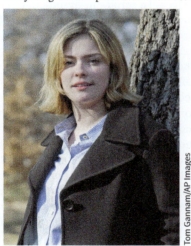

In her book, *Brain on Fire: My Month of Madness*, Susannah Cahalan described her experiences with a rare condition that has symptoms very similar to those of schizophrenia.

In her beautifully written book, *Brain on Fire: My Month of Madness*, Susannah Cahalan (2012) writes about her experience with these symptoms over the course of a month. She did not remember many of these experiences and instead had to piece together what happened to her based on reports from family and friends who cared for her, as well as medical records that were collected once she was hospitalized because she was considered a danger to herself. When Susannah later watched these videotapes of her disorganized and bizarre behavior and ramblings, she did not recognize herself.

She was under the care of neurologists in the hospital who were concerned she had a seizure disorder or some other neurological condition. Yet they did not fully rule out a psychological disorder because her paranoia, hallucinations, and disorganization were so profound. And her MRIs and CT scans came back normal, as did her blood tests, suggesting that she did not have an infection or a disease that had attacked the brain. The neurologists consulted psychiatrists who felt certain that she had some type of psychotic disorder. She was given antipsychotic medications and began to develop motor symptoms that looked like catatonia. She wasn't getting any better.

Finally, the results of a second lumbar puncture (spinal tap) pointed to a possible clue. She had a very high number of white blood cells in her cerebrospinal fluid. Susannah's brain was quite literally inflamed, or "on fire," as the title of her book indicates. Further neuropsychological testing (discussed later in this chapter) revealed that she was experiencing left neglect, an indication that it was the right side of her brain that was inflamed. Her immune system was not responding to an infection; instead, it was attacking her healthy neurons as if they were infectious agents. Additional testing revealed that her immune system was attacking specific neurons with NMDA (N-methyl-D-aspartic acid) receptors. Susannah was having what is called an *autoimmune reaction*, in which the immune system automatically activates for no identifiable reason, and the reaction was wreaking havoc on neurons with NMDA receptors, causing the paranoia, hallucinations, catatonia, and other symptoms. Her official diagnosis was anti-NMDA-receptor-autoimmune encephalitis, an extremely rare condition that was not identified until 2005 (Dalmau, Tüzün, et al., 2007; Vitaliani, Mason, et al., 2005).

At the time of her diagnosis, Susannah was just the 217th person to receive that diagnosis, and it took her doctors nearly a month to make it. Cahalan poignantly wonders, "If it took so long for one of the best hospitals in the world to get to this step, how many other people were going untreated, diagnosed with a mental illness or condemned to a life in a nursing home or a psychiatric ward?" (Cahalan, 2012, p. 151).

Given that anti-NMDA-receptor-autoimmune encephalitis is so rare, it is unlikely that a huge number of people with schizophrenia are misdiagnosed. In fact, recent research has found that some people early in the course of schizophrenia have the NMDA antibodies but not anti-NMDA-receptor-autoimmune encephalitis (Steiner, Walter, et al., 2013). Still, Cahalan's experience presents an important cautionary tale about diagnosis of psychological disorders. Since we do not yet have a blood or brain test for schizophrenia, the diagnosis is made based on the set of observed behavioral symptoms. Yet, as we have seen, these symptoms can occur in other disorders besides the psychological disorders we cover in this book. Thus, mental health professionals would do well not to be too quick to make a diagnosis of schizophrenia or bipolar disorder or any other psychological disorder and instead consider that other factors might be contributing to the symptoms.

In Susannah's case, she was successfully treated over the course of several months with a combination of steroids to reduce the brain inflammation, plasma exchange (taking blood out of the body, treating the plasma to get rid of anti-NMDA antibodies, and returning the blood), and an intravenous immunoglobulin treatment. She also attended several cognitive rehabilitation sessions to help restore cognitive functions like planning, memory, and attention that were disrupted by the inflammation in her brain. She returned to work 7 months after her hospitalization, and she wrote a newspaper article 8 months after her diagnosis. Her book was published 3 years later.

Tom Gannam/AP Images

young woman who had these symptoms but who most definitely did not have schizophrenia. This case points to the importance of conducting thorough assessments, as we discuss later, in the section on assessment.

Does the prevalence of comorbidity indicate that we should lump some of the disorders into one category? Beliefs about lumping versus splitting differ. Some think we should keep the finer distinctions, whereas others believe we should lump (Caspi, Houts, et al., 2014).

In support of lumping, many risk factors relate to more than one disorder, and many treatments are helpful for multiple disorders. For example, in one study of more than 600 adolescents, neuroticism was highly correlated with tendencies toward internalizing disorders. The association with internalizing disorders (as a group) was much stronger than the association of neuroticism with any one of the internalizing disorders (Griffith, Zinbarg, et al., 2009). These findings suggest that risk factors may set the stage for internalizing disorders as a whole. Neuroticism is not the only risk variable that predicts the onset of multiple disorders. For example, some genes are associated with an increase in the risk of externalizing disorders as a whole (Kendler, Prescott, et al., 2003). Anxiety and mood disorders overlap in genetic risk (Kendler, Jacobson, et al., 2003). Tendencies to attend to and remember negative information about the self increase risk for many different internalizing disorders (Harvey, Watkins, et al., 2004). Similarly, as we will see throughout this book, selective serotonin reuptake inhibitors (SSRIs), such as Prozac, often relieve symptoms of depression, anxiety, and many other diagnoses. Different diagnoses do not seem to be distinct in their causes or treatment.

To take the idea of lumping a step further, consider the fact that people who have an internalizing disorder are at higher risk for an externalizing disorder, and vice versa. Some researchers have suggested that we consider a general "psychopathology" factor, or "p" factor (Caspi et al., 2014). According to this perspective, some risk factors are probably related to all of the psychopathologies; other risk factors may predict more specific syndromes. In this book, we will focus on some risk factors that help explain a specific disorder, but you will see that some of the same risk factors—such as early adversity, serotonin dysfunction, poor function of the prefrontal cortex, and the personality trait neuroticism—appear in multiple chapters because they relate to many different disorders.

Two different approaches are being taken to eventually develop improved diagnostic systems. The **HiTOP model** (short for Hierarchical Taxonomy of Psychopathology) focuses on how symptoms and syndromes co-occur, using data available from studies with thousands of patients. Within the HiTOP model, syndromes that frequently co-occur are assembled into subfactors, and subfactors are assembled into higher-order dimensions. For example, adult antisocial personality disorder, alcohol use disorder, and substance use disorder co-occur so often that they could be considered different manifestations of one underlying vulnerability and jointly labeled as disinhibited **externalizing disorders** (Krueger, Markon, et al., 2005). Similarly, anxiety disorders, posttraumatic stress disorder, and depressive disorders, which often co-occur, could be considered to be **internalizing disorders**. Symptoms of different psychotic disorders often co-occur and could be considered indicators of a broader category of thought disorders (Kotov, Krueger, et al., 2017). Within HiTOP, syndromes that frequently co-occur are clustered together into the six domains shown in **Figure 3.4**: somatoform, internalizing, thought disorder, detachment, disinhibited externalizing, and antagonistic externalizing. This model, thus, uses patterns of comorbidity to consider how to refine the diagnostic system.

In contrast, the National Institute of Mental Health has developed the **Research Domain Criteria**, or RDoC (https://www.nimh.nih.gov/research-priorities/rdoc/index.shtml). The RDoC domains focus on risk variables that are relevant for many different conditions, such as problems in responses to negative stimuli or contexts, problems in responses to positive stimuli or contexts, cognitive problems, social problems, and lack of ability to regulate emotion or behavior. Funding is being invested in identifying the genetic and neuroscience correlates of these dimensions. The hope is that basic science advances will allow the field to develop a new classification system that is based on these psychological, neuro imaging, and genetic dimensions of risk rather than just clinical symptoms (Insel, 2014).

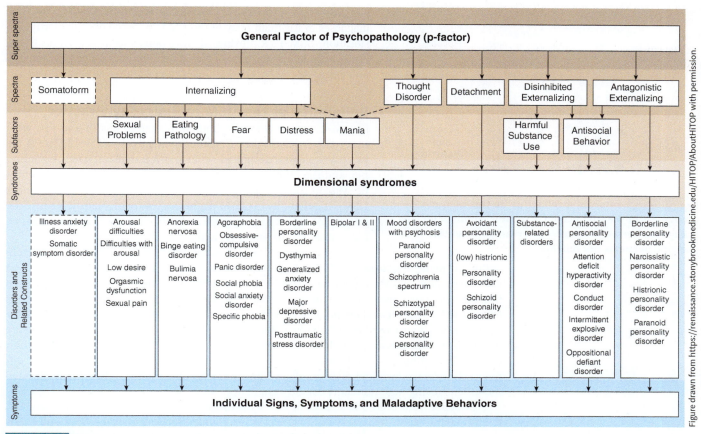

Figure drawn from https://renaissance.stonybrookmedicine.edu/HITOP/AboutHITOP with permission.

FIGURE 3.4 HiTOP Diagnostic Classification System Recommendations to Date.

⬤ INTERACTIVE
FIGURES, CHARTS, & TABLES

Categorical Classification Versus Dimensional Classification

In DSM-5-TR, clinical diagnoses are based on **categorical classification**. Does the person have schizophrenia or not? Do the symptoms fit the category of mania or not? For example, in Table 3.1 we see that the diagnosis of mania requires the presence of three symptoms plus high mood and excessive energy. But why require three symptoms rather than two or five? A categorical system defines one threshold as "diagnosable." There is often little research support for the DSM diagnostic threshold, and there is a good deal of evidence that many people with subthreshold symptoms are experiencing considerable distress and difficulty with functioning (Rodriguez-Seijas, Eaton, & Krueger, 2015). Categorical diagnoses foster a false impression that psychological disorders have actual, hard boundaries.

It may be more helpful to know the severity of symptoms as well as whether they are present. In contrast to a categorical system, a **dimensional diagnostic system** describes the *degree* to which an entity is present (e.g., a 1-to-10 scale of anxiety, where 1 represents minimal and 10, extremely severe). See **Figure 3.5** for an illustration of the difference between dimensional and categorical approaches. Dimensional systems provide a way to describe subthreshold symptoms, as well as symptoms that are particularly severe.

One reason categorical systems are popular is that they define a threshold for treatment. Consider high blood pressure (hypertension). Blood pressure measurements form a continuum, which clearly fits a dimensional approach; yet defining a threshold for high blood pressure allows doctors to feel more certain about when to offer treatment. Similarly, a threshold for clinical depression may help demarcate a point where treatment is recommended. Although the cutoffs are likely to be somewhat arbitrary, they can provide helpful guidance.

Categorical Classification

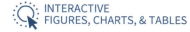

Dimensional Classification

© John Wiley & Sons, Inc.

FIGURE 3.5 **Categorical versus dimensional systems of diagnosis.**

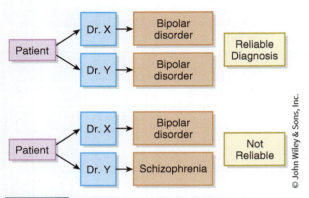

© John Wiley & Sons, Inc.

FIGURE 3.6 **Inter-rater reliability. In this example, the diagnosis of the first person is reliable—both clinicians diagnose bipolar disorder—whereas the diagnosis of the second person is not reliable.**

DSM-5-TR preserved a categorical approach to diagnosis. The diagnoses in the main body of the DSM are based on categorical classification. DSM-5-TR provides severity ratings for nearly all disorders, however, as a first step toward including dimensions alongside the current categories.

Reliability of the DSM in Everyday Practice Suppose you were concerned about your mental health and you went to see two psychologists. Consider the distress you would feel if the two psychologists disagreed—one told you that you had schizophrenia, and the other told you that you had bipolar disorder. Diagnostic systems must have high inter-rater reliability to be useful. Before DSM-III, reliability for DSM diagnoses was poor, mainly because the criteria for making a diagnosis were not clear (see **Figure 3.6** for an illustration of inter-rater reliability).

The increased explicitness of the DSM criteria has improved reliability for many diagnoses (see Table 3.1). Nonetheless, because clinicians might not rely on the criteria precisely, the reliability of the DSM in everyday usage may be lower than that seen in research studies that use structured interviews to assess diagnoses. Even when clinicians follow the DSM criteria, there is some room for disagreement. For example, in the criteria for mania, mood is supposed to be "abnormally" elevated. What is abnormal? When criteria are vague, diagnosticians are more likely to insert their personal biases—or those based on their cultural background—into deciding what the average person should be doing. Because different clinicians may adopt different definitions for symptoms such as "abnormally elevated mood," achieving high reliability can be a challenge.

Evidence from DSM-5 field trials in which the diagnostic criteria were tested at several different mental health treatment facilities across the country suggests that the DSM still needs work when it comes to reliability (see **Table 3.3**). Some have argued that expecting high reliability is unrealistic, particularly since the reliability of these diagnoses is comparable to that of most medical diagnoses (Kraemer, 2014). Later in the chapter, we will discuss how inter-rater reliability is improved using structured diagnostic interviews.

How Valid Are Diagnostic Categories? The DSM diagnoses are based on a pattern of symptoms. A diagnosis of schizophrenia, then, does not have the same status as a diagnosis of, say, diabetes, for which we have laboratory tests.

One way of thinking about diagnosis is to ask whether the system helps organize different observations (see Figure 3.1). Diagnoses have construct validity if they help in making accurate predictions. What types of predictions should a good diagnostic category facilitate? One would hope that a diagnosis would inform us about related clinical characteristics and about functional impairments. The DSM specifies that impairment or distress must be present to meet criteria for a diagnosis, so perhaps it is not surprising that diagnoses are related to functional impairments such as marital distress and missed days at work (see **Table 3.4**). Beyond capturing the most common difficulties for a person with the diagnosis, one would hope that a diagnosis would inform us about what to expect next—the likely course of the disorder and response to different treatments. Perhaps most importantly, one would hope that the diagnosis relates to possible causes of the disorder—for example, a genetic predisposition or a history of trauma. A diagnosis with strong construct validity should help predict a broad range of characteristics.

We have organized this book around the major DSM diagnostic categories because we believe that they do

TABLE 3.3 **Reliability Data from DSM-5 Field Trials**

Diagnosis	Pooled Reliability Estimate
Schizophrenia	.46
Bipolar I disorder	.56
Major depressive disorder	.28
Posttraumatic stress disorder	.67
Borderline personality disorder	.54
ADHD	.61
Autism spectrum disorder	.69

Numbers are kappa statistics—the closer to 1.0, the better the reliability. Kappa scores between .40 and .60 are generally considered moderate (Altman, 1991).

Source: Adapted from Narrow, Clarke, et al. (2013) and Regier, Narrow, et al. (2013).

TABLE 3.4	Rates of Marital Distress and Missed Work Days Among People with Psychological Disorders in the Past Year	
Disorder	**Odds of Marital Distress for a Given Diagnosis Compared to No Psychological Disorder**	**Odds of Missed Work Days for a Given Diagnosis Compared to No Psychological Disorder**
Panic disorder	1.28	3.32
Specific phobia	1.34	2.82
Social phobia	1.93	2.74
Generalized anxiety disorder	2.54	1.15
Posttraumatic stress disorder	2.30	2.05
Major depressive disorder	1.68	2.14
Bipolar I or II disorder	3.60	Not assessed
Alcohol use disorder	2.78	2.54

possess some construct validity. Certain categories have less validity than others, however, and we will discuss gaps in the validity of specific diagnostic categories in later chapters.

General Criticisms of Diagnosing Psychological Disorders

Although we described some advantages of diagnosis in the beginning of this chapter, it is also clear that diagnoses can have negative effects. Consider how your life might be changed by receiving the diagnosis of schizophrenia. You might become worried that someone will recognize your disorder. Or you might fear the onset of another episode. You might worry about your ability to deal with new challenges. The fact that you have a diagnosis of a psychological disorder could have a stigmatizing effect. Friends and loved ones might treat you differently, and employment might be hard to find.

Without doubt, receiving a diagnosis can be difficult. Research shows that psychological disorders are widely viewed negatively (Evans-Lacko, Brohan, et al., 2011), and people with psychological disorders and their families often encounter stigma as a result (Wahl, 1999), which remains a huge problem. Many have raised concerns that a diagnosis might contribute to stigma. To study this problem, researchers have given people brief written descriptions of a person. Beyond including a bit of information about the person's life and personality, the descriptions include either a psychological disorder diagnosis (such as schizophrenia or bipolar disorder), a description of their symptoms (such as periods of high moods, decreased sleep, and restlessness), both (a diagnosis and symptoms), or neither. In this way, researchers can examine whether people tend to be more negative about diagnostic category labels or symptomatic behavior. Research suggests that people tend to view the behaviors more negatively than the diagnostic labels. Sometimes labels may actually relieve stigma by providing an explanation for the symptomatic behavior (Lilienfeld, Lynn, et al., 2010). Of course, making a diagnosis is still a serious process that warrants sensitivity and privacy. But it may not be fair to presume that diagnostic labels are the major source of stigma.

Another concern is that when a diagnostic category is applied, we may focus less on the uniqueness of that person. Because of this concern, the American Psychological Association recommends that people avoid using words like *schizophrenic* or *depressive* to describe people. After all,

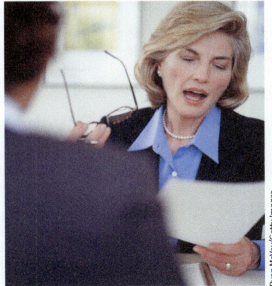

Ryan McVay/Getty Images

Although it is illegal to discriminate against those with psychological disorders, many employers do so. Stigma must be considered when giving a person a diagnosis of a psychological disorder.

we do not call people with medical illnesses by their disease (e.g., you aren't likely to hear someone with cancer described as the *canceric*). Rather, psychologists are encouraged to use phrases such as *a person with schizophrenia*.

Quick Summary

Diagnostic systems for psychological disorders have changed a great deal in the past 100 years.

The DSM provides specific criteria for each disorder, as well as a summary of research on prevalence, comorbidity, and other features. The DSM also provides guidance to enhance sensitivity to culturally specific expressions of symptoms and to help clinicians consider the cultural influences on diagnoses.

There are several concerns about DSM-5-TR. Some argue that there are too many diagnoses. Others challenge the use of a categorical rather than a dimensional approach. Reliability is higher than it was for earlier editions of the DSM, but clinicians still disagree regarding some diagnoses, and the reliability achieved in practice may be lower than that attained with structured diagnostic interviews. Researchers are focused on validating DSM-5-TR by identifying the course of symptoms over time, causal factors, and treatment outcomes predicted by a given diagnosis, but it is clear that there is considerable overlap in the causes and treatments for different DSM diagnoses. The HiTOP and RDoC systems are efforts to reconsider the general approach to diagnosis; HiTOP focuses on overlap among symptoms, while RDoC seeks to understand the basic building blocks of different risk factors.

Regardless of which diagnostic system is used, certain problems are inherent in diagnosing people with psychological disorders. The American Psychological Association recommends using phrases such as *person with schizophrenia* rather than *schizophrenic* as one way to acknowledge that a person is much more than their diagnosis. Although many worry that applying labels may increase stigma, diagnoses can sometimes relieve stigma by providing a way to understand symptoms.

3.2 Check Your Knowledge

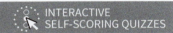
INTERACTIVE
SELF-SCORING QUIZZES

(Answers are at the end of the chapter.)

Answer the following questions.

1. Describe three ways in which DSM-5-TR considers the role of culture in the assessment of psychological disorders.

2. List three reasons why some think the DSM should lump diagnoses.

3. What are three broad types of characteristics that a valid diagnosis should help predict?

4. What are the chief ways in which the HiTOP model and the RDoC system differ from each other?

Psychological Assessment

To make a diagnosis, mental health professionals can use a variety of assessment measures and tools. Beyond helping to make a diagnosis, psychological assessment techniques are used in other important ways. For example, assessment methods are often used to identify appropriate therapeutic interventions. And repeated assessments are very useful in monitoring the effects of treatment over time. In addition, assessments are fundamental to conducting research on the causes of disorder.

Here we discuss clinical interviews for symptoms, diagnoses, and stress; personality tests; cognitive and neuropsychological tests; behavioral observation; experience sampling; and self-report questionnaires. Although we present these methods individually, a complete psychological assessment of a person will often entail combining several assessment techniques. The sets of data from the various techniques complement each other and provide a more complete picture of the person. In short, there is no one best assessment measure. Rather, using multiple techniques and multiple sources of information will provide the best assessment.

Clinical Interviews

Mental health professionals use both formal and structured as well as informal and less structured clinical interviews in assessing psychological disorders. Carrying out a good **clinical interview** requires great skill. Clinicians must recognize the importance of establishing rapport with a person who seeks their professional help and obtaining the trust of the person; it is naive to assume that a person will easily reveal information to another, even to someone with the title "Doctor." And even a person who sincerely, perhaps desperately, wants to recount intensely personal problems to a professional may not be able to do so without help. Most clinicians show empathy to encourage interviewees to elaborate on their concerns. An accurate summary statement, or reflection, of what a person has been saying can help sustain the momentum of talk about painful and possibly embarrassing events and feelings and convey an accepting attitude toward personal disclosures.

Unstructured Interviews

Interviews vary in the degree to which they are structured. In practice, most clinicians probably operate from only the vaguest outlines. Exactly how information is collected is determined largely by the particular interviewer and depends, too, on the responsiveness and responses of the interviewee. Through years of training and clinical experience, clinicians develop ways of asking questions that they are comfortable with and that seem to draw out the information that will be of maximum benefit to the person. Thus, to the extent that an interview is unstructured, the interviewer must rely on intuition and general experience.

Structured Interviews

To help determine whether a person meets diagnostic criteria for a disorder, a mental health professional can use a **structured interview**, in which the questions are set out in a prescribed fashion for the interviewer. One example of a commonly used structured interview is the Structured Clinical Interview (SCID) (First, Williams, et al., 2015). The general format of this interview is shown in **Figure 3.7**.

The SCID is a branching interview; that is, a person's response to one question determines the next question that is asked. It contains detailed instructions to the interviewer concerning when and how to probe in detail and when to go on to questions about another diagnosis. Most symptoms are rated on a three-point scale of severity, with instructions in the interview for translating the symptom ratings into diagnoses. The initial questions pertaining to obsessive-compulsive disorder (discussed in Chapter 7) are presented in **Figure 3.8**. The interviewer begins by asking about obsessions. If the responses elicit a rating of 1 (absent), the interviewer turns to questions about compulsions. If the person's responses again elicit a rating of 1, the interviewer is instructed to go to the questions for the next disorder. On the other hand, if positive responses (rating of 2 or 3) are elicited about obsessive-compulsive disorder, the interviewer continues with further questions about that problem. In practice, most clinicians review the DSM symptoms in an informal manner without using a structured interview. Inter-rater reliability is higher when clinicians use the SCID than it is when they conduct an unstructured interview.

Assessing Stress

Given its centrality to nearly all psychological disorders, stress is clearly important to measure. To understand the role of stress, we must first be able to define and measure it. Neither task is simple, as stress has been defined in many ways. See **Focus on Discovery 3.2** for influential antecedents to our current conceptualizations of stress. Although stress can be assessed with a self-report questionnaire, these tools are limited in coverage and have limited validity (Harkness & Monroe, 2016). Here, we examine the most comprehensive interview measure of life stress: the Bedford College Life Events and Difficulties Schedule.

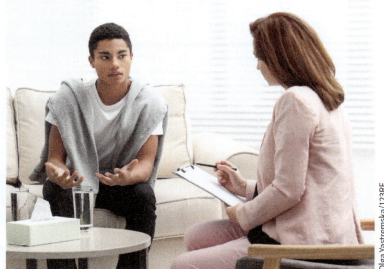

Olga Yastremska/123RF

Structured interviews are widely used to make reliable diagnoses.

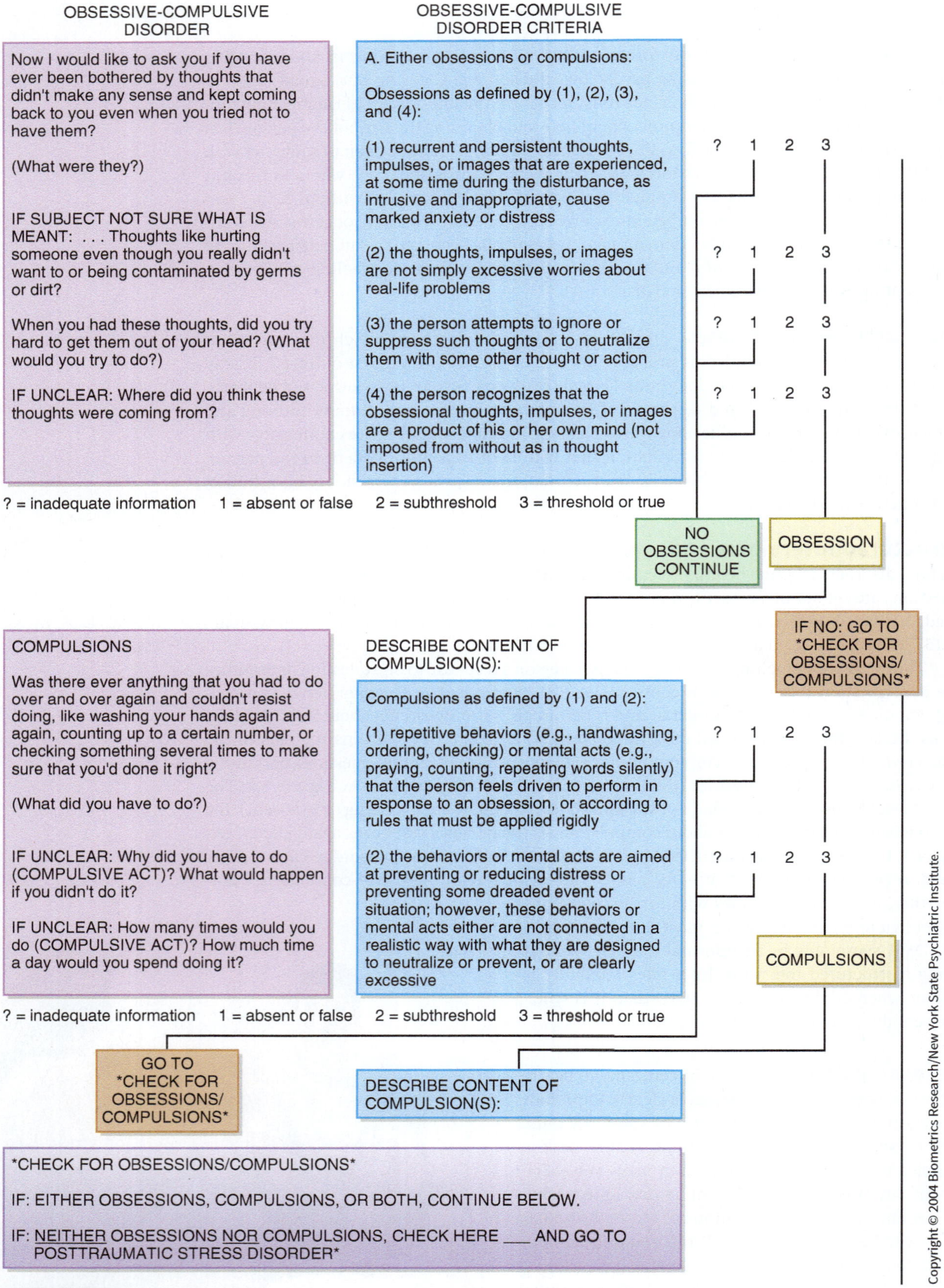
OBSESSIVE-COMPULSIVE DISORDER
Now I would like to ask you if you have ever been bothered by thoughts that didn't make any sense and kept coming back to you even when you tried not to have them?
(What were they?)
IF SUBJECT NOT SURE WHAT IS MEANT: . . . Thoughts like hurting someone even though you really didn't want to or being contaminated by germs or dirt?
When you had these thoughts, did you try hard to get them out of your head? (What would you try to do?)
IF UNCLEAR: Where did you think these thoughts were coming from?
OBSESSIVE-COMPULSIVE DISORDER CRITERIA
A. Either obsessions or compulsions:
Obsessions as defined by (1), (2), (3), and (4):
(1) recurrent and persistent thoughts, impulses, or images that are experienced, at some time during the disturbance, as intrusive and inappropriate, cause marked anxiety or distress
? 1 2 3
(2) the thoughts, impulses, or images are not simply excessive worries about real-life problems
? 1 2 3
(3) the person attempts to ignore or suppress such thoughts or to neutralize them with some other thought or action
? 1 2 3
(4) the person recognizes that the obsessional thoughts, impulses, or images are a product of his or her own mind (not imposed from without as in thought insertion)
? 1 2 3
? = inadequate information 1 = absent or false 2 = subthreshold 3 = threshold or true
NO OBSESSIONS CONTINUE
OBSESSION
IF NO: GO TO *CHECK FOR OBSESSIONS/ COMPULSIONS*
COMPULSIONS
Was there ever anything that you had to do over and over again and couldn't resist doing, like washing your hands again and again, counting up to a certain number, or checking something several times to make sure that you'd done it right?
(What did you have to do?)
IF UNCLEAR: Why did you have to do (COMPULSIVE ACT)? What would happen if you didn't do it?
IF UNCLEAR: How many times would you do (COMPULSIVE ACT)? How much time a day would you spend doing it?
DESCRIBE CONTENT OF COMPULSION(S):
Compulsions as defined by (1) and (2):
(1) repetitive behaviors (e.g., handwashing, ordering, checking) or mental acts (e.g., praying, counting, repeating words silently) that the person feels driven to perform in response to an obsession, or according to rules that must be applied rigidly
? 1 2 3
(2) the behaviors or mental acts are aimed at preventing or reducing distress or preventing some dreaded event or situation; however, these behaviors or mental acts either are not connected in a realistic way with what they are designed to neutralize or prevent, or are clearly excessive
? 1 2 3
COMPULSIONS
? = inadequate information 1 = absent or false 2 = subthreshold 3 = threshold or true
GO TO *CHECK FOR OBSESSIONS/ COMPULSIONS*
DESCRIBE CONTENT OF COMPULSION(S):
CHECK FOR OBSESSIONS/COMPULSIONS
IF: EITHER OBSESSIONS, COMPULSIONS, OR BOTH, CONTINUE BELOW.
IF: NEITHER OBSESSIONS NOR COMPULSIONS, CHECK HERE ___ AND GO TO POSTTRAUMATIC STRESS DISORDER*
Copyright © 2004 Biometrics Research/New York State Psychiatric Institute.

FIGURE 3.7 **Sample item from the SCID. Reprinted by permission of New York State Psychiatric Institute Biometrics Research Division.**

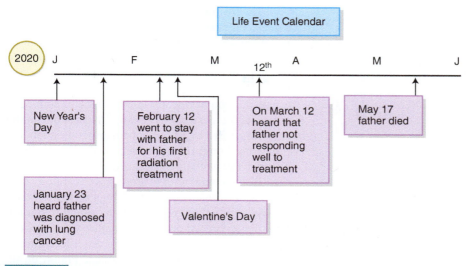

FIGURE 3.8 **Example of a life events timeline. The LEDS interview is designed to capture the major stressors a person has encountered in the past year.**

The Life Events and Difficulties Schedule, or LEDS (Brown & Harris, 1978), is an interview that covers over 200 different kinds of stressors. Because the interview is only semi-structured, the interviewer can tailor questions to cover stressors that might occur only to a few people. The interviewer and the interviewee work collaboratively to produce a calendar of each of the major events within a given time period (see Figure 3.8 for an example). After the interview, raters evaluate the severity and several other dimensions of each stressor. The LEDS was designed to address several problems in life stress assessment, including the need to

VIDEO CONTENT

Stress

Focus on Discovery 3.2

A Brief History of Stress

The pioneering work by the physician Hans Selye set the stage for our current conceptualizations of stress. He introduced the term *general adaptation syndrome* (GAS) to describe the biological response to sustained and high levels of stress (see **Figure 3.9**). In Selye's model, there are three phases of the response:

1. During the first phase, the alarm reaction, the autonomic nervous system is activated by the stress.

2. During the second phase, resistance, the organism tries to adapt to the stress through available coping mechanisms.

3. If the stressor persists or the organism is unable to adapt effectively, the third phase, exhaustion, follows, and the organism dies or suffers irreversible damage (Selye, 1950).

Phase 1 The Alarm Reaction	Phase 2 Resistance	Phase 3 Exhaustion
ANS activated by stress	Damage occurs or organism adapts to stress	Organism dies or suffers irreversible damage

FIGURE 3.9 Selye's general adaptation syndrome.

In Selye's syndrome, the emphasis was on the body's response, not the environmental events that trigger that response. Psychological researchers later broadened Selye's concept to account for the diverse stress responses that people exhibited, including emotional upset, deterioration of performance, or physiological changes such as increases in the levels of certain hormones. The problem with these response-focused definitions of stress is that the criteria are not clear-cut. Physiological changes in the body can occur in response to many things that we would not consider stressful (e.g., anticipating a pleasurable event).

Other researchers defined stress as exposure to a difficult life event, often referred to as a stressor. Stressors can be acute (failing an exam) or chronic (a persistently unpleasant work environment). For the most part, they are experiences that people regard as unpleasant, but they can also be pleasant events (a wedding).

It is important to acknowledge that people vary widely in how they respond to life's challenges. A given event does not elicit the same amount of stress in everyone. For example, one person may be devastated by a failing grade, and another may shrug off the disappointment. Current conceptualizations of stress emphasize that how we perceive the environment shapes our response to a stressor. This raises the very important point that the life stressors and the response to life stressors are two different variables (Harkness & Monroe, 2016). Both of these variables appear important to the study and treatment of psychological disorders.

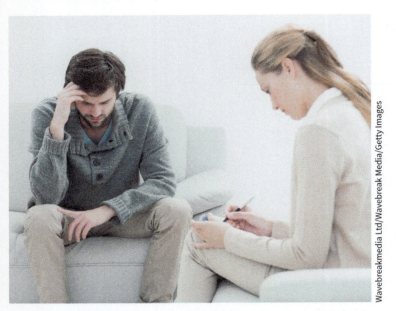

Assessing stressors, such as job losses, romantic breakups, early childhood experiences, or discrimination experiences, is often done using clinical interviews.

evaluate the importance of any given life event in the context of a person's life circumstances. For example, pregnancy might have quite a different meaning for an unmarried 14-year-old girl and a 38-year-old woman who has been trying to conceive for a long time. A second goal of the LEDS is to exclude life events that might be consequences of symptoms. For example, if a person misses work because he or she is too depressed to get out of bed, any consequent job problems should really be seen as symptoms of the disorder rather than a triggering life event. Finally, the LEDS includes a set of strategies to carefully date when a life stressor occurred. Using this more careful assessment method, researchers have found that life stressors are robust predictors of episodes of anxiety, depression, schizophrenia, and even the common cold (Brown & Harris, 1989; Cohen, Frank, et al., 1998).

It is also important to assess for childhood stress and trauma in psychological assessments. One metric that is often used is called "Adverse Childhood Experiences" or ACEs (Felitti, Anda, et al., 1998). ACEs include physical, psychological, or sexual abuse; psychological disorders, family conflict, parental death, violence, or illegal behavior in the household; witnessing or exposure to community violence or war; ACEs can be assessed using a semi-structured interview, such as the ACE International Questionnaire (ACE-IQ; World Health Organization, 2018), or the Centers for Disease Control ACEs measure (Felitti et al., 1998; Centers for Disease Control, 2023). The total number of ACEs is computed following the interview. A higher number of ACEs increases the risk for health problems and psychological disorders (Hughes, Bellis, et al., 2017).

Another important domain for clinicians to assess is stress associated with minority status, including racial and sexual/gender minority status (Rodriguez-Seijas, Eaton, & Paychankis, 2019). Experiences of discrimination, stereotyping, stigma, bias, and inequality can be assessed during clinical interviews and with self-report questionnaires. For some people of color, particularly Black people, talking about distress or psychological symptoms can itself be emotionally fraught and stressful given that some symptoms continue to be wrongly linked to violence among Black Americans (Villarosa, 2022). The American Academy of Pediatrics released a policy statement in 2019 documenting how racism adversely impacts the mental health of children and adolescents (Trent, Dooley, et al., 2019), and emphasized the importance of assessing stress that is associated with racism and training clinicians to deliver culturally competent care (a topic we discuss further later in the chapter).

Personality Tests

Personality tests are a type of self-report questionnaire that includes statements to assess behavioral and emotional tendencies. When these tests are developed, they are typically administered to many people to analyze how certain kinds of people tend to respond. Statistical norms for the test can thereby be established. This process is called **standardization**. The responses of a particular person can then be compared with the statistical norms. In **Focus on Discovery 3.3**, we discuss historical personality measures called projective tests.

One well-known personality test is the Minnesota Multiphasic Personality Inventory. The current version was released in 2020 and is known as the **MMPI-3** (Ben-Porath & Tellegen, 2020). The MMPI-3 is called multiphasic because it was designed to detect several psychological problems. Hundreds of items were tested in very large samples of people with and without a diagnosis. Sets of these items were established as scales. If a person answers many of the items in a scale in the same way as did people from a certain diagnostic group, their behavior is expected to resemble that of the particular diagnostic group. The MMPI-3F includes several "validity scales" designed to detect over- or underreporting of symptoms or experiences and other types of biased responses. For example, an item for this purpose might read "I read the newspaper editorials every day." The assumption is that few people would be able to endorse such a statement honestly. People who endorse many of the statements might be attempting to present themselves in a good light. The MMPI-3 is comparable to the previous version, the MMPI-2-RF (Hall, Menton, & Ben-Porath, 2022). Additional work is under way to confirm that its reliability and validity remain as strong as prior versions. The MMPI-3 also agrees well with the HiTOP model described earlier and shown in Figure 3.5 (Sellbom, Kremyar, & Wygant, 2021).

Focus on Discovery 3.3

Projective Tests: Another Type of Personality Test

A projective test is an older psychological assessment tool in which a person is presented with a set of standard stimuli—inkblots or drawings—ambiguous enough to allow variation in responses. The assumption is that because the stimulus materials are unstructured and ambiguous, the person's responses will be determined primarily by unconscious processes and will reveal their "true" attitudes, motivations, and modes of behavior.

The use of projective tests assumes that the person would be either unable or unwilling to express their true feelings if asked directly. As you might have guessed, projective techniques are derived from the work of Freud and his followers (see Chapter 1).

In the Thematic Apperception Test (TAT), a person is shown a series of black-and-white pictures one by one and asked to tell a story related to each. If, for example, a person seeing a picture of a boy observing a youth baseball game from behind a fence tells a story that contains angry references to the boy's parents, the clinician may infer that the person harbors resentment toward their parents. There are few reliable scoring methods for this test, and the norms are based on a small and limited sample (i.e., there are few norms for people of different ethnic or cultural backgrounds). The construct validity of the TAT is also limited (Lilienfeld, Wood, & Garb, 2000).

The Rorschach Inkblot Test is perhaps the best-known projective technique. In the Rorschach test, a person is shown 10 inkblots (for similar inkblots, see **Figure 3.10**), one at a time, and asked to tell what the blots look like.

Projective tests like the Rorschach or TAT are not as widely used today, due to their poor validity (Lilienfeld et al., 2000).

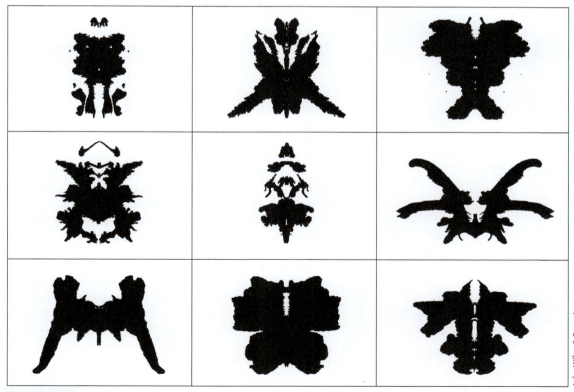

John Wiley & Sons, Inc.

FIGURE 3.10   In the Rorschach test, the person is shown a series of inkblots and is asked what the blots look like.

A highly influential model of personality focuses on five broad domains, known as "the big 5": openness to experience, conscientiousness, extraversion, agreeableness, and neuroticism (often recalled by the acronym *ocean*, with each letter representing one of the personality domains). Two measures commonly used to assess the big 5 are the NEO Personality Inventory (NEO-PI) (McCrae, Costa, & Martin, 2005) and the Big Five Inventory-2 (BFI-2) (John, Naumann, & Soto, 2008; Soto & John, 2016). The five broad domains of personality are central to dimensional approaches to personality disorders (Chapter 15) but are also important in mood and anxiety disorders (Chapters 5 and 6). Like the MMPI-3, the BFI-2 has measurement properties that allow clinicians and researchers to identify respondents who show a different response style, such as tendencies to minimize concerns.

Cognitive and Neuropsychological Tests

Psychological assessments often involve the use of different cognitive tests. These tests are designed to assess different aspects of cognitive functioning, such as intellectual functioning, memory, reasoning, spatial and motor skills, and perception. Here we review intelligence tests and neuropsychological tests.

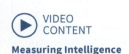

VIDEO CONTENT

Measuring Intelligence

Intelligence Tests

An intelligence test, often referred to as an IQ test, is a way of assessing a person's current cognitive ability. IQ tests are based on the assumption that a detailed sample of a person's current intellectual functioning can predict how well they will perform in school, and most such tests are individually administered. The most commonly administered tests include the Wechsler Adult Intelligence Scale, 4th edition (WAIS-IV, 2008); the Wechsler Intelligence Scale for Children, 5th edition (WISC-V, 2014); the Wechsler Preschool and Primary Scale of Intelligence, 4th edition (WPPSI-IV, 2012); and the Stanford-Binet, 5th edition (SB5, 2003). IQ tests are regularly updated and, like personality inventories, they are standardized.

IQ tests tap several functions believed to constitute intelligence, including language skills, abstract thinking, nonverbal reasoning, visual-spatial skills, attention and concentration, and speed of processing. In addition to predicting school performance, intelligence tests are used to diagnose learning disorders or intellectual ability (discussed in Chapter 13) and as part of neuropsychological evaluations (discussed in the next subsection).

IQ tests are highly reliable and have good validity (Drozdick, Raiford, et al., 2018). Although IQ and educational attainment are positively correlated (see Chapter 4 for a discussion of correlational methods), what remains less clear is whether more education causes an increase in IQ or whether IQ causes one to attain more education (Deary & Johnson, 2010). Furthermore, although correlations between IQ scores and school performance are statistically significant, IQ tests explain only a small part of school performance; much more is unexplained by IQ test scores than is explained.

Regarding construct validity, it is important to keep in mind that IQ tests measure only what psychologists consider intelligence. Factors other than what we think of as intelligence, however, also play an important role in how people will do in school, such as family and circumstances, motivation to do well, expectations, performance anxiety, and difficulty of the curriculum. Another factor relevant to IQ test performance is called *stereotype threat*. This refers to the notion that calling attention to stereotypes (e.g., Black people do poorly on IQ tests; women perform worse than men on mathematics tests) actually interferes with performance on these tests.

Unfortunately, awareness of these stereotypes develops early. For example, a study revealed that children develop awareness of stereotypes regarding race and ability between the ages of 6 and 10, with 93% of children being aware of such stereotypes by age 10

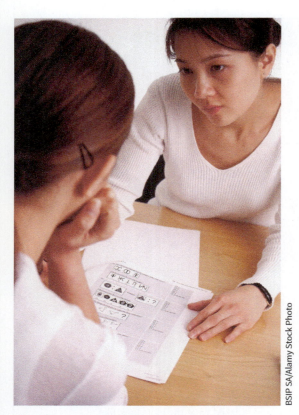

IQ tests have many subtests, including this test to assess spatial ability.

BSIP SA/Alamy Stock Photo

(McKown & Weinstein, 2003). This awareness seems to influence stereotype threat (and performance). In the McKown and Weinstein study, children were asked to complete a puzzle task. Half of the children received instructions that the task reflected their ability (stereotype threat condition), and half the children received instructions that the test did not reflect their ability. Black children who were aware of the stereotype about ethnicity and ability showed evidence of stereotype threat. Specifically, among Black children, those who received the ability instructions performed more poorly on the puzzle task than the children who did not, suggesting that the instructions activated the stereotype and thus influenced their performance.

Neuropsychological Tests
Neuropsychological tests are often used to help pinpoint specific areas of cognitive functioning impairment. Neuropsychological tests are based on the idea that different cognitive functions (e.g., motor speed, memory, language) rely on different areas of the brain. Thus, for example, neuropsychological testing might help identify the extent of cognitive impairment suffered during a stroke, and it can provide clues about where in the brain the damage may have occurred, which can then be confirmed with more expensive brain-imaging techniques.

Examples of neuropsychological tests include:

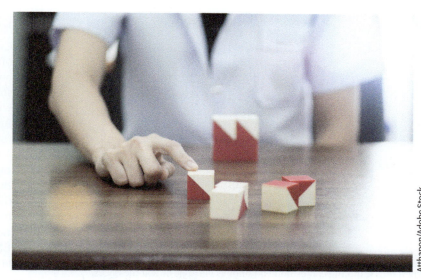

Neuropsychological tests assess cognitive functions such as memory, language, perception, and motor movement.

- **Trail Making Test:** The person is asked to draw connecting lines (trails) between numbers or letters.
- **California Verbal Learning Test** (CVLT-3; Delis, Kramer, et al., 2017): For this test of verbal memory, a person listens to lists of words and recalls as many as possible.

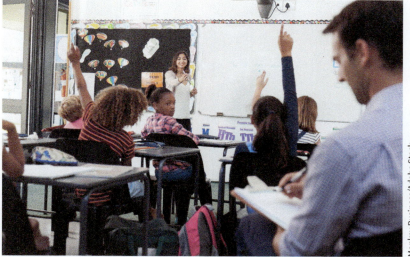

Behavioral assessment often involves direct observation of behavior, as in this case, where the examiner observes a child's behavior in a classroom.

- **Rey Complex Figure Test:** This is a test of visual memory in which an intricate figure drawing is shown to a person and the person is asked to copy the figure. Memory for the figure is also assessed.
- **Digit Span:** The person is asked to repeat a series of numbers back to the examiner both forwards and backwards.

Direct Observation of Behavior

In direct behavioral observation, the observer divides a sequence of behaviors into various parts that make sense within a learning framework, including such things as the antecedents and consequences of particular behaviors.

Direct observation is most frequently done in child assessments. For example, an examiner might go to a child's school and observe the child's behavior in the classroom. The examiner may observe how frequently a child disrupts the other students by talking out of turn or moving around the room.

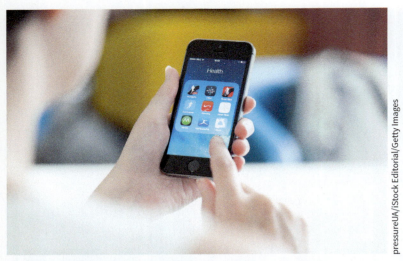

Experience sampling can be done on phones via apps or text messages.

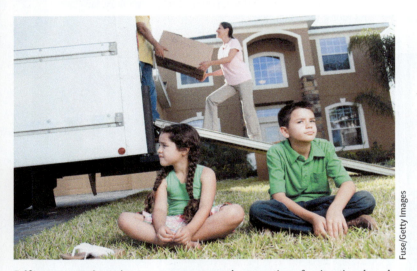

Self-report questionnaires can assess a person's perception of a situation, based on the assumption that the same event can be perceived differently. For example, moving could be regarded as a very negative event or a very positive one, resulting in different levels of stress.

Experience Sampling

Cognitive behavior therapists and researchers often ask people to monitor and record their own behavior and responses. Such sampling of a person's daily experience is used to collect data on a wide variety of topics, including emotions, stressful experiences, coping behaviors, and thoughts (Stone, Schneider, & Smyth, 2023).

Experience sampling is also called **ecological momentary assessment (EMA)**. EMA involves the collection of data in real time as opposed to the more usual method of having people reflect back over some time period and report on recently experienced thoughts, emotions, or stressors. With EMA, a person is signaled (via text message or an app alert on a smartphone alert most typically) several times a day and asked to enter responses directly into the device. Self-monitoring with portable electronic devices like smartphones has also been included effectively in cognitive behavior therapy for different anxiety disorders (Przeworski & Newman, 2006).

Self-Report Questionnaires

In addition to personality tests, mental health professionals use other self-report questionnaires to assess a person's internal experiences of emotion, thoughts about the self, past experiences, or symptoms. These assessments can be used to help plan targets for treatment, as well as to determine whether clinical interventions are helping to change the focus of treatment. In format, these questionnaires are similar to the personality tests we have already described, but they typically have fewer questions than personality tests because they are focused on a particular domain (e.g., emotion, depression symptoms).

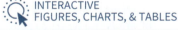
INTERACTIVE
FIGURES, CHARTS, & TABLES

TABLE 3.5   Psychological Assessment Methods

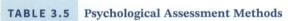

Clinical Interviews	Unstructured interviews	The clinician learns about the person's problems through conversation.
	Structured interviews	Questions to be asked are spelled out in detail. The Structured Clinical Interview is a structured interview that is commonly used to help make a diagnosis.
	Stress interviews	Interviews like the LEDS assess stressful events and responses to these events.
Personality and Cognitive Tests	Personality tests	These measures are used to assess a broad range of traits, as in the BFI-2 or NEO PI.
	Intelligence tests	These assessments of current cognitive functioning are used to predict school performance and identify cognitive strengths and weaknesses.
	Neuropsychological tests	These tests assess abilities such as motor speed, memory, and spatial ability.
Direct Observation of Behavior		This method is used by clinicians to identify problem behaviors as well as antecedents and consequences.
Experience Sampling		People monitor and record their feelings, thoughts, and behaviors, often several times a day, as in ecological momentary assessment.
Self-Report Questionnaires		This method is used to assess a person's internal experiences of emotions, thoughts about the self, past experiences, or symptoms.

Quick Summary

The psychological assessments we have described are summarized in **Table 3.5**. A comprehensive psychological assessment draws on many different methods and tests. Interviews can be structured, with the questions predetermined and followed in a certain order, or unstructured, to follow more closely what the person tells the interviewer. Rapport is important to establish, regardless of the type of interview. Stress is best assessed via a semistructured interview that captures the importance of any given life event in the context of a person's life circumstances, as is done with the LEDS.

The MMPI-3, BFI-2, and NEO-PI are standardized personality tests. They have good reliability and validity and are widely used. Intelligence tests have been used for many years and are quite reliable. As with any test, there are limits to what an IQ test can tell a clinician or researcher. Neuropsychological tests can assess different aspects of cognitive function, such as memory, reasoning, motor functioning, and perception.

Direct observation of behavior can be useful, particularly in child assessments, though it generally takes more time than a self-report questionnaire. Other assessment methods include ecological momentary assessment (EMA).

3.3 Check Your Knowledge

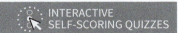

INTERACTIVE
SELF-SCORING QUIZZES

(Answers are at the end of the chapter.)

True or false?

1. If conducted properly, a psychological assessment can include only one measure most appropriate to the person.
2. Unstructured interviews can be valuable in a psychological assessment.
3. The BFI-2 assesses five broad domains of personality.
4. A neuropsychological test assesses performance on tasks thought to rely on certain regions of the brain.
5. Intelligence tests are highly reliable.
6. EMA is a method to assess unwanted impulses.

Neurobiological Assessment

Recall from Chapters 1 and 2 that, throughout history, people interested in psychological disorders have assumed, quite reasonably, that some symptoms are likely to be due to problems in the brain. We turn now to contemporary work in neurobiological assessment. We'll look at two areas in particular: brain imaging and brain stimulation (see **Table 3.6** for a summary of these methods). As important as these assessment methods are, they are not often used outside of research settings, given the expertise required to use them and their cost.

TABLE 3.6 **Neurobiological Assessment Methods**	INTERACTIVE FIGURES, CHARTS, & TABLES
Brain imaging	MRI scans reveal the structure of the brain. PET and SPECT reveal brain function and, to a lesser extent, brain structure. fMRI is used to assess both brain structure and brain function.
Brain stimulation	Transcranial magnetic stimulation (TMS) and transcranial direct current stimulation (tDCS) are two methods to stimulate brain activity either by applying an electronic pulse (TMS) or mild current (tDCS).

Brain Imaging: "Seeing" the Brain

Several different types of brain-imaging techniques allow clinicians and researchers to get a direct look at both the structure and the functioning of the brain.

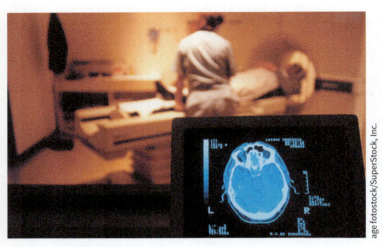

A person entering an fMRI scanner.

age fotostock/SuperStock, Inc.

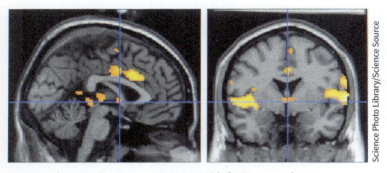

Functional magnetic resonance images. With fMRI, researchers can measure how brain activity changes when a person is doing different tasks, such as viewing an emotional film, completing a memory test, looking at a visual puzzle, or hearing and learning a list of words.

Science Photo Library/Science Source

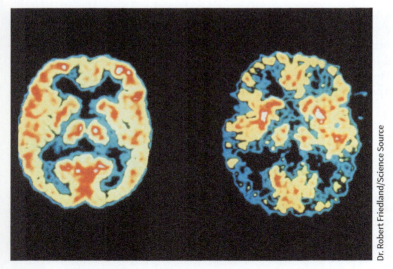

The PET scan on the left shows a normal brain; the one on the right shows the brain of a person with Alzheimer's disease.

Dr. Robert Friedland/Science Source

One method for seeing brain structure is **magnetic resonance imaging (MRI)**. In an MRI, the person is placed inside a large, circular magnet, which causes the hydrogen atoms in the body to change their alignment. When the magnetic force is turned off, the atoms return to their original alignments and thereby produce an electromagnetic signal. These signals are then read by the computer and translated into pictures of brain tissue.

Another brain-imaging technique, called **functional MRI (fMRI)**, allows researchers to measure both brain structure and brain function. This technique involves taking MRI pictures so quickly that metabolic changes can be measured, providing a picture of the brain at work rather than of its structure alone. fMRI measures blood flow in the brain, using what is called the **BOLD (blood oxygenation level dependent)** signal. As neurons fire, presumably blood flow increases to that area. Therefore, blood flow in a particular region of the brain is a reasonable proxy for neural activity in that brain region.

Positron emission tomography, which yields a **PET scan**, is a more invasive procedure that also allows measurement of both brain structure and brain function, although the measurement of brain structure is not as precise as with MRI or fMRI. A substance used by the brain is labeled with a short-lived radioactive isotope and injected into the bloodstream. The radioactive molecules of the substance emit a particle called a positron, which quickly collides with an electron. A pair of high-energy light particles shoot out in opposite directions from the location of the collision and are detected by the scanner. The computer analyzes millions of such recordings and converts them into a picture of the functioning brain. The images are in color; fuzzy spots of lighter and warmer colors are areas in which metabolic rates for the substance are higher. Because a PET is more invasive than a fMRI, it is used less often as a measure of brain function. Nevertheless, this method is useful for assessing neurotransmitter functioning in the brain.

Another way to measure neurotransmitter activity in the living brain is with single photon emission computed tomography, or **SPECT**. Like PET, this method involves injecting a radioisotope into the bloodstream. However, this method is less expensive because the isotopes it uses are more readily available. SPECT directly measures gamma rays that are produced by the injected radioisotopes and generates images of activity in different regions of the brain.

Researchers in many disciplines are currently using brain-imaging assessment techniques both to discover previously undetectable brain problems and to conduct inquiries into the neurobiological contributions to thought, emotion, and behavior. This area of research and application is a very lively and exciting one. Results to date, however, are not strong enough for these methods to be used in diagnosing psychological disorders. For example, the problems in some disorders are so widespread that finding the contributing brain dysfunction is a daunting task. Take, for example, schizophrenia, which affects thinking, feeling, and behavior. Where in the brain might there be dysfunction? Looking for areas that influence thinking, feeling, and behavior requires looking at the entire brain.

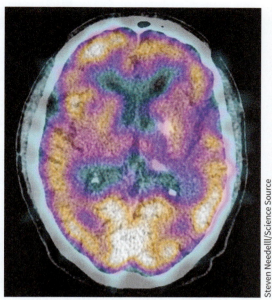

SPECT image. This type of image can show neurotransmitter activity.

Brain Stimulation

Recent advances in technology have allowed clinicians and researchers to stimulate different areas of the brain noninvasively. These tools allow us to test hypotheses about how our behavior is linked to brain regions. In addition, these methods have begun to be used as interventions. Two techniques we discuss here are **transcranial magnetic stimulation (TMS)** and **transcranial direct current stimulation (tDCS)**. These are often referred to as rTMS or rtDCS, where "r" stands for *repetitive*, indicating that there are many sessions of stimulation.

TMS involves placing an electromagnetic coil, often shaped like a figure 8, on the scalp. The coil is attached to an electronic pulse generator that is plugged into an electrical outlet and emits electric pulses to the areas of the brain near where the coil is placed. TMS can apply one pulse or multiple pulses. The TMS apparatus is large and is typically on a rolling cart that can be wheeled close to the person receiving the stimulation. By contrast, tDCS is administered with a smaller device, worn on the head, that is battery-powered. The device contains electrodes, and a current weaker than that used in TMS is applied over several minutes.

One exciting advantage of these tools is that they allow researchers to test hypotheses about brain–behavior relationships. That is, a researcher can stimulate an area of the brain and immediately examine the impact on behavior. For example, stimulation can be applied to the motor areas of the brain, causing a finger to twitch. Stimulation can be applied while a person is doing a behavioral task (e.g., speaking out loud), and the behavior can be temporarily stopped. Similar to neuropsychological tests, these methods can help assess areas of the brain and behavior that are disrupted in psychological disorders.

Using rTMS and fMRI together can help identify brain networks (see Chapter 2). For example, stimulating one area of the brain, such as the occipital cortex that is associated with vision, using rTMS can show effects not only in the occipital cortex but in other brain regions involved in networks that include this region but are not able to be stimulated directly (e.g., a subcortical structure such as the amygdala). rTMS and fMRI can also identify problems in functional connectivity (see Chapter 2) in the brain, and this has been done in studies of depression as well as in studies of the aging brain (Pitcher, Parkin, & Walsh, 2021).

Also exciting is the potential these tools have for treatment of psychological disorders (George, 2019). In the United States, the Food and Drug Administration (FDA) has approved rTMS as a treatment for depression for people who have not responded to other types of treatment and for obsessive-compulsive disorder. Investigations of other disorders, including Alzheimer's disease and schizophrenia (Lefaucheur, André-Obadia, et al., 2014), are under way, but the evidence is limited so far (Chou, Ton That, & Sundman, 2020; Dougall, Maayan, et al., 2015; Weiler, Stieger, et al., 2020). tDCS has shown promise as a treatment for depression and schizophrenia (Bennabi & Haffen, 2018; Cheng, Louie, et al., 2020).

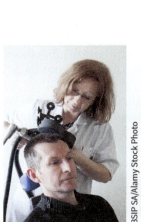
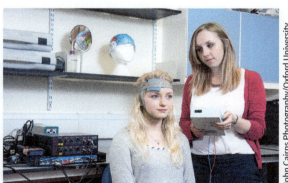

These photos illustrate brain stimulation techniques. The photo on the left shows TMS, and the photo on the right shows tDCS.

Quick Summary

Brain-imaging methods allow clinicians and researchers to "see" the living brain. Different imaging techniques, such as fMRI, PET, and SPECT, have the potential to show areas of the brain that might not be working optimally. Noninvasive brain stimulation techniques including TMS and tDCS are promising treatments for psychological disorders and can be used to test hypotheses about how the brain supports different behaviors.

3.4 Check Your Knowledge

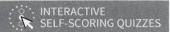
INTERACTIVE
SELF-SCORING QUIZZES

(Answers are at the end of the chapter.)

True or false?

1. MRI is a technique that shows both the structure and the function of the brain.
2. SPECT is invasive but less expensive than PET and can be used to examine neurotransmitter function in the brain.
3. tDCS delivers a weaker electric current to the brain than does TMS.
4. Brain imaging methods such as fMRI are useful in the diagnosis of psychological disorders.

Diversity and Assessment

Studies of the influences of culture, race, and ethnicity on psychological disorders and its assessment are essential to the field (López & Guarnaccia, 2016). As you read about some of this research, keep in mind that there are typically more differences within cultural, ethnic, and racial groups than between them. Remembering this important point can help you avoid stereotyping members of a culture, racial, or ethnic group.

We should also note that the reliability and validity of various forms of psychological assessment have been rightly questioned on the grounds that their content and scoring procedures reflect the culture of White Americans and so may not accurately assess people from other races or cultures. In this section, we discuss problems of cultural and racial bias and what can be done about them.

Cultural and Racial Bias in Assessment

The issue of bias in assessment refers to the notion that a measure developed for one cultural, ethnic, or racial group may not be equally reliable and valid with a different group. Some tests that were developed in the United States have been translated into different languages and used in different cultures and countries successfully. For example, Spanish-language versions of the WAIS and WISC have been available for over 50 years. The WISC-IV Spanish includes not just a translation from English to Spanish but also norms for Spanish-speaking children and items designed explicitly to minimize cultural bias. The MMPI-3 has been translated into Spanish, and the BFI-2 has been translated into 12 other languages, with many other translations under way.

Simply translating words into a different language, however, does not ensure that the meaning of those words will be the same across different cultures. Several steps in the translation process, including working with multiple translators, back-translating, and testing with multiple native speakers, can help to ensure that the test is similar in different languages. The International Test Commission publishes an important guide called *The ITC Guidelines for Translating and Adapting Tests*. These guidelines cover the context of a test, the development and adaption of a test to a different language, administration, and scoring interpretations (International Test Commission, 2017).

Although translations of assessment measures is helpful, the field still has a way to go in reducing cultural, ethnic, and racial bias in clinical assessment. First, the guidelines are not always followed. One review of 61 articles of test translations found that the majority of the studies did not follow the guidelines (Rios & Sireci, 2014). More systemically, cultural assumptions or biases may cause clinicians to over- or underestimate psychological problems in members of other cultures and racial groups (López, 1989, 1996). For decades, researchers have shown that Black Americans are more likely to receive a diagnosis of schizophrenia than are White Americans; this does not likely reflect an actual difference but instead a form of racial bias on the part of clinicians (Arnold, Keck, et al., 2004; Gara, Minsky, et al., 2019; Trierweiler, Neighbors, et al., 2000). Racial bias has also been shown to occur in the diagnosis of conduct disorder, antisocial personality disorder, eating disorders, and posttraumatic stress disorder (Garb, 2021).

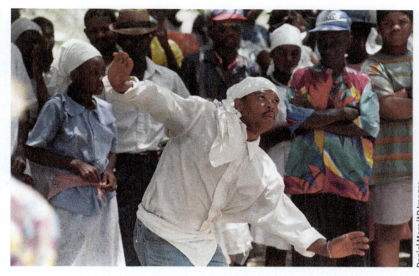

Assessment must take the person's cultural background into account. Belief in spirit possession should not always be taken to mean that the believer is psychotic, as it is common in some cultures.

Clinicians can also make mistakes based on assumptions they hold about culture and emotion. For example, a clinician may assume that an Asian man who reports that he does not want to feel happy or excited is depressed. Yet, as we discussed in Chapter 2, we know that people from East Asian cultures are more inclined to want to feel low-arousal positive emotions, such as calmness and contentment (Tsai, 2017). By contrast, people from European cultures are more likely to want to feel high arousal positive emotions like happiness, enthusiasm, and excitement. Thus, someone from an Asian background who does not want to feel happy is not necessarily experiencing depression. Instead, research with people from different cultures has found that a greater discrepancy between what one wants to feel and what one currently feels—that is, a discrepancy between ideal and current affect—is associated with depression (Tamir, Schwartz, et al., 2017).

Cultural and racial differences in psychological disorders must be examined more closely. Unfortunately, the cultural and racial biases that can creep into clinical assessment do not necessarily yield efforts to compensate for them. There is no simple answer. The DSM-5-TR's emphasis on cultural factors in the discussion of every category of disorder, along with its new cultural formulation interview, may well sensitize clinicians and researchers to the issue. When practitioners were surveyed, they overwhelmingly reported taking culture into account in their clinical work (López, 1994), so it appears that the problem, if not the solution, is clearly in focus.

Strategies for Avoiding Cultural and Racial Bias in Assessment

Clinicians can—and do—use various methods to minimize the negative effects of biases when conducting assessments. One place to begin is with graduate training programs (Galán, Bekele, et al., 2021; Rodriguez-Seijas, McClendon, et al., in press). Perhaps most important to instill at the outset of graduate training in clinical psychology are the concepts of cultural competence cultural humility. *Cultural competence* refers to training that helps prepare psychologists to work with people from different cultural, racial, and ethnic groups. *Cultural humility* is multifaceted and includes:

a. having an awareness of own's own culture and biases;

b. recognizing differences, imbalances, and inequities that may occur in clinical contexts; and

c. a commitment to continue learning about cultural and racial biases that may impact clinical work.

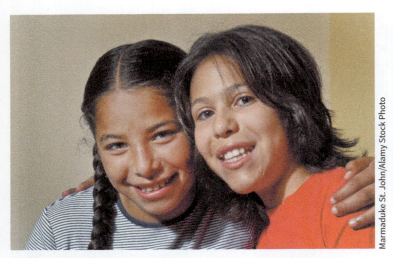

Cultural differences can lead to different results on an aptitude or IQ test. For example, Native American children may not recognize the need to perform quickly on some tests even if that causes them to make mistakes.

López (2002) discussed three important issues that should be taught to graduate students in clinical psychology programs. First, students must learn about basic issues in assessment, such as reliability and validity. Second, students must become informed about the specific ways in which culture, race, or ethnicity may impact assessment (i.e., cultural competence). Third, students must consider that culture, race, or ethnicity may not impact assessment in every individual case.

Assessment procedures can be modified to ensure that all people truly understand the requirements of the task. For example, suppose that a Native American child performed poorly on a test measuring psychomotor speed. The examiner's hunch is that the child did not understand the importance of working quickly and was overly concerned with accuracy instead. The test could be administered again after a more thorough explanation of the importance of working quickly without worrying about mistakes. If the child's performance improves, the examiner gains an important understanding of the child's test-taking strategy and avoids diagnosing psychomotor speed deficits.

As López (1994) points out, however, "the distance between cultural responsiveness and cultural stereotyping can be short" (p. 123). To minimize such problems, clinicians are encouraged to be very cautious about drawing conclusions regarding people from different cultural and ethnic backgrounds. Rather, they are advised to approach assessments with cultural humility, to make hypotheses about the influence of culture on a person, entertain alternative hypotheses, and then test those hypotheses.

Training is truly important, as a clinician's biases can influence diagnosis. For example, research indicates that schizophrenia is often overdiagnosed among Black Americans, and this bias contributes to higher dosages of antipsychotic medications than may be necessary (Alarcon, Becker, et al., 2009). One way to combat such biases is to use structured diagnostic interviews, like the SCID described earlier. When clinicians use structured interviews, they are less likely to overdiagnose people from different ethnic or racial groups (Garb, 2021).

Summary

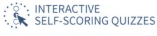

INTERACTIVE
SELF-SCORING QUIZZES

Chapter 3 Practice Quiz

Reliability and Validity

In gathering diagnostic and assessment information, clinicians and researchers must be concerned with both reliability and validity. Reliability refers to whether measurements are consistent and replicable, and validity refers to whether assessments are tapping into what they are meant to measure. Assessment procedures vary greatly in their reliability and validity.

Diagnosis

- Diagnosis is the process of assessing whether a person meets the criteria for a psychological disorder. Having an agreed-on diagnostic system allows clinicians to communicate effectively with each other and facilitates the search for causes and treatments. Clinically, diagnosis provides the foundation for treatment planning.

- The *Diagnostic and Statistical Manual of Mental Disorders* (DSM), published by the American Psychiatric Association,

is an official diagnostic system widely used by mental health professionals. The latest edition of the manual, referred to as DSM-5-TR, was published in 2022.

- Reliability of diagnosis has been improved by including specific criteria for each diagnosis. Criticisms of the DSM include the large number of diagnoses that are often related to the same risk factors and tend to co-occur; the reliance on a categorical rather than a dimensional approach to classification; the fact that reliability in practice may be lower than that achieved in research studies; and the ongoing need to validate diagnoses against causes, course, and treatment. Most researchers and clinicians, though, recognize that the DSM is an enormous advance compared to previous systems.

- HiTOP and RDoC are new approaches to building a diagnostic system; HiTOP focuses on overlap among symptoms, while RDoC focuses on systematically understanding risk factors for psychological disorders.

- Some critics of the DSM argue against diagnosis in general. They point out that diagnostic classifications may ignore important information. Although many worry that diagnostic labels will increase stigma, some data suggest that a diagnosis can reduce stigma by providing an explanation for worrisome behavior.

Assessment

- Clinicians rely on several types of assessment in trying to find out how best to describe an individual, search for the reasons the person is troubled, arrive at an accurate diagnosis, and implement effective treatments. The best assessment involves multiple types of methods.

- Clinical interviews are structured or relatively unstructured conversations in which the clinician asks the person for information about symptoms, stress, and other problems. The LEDS is a useful and valid method for assessing stress.

- Personality assessments include empirically derived self-report questionnaires, such as the Minnesota Multiphasic Personality Inventory-3, the Big Five Inventory-2, and the NEO Personality Inventory.

- Intelligence tests, such as the Wechsler Adult Intelligence Scale, evaluate a person's intellectual ability and can predict how well he or she will perform academically. Neuropsychological tests, such as the Trail Making Test and the California Verbal Learning Test, assess different cognitive functions that are associated with different brain regions.

- Behavioral and self-report assessments are concerned with how people act, feel, and think in particular situations. Approaches include direct observation of behavior, experience sampling, and self-report questionnaires that are situational in their focus.

- Neurobiological assessments include brain-imaging techniques, such as fMRI, that enable clinicians and researchers to see various structures and access functions of the living brain, and brain stimulation techniques that are used to assess brain and behavior relationships.

- Cultural, ethnic, and racial factors play a role in clinical assessment. Assessment techniques developed on the basis of research with white, U.S. populations may be inaccurate when used with people of differing ethnic, racial, or cultural backgrounds. Clinicians can have biases that come into play when they are evaluating people from different racial and cultural groups, and these can lead to minimizing or exaggerating a person's symptoms. Clinicians use various methods to guard against the negative effects of these biases in assessment.

Answers to Check Your Knowledge Questions

3.1 1. b; 2. c; 3. d; 4. a; 5. a; 6.c.

3.2 1. Culture-related issues are described for most of the specific disorders; a cultural formulation interview is provided; an appendix describes cultural concepts of distress, culturally specific ways of expressing distress, and cultural explanations of symptoms; 2. high comorbidity, many different diagnoses are related to the same causes, symptoms of many different diagnoses respond to the same treatments; 3. any three of the following: causes, course, social functioning, treatment; 4. HiTOP focuses on overlap in symptoms and syndromes, whereas RDoC focuses on risk variables.

3.3 1. False; 2. True; 3. True; 4. True; 5. True; 6. False

3.4 1. False; 2. True; 3. True; 4. False

Key Terms

CHAPTER 4

Research Methods in the Study of Psychological Disorders

1. Describe issues in defining *theory* and *hypothesis*.
2. Discuss the advantages and disadvantages of case studies, correlational designs, and experimental designs, and identify common types of correlational and experimental designs.
3. Explain the standards and issues in conducting psychotherapy outcome research.
4. Describe the types of analogues that are most common in research on psychological disorders, and identify concerns about the use of analogues.
5. Discuss the current debate concerning replicability in science, and list the basic steps in conducting a meta-analysis.

The ability to conceptualize and treat psychological disorders has improved vastly over the past 50 years. Nonetheless, important questions remain unanswered about the causes and treatments of psychological disorders. Therefore, it is important to pursue new discoveries using scientific research methods.

In this chapter, we discuss key issues in designing and evaluating research on psychological disorders. We begin with defining *theory* and *hypothesis*. Then we discuss the pros and cons of common research designs, and we provide examples of how these different types of designs are used in research on psychological disorders. We discuss several types of analogue research that are used to overcome ethical and pragmatic barriers in the study of psychological disorders. We then consider another core facet of the scientific process—the need to replicate findings and to integrate findings from multiple studies. As we discuss these elements of the research process, bear in mind that researchers also must consider ethical issues in the conduct of research, as discussed in Chapter 16.

Even with carefully designed research on the causes of and treatments for psychological disorders, we will often encounter shortcomings in the predictive power of our research findings. Even if we knew all the variables controlling behavior—and no one would claim that we do—our ability to predict behavior would be limited by the many unexpected and uncontrollable factors that are likely to affect a person over time. People do not behave in a social vacuum. Research participants and therapy clients live moment to moment in exquisitely complex interaction with others who themselves are affected on a moment-to-moment basis by hundreds of factors that are impossible to anticipate. We want to counsel humility, even awe, in an enterprise that tries to understand how things go awry with mental health.

Science, Theory, and Hypotheses

The term *science* comes from the Latin *scire*, meaning "to know." At its core, science is a way of knowing. More formally, it is the systematic pursuit of knowledge through observation. Science involves forming a theory and then systematically gathering data to test the theory.

A **theory** is a set of propositions meant to explain a class of observations. Usually, the goal of scientific theories is to understand cause–effect relationships. A theory permits the generation of more specific hypotheses—expectations about what should occur if a theory is true. For example, if the original classical conditioning theory of phobias is valid, people with dog phobias should be more likely than those without dog phobias to have had traumatic experiences with dogs. By collecting such data, you could test this **hypothesis**.

What makes a good theory? A scientific approach requires that the theory and hypotheses be stated clearly and precisely so that scientific claims can be exposed to systematic tests that could negate the scientist's expectations. That is, regardless of how plausible a theory seems, it must be subject to disproof. Science proceeds by disproving theories, never by "proving theories." Consequently, it is not enough to assert that traumatic experiences during childhood cause psychological maladjustment in adulthood. This is no more than a possibility. According to a scientific point of view, a hypothesis must be amenable to systematic testing that could show it to be false. That is, the focus of testing is on disproving rather than proving a theory.

Researchers must consider a set of principles in testing a theory. They must choose assessments with strong reliability and validity, as discussed in Chapter 3. They also must consider whether their sample adequately reflects the real-world people they are interested in understanding. In addition to selecting measures carefully, researchers must recruit representative samples. They also must choose among different types of research designs, a topic we turn to next.

Quick Summary

Science is the systematic pursuit of knowledge through observation. The first step of science is to define a theory and related hypotheses. A good theory is precise and could be disproven.

4.1 Check Your Knowledge

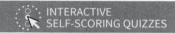 INTERACTIVE
SELF-SCORING QUIZZES

(Answers are at the end of the chapter.)

True or false?

1. A good theory can be proven.
2. Good research depends on the validity, but not reliability, of measures.
3. Hypotheses are broader and more abstract than theories.

Research Designs in the Study of Psychological Disorders

In this section, we describe the most common research methods in the study of psychological disorders: the case study, correlational methods, and experimental methods. You will learn how these methods are applied in studies described throughout this book. In this chapter, we will describe some of the typical ways these different research methods are used in psychological research. **Table 4.1** provides a summary of the strengths and weaknesses of each.

The Case Study

The **case study**, perhaps the most familiar method of observing human behavior, involves recording detailed information about one person at a time. Case studies are often used before more quantitative studies are conducted.

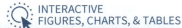

TABLE 4.1   **Research Methods in the Study of Psychological Disorders**

Method	Description	Evaluation
Case study	Collection of detailed biographical information	Excellent source of hypotheses
		Can provide information about novel cases or procedures
		Can disconfirm a relationship that was believed to be universal
		Cannot provide causal evidence because alternative hypotheses cannot be eliminated
		May be biased by observer's theoretical viewpoint
Correlation	Study of the relationship between two or more variables, measured as they exist in nature	Widely used because we cannot manipulate many risk variables (such as personality, trauma, or genes) or diagnoses in psychopathology research with humans
		Often used by epidemiologists to study the incidence, prevalence, and risk factors of disorders in a representative sample
		Often used in behavioral genetics research to study the heritability of different disorders
		Directionality and third-variable problems can interfere with determining causality
Experiment	Includes a manipulated independent variable, a dependent variable, preferably at least one control group, and random assignment	Most powerful method for determining causal relationships
		Often used in studies of treatment
		Single-case experimental designs common but can have limited external validity
		Can also examine analogue versions of risk factors

Source: National Academy of Science, Engineering, and Medicine (2022).

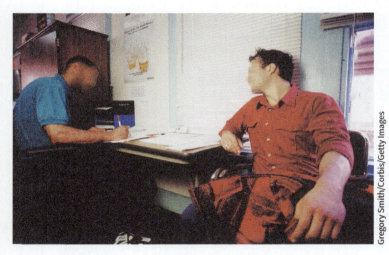

Although the information yielded by a case study does not provide strong support for a theory, it is an important source of hypotheses.

Gregory Smith/Corbis/Getty Images

There are several problems in interpreting case studies. First, the objectivity of case studies is limited because the author's views will shape the kinds of information reported in a case study. Second, case studies do not provide good evidence in support of a theory because they do not rule out alternative hypotheses. As an illustration of this problem, consider a case study that describes a client who responds well to a novel therapy. Although it would be tempting to conclude that the therapy is effective, such a conclusion cannot be drawn legitimately because other factors could have produced the change. A stressful situation in the client's life may have resolved during the time period of the intervention. Thus, rival hypotheses could account for the clinical improvement. The data yielded by the case study do not allow us to determine the true cause of the change.

Despite their relative lack of control, case studies still play an important role in the study of psychological disorders. Specifically, the case study can be used:

1. to provide a rich description of a new or unusual clinical phenomenon or treatment,
2. to disprove an allegedly universal hypothesis, and
3. to generate hypotheses that can be tested through quantitative research.

The Correlational Method

A great deal of research relies on the **correlational method**. Correlational studies address questions of the form "Do variable X and variable Y vary together (co-relate)?" In correlational research, variables are measured as they exist in nature. This is distinct from experimental research (discussed later in this chapter), in which the researcher manipulates variables.

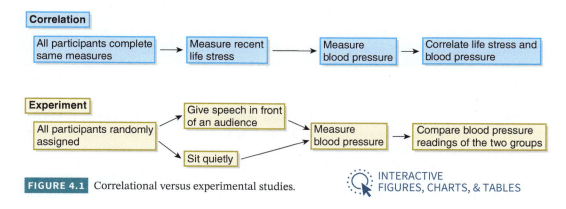

Correlation

| All participants complete same measures | → | Measure recent life stress | → | Measure blood pressure | → | Correlate life stress and blood pressure |

Experiment

All participants randomly assigned → Give speech in front of an audience / Sit quietly → Measure blood pressure → Compare blood pressure readings of the two groups

FIGURE 4.1 Correlational versus experimental studies.

INTERACTIVE
FIGURES, CHARTS, & TABLES

As an illustration of the difference, consider research on the role of stress in hypertension (high blood pressure), which can be assessed with either a correlational or an experimental design. In a correlational study, we might measure stress levels by interviewing people about their recent stressful experiences. Stress would then be correlated with blood pressure measurements collected from these same people. In an experimental study, in contrast, the experimenter might create stress in the laboratory; for example, half of the participants might be asked to give a speech to an audience about the aspect of their personal appearance that they find least appealing, and the other half might be assigned to a nonstressful condition (see **Figure 4.1**). The key difference between correlational and experimental designs is whether or not a variable is manipulated. Researchers will rely on correlational methods when there are ethical reasons not to manipulate a variable; for example, no researcher would try to manipulate genes, trauma, severe stressors, or neurobiological deficits in humans.

Numerous examples of **correlation** can be drawn from research on psychological disorders. For example, depression tends to correlate with anxiety; people who feel depressed tend to report feeling anxious. Comparisons of people with and without a diagnosis can be correlational as well. See **Table 4.2** for a description of how data might be coded if, for example, two diagnostic groups were being compared to see how much stress was experienced before the onset of a disorder. In correlational studies, questions are asked about the relationship between a given diagnosis and some other variable—for example, "Is schizophrenia related to social class?" or "Are anxiety disorders related to neurotransmitter function?"

TABLE 4.2   Data for a Correlational Study with Diagnosis

Participant	Diagnosis	Stress Score
1	1	65
2	1	72
3	0	40
4	1	86
5	0	72
6	0	21
7	1	65
8	0	40
9	1	37
10	0	28

Note: Diagnosis of an anxiety disorder is coded as 1 if present and 0 if not present. Recent life stress is assessed on a 0–100 scale. Higher scores indicate greater recent stress. This illustration includes a smaller sample of cases than would be used in an actual research study. Notice that diagnosis is correlated with recent life stress. Patients with an anxiety disorder tend to have higher stress scores than people without an anxiety disorder. In this example, the correlation between stress and anxiety scores is +.60.

In the next sections, we discuss how to measure the relationship (correlation) between two variables, how to test whether the relationship is statistically and clinically significant, and some issues involved in determining whether variables are causally related. Then we discuss two specific fields in which researchers tend to use correlational designs: epidemiology and behavior genetics.

Measuring Correlation   The first step in determining a correlation is to obtain pairs of observations of the two variables in question. One example would be the height and weight of each participant. Another example would be the intelligence of mothers and daughters. Once such pairs of measurements have been obtained, the strength of the relationship between the paired observations can be computed to determine the **correlation coefficient**, denoted by the symbol r. This statistic may take any value between −1.00 and +1.00, and it measures both the magnitude and the direction of a relationship. The higher the absolute value of r, the stronger the relationship between the two variables. That is, an r of either +1.00 or −1.00 indicates the strongest possible, or perfect, relationship, whereas an r of .00 indicates that the variables are unrelated. If the sign of r is positive, the two variables are said to be positively related; in other words, as the values for variable X increase, those for variable Y also tend to increase. Table 4.3 shows data for a correlation of +.88 between height and weight, indicating a very strong positive relationship; as height increases, so does weight. Conversely, when the sign of r is negative, variables are said to be negatively related; as scores on one variable increase, those for the other tend to decrease. For example, the number of hours spent watching television is negatively correlated with grade point average.

One way to think about the strength of a correlation is to plot the two variables. In Figure 4.2, each point represents the scores for a given person on variable X and variable Y. In a perfect correlation, all the points fall on a straight line; if we know the value of only one of the variables for a person, we can know the value of the other variable. Similarly, when the correlation is relatively large, there is only a small degree of scatter about the line of perfect correlation. The values tend to scatter increasingly far from the line as the correlations become lower. When the correlation is .00, knowledge of a person's score on one variable tells us nothing about their score on the other.

Statistical and Clinical Significance   Thus far, we have established that the magnitude of a correlation coefficient tells us the strength of a relationship between two variables. But scientists use **statistical significance** for a more rigorous test of the importance of a relationship. (Although we focus on correlation coefficients here, significance

TABLE 4.3   **Data for Determining a Correlation**

	Height in Inches	Weight in Pounds
John	70	170
Asher	70	140
Eve	64	112
Gail	63	105
Jerry	70	177
Gayla	62	100
Steve	68	145
Margy	65	128
Gert	66	143
Sean	70	140
Kathleen	64	116

Note: For this data set, the r of height and weight = +.88.

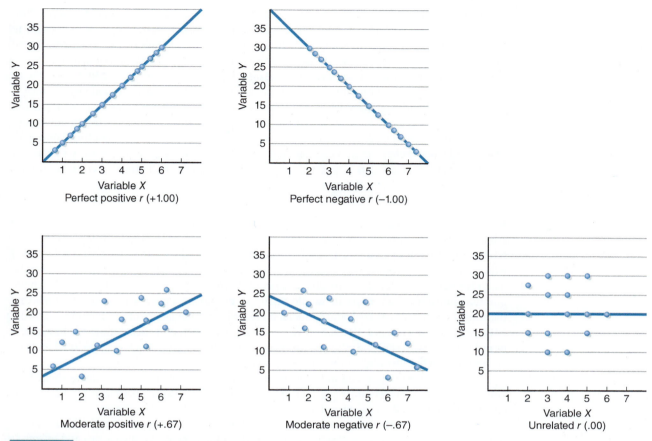

FIGURE 4.2 Scatter diagrams showing various degrees of correlation.

is assessed with statistics other than correlation coefficients as well.) Imagine that a researcher conducted the same study again and again. You would not expect to see exactly the same results every time. For example, differences in who signed up for the study might influence the pattern of findings. This random variation, or chance, must be considered in evaluating the findings of any study. Significance testing begins with the assumption that there is no true relationship between X and Y in the population—an assumption known as the *null hypothesis*. Even if it is true, one would expect some samples, by chance alone, to show a larger correlation. A statistically significant correlation indicates that the correlation observed is unlikely when the null hypothesis is true. When a correlation is not statistically significant, it is highly likely that no significant relationship would be observed if the study were repeated. A nonsignificant correlation does not provide evidence for an important relationship.

A statistical finding is usually considered significant if the probability that the null hypothesis is true is 5 or less in 100. This level of significance is called the *alpha level*, commonly written as $p < .05$ (the p stands for probability). We will discuss the p value later in this chapter as we consider replicability of studies. In general, as the absolute size of the correlation coefficient increases, the result is more likely to be statistically significant. For example, a correlation of .80 (or −.80) is more likely to be significant than a correlation of .40.

Statistical significance is influenced not only by the size of the relationship between variables but also by the number of participants in a study. The fewer people studied, the larger the correlation must be to reach statistical significance. For example, a correlation of $r = .30$ is statistically significant when the number of observations is large—say, 300—but is not significant if only 20 observations were made. Thus, if the alcohol consumption of 20 men was studied and the correlation between depression and drinking was found to be .30, the correlation would not be statistically significant. The same correlation, however, would be significant if 300 men were studied.

Beyond statistical significance, it is important to consider **clinical significance**. Clinical significance is defined by whether a relationship between variables is large enough to matter. In a survey as large as the U.S. Census, almost every correlation you could conceive of would be statistically significant; thus, researchers need to attend to whether a correlation is large enough to be clinically significant. For example, one might want to see that a risk factor has a moderately strong relationship with the severity of symptoms. Clinical significance is also considered with statistics other than correlations. For a treatment effect to be considered clinically significant, a researcher might want to see that, at the end of active treatment, symptoms were decreased by 50% or patients appeared comparable to those without the disorder. In other words, researchers should evaluate not only whether an effect is statistically significant but also whether the effect is large enough to be meaningful in predicting or treating a psychological disorder (Jacobson, Roberts, et al., 1999).

Problems of Causality

Even though correlational designs are common, they have a critical drawback: They do not allow determination of cause–effect relationships. A large correlation between two variables tells us only that they are related to each other; we do not know if either variable is the cause of the other. For example, there is a moderate correlation between the diagnosis of schizophrenia and social class; people with less income are diagnosed with schizophrenia more often than people in middle and upper classes are. One possible explanation is that the stress of living in poverty could cause an increase in the prevalence of schizophrenia (Kwok, 2014). But a second hypothesis has been supported: It may be that the disorganized behavior patterns of people with schizophrenia cause them to perform poorly in their occupational endeavors and thus to become impoverished (Dohrenwend & Dohrenwend, 1974).

The **directionality problem** is present in most correlational research designs—hence the often cited dictum "correlation does not imply causation." One way of overcoming the directionality problem is based on the idea that causes must precede effects. In a **longitudinal design**, the researcher tests whether causes are present before a disorder has developed. This is in contrast to a **cross-sectional design**, in which the researcher measures the causes and effects at the same point in time. The ABCD study, for example, is a longitudinal study in which over 10,000 children are being assessed repeatedly until they reach adulthood, to assess predictors of health outcomes. Longitudinal studies of rare disorders, though, are prohibitively expensive, for only about 1 person in 100 eventually develops schizophrenia or bipolar I disorder.

The **high-risk method** overcomes this problem; with this approach, researchers study only people with above-average risk of developing a rare condition. For example, many research programs involve studying people who have a parent diagnosed with schizophrenia (having a parent with schizophrenia increases a person's risk for developing schizophrenia). The high-risk method is used to study the onset of several disorders, and we will examine these findings in subsequent chapters.

Even if a longitudinal study identifies a variable that precedes schizophrenia, a researcher still faces the **third-variable problem**: A third factor may have produced the correlation. Such factors are labeled as *confounds*. Research on psychological disorders offers numerous examples of third variables. Researchers often report biochemical differences between people with and without schizophrenia. These differences could reflect the influence of medications used for schizophrenia or even dietary differences between groups; the differences might not reveal anything about the nature of schizophrenia. Are there ways to resolve the third-variable problem? Although some strategies can help address some of the confounds, the solutions are only partially satisfactory. Take the example of diet as a potential confound in biochemical differences in schizophrenia. Researchers can try to control for diet in statistical analyses, but they may not measure the most important aspects of diet. It is not feasible to measure every possible confound. Because of the third-variable problem, causal claims cannot be made from correlational data.

One Example of Correlational Research: Epidemiologic Research

Epidemiology is the study of the distribution of disorders in a population. That is, data are gathered about the rates of disorder and the correlates of disorder in a large sample. Epidemiologic research focuses on three features of a disorder:

1. **Prevalence.** The proportion of people with the disorder either currently or during their lifetime

2. **Incidence.** The proportion of people who develop *new* cases of the disorder in some period, usually a year

3. **Correlates.** Variables that are correlated with the presence of the disorder

Epidemiologic studies are usually correlational studies because they examine how variables relate to each other without manipulating any of the variables.

Epidemiologic studies are designed to be *representative* of the population being studied—researchers test a group of people who match the population on key characteristics, like gender, economic status, and ethnicity. Unfortunately, much of the research on psychological disorders draws on samples that are not representative. For example, many studies use undergraduate samples. Undergraduates, though, are likely to be wealthier and more educated than the general population. If we only studied undergraduates with anxiety disorders, we could end up concluding that people with anxiety disorders are above average in intelligence. Other studies use samples drawn from treatment centers, but people who seek treatment tend to be those with the more severe forms of disorders. For example, estimates of suicide rates for a given disorder measured in hospitalized samples are much higher than rates in representative community samples. These types of bias can skew our perceptions of factors related to psychological disorders. Epidemiologic studies, then, are needed to carefully identify the correlates of and outcomes for disorders.

The National Comorbidity Survey Replication (NCS-R) is an example of one large-scale national survey that used structured interviews to collect information on the prevalence of several diagnoses (Kessler, Berglund, et al., 2005). In the World Mental Health Survey, interviews that were parallel with those used in the NCS-R were conducted in dozens of countries to allow cross-national comparison of the prevalence of psychological disorders (Kessler, Angermeyer, et al., 2007). **Table 4.4** shows some of the survey data gathered in the United States. The table presents lifetime prevalence rates—the proportion of people who experienced a disorder during their lifetime. From the table, we can see that major depressive disorder, alcoholism, and anxiety disorders are very common—so common, in fact, that about one out of every two people (46.4%) in the United States describes meeting criteria for a psychological disorder at some point during their lives.

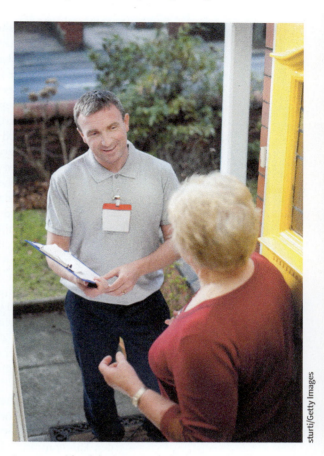

In some epidemiologic research, interviewers go door to door to conduct interviews.

TABLE 4.4   Lifetime Prevalence Rates of Selected Diagnoses in the United States

Disorder	Male	Female	Total
Major depressive disorder	13.2	20.2	16.6
Bipolar I or II disorder	na	na	3.9
Dysthymia	1.8	3.1	2.5
Panic disorder	3.1	6.2	4.7
Specific phobia	11.1	13.0	12.1
Social phobia	8.9	15.8	12.5
Generalized anxiety disorder	na	na	5.7
Alcohol abuse	19.6	7.5	13.2
Drug abuse	11.6	4.8	7.9

Source: Data from Kessler, R. C., Berglund, P., Demler, O., Jin, R., Merikangas, K. R., & Walters, E. E. (2005). Lifetime prevalence and age-of-onset distributions of DSM-IV disorders in the National Comorbidity Survey Replication. *Archives of General Psychiatry, 62*(6), 593–602.

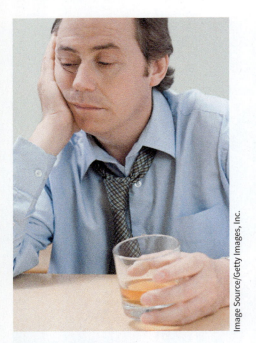

Epidemiologic research has shown that mood disorders, anxiety disorders, and substance abuse are extremely common.

Although the estimate that almost half of people will meet diagnostic criteria may seem high, even this number may be an underestimate. In one study, researchers interviewed participants about psychological symptoms during their lifetime four different times—at ages 18, 21, 26, and 32. At any one of those four interviews, the rates of depressive and anxiety disorders appeared similar to the levels reported in the NCS-R study and observed in multiple other epidemiologic studies. But about half of people who endorsed a given disorder in any one interview did not do so in other interviews (Moffitt, Caspi, et al., 2010). Because of this inaccuracy in any one interview, the researchers tallied how many people reported a psychological disorder in at least one interview. Using these tallies, the researchers estimated that 60% or more of people will meet criteria for a psychological disorder during their lifetime, findings that have been replicated in several longitudinal epidemiologic studies (Schaefer, Caspi, et al., 2017).

Knowing that psychological disorders will strike so many people should help reduce stigma. People who experience the disorders may take comfort in knowing that so many other people struggle with similar issues.

Knowledge about the correlates of disorder may provide clues to the causes of disorders. For example, depression is about twice as common in women as in men. In Chapter 5, we will review theories about this gender difference. Trauma, poverty, and income inequality also are tied to many different psychological disorders. The results of epidemiologic research may inform us about correlates of disorder (like gender, trauma, poverty, and income inequality) that can be more thoroughly investigated using other research methods.

Another Example of Correlational Research: Behavior Genetics

Behavior genetics estimates genetic predisposition for a disorder by considering whether relatives demonstrate similarity (correlations) in their patterns of disorder. This contrasts with the focus of molecular genetics (see Chapter 2) on identifying specific genes that contribute to the presence of a disorder. Both behavior genetics and molecular genetics rely on correlational techniques in the study of psychological disorders in humans. Here we will focus on three common methods used in behavior genetics to examine the genetic contribution to psychological disorders—comparison of members of a family, comparison of pairs of twins, and investigation of adoptees.

The **family method** can be used to study a genetic predisposition among members of a family because the average number of genes shared by two blood relatives is known. Children receive a random sample of half their genes from one parent and half from the other, so, on average, siblings as well as parents and their children share 50% of their genes. People who share 50% of their genes with a given person are called *first-degree relatives* of that person. Relatives who are not as closely related share fewer genes. For example, nephews and nieces share 25% of the genes of an uncle and are called *second-degree relatives*. If a predisposition for a psychological disorder can be inherited, a study of the family should reveal a relationship between the proportion of shared genes and the **concordance** of the disorder in relatives. When relatives are matched on presence or absence of a disorder, they are said to be concordant.

The starting point in such investigations is the recruitment of a sample of people with the diagnosis in question. These people are referred to as **index cases** or **probands**. Then relatives are studied to determine the frequency with which the same diagnosis might be applied to them. If a genetic predisposition to the disorder being studied is present, first-degree relatives of the index cases should have the disorder at a rate higher than that found in the general population. This is the case with schizophrenia: About 10% of the first-degree relatives of index cases with schizophrenia can be diagnosed as having this disorder, compared with about 1% of the general population.

Although the methodology of family studies is clear, the data they yield are not easy to interpret. For example, children of parents with agoraphobia—people suffering from a fear of being in places from which it would be hard to escape if they were to become highly anxious—are themselves more likely than average to have agoraphobia. Does this mean that a predisposition for this anxiety disorder is genetically transmitted? Not necessarily. The greater number of family members with agoraphobia could reflect the child-rearing practices and modeling of the agoraphobic parents. In other words, family studies show that agoraphobia runs in families but not necessarily that a genetic predisposition is involved.

In the **twin method**, both **monozygotic (MZ) twins** and **dizygotic (DZ) twins** are compared. MZ, or identical, twins develop from a single fertilized egg and are genetically the same. DZ, or fraternal, pairs develop from separate eggs and are on average 50% alike genetically, no more alike than are any two siblings. MZ twins are always the same sex, but DZ twins can be either the same sex or opposite in sex. Twin studies begin with diagnosed cases and then assess the presence of the disorder in the other twin. To the extent that a predisposition for a psychological disorder can be inherited, concordance for the disorder should be greater in genetically identical MZ pairs than in DZ pairs. When the MZ concordance rate is higher than the DZ rate, the characteristic being studied is said to be heritable. As described in Chapter 2, heritability estimates range from 0 (no genetic contribution) to 1 (100% genetic contribution). We will see in later chapters that the concordance for most psychological disorders is higher in MZ twins than in DZ twins.

The **adoptees method** studies children who were adopted and reared completely apart from their biological parents. Though infrequent, findings from this method are more clear-cut because the child is not raised by the parent with a disorder. If a high frequency of agoraphobia was found in children reared apart from their parents who also had agoraphobia, we would have convincing support for the heritability of the disorder. In another adoptee method called **cross-fostering**, researchers assess children who are adopted and reared completely apart from their biological parents. In this case, however, the adoptive parent has a particular disorder, not the biological parent. The adoptees method is also used to examine gene–environment interactions. For example, one study found that adoptees who had a biological parent with antisocial personality disorder (APD) and were raised in an unhealthy adoptive family (e.g., parental conflict, abuse, alcohol/drugs in the adoptive family) were more likely to develop APD than two other groups of adoptees: (1) adoptees who had a biological parent with APD but were raised in a healthy family and (2) adoptees who had no biological parent with APD but were raised in an unhealthy adoptive family (Cadoret, Yates, et al., 1995). Thus, genes (APD in a biological parent) and environment (unhealthy adoptive family) worked together to increase the risk for developing antisocial personality disorder.

The Experiment

The **experiment** is the most powerful tool for determining causal relationships. It involves the **random assignment** of participants to conditions, the manipulation of an **independent variable**, and the measurement of a **dependent variable**. We will begin with a brief overview of the basic features of an experiment.

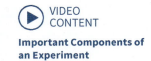

VIDEO CONTENT

Important Components of an Experiment

To illustrate the basics of experimental research, let's consider a study designed to assess whether a specific form of cognitive behavior therapy called dialectical behavior therapy (DBT) has efficacy in reducing suicidal behavior (Linehan, Comtois, et al., 2006). In this study, researchers recruited women who had engaged in recent suicidal behavior and randomly assigned them to receive either 1 year of DBT or treatment as usual by experts in the community. The researchers interviewed patients about their suicidal behavior at baseline before the treatment began, and then every 4 months for 2 years. At baseline, the patients in the two groups did not differ in the number or severity of their previous suicide attempts. During the 2 years of the study, patients assigned to receive DBT were less likely to make a suicide attempt (23.1%) than were those in the treatment as usual condition (46%).

Basic Features of Experimental Design   The treatment study just discussed illustrates many of the basic features of an experiment:

1. The investigator manipulates an independent variable. In this study, the independent variable was the treatment condition.

2. Participants are allocated to the two conditions (DBT versus treatment as usual) by random assignment. To randomly assign participants in a two-group experiment, for example, the researchers could toss a coin for each participant. If the coin turned up heads, the participant would be assigned to one group; if tails, to the other group.

3. The researcher measures a dependent variable that is expected to vary with conditions of the independent variable. The dependent variable in this study was the presence or absence of a suicide attempt.

4. Differences between conditions on the dependent variable are called the **experimental effect**. In this example, the experimental effect was the difference in the probability of suicide attempts for those assigned to receive DBT compared to those assigned to treatment as usual.

Internal Validity

Internal validity refers to the extent to which the experimental effect can be attributed to the independent variable. For a study to have internal validity, the researchers must include at least one **control group**. The control group does not receive the experimental treatment and is needed for the researchers to claim that the effects of the experiment are due to the independent variable. The data from a control group provide a standard against which the effects of an independent variable can be assessed. In the study described, the control group—treatment as usual—allows for a test of whether DBT was more efficacious than standard care in the community. We will describe control groups in more detail as we discuss treatment outcome studies.

The inclusion of a control group does not ensure internal validity, however. Random assignment is also important. Random assignment helps ensure that groups are similar on variables other than the independent variable. Consider a treatment study in which participants can choose to enroll in one of two experimental conditions—psychotherapy or medication. In this study, the researchers cannot claim that group differences are the result of treatment because a competing hypothesis cannot be disproven: Patients in the two conditions might have differed in baseline characteristics such as their willingness to discuss difficult emotional issues or their beliefs about medications. This study design is poor because the researchers did not use random assignment. Without true random assignment, potential confounds make results hard to interpret, so internal validity can be limited.

External Validity

External validity is defined as the extent to which results can be generalized beyond the study. If investigators find that a treatment helps a particular group of patients, they will want to conclude that this treatment will be effective for other similar patients at other times and in other places. For example, Linehan and her colleagues would hope that their findings would generalize to men. Determining the external validity of the results of an experiment is extremely difficult. One problem is that participants in studies often behave in certain ways because they are being observed, and thus results that are produced in the laboratory may not be reproduced in the natural environment.

Perhaps the largest threat to external validity comes from the narrow range of participants in most psychological research—external validity may be threatened by including only a select group of persons in a study, such as college students or White middle-class Americans. This is a concern in correlational and experimental studies. The National Institute of Mental Health has mandated for 40 years that researchers consider gender, race, and ethnicity in studies that they fund. Nonetheless, it remains the case that individuals from minority groups are under-represented in research. Indeed, in a review of articles published in six journals of the American Psychological Association between 2003 and 2007, 68% of participants in studies were from the United States and 96% from Western industrialized countries (Arnett, 2008). Findings from a specific group, such as college students in the United States, may not generalize to people from other contexts (Hanel & Vione, 2016). Improving the diversity of samples, so that we can determine whether findings generalize across people from varied cultural and racial backgrounds, is an urgent priority (National Academy of Science, Engineering, and Medicine, 2022). We will discuss these concerns further as we consider treatment outcome research.

Single-Case Experiments

We have been discussing experimental research with groups of participants, but experiments are not always conducted on groups. In a **single-case experimental design**, the experimenter studies how one person responds to manipulations of the independent variable (Kazdin, 2011). Unlike the traditional case studies described earlier, single-case experimental designs can have high internal validity. For an example of a single-case experiment with high internal validity, see **Focus on Discovery 4.1**.

Focus on Discovery 4.1

An Example of a Single-Case Experiment

Chorpita, Vitali, and Barlow (1997) provide an example of how single-case experimental studies can provide well-controlled data. They describe their treatment of a 13-year-old girl with a phobia (intense fear) of choking, such that she was no longer able to eat solid foods. At times, her fear was so intense that she would experience a fast heart rate, chest pain, and dizziness. She reported that the most frightening foods were hard foods, such as raw vegetables.

A behavioral treatment was designed based on exposure, a common strategy for treating anxiety. During the first 2 weeks, baseline assessments were taken of the amount of different foods eaten, along with her level of discomfort in eating those foods. Discomfort ratings were made on the Subjective Units of Distress Scale (SUDS), ranging from 0 to 9. **Figure 4.3** shows her SUDS ratings and eating behavior over time for each food group. During week 3, she was asked to begin eating foods she described as mildly threatening—crackers and cookies—in three 4-minute blocks each day. The authors hoped that exposure to feared foods would reduce her anxiety. Despite this intervention, the patient's SUDS ratings and food consumption did not improve. When the therapist talked with the client and her parents, he discovered that the client was eating

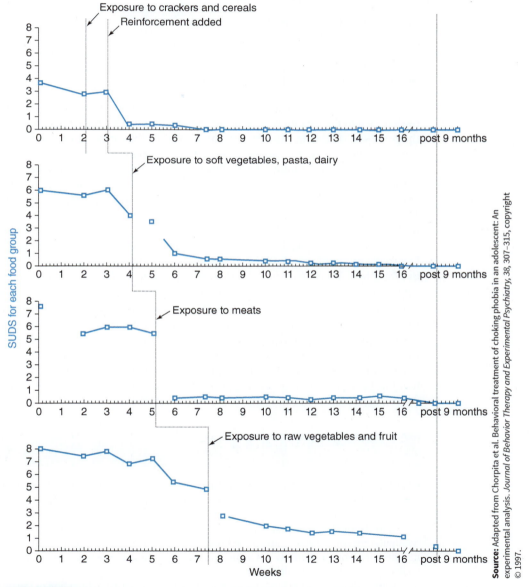

Source: Adapted from Chorpita et al. Behavioral treatment of choking phobia in an adolescent: An experimental analysis. *Journal of Behavior Therapy and Experimental Psychiatry, 38,* 307–315, copyright © 1997.

FIGURE 4.3 Effects of exposure treatment and reinforcement for food phobia in a single-case design. Note the rapid shifts in SUDS ratings as exposure for each new food group is introduced.

only the absolute minimum of foods, such that she was not getting enough exposure to the feared stimulus. To increase her exposure to foods, he added reinforcement to the program—he instructed her parents to give her ice cream at the end of any day in which she had consumed at least three servings of the target food. Within a week, she reported being able to consume crackers and cereals without distress. Gradually, she was asked to begin eating more frightening foods. One week she was asked to begin consuming soft vegetables, pasta, and cheese; followed

the next week by meat; and the next week by raw vegetables, salad, and hard fruit. As shown by the graphs, as exposure to each new food group was introduced, the client experienced a reduction in SUDS ratings within the next week; these effects do not appear to have been due simply to time or maturation, as anxiety was reduced only after the client was first exposed to the new food group. The repeated decrements in anxiety are hard to explain using any variable other than treatment. Gains were maintained through a 9-month follow-up.

In one form of single-case design, referred to as a **reversal design** or an **ABAB design**, the participant's behavior is carefully measured in a specific sequence:

1. An initial time period, the baseline (A)
2. A period when a treatment is introduced (B)
3. A reinstatement of the conditions of the baseline period (A)
4. A reintroduction of the treatment (B)

If behavior in the experimental period is different from that in the baseline period, reverses when the treatment is removed, and resumes when the treatment is again introduced, there is little doubt that the manipulation, rather than chance or uncontrolled factors, has produced the change. Hence, "A" time periods serve as control comparisons for the treatment.

The reversal technique cannot always be employed, however, because the initial state of a participant may not be recoverable. Remember that most treatments aim to produce enduring change, so just removing an intervention may not return a person to the pretreatment state. This reversal technique, then, is most applicable when researchers believe that the effects of their manipulation are temporary.

The biggest drawback of single-case designs is the potential lack of external validity. The fact that a treatment works for a single person does not necessarily imply that it will be effective for others. Findings may relate to a unique aspect of that one person. Some researchers use single-case experimental research to decide whether research with larger groups is warranted. Other researchers conduct a series of single-case experiments to see if findings generalize. In doing so, it is important to include participants who differ. With replication across diverse participants, single-case designs can provide a strong test of hypotheses. Indeed, single-case experimental research can be used as evidence that a treatment is efficacious. The APA (Task Force on Promotion and Dissemination of Psychological Procedures, 1995) considers a treatment to have gained empirical support if it has shown success compared to a well-designed control condition in at least nine single-case experiments.

Quick Summary

Case studies can provide detailed information about a novel phenomenon or treatment technique, and they can disprove a hypothesis. They do not provide good evidence for cause and effect, and they can be biased.

Correlational studies examine the strength of relation between variables, and they do not involve manipulating any variable. Correlation does not imply causation. Longitudinal studies can help address the directionality problem by assessing whether one variable precedes the other, but third variables (called confounds) could still explain any observed relationship.

Correlation coefficients provide an estimate of the strength and direction of the relationship. A correlation coefficient of −1.00 or +1.00 indicates a perfect relationship, and a correlation coefficient of .00 indicates that there is no systematic relationship between two variables.

A statistically significant correlation indicates that the correlation observed is unlikely when the null hypothesis is true. Statistical significance is influenced by the size of the sample.

A clinically significant finding is one in which the relationship is large enough to matter.

Epidemiology and behavior genetics are correlational approaches that are commonly used in research on psychological disorders.

Epidemiology is the science of obtaining and testing representative samples drawn from the community. Epidemiology is used to estimate the prevalence and incidence of disorders, and the correlates of those disorders.

Behavior genetics involves the study of concordance among first-degree relatives, MZ versus DZ twins, and adoptees as a way to estimate the heritability of disorders and to evaluate interactions between genetic and environmental contributions to disorders.

The experimental method entails manipulating an independent variable and measuring the effect on a dependent variable. Generally, participants are randomly assigned to one of at least two groups: an experimental group, which experiences the active condition of the independent variable, and a control group, which does not. The researcher tests to see if the independent variable had an effect (the experimental effect) by looking for differences between the experimental and control groups on the dependent variable.

Internal validity refers to whether an effect can be confidently attributed to the independent variable. External validity refers to whether experimental effects can be generalized to situations and people outside this specific study. Experimental designs can provide internal validity, but external validity is sometimes a concern. Correlational studies can provide solid external validity but poorer internal validity.

In single-case experimental designs, the researcher examines the effects of manipulating an independent variable in a single person. These designs can have high internal validity, particularly if reversal designs are employed. External validity can be limited for single-case experimental designs.

4.2 Check Your Knowledge

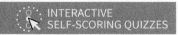
INTERACTIVE
SELF-SCORING QUIZZES

(Answers are at the end of the chapter.)

Answer the following questions.

1. Which of the following are good uses of case studies (circle all that apply)?

    a. to illustrate a rare disorder or treatment

    b. to show that a theory does not fit everyone

    c. to prove a model

    d. to show cause and effect

2. Correlational studies involve:

    a. manipulating the independent variable

    b. manipulating the dependent variable

    c. manipulating the independent and dependent variables

    d. none of the above

3. What central problem is unique to correlational studies as compared to experimental studies, regardless of how carefully researchers design them?

    a. Findings are qualitative rather than statistical.

    b. It is impossible to know which variable changes first.

    c. Third variables may explain a relationship observed.

    d. Findings may not be generalized.

4. *Incidence* refers to:

    a. the number of people who will develop a disorder during their lifetime

    b. the number of people who report a disorder at the time of an interview

    c. the number of people who develop a disorder during a given time period

    d. none of the above

5. In behavior genetics research, researchers can most effectively rule out the influence of parenting variables if they conduct studies using the:

    a. correlational method

    b. family method

    c. twin method

    d. adoptees method

One Example of Experimental Research: Treatment Outcome Research

Treatment outcome research is designed to address a simple question: Does treatment work? The clear answer is yes. Here we will focus on the issues in testing psychotherapy, but many of these same issues must be considered in evaluating medication treatments.

Treatment outcome studies are the most common form of experiment in the mental health field. Hundreds of studies have examined whether people who receive psychotherapy fare better than those who do not. In meta-analyses of more than 300 studies, researchers have found that there is a moderately positive effect of treatment. About 75% of people who enter treatment achieve at least some improvement (Lambert & Ogles, 2004). As shown in **Figure 4.4**, the effects of psychotherapy appear to be more powerful than the passage of time or support from friends and family. On the other hand, it is also clear from this figure that therapy does not always work. That is, about 25% of people do not improve in therapy (Lambert, 2004).

What standards must treatment outcome research meet to be valid? Several different working groups have come up with slightly different answers to this question. At a minimum, most researchers agree that a treatment study should include the following criteria:

- A clear definition of the sample being studied, such as a description of diagnoses or problem behavior to be addressed
- A clear description of the treatment being offered, as in a treatment manual (described in a later section)
- Inclusion of a control or comparison treatment condition
- An experimental design that involves random assignment of clients to treatment or comparison conditions
- Reliable and valid outcome measures (see Chapter 3 for definitions of reliability and validity)
- Evaluation of outcomes by a rater who is unaware of the patient's treatment assignment
- A large enough sample size

Studies in which clients are randomly assigned to receive active treatment or a comparison (either no treatment, a placebo, or another treatment) are called **randomized controlled trials (RCTs)**. In this type of experiment, the independent variable is the treatment condition and the dependent variable is the client's outcome.

The American Psychological Association (APA) publishes a report on the therapies that have received empirical support based on standards like those just listed. The APA standards

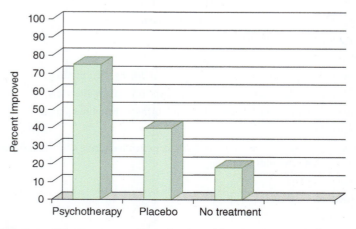

FIGURE 4.4   Summary of the percentage of people who achieve improvement after psychotherapy, placebo, and no treatment across treatment outcome studies. Drawn from Lambert (2004).

also require that two independent research teams must find positive effects for a treatment before it is considered to be empirically supported (Task Force on Promotion and Dissemination of Psychological Procedures, 1995). The goal is to help clinicians, consumers, managed care agencies, and insurance companies draw more easily on the rapidly growing literature about **empirically supported treatments (ESTs)**. A division of the APA publishes a list of therapies that have met these criteria, and some of the therapies from that list of ESTs are shown in **Table 4.5**. We will describe empirically supported treatments throughout this book when we discuss specific psychological disorders.

Some have hotly debated aspects of the APA criteria for ESTs. Of concern, these criteria do not consider whether treatments cause harm (see **Focus on Discovery 4.2**) (American Psychological Association, 2002). Of course, a treatment's failure to appear on the list of ESTs in Table 4.5 could simply reflect a lack of careful studies. As you can see, most of the treatments listed are cognitive behavioral. Research on other treatments had not met the APA's criteria at the time the report was published. In 2017 and 2019, the APA released updated guidelines for PTSD and depression, and psychodynamic treatment was listed as one treatment option for depression (American Psychological Association, 2017, 2019).

We now turn to some of the major decisions researchers face as they design treatment outcome studies. The issues include defining the treatment procedures, choosing the best possible control group, and recruiting an appropriate sample of patients. Once a treatment has been shown to work well in a tightly controlled treatment outcome study, effectiveness research

TABLE 4.5   **Examples of Empirically Supported Treatments for Adult Disorders**

Generalized anxiety disorder	*Depression*
Cognitive therapy	Cognitive therapy
Applied relaxation	Behavior therapy
Social phobia	Interpersonal psychotherapy
Exposure	Problem-solving therapy
Cognitive behavioral group therapy	Self-management/self-control therapy
Systematic desensitization	*Schizophrenia*
Simple phobia	Family psychoeducation
Exposure	Cognitive behavior therapy
Guided mastery	Social learning/token economy programs
Systematic desensitization	Cognitive remediation
Obsessive-compulsive disorder	Social skills training
Exposure and response prevention	Behavioral family therapy
Cognitive therapy	Supported employment programs
Agoraphobia	Assertive community treatment
Exposure	*Alcohol abuse and dependence*
Cognitive behavior therapy	Community reinforcement approach
Panic	*Relationship distress*
Cognitive behavior therapy	Behavioral couples therapy
Posttraumatic stress disorder	Emotion-focused therapy
Prolonged exposure	Insight-oriented couples therapy
Cognitive processing therapy	*Sexual dysfunctions*
Bulimia	Partner-assisted sexual skills training
Cognitive behavior therapy	*Borderline personality disorder*
Interpersonal psychotherapy	Dialectical behavior therapy
Anorexia nervosa	
Family-based treatment	

Source: Based on the Division 12 of APA, Society of Clinical Psychology report available at https://div12.org/psychological-treatments/.

Focus on Discovery 4.2

Can Therapy Be Harmful?

Although there is substantial evidence that therapies, on average, tend to be helpful, this does not mean that they help everyone. Indeed, a small number of people may be in worse shape after therapy. Estimating how often therapy is harmful is not easy. Up to 10% of people are more symptomatic after therapy than they were before therapy began (Lilienfeld, 2007). Does this mean that therapy harmed them? Maybe not. Without a control group, it is hard to know whether symptoms would have worsened even without therapy. Unfortunately, few researchers report the

percentage of people who worsened in the different branches of treatment trials.

Nonetheless, it is important to be aware that several treatments have been found to be harmful to some people. Table 4.6 lists treatments identified as resulting in worsened outcomes in randomized controlled trials or in multiple case reports (Lilienfeld, 2007). We should note that harmful effects are not exclusive to therapy; the U.S. Food and Drug Administration has issued warnings that antidepressants and antiseizure medications can increase the risk of suicidal behavior in some groups and that antipsychotic medications can increase the risk of death among older adults.

TABLE 4.6   **Examples of Treatments Found to Be Harmful in Multiple Studies or Case Reports**

Treatment	Negative Effects
Critical incident stress debriefing	Heightened risk for posttraumatic symptoms
Scared Straight programs	Exacerbation of conduct problems
Facilitated communication	False accusations of child abuse against family members
Attachment therapies (e.g., rebirthing)	Death and serious injury to children
Recovered-memory techniques	Production of false memories of trauma
Dissociative identity disorder–oriented therapy	Induction of "alter" personalities
Grief counseling for people with normal bereavement reactions	Increases in depressive symptoms
Expressive-experiential therapies	Exacerbation of painful emotions
Drug Abuse Resistance Education (DARE) programs	Increased intake of alcohol and cigarettes

Source: From Lilienfeld, S. O. Psychological treatments that cause harm. *Perspectives on Psychological Science,* 2, 53–70. © 2007 SAGE Publications. Reproduced with permission of Sage Publications.

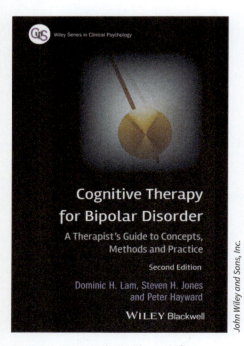

A treatment manual provides specific procedures for a therapist to use in working with a client. Such manuals are standard in treatment outcome studies.

John Wiley and Sons, Inc.

is designed to test how well the treatment fares in the real world. As evidence accrues that a treatment works, dissemination encourages therapists in the community to adopt the treatment.

Defining the Treatment Condition

There are different ways to define the goals of psychological treatments. For several decades, most researchers have focused on designing treatments to address a given diagnosis, such as major depressive disorder. More recently, the National Institute of Mental Health (NIMH) has prioritized funding treatment studies designed to target a mechanism involved in psychological disorders (e.g., low motivation) (Insel, 2015). This NIMH approach differs in that some mechanisms may be involved across a broad range of diagnoses.

Regardless of whether a treatment aims to address a diagnostic condition or a mechanism, treatment manuals are widely recommended for psychotherapy research (e.g., Nathan & Gorman, 2015) and for training therapists (Crits-Christoph, Frank, et al., 1995). Treatment manuals are books that provide details on how to conduct a particular psychological treatment, including procedures for the therapist to follow at each stage of treatment. Manuals make it possible for someone reading a psychotherapy study to have an idea of what happened in therapy sessions. A good manual provides enough freedom that therapists will not feel constrained—for example, it may describe ways to use exposure treatment to reduce conditioned fears in anxiety disorders but also give a menu of options of how to conduct exposure (Kendall & Beidas, 2007).

Defining Control Groups

For an illustration of the importance of a control group, consider a study of a particular therapy for anxiety. Let us assume that persons with anxiety disorders receive therapy and that, from the start to the end of a 16-week program, their anxiety symptoms diminish. With no control group against which to compare the improvement, we cannot argue that changes are due to the treatment. The improvement in anxiety could have been due to factors other than the treatment, such as the passage of time or support from friends. Without a control group, any changes during treatment are difficult to interpret.

Researchers use many different types of control groups in treatment outcome research. A no-treatment control group allows researchers to test whether the mere passage of time helps as much as treatment does. A treatment-as-usual control group allows for a comparison against standard treatment in the community. A stricter test compares the treatment to a more carefully specified control condition. In psychotherapy research,

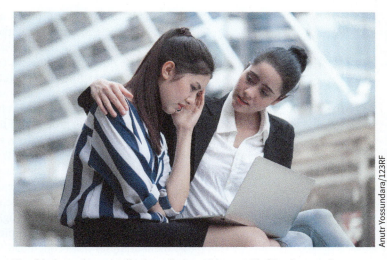

Troubled people may talk about their problems with friends or seek professional therapy. Treatment is typically sought by those for whom the advice and support of family or friends have not provided relief.

the control condition might be a therapy that consists of support and encouragement (the "attention" component) but not the active ingredient of the therapy under study (e.g., exposure to a feared stimulus in a behavioral treatment of a phobia). In medication studies, a **placebo** might be a sugar pill that is described to the patient as a proven treatment. A placebo condition allows researchers to control for expectations of symptom relief. The strictest type of design includes an active-treatment control group in which researchers compare the new treatment against a well-tested treatment. This type of design allows researchers to make comparative statements about two treatments.

The **placebo effect** refers to a physical or psychological improvement that is due to a patient's expectations of help rather than to any active ingredient in a treatment. The placebo effect is often significant and even long-lasting. Indeed, placebos have been shown to influence activity of key brain regions and neurotransmitters implicated in psychological disorders (Benedetti, 2008). Perhaps not surprisingly, symptoms improve for many patients after they receive a placebo or if they take part in a psychotherapy control condition (Faltinsen, Todorovac, et al., 2022). Because patients often improve while taking part in these control conditions, many researchers believe it is important to include a placebo or attention control condition.

In contrast, some have argued that placebos and no-treatment controls are unethical, in that withholding active treatment—which one would expect to be even more powerful than a placebo—might cause patients to suffer (Wolitzky, 1995). An active-treatment control group may not raise ethical concerns, but it can be hard to show a difference between different types of active treatments. Choosing the best control group, then, is a difficult decision!

When outcomes in a treatment trial are evaluated, it is important that the rater doing the evaluating be unaware of the treatment condition, so as to reduce bias. In medication trials, researchers use a **double-blind procedure**. That is, the psychiatrist and the patient are not told whether the patient is receiving active medication or a placebo. A double-blind procedure can be hard to implement. Treatment providers and patients may guess who is getting the active treatment because medications are much more likely to produce side effects than are placebos (Salamone, 2000). Researchers often measure whether participants guessed that they were in the placebo condition, as well as how much they expected their treatment to help them.

Defining a Sample

Many treatment studies exclude groups of potential participants—for example, those with acute suicidality might be excluded for ethical reasons. These exclusions can limit the external validity of findings. As researchers have become willing to include a broader range of individuals in studies, no decay in outcomes has been observed (Foa, Gillihan, & Bryant, 2013). Nonetheless, some participants might be unwilling to enroll in a study in which they might be assigned to an ineffective treatment (the control condition).

As with other psychological research, one major concern in treatment outcome studies has been whether findings are relevant to people from different cultural backgrounds. As shown in **Table 4.7**, there are dramatic differences between countries in rates of treatment seeking among people with psychological disorders (Wang, Aguilar-Gaxiola, et al., 2007). Members of minority groups and those from non-Western cultures are less likely to seek or to receive treatment than are White, non-Hispanic adults in the United States (U.S. Department of Health and Human Services, 2014; Snowden, 2012). A lack of cultural and ethnic representation in treatment studies can limit the relevance of findings to minority populations. In an analysis of over 4,000 clinical trials for medical and psychological conditions, over 40% of trials included no Black participants, and 10% of trials included only White participants (Turner, Steinberg, 2022). Although many studies fail to consider diversity, many researchers are studying psychological therapies in minority populations. Indeed, at this point, more than 20 meta-analyses have concluded that the effects of psychotherapy are as powerful for racial and ethnic minorities as they are for Whites (Cougle & Grubaugh, 2022). A growing body of research also focuses on how to improve therapies to address concerns from people from varied cultural backgrounds (Huey, Tilley, et al., 2014). See **Focus on Discovery 4.3** for other ways to consider culture and ethnicity in treatment.

TABLE 4.7	Percentage of People Who Sought Treatment in the Past 12 Months for Emotions, Nerves, Mental Health, or Drug/Alcohol Concerns by Country ($N = 84{,}850$)
Country	**Percentage of People Seeking Treatment**
Nigeria	1.6
China	3.4
Italy	4.3
Lebanon	4.4
Mexico	5.1
Colombia	5.5
Japan	5.6
Spain	6.8
Ukraine	7.2
Germany	8.1
Israel	8.8
Belgium	10.9
Netherlands	10.9
France	11.3
New Zealand	13.8
South Africa	15.4
United States	17.9

Source: Based on Wang, P. S., Aguilar-Gaxiola, S., Alonso, J., Angermeyer, M. C., Borges, G., Bromet, E. J., et al. (2007). Use of mental health services for anxiety, mood, and substance disorders in 17 countries in the WHO World Mental Health Surveys. *The Lancet, 370*, 841–850.

The Importance of Culture and Ethnicity in Psychological Treatment

We have already mentioned that members of racial and ethnic minority groups are less likely to seek mental health care (Wang, Lane, et al., 2005). Even when they do seek care, they are less likely to see a mental health expert, more likely to stop treatment prematurely, and less likely to receive state-of-the-art effective treatments. A growing body of research is considering how to make treatments more accessible and effective for people from diverse backgrounds (Lopez, Barrio, et al., 2012; Snowden, 2012). As we consider this area, we want to raise one caveat about the risks of stereotyping: People from minority groups can differ as much from each other as their racial or ethnic group differs from another racial or ethnic group.

Many minority clients report that they would prefer to see someone from a similar background (Lopez, Lopez, & Fong, 1991). Many clients believe that therapists of similar background, perhaps even of the same gender, will understand their life circumstances better and more quickly. Indeed, minority individuals are more likely to continue past the first session of therapy when their therapist is of a similar ethnicity (Ibaraki & Nagayama Hall, 2014). Despite this benefit of race or ethnic matching, such matching does not seem to have much effect on the more distal outcome of symptom relief (Griner & Smith, 2006).

Cultural competence matters more than ethnic matching. A therapist who is culturally competent has an appreciation for and understanding of cultural differences and similarities, appreciates sociopolitical events that may have been salient for some cultural groups, and has an awareness of his or her own culturally based assumptions and biases. A large body of research indicates that therapists who are more culturally competent are more likely to have clients who feel satisfied and see the therapeutic relationship positively. Cultural competence also has small positive effects on the degree of symptom relief that clients achieve (Tao, Owen, et al., 2015).

As part of developing cultural competence, therapists need to consider that many members of minority groups have encountered prejudice and racism (Comas-Díaz, Hall, & Neville, 2019), and many have been subjected to hate crimes (Sue, Zane, et al., 2009). Families often immigrate to new countries to escape political turmoil and persecution, and these traumas may intensify the risks of posttraumatic stress disorder and emotional distress. Cultural background may shape values and beliefs about emotion (Boiger & Mesquita, 2012), as well as beliefs about how to interact with authorities like treatment providers. These values and beliefs will influence the therapeutic interview. For example, Asian Americans may place value on modulation of emotion to avoid negative consequences for others, and so may express distress less directly (Nagayama Hall & Huang, 2020). Native American spiritual beliefs shape beliefs and rituals around healing that are not reflected in standard treatments developed for Western majority individuals (Walker & Bigelow, 2015). Hence, cultural background may shape not only experiences relevant to the development of symptoms but also how people will communicate and set expectations in treatment.

Even though there is evidence that established treatments are helpful for minority populations, many argue that treatments should be adapted to be more culturally sensitive. There are several ways researchers have made culturally sensitive adaptations to treatments. One is to adjust treatment content to fit culturally driven beliefs, as culture can influence beliefs about illness, manifestation of symptoms, social consequences of symptoms, and expectations about treatment (Benish, Quintana, & Wampold, 2011). Another approach to developing culturally sensitive interventions is to draw on the strengths of a given culture. For example, Latino culture emphasizes family values and spirituality. One team modified CBT for depression to incorporate more emphasis on family values. Puerto Rican adolescents who received culturally sensitive CBT demonstrated significantly more decrease in depressive symptoms than did those who received interpersonal psychotherapy or were assigned to a control condition (Rossello, Bernal, & Rivera-Medina, 2008).

Across dozens of studies, culturally adapted interventions have been found to be beneficial compared to control conditions (Hall, Ibaraki, et al., 2016). Researchers have also considered a more difficult test—do these culturally sensitive interventions work better than empirically supported psychotherapies? Evidence on this front is more mixed. Cultural tailoring appears to be more helpful when clients are less acculturated into the majority culture (Huey, Tilley, et al., 2014). Despite many positive examples of culturally sensitive interventions, there is some evidence that too much focus on how a given cultural group differs from others can backfire—perhaps because of the risk that individuals feel stereotyped (Huey et al., 2014). Researchers are continuing to consider the best ways to provide accessible and effective interventions for people from different backgrounds.

milkos/123RF

Although many minority clients report that they would like to see a minority therapist, cultural sensitivity appears to be more important to outcome than a match of ethnicity between client and therapist.

Assessing and Implementing Treatments in the Real World

RCTs, typically conducted in academic research settings, are designed to determine the **efficacy** of a treatment—that is, whether a treatment works under the purest of conditions. Because of the kinds of concerns just raised, some RCTs might not inform us about how these treatments work with broader samples in the hands of nonacademic therapists. That is, the external validity of RCTs is sometimes criticized. We need to determine not just the efficacy of a treatment but also its **effectiveness**—that is, how well the treatment works in the real world. Studies of effectiveness might include clients with a broader range of problems and provide less intensive supervision of therapists. Effectiveness studies often rely on briefer assessments as well. As you might expect, when clients have more serious diagnostic complications and providers have less support, psychotherapies and even medications tend to look less powerful than they do in efficacy studies (Rush, Trivedi, et al., 2006).

Dissemination is the process of facilitating adoption of efficacious treatments in the community, most typically by providing guidelines about the best available treatments, along with training for clinicians on how to conduct those treatments. For example, mental health outcomes were improved in the U.S. Veterans Health Care System by training thousands of mental health providers to provide ESTs for anxiety, depression, pain, and PTSD (Karlin & Cross, 2014). In Britain, a major dissemination initiative provides ESTs by phone, with over a million persons screened so far (Carey, 2017). Other dissemination research considers how to tailor empirically supported treatments to make their delivery feasible in countries with few mental health professionals—for example, by creating short versions of these treatments that can be offered online or by those without advanced degrees (Patel, Chisholm, et al., 2016). Dissemination is highly important because too few clients are offered ESTs.

Quick Summary

Treatment outcome studies are the most common form of experiment in research on psychological disorders. These studies focus on whether a given treatment works well.

Many groups have attempted to provide standards for psychotherapy research and to identify psychotherapies that have received empirical support. It is generally agreed that treatment outcome researchers should use treatment manuals, randomly assign participants to the treatment or control condition, clearly define the sample, and include reliable and valid measures of outcome.

Treatment manuals provide detailed guidance about how to conduct each phase of a psychotherapy.

There is some debate about the best type of control condition, in that the use of no-treatment and placebo-condition control groups involves withholding active treatments for those who may be suffering. Placebo conditions, however, are informative in that many people demonstrate symptom reduction after taking a placebo.

The external validity of randomized controlled trials (RCTs) has been criticized because so many people are excluded or do not take part in studies. A growing body of research, though, shows that empirically supported treatments are helpful in addressing the concerns of people from different ethnic and cultural backgrounds. Effectiveness studies focus on whether treatment findings generalize to the real world.

4.3 Check Your Knowledge

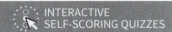
INTERACTIVE SELF-SCORING QUIZZES

(Answers are at the end of the chapter.)

Answer the following questions.

1. What is an RCT?

2. Describe the major pro and major con of placebo-controlled designs.

3. Why are treatment manuals recommended in psychotherapy outcome research?

True or false?

4. Very little research is available on whether empirically supported treatments work well for minority individuals.

Match the word to the definition.

5. Efficacy

6. Effectiveness

7. Dissemination

    a. The process of encouraging treatment providers in the community to adopt a treatment

    b. The degree to which a treatment appears to work well in a carefully controlled RCT

    c. The degree to which a treatment appears to work well when administered in a less controlled study in the community

---

Analogues in Mental Health Research

In conducting research on psychological disorders, researchers are often confronted with ethical and pragmatic barriers. Here we describe several types of analogue research that are commonly used to overcome those barriers.

Using the experimental method is the clearest way to determine cause–effect relationships. There are many situations, however, in which the experimental method cannot be used to understand the causes of psychological disorders. Why? Suppose that a researcher has hypothesized that emotionally charged, overly dependent maternal relationships cause generalized anxiety disorder. An experimental test of this hypothesis would require randomly assigning infants to one of two groups of mothers. The mothers in one group would undergo an extensive training program to ensure that they would be able to create a highly emotional atmosphere and foster overdependence in children. The mothers in the second group would be trained not to create such a relationship with their children. The researcher would then wait until the participants in each group reached adulthood and determine how many of them had developed generalized anxiety disorder. Clearly, this would be unethical.

To take advantage of the power of the experimental method, researchers sometimes use an **analogue experiment**. Investigators attempt to create or observe a related but less severe phenomenon—that is, an analogue of the risk variable—in the laboratory. Because a true experiment is conducted, results with good internal validity can be obtained. The problem of external validity arises, however, because the researchers are no longer studying the actual phenomenon of interest.

In one type of analogue experiment, temporary symptoms are produced through experimental manipulations. For example, lactate infusion can elicit a panic attack, and threats to self-esteem can produce anxiety or sadness. The success of experimental manipulations in producing mild symptoms provides clues into the causes of more severe symptoms.

In addition to analogue experiments, researchers sometimes use analogue samples, in which participants are selected because they are similar to people with certain diagnoses. Thousands of studies, for example, have been conducted with college students who received high scores on questionnaire measures of anxiety or depression. These samples may be assessed in either experimental or correlational designs.

A third type of analogue study involves using animals to understand human behavior. For example, researchers found that dogs that were exposed to electrical shocks that the dogs could not control developed many of the symptoms of depression, including seeming despair, passivity, and decreased appetite (Seligman, Maier, & Geer, 1968). Similarly, researchers often rely on

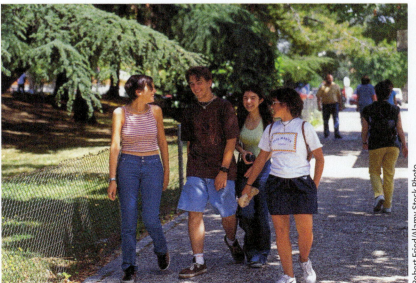

Studies of college students with mild symptoms may not provide a good analogue for major psychological disorders.

Robert Fried/Alamy Stock Photo

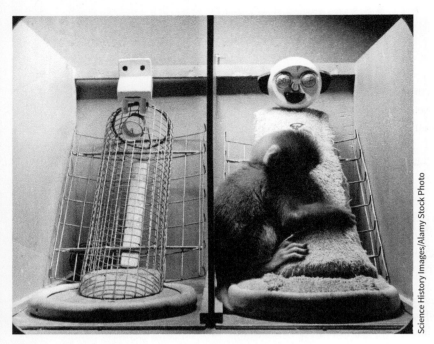

Harlow's famous analogue research examined the effects of early separation from the mother on infant monkeys. Even a cloth surrogate mother is better than isolation for preventing subsequent emotional distress and depression.

animal models in the development of novel pharmacological treatments for psychological disorders (Micale, Kucerova, & Sulcova, 2013). Such animal models have helped us understand more about the neurobiology of depression, anxiety, and other disorders in humans. Sometimes, animal researchers use an experimental design, as when researchers manipulate stress; other times, animal researchers use correlational designs.

The key to interpreting such studies lies in the validity of the analogue. Is a stressor encountered in the laboratory fundamentally similar to a serious stressor such as the death of a parent? Are distressed college students similar to people with clinically diagnosable depression? Are lethargy and decreased eating in dogs akin to depressive symptoms in humans? Some argue against analogue research, even when researchers are careful to discuss the limits of generalizability. For example, Coyne (1994) has argued that clinical depression is caused by different processes from those that cause common distress, and that analogue studies of mild symptoms among undergraduates have poor external validity.

We believe that analogue studies can be very helpful but that findings from these types of studies must be considered conjointly with those from studies that do not rely on analogues. Science often depends on comparing the results of experimental analogue studies to those of longitudinal correlational studies. For example, analogue studies have shown that people with depression respond more negatively to laboratory stressors (an analogue of life stress) than do those without depression, and correlational studies have shown that severe life events predict the onset of clinical depression. Because the findings from correlational and analogue studies complement each other, they provide strong support for life event models of depression. The analogue studies of life stress provide the precision of an experiment (high internal validity), whereas correlational studies provide the ability to study very important influences that cannot be manipulated, like the influence of death and trauma (high external validity).

Quick Summary

Several types of analogues are commonly used in research on psychological disorders.

Analogue experiments rely on a milder version of a risk variable; the milder version of the risk variable is manipulated as the independent variable within the laboratory. Analogue experiments are helpful when a risk variable cannot be ethically manipulated.

Other types of analogue research rely on assessment of milder symptoms, rather than full-blown diagnoses, or on the use of animal rather than human models.

4.4 Check Your Knowledge

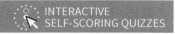
INTERACTIVE
SELF-SCORING QUIZZES

(Answers are at the end of the chapter.)

Answer the following questions.

1. A researcher decides to use an analogue experiment to study the effects of 1 hour of social separation on anxiety. What are the pros and cons of this type of analogue experiment as compared to a correlational study of the effects of maternal loss?

2. Which of the following are analogue studies? (Circle all that apply.)

a. A researcher exposes dogs to uncontrollable stress as a way of understanding human depression.

b. A researcher conducts an online survey to assess how long the typical experience of sadness lasts.

c. A researcher asks participants about their most recent experience of sadness as a way to understand clinically diagnosable depression.

d. A researcher interviews 25 people each month for 3 years after their spouse dies to estimate the duration of bereavement.

Integrating the Findings of Multiple Studies

Understanding the pros and cons of different research designs suggests a natural conclusion—there is no perfect research study. Rather, a body of research studies is needed to test a theory. After an important research finding emerges, dozens of studies may be published on the same topic. Sometimes the results of different studies will be similar, but more often, differences will arise across studies. Indeed, there has been growing concern throughout the scientific community, not just in psychology, about failures to replicate findings and techniques for aggregating findings across multiple studies.

Replication

In a successful **replication**, findings from one research study hold up when that study is repeated a second time. Findings are considered more believable when other researchers have independently replicated them, ideally more than once. Replication is a core aspect of the scientific method.

In recent years, a spotlight has been placed on replication failures across the sciences (National Academies of Sciences, Engineering, and Medicine, 2019). In one report, Ioannidis (2005a) identified 49 articles that had been published in influential medical journals and had each been cited more than 1,000 times. Many of these studies described interventions that had been widely adopted by the medical community—for example, hormone replacement for menopausal women and vitamin E to reduce risk of cardiovascular disease. Ioannidis then identified 34 studies that had attempted to replicate the original findings. In those replication studies, 20% of the interventions had not been replicated at all, and another 20% had shown significantly smaller effects (Ioannidis, 2005a). The mental health field has not been immune from problems with replicability. In a review of highly cited psychopharmacological treatment findings published in top psychiatry journals, the authors identified 43 attempts at replication; of the 43, a full 16 of the replication attempts contradicted the initial findings (Tajika, Ogawa, et al., 2015). In one test of replicability in psychology, researchers selected 100 studies published in top-tier psychology journals and conducted new studies to see if those findings replicated. Only 39% of the findings replicated (Open Science Collaboration, 2015).

Obviously, lack of replicability is a major concern—after all, if we cannot believe the findings from our research, they are not of much value for advancing our understanding and improving treatments. Consistent failures to replicate reduce public trust and investment in science. Because many scientists build their work on previous findings, inaccurate publications also misguide the next wave of science.

Replicability may be overestimated when we rely only on published articles. Scientific journals tend to prioritize the publication of new and positive findings over negative results, which are regarded as uninteresting. Also, there is always the possibility that negative findings are due to methodological problems. For example, an effect for a given treatment might be observed with longer duration of treatment, more skilled therapists, or a better outcome measure. The tendency to publish only positive results is referred to as **publication bias**. Publication bias is widespread across the sciences. It has been estimated that positive findings are more than twice as likely as negative findings to be published (Franco, Malhotra, & Simonovits, 2014). In one analysis, researchers examined the data from trials designed to assess psychological treatments for major depressive disorder that were funded by the National Institutes of Health. Almost a quarter of the grants had yielded no publications. When the researchers sought the data from the unpublished trials, they found that treatment effects in the unpublished studies were half as strong as those from the published studies (Driessen, Hollon, et al., 2015). Of course, we don't know whether those studies were unpublished because of the poor effects or because of other quality issues in the data. Nonetheless, publication bias may keep the scientific community unaware of replication failures and may inflate our sense of how well our treatments work (Hengartner, 2018).

There are many reasons studies may fail to replicate. One explanation is that statistical analyses rely on probability. Earlier, we described how a finding is considered statistically significant when statistics indicate that there is 5% or less probability that the finding would have been observed by chance alone if the null hypothesis were true (i.e., $p < .05$). This means that 5% of the time, purely by chance, a positive finding would not be expected to replicate in a second study. However, the estimates we describe here suggest that nonreplication happens much more than 5% of the time. Other factors must be involved. One possibility is fraud, but most believe that fraud is too rare to explain the low rates of replication.

Several issues in research methods can contribute to replication failures:

- Small samples, which are often used in clinical psychology, are more likely to yield unusual patterns of results (Ioannidis, 2005b). Findings are generally more believable when they come from studies with larger sample sizes. Sample sizes have been increasing over time in clinical psychology studies but generally remain too small for testing more complex statistical models (Reardon et al., 2019).
- Findings are less likely to replicate if unreliable measures are used.
- Replication failures are more likely when the methods of the original research study are not described well.
- Differences in methods, such as measures or sample characteristics, may diminish the likelihood of replication (Gilbert, King, et al., 2016). For example, findings observed among people who are hospitalized may not generalize to outpatient or community samples.

In addition to these issues, **questionable research practices** contribute to replication failures (Simmons, Nelson, & Simonsohn, 2011). Let's consider a hypothetical study of neuroticism and depression to illustrate questionable research practices. Imagine that researchers collect two different measures of depression (a self-rating and an interviewer rating). After the data are collected, the researchers may decide to include either or both measures in their analyses. When the researchers examine the data, they see that several participants have extremely high neuroticism scores; analyses could be conducted with or without these high scorers (doubling the number of potential analyses). In total, the investigators have the opportunity to conduct their analyses in six different ways depending on the measures they include (self-rating, interview rating, or both measures of depression) and the participants they include (with or without the high scorers). Although the probability of a false positive finding is only 5% in each separate analysis, the probability of at least one false positive finding is much higher when the researchers conduct analyses six different ways. In other words, simply by taking a flexible approach to data analysis the researchers can dramatically increase their chances of obtaining a positive result.

The situation gets even more complex if some of the six results are positive and others are negative, as often happens. Researchers tend to be biased to believe the findings that fit their hypotheses and to disregard the negative results, a phenomenon referred to as *confirmation bias*. Confirmation bias, along with awareness of publication bias, may tempt the researchers to report only the analyses that support their hypotheses without acknowledging negative results. Researchers may also be motivated to continue to tweak their analyses or comb through their data until they arrive at a significant (and thus more publishable) result, a process known as **p-hacking.** The need to publish work to obtain promotions and future grant funding is likely to intensify the temptation to present only the significant results. Some people, then, suggest that questionable research practices, driven by problematic systems that reward people for focusing on significant findings, are a major contributor to the lack of replicability in science (Ioannidis, 2005b).

Several policies have been recommended to address these issues in replication (Tackett, Brandes, et al., 2019):

- Many scientists now *preregister* their hypotheses, measures, and analysis plan before conducting a study. This promotes a more honest presentation of which analyses did and did not support hypotheses. The National Institutes of Health requires that the clinical trials they fund be preregistered.

- Once a study is completed, many researchers now make their data publicly available (with all personally identifiable information about participants removed). The National Institute of Mental Health requires data from their funded studies to be uploaded into a repository that is accessible to other researchers.

- To improve the odds that negative findings will be published, some journals ask reviewers to weight the rationale and methods of a study more heavily than the statistical results in evaluating a manuscript for potential publication. This removes rewards for p-hacking.

- Editors now often demand that scientists use large sample sizes. There is a push to use parallel measures across studies, so that researchers can compile large integrated data sets. This practice has progressed rapidly in molecular genetic studies, where researchers now routinely use sample sizes in excess of 5,000 persons (although findings from these studies often still fail to replicate!).

- Consumers of science are advised to consider whether findings have been replicated. For example, the APA standards for empirically supported treatments, described previously, specify that findings must be replicated.

Thousands of psychologists have begun to implement these practices to improve replicability in science (Nelson, Simmons, & Simonsohn, 2018). We hope that this movement continues to foster change at the level of individual scientists, in social systems guiding science, and among consumers of science.

Meta-Analysis

How does a researcher go about drawing conclusions from a series of investigations, especially when some findings are positive and others are negative? One could read individual studies, mull them over, and decide what they mean overall. The disadvantage of this approach is that the researcher's biases and subjective impressions can play a significant role in determining what conclusion is drawn. It is common for two scientists to read the same set of studies and reach very different conclusions.

Meta-analysis was developed as a partial solution to this problem (Smith, Glass, & Miller, 1980). The first step in a meta-analysis is a thorough literature search, to identify all relevant studies. Because these studies have typically used different statistical tests, meta-analysis then puts all the results into a common scale, using a type of statistic called an *effect size*. In treatment studies, for example, the effect size offers a way of standardizing the differences in improvement between a therapy group and a control group so that the results of multiple studies can be averaged. **Figure 4.5** summarizes the steps in a meta-analysis.

As the effect sizes across studies are compiled, researchers also try to estimate publication bias—the tendency for negative findings not to be published. To do so, they may ask members of the research community to share unpublished findings. They also may examine the proportion of effect sizes that are barely above the threshold for statistical significance; if many effect sizes are in this range, there is a stronger chance that there are unpublished findings that were not significant.

In their often-cited report, Smith and colleagues (1980) meta-analyzed 475 psychotherapy outcome studies involving more than 25,000 patients and 1,700 effect sizes. Most importantly, they concluded that psychotherapies produce more improvement than does no treatment. Specifically, treated patients were found to be better off than almost 80% of untreated patients. Subsequent meta-analyses have confirmed that therapy appears to be effective (Lambert & Ogles, 2004).

Meta-analysis has been criticized primarily because researchers sometimes include studies that are of poor quality. For example, Smith and colleagues gave equal weight to all studies,

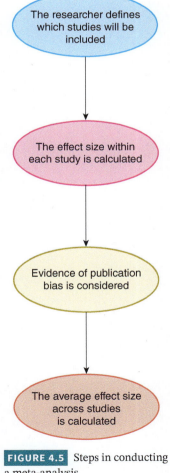

FIGURE 4.5 Steps in conducting a meta-analysis.

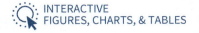
INTERACTIVE
FIGURES, CHARTS, & TABLES

| TABLE 4.8 | An Example of a Meta-Analysis: 12-Month Prevalence Rates for Psychological Disorders Across 27 European Studies |

DSM-IV Diagnosis	Number of Studies	Combined *N*	12-Month Prevalence (as a Percentage) Across the Combined Sample	Range of Prevalence Estimates Within Different Studies
Alcohol dependence	12	60,891	3.3	0.1–6.6
Illicit substance dependence	6	28,429	1.1	0.1–2.2
Psychotic disorders	6	27,291	0.9	0.2–2.6
Major depressive disorder	17	152,044	6.4	3.1–10.1
Bipolar I disorder	6	21,848	0.8	0.2–1.1
Anxiety disorders	12	53,597	1.6	0.7–3.1
Somatic symptom disorders	7	18,894	6.4	1.1–11
Eating disorders	5	19,761	4.8	0.2–0.7

Source: Adapted from Wittchen, H. U., & Jacobi, F. (2005). Size and burden of mental disorders in Europe—A critical review and appraisal of 27 studies. *European Neuropsychopharmacology*, *15*, 357–376.

so a poorly controlled outcome study (such as one that did not evaluate what the therapists actually did in each session) received as much weight as a well-controlled one (such as a study in which therapists used a manual that specified what they did with each research participant). When Smith and colleagues attempted to address this problem by comparing the effect sizes of good versus poor studies and found no differences, they were further criticized for the criteria they employed in separating the good from the not so good (Rachman & Wilson, 1980). The ultimate problem is that someone has to make a judgment of good versus poor quality in research, and others can find fault with that judgment. A good meta-analysis, though, will be clear about the criteria for including and excluding studies and will systematically consider several indicators of study quality.

Table 4.8 provides another example of a meta-analysis. In this meta-analysis, researchers integrated the findings of 27 epidemiologic studies conducted in Europe on the 12-month prevalence rate of psychological disorders (Wittchen & Jacobi, 2005). Across these studies, more than 155,000 participants were interviewed. Prevalence estimates from the different studies varied. Tallying the findings across studies should give a stronger estimate of how common the disorders are.

4.5 Check Your Knowledge

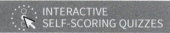
INTERACTIVE
SELF-SCORING QUIZZES

(Answers are at the end of the chapter.)

Answer the following questions.

1. In the 2015 Open Science Collaboration project to examine replicability in psychological science, researchers had success with only __% of the psychological studies they attempted to replicate.

2. Describe approaches recommended to improve replicability.

Choose the best answer.

3. The step in meta-analysis that has received extensive criticism is:
   a. determining which studies should be included
   b. calculating the effect size of each study
   c. calculating the average effect size across studies
   d. none of the above

Summary

Science, Theory, and Hypotheses

- Science involves forming a theory, developing hypotheses based on that theory, and then systematically gathering data to test the hypotheses. Good science requires reliable and valid measures.

Research Designs in the Study of Psychological Disorders

- Common methods for studying psychological disorders include case studies, correlational studies, and experimental studies. Each method has strengths and weaknesses.

- Case studies provide detailed descriptions of rare phenomena or novel procedures. Case studies can disconfirm that a relationship is universal and can generate hypotheses to be tested through controlled research. Case studies, however, may be biased by the researcher's perspective, and they are of limited value in providing evidence to support a theory.

- Correlational methods are the most common way to study the causes of psychological disorders, because we cannot manipulate most of the major risk factors for psychological disorders.

- Cross-sectional correlational studies do not provide evidence for cause and effect because of the directionality problem. Longitudinal studies help address which variable came first but can still suffer from the third-variable problem.

- One form of correlational study, epidemiologic research, involves gathering information about the prevalence and incidence of disorders in populations and about the correlates of disorders. Epidemiologic studies avoid the sampling biases seen in studies of participants drawn from undergraduate psychology classes or from treatment clinics.

- Studies of behavior genetics typically rely on correlational techniques as well. The goal of behavior genetics is to understand the magnitude of genetic and environmental contributions and the interaction of genetic and environmental contributions to disease and related risk variables. The most common behavior genetic methods include the family method, the twin method, and the adoptees method.

- In the experimental method, the researcher randomly assigns people to one of at least two groups: an experimental group or a control group. The effects of the independent variable on a dependent variable are then tested. Treatment outcome studies and analogue studies are common types of experimental research in the study of psychological disorders. Single-case experimental designs can provide well-controlled data.

- Generally, experimental methods help enhance internal validity, but correlational methods sometimes offer greater external validity.

One Example of Experimental Research: Treatment Outcome Research

- Research on the efficacy of various forms of psychological treatments has been conducted for many decades. Overall, this research suggests that about 80% of people gain some improvement from therapy. Therapy seems to be more helpful than a placebo or the passage of time.

- Scientists have defined standards for research on psychotherapy trials. These standards typically include the need to use a treatment manual, to randomly assign participants to a treatment or a control condition, to define the sample carefully, and to use reliable and valid outcome measures. Guidelines suggest that positive findings should be observed from more than one research team before a treatment is considered empirically supported. Scientists have used these standards to identify empirically supported treatments (ESTs).

- Researchers are urged to evaluate whether treatments may cause harm.

- External validity is a concern in treatment research, in that many people are excluded from or will not take part in clinical trials. A growing number of studies, though, demonstrate that empirically supported psychotherapies are helpful for people from diverse racial, ethnic, and cultural backgrounds.

- A broader concern is that a gap exists between what happens in the research world and in the real world. Efficacy research focuses on how well therapies work in carefully controlled experiments, whereas effectiveness research focuses on how well therapies work in the real world with a broader array of clients and therapists. Dissemination refers to the process of implementing empirically supported treatments in community settings.

Analogues in Research on Psychological Disorders

- Analogue experiments allow researchers to study a minor variant of a risk factor related to psychological disorders, such as stressors. Although the stressor used in an analogue study is typically much milder than the types of stressors that might trigger the onset of a psychological disorder, the experimental method provides greater control. Analogue samples are composed of people with mild symptoms. Animal studies can also provide an analogue to human disorders.

Integrating the Findings of Multiple Studies

- Replication refers to obtaining parallel findings when a study is repeated. There has been growing concern about a lack of replicability of scientific findings. Policy reforms are beginning to address this concern.

- Meta-analysis is an important tool for reaching conclusions from a group of research studies. It entails putting the statistical comparisons from single studies into a common format—the effect size—so that scientists can average the results of many studies.

Answers to Check Your Knowledge Questions

4.1 1. False; 2. False; 3. False

4.2 1. a and b; 2. d; 3. c; 4. c; 5. d

4.3 1. An RCT is a randomized controlled trial—a form of treatment outcome study in which the active treatment is compared to at least one comparison condition (controlled) and people are assigned to treatments randomly; 2. Pro: Placebos allow for a control of the effects of treatment expectations, and research suggests that the placebo effect can be large; Con: Placebo trials involve withholding active treatment from people who may have serious symptoms and distress, which is an ethical concern; 3. Treatment manuals provide specific guidance to therapists, so that researchers can be more confident that therapists are providing the same type of intervention; 4. False (explanation: Hundreds of trials have been conducted to test empirically supported treatments with minority individuals and those from differing ethnic and racial backgrounds); 5. b; 6. c; 7. a

4.4 1. Pro: The analogue study has the advantage of experimental manipulation, which provides internal validity. Con: Brief periods of social separation may not invoke even minor temporary symptoms that are similar to those from losing one's mother, and so external validity may be limited; 2. a, c

4.5 1. 39; 2. Preregistering study hypotheses, measures, and analyses before the study begins; making data available; placing more emphasis on the importance of hypotheses and the quality of study methods than on the results of a study when reviewing a manuscript to consider potential publication; using larger samples; routinely considering whether a finding has been replicated; 3. a

Key Terms

Mood Disorders

LEARNING GOALS

1. Describe the symptoms of depression, the diagnostic criteria for depressive disorders, and the epidemiology of depressive disorders.

2. Explain the symptoms of mania, the diagnostic criteria for bipolar disorders, and the epidemiology of bipolar disorders.

3. Discuss the genetic, neurobiological, social, and psychological influences that contribute to the mood disorders.

4. Describe the biological and psychological treatments of mood disorders as well as the current views of electroconvulsive therapy.

5. Explain the epidemiology of suicide, the risk factors for suicide, and methods for preventing suicide.

Clinical Case

Mary

Mary M., a 38-year-old mother of four children, had been deeply depressed for about 2 months when she first went to see a psychologist. About 7 months earlier, she was laid off from her job as an administrative assistant, which was a serious blow to the family's finances. She felt guilty about the loss of her job and became preoccupied with signs of her overall incompetence. Each night, she struggled for more than an hour to fall asleep, only to wake up frequently throughout the night. She had little appetite and as a result had lost 10 pounds. She also had little energy for and no interest in activities that she had enjoyed in the past. Household chores felt impossible for her to complete, and her husband began to complain. Their marriage had already been strained for 2 years, and her negativity and lack of energy contributed to further arguments. Finally, realizing that Mary's symptoms were serious, Mr. M. cajoled her into making an appointment with a psychologist. (You will read about the outcome of Mary's treatment later in this chapter.)

Mood disorders involve profound disturbances in emotion—from the deep sadness and disengagement of depression to the extreme elation and irritability of mania. In this chapter, we begin by discussing the clinical description and the epidemiology of the different mood disorders. Next, we consider various perspectives on the causes of these disorders, and then we consider approaches to treating them. We conclude with an examination of suicide, an action far too often associated with mood disorders.

The DSM-5-TR recognizes two broad types of mood disorders: those that involve only depressive symptoms (unipolar depressive disorders) and those that involve manic symptoms (bipolar disorders). Table 5.1 presents a summary of the symptoms of each of these disorders. We will begin by discussing the depressive disorders, and then we will turn to the bipolar disorders. Within each group, we will describe the core signs, the formal criteria for the specific disorders, and then the epidemiology and consequences of the disorders.

TABLE 5.1 Overview of the Major DSM-5-TR Mood Disorders

Unipolar Depressive Disorders	
DSM-5-TR Diagnoses	**Major Features**
Major depressive disorder	Five or more depressive symptoms, including sad mood or anhedonia, for 2 weeks
Persistent depressive disorder	Low mood and at least two other symptoms of depression at least half of the time for 2 years
Premenstrual dysphoric disorder	Mood symptoms in the week before menses
Disruptive mood dysregulation disorder	Severe recurrent temper outbursts and persistent negative mood for at least 1 year beginning before age 10

Bipolar Disorders	
DSM-5-TR Diagnoses	**Major Features**
Bipolar I disorder	At least one lifetime manic episode
Bipolar II disorder	At least one lifetime hypomanic episode and one major depressive episode No lifetime manic episode
Cyclothymia	Recurrent mood changes from high to low for at least 2 years, without hypomanic or depressive episodes

Clinical Descriptions and Epidemiology of Depressive Disorders

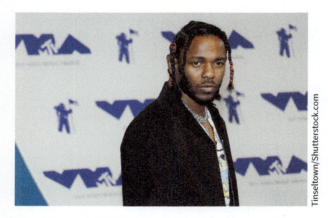

In an interview with MTV, Kendrick Lamar, a rapper who has won 13 Grammy awards and 5 Billboard music awards, discussed his struggles with depression.

Tinseltown/Shutterstock.com

The cardinal symptoms of depression include profound sadness and/or an inability to experience pleasure. The inability to experience pleasure is called **anhedonia,** and as we will describe, this symptom is a major focus of research. Most of us experience sadness during our lives, and most of us say that we are "depressed" at one time or another. But most of these experiences do not have the intensity and duration to be diagnosable. The author William Styron (1992) wrote about his depression: "Like anyone else I have always had times when I felt deeply depressed, but this was something altogether new in my experience—a despairing, unchanging paralysis of the spirit beyond anything I had ever known or imagined could exist."

The symptoms of depression are varied. When people develop a depressive disorder, their heads may reverberate with self-recriminations. Like Mary, described in the Clinical Case, they may become focused on their flaws. Paying attention can be so exhausting that they have difficulty absorbing what they read and hear. They often view things in a very negative light, and they tend to lose hope. Initiative may disappear. Social withdrawal is common; many prefer to sit alone and be silent. Some people with depression neglect their appearance. When people become utterly dejected and hopeless, thoughts about suicide are common.

Physical symptoms of depression are also common, including fatigue and low energy as well as physical aches and pains. These symptoms can be profound enough to convince afflicted persons that they must be suffering from some serious medical condition, even though the symptoms have no apparent physical cause. Although people with depression typically

Defining Symptoms of Major Depressive Disorder

Sad mood or anhedonia (loss of pleasure in usual activities).
At least five symptoms (counting sad mood and anhedonia):

- Sleeping too much or too little
- Psychomotor retardation or agitation
- Weight loss or change in appetite
- Loss of energy

- Feelings of worthlessness or excessive guilt
- Difficulty concentrating, thinking, or making decisions
- Recurrent thoughts of death or suicide

Symptoms are present nearly every day, most of the day, for at least 2 weeks. Symptoms are distinct from and more severe than a normative response to significant loss.

---

feel exhausted, they may find it hard to fall asleep and may wake up frequently. Other people sleep throughout the day. They may find that food tastes bland or that their appetite is gone, or they may experience an increase in appetite. Sexual interest disappears. Some may find their limbs feel heavy. Thoughts and movements may slow for some (**psychomotor retardation**), but others cannot sit still—they pace, fidget, and wring their hands (**psychomotor agitation**).

It is worth pausing to consider how many different symptoms of depression we have described. Most people who are struggling with depression experience only some of these symptoms, not all of them. Indeed, in one study, researchers identified more than 1,000 different profiles of depressive symptoms, with no one profile occurring in more than 2% of patients (Fried & Nesse, 2015). For example, some patients report suicidal ideation while others don't, and some are tortured by insomnia while others sleep well. As we will describe, some symptoms may be more closely tied to specific risk factors than others are.

The DSM-5-TR includes several depressive disorders. Here, we focus on major depressive disorder and persistent depressive disorder because both diagnoses are well researched. We will briefly discuss a newly defined diagnosis specific to children and adolescents, disruptive mood dysregulation disorder, in Chapter 13.

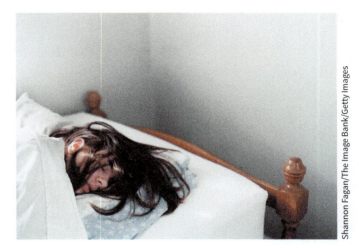

Some people with depression have trouble falling asleep and staying asleep. Others find themselves sleeping for more than 10 hours but still feeling exhausted.

Major Depressive Disorder

Major depressive disorder (MDD) is an **episodic disorder**, because symptoms tend to be present for a period and then clear. Even though episodes tend to dissipate over time, an untreated episode may persist for 6 months or even longer. Major depressive episodes often recur—once a given episode clears, a person is likely to experience another episode. To estimate the course of this disorder, researchers have used representative community samples (rather than patient samples, which may have a more severe course of disorder). In one such study in which researchers conducted annual interviews of people who had experienced a first episode of MDD, about 15% of people reported depressive symptoms that persisted for 10 years. About 40–50% of people who recovered from a first episode of MDD experienced at least one more episode across the 10 years of follow-up (Eaton, Shao, et al., 2008).

Although the DSM criteria require five symptoms of depression to be present to diagnose MDD, there is little evidence to support this threshold. Rather, depressive severity appears to operate as a continuum, with increases in functional impairment and suicidality as the number of symptoms increases. That is, people with seven to nine depressive symptoms often report more problems in daily functioning and more suicidal behavior than do those with five or six symptoms (Ruscio, 2019).

Defining Symptoms of Persistent Depressive Disorder

Depressed mood for most of the day more than half of the time for 2 years (or 1 year for children and adolescents).
At least two of the following during that time:

- Sleeping too much or too little
- Poor appetite or overeating
- Low energy

- Poor self-esteem
- Trouble concentrating or making decisions
- Feelings of hopelessness

    The symptoms do not clear for more than 2 months at a time. Bipolar disorders are not present.

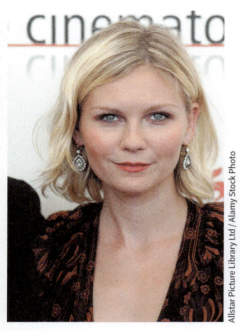

Kirsten Dunst's personal experience with major depressive disorder (MDD) provided her with insight for her role as an actress in the award-winning film *Melancholia*. One out of every five women will experience an episode of depression during her lifetime.

Persistent Depressive Disorder

People with **persistent depressive disorder** are chronically depressed—more than half of the time for at least 2 years, they feel blue or obtain little pleasure from activities and pastimes. In addition to these mood changes, they have at least two of the other symptoms of depression. The central feature of this diagnosis is the chronicity of symptoms, which is a stronger predictor of poor outcome than the number of symptoms. Among people who have experienced depressive symptoms for at least 2 years, those who do and do not have a history of major depressive disorder appear similar in their treatment response (McCullough, Klein, et al., 2000).

Epidemiology and Consequences of Depressive Disorders

MDD is one of the most common psychological disorders. One large-scale epidemiologic study estimated that 16.2% of people in the United States met the criteria for diagnosis of MDD at some point in their lives (Kessler, Berglund, et al., 2003). This may be an underestimate because researchers asked people to recall depressive episodes that happened any time in their life, and people may forget episodes of depression that happened many years ago (Moffitt, Caspi, et al., 2010). About 5% of people report experiencing depressive episodes that persisted for more than 2 years (Murphy & Byrne, 2012).

    MDD and persistent depressive disorder are both twice as common among women as among men (Seedat, Scott, et al., 2009); see **Focus on Discovery 5.1** for a discussion of possible reasons for this gender difference. Rates of depression are also high for Socioeconomic status also matters—that is, MDD is three times as common among people who are impoverished compared with those who are not (Kessler, Birnbaum, et al., 2010).

    The prevalence of depression varies considerably across cultures. In a major cross-cultural study using the same diagnostic criteria and structured interview in each country, the prevalence of MDD varied from a low of 6.5% in China to a high of 21% in France (Bromet, Andrade, et al., 2011). It is tempting to assume that differences in prevalence rates by country indicate a strong role for culture. It turns out that differences among countries in rates of depression are complex. For example, higher national income inequality levels appear to be tied to higher prevalence of depression (Pickett & Wilkinson, 2010). Undoubtedly, cultural influences, such as family cohesion and mental health stigma, play an important role in rates of depression as well.

    In most countries, the age of onset for MDD has become earlier over the past 60 years (Daly, 2022; Kessler, et al., 2010). The rates of depression among adolescents have risen to the point that currently, an estimated 15.8% of adolescents and 20% of college students have experienced at least one episode of major depressive disorder (Auerbach, Alonso, et al., 2016; Daly, 2022).

Focus on Discovery 5.1

Gender Differences in Depression

Women are twice as likely as men are to experience MDD and persistent depressive disorder, and the gender ratio is observed in large-scale studies around the world, even in countries with relatively equitable gender roles (Salk, Hyde, & Abramson, 2017). The gender gap typically begins to emerge during early adolescence and is fully present by late adolescence (Avenevoli, Swendsen, et al., 2015). (Rates of depression are even higher among gender minorities; Reisner et al., 2016). Some of you might wonder if these findings just reflect a tendency for men not to disclose symptoms. Evidence does not support that idea (Kessler, 2003). Several factors may help explain this gender difference (Hilt & Nolen-Hoeksema, 2014):

Biological Influences

- Fluctuations in gonadal hormones, experienced at puberty, premenstrually, postpartum, and at menopause, may increase stress reactivity for some women. This may explain only a small portion of the gender difference, as hormone findings are mixed.

Social Influences

- Twice as many girls as boys are exposed to childhood sexual abuse.
- During adulthood, women are more likely than men to be exposed to chronic stressors such as poverty and caretaker responsibilities.
- Women tend to provide more support to others facing stress. This exposure to others' stress has been called "the cost of caring."

Stress Reactivity

- Traditional social roles among girls may intensify self-critical attitudes about appearance. Adolescent girls worry more than adolescent boys about their body image, and this worry is tied to depression (Hankin & Abramson, 2001).
- Exposure to childhood and chronic stressors, as well as the effects of female hormones, could change the reactivity of the hypothalamic-pituitary-adrenal (HPA) axis, a biological system guiding reactions to stress.
- A focus on gaining approval and closeness within interpersonal relationships, which is more commonly endorsed by women, may intensify reactions to interpersonal stressors

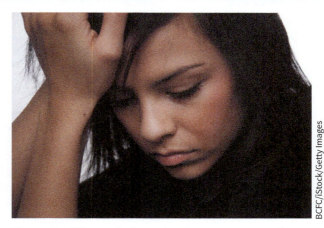

BCFC/iStock/Getty Images

The gender difference in depression does not emerge until adolescence. At that time, young women encounter many stressors and more pressure concerning social roles and body image, and they tend to ruminate about the resulting negative feelings.

(Hankin, Young, et al., 2015). Men are more likely than women to become depressed after life events involving financial or occupational stress, whereas women are more likely than men to become depressed after interpersonal life events (Kendler & Gardner, 2014).

- Social roles promote emotion-focused coping among women, which may then extend the duration of sad moods after major stressors. More specifically, women tend to spend more time ruminating about sad moods or wondering about why unhappy events have occurred. Men tend to spend more time using distracting or action-focused coping, such as playing a sport or engaging in other activities that shake off the sad mood. As we discuss when we review cognitive influences on depression later in this chapter, a fair amount of research suggests that rumination prolongs sad moods and can predict the onset of MDD.

It's pretty clear that gender differences in depression are related to multiple factors. In considering these issues, bear in mind that men are more likely to demonstrate other types of disorders, such as alcohol use disorder, substance use disorder, and antisocial personality disorder (Seedat, et al., 2009). Hence, understanding gender differences in psychological disorders is likely to require attending to many different risk factors and syndromes.

Although MDD and persistent depressive disorder are considered separate disorders in the DSM-5-TR, they tend to be highly comorbid. Most people with persistent depressive disorder will experience episodes of MDD (Vandeleur, Fassasi, et al., 2017). About 30% of those with MDD will have symptoms that persist for at least 2 years and so will then qualify for a diagnosis of persistent depressive disorder (Murphy & Byrne, 2012).

Both MDD and persistent depressive disorder are often comorbid with other psychological disorders. About 60% of people who meet the criteria for diagnosis of MDD

VIDEO CONTENT

Case Study: Depression Pause and Ponder

during their lifetime also will meet the criteria for diagnosis of an anxiety disorder at some point (Kessler, et al., 2003). (See **Focus on Discovery 5.2** later in the chapter for more discussion of the overlap of anxiety disorders and depressive disorders.) Other common comorbid conditions include substance-related disorders, sexual dysfunctions, and personality disorders.

Depression has many serious consequences. From the depths of a depression, getting to work may require overwhelming effort, parenting can feel like a burden, and suicide can seem like an option. As we will discuss later in this chapter, suicide is a real risk. MDD is also the second leading cause of mental health-related disability worldwide (Ferrari, 2022). MDD also has important effects for the next generation: Offspring who are exposed to a mother's MDD during early childhood are at high risk for developing depression (Hammen, Hazel, et al., 2012).

MDD is also related to a high risk of other health problems (Gold, Köhler-Forsberg, et al., 2020). There is particularly strong evidence that depression is related to the onset and more severe course of cardiovascular disease (Carney & Freedland, 2017). Depression is related to a more than twofold increase in the risk of death from cardiovascular disease, even after controlling for baseline cardiovascular health (Meijer, Conradi, et al., 2011).

Although the diagnostic criteria for persistent depressive disorder include fewer symptoms than those for MDD do, do not make the mistake of thinking that persistent depressive disorder is a less severe disorder than MDD. Chronic depressive symptoms persist on average for 10 years (Klein & Kotov, 2016). The chronicity of these symptoms takes a toll. Indeed, in a study following patients for 5 years, people with chronic depressive symptoms were more likely to require hospitalization, to attempt suicide, and to be impaired in their functioning than were people with MDD (Klein, Schwartz, et al., 2000). Functioning declines as depressive symptoms persist for more years (Klein, Shankman, & Rose, 2006).

Quick Summary

The DSM-5-TR contains two broad types of mood disorders: unipolar depressive disorders and bipolar disorders.

Depressive disorders include major depressive disorder (MDD) and persistent depressive disorder as well as two more recently recognized disorders: premenstrual dysphoric disorder and disruptive mood dysregulation disorder.

MDD is characterized by episodes involving at least five symptoms that last at least 2 weeks, whereas persistent depressive disorder is characterized by at least three symptoms that last at least 2 years.

MDD is one of the most common psychological disorders. Among adolescents and adults, MDD and persistent depressive disorder affect twice as many females as males. From 40% to 50% of people with MDD will experience another episode within 10 years.

5.1 Check Your Knowledge

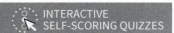
INTERACTIVE SELF-SCORING QUIZZES

(Answers are at the end of the chapter.)

Fill in the blanks.

1. Major depressive disorder is diagnosed based on at least _____ symptoms lasting at least 2 weeks.

2. Approximately _____ % of people will experience major depressive disorder during their lifetime.

Answer the question.

3. What is the key difference between the diagnostic criteria for major depressive disorder and persistent depressive disorder?

Clinical Descriptions and Epidemiology of Bipolar Disorders

The DSM-5-TR recognizes three forms of bipolar disorders: bipolar I disorder, bipolar II disorder, and cyclothymic disorder. Manic symptoms are the defining feature of each of these disorders. Bipolar disorders are differentiated by how severe and long-lasting the manic symptoms are.

These disorders are labeled "bipolar" because most people who experience mania will also experience depression during their lifetime (mania and depression are considered opposite poles). Contrary to what people may believe, an episode of depression is not required for a diagnosis of bipolar I disorder. At least a quarter of people with bipolar I disorder report never having an episode of depression; Angst, Rössler, et al., 2019). Depression is required for a diagnosis of bipolar II disorder.

Bipolar I Disorder

The criteria for diagnosis of **bipolar I disorder** (formerly known as manic-depressive disorder) include at least one episode of mania during a person's life. Note, then, that a person who is diagnosed with bipolar I disorder may or may not be experiencing current symptoms of mania. In fact, even someone who experienced only 1 week of manic symptoms years ago is still diagnosed with bipolar I disorder.

Mania is a state of intense elation or irritability, along with abnormally increased activity and other symptoms shown in the diagnostic criteria. During manic episodes, people will act and think in ways that are highly unusual compared to their typical selves. They may become louder and make an incessant stream of remarks, sometimes full of puns, jokes, rhymes, and interjections about nearby stimuli that attract their attention. They may be difficult to interrupt and may shift rapidly from topic to topic, reflecting an underlying **flight of ideas**. During mania, people may become sociable to the point of intrusiveness. They can also become excessively self-confident. They may stop sleeping even as they become incredibly energetic. Attempts by others to curb such excesses can quickly bring anger and even rage. Mania often comes on suddenly over a period of a day or two. For many, the boundless energy, bursts of joy, and incredible surge in goal pursuit are welcome, so some fail to recognize the sudden changes as a sign of disorder.

In 2018, Mariah Carey discussed her bipolar disorder, and the heavy burden she felt in hiding the diagnosis for many years (Cagle, J., 2018).

Featureflash Photo Agency/Shutterstock.com

 VIDEO CONTENT

Case Study: Bipolar Disorder Pause and Ponder

Defining Symptoms of Manic and Hypomanic Episodes

Distinctly elevated or irritable mood.
Abnormally increased activity or energy.
At least three of the following are noticeably changed from baseline (four if mood is only irritable):

- Increase in goal-directed activity or psychomotor agitation

- Unusual talkativeness; rapid speech

- Flight of ideas or subjective impression that thoughts are racing

- Decreased need for sleep

- Increased self-esteem; belief that one has special talents, powers, or abilities

- Distractibility; attention easily diverted

- Excessive involvement in pleasurable activities that are likely to have painful consequences, such as reckless spending, sexual indiscretions, or unwise business investments

- Symptoms are present most of the day, nearly every day

For a manic episode:

- Symptoms last at least 1 week, require hospitalization, or include psychosis

- Symptoms cause significant distress or functional impairment

For a hypomanic episode:

- Symptoms last at least 4 days

- Clear changes in functioning are observable to others, but impairment is not marked

- No psychotic symptoms are present

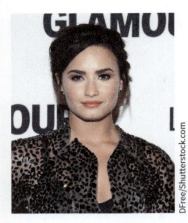

Demi Lovato, the highly successful singer, songwriter, and actress, has drawn from her own experiences with bipolar disorder to become a mental health advocate (Washington, 2017).

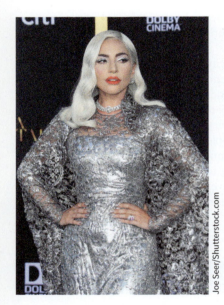

Lady Gaga has been a strong advocate for mental health and well-being, arguing that we should do more to offer compassion to those who struggle with depression and other conditions (Weisholz, D., 2020).

Unfortunately, as symptoms escalate into mania, people can be unaware to the potentially disastrous consequences of their symptoms, which can include risky sexual activities, overspending, and reckless driving. The following quote illustrates some of the impulsivity of this state.

When I am high I couldn't worry about money if I tried. So I don't. The money will come from somewhere; I am entitled; God will provide … So I bought twelve snakebite kits, with a sense of urgency and importance. I bought precious stones, elegant and unnecessary furniture, three watches within an hour of one another (in the Rolex rather than Timex class: champagne tastes bubble to the surface, are the surface, in mania), and totally inappropriate siren-like clothes. During one spree in London I spent several hundred pounds on books having titles or covers that somehow caught my fancy: books on the natural history of the mole, twenty sundry Penguin books because I thought it could be nice if the penguins could form a colony. Once I think I shoplifted a blouse because I could not wait a minute longer for the woman-with-molasses feet in front of me in line. Or maybe I just thought about shoplifting, I don't remember, I was totally confused. I imagine I must have spent far more than thirty thousand dollars during my two major manic episodes, and God only knows how much more during my frequent milder manias. But then back on lithium and rotating on the planet at the same pace as everyone else, you find your credit is decimated, your mortification complete. (Jamison, 1995, p. 75)

Bipolar II Disorder

Bipolar II disorder is defined by at least one hypomanic episode and at least one depressive episode during a person's life. **Hypomania** (see the defining symptoms of manic and hypomanic episodes) is milder than mania. *Hypo-* comes from the Greek for "under"; hypomania is "under"—or less extreme than—mania. Although mania involves significant impairment, hypomania does not. Rather, hypomania involves a change in functioning that does not cause serious problems. The person with hypomania may feel more social, energized, productive, and sexually alluring, as captured in this passage:

When you're high it's tremendous. The ideas and feelings are fast and frequent like shooting stars, and you follow them until you find better and brighter ones. Shyness goes, the right words and gestures are suddenly there, the power to captivate others a felt certainty. There are interests found in uninteresting people. Sensuality is pervasive and the desire to seduce and be seduced irresistible. Feelings of ease, intensity, power, well-being, financial omnipotence, and euphoria pervade one's marrow. (Jamison, 1993, pp. 67–68)

Cyclothymic Disorder

Also called *cyclothymia*, **cyclothymic disorder** is a chronic mood disorder. In cyclothymic disorder, the person has frequent but mild symptoms of depression alternating with mild symptoms of mania. Although the symptoms do not reach the severity of full-blown hypomanic or depressive episodes, people with the disorder and those close to them typically notice the ups and downs.

Defining Symptoms of Cyclothymic Disorder

For at least 2 years (or 1 year in children or adolescents):

- Numerous periods with hypomanic symptoms that do not meet criteria for a hypomanic episode
- Numerous periods with depressive symptoms that do not meet criteria for a major depressive episode

The symptoms are present at least half the time and do not clear for more than 2 months at a time.

Criteria for a major depressive, manic, or hypomanic episode have never been met.

Symptoms cause significant distress or functional impairment.

Epidemiology and Consequences of Bipolar Disorders

Bipolar disorder is much rarer than MDD. In the World Mental Health Survey, an epidemiologic study that involved structured diagnostic interviews with a representative sample of 61,392 people across 11 countries, about 0.6% of people met the criteria for bipolar I disorder (Merikangas, Jin, et al., 2011). Rates of bipolar disorder appear to be higher in the United States than in other countries. In the United States, about 1% of people experience bipolar I disorder. Findings of large-scale epidemiologic studies suggest that bipolar II disorder affects somewhere between 0.4% and 2% of people (Merikangas, et al., 2011). Although less is known about cyclothymic disorder, it is estimated that about 4% of people experience it (Regeer, Ten Have, et al., 2004).

Like depression, bipolar disorders are being seen with increasing frequency among children and adolescents (Kessler, et al., 2003). More than half of those with bipolar disorders report onset before age 25 (Merikangas, et al., 2011). Although bipolar disorders occur equally often in men and women, women diagnosed with bipolar disorder experience more episodes of depression than do men with this diagnosis (Altshuler, Kupka, et al., 2010). Even more than episodes of MDD, bipolar episodes tend to recur. More than half of people with bipolar I disorder experience four or more episodes during their lifetime (Goodwin & Jamison, 2007). Across the forms of bipolar disorder, a meta-analysis of eight studies found that 41% of people with bipolar disorder experienced a recurrence in the first year and 60% experienced one in the first 4 years after the first episode of bipolar disorder (Gignac, McGirr, et al., 2015). About two-thirds of people diagnosed with bipolar disorder meet diagnostic criteria for a comorbid anxiety disorder, and many meet criteria for comorbid substance use disorder.

Bipolar I disorder is among the most severe forms of psychological disorders. In a large community sample, less than 15% of people with bipolar disorder had been employed full time in the past year. Functional outcomes were particularly low for those with ongoing symptoms (Morgan, Mitchell, & Jablensky, 2005).

In the World Mental Health Survey, one in four persons diagnosed with bipolar I disorder reported a suicide attempt during their lifetime and more than half reported suicidal ideation within the past year (Merikangas, et al., 2011). In a national cohort of individuals who were followed for 36 years after psychiatric hospitalization, bipolar disorder was the psychiatric condition with the highest rate of suicide (Nordentoft, Mortensen, & Pedersen, 2011). Even in countries with accessible medical care for all, bipolar disorder has been found to relate to dying an average of 8.5 to 9 years earlier than those in the general population (Crump, Sundquist, et al., 2013). Increased risk of death from cardiovascular disease has been particularly well documented, with estimates that the risk of death from cardiovascular disease is twice as high for those with bipolar disorder compared with the general population. Risks, though, are not restricted to cardiovascular disease—large national cohort studies suggest higher mortality from a range of medical conditions (Westman, Hällgren, et al., 2013). These sad consequences of bipolar disorders are not offset by evidence that bipolar individuals and their family members possess heightened creativity (see **Read More About It 5.1**).

People with cyclothymia are at elevated risk for developing episodes of mania and major depression. Even if full-blown manic episodes do not emerge, the chronicity of cyclothymic symptoms takes its toll.

Quick Summary

Bipolar disorders include bipolar I disorder, bipolar II disorder, and cyclothymic disorder.

Bipolar I disorder is diagnosed on the basis of a single lifetime manic episode, and bipolar II disorder is diagnosed on the basis of hypomania and major depression. Cyclothymia is defined by frequent shifts between mild depressive and manic symptoms that last at least 2 years.

Bipolar I disorder affects 1% or less of the population.

About half of people with bipolar I disorder experience four or more episodes.

Read More About It 5.1

Touched with Fire: Manic-Depressive Illness and the Artistic Temperament

In her book *Touched with Fire: Manic-Depressive Illness and the Artistic Temperament* (1993), Kay Redfield Jamison assembled evidence linking mood disorders, especially bipolar disorder, to artistic creativity. Of course, most people with mood disorders are not exceptionally creative, and most creative people do not have mood disorders—but the list of visual artists, composers, and writers who seem to have experienced mood disorders is impressive. Jamison's list includes Michelangelo, van Gogh, Tchaikovsky, Schumann, Gauguin, Tennyson, Shelley, Faulkner, Hemingway, F. Scott Fitzgerald, Whitman, and Robert Lowell.

Following publication of Jamison's book, many different researchers began to study the objective links between bipolar disorder and creativity. In a population-based study of more than a million people, researchers found that those with bipolar disorder and their unaffected family members were overrepresented in creative occupations compared to the general population (Kyaga, Landen, et al., 2013). In recent years, many actors and musicians have spoken out about their history of mania, including Stephen Fry, Carrie Fisher, Linda Hamilton, and Bebe Rexha.

Many people assume that the manic state itself fosters creativity through elated mood, increased energy, rapid thoughts, and a heightened ability to make connections among seemingly unrelated events. Extreme mania, however, lowers creative output, and even if people produce more work during a manic period, the quality of that work might suffer, as seems to have been the case for the composer Robert Schumann (Weisberg, 1994). Moreover, studies have shown that people who have experienced episodes of mania tend to be less creative than those who have had the milder episodes of hypomania, and both groups tend to produce less creative output than do non-ill family members (Richards, Kinney, et al., 1988). Although many people with bipolar disorder worry that taking medications may limit their creativity, these findings suggest that reducing manic symptoms should help, rather than hurt, creativity.

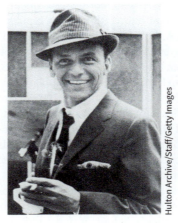

Frank Sinatra is quoted as having said this about himself: "Being an 18-karat manic depressive, and having lived a life of violent emotional contradictions, I have an over-acute capacity for sadness as well as elation" (Summers & Swan, 2006, p. 218).

Hulton Archive/Staff/Getty Images

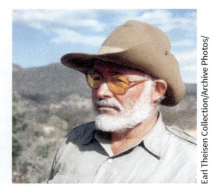

Earl Theisen Collection/Archive Photos/Getty Images

Mood disorders are common among artists and writers. Author Ernest Hemingway was affected.

5.2 Check Your Knowledge

INTERACTIVE SELF-SCORING QUIZZES

(Answers are at the end of the chapter.)

Fill in the blank.

1. Bipolar I is defined by _____.

Answer the following question.

2. What is the key difference between the diagnostic criteria for bipolar I disorder and bipolar II disorder?

Influences on Mood Disorders

When we think of the profound extremes embodied in the mood disorders, it is natural to ask why these extremes happen. How can we explain Mary sinking into the depths of depression? What factors combined to drive Kay into her racing thoughts and reckless shopping? No single cause can explain mood disorders. A number of different influences combine to explain their onset.

Although the DSM includes several different depressive disorders and bipolar disorders, the research on causes and treatment has tended to focus on major depressive disorder and bipolar I disorder. For simplicity, we refer to these conditions as *depression* and *bipolar disorder* through the remainder of this chapter.

We begin by discussing biological influences involved in depression and bipolar disorder. As **Table 5.2** shows, many different biological approaches have been applied to mood disorders, and we will describe genetic and brain-imaging research, and then discuss research on cytokines. After describing these biological influences, we discuss sleep and circadian rhythm disturbances in depression and bipolar disorder. Then, we discuss psychosocial predictors, first for depression and then for bipolar disorder.

Genetic Influences

As described in Chapter 2, heritability can be interpreted as the proportion of the variance in depression (within the population) that is explained by genes. The most careful studies of heritability involve interviews with representative samples of twins selected from the community (rather than focusing only on people who seek treatment, who may have more severe cases of the disorder than those who are not treated). These more careful studies of MZ (identical) and DZ (fraternal) twins yield a heritability estimate of 0.37 for MDD (Sullivan, Neale, & Kendler, 2000). Heritability estimates are higher when researchers study more severe samples (e.g., when the people in the study are recruited from inpatient hospitals rather than outpatient clinics).

Bipolar disorder is among the most heritable of disorders. One community-based twin sample that used structured interviews to verify diagnoses obtained a heritability estimate of 0.93 (Kieseppa, Partonen, et al., 2004). Adoption studies also confirm the importance of heritability in bipolar disorder (Wender, Kety, et al., 1986). Bipolar I and bipolar II disorders are both highly heritable (Edvardsen, Torgersen, et al., 2008).

Molecular genetics research (see Chapter 2) aims to identify the specific genes involved in mood disorders. In GWAS studies of more than 185,000 mood disorder cases and 439,000 control cases, researchers identified 39 single nucleotide polymorphisms (SNPs) related to major depressive disorder and four related to bipolar disorder that showed replicable effects across multiple data sets (Coleman, Gaspar, et al., 2020). Many of the SNPs related to bipolar disorder overlap with those involved in schizophrenia (Bipolar Disorder and Schizophrenia Working Group of the Psychiatric Genomics Consortium, 2018). SNPs are more closely tied to depression when researchers used careful diagnostic interviews as opposed to self-report scales or medical diagnoses to identify major depressive disorder (Cai, Revez, et al., 2020).

Neural Regions Involved in Emotion and Reward Processing

Functional brain-imaging studies suggest that MDD is associated with changes in the activity patterns of brain regions involved in experiencing and regulating emotion and in responding to rewards (Treadway & Pizzagalli, 2014). Many of these studies examine neural responses to stimuli that would likely induce emotion, such as pictures of positive or negative scenes, or to rewards, such as earning money. **Table 5.3** summarizes five primary brain structures that have been most studied in depression: the amygdala, the **anterior cingulate**, the prefrontal cortex, the hippocampus, and the **striatum** (see also **Figure 5.1**). Several different regions of the prefrontal cortex, including the medial prefrontal cortex, the orbitofrontal cortex, and the **dorsolateral prefrontal cortex**, are involved in the mood disorders. We will discuss each of these regions, beginning with the amygdala.

The amygdala is engaged when people perceive salient and emotionally important stimuli. For example, the amygdala activates when people are shown pictures of threatening stimuli. Animals with damage to the amygdala fail to react with fear to threatening stimuli and also fail to respond positively to food. In functional

TABLE 5.2	Summary of Neurobiological Hypotheses About MDD and Bipolar Disorder	
Neurobiological Hypothesis	**MDD**	**Bipolar Disorder**
Genetic contribution	Moderate	High
Changes in activation of regions in the brain in response to emotion stimuli	Present	Present
Activation of the striatum in response to reward	Diminished	Elevated

TABLE 5.3   Neural Regions Associated with Mood Disorders

Brain Structure	Activity Level in Depression	Activity Level in Mania
Amygdala	Elevated	Elevated
Anterior cingulate	Elevated	Elevated
Regions of the prefrontal cortex	Diminished	Diminished
Hippocampus	Atypical, but studies differ in whether it is elevated or diminished	Diminished
Striatum	Diminished	Elevated

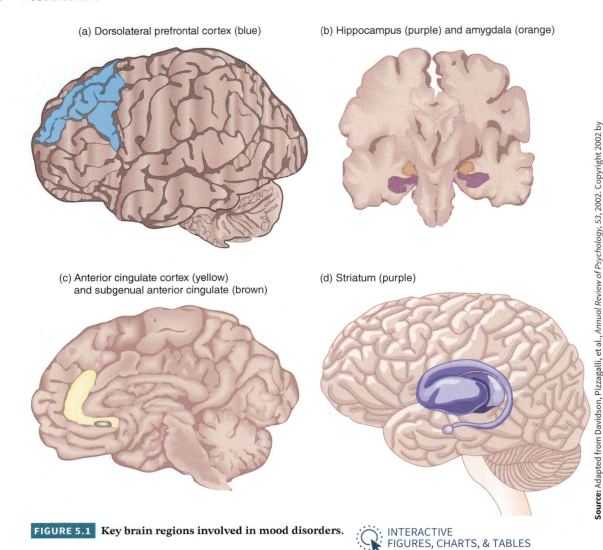

(a) Dorsolateral prefrontal cortex (blue)

(b) Hippocampus (purple) and amygdala (orange)

(c) Anterior cingulate cortex (yellow)
and subgenual anterior cingulate (brown)

(d) Striatum (purple)

FIGURE 5.1   **Key brain regions involved in mood disorders.**   INTERACTIVE FIGURES, CHARTS, & TABLES

MRI (fMRI) studies, people with MDD show elevated activity of the amygdala when responding to emotion-relevant stimuli, such as negative words or pictures of sad or angry faces. This profile of amygdala overreactivity to negative emotion stimuli was supported in a meta-analysis of 79 fMRI studies (McTeague, Rosenberg, et al., 2020). Amygdala overreactivity to negative stimuli is also shown among relatives of people with depression who have no personal history of MDD, suggesting this might be part of the vulnerability to depression rather than just the aftermath of being depressed (Pilhatsch, Vetter, et al., 2014; Swartz, Williamson, & Hariri, 2015). Amygdala hyper-reactivity is shown in other emotion-related disorders, including anxiety disorders (McTeague, et al., 2020).

In addition to elevated activity of the amygdala, MDD is associated with greater activation of the anterior cingulate (Hamilton, Etkin, et al., 2012), lowered activation of several regions of the prefrontal cortex, and differential activation of the hippocampus when people are viewing negative stimuli (McTeague, et al., 2020). Disturbances in these regions are believed to interfere with effective emotion regulation and cognitive control, and are observed across many disorders (McTeague, et al., 2020). Caution is warranted, in that the direction of effects for the hippocampus has varied across studies, with some studies suggesting greater activation, but others suggesting less activation (Hamilton, et al., 2012; McTeague et al., 2020).

How might these findings fit together? One theory is that the overactivity in the amygdala during depression is related to oversensitivity to emotionally relevant stimuli. At the same time, systems involved in regulating emotions are compromised (the anterior cingulate, the hippocampus, and regions of the dorsolateral prefrontal cortex).

In addition to these findings about emotion reactivity and regulation, research has suggested that neural regions involved in responding and mobilizing to rewards may be underactive in depression. For example, people with depression demonstrate diminished activation of the striatum during exposure to emotional stimuli (Hamilton, et al., 2012), and particularly to cues of potential reward, such as money (Ng, Alloy, & Smith, 2019). A specific region of the striatum (called the *nucleus accumbens*) is a central component of the reward system in the brain and plays a key role in motivation to pursue rewards (Salamone & Correa, 2012). The lack of activity of the striatum in response to cues of reward, then, may help explain why people with depression feel less motivated by the positive events in their lives. We will discuss this lack of motivation to pursue rewards again, later in this chapter.

Many of the brain structures implicated in MDD also appear to be involved in bipolar disorder. Bipolar I disorder is associated with elevated activity of the amygdala during when viewing emotion-related stimuli and in some studies, with diminished activity of the hippocampus and dorsolateral prefrontal cortex (McTeague, et al., 2020; Schumer, Chase, et al., 2023).

Although these patterns of neural activation parallel those observed among people with MDD, there are some differences in the neural activation patterns of people with bipolar disorder as compared to MDD. These differences are observed in fMRI studies involving responses to potential rewards. In some fMRI studies, people with bipolar disorder tend to show high activation of the striatum (Bart, Titone, et al., 2021), in contrast with the low activity observed for those with MDD. They also tend to show differential activation of the orbitofrontal cortex in response to reward when compared to persons without mood disorders. Caution is warranted, though, because the findings are mixed regarding neural responses to reward cues for those with bipolar disorder (Bart, et al., 2021; Johnson, Mehta, et al., 2019).

Many researchers have used functional connectivity analyses to examine the strength of connection between brain regions or the coupling of activity across regions. Rather than assume that any one region is a causal factor in depression, these models focus on the idea that dysfunction may involve a network of regions. Researchers examine connectivity when individuals are resting and while they are doing tasks. Findings indicate depression may be tied to differences in the functional connectivity of many different networks involved in responding to negative or positive stimuli, emotion responsivity, emotion regulation, cognitive control, and thinking about one's past and future (Disabato, Bauer, et al., 2016; Williams, 2017). In a meta-analysis of 68 studies of resting state functional connectivity, two networks showed hyperconnectivity in depression as compared to anxiety or chronic pain: the default-mode network, involved in self-referential processing, and frontoparietal network, involved in cognitive control and emotion regulation (Brandl, Weise, et al., 2022). Across 40 studies of resting state functional connectivity in bipolar disorder, atypical connectivity within these two networks is frequently observed, along with disrupted connectivity of the salience network, which is involved in responses to emotionally salient stimuli (Yoon, Kim, et al., 2021).

Cytokines

As described in Chapter 2, cytokines are proteins that are released as part of an immune response. One set of these cytokines, pro-inflammatory cytokines, play a vital role in wound healing and fighting off infection by triggering inflammation. In the short term, this inflammation is adaptive. Problems arise, though, when the inflammation becomes prolonged. Current theory is that people vary in how well and quickly they recover from the influence of pro-inflammatory cytokines and that this prolonged response might be tied to depression.

Three of these pro-inflammatory cytokines, IL-1 beta, IL-6, and TNF alpha, have been shown to cause a syndrome called **sickness behavior**, which includes many of the symptoms that are seen in depression: decreased motor activity, reduced food consumption, social withdrawal, changes in sleep patterns, and reduced motivation to pursue rewards (like sugar, in the case of rats). Of course, when one is fighting off physical illness, these changes are adaptive in promoting rest and recovery. A wide range of studies support the idea that pro-inflammatory cytokines can cause sickness behavior. For example, experimental administration of pro-inflammatory cytokines to animals triggers the symptoms of sickness behavior. One way that these cytokines may promote rest is to reduce activity in brain regions involved in motivation to pursue rewards (Bekhbat, Treadway, & Felger, 2022).

Several types of evidence support the idea that these pro-inflammatory cytokines are related to depression. Sickness behavior symptoms in animals can be relieved by administering antidepressant medications. In humans, drugs such as interferon, which are used for severe medical conditions such as cancer, also increase levels of pro-inflammatory cytokines. Between a third and a half of patients treated with interferon develop the symptoms of MDD (Raison, Capuron, & Miller, 2006).

In naturalistic studies without experimental manipulation, people with repeated episodes of depression and those with bipolar disorder tend to show high levels of some pro-inflammatory cytokines, including IL-6 and TNF-alpha, despite some nonreplications (Goldsmith, Rapaport, & Miller, 2016; Köhler, Freitas, et al., 2017). High levels of IL-6, but not TNF-alpha, predict modest increases in depressive symptoms over time (Mac Giollabhui, Ng, et al., 2021).

Given these effects, many investigators are considering whether anti-inflammatory medications may be helpful in relieving depression (Bai, Guo, et al., 2020), but findings of a study of 19,000 older adults showed no benefits of the anti-inflammatory drug aspirin in preventing depressive symptoms (Berk, Woods, et al., 2020). Although researchers do not think that all depressions are related to cytokines, cytokines may be important for understanding some depressions (Slavicj & Irwin, 2014).

Circadian Rhythms and Sleep

Sleep is central to healthy emotion regulation, cognitive ability, health, and immune function. The timing of sleep is shaped by underlying **circadian rhythms**—24-hour biological rhythms that guide activity, alertness, and body functions to keep us in sync with day/night rhythms (See **Figure 5.2**). Some of the studies of day/night activity patterns use **actigraphy** devices worn on the wrist to capture movement levels every second around the clock. With actigraphy, researchers can estimate sleep periods by looking for long windows without movement, and they can graph the level of daytime versus nighttime activity as well. A large body of work links circadian rhythm and sleep disruptions to many forms of psychological disorders (Goldstone, Javitz, et al., 2020; Wellcome Trust, 2022).

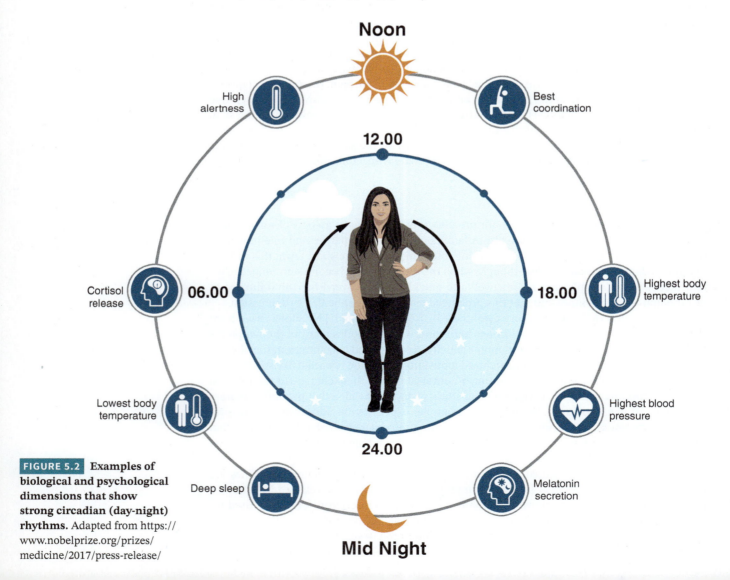

FIGURE 5.2 **Examples of biological and psychological dimensions that show strong circadian (day-night) rhythms.** Adapted from https://www.nobelprize.org/prizes/medicine/2017/press-release/

Many findings suggest that circadian rhythm and sleep disruptions are key to depression and bipolar disorder. Among people with depression, several circadian rhythm and sleep disruptions are common, including insomnia, relatively low levels of daytime activity compared to nighttime activity, and patterns of later and more varied bedtimes. People with bipolar disorder show similar circadian rhythm and sleep problems, even during well periods (Ng, Chung, et al., 2015).

Circadian and sleep disruptions also can predict more severe depression over time. Insomnia, sleep disruptions, and actigraphy profiles of diminished day versus night activity can each predict depression symptoms and onset over time (Li, Wu, et al., 2016; Wellcome Trust, 2022). Poor sleep also predicts depression relapse as well as increases in suicidal ideation (Littlewood, Kyle, et al., 2019). Poor sleep has been tied to many other factors involved in mood disorders, including greater emotional reactivity, increased inflammation, and changes in neurocircuitry (Wellcome Trust, 2020).

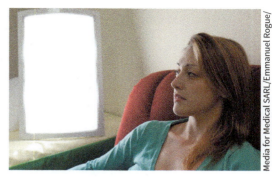

This woman is having light therapy, which is an effective treatment for unipolar and bipolar depression.

Just as with depression, sleep and circadian disruptions also can predict manic symptoms (Ritter, Höfler, et al., 2015; Wellcome Trust, 2022). Experimental studies indicate that sleep deprivation can trigger manic episodes. In one study, participants who were experiencing bipolar depression were asked to stay at a sleep center, where they were kept awake all night. By the next morning, about 10% were experiencing at least mild symptoms of mania (Colombo, Benedetti, et al., 1999).

Researchers are testing the idea that the genetic vulnerability for mood disorder may overlap with the genetic vulnerability to

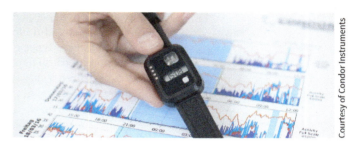

Actigraph watches that measure movement are frequently used for studying circadian rhythms.

sleep and circadian problems. Some of the genetic polymorphisms that are related to depression are also common among people who experience insomnia (Coleman, et al., 2020). In addition, people with bipolar disorder often show polymorphisms of "**clock genes**," which regulate circadian rhythms (Wellcome Trust, 2022).

Sleep and circadian problems might help explain the increasingly high rates of depression among adolescents. Sleep and circadian problems are common among adolescents—less than 40% of adolescents meet recommendations to sleep at least 7 hours per night (Keyes, Maslowsky, et al., 2015). Not only are sleep problems common in this age group, but lack of sleep can predict the onset of depression among adolescents (Goldstone, et al., 2020; Wellcome Trust, 2022). Poor sleep can also increase the risk of bipolar disorder onset in youth (Ritter, et al., 2015).

Profiles of sleep and circadian problems are relevant for treatment. The medicines that are used to treat mood disorders also help improve circadian rhythms and sleep (Wellcome Trust, 2020). Cognitive behavioral treatment for insomnia for those with comorbid depression or bipolar disorder leads to short-term relief from depression and mania (Harvey, Dong, et al., 2021; Harvey, Soehner, et al., 2015). Light therapy, which is a treatment to improve circadian rhythms by exposing individuals to bright light for 30 minutes each morning, has shown success for the treatment of MDD and bipolar depression (Wellcome Trust, 2022).

Social Influences on Depression: Childhood Adversity, Life Events, and Interpersonal Difficulties

Interpersonal problems are very common for those with depression, but showing cause and effect takes much more than just documenting this correlation. The depressive symptoms could easily contribute to interpersonal difficulties, as the person withdraws, begins to feel irritable, and finds no joy when engaging with others. To show that interpersonal concerns are not just an effect of the depressive symptoms, longitudinal studies are extremely important in order to establish that an interpersonal factor is present before onset. Fortunately, many large longitudinal studies are available, and we will focus on social variables that have been shown to precede and predict the onset of depressive episodes, including childhood adversity, negative life events, lack of social support, and family criticism.

Childhood adversity, such as early parental death, physical abuse, or sexual abuse, increases the risk that depression will develop in adolescence or adulthood (Daley, Hammen,

& Rao, 2000) and that those depressive symptoms will be long-lasting and severe (Vallati, Cunningham, et al., 2020). Childhood abuse can also set the stage for other risk factors in depression, including a negative cognitive style (Lumley & Harkness, 2007), poorer marital relationship quality (DiLillo, Giuffre, et al., 2001), and increased rates of life stress (Harkness, Bagby, & Kennedy, 2012). Child abuse, though, is also strongly tied to anxiety disorders (Kessler, McLaughlin, et al., 2010). This suggests that child abuse may increase the risk for several different disorders, whereas other influences may more uniquely contribute to depression.

Beyond childhood adversity, the role of recent stressful life events in triggering episodes of depression is well established. Prospective studies have shown that negative life events often precede a depressive episode (Mineka, Williams, et al., 2020). Even with a prospective study, though, it remains possible that some life events are caused by early symptoms of depression that have not yet developed into a full-blown disorder. Remember the case of Mary, who developed symptoms after she was laid off from her job. Maybe Mary lost her job because her trouble waking in the morning caused her to arrive at work late; disturbed sleep patterns can be an early sign of depression. To disentangle these issues, researchers conduct analyses in which they exclude stressful life events that could have been caused by mild depressive symptoms. Even when those types of events are excluded, evidence consistently indicates that stressful life events can cause depression. In careful prospective studies, 42–67% of people report that they experienced a very serious life event that was not caused by symptoms in the year before their depression began. Common events include losing a job, a key friendship, or a romantic relationship (Brown & Harris, 1989).

Why do some people, but not others, become depressed after stressful life events? The obvious answer is that some people must be more vulnerable to stress than others. Some of the disturbances in neural circuitry that we described earlier could increase reactivity to stress. Social, psychological, and cognitive characteristics also are important and could be vulnerability factors. The most common models, then, consider both vulnerabilities and stressors. Social, psychological, and cognitive vulnerability factors may also shape the development of depression for some people who become depressed in the absence of a life event (Monroe & Harkness, 2019).

One vulnerability may be a lack of social support. People who are depressed tend to have sparse social networks and to regard those networks as providing little support. Low social support may lessen a person's ability to handle stressful life events. One study showed that women experiencing a severely stressful life event without support from a confidant had a 40% risk of developing depression, whereas those with a confidant's support had only a 4% risk (Brown & Andrews, 1986). Social support, then, seems to buffer against the effects of severe stressors.

Family problems are another important interpersonal predictor of depression. A long line of research has focused on **expressed emotion (EE)**—defined as a family member's critical or hostile comments toward or emotional overinvolvement with the person with depression. High EE strongly predicts relapse in depression. Indeed, one review of six studies found that 69.5% of patients in families with high EE relapsed within 1 year, compared to 30.5% of patients in families with low EE (Butzlaff & Hooley, 1998). Marital discord also can predict the onset of depression (Whisman & Bruce, 1999).

Clearly, interpersonal problems can trigger the onset of depressive symptoms, but consider the flip side of the coin. Once depressive symptoms emerge, they can create interpersonal problems—that is, depressive symptoms often elicit negative reactions from others (Coyne, 1976). Taken together, it is clear that interpersonal loss, isolation, and relationship concerns can trigger depression, but it is good to be aware that the depression and the related vulnerability can also create challenges in interpersonal relationships.

Psychological Influences on Depression

Many different psychological factors play a role in depressive disorders. In this section, we discuss personality and cognitive factors that increase the risk of depression in the context of stress. Here again, we will focus on some of the longitudinal research documenting factors that predict increases in depressive symptoms over time.

Neuroticism   Several longitudinal studies suggest that **neuroticism**, a personality trait that involves the tendency to experience frequent and intense negative affect, predicts the onset of depression (Jorm, Christensen, et al., 2000). A large study of twins suggests that neuroticism explains at least part of the link of genetic vulnerability with depression (Fanous,

Focus on Discovery 5.2

Understanding the Overlap in Anxiety and Depression

There are several reasons to question whether anxiety disorders are separable from depressive disorders. Chief among these reasons is the high rate of comorbidity. At least 60% of people with an anxiety disorder will experience MDD during their lifetime, and similarly—about 45% of those with depression will experience an anxiety disorder (Kessler, Sampson, et al., 2015; Moffitt, Caspi, et al., 2007). Given the high rates of co-occurrence, many researchers have argued that we should consider depression and anxiety disorders conjointly in an overarching category of internalizing disorders (Wright, Krueger, et al., 2013).

Beyond patterns of comorbidity, there is overlap in the causes of anxiety and depression. The genetic risk for anxiety and depression

overlap substantially (Kendler, Aggen, et al., 2011), and the brain regions involved in anxiety and depression also show substantial overlap (McTeague, et al., 2020; Zhukovsky, Wainberg, et al., 2022). Many psychological and social risk factors, such as neuroticism (Ormel, Jeronimus, et al., 2013) and childhood adversity (Kessler, et al., 2010), are tied to both depressive disorders and anxiety disorders.

Rather than lumping the anxiety and depressive symptoms together, the DSM-5-TR includes a specifier (subtype) "with anxious distress" to be used when depressive episodes are accompanied by at least two anxiety symptoms. Many patients meet the criteria for this specifier. The presence of anxiety among people who are seeking treatment for depression predicts a poor response to antidepressant treatment (Saveanu, Etkin, et al., 2015), suggesting the need to understand much more about people who experience both depression and anxiety.

Prescott, & Kendler, 2004). As you would expect, neuroticism also predicts the onset of anxiety (Zinbarg, Mineka, et al., 2016), an overlap we discuss in **Focus on Discovery 5.2**.

Cognitive Theories
Pessimistic and self-critical thoughts can torture the person with depression. In cognitive theories, these negative thoughts and beliefs are seen not just as symptoms, but as major causes of depression. We will describe three cognitive theories. These models are not incompatible with the interpersonal and life stress research discussed earlier; a person's negative thoughts may sometimes reflect genuinely stressful life circumstances. In cognitive models, though, cognitions are seen as the most important force driving depression.

Beck's Theory
Aaron Beck (1967) argued that depression is associated with a **negative triad**: negative views of the self, the world, and the future. According to this model, in childhood, people with depression acquired negative schemas through experiences such as loss of a parent, the social rejection of peers, or the depressive attitudes of a parent. Schemas are different from conscious thoughts—they are an underlying set of beliefs that operate outside a person's awareness to shape the way a person makes sense of his, her, or their experiences. A negative schema is activated whenever the person encounters situations like those that originally caused the schema to form. Once activated, negative schemas are believed to cause negative **information-processing biases**, or tendencies to process information in certain negative ways. That is, people with depression might attend to and remember even the smallest negative feedback about themselves, while at the same time failing to notice or remember positive feedback about themselves. People with a schema of ineptness might readily notice and remember signs that they are inept, while ignoring or forgetting signs that they are competent. Together, these errors in attention, interpretation, and recall lead people with depression to draw conclusions that are consistent with their underlying schema, which then maintain the schema (a vicious cycle shown in **Figure 5.3**).

How has Beck's theory been tested? One widely used instrument in studies of Beck's theory is a self-report scale called the Dysfunctional Attitudes Scale (DAS), which includes items concerning whether people consider themselves worthwhile or lovable. Hundreds of studies have shown that people who are depressed endorse patterns of negative thinking on scales like the DAS (Haaga, Dyck, & Ernst, 1991). These findings, though, are hard to interpret, as negative thoughts could be a symptom or a cause of the depression. More compelling evidence comes from longitudinal findings that negative cognitive styles can predict the onset of a first episode of MDD (Carter & Garber, 2011) and depressive relapse (Segal, Kennedy, et al., 2006).

Beyond studies with self-report scales to measure cognition, researchers have tested whether depression relates to information processing biases. Findings have been mixed for whether depression relates to more attention to negative stimuli or to more negative interpretations of ambiguous stimuli, but depression does tend to be associated with memory for negative and positive information (LeMoult & Gotlib, 2019). In a meta-analysis of 25 studies, Mathews and

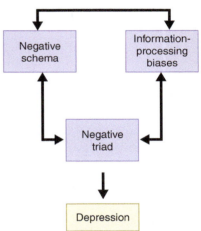

FIGURE 5.3 The interrelationships among different kinds of cognitions in Beck's theory of depression.

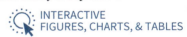
INTERACTIVE
FIGURES, CHARTS, & TABLES

MacLeod (2002) described evidence that most people who are not depressed will remember more positive than negative information. For example, if presented with a list of 20 negative and 20 positive self-descriptive adjectives, most people will remember more of the positive than the negative words when queried later in a session. People with MDD, though, tend to remember about 10% more negative words than positive words. This tendency to remember more negative words is more pronounced if they were asked to consider whether the words were self-descriptive—that is, memories appear more biased for self-referential material (Everaert, Vrijsen, et al., 2022). While people who are not depressed seem to wear rose-colored glasses, those with depression tend to have a negative bias in the way that they recall information about the self. Although these recall biases tend to be less present after recovery from a depressive episode, the recall biases can re-emerge when the person experiences a negative mood or a stressor (Everaert, et al., 2022).

One important caveat has been raised about the link of recall bias with depression, however. Researchers examined whether this form of information processing related to all symptoms of depression. Negative recall biases were found to be related to some of the symptoms of depression, including sadness, self-dislike, punishment, and pessimism, but not to physical symptoms such as loss of appetite, low energy, or sleep disturbance (Beevers, Mullarkey, et al., 2019). This suggests that other variables may be important to consider in predicting physical symptoms of depression. Nonetheless, across a very broad range of measures, researchers have generally shown support for Beck's model.

Hopelessness Theory According to **hopelessness theory** (see **Figure 5.4**; Abramson, Metalsky, & Alloy, 1989), the most important trigger of depression is hopelessness, which is defined by the belief that desirable outcomes will not occur and that there is nothing a person can do to change this. The model places emphasis on two key dimensions of **attributions**—the explanations a person forms about why a stressor has occurred (Weiner, Frieze, et al., 1971):

- Stable (permanent) versus unstable (temporary) causes
- Global (relevant to many life domains) versus specific (limited to one area) causes

Table 5.4 illustrates these dimensions by considering how different people might explain their low score on the Graduate Record Examination (GRE). People whose **attributional style** leads them to believe that negative life events are due to stable and global causes are likely to become hopeless, and this hopelessness will set the stage for depression.

Many studies have been conducted on the hopelessness model of depression. These studies consistently show that people who are depressed tend to endorse making stable, global attributions for negative events. Among those who are not depressed at baseline, tendencies to make stable, global attributions predict the onset of a first episode of MDD and increases in depressive symptoms over time (Mac Giollabhui, Hamilton, et al., 2018).

Rumination Theory While Beck's theory and the hopelessness model tend to focus on the nature of negative thoughts, Susan Nolen-Hoeksema (1991) suggested that a way of thinking called **rumination** may increase the risk of depression. Rumination is defined as a tendency to repetitively dwell on sad experiences. The most detrimental form of rumination may be a tendency to brood regretfully about why a sad event happened (Treynor, Gonzalez, & Nolen-Hoeksema, 2003).

Tendencies to ruminate, as measured using self-report scales, have been found to predict the onset of major depressive episodes among initially nondepressed persons (Nolen-Hoeksema, 2000). As described in **Focus**

INTERACTIVE FIGURES, CHARTS, & TABLES

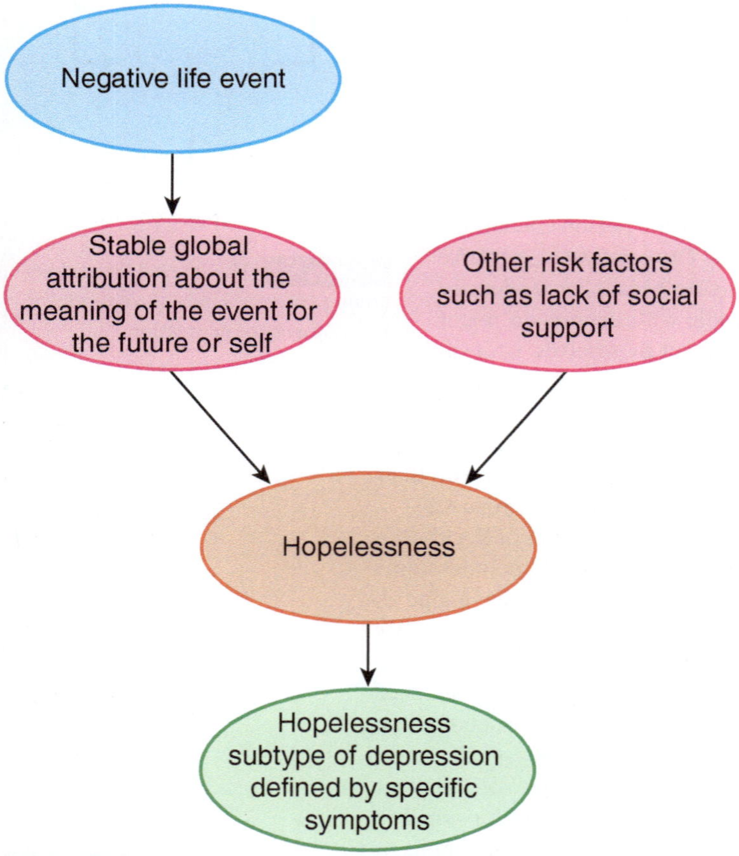

FIGURE 5.4 Major elements of the hopelessness theory of depression.

TABLE 5.4	**An Example of Attributions: Why I Failed My GRE Math Exam**	
	Stable	**Unstable**
Global	I lack intelligence.	I am exhausted.
Specific	I lack mathematical ability.	I am fed up with math right now.

on Discovery 5.1, one interesting aspect of this theory is that women tend to ruminate more than men do, perhaps because they are exposed to more interpersonal stress that can be difficult to solve (Hamilton, Stange, et al., 2015). The tendency for women to ruminate more may help explain the higher rates of depression among women than among men (Nolen-Hoeksema, 2000).

Dozens of experimental studies have been conducted to examine how inducing rumination affects moods. Typically, in the rumination-induction condition, participants are exposed to stress and then asked to dwell on their current feelings and on themselves (e.g., "Think about the way you feel inside"), whereas in a distraction (control) condition, participants are asked to think about topics unrelated to their self or feelings (e.g., "Think about a fire darting round a log in a fireplace"). The findings of these experimental studies indicate that rumination increases negative moods, particularly when people focus on negative aspects of their mood and their self (Watkins, 2008).

If rumination leads to such negative feelings, one might wonder why some people tend to ruminate more. There are different explanations of why people ruminate. According to the meta-cognitive model, some people ruminate more because they believe it will help them solve problems (Papageorgiou & Wells, 2003). Consistent with this model, dozens of studies show that people who believe in the utility of rumination tend to ruminate more (Cano-López, García-Sancho, et al., 2022). According to another model, people ruminate because they have poor cognitive control that makes it hard for them to remove negative information from their working memory (Joormann, Levens, & Gotlib, 2011). Findings of a meta-analysis of dozens of studies indicate that those with depression do have difficulty with the cognitive control of negative information (Quigley, Thiruchselvam, & Quilty, 2022). In turn, poor cognitive control over negative information has been tied to rumination (LeMoult & Gotlib, 2019). Taken together, people may ruminate for more than one reason—sometimes because they think it is useful, and sometimes because they cannot stop themselves from doing so.

Putting It All Together: Integrating Biological and Social Influences on Depression

We have considered evidence for biological, psychological, and social risk factors for depression separately. But here, we focus on a risk factor that can be measured biologically and psychologically, and is influenced by the social environment: dampened reward sensitivity.

Reward sensitivity is defined as the extent to which a person is motivated by potentially rewarding events and experiences pleasure when they do experience rewards. Reward sensitivity can be measured using behavioral and biological measures. On behavioral tasks, people with MDD show deficits in the motivation to pursue rewards (Treadway, Bossaller, et al., 2012). For example, if given a choice about whether to work harder to earn more money, they are less likely to choose the harder task than are people without depression. As we described, in neuroimaging studies, people with depression often show diminished activation of the nucleus accumbens and other regions involved in reward processing when engaging in tasks in which they could earn rewards. They also show a blunted EEG response, called the Reward Positive (RewP) index, when shown reward feedback as compared to negative or neutral feedback (Proudfit, 2015). Behavioral measures of motivation to pursue rewards correlate with these neural and EEG indices of reward responses (Crane, Burkhouse, et al., 2022). That is, the lack of response to reward cues can be measured with behavioral tasks, fMRI, or EEG.

This blunted response to reward does not appear to be just an after-effect of depression. Lower motivation on behavioral measures is seen even after recovery from depression (Yang,

Huang, et al., 2014). Reduced RewP is seen among the children of mothers with MDD. EEG and fMRI measures of reward sensitivity both predict increases in depressive symptoms over time (Pagliaccio, Pizzagalli, et al., 2023; Weinberg, Kujawa, & Riesel, 2022).

People who are depressed often experience anhedonia, defined as an absence of pleasure in typically enjoyable activities. The severity of anhedonia is related to less reward sensitivity, when assessed with behavioral, neural, and EEG measures (Foti, Carlson, et al., 2014; Moran, Prevost, et al., 2023; Yang et al., 2014). This suggests that reward sensitivity might help explain anhedonia-related symptoms of depression more than other symptoms.

Stress matters in considering reward sensitivity and depression. Several studies show that people with low RewP are more vulnerable to developing depressive symptoms when faced with stressors, such as the COVID pandemic (Freeman, Carpentier, & Weinberg, 2023). At the same time, stress may actually lower reward sensitivity, as measured in several fMRI studies of reward (Ironside, Kumar, et al., 2018).

Taken together, a growing body of work shows that many people who experience MDD show low reward sensitivity on self-report, biological, and behavioral indices. In addition, reward sensitivity is lowered by stress and predicts depressive and anhedonic symptoms in the context of stress. These findings highlight that social influences, such as stress, may shape the biological influences on depression and anhedonia.

Social and Psychological Influences on the Course of Bipolar Disorder

Most people who experience a manic episode during their lifetime will also experience a major depressive episode, but not everyone will. For this reason, researchers often study the triggers of manic and depressive episodes separately within bipolar disorder.

Depression in Bipolar Disorder
The triggers of depressive episodes in bipolar disorder are similar to the triggers of major depressive episodes (Johnson, Cuellar, & Peckham, 2014). As in MDD, early adversity, negative life events, neuroticism, negative cognitive styles, family criticism, and lack of social support predict depressive symptoms in bipolar disorder. Not only do these variables predict bipolar depression, but sadly, people with bipolar disorder all too often experience early adversity, negative life events, and high levels of criticism from their loved ones (Johnson & Miklowitz, 2017).

Predictors of Mania
In addition to the evidence for sleep and circadian problems we discussed above, reward sensitivity has been found to predict increases in manic symptoms over time.

Previously, we discussed evidence that reward sensitivity is often low in depression. One model suggests that mania reflects heightened activity in the reward system of the brain (Depue, Collins, & Luciano, 1996). Several types of evidence support this model. To begin, dopamine plays a major role in reward sensitivity. Among people with bipolar disorder, drugs that increase dopamine levels have been found to trigger manic symptoms (Anand, Verhoeff, et al., 2000; Burdick, Braga, et al., 2014). Previously, we discussed differential profiles of activation of the striatum and other neural pathways to reward among those with bipolar disorder.

At a behavioral level, findings of many studies indicate that people with bipolar disorder tend to describe themselves on self-report scales as highly responsive to rewards (Johnson, Edge, et al., 2012). Being highly reward-sensitive has also been shown to predict the onset of bipolar disorder (Alloy, Abramson, et al., 2008) and a more severe course of mania after onset (Meyer, Johnson, & Winters, 2001). In addition, a particular kind of life event predicts increases in manic symptoms among people with bipolar I disorder—specifically, life events that involve attaining goals, such as gaining acceptance to graduate school or getting married. How could successes like these promote increases in symptoms? Researchers have proposed that life events involving success may trigger cognitive changes in confidence, which then spiral into excessive goal pursuit (Johnson, et al., 2012). This excessive goal pursuit may help trigger manic symptoms among people who are biologically vulnerable to bipolar disorder.

Quick Summary

Bipolar disorder is highly heritable. MDD is modestly heritable. GWAS studies have identified specific genetic loci that are related to MDD and bipolar disorder. Many of the genetic loci identified for bipolar disorder also relate to schizophrenia.

Neuroimaging studies suggest that depression and bipolar disorder are both associated with changes in regions of the brain that are involved in emotion and in responding to reward. These changes are consistent with greater emotional reactivity (heightened activity of the amygdala) but less ability to regulate emotion (differential activity of the hippocampus, diminished activity in regions of the prefrontal cortex, and greater activity of the anterior cingulate). Depression is related to lower activity of the striatum, whereas striatum activity and orbitofrontal cortex activity in response to reward cues is high among some with bipolar disorder. Connectivity research has shown that circuits involved in self-referential processing (the default mode network), cognitive control, and emotion regulation (the frontoparietal network) are involved in depression and bipolar disorder.

Pro-inflammatory cytokines are sometimes elevated in depression and in bipolar disorder, some of these cytokines can trigger a syndrome known as sickness behavior, and high levels of one of these pro-inflammatory cytokines (IL-6) predict increases in depression.

Social research strongly suggests that childhood adversity and recent negative life events increase the risk for MDD. Because many people do not become depressed after a life event, researchers have studied factors that could explain vulnerability to life events. Social influences on depression include low social support, high expressed emotion, and marital discord.

Sleep and circadian problems are risk factors for depression and bipolar disorder. Insomnia and circadian problems can predict the onset and worsening of depression and bipolar disorder. There is evidence that the genetic vulnerabilities for mood disorders and sleep/circadian problems have some overlap. Many treatments can be helpful when insomnia is comorbid with mood disorders.

Neuroticism, which involves frequent and intense negative affect, predicts the onset of depression. Several cognitive models have been proposed. Beck proposed that cognitive schemas guide information-processing biases in attention and memory that sustain the negative cognitive triad. Alloy and colleagues proposed that global and stable attributions for negative events guide hopelessness. Nolan-Hoeksema proposed that tendencies to ruminate about negative feelings contribute to depression and may help explain the gender difference in depression. Prospective evidence supports each of these cognitive models.

Biological, psychological, and social influences on depression interact, and the blunted reward sensitivity of depression gives one example of how these various influences might contribute to risk. Biological and behavioral measures both show that reward sensitivity is low among people with depression and predicts more depression over time. Stress can dampen reward sensitivity.

Many of the variables that predict MDD also predict depressive symptoms within bipolar disorder. Mania is predicted by tendencies to be highly reward sensitive and by life events involving goal attainment.

5.3 Check Your Knowledge

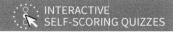
INTERACTIVE
SELF-SCORING QUIZZES

(Answers are at the end of the chapter.)
Answer the following questions.

1. Estimates of heritability are approximately _____ for MDD and approximately _____ for BD.
    a. 0.60, 0.65
    b. 0.20, 0.55
    c. 0.37, 0.93
    d. 0.10, 0.93

2. One brain region that appears to be overly active in response to emotion stimuli among people with mood disorders is the:
    a. hippocampus
    b. prefrontal cortex
    c. cerebellum
    d. amygdala

3. Describe key elements of the three cognitive models of depression.

Treatment of Mood Disorders

Many episodes of depression end in a year or less, but the time may seem immeasurably longer to people with the disorder and to those close to them. With mania, even a few days of acute symptoms can create troubles with relationships and jobs. Moreover, suicide is a risk for people with mood disorders. Thus, it is important to treat mood disorders.

In the United States, about two-thirds of people who experience major depressive disorder receive treatment for their symptoms (SAMHSA, 2020). Most commonly, treatment consists of antidepressants. More than 13% of adults in the United States currently take antidepressant medication (Brody & Gu, 2020).

For those with bipolar disorder, receipt of appropriate treatment is often delayed by the failure to recognize the diagnosis. Because patients are more likely to seek treatment during depression than during mania and providers often do not ask about prior mania, it typically takes about 6 years after the first manic episode for those with bipolar disorder to receive the correct diagnosis and begin to receive appropriate treatment (Scott, Graham, et al., 2022). Even once treatment begins to address bipolar disorder, more than half of people will discontinue that treatment (Merikangas, et al., 2011). Minorities are particularly unlikely to receive good care for bipolar disorder. In one large epidemiologic sample, none of the Black persons who were diagnosed with bipolar disorder were receiving adequate pharmacological treatment (Johnson & Johnson, 2014). With these concerns about treatment availability in mind, we turn to evidence concerning the best treatments for the mood disorders.

Psychological Treatment of Depression

Several different forms of psychological treatment have been shown to help relieve depression. These treatments are similar in being relatively brief (3–4 months of weekly sessions) and focused on the here and now. As with studies of causes, most of the research has focused on MDD, but similar treatments can be helpful when depressive symptoms are chronic (Schramm, Kriston, et al., 2017).

Interpersonal Psychotherapy

As we described in Chapter 2, interpersonal psychotherapy (IPT) builds on the evidence that depression is closely tied to interpersonal problems (Klerman, Weissman, et al., 1984). The core of the therapy is to examine major interpersonal problems, such as role transitions, interpersonal conflicts, grief, and interpersonal isolation. Typically, the therapist and the patient focus on one or two such issues, with the goal of helping the person identify their feelings about these issues, make important decisions, and effect changes to resolve problems related to these issues. Techniques include discussing interpersonal problems, exploring negative feelings and encouraging their expression, improving communications, problem solving, and suggesting new and more satisfying modes of behavior.

IPT has fared well in a series of randomized controlled trials. Several studies have found that in relieving MDD, IPT is more efficacious than placebo or usual care and that IPT achieves results as powerful as those observed for cognitive therapy (van Hees, Rotter, et al., 2013). Research also indicates that IPT prevents relapse when continued after recovery (Frank, Kupfer, et al., 1990).

IPT also works well outside the confines of carefully controlled university studies. In a dissemination trial, over 100 therapists in the Veterans Administration (VA) system were taught to administer IPT. Clients who received IPT treatment from those therapists showed large decreases in their depressive symptoms during the course of treatment (Stewart, Raffa, et al., 2014).

Cognitive Therapy

In keeping with their theory that depression is caused by negative schema and information-processing biases, Beck and associates developed a cognitive therapy (CT) aimed at altering maladaptive thought patterns. To begin, the client is taught to understand that our thoughts influence our moods powerfully and that the negative self-talk they engage in day by day contributes to low mood. To help increase awareness of the connection between thoughts and mood, the client might be asked to complete daily homework that involves recording negative thoughts. The therapist then tries to help the person with depression to change their self-beliefs. When a person states that they are worthless because "nothing goes right, and everything I do ends in a disaster," the therapist helps the person look for evidence that contradicts this overgeneralization, such as abilities that the person is overlooking or discounting.

TABLE 5.5	An Example of a Daily Thought-Monitoring Log, a Strategy Commonly Used in Cognitive Therapy						
Date and Time	Situation *What was happening?*	Negative Emotion *Note type of emotion (e.g., sad, nervous, angry) and the intensity of the emotion (0–100).*	Automatic Negative Thought	How Much Did You Believe This Initial Thought (0–100)?	Alternative Thought *Is there another view of the situation?*	Re-rate Your Belief in the Initial Thought	Outcome *Note type of emotion felt and emotion intensity (0–100) after considering the alternative.*
Tuesday 9:30 A.M.	I made a mistake on a report at work.	Sad–90 Embarrassed–80	I always mess things up. I'm never going to be good at anything.	90	My boss didn't give me enough time to prepare the report. I could have done a better job with more time.	50	Relief–30 Sad–30
Wednesday 7 P.M.	Eating dinner at a restaurant. An old friend from high school was at the next table and didn't recognize me.	Sad–95	I'm a nobody.	100	I've changed my hair drastically since then. Many people don't recognize me, but maybe she would have been happy to see me if I had reminded her of who I was.	25	Sad–25
Thursday 8:30 A.M.	My husband left for work without saying goodbye to me.	Sad–90	Even the people I love don't seem to notice me.	100	I know that he had a huge presentation, and he gets stressed.	20	Sad–20

The therapist then teaches the person to challenge negative beliefs and to learn strategies that promote making realistic and positive assumptions. Often, the client is asked to practice challenging overly negative thoughts in their day-to-day life, recording an initially negative thought and then reconsidering whether this is the most accurate lens on the situation (see **Table 5.5** for an example of a thought-monitoring homework assignment). Beck's emphasis is on cognitive restructuring (i.e., persuading the person to think less negatively).

Beck's therapy also includes a behavioral technique called behavioral activation (BA), in which people are encouraged to engage in pleasant activities that might bolster positive thoughts about one's self and life. For example, the therapist encourages patients to schedule positive events, such as going for a walk and talking with friends.

More than 100 randomized controlled trials, including 11 trials that involved careful steps to avoid potential bias in the results, have provided support for the efficacy of CT for depression (Cuijpers, Berking, et al., 2013; Cuijpers, Cristea, et al., 2016). CT has been adapted for cultural groups, including Latino and Chinese individuals (Aguilera, Bruehlman-Senecal, et al., 2018; Ren, Qiu, et al., 2019). CT is as helpful as antidepressant medication for severe depression. CT has two advantages over medication: It is more affordable, and it helps protect against relapse after treatment is finished (Hollon, DeRubeis, et al., 2014).

As with IPT, the findings of a large-scale dissemination trial, in which therapists in the VA system were taught to administer CT, showed that clients who received CT experienced large reductions in their depressive symptoms (Karlin, Brown, et al., 2012). Given how common relapse is in MDD, it is important that the strategies that clients learn in CT help diminish the risk of relapse even after therapy ends (Vittengl, Clark, et al., 2007). Offering even eight sessions of CT after remission reduces the risk of relapse among patients with recurrent MDD (De Jonge, Bockting, et al., 2019).

Clinical Case

An Example of Challenging a Negative Thought in Cognitive Therapy

The following dialogue is an example of one way a therapist might begin to challenge a person's negative thoughts in CT, although it would take several sessions to help a client learn the cognitive model and to identify overly negative thoughts (Leahy, 2003, 2017).

Therapist: You said that you are a "loser" because you and Roger got divorced. Now we already defined what it is to be a loser—not to achieve anything.

Patient: *Right. That sounds extreme.*

Therapist: OK. Let's look at the evidence for and against the thought that you have achieved something. Draw a line down the center of the page. On the top, I'd like you to write, "I have achieved some things."

Patient: *[draws line and writes statement]*

Therapist: What is the evidence that you have achieved some things?

Patient: *I graduated from college, I raised my son, I worked at the office, I have some friends, and I exercise. I am reliable. I care about my friends.*

Therapist: OK. Let's write all that down. Now, in the right column, let's write down evidence against the thought that you have achieved some things.

Patient: *Well, maybe it's irrational, but I would have to write down that I got divorced.*

Therapist: OK. Now, in looking at the evidence for and against your thought that you have achieved some things, how do you weigh it out? 50–50? Differently than 50–50?

Patient: *I'd have to say it's 95% in favor of the positive thought.*

Therapist: So, how much do you believe now that you have achieved some things?

Patient: *100%.*

Therapist: And how much do you believe that you are a failure because you got divorced?

Patient: *Maybe I'm not a failure, but the marriage failed. I'd give myself about 10%.*

Quoted from Leahy, R. L. (2003, 2017). *Cognitive Therapy Techniques: A Practitioner's Guide*, pp. 46, 64–65. Published by Guilford Press.

Note: As is typical, this dialogue challenges some, but not all, negative thoughts. Future sessions are likely to examine other negative thoughts.

Dozens of randomized controlled trials also provide evidence that CT when offered by internet is more effective than treatment as usual or waitlist control is for patients with MDD (Andrews, Basu, et al., 2018). Internet-based CT is more helpful when clinicians are available to review the material with the patient not only at baseline but intermittently throughout the intervention (Krieger, Bur, et al., 2023).

An adaptation of CT called **mindfulness-based cognitive therapy (MBCT)** is based on the idea that when people who are vulnerable to depression become sad, they begin to think negatively, and these patterns of thinking in turn intensify the sadness (Segal, Williams, & Teasdale, 2001). The goal of MBCT is to teach people to recognize when they start to feel sad and to try adopting what can be called a "decentered" perspective—viewing their thoughts merely as "mental events" rather than as core aspects of the self or as accurate reflections of reality. For example, the person might say to themself such things as "thoughts are not facts" and "I am not my thoughts" (Teasdale, Segal, et al., 2000, p. 616). In other words, using a wide array of strategies, including meditation, the person is taught over time to develop a detached relationship to depression-related thoughts and feelings. This perspective, it is believed, can prevent the escalation of negative thinking patterns that may cause depression.

Across multiple randomized clinical trials, MBCT has been shown to be more efficacious than treatment as usual and as helpful as other forms of active treatments (Goldberg, Tucker, et al., 2019). MBCT appears to be comparable to antidepressants in treatment efficacy for those with three or more episodes of MDD (Kuyken, Hayes, et al., 2015).

Behavioral Activation (BA) Therapy   Earlier, we mentioned that BA is one component of Beck's therapy. BA was originally developed as a stand-alone treatment, and it is based on the idea that many of the risk factors for depression interfere with receiving positive reinforcement (Lewinsohn, 1974). Poverty, negative life events, low social support, marital distress, and individual differences in social skills, personality, and coping may all lead to low levels of positive reinforcement. As depression begins to unfold, inactivity, withdrawal, and inertia are common symptoms, and these symptoms diminish the already low levels of positive reinforcement even further. Consequently, the goal of BA therapy is to increase participation in positively reinforcing activities so as to disrupt the spiral of depression, withdrawal, and avoidance (Martell, Addis, & Jacobson, 2001).

Returning to Clinical Case

Treatment Decisions for Mary

Mary, the woman described at the beginning of this chapter, reported increasing problems because of her depression. Accordingly, her therapist referred her to a psychiatrist, who prescribed fluoxetine (Prozac). Both the psychologist and the psychiatrist agreed that medication might help by quickly relieving her symptoms. But after 2 weeks, Mary decided she did not want to continue taking Prozac because she found the side effects uncomfortable and did not like the idea of taking medication over the long term. She had not gotten much relief, maybe because her concerns about medication had led her to skip many doses.

With so many different types of treatment available, determining the best therapy for a given client can be a challenge. Mary had experienced a major life event and transition, suggesting that interpersonal psychotherapy might fit. That she was blaming herself for her job loss and other issues suggested that CT might help.

Marital conflicts suggested that behavioral couples therapy could be appropriate. How does a therapist choose which approach to use? Sometimes this decision reflects the personal preferences and training of the therapist. Ideally, the approach incorporates the treatment preferences of the client as well.

Her therapist began CT, in the belief that Mary's tendency to blame herself excessively when things went wrong was contributing to her depression. CT helped her learn to identify and challenge irrationally negative cognitions about herself. Therapy began by helping her identify times in her day-to-day life when her sad moods could be explained by overly negative conclusions about small events. For example, when her children would misbehave, Mary would quickly assume this was evidence that she was a bad mother. Over time, Mary began to examine and challenge long-held beliefs about her lack of competence. By the end of 16 weeks of treatment, she had obtained relief from her depression.

The BA component of CT is more affordable to implement than the full CT package (Richards, Ekers, et al., 2016) and has been found to perform as well as the full CT package does in relieving MDD and preventing relapse over a 2-year follow-up period (Dobson, Hollon, et al., 2008). Group versions of BA also are efficacious (Chan, Sun, et al., 2017), and the treatment has been successful in many different settings for clients from a diverse range of backgrounds (Oei & Dingle, 2008). These findings challenge the notion that people must directly modify their negative thinking to alleviate depression, suggesting instead that engaging in rewarding activities may be enough.

Psychological Treatment of Bipolar Disorder

Medication is a necessary part of treatment for bipolar disorder, but psychological treatments can supplement medication to help patients understand the disorder and treatments, learn to avoid symptom triggers, and to recover from the social and psychological problems caused by the episodes. Psychological treatment has been shown to reduce relapse and risk of hospitalization among those with bipolar disorder (Miklowitz, Efthimiou, et al., 2021).

Educating people about their illness is a common component of treating many disorders, including bipolar disorder and schizophrenia. **Psychoeducation** is designed to help people learn about the symptoms of the disorder, the expected time course of symptoms, the triggers for symptoms, and treatment strategies. Studies confirm that education about bipolar disorder can help people adhere to treatment with medications such as lithium (Colom, Vieta, et al., 2003). This is an important goal because as many as half of people being treated for bipolar disorder do not take medication consistently (Merikangas, et al., 2011). Psychoeducation can help clients understand the rationale for taking their medications even after symptoms dissipate and can foster hope that the medications will help. Most importantly, psychoeducation lowers the risk of relapse (Bond & Anderson, 2015).

Several other types of therapy are used to build skills, reduce symptoms, and decrease the risk of relapse for those with bipolar disorder. CT draws on the types of techniques that are used in MDD, with some additional content designed to address the early signs of manic episodes (Lam, Jones, & Hayward, 2010). One component of CT for bipolar disorder focuses on the broader goal of fostering a satisfying and hopeful life even if some symptoms persist (Jagfeld, Lobban, et al., 2021). Family-focused therapy aims to educate the family about the illness, enhance family communication, and develop problem-solving skills (Miklowitz & Goldstein, 1997). IPT has been adapted for bipolar disorder to include more focus on enhancing stability in social activity patterns.

CT, family-focused therapy, or IPT have each been found to be more helpful than collaborative care for those experiencing bipolar depression, and in a large trial, their effects on depression did not differ (Miklowitz, Otto, et al., 2007). Across dozens of randomized clinical trials, these psychotherapies appear to be more helpful for bipolar depressive symptoms than they are for the manic symptoms (Miklowitz, et al., 2021).

Biological Treatment of Mood Disorders

Antidepressants are the major biological treatments used for depression. As we will discuss, though, some depressions do not respond to antidepressants, and so we will describe three treatments that are considered when depression has not responded to an adequate dose of antidepressant: esketamine, electroconvulsive therapy, and transcranial magnetic stimulation. Then, we will turn to the medications used for bipolar disorder.

Medications for Depressive Disorders Drugs are the most common and best-researched treatment—biological or otherwise—for depressive disorders (and, as we will discuss, for bipolar disorders as well). Antidepressants provide relief from depressive symptoms more quickly than psychotherapy does. As shown in Table 5.6, there are six major categories of **antidepressant** drugs. **Monoamine oxidase inhibitors (MAOIs)** and **tricyclic antidepressants** were developed earlier than the others. **Selective serotonin reuptake inhibitors (SSRIs)** and **serotonin-norepinephrine reuptake inhibitors (SNRIs)** have become the more widely used antidepressants because they tend to produce fewer side effects, even though the effectiveness of all four classes of antidepressants is about the same (Depression Guidelines Panel, 1993; Gartlehner, Gaynes, et al., 2008). About 60% of people who take antidepressants report at least one side effect (Gartlehner, et al., 2008). Many stop taking the medications because of these side effects. Although most of the side effects are minor, the FDA requires manufacturers to include packaging information to warn people that SSRIs have been associated with suicidality among those younger than age 25, particularly early in treatment or after dosage increases (Fergusson, Doucette, et al., 2005).

In 2023, the FDA approved two new antidepressant approaches: a **serotonin 1A agonist** and an **N-methl D-asparate (NMDA) receptor**. The serotonin 1A agonist, Gepirone (Exxua), is expected to have fewer side effects compared to other antidepressant medications. Dextromethorphan-bupropion (Auvelity) is unique compared to other antidepressants in that it targets N-methyl D-aspartate (NMDA) receptors rather than directly targeting serotonin. It has been shown to provide more rapid relief from depression than other antidepressants, with symptoms beginning to decrease in the first week of treatment.

TABLE 5.6   **Most Commonly Used Medications for Treating Mood Disorders**

Antidepressants		
Category	**Generic Name (Examples)**	**Trade Name**
MAO inhibitors	tranylcypromine	Parnate
Tricyclic antidepressants	imipramine, amitriptyline	Tofranil, Elavil
Selective serotonin reuptake inhibitors (SSRIs)	fluoxetine, sertraline	Prozac, Zoloft
Serotonin–norepinephrine reuptake inhibitors (SNRIs)	venlafaxine, duloxetine	Effexor, Cymbalta
Serotonin 1A Agonist	gepirone	Exxua
N-methyl D-aspartate (NMDA) receptor antagonist	dextromethorphan-bupropion	Auvelity
Mood Stabilizers		
Category	**Generic Name (Examples)**	**Trade Name**
	lithium	Lithium
Anticonvulsants	divalproex sodium	Depakote
Antipsychotics	olanzapine	Zyprexa

More than 150 double-blind studies have been conducted on antidepressant medications for depressive disorders. In published studies, about 60% of people who complete treatment show at least a 50% drop in symptom levels and about 40–50% achieve full remission of their symptoms (Gartlehner, et al., 2008).

Treatment guidelines recommend continuing antidepressant medications, without lowering the dosage, for at least 6 months after a depressive episode ends—and longer if a person has experienced several episodes. Continuing antidepressants after remission lowers the risk of recurrence from approximately 40% to about 20% (Kato, Hori, et al., 2021).

Of concern is that published studies may overestimate how many people respond well to antidepressant medications. When pharmaceutical companies apply for either initial approval to market a medication or a change in the use of a medication in the United States, their relevant data must be filed with the Food and Drug Administration (FDA). One research team examined what happened to the data from antidepressant studies conducted between 1987 and 2004 (Turner, Matthews, et al., 2008). Of the 74 studies conducted, almost all of the studies with positive findings were published, whereas less than half of the neutral or negative findings were published.

In one analysis, researchers examined the data shared with the FDA for 232 studies of antidepressants for MDD (Stone, Yaseen, et al., 2022). Among those who took antidepressants, 88% of people showed at least some drop in symptoms, and about 25% showed large drops in their symptoms. Although this sounds very promising, people who took placebos showed similar improvements. Antidepressants showed only a minor benefit compared to the placebo, in that the average scores at the end of treatment for those who were taking antidepressants were only a little lower than those for people who took placebos (1.6 points on a scale ranging from 0 to 53). Overall, then, the published reports are much more positive than the data in the FDA files. In the FDA data set, antidepressants were more powerful for those with more severe depression. Some treatment guidelines suggest that clients with mild depression should be offered psychotherapy, unless they prefer medication (Kendrick, Pilling, et al., 2022).

Even among those with severe depression, though, many people still experience symptoms after taking an antidepressant. Will a different antidepressant be helpful for them? To answer this question, the STAR*D (Sequenced Treatment Alternatives to Relieve Depression) trial examined antidepressant responses among 3,671 patients (Rush, Trivedi, et al., 2006). In sharp contrast to the types of clean, non-comorbid depression histories reported in most medication trials, most of the patients enrolled in STAR*D suffered from chronic or recurrent depression, had comorbid psychiatric conditions, and had already received some (unsuccessful) treatment for the current episode. Patients were all started on citalopram (Celexa), an SSRI. If they did not respond to citalopram, they were offered (1) a choice of a different medication to replace the citalopram, (2) a chance to add a second medication to the citalopram, or (3) CT if they were willing to pay part of the cost. The researchers provided patients who did not respond to the second form of treatment with a third type of antidepressant and, if needed, even a fourth.

The findings were sobering. Only about one-third of patients achieved full symptom relief when treated with citalopram (Trivedi, Rush, et al., 2006). Among those who did not respond to citalopram, very few wanted to pay for CT and only 30.6% who received a second medication (either alone or as a supplement to citalopram) achieved remission. Even with the complex array of treatments offered, remission rates were low and relapse rates were high; only 43% of people achieved sustained recovery (Nelson, 2006).

When symptoms are not relieved by an antidepressant, several other biological treatment approaches can be considered. We turn to those next.

Biological Approaches for Depression That Is Not Relieved by an Antidepressant

The FDA has approved several medications as add-ons to an antidepressant. They have also approved two forms of transcranial magnetic stimulation. After discussing these options, we discuss electroconvulsive therapy (ECT), which is typically used only to treat MDD that has not responded to medication.

Among the several FDA-approved antidepressant add-on medications, one has received a large amount of attention: **Esketamine (Spravato)**. Esketamine is a nasal spray that is approved as an add-on to antidepressants only if two antidepressant trials have failed. It affects glutamate, and the effects are often observed within hours. Despite mixed evidence about the long-term efficacy from early trials (Food and Drug Administration [FDA], 2019), the combination of ongoing Spravato and oral antidepressant treatment has been shown to help reduce depression over

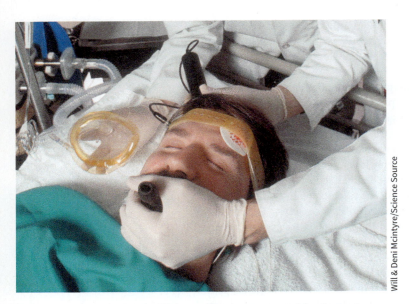

Will & Deni Mcintyre/Science Source

Electroconvulsive therapy (ECT) is an efficacious treatment for depression that has not responded to medication. Using unilateral shock and muscle relaxants has reduced undesirable side effects.

a 6-month period as compared to a placebo and oral antidepressant (Daly, Trivedi, et al., 2019).

In addition to add-on medications, two forms of repetitive transcranial magnetic stimulation (rTMS) are FDA-approved for adults whose depression has failed to respond to antidepressant treatment during the current episode. In the most typical rTMS approach, an electromagnetic coil is placed against the scalp, and intermittent pulses of magnetic energy are used to increase activity in the left dorsolateral prefrontal cortex. Typical treatment sessions last 30 to 60 minutes, with daily doses delivered for 10 to 30 days. In most randomized controlled trials, researchers have compared the treatment with a sham treatment in which the device is placed against the scalp at enough of an angle that the magnetic pulse will not increase brain activity. Multiple randomized controlled trials suggest that rTMS can help relieve treatment-resistant depression compared with the sham treatment (Sehatzadeh, Daskalakis, et al., 2019). Treatment gains persist at 1 year after treatment (Dunner, Aaronson, et al., 2014).

A new form of TMS, Stanford neuromodulation therapy (SNT), uses neuroimaging to accurately target the dorsolateral prefrontal cortex and delivers more powerful magnetic stimulation. The timing of treatments also differs from traditional rTMS, as SNT is delivered in 3-minute doses 10 times per day for 5 consecutive days. In one randomized controlled trials and three small trials, rapid and meaningful symptom reduction was observed within 5 days for more than 75% of people treated with SNT. Benefits lasted through a 1-month follow-up (Cole, Stimpson, et al., 2020), and researchers are now testing the durability of effects.

Perhaps the most controversial treatment for MDD is ECT. ECT entails deliberately inducing a momentary seizure by placing an electrode on the nondominant side of the forehead and passing a 70- to 130-volt current through the patient's brain. A muscle relaxant is given before the current is applied so that the patient sleeps through the procedure and the convulsive spasms of muscles are barely perceptible. The patient awakens a few minutes later, remembering nothing about the treatment. Typically, patients receive between 6 and 12 treatments, spaced several days apart.

Inducing a seizure is drastic treatment. Why should anyone agree to undergo such radical therapy? The answer is simple. ECT is more powerful than antidepressant medications for the treatment of depression (UK ECT Review Group, 2003), particularly when psychotic symptoms are present or the patient is an older adult (Van Diermen, Van Den Ameele, et al., 2018). Most professionals acknowledge that people undergoing ECT face some risks of short-term confusion and memory loss. It is common for patients to have no memory of the period during which they received ECT and sometimes for the weeks surrounding the procedure. For the vast majority of people, these problems remit quickly and cognition improves compared to levels before ECT (Obbels, Vansteelandt, et al., 2019; Semkovska & McLoughlin, 2010). Because of the initial cognitive side effects, clinicians typically resort to ECT only if less drastic treatments have failed. Given that suicide is a real possibility among people who are depressed, many experts regard the use of ECT after other treatments have failed as a responsible approach, and ECT continues to be a common approach.

Medications for Bipolar Disorder
Medications that reduce manic symptoms are called *mood-stabilizing medications*. Even though symptoms are usually decreased substantially with medications, most patients continue to experience at least mild manic and depressive symptoms. It is recommended that mood-stabilizing medications be used continually for the person's entire life (American Psychiatric Association [APA], 2002).

Lithium, a naturally occurring chemical element, was the first mood stabilizer identified. Up to 80% of people with bipolar I disorder experience at least a mild benefit from taking this drug (Prien & Potter, 1993). Across studies, 40% of people relapsed while taking lithium, compared with 60% while taking a placebo (Geddes, Burgess, et al., 2004), and relapse was less likely among those with relatively higher lithium levels (Hsu, Tsai, et al., 2022). Lithium also appears to decrease the severity of relapse. Because of possibly serious side effects, lithium must be prescribed and used very carefully. Lithium levels that are too high can be toxic, so patients taking lithium must have regular blood tests.

Two classes of medications other than lithium have been approved by the FDA for the treatment of acute mania: anticonvulsant (antiseizure) medications such as divalproex sodium (Depakote) and antipsychotic medications such as olanzapine (Zyprexa). These other treatments are recommended for people who are unable to tolerate lithium's side effects. Like lithium, these medications help reduce mania and, to some extent, depression.

Typically, lithium is used in combination with other medications. Because lithium takes effect gradually, treatment for acute mania often begins with both lithium and an antipsychotic medication, such as olanzapine, which has an immediate calming effect (Scherk, Pajonk, & Leucht, 2007).

The mood-stabilizing medications used to treat mania also help relieve depression. Nonetheless, many people continue to experience depression even when taking a mood-stabilizing medication such as lithium. For these people, an antidepressant medication is often added to the regimen, but two potential issues are associated with this practice. First, it is not clear whether antidepressants help reduce depression among persons who are already taking a mood stabilizer. Second, among people with bipolar disorder, antidepressants are related to a modest increase in the risk of a manic episode if taken without a mood stabilizer (Pacchiarotti, Bond, et al., 2013). The FDA has approved several atypical antipsychotic medications for the treatment of bipolar depression (McIntyre, Berk, et al., 2020).

Quick Summary

Many different treatments are available for depression. Cognitive therapy (CT), interpersonal psychotherapy (IPT), and behavioral activation (BA) therapy have all received support. The classes of antidepressants are similarly efficacious; SSRIs and SNRIs are more popular because they have fewer side effects than MAOIs and tricyclic antidepressants. In 2023, the FDA approved two new forms of antidepressants: a serotonin 1A receptor partial agonists expected to have fewer side effects, and an NMDA receptor antagonist that has been shown to provide rapid relief from symptoms. Antidepressant medications appear to be helpful for severe, but not mild, depression. When depression is not relieved by antidepressants, treatment options include an add-on medication, ECT, and rTMS.

Medication treatment is the first line of defense against bipolar disorder. The best-researched mood stabilizer is lithium, but anticonvulsants and antipsychotic medications are also effective mood stabilizers. Atypical antipsychotic medications also provide relief from bipolar depression. Some psychological treatments may help when offered as supplements to medications for the treatment of bipolar disorder. The best-validated approaches include psychoeducation, CT, family-focused therapy, and IPT. These psychological treatments help improve adherence to medication regimens, relieve symptoms of bipolar disorder, and reduce the risk of relapse and hospitalization.

5.4 Check Your Knowledge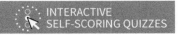

(Answers are at the end of the chapter.)
Circle all answers that apply.

1. Which of the following psychotherapies have obtained the strongest support from randomized controlled trials in the treatment of MDD?
    a. interpersonal psychotherapy
    b. behavioral activation therapy
    c. psychoanalytic therapy
    d. cognitive therapy

2. The most efficacious treatment for MDD with psychotic features is:

    a. Prozac

    b. any antidepressant medication

    c. ECT

    d. psychotherapy

3. Selective serotonin reuptake inhibitors (SSRIs) and serotonin–norepinephrine reuptake inhibitors (SNRIs) are more popular than older antidepressants because they:

    a. are more efficacious

    b. have fewer side effects

    c. are cheaper

Suicide

The effects of suicide on the surviving friends and relatives are profound. Survivors have an especially high mortality rate in the months after the suicide of a loved one (Mogensen, Möller, et al., 2016). In one population-based study of the offspring of more than 40,000 parents who died from suicide, researchers found that offspring who were younger than 18 at the time of the death showed a threefold greater risk of dying from suicide compared to the general population. This higher risk of suicide appeared to be specific, in that suicide rates were not elevated among offspring who were older at the time of parental suicide or whose parents died from causes other than suicide (Niederkrotenthaler, Fu, et al., 2012). Suicide is a profoundly distressing event.

We will focus on quantitative research on suicide, but those who study suicide learn from many different sources. A number of philosophers have written searchingly on the topic, including Descartes, Voltaire, Kant, Heidegger, and Camus. Increasingly, those who have survived suicide attempts have joined public advocacy and support movements to help inform this field, and their perspectives enhance our ability to understand factors that lead up to suicide attempts (see **https://www.livethroughthis.org**).

We begin by defining terms (see **Table 5.7**). **Suicidal ideation** refers to thoughts of killing oneself and is much more common than attempted suicide. **Suicide attempts** involve behaviors that are intended to cause death. Most suicide attempts do not result in death. **Suicide** involves behaviors that are intended to cause death and do so. **Nonsuicidal self-injury (NSSI)** involves behaviors that are meant to cause immediate bodily harm but are not intended to cause death (see **Focus on Discovery 5.3**).

Clinical Case

Steven

"Shannon Neal can instantly tell you the best night of her life: Tuesday, December 23, 2003, the Hinsdale Academy debutante ball. Her father, Steven Neal, a 54-year-old political columnist for The Chicago Sun-Times, *was in his tux, white gloves, and tie. 'My dad walked me down and took a little bow,' she said, and then the two of them goofed it up on the dance floor as they laughed and laughed. A few*

weeks later, Mr. Neal parked his car in his garage, turned on the motor and waited until carbon monoxide filled the enclosed space and took his breath, and his life, away."

"Those who knew him were blindsided. 'If I had just 30 seconds with him now,' Ms. Neal said of her father, 'I would want all these answers.'"

(Cohen, 2008, p. 1)

TABLE 5.7   Key Terms in the Study of Suicidality

Suicidal ideation: thoughts of killing oneself

Suicide attempt: behavior intended to kill oneself

Suicide: the act of intentionally ending one's own life

Nonsuicidal self-injury (NSSI): behaviors intended to cause immediate injury to oneself without intent to cause death

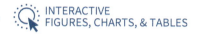

INTERACTIVE
FIGURES, CHARTS, & TABLES

Focus on Discovery 5.3

Nonsuicidal Self-Injury

Nonsuicidal self-injury (NSSI) is more common than previously thought, and contrary to previous thinking, it is practiced by many who do not have borderline personality disorder (Nock, 2010). Here we define this behavior and give some reasons it occurs.

There are two key issues to consider in defining NSSI. The first is that the person did not intend to cause death. The second is that the behavior is designed to cause immediate injury. Most commonly, people cut, hit, or burn their body (Franklin, Hessel, et al., 2010). When surveyed, 12–24% of adolescents report having engaged in NSSI (Muehlenkamp, Claes, et al., 2012), but the higher estimates may be due to overly broad definitions. For example, some studies will include "scratching to the point of bleeding," without ruling out poison ivy or other reasons people might be scratching. Without a doubt, though, there is a group of people who engage in serious attempts to hurt themselves. NSSI is most common in early adolescence, and most who try NSSI do so less than 10 times (Nock, 2009). Some people persist in self-injury, sometimes reporting more than 50 incidents of self-injury per year, and this persistent NSSI is a risk factor for suicidal ideation and behavior (Ribeiro, Franklin, et al., 2016). Social factors, emotionality, and self-critical beliefs influence whether people engage in repetitive NSSI.

Many different social influences may be involved in the onset and perpetuation of NSSI. Social modeling may influence whether NSSI begins—in one longitudinal study, adolescent girls were found to be more likely to try NSSI if their best friend had engaged in NSSI (Prinstein, Heilbron, et al., 2010). Among those who engage in NSSI, social stress may trigger the behavior in the moment. People who engage in self-injury often report that it is hard for them to manage their relationships and that their bouts of self-injury often occur after interpersonal rejection (Nock, Prinstein, & Sterba, 2009). After NSSI occurs, some may receive reinforcement for engaging in the behavior—friends and family members may respond by offering support or by reducing aggression. Hence, social factors may be important in initiation and maintenance of NSSI.

Problems with emotion also appear important (Nock, 2010). For some, the injury seems to help quell negative emotions, such as anger. Several studies provide evidence that those who are prone to self-injury experience more intense emotions and more intense psychophysiological responses to stress than others do (Nock & Mendes, 2008).

Even when social and emotional risk factors are present, why would people want to inflict pain on themselves? Self-critical beliefs are an important part of this puzzle. Some people report that self-injury satisfies a need for punishment that they believe they deserve. In a study in which people who engaged in NSSI were asked to record feelings, events, and NSSI incidents daily over time, feelings of self-hatred and of being rejected were common just before incidents of self-injury took place (Nock, Prinstein, & Sterba, 2009). These self-critical beliefs may help explain why people would engage in a behavior that involves pain. In one study, people who engage in NSSI were asked to take part in a laboratory experiment in which they were instructed to place their finger in a device that created pain by applying pressure; participants could choose the level and duration of the pressure. Those who engaged in NSSI chose to apply more pressure and left their finger in the device for longer than did those with no history of NSSI. Self-critical beliefs were highly related to this willingness to endure more pain (Glenn, Michel, et al., 2014). Hence, self-critical beliefs may provide a reason to engage in behaviors that cause pain, as a form of self-punishment. Consistent with this idea, when researchers provided a brief cognitive intervention designed to reduce self-critical beliefs, people who engage in NSSI became less willing to tolerate pain (Hooley & St. Germain, 2013).

Taken together, social modeling and reinforcement, difficulties in coping with emotions, and self-critical beliefs may drive NSSI. We will need to consider social, emotional, and cognitive factors to fully understand this complex behavioral pattern.

Epidemiology of Suicide and Suicide Attempts

Suicide rates may be grossly underestimated because the circumstances of some deaths are ambiguous; for example, a seemingly accidental death may have involved suicidal intentions. Nonetheless, worldwide, it is estimated that more than 700,000 people die from suicide each year (World Health Organization [WHO], 2021).

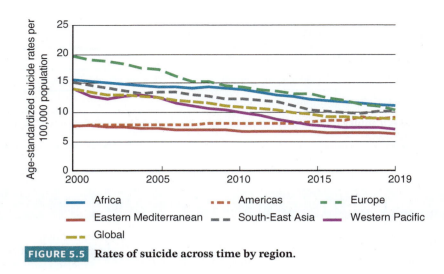

FIGURE 5.5 Rates of suicide across time by region.

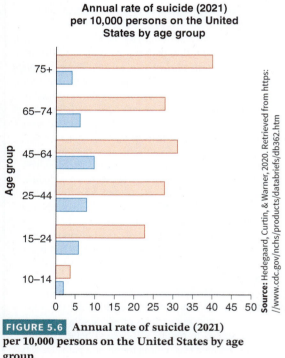

Annual rate of suicide (2021) per 10,000 persons on the United States by age group

Source: Hedegaard, Curtin, & Warner, 2020. Retrieved from https://www.cdc.gov/nchs/products/databriefs/db362.htm

FIGURE 5.6 Annual rate of suicide (2021) per 10,000 persons on the United States by age group.

Source: Hedegaard, Curtin, & Warner, 2020. https://www.cdc.gov/nchs/products/databriefs/db362.htm

Studies on the epidemiology of suicidality suggest the following:

- Worldwide, about 9% of people report suicidal ideation at least once in their lives, 2.5% have made at least one suicide attempt, and about 1 in every 100 deaths is due to suicide (WHO, 2021).
- Worldwide, men are 2.3 times more likely than women to kill themselves (WHO, 2021), and in the United States, men are 4 times more likely than women to kill themselves.
- Women are more likely than men to make suicide attempts that do not result in death (Nock & Mendes, 2008).
- Suicide rates have been decreasing over time in most regions of the world over the past 20 years (WHO, 2021), with the exception of the Americas and the Eastern Mediterranean region (see **Figure 5.5**). In the United States, suicide rates have increased by an estimated 36% over the past 20 years (Center for Disease Control [CDC], 2023).
- The rates of suicide for adolescents and children in the United States are increasing but are still below the rates for adults (see **Figure 5.6**). People age 85 and older have higher rates of suicide than any other age group (CDC, 2023). Because young people are less likely to die from other causes, suicide ranks as the second-leading cause of death among those aged 10 to 24 (Hedegaard, Curtin, & Warner, 2020).
- Suicide rates are higher in states, regions, and countries where more people own guns. Guns are by far the most common means of suicide in the United States, accounting for more than 50% of all suicides (CDC, 2023; Kochanek, Murphy, et al., 2016). People who live in homes with guns have more than twice the general risk of death by suicide (Azrael & Miller, 2016).
- Suicide rates are higher among Native American/Alaska Native and among non-Hispanic Whites compared to other ethnic groups in the United States (CDC, 2023).
- Suicide rates are elevated among LGBTQIA+ and particularly transgender individuals (CDC, 2023; Erlangsen, Jacobsen, et al., 2023).

Risk Factors for Suicide

Suicide is such a complex and multifaceted act that no single model can hope to explain it. Even our best current models leave many questions unanswered (Franklin, Ribeiro, et al., 2017).

Psychological Disorders   Many people who attempt suicide have a history of psychological disorder. Among those who have psychological symptoms severe enough to lead to hospitalization, about 6–8% of people diagnosed with MDD, with bipolar disorder, and with schizophrenia eventually die from suicide (Nordentoft, Mortensen, & Pedersen, 2011). Mood disorders, schizophrenia, impulse control disorders, substance use disorders, anxiety disorders, PTSD, and borderline personality disorder are each related to a higher-than-average risk of suicide attempt (Chesney, Goodwin, & Fazel, 2014; Nock, Hwang, et al., 2009; Paris, 2019). Although understanding the effects of psychological disorders on suicidality is extremely important, most people with psychological disorders do not die from suicide. Suicide is discussed in this chapter because many people with mood disorders have suicidal thoughts, and some engage in suicidal behaviors (Nock, et al., 2009).

Neurobiological Factors   Twin studies suggest that heritability may explain about half of the variance in suicide attempts and in suicide deaths (Edwards, Ohlsson, et al., 2021). PET imaging indicates disruptions of the serotonin system are more likely to be present among people with a history of a suicide attempt than among people with depression who have not made a suicide attempt, despite some nonreplications (Bartlett, Zanderigo, et al., 2023).

Social Influences   Economic and social events have been shown to influence suicide rates. For example, across the past 100 years, suicide rates have been shown to increase modestly during economic recessions (Luo, Florence, et al., 2011).

Suicide clusters, in which a group of suicides or suicide attempts occur closer together in time and space than would normally be expected, are another indicator that there are social influences on suicide. Sometimes, a cluster of suicides occurs after media reports of the suicide of a celebrity (Jeong, Shin, et al., 2012). In one example of this effect, suicides rose 12% in the month after Marilyn Monroe's suicide (Phillips, 1985). Across hundreds of studies, media coverage of a celebrity suicide has been shown to be much more likely to spark an increase in suicidality than coverage of a noncelebrity suicide (Stack, 2000). Media reports of natural deaths of famous people are not followed by increases in suicide, suggesting that it is not grief per se that is the influential factor (Phillips, 1974).

When clusters occur, they tend to grab attention and become a focus of media coverage. Suicide clusters, though, are rare—they appear to account for less than 2% of suicide deaths. Nonetheless, clusters are more common in schools, where they may account for up to 5% of adolescent deaths from suicide. Clusters are also more common in prisons, in the military, among groups living in remote rural regions, and among indigenous groups. Because the chances of cluster suicides are thought to be worsened when media accounts are overly detailed, appear frequently, or glamorize the suicide (Robinson, Pirkis, & O'Connor, 2016), guidelines for reporters suggest providing mental health resource information rather than publicizing details such as the method or the location. Reporters are also encouraged not to normalize suicide by describing rates as epidemic or growing (Montgomery, 2018).

Social factors that are more directly relevant to the individual are also powerful predictors of suicidality. For example, being divorced or widowed elevates suicide risk more than fourfold. In a large-scale study, a history of multiple physical and sexual assaults was found to be related to suicide attempts (Nock & Kessler, 2006). Joiner (2005) has suggested that suicidality is closely tied to two key issues: a perceived sense of burden to others and a lack of belongingness. According to this theory, the sensation of being alone, without others to turn to, is a major factor in the development of suicidality and this effect is amplified when people feel as though they are a burden to others. Dozens of studies show that people who experience suicidal ideation endorse high levels of burdensomeness and lack of belonging (Chu, Buchman-Schmitt, et al., 2017). Consistent with this idea, adolescents often describe social isolation, interpersonal conflict, and peer victimization as triggers of suicidal behavior, and peer ratings of interpersonal status have been found to predict the onset of suicidality over a 2-year period (Prinstein, et al., 2010). Conversely, many studies suggest the protective value of connectedness, whether measured by marital or parenting status, quality of family relationships, social support, quality of one's relationship with a therapist, or social roles that provide a sense of purpose

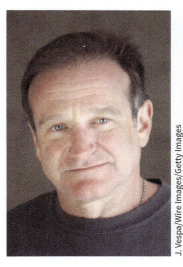

J. Vespa/Wire Images/Getty Images

Robin Williams, a highly acclaimed actor and comedian, died from suicide in 2014 (Williams, 2016). Researchers have shown that suicide rates increase in the month after a celebrity dies from suicide. These findings provide evidence that the social environment is an influence on suicide.

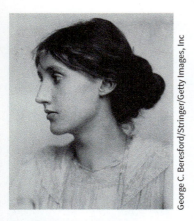

George C. Beresford/Stringer/Getty Images, Inc

English novelist and critic
Virginia Woolf (1882–1941).

On March 28, 1941, at the age of 59, Virginia Woolf drowned herself in the river near her Sussex home. Two suicide notes were found in the house, similar in content; one may have been written 10 days earlier, and it is possible that she may have made an unsuccessful attempt then, for she returned from a walk soaking wet, saying that she had fallen. The first was addressed to her sister Vanessa and the second to her husband, Leonard. To him, she wrote:

Dearest, I feel certain I am going mad again. I feel we can't go through another of those terrible times. And I shan't recover this time. I begin to hear voices, and I can't concentrate. So I am doing what seems the best thing to do. You have given me the greatest possible happiness. You have been in every way all that anyone could be. I don't think two people could have been happier till this terrible disease came. I can't fight it any longer. I know that I am spoiling your life, that without me you could work. And you will I know. You see I can't even write this properly. I can't read. What I want to say is I owe all the happiness of my life to you. You have been entirely patient with me and incredibly good. I want to say that—everybody knows it. If anybody could have saved me it would have been you. Everything has gone from me but the certainty of your goodness. I can't go on spoiling your life any longer. I don't think two people could have been happier than we have been. V.

Quoted from pp. 400–401, Briggs, J. (2005). Virginia Woolf: An Inner Life. Orlando, Fl: Harcourt, Inc.

and meaning (Zareian & Klonsky, 2020). Taken together, social influences are important to understanding suicidality.

Psychological Influences   Almost all individuals who have attempted suicide and yet lived to be interviewed describe wanting to escape from a sense of unbearable pain at the time of their attempt (Wenzel & Spokas, 2014). What factors lead a person to reach that point at which life seems so unbearable?

Suicidal ideation appears tied to the sense that one has been defeated and that the problems that led to defeat seem inescapable (Dhingra, Boduszek, & O'Connor, 2015). For some, inability to engage in effective problem solving may cause problems to seem inescapable. People who express suicidal ideation not only describe themselves as poor problem solvers but also have more difficulty than others in solving puzzles presented to them in laboratory experiments (Wenzel & Spokas, 2014). Problem-solving deficits also predict suicide attempts prospectively (Dieserud, Roysamb, et al., 2003). In keeping with the sense of defeat and lack of solutions to key problems, hopelessness—the expectation that life will be no better in the future than it is in the present—is strongly tied to suicidal ideation in both cross-sectional and longitudinal studies (May & Klonsky, 2016; Wenzel & Spokas, 2014).

Differentiating Ideation from Action   Although many people think about suicide, relatively few engage in suicidal actions. A key question, then, is which variables help explain suicidal behavior among those who think about suicide (Klonsky, May, & Saffer, 2016). It is much harder to predict suicidal behavior than it is to predict ideation (May & Klonsky, 2016). Social and psychological variables including lack of belonging, burdensomeness, and hopelessness are closely tied to suicidal ideation but provide little additional information about which people with ideation are likely to engage in suicidal behavior (Chu, et al., 2017; May & Klonsky, 2016). A growing body of work suggests that, among those who are experiencing suicidal ideation, people who have a blunted fear of bodily harm and death are more likely to engage in suicidal action (Klonsky, May, & Saffer, 2016).

Preventing Suicide

Many people worry that talking about suicide will make it more likely to happen. But researchers have shown that it is helpful to talk about suicide in an open manner (Dazzi, Gribble, et al., 2014). Most people who think about suicide are ambivalent, and talking can relieve the sense of isolation, as well as help identify other ways to relieve the pain that is driving the suicidality. Among those who attempt suicide but do not die, 80% report that within the next 2 days they are either glad to be alive or ambivalent about whether they want to die (Henriques, Wenzel, et al., 2005).

Treating the Associated Psychological Disorder   One approach to suicide prevention builds on our knowledge that most people who kill themselves are suffering from a psychological disorder. Thus, when Beck's cognitive approach successfully lessens a patient's depression, that patient's suicidal risk is also reduced.

Medications for psychological disorders reduce the risk of suicidality (Angst, Stassen, et al., 2002). Specifically, lithium reduces suicidality among people with bipolar disorder (Cipriani, Pretty, et al., 2005). Among people who have been diagnosed with depressive disorders, ECT and antidepressants reduce suicidality (Bruce, Ten Have, et al., 2004; Kellner, Fink, et al., 2005). Ketamine has been shown to provide same-day relief from suicidal ideation (Wilkinson, Ballard, et al., 2018). Antipsychotic medication can reduce the risk of suicide attempts among people with schizophrenia (Meltzer, 2003). These effects, though, are small enough that it is important to treat suicidality directly.

Treating Suicidality Directly

Several approaches directly target suicidal thoughts and behavior. The three that have been most carefully researched are cognitive behavior therapy (CBT), dialectical behavior therapy (DBT), and collaborative assessment and management of suicidality (CAMS). Let's review the principles and evidence for each.

CBT encompasses a set of strategies to prevent suicide. Early in treatment, therapists and clients collaborate to develop a safety plan of coping strategies that could be used if a suicidal crisis occurs. Therapists help clients understand the emotions and thoughts that trigger suicidal urges. Therapists work with clients to challenge their negative thoughts and to provide new ways to tolerate emotional distress. They also help clients solve the problems they are facing. The goal is to improve problem solving and social support and thereby to reduce the feelings of hopelessness that often precede these episodes.

In a meta-analysis of 28 treatment trials, adults who received CBT reported less hopelessness, suicidal ideation, and suicidal behavior than those who received no treatment or other forms of treatment (Tarrier, Taylor, & Gooding, 2008). Among those who have tried to kill themselves, CBT has been found to halve the risk of a future attempt associated with treatment as usually offered in the community (Brown, Ten Have, et al., 2005). CBT also has been found to reduce NSSI (Hawton, Witt, et al., 2016). Even brief interventions can make a difference. In one study, researchers randomly assigned patients who were seen in emergency rooms with suicide-related concerns to receive either standard care or a safety intervention that included reviewing possible coping plans and strategies, with at least two telephone follow-ups. Those who received the safety intervention showed 45% fewer suicidal behaviors in the next 6 months than did those in the control condition (Stanley, Brown, et al., 2018).

DBT is a version of CBT that was developed specifically for patients engaging in recurrent self-harm. It has been used widely in the treatment of borderline personality disorder (see Chapter 15). The treatment integrates Eastern philosophy and techniques, such as mindfulness and acceptance, with more traditional CBT strategies focused on emotion regulation, through a combination of individual and group therapy (Linehan, 1993). Early in the treatment, the therapist and client focus on helping the client identify triggers for self-harm and on creating a safety plan for responding to self-harm urges. Six studies have now shown that DBT can provide more relief from suicidal ideation or behavior than does treatment as usual (Chang, Jager-Hyman, et al., 2016).

CAMS is an overarching therapeutic framework for working with suicidal clients. CAMS therapists strive to understand the client's perspective on the factors that drive their suicidal ideation. CAMS provides an outline that therapists and clients can use to identify possible drivers of suicidal thoughts and then flexibly draw from a range of techniques to target those concerns. Several studies have shown that patients assigned to receive 6–8 weeks of CAMS treatment exhibit declines in suicidal ideation, and some work suggests that those declines are larger than declines shown among patients engaged in treatment as usual (Jobes, Comtois, et al., 2016; Pistorello, Jobes, et al., 2020; Ryberg, Zahl, et al., 2019). However, CAMS has not been found to reduce suicidal behavior specifically.

Professional organizations such as the American Psychiatric Association, the National Association of Social Workers, and the American Psychological Association charge their members with protecting people from suicide even if doing so requires breaking the confidentiality of the therapist–patient relationship. Therapists are expected to take reasonable precautions when they learn a patient is suicidal. One approach to keeping such patients alive is to hospitalize them as a short-term means of keeping them safe until they can begin to consider ways of improving their lives.

Broader Approaches to Suicide Prevention

One of the most common approaches to suicide prevention is to offer hotlines. In 2022, a national suicide hotline number, 988, was created, so that people could phone, text, or chat from anywhere in the United States to receive free, anonymous support 24 hours a day. In the first year of operation, the service received 2.6 million calls, over 740,000 chats, and more than 600,000 texts, indicating a substantial need.

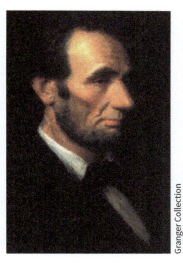

Granger Collection

After a broken engagement at age 31, Abraham Lincoln developed symptoms of depression so severe that his friends feared he would hurt himself, and they removed any sharp objects from his room. "I am now the most miserable man living," he confessed. "Whether I shall ever be better I cannot tell; I awfully forebode I shall not. To remain as I am is impossible; I must die or be better" (cited in Goodwin, 2003).

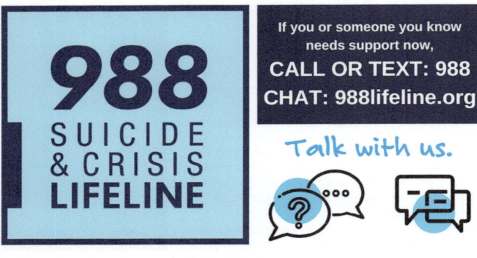

The National suicide hotline, 988, was launched in July 2022.

It is exceedingly difficult to do controlled research on suicide prevention because the base rates are so low. One approach has been to study suicide prevention within the military, where rates of suicide are much higher than in the general population (Schoenbaum, Kessler, et al., 2014), programs can be offered to the entire community, and outcomes can be tracked carefully. In one study, researchers examined suicide rates in the Air Force before and after implementation of a comprehensive suicide prevention program. The program provided training for military leaders and for soldiers to encourage and destigmatize seeking help, to normalize the experience of distress, and to promote effective coping. After the program, rates of death by suicide in the military units dropped by 25% (Knox, Pflanz, et al., 2010). It appears that prevention efforts can reduce suicide rates.

Beyond prevention programs that target high-risk individuals, another approach to suicide prevention is **means restriction**, which involves making highly lethal methods less available. This idea draws from the well-established findings that many suicidal urges are fleeting and that people often make a suicide attempt very quickly without much forethought. In one study, researchers interviewed people within 3 days of a hospitalization for a suicide attempt. Participants were asked to think back to the suicidal thought that had started the episode. Half the participants reported that they had made their suicide attempt within 10 minutes after the suicidal thought entered their mind (Deisenhammer, Ing, et al., 2009). Given this evidence, any type of delay or barrier in gaining access to means may help save lives.

Means restriction strategies often involve large-scale changes across a geographical region. Reduction in the use of coal ovens in Britain provides one example of how a national reduction in availability of a method can make a difference. For decades, the most common ovens in Britain relied on coal gas. Coal gas was cheap and widely available, but before it was burned, it released levels of carbon monoxide that were so high as to be deadly if one put one's head into a coal gas oven for even a couple of minutes. By the late 1950s, about 2,500 suicides per year (almost half of the suicides in Britain) were occurring in this manner. The British government phased out coal gas, and by the 1970s, almost no coal gas ovens remained. Over the course of those years, the British suicide rate dropped by a third, and it has remained at this lower level.

Several means restriction strategies have been used to reduce suicide, with positive effects. For example, erecting a barrier on a bridge so that people cannot jump off the bridge on a moment's impulse can be highly successful (Beautrais, Gibb, et al., 2009). In Israel, higher rates of suicide were noticed among those in the Israel Defense Force during the weekends when soldiers returned home with their guns. In response to this discovery, soldiers were required to leave their guns on the base when they returned home. With this change, rates of suicide dropped by 40% (Lubin, Werbeloff, et al., 2010). Reducing the lethality of formulations and the availability of drugs and poisons has also been shown to reduce suicide deaths (Chen, Wu, et al., 2016). Hence, these targeted public health approaches can have powerful effects.

The Golden Gate Bridge is one of the most popular locations in the world for suicide; more than 1,700 people have jumped to their death from its heights. Drawing on evidence showing that means restriction programs can be highly effective, a suicide barrier was installed on the bridge.

vicm/iStock/Getty Images

5.5 Check Your Knowledge

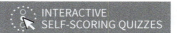

INTERACTIVE SELF-SCORING QUIZZES

(Answers are at the end of the chapter.)

True or false?

1. Men have higher rates of suicide than women.

2. Adolescents have higher rates of suicide than adults.

3. Suicide rates increase after media reports of both noncelebrity and celebrity suicides.

Answer the following question.

4. What psychological factor seems to buffer against suicidal action among those who are experiencing suicidal ideation?

Summary

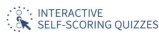

INTERACTIVE SELF-SCORING QUIZZES
Chapter 5 Practice Quiz

Clinical Descriptions and Epidemiology of Depressive Disorders

- Depressive disorders include major depressive disorder (MDD) and persistent depressive disorder, along with the newer diagnoses of premenstrual dysphoric disorder and disruptive mood dysregulation disorder.
- MDD is episodic, and recurrence is common.
- Persistent depressive disorder is characterized by low levels of symptoms that last at least 2 years.
- MDD is one of the most common psychological disorders, affecting at least 16.2% of people during their lifetime.

Clinical Descriptions and Epidemiology of Bipolar Disorders

- Bipolar disorders include bipolar I disorder, bipolar II disorder, and cyclothymia. Bipolar I disorder is defined by mania. Bipolar II disorder is defined by hypomania and episodes of depression. Cyclothymic disorder is characterized by low levels of manic and depressive symptoms that last at least 2 years.
- Bipolar I disorder and bipolar II disorder are episodic. Recurrence is even more common in these disorders than it is in major depressive disorder.
- Bipolar I disorder affects less than 1% of the population. Estimates of the prevalence of bipolar II disorder are varied (from 0.4% to 2%). Cyclothymic disorder may affect 4% of the population.

Influences on Mood Disorders

- Bipolar disorder is strongly heritable, and MDD is somewhat heritable.
- Bipolar disorders and unipolar depression are tied to elevated activity of the amygdala and the anterior cingulate, to diminished activity in regions of the prefrontal cortex, and to altered activity in the hippocampus during tasks that involve emotion and emotion regulation. Bipolar disorder is related to heightened activity of the striatum and orbitofrontal cortex in response to reward in some studies, in contrast with the low striatal activity in response to reward among those with depression.
- Pro-inflammatory cytokines are sometimes elevated in people with unipolar depression and those with bipolar disorder.

- Sleep and circadian problems are common in depression and bipolar disorder and can predict worsening depression and mania over time.
- Socioenvironmental models focus on the role of childhood adversity, recent negative life events (and particularly negative interpersonal life events), lack of social support, marital discord, and expressed emotion as triggers for episodes.
- The personality trait that is most closely related to depression is neuroticism. Neuroticism predicts the onset of depression.
- Influential cognitive theories include Beck's cognitive theory, hopelessness theory, and rumination theory. All posit that depression can be caused by cognitive factors, but the nature of the cognitive factors differs across theories. Beck's theory focuses on the cognitive triad, negative schemas, and information-processing biases. According to hopelessness theory, beliefs that a life event will have stable global consequences can instill a sense of hopelessness, which in turn results in depression. Rumination theory focuses on the negative effects of repetitively dwelling on the reasons for a sad mood. Prospective evidence is available for each model.
- Biological and behavioral measures indicate that reward sensitivity is often dampened among people who are depressed and among their first-degree relatives. Reward sensitivity can be suppressed by stress but can also predict greater reactivity to stress.
- Psychological theories of depression in bipolar disorder are similar to those proposed for unipolar depression. Some researchers have suggested that manic symptoms arise because of dysregulation in the reward system in the brain. Mania can be triggered by life events involving goal attainment.

Treatment of Mood Disorders

- Several psychological therapies are effective for depression, including interpersonal psychotherapy, cognitive therapy, and behavioral activation therapy.
- Psychoeducation, family therapy, interpersonal psychotherapy, and cognitive therapy are helpful adjuncts to medication for bipolar disorder.
- Antidepressant drugs (tricyclics, MAOIs, selective serotonin reuptake inhibitors, serotonin–norepinephrine reuptake inhibitors, a serotonin receptor 1A partial agonist, and a N-methyl D-aspartate (NMDA) receptor antagonist) have been shown to

be helpful in lifting depression, particularly when symptoms are severe. Add-on medications and two forms of repetitive transcranial magnetic stimulation are FDA-approved for people with antidepressant-resistant depression. Electroconvulsive shock has proved its worth in lifting depression.

- Lithium is the best-researched treatment for bipolar disorder, but antipsychotic and anticonvulsant medications also help decrease manic symptoms. Antipsychotic medications are FDA-approved for the treatment of bipolar depression.

Suicide

- Rates of suicide have been increasing in the United States over time while declining in many other countries. Men, older adults, Native Americans and non-Hispanic Whites, and sexual minorities are at higher risk for suicide than are other groups. Gun ownership is a risk factor for suicide.

- Many people who make suicide attempts meet diagnostic criteria for psychological disorders. Suicide is at least partially heritable,

and neurobiological models focus on serotonin. Social influences are also important: Sociocultural events such as celebrity suicides and economic recessions can influence rates of suicide in the population, and a lack of social belonging is a robust predictor of suicide. Psychological influences on suicidal ideation include poor problem solving and hopelessness. Among those with suicidal ideation, suicidal action appears related to a lack of fear of bodily harm.

- Several approaches have been taken to suicide prevention. For people with a psychological disorder, medications and psychotherapies targeting those symptoms help reduce suicidality. It is also important to address suicidality more directly. CBT and DBT can help reduce suicidal ideation and behavior, and CAMS can help reduce suicidal ideation. Research suggests that suicide prevention can work. Public health interventions that reduce the availability of means for suicide, such as guns, can have powerful effects.

Answers to Check Your Knowledge Questions

5.1 1. five; 2. 16.2; 3. Chronicity; MDD is diagnosed on the basis of five symptoms lasting at least 2 weeks; persistent depressive disorder requires only two symptoms, but they must be present for 2 years (or 1 year in children and adolescents).

5.2 1. mania; 2. Bipolar I disorder is diagnosed on the basis of manic episodes, which are more severe than the hypomanic episodes that are the core criterion for bipolar II disorder.

5.3 1. c. 0.37, 0.93; 2. d. amygdala; 3. Beck's model of cognitive schemas guiding information-processing errors in attention and memory that sustain the negative cognitive triad, Alloy's model of global and stable attributions guiding hopelessness, and Nolen-Hoeksema's theory of rumination in which tendencies to chew on negative events can trigger depression.

5.4 1. a,b,d; 2. c; 3. b.

5.5 1. True; 2. False; 3. False; 4. fear of bodily harm

Key Terms

Anxiety Disorders

LEARNING GOALS

1. Define the emotions of anxiety and fear and their adaptive benefits.

2. Describe the clinical features of the anxiety disorders, the prevalence of the anxiety disorders, and how the anxiety disorders co-occur with each other.

3. Discuss how gender and culture influence the prevalence of anxiety disorders.

4. Explain commonalities in causes across the anxiety disorders.

5. Describe the influences on the expression of specific anxiety disorders.

6. Discuss psychological and medication treatment approaches that are common across the anxiety disorders and how psychological treatment approaches are modified for the specific anxiety disorders.

Clinical Case

Jenny

Jenny was a 23-year-old student completing her first year of medical school. The year had been a hard one, not only because of the long hours and academic challenges of medical school but also because her mother had been diagnosed with cancer. One day, while attending rounds, Jenny found herself feeling lightheaded and dizzy. During rounds, the attending physician would ask students to diagnose and explain a given case, and on that day, Jenny became extremely worried about whether she would be able to answer these questions when her turn came. As she thought about all this, her heart began to pound, and her palms began to sweat. Overwhelmed by fear and a deep sense that something was horribly wrong, she abruptly fled the room without explaining her departure.

Later in the day, she wanted to explain leaving rounds but could not think of a good way to describe the situation to the attending physician. That night, she could not sleep, wondering what had happened and worrying about whether it would happen again. She worried about how this would affect her ability not only to take part in rounds but also to perform well in other roles, such as leading a small research group and meeting with other medical staff and clients. One week later, while driving to school, she experienced a sudden attack of similar symptoms, which forced her to pull off to the side of the road. She took the day off from school. Over the next several weeks, she began to avoid public situations as much as possible because she feared being humiliated by the return of these symptoms. She avoided study groups and going out with friends, and she turned down opportunities for training that involved public interviews of patients. She resigned from the choir that she had enjoyed being a part of for several years. Despite her withdrawal, she experienced three more attacks, each in an unexpected situation. She began to think that maybe medical school was a poor choice for her because she had such deep fears about experiencing another attack during rounds. After she read about panic disorder in one of her textbooks, she decided to visit a psychologist. The psychologist confirmed that she was experiencing panic disorder, and they started cognitive behavioral therapy.

Very few of us go through even a week of our lives without experiencing anxiety or fear. In this chapter, we focus on a group of disorders called **anxiety disorders**. Both anxiety and fear play a significant role in these disorders, so we begin with a description of these two emotions. After discussing normative experiences of anxiety and fear, we turn to the core clinical features of anxiety disorders and the outcomes of anxiety disorders before discussing specific anxiety disorders. Then, we turn to the common influences of anxiety disorders as a group. We then describe influences that shape whether a specific anxiety disorder develops. As with most disorders, many different influences contribute to the development of anxiety

VIDEO CONTENT
Anxiety Disorders

disorders. Therefore, throughout our discussions of causes we examine various perspectives, including genetic, neurobiological, personality, cognitive, and behavioral research. Finally, we consider the treatment of the anxiety disorders. We describe commonalities in the psychological treatment of various anxiety disorders, and then we describe how these general treatment principles are modified to address specific anxiety disorders. Finally, we discuss biological treatments of anxiety disorders.

Emotions of Anxiety and Fear

Anxiety is defined as apprehension over an anticipated problem. In contrast, **fear** is defined as a reaction to immediate danger. Fear tends to be about a threat that is happening now, whereas anxiety tends to be about a future threat. Thus, a person facing a bear experiences fear, whereas a college student concerned about the possibility of unemployment after graduation experiences anxiety.

Both anxiety and fear can involve arousal, or sympathetic nervous system activity (see **Focus on Discovery 2.1** for an overview of the sympathetic nervous system). Anxiety often involves moderate arousal, and fear involves higher arousal. At the low end, a person experiencing anxiety may feel no more than restless energy and physiological tension; at the high end, a person experiencing fear may sweat profusely, breathe rapidly, and feel an overpowering urge to run.

Anxiety and fear are not necessarily "bad"; in fact, both are adaptive. Anxiety helps us notice and plan for future threats—that is, to increase our preparedness, to help us avoid potentially dangerous situations, and to think through potential problems before they happen. "Without anxiety, little would be accomplished. ... The performance of athletes, entertainers, executives, artisans, and students would suffer; creativity would diminish; crops might not be planted" (Barlow, 2004, p. 12). In laboratory studies first conducted 100 years ago and since verified many times over, a small degree of anxiety has been found to improve performance on laboratory tasks (Yerkes & Dodson, 1908). Ask anyone with extreme test anxiety, though, and that person will tell you that too much anxiety interferes with performance. Anxiety, then, provides a classic example of an inverse U-shaped curve when plotted against performance—an absence of anxiety is a problem, a little anxiety is adaptive, and a lot of anxiety is detrimental.

Fear is fundamental for "fight-or-flight" reactions—that is, fear triggers rapid changes in the sympathetic nervous system to prepare the body for escape or fighting. In the right circumstance, fear saves lives. (Imagine a person who faces a bear and doesn't marshal energy to run quickly!) In some anxiety disorders, though, the fear system seems to misfire—a person experiences fear even when no danger is present in the environment. This is most vividly seen in panic attacks, which we will discuss later in this chapter.

Quick Summary

Anxiety is defined as apprehension over an anticipated problem, and fear is defined as a reaction to immediate danger. Anxiety helps us prepare for future threats and motivates us to think through potential problems before they happen. Fear drives a fight-or-flight response. The anxiety disorders involve excessive amounts of anxiety and fear.

6.1 Check Your Knowledge

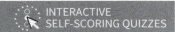 INTERACTIVE
SELF-SCORING QUIZZES

(Answers are at the end of the chapter.)
True or false?

1. Both anxiety and fear play a significant role in anxiety disorders.

2. Fear often involves moderate arousal, and anxiety involves higher arousal.

3. Anxiety and fear are usually adaptive.

4. Describe the inverse U-shaped curve of anxiety.

Clinical Descriptions of the Anxiety Disorders

In this chapter, we examine the major anxiety disorders included in DSM-5-TR: specific phobias, social anxiety disorder, panic disorder, agoraphobia, and generalized anxiety disorder (see **Table 6.1** for key features of each of these). All of these anxiety disorders involve excessively high anxiety, and with the exception of generalized anxiety disorder, all involve tendencies to experience unusually intense fear (Kotov, Krueger, et al., 2017). **Read More About It 6.1** provides a glimpse of how intense these feelings of anxiety and fear can be.

Anxiety disorders as a group are the most common type of psychological disorder. For example, in the NCS-R study of over 8,000 adults in the United States, about 28% of people endorsed having experienced symptoms at some point during their lives that met criteria for diagnosis of an anxiety disorder (Kessler, Petukhova, et al., 2012). See **Table 6.2** for the prevalence estimates for specific anxiety disorders. A prevalence estimate of more than a quarter of the adult population may seem very high, but this may be an underestimate. In the NCS-R study, researchers conducted only one diagnostic interview to cover anxiety that occurred at any time during participants' lives. Research indicates that many people forget about their anxiety symptoms over the years, particularly if symptoms were short-lived (Moffitt, Caspi, et al., 2010). This indicates that prevalence estimates of 28% are likely too low.

The onset of anxiety disorders tends to be early in life. In a study of people who had developed anxiety disorders by age 32, more than a third had met criteria for an anxiety disorder before the age of 15, and about two-thirds had met the criteria for an anxiety disorder by age 21 (Gregory, Caspi, et al., 2007). Those who develop anxiety disorders tend to experience chronic or intermittent symptoms. In a 9-year follow-up of people diagnosed with anxiety disorders, only 10–20% showed consistent remission of their symptoms across the 9 years (Solis, van Hemert, et al., 2021).

Anxiety disorders are very costly to society and to people with the disorders. Anxiety disorders were ranked as the eighth leading cause of medical disability worldwide in 2019 (Ferrari & GBD 2019 Mental Disorders Collaborators, 2022). Those with anxiety disorders have twice the rate of unemployment of other people. While anxiety disorders predict unemployment over time, it is also the case that unemployment predicts increased risk of developing an anxiety disorder (Mojtabai, Stuart, et al., 2015). These disorders are related to an elevated risk of marital discord (Whisman, 2007), more than a fourfold higher risk of suicide attempts (Nock, Hwang, et al., 2010), and high risk of developing medical conditions (Scott, Lim, et al., 2016; Stein, Aguilar-Gaxiola, et al., 2014). Each disorder, though, is defined by a different set of symptoms related to anxiety or fear (see Table 6.1 for a brief summary). In the next sections, we discuss the symptoms of the specific anxiety disorders.

TABLE 6.1   **Overview of the Major Anxiety Disorders**   INTERACTIVE FIGURES, CHARTS, & TABLES

Disorder	Description
Specific phobia	Fear of objects or situations that is out of proportion to any real danger
Social anxiety disorder	Fear of unfamiliar people or social scrutiny
Panic disorder	Anxiety about recurrent panic attacks
Agoraphobia	Anxiety about being in places where escaping or getting help would be difficult if anxiety symptoms occurred
Generalized anxiety disorder	Uncontrollable worry

Read More About It 6.1

My Age of Anxiety: Fear, Hope, Dread, and the Search for Peace of Mind

In this book, Scott Stossel, the editor of *The Atlantic* magazine, writes about his personal history of anxiety, provides a quick tour of the history of these syndromes, and succinctly recaps major themes that emerge in the thousands of articles per year published on the topic of anxiety. The author has plenty of experience to draw on—beyond his own anxiety, his great-grandfather was hospitalized for anxiety; his mother struggled with worries, phobias, and panic attacks; and his younger sister experiences intense anxiety. He shares his own experience of anxiety, writing:

> *On ordinary days, doing ordinary things—reading a book, lying in bed, talking on the phone, sitting in a meeting, playing tennis—I have thousands of times been stricken by a pervasive sense of existential dread and been beset by nausea, vertigo, shaking, and a panoply of other physical symptoms. In these instances, I have sometimes been convinced that death, or something somehow worse, was imminent.* (Stossel, 2014, p. 2)

In another passage, he describes the range of worries that haunted him, including his health, his family members' health, finances, work, his car, his house, and even "the encroachment of old age and the inevitability of death ... everything and nothing." His symptoms extended far beyond the worries of generalized anxiety disorder, though. He describes the physical symptoms of panic disorder; phobias of enclosed spaces, heights, fainting, airplanes, germs, and cheese; and the social anxiety symptom of fear of public speaking. He shares how these symptoms interfered with daily life, as his anxiety would surface during exams, job interviews, public lectures, plane flights, car rides, and dates. At times, his anxiety led him to flee the scene at critically important moments, including leaving the stage during his own presentations.

His symptoms started early in his childhood with fears about being separated from his parents, and by grade school, his symptoms escalated to headaches and stomach aches, germ phobia, separation anxiety, and phobia of vomiting. When he was 10 years old, his parents took him to see a psychiatrist, the first of many rounds of treatment over the years. Nonetheless, anxiety continued to hound him during adolescence as he struggled with sports and dating.

One of the many ways he pursued treatment and coping strategies was by visiting the highly regarded Center for Anxiety and Related Disorders at Boston University. He describes firsthand the experience of imaginal exposure. Any myth that imagining threatening scenarios is easy will be dispelled as he discusses the experience of sweating and hyperventilating to his mental images.

Beyond his personal experiences, he considers core issues in anxiety research, such as the following: How valid are these diagnoses? What does it mean that a person can have so many different anxiety diagnoses? How much does neuroscience explain about these syndromes? Do medications or psychotherapy fully cure the symptoms? The book provides a masterful summary of current findings while highlighting the need for more science.

TABLE 6.2	Percent of Adults Ages 18–64 in the General Population Who Meet Diagnostic Criteria for Anxiety Disorders in the Past Year and in Their Lifetime	
	12-Month Prevalence Estimate	**Lifetime Prevalence Estimate**
Anxiety Disorder		
Specific phobia	10.1	13.8
Social anxiety disorder	8.0	13.0
Panic disorder	3.1	5.2
Agoraphobia	1.7	2.6
Generalized anxiety disorder	2.9	6.2

Source: Based on Kessler, R. C., Petukhova, M., Sampson, N. A., Zaslavsky, A. M., & Wittchen, H. U. (2012). Twelve-month and lifetime prevalence and lifetime morbid risk of anxiety and mood disorders in the United States. *International Journal of Methods in Psychiatric Research, 21*, 169–184.

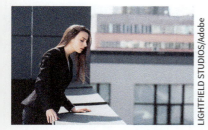

Acrophobia, or phobia of heights, is common. People with this fear would find a glass elevator terrifying. Other common specific phobias include fears of animals, injections, and enclosed spaces.

LIGHTFIELD STUDIOS/Adobe Stock

Specific Phobias

A **specific phobia** is a consistent tendency to experience extreme fear of an object or situation, such as flying, snakes, or heights. The person recognizes that the fear is excessive but still goes to great lengths to avoid the feared object or situation. The names for these fears consist of a Greek word for the feared object or situation followed by the suffix -*phobia* (derived from the name of the Greek god Phobos, who frightened his enemies). Phobias have been recognized for a very long time—an Islamic text from the 9th century describes phobia as a distinct mental health syndrome (Awaad & Ali, 2016). Two of the more common phobias are claustrophobia (fear of closed spaces) and acrophobia (fear of heights). Specific phobias tend to cluster around a small number of feared objects and situations (see **Table 6.3**). One form of phobia, to blood, injections, and injury, is unique in that the specific fears tend to run in families, and people who are affected by this form of phobia tend to show a profile of heart rate slowing and possible fainting when facing the feared stimuli (LeBeau, Glenn, et al., 2010). As with Scott Stossel's experience, described in **Read More About It 6.1**, a person with a specific phobia for one type of object or situation is very likely to have a specific phobia for a second object or situation—that is, specific phobias are highly comorbid (Kendler, Myers, & Prescott, 2002). The **Clinical Case of Jan** provides a glimpse of how a specific phobia can interfere with important life goals.

Defining Symptoms of Specific Phobia

- Disproportionate fear consistently triggered by specific objects or situations, typically lasting 6 months or more

- The object or situation is avoided or else provokes intense anxiety or fear

TABLE 6.3   Types of Specific Phobias

Type of Phobia	Examples of the Feared Object
Animal	Snakes, insects
Natural environment	Storms, heights, water
Blood, injection, injury	Blood, injury, injections, or other invasive medical procedures
Situational	Public transportation, tunnels, bridges, elevators, flying, driving, closed spaces
Other	Choking, contracting an illness, etc. Children's fears of loud sounds, clowns, etc.

Clinical Case

Jan

Jan, a 42-year-old woman, had been offered a high-paying job in Florida. She was considering declining the offer because it would force her to live in an area known for having snakes. Before making this decision, she decided to see a therapist. During her first meeting with the therapist, she described a litany of ways she had avoided any contact with anything remotely resembling a snake. She had steered clear of outdoor activities, TV programs on nature, and even her children's books on nature. Although her fears had not interfered with meaningful life goals so far, the idea of living in an area with snakes had greatly increased her apprehension. Aside from her phobia, Jan reported that she had always been a bit of a nervous person, a trait she shared with her mother.

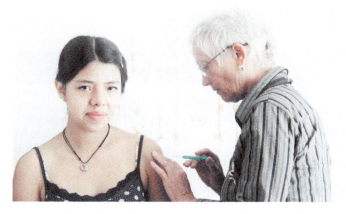

Sigrid Gombert/Cultura/Getty Images

One form of specific phobia is an intense fear of blood, injection, or injuries.

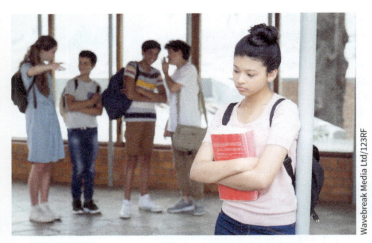

Social anxiety disorder typically begins in adolescence and interferes with developing friendships.

Wavebreak Media Ltd/123RF

Social Anxiety Disorder

The core feature of **social anxiety disorder** is a persistent, unrealistically intense fear of social situations that might involve being scrutinized by, or even just exposed to, unfamiliar people. In interpersonal interactions, people with social anxiety disorder are deeply concerned that they will do or say embarrassing things and that others will judge them harshly as a result. Although this may sound like shyness, people with social anxiety disorder experience intense feelings of shame and humiliation, and these feelings are more chronic than they are for people who are shy (Burstein, Ameli-Grillon, & Merikangas, 2011). Many fear that their anxiety will become apparent to others and that they will be judged as inferior to others (McEwan, Gilbert, & Duarte, 2012). The intense anxiety leads most with social anxiety disorder to avoid social situations, as illustrated by Maureen in the next **Clinical Case**. The most common fears for those with social anxiety include public speaking, speaking in meetings or group settings, meeting new people, and talking to people in authority (Ruscio, Brown, et al., 2008). Forced to engage in one of these feared activities, the person may spend days in advance thinking about all the possible ways things that could go wrong, and then spend days after the event feeling ashamed about any small moments that did go badly.

The manifestations and outcomes of social anxiety disorder vary greatly. Social anxiety disorder can range in severity from a few specific fears to a generalized host of fears. For example, some people might be anxious about speaking in public but not about other social situations. In contrast, others fear most social situations. Those with a broader array of fears are more likely to experience comorbid depression and alcohol abuse (Acarturk, de Graaf, et al., 2008), along with other negative outcomes. People with social anxiety disorder often work in occupations far below their talents because of their extreme social fears. Many would rather work in an unrewarding job with limited social demand than deal with social situations every day.

Among people with social anxiety disorder, at least a third also meet the criteria for a diagnosis of avoidant personality disorder (see Chapter 15). The symptoms of the two conditions overlap a great deal, as does the genetic vulnerability for the two conditions (Torvik, Welander-Vatn, et al., 2016). Avoidant personality disorder, though, is a more severe disorder with more pervasive symptoms.

Defining Symptoms of Social Anxiety Disorder

- Marked and disproportionate fear consistently triggered by exposure to potential social scrutiny
- Exposure to the trigger leads to intense anxiety about being evaluated negatively

- Trigger situations are avoided or else endured with intense anxiety
- Symptoms typically last 6 months or more

Clinical Case

Maureen

Maureen, a 30-year-old accountant, sought psychotherapy after reading a notice advertising group therapy for people with difficulties in social situations. Maureen appeared nervous during the interview and described feeling intensely anxious in conversations with others. She described the anxiety as worsening over the years, to the point where she no longer interacted socially with anyone other than her husband. She would not even go to the supermarket for fear of having to interact with people. Maureen deeply feared being perceived as stupid. This fear made her so nervous that she would often stammer or forget what she was going to say while talking to others, thus adding to her apprehension that others would view her as stupid and creating a vicious circle of ever-increasing fear.

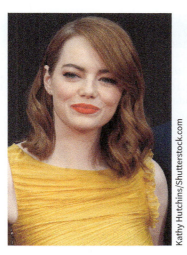
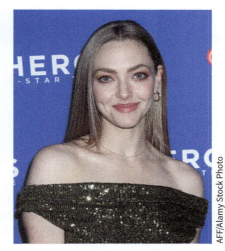

Emma Stone and Amanda Seyfried have both described experiencing panic attacks when younger (Garner, 2021; Mazziotta, 2018).

Panic Disorder

Panic disorder is characterized by recurrent panic attacks that are unrelated to specific situations and by worry about having more panic attacks (see the **Clinical Case of Jenny** at the beginning of this chapter). A **panic attack** is a sudden experience of intense apprehension, terror, or feelings of impending doom, accompanied by at least four other symptoms. Physical symptoms can include shortness of breath, heart palpitations, nausea, upset stomach, chest pain, feelings of choking and smothering, dizziness, lightheadedness, faintness, sweating, chills, heat sensations, numbness or tingling sensations, and trembling. Other symptoms that may occur during a panic attack include **depersonalization** (a feeling of being outside one's body); **derealization** (a feeling of the world not being real); and fears of losing control, of "going crazy," or even of dying. Not surprisingly, people often report that they have an intense urge to flee whatever situation they are in when a panic attack occurs. The symptoms tend to come on very rapidly and reach a peak of intensity within 10 minutes. Many people seek emergency medical care when they first experience a panic attack because they are terrified that they are having a heart attack.

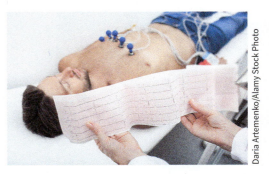

People with panic disorder often seek cardiac tests because they are frightened by changes in their heart rate.

As noted, we can think about a panic attack as a misfire of the fear system: Physiologically, the person experiences a level of sympathetic nervous system arousal matching what most people might experience when faced with an immediate threat to life. Because the symptoms are inexplicable, the person tries to make sense of the experience. A person who begins to think that they are dying, losing control, or going crazy is likely to feel even more fear. Among people with panic disorder, 90% report these types of beliefs when panic attacks occur.

The diagnostic criteria for panic disorder require more than the presence of recurrent panic attacks. A person must experience recurrent panic attacks that are unexpected. That is, panic attacks triggered by specific situations, such as seeing a snake for a person with snake phobia, should not be considered in diagnosing panic disorder. Beyond the occurrence of unexpected panic attacks, the person must worry about the attacks or change his, her or their behavior because of the attacks for at least 1 month. Hence, in making this diagnosis, the response to panic attacks is as important as the attacks themselves. The ongoing worry about possible attacks interferes with daily life as people begin to avoid more and more situations that could trigger panic attacks.

Defining Symptoms of Panic Disorder

- Recurrent unexpected panic attacks
- At least 1 month of concern about the possibility that more attacks could occur or the possible consequences of an attack, or problematic behavioral changes to avoid attacks or their consequences

Defining Symptoms of Agoraphobia

Disproportionate and marked fear or anxiety about at least two situations where it would be difficult to escape or receive help in the event of incapacitation, embarrassing symptoms, or panic-like symptoms, such as being outside the home alone; traveling on public transportation; being in open spaces such as parking lots, bridges, and marketplaces; being in enclosed spaces such as shops, theatres, or cinemas; or standing in line or being in a crowd.

- These situations consistently provoke fear or anxiety
- These situations are avoided, require the presence of a companion, or are endured with intense fear or anxiety
- Symptoms typically last 6 months or more

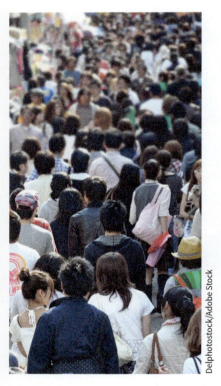

Delphotostock/Adobe Stock

People with agoraphobia often find crowds very distressing because escape would be difficult if anxiety symptoms occurred.

Remember that the criteria for panic disorder specify that panic attacks must be recurrent. It is fairly common for people to experience a single panic attack—more than a quarter of people in the United States report that they have experienced at least one panic attack during their lifetime (Kessler, Chiu, et al., 2006). As Table 6.2 shows, though, many fewer people develop full-blown panic disorder.

Agoraphobia

Agoraphobia (from the Greek *agora,* meaning "marketplace") is defined by anxiety about situations from which it would be embarrassing or difficult to escape if anxiety symptoms occurred. Commonly feared situations include crowds and crowded places such as grocery stores, malls, and theaters. Sometimes the situations are those that are difficult to escape from, such as trains, bridges, or long road trips. Due to their fear of these situations, many people with agoraphobia are virtually unable to leave their house, and even those who can leave do so only with great distress. The effects of agoraphobia on quality of life are as severe as those observed for the other anxiety disorders (Wittchen, Gloster, et al., 2010).

Generalized Anxiety Disorder

The central feature of **generalized anxiety disorder (GAD)** is worry. Like Joe in the **Clinical Case**, people with GAD are persistently worried, often about minor things. The term *worry* refers to the cognitive tendency to chew on a problem and to be unable to let go of it (Mennin, Heimberg, & Turk, 2004). Often, worry continues because a person cannot settle on a solution to the problem. Most of us worry from time to time, but the worries of people with GAD are excessive, uncontrollable, and long-lasting. The worries of people with GAD center on the same types of threats that worry most of us: They worry about relationships, health, finances, and daily hassles—but they worry more about these issues, and the worry is accompanied by arousal-related symptoms, as illustrated by the following passage:

> *I had graduated from college the year before, with honors. I had a prestigious job, loyal friends, a good apartment I shared with a bright and beautiful girlfriend, and as much money as I needed. Yet every day was torture. I slept fitfully, with recurring nightmares—tsunamis, feral animals, the violent deaths of loved ones. I had intestinal cramps and nausea and headaches. A sense of impending catastrophe colored every working moment. Worse, I had the distinct sense that catastrophe had already occurred. I had made the wrong decisions, gone down the wrong path, screwed up in a ruinous, irrevocable, epoch-making way.* (Smith, 2012, pp. 3–4)

GAD has a major impact on relationships. People with GAD are more likely to report marital distress and an absence of friendships than are those with any other anxiety disorder (Whisman, 2007; Whisman, Sheldon, & Goering, 2000).

Comorbidity in Anxiety Disorders

More than half of people with one anxiety disorder meet the criteria for another anxiety disorder during their lives (Wright, Krueger, et al., 2013). Anxiety disorders are also highly comorbid with other disorders: Three-quarters of people with an anxiety disorder meet the diagnostic criteria for

Defining Symptoms of Generalized Anxiety Disorder

- Excessive anxiety and worry about multiple events or activities (e.g., family, health, finances, work, and school)
- The person finds it hard to control the worry
- The anxiety and worry are associated with at least three (or one in children) of the following:
  - restlessness or feeling keyed up or on edge
    - tiring easily
    - difficulty concentrating or mind going blank
    - irritability
    - muscle tension
    - sleep disturbance
- Symptoms are present at least 50% of days for at least 6 months

Clinical Case

Joe

Joe, a 24-year-old mechanic, was referred for psychotherapy by his physician, whom he had consulted because of difficulty falling asleep. He was visibly distressed during the entire initial interview, with a furrowed brow and continuous fidgeting. Although he first described worries about his health, a picture of pervasive anxiety soon emerged. He reported that he nearly always felt tense and he seemed to worry about everything. He was apprehensive of disasters that could befall him as he interacted with people and worked, and he described worrying much of the time about his finances, his inability to establish a romantic relationship, and other issues. He reported a long history of difficulties relating to others, which had led to his being fired from several jobs. As he put it, "I really like people and try to get along with them, but I fly off the handle too easily. Little things upset me too much." Joe reported that he had always felt more nervous than other people but that his anxiety had become much worse after his girlfriend broke up with him 1 year ago.

at least one other psychological disorder (Kessler, Chiu, et al., 2005). More specifically, about 60% of people in treatment for anxiety disorders meet the diagnostic criteria for major depression in their lifetime. We discuss this overlap in Focus on Discovery 5.5. Obsessive compulsive disorder also commonly co-occurs with anxiety disorders (Wright et al., 2013). As with many disorders, comorbidity is associated with greater severity and poorer outcomes of the anxiety disorders.

Quick Summary

As a group, anxiety disorders are the most common type of psychological disorder. Large-scale epidemiologic studies suggest that 28% of people will experience an anxiety disorder during their lifetime, and some research suggests that this may be an underestimate. The age of onset for anxiety disorders is typically before age 21.

Specific phobia is defined by an intense fear of an object or situation, social anxiety disorder by an intense fear of strangers or social scrutiny, panic disorder by anxiety about recurrent panic attacks, agoraphobia by a fear of places where escaping or getting help would be difficult if anxiety symptoms were to occur, and generalized anxiety disorder by worries lasting at least 6 months.

People with one anxiety disorder are very likely to experience a second anxiety disorder during their lives. About 60% of people with anxiety disorders will experience major depression during their lives.

6.2 Check Your Knowledge

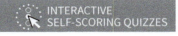 INTERACTIVE SELF-SCORING QUIZZES

(Answers are at the end of the chapter.)
Match the word to the definition.

a. an emotional response to immediate danger

b. an excessive fear of a specific object or situation that causes distress or impairment

c. a state of apprehension often accompanied by mild autonomic arousal

d. thinking about potential problems, often without settling on a solution

1. Fear

2. Anxiety

3. Worry

4. Phobia

Fill in the blank.

5. In epidemiologic studies that conduct just one interview with people about whether they met diagnostic criteria for an anxiety disorder, the estimated lifetime prevalence of anxiety disorders is: _____

6. The key symptom of GAD is: _____

Gender and Cultural Influences on the Anxiety Disorders

It is well known that gender and culture influence the risk for anxiety disorders and the specific types of symptoms that a person develops. As you will learn however, there are still some puzzles about why these patterns exist.

Gender

Women are almost twice as likely to experience anxiety disorders as men are (Baxter, Scott, et al., 2013). When present, anxiety disorders also appear related to more functional impairment for women compared with men (McLean, Asnaani, et al., 2011). Many different theories have been proposed to explain these gender differences. First, women may be more likely to report their symptoms. Social influences, such as gender roles, are also involved. For example, men may experience more social pressure than women to face fears—as we will discuss, facing fears is the basis for one of the most effective treatments available. Women may also experience different life circumstances than do men. For example, women are much more likely than men to be sexually assaulted during childhood and adulthood (Tolin & Foa, 2006). These traumatic events may interfere with developing a sense of control over one's environment, and, as we will see when we discuss cognitive influences, having less perceived control over one's environment may set the stage for anxiety disorders. Men may be raised to believe more in their personal control over situations than women are. It also appears that women show higher neuroticism levels (De Bolle, De Fruyt, et al., 2015) and more biological reactivity to stress than do men (Olff, Langeland, et al., 2007), perhaps as a result of these social and psychological influences. Although the gender gap is not fully understood, it is an important phenomenon. Newer research is also beginning to examine the high rates of anxiety disorders among gender minorities (White et al., 2023).

Culture

People in every culture seem to experience problems with anxiety disorders, but culture and environment influence what people come to fear (Kirmayer, 2001). "If you live near a volcano, you're going to fear lava. If you live in the rainforest, you're going to fear malaria" (Smith, 2012, p. 72). *Kayak-angst*, a disorder that is similar to panic disorder, occurs among the Inuit people of western Greenland; seal hunters who are alone at sea may experience intense fear, disorientation, and concerns about drowning.

Several cultural concepts of distress (see Chapter 3) provide examples of how culture and environment may shape the expression of an anxiety disorder. For example, in Japan, a syndrome called *taijin kyofusho* involves fear of displeasing or embarrassing others; people with this syndrome typically fear making direct eye contact, blushing, having body odor, or having a bodily deformity. The symptoms of this disorder overlap with those of social anxiety disorder, but the focus on others' feelings is distinct (Hofmann & Hinton, 2014). Perhaps this focus is related to characteristics of traditional Japanese culture that encourage deep concern for the feelings of others. Other syndromes, such as *dhat syndrome* (anxiety or distress attributed to the loss of semen—reported in South Asia), and *susto* (fright-illness, the belief that a severe fright has caused the soul to leave the body—reported in Latin America and among Latinos in the United States), also involve symptoms similar to those of the anxiety disorders defined in the DSM. As with the Japanese syndrome *taijin kyofusho*, the objects of anxiety and fear in these syndromes relate to environmental challenges as well as to attitudes that are prevalent in the cultures where the syndromes occur.

Beyond cultural concepts of distress, the prevalence of anxiety disorders varies dramatically across cultures, ranging, for example, from 3% to 19% in the World Mental Health Study (Kessler, Aguilar-Gaxiola, et al., 2009). This is not surprising given that cultures differ with regard to variables such as stress levels, the nature of family relationships, the presence of war, and the prevalence of poverty—all of which are known to play a role in the occurrence of anxiety disorders. Countries with recent war, revolution, or large-scale persecution have higher rates of anxiety disorders than do those without such conflicts (Baxter et al., 2013). Countries with higher rates of COVID-19 during the first year of the pandemic showed greater increases in the prevalence of anxiety disorders (Santomauro et al., 2021). Cultural attitudes may also guide how comfortable people are with disclosing psychological symptoms. In some countries, cultural concepts of distress related to anxiety may be more common than the anxiety disorders listed in the main body of the DSM, meaning that prevalence estimates that omit cultural concepts of distress may be misleading (Steel, Silove, et al., 2009).

One important difference across countries is the level of income inequality—the gap between the highest and lowest incomes in a country. Countries with high levels of income inequality, such as European countries and the United States, have much higher rates of anxiety disorders than do most other regions of the world (see **Table 3.2**). Indeed, in some studies, about half of the variance across countries in the prevalence of anxiety disorders appears tied to income inequality. It has been argued that seeing wealthy people enjoying high levels of luxury and success can instill competition and insecurity about how one compares, which in turn increases the risk for anxiety (Wilkinson & Pickett, 2018). Testing these models, though, is difficult, as countries vary on so many dimensions beyond income inequality.

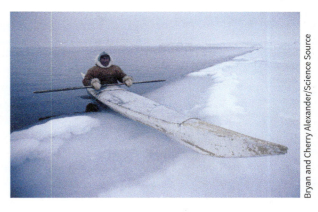

Disorders with symptoms similar to panic attacks occur cross-culturally. Among the Inuit, kayak-angst is defined by intense fear in lone hunters.

Quick Summary

Women are much more likely than men to report an anxiety disorder. Culture influences the focus of fears, the ways that symptoms are expressed, and even the prevalence of different anxiety disorders. Countries with recent histories of war or persecution and those with more income inequality show a higher prevalence of anxiety disorders. The prevalence of anxiety disorders increased more during the first year of the COVID-19 pandemic in countries with higher rates of infection.

6.3 Check Your Knowledge INTERACTIVE SELF-SCORING QUIZZES

(Answers are at the end of the chapter.)
Answer the following questions.

1. What is the size of the gender ratio in anxiety disorders?
2. Which countries have the highest rates of anxiety disorders?

True or false?

3. Cultural concepts of distress are less common than the DSM-5-TR anxiety disorders in every country where prevalence estimates are available.

Common Influences Across the Anxiety Disorders

In considering the causes of the anxiety disorders, we begin by describing several influences that seem to increase risk for all of the anxiety disorders. The existence of such influences may help explain why people with one anxiety disorder are likely to develop a second one—that is, some risk factors increase the odds of having more than one anxiety disorder. For example, the factors that increase risk for social anxiety disorder may also increase risk for panic disorder.

Unlike the way we have organized most of the other chapters in this book, we have chosen to begin here with the behavioral model, which focuses on classical conditioning of fear responses. We do this because classical conditioning of fear is at the heart of many anxiety disorders. Many of the other influences, including genetic vulnerability, neurobiological

TABLE 6.4	Influences That Increase General Risk for Anxiety Disorders

Cultural and cross-national influences: exposure to war, persecution, and income inequality

Behavioral conditioning (classical and operant conditioning)

Genetic vulnerability

Disturbances in the activity of the amygdala, the medial prefrontal cortex, and other brain regions involved in processing fear and emotion

Decreased functioning of gamma-aminobutyric acid (GABA) and serotonin; increased norepinephrine activity

Behavioral inhibition

Neuroticism

Cognitive influences, including sustained negative beliefs, perceived lack of control, overattention to cues of threat, and intolerance of uncertainty

correlates, personality traits, and cognition, shape sensitivity to threat and how readily a person can be conditioned to develop a new fear response (Craske, Rauch, et al., 2009). **Table 6.4** summarizes the influences that operate across the anxiety disorders.

Fear Conditioning

Earlier we mentioned that most anxiety disorders involve fears that are more frequent or intense than what most people experience. Where do these fears come from? The behavioral theory of anxiety disorders focuses on conditioning. **Mowrer's two-factor model** of anxiety disorders, published in 1947, continues to influence thinking in this area. Mowrer's model suggests two steps in the development of an anxiety disorder (Mowrer, 1947):

1. Through *classical conditioning* (see Chapter 1), a person learns to fear a neutral stimulus (the conditioned stimulus, or CS) that is paired with an intrinsically aversive stimulus (the unconditioned stimulus, or UCS).

2. A person gains relief by avoiding the CS. Through *operant conditioning* (also discussed in Chapter 1), this avoidant response is maintained because it is reinforcing (it reduces fear).

Consider the example shown in **Figure 6.1**. Imagine that a man is bitten by a dog and then develops a phobia of dogs. Through classical conditioning, he has learned to associate dogs (the CS) with painful bites (the UCS). This corresponds to step 1. In step 2, the man reduces his fear by avoiding dogs as much as possible; the avoidant behavior is reinforced by the reduction in fear. This second step explains why the phobia isn't extinguished. With repeated exposure to dogs that don't bite, the man would have lost his fear of dogs, but by avoiding dogs, the man gets little or no such exposure.

We should note that Mowrer's early version of the two-factor model does not actually fit the evidence very well, for two reasons. First, many people who have anxiety disorders cannot remember any threatening event that triggered their symptoms. Second, many people who do experience serious threats do not develop anxiety disorders. Let's consider several extensions of this model that were developed to explain these gaps.

We begin with an extension to the model to explain why some people with anxiety disorders do not remember any conditioning experience (Mineka & Zinbarg, 1998). According to this extension, classical conditioning could occur in different ways (Rachman, 1977), including:

- Direct experience (like the dog bite the example)

- Modeling (e.g., seeing a dog bite a man or watching a video of a vicious dog attack)

- Verbal instruction (e.g., hearing a parent warn that dogs are dangerous).

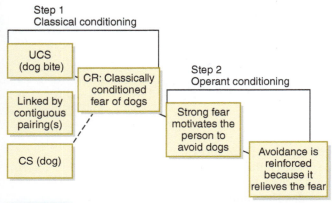

FIGURE 6.1 **Two-factor model of conditioning as applied to dog phobia.**

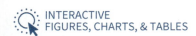
INTERACTIVE FIGURES, CHARTS, & TABLES

In any of these ways, a person could learn to associate a stimulus with fear.

The second major problem with Mowrer's model is that many people who are exposed to major threats (e.g., a dog bite) do not develop anxiety disorders. That is, some people are more vulnerable to developing anxiety disorders than others. Researchers have shown in carefully controlled tests in laboratory settings that people with anxiety disorders are more responsive to threats.

Most centrally, many studies have used classical conditioning to test how people with anxiety disorders acquire and sustain fears. Findings of these studies suggest that people with anxiety disorders seem to be slower to extinguish fears once they are conditioned (Beckers, Hermans, et al., 2023). In one study, researchers conditioned people to fear a neutral picture of a Rorschach card (see Figure 3.11) by pairing the card with a shock six times (Michael, Blechert, et al., 2007). After receiving six shocks, most participants learned to fear the Rorschach card, as measured by skin conductance responses to seeing the card—even those without an anxiety disorder developed this conditioned response. However, participants with and without an anxiety disorder (in this study, panic disorder) differed in the extinction phase of the study, when the card was shown without any shock being provided. People who were not diagnosed with panic disorder showed a quick drop in their fear responses during the extinction phase, but people with panic disorder showed very little decrease in their fear response. Thus, for a person with an anxiety disorder, once a fear is conditioned, that fear may stubbornly persist and be difficult to unlearn despite evidence to the contrary. Findings from a meta-analysis of 44 studies suggest that anxiety disorders are related to slowed extinction of fears (Duits et al., 2015). Research also suggests that the offspring of those with anxiety disorders show slow extinction of conditioned fears (Waters, Peters, et al., 2014). These findings help explain why some people are more likely to develop an anxiety disorder after a threatening event, whereas other people seem not to do so.

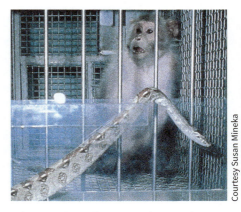

When monkeys observe another monkey display fear of a snake, they also acquire the fear (Cook & Mineka, 1989). This finding supports the idea that modeling influences the development of phobias.

One body of research suggests that people with anxiety disorders are particularly sensitive to unpredictable, diffuse, or remote threats, rather than acute, immediate, well-defined threats (Shackman, Tromp, et al., 2016). In a careful experimental approach to testing responses to unpredictable threats, participants are assigned to undergo three different conditions of a behavioral task called the **neutral predictable unpredictable (NPU) threat task**: (1) a neutral condition in which they do not experience an aversive stimulus, (2) a predictable condition in which they experience an aversive stimulus and receive a warning beforehand, and (3) an unpredictable condition in which they experience an aversive stimulus without prior warning. The threat in the predictable and unpredictable threat condition is the same—for example, participants could receive identical electric shocks in both threat conditions. The difference is that in the predictable threat condition, it is clear when the threat will happen, but in the unpredictable threat condition, the timing of the threat is unclear (Schmitz & Grillon, 2012). Anxiety disorders are specifically related to increased affective and psychophysiological response to the *unpredictable* threat condition compared with the predictable threat condition. That is, people with social anxiety disorder, specific phobias, panic disorder, and PTSD have been found to show particularly high psychophysiological arousal levels during the unpredictable threat condition compared with healthy controls (Gorka, Lieberman, et al., 2017; Grillon, Lissek, et al., 2008). This profile appears to be specific to anxiety disorders, in that people with major depressive disorder respond as healthy controls do to unpredictable threat (Gorka et al., 2017). Unpredictable threat, then, seems to be key in anxiety disorders.

In sum, although Mowrer's two-factor model continues to shape our understanding of the processes through which anxiety disorders develop, clearly not everyone who is bitten by a dog will go on to develop a phobia. So, what factors seem to distinguish individuals with anxiety disorders from those without? People with anxiety disorders seem to sustain conditioned fears longer, particularly to unpredictable threats. How might this look in everyday life? Imagine a child who is bullied on the playground. Because it is hard to know when the bully will target the child, the threat is unpredictable. The child with an anxiety disorder might experience more fear of the bullying (an unpredictable threat). Although most kids might feel safe again if they were able to play in that area without bullying happening (extinction), this process is slow for the child with an anxiety disorder.

As you can see, fear-conditioning models consider many different aspects of how people learn fears and how those fears are sustained. Many of the variables we describe next have been shown to influence this sensitivity to fear conditioning.

Genetic Vulnerability

A large-scale twin study suggested a heritability estimate of 0.5 to 0.6 for anxiety disorders (Kendler, Aggen, et al., 2011). That is, genetic vulnerability may explain about 50–60% of the risk for anxiety disorders in the population. Some genes may elevate risk for several different types of anxiety disorder. For example, genetic vulnerability to phobia is related to increased risk of developing other anxiety disorders as well (Purves et al., 2020, Czajkowsky, et al., 2009). Other genes may elevate risk for a specific type of anxiety disorder (Hettema, Prescott, et al., 2005). Genetic vulnerability to anxiety disorders, and particularly to GAD, also appears to overlap with major depressive disorder (Purves et al., 2020). Some research helps explain how genetic vulnerability could contribute to depression and multiple anxiety disorders. For example, genetic vulnerability is tied to higher neuroticism, which in turn predicts the onset of depressive disorders and multiple anxiety disorders (Dao, Mahon, et al., 2010; Kendler, Gardner, et al., 2007).

Neurobiological Correlates: Brain Regions and Activity of Neurotransmitters

A set of brain structures is engaged when people feel anxious or fearful. Although some have referred to this set of regions as the **fear circuit**, this label has been criticized because these structures are also activated during processing of other types of salient stimuli (Feldman Barrett, 2017) and are also implicated in other disorders involving emotion disturbances, such as the mood disorders. Key regions of this circuit, shown in **Figure 6.2**, are related to anxiety disorders. One important part of this circuit is the amygdala. The amygdala is a small, almond-shaped structure in the temporal lobe that appears to be involved in assigning emotional significance to stimuli. In animals, the amygdala has been shown to be critical for the conditioning of fear. The amygdala sends signals to a range of different brain structures involved in processing threats. Studies suggest that when shown pictures of angry faces (one signal of a threat), people with several different anxiety disorders respond with greater activity in the amygdala than do people without anxiety disorders (Fox, Oler, et al., 2015). Hence, elevated activity in the amygdala may be related to many different anxiety disorders.

The **medial prefrontal cortex** helps to regulate amygdala activity—it is involved in extinguishing fears, in conscious processing of anxiety and fear, and in regulation of emotions (Indovina, Robbins, et al., 2011; Kim, Loucks, et al., 2011; LeDoux & Pine, 2016). Researchers have found that adults who meet diagnostic criteria for anxiety disorders display less activity in the medial prefrontal cortex when viewing and appraising threatening stimuli (Britton, Grillon, et al., 2013), when asked to regulate their emotional responses to threatening stimuli (Goldin, Manber-Ball, et al., 2009), and during extinction of conditioned fear responses (Marin, Zsido, et al., 2017).

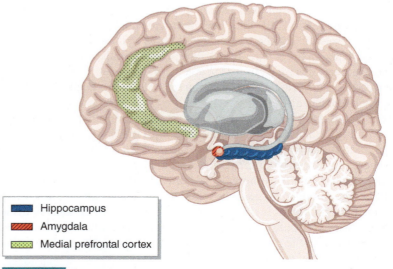

Hippocampus
Amygdala
Medial prefrontal cortex

FIGURE 6.2 The anxiety disorders appear to be related to heightened activity in the amygdala and diminished activity of the medial prefrontal cortex in response to threatening stimuli.

Much current work in anxiety disorders focuses on connectivity among neural regions (Pessoa, 2023). For example, the medial prefrontal cortex shows important connectivity with other key regions involved in anxiety (Kenwood, Kalin, et al., 2022). One pathway from the medial prefrontal cortex is involved in inhibiting activity of the amygdala. This connectivity of the medial prefrontal cortex with the amygdala is weaker among those with anxiety disorders, and this may interfere with the effective regulation and extinction of anxiety.

Although we focus on the amygdala and the medial prefrontal cortex here, other brain regions interface with the amygdala to process threat-related stimuli (Chavanne & Robinson, 2021). The bed nucleus of the stria terminalis, considered an extended part of the amygdala, is also engaged by cues of threat (Fox & Shackman, 2019). The anterior cingulate cortex appears involved in the allocation of attention and the anticipation of threat, and the insula appears related to awareness of and processing of bodily cues, such as the high arousal invoked by threat. In a meta-analysis of 181 fMRI studies measuring responses to threat stimuli, participants with anxiety disorder showed higher activity in both of these regions as compared to those without anxiety disorders (Chavanne & Robinson, 2021). The hippocampus plays a role in encoding the context in which feared stimuli occur (Vervliet, Craske, & Hermans, 2013). We'll consider the hippocampus more in the discussion of PTSD in Chapter 7. We will consider another part of this circuit, the locus coeruleus, when we discuss the causes of panic disorder. Beyond these areas, researchers now believe that many other brain regions are involved in anxiety disorders (Pessoa, 2023). With the complexity of these neurobiological systems, researchers worldwide are developing ways to integrate data sets and examine neurobiological models using large sample sizes (Bas-Hoogendam, Groenewold, et al., 2022).

Multiple neurotransmitters and neuropeptides are implicated in anxiety disorders, and many different techniques have been used to test their roles. PET and SPECT imaging studies link anxiety disorders to disruptions in serotonin levels (Hjorth et al., 2021). Serotonin is believed to help modulate emotions and responses to threat (Carver, Johnson, & Joormann, 2008). PET and SPECT imaging studies also suggest changes in the function of the GABA system in the anxiety disorders (Bandelow, Baldwin, et al., 2016). GABA is widely distributed throughout the brain and is involved in modulating activity in the amygdala and other regions involved in processing threats (Nuss, 2015). Researchers have also used drug manipulation studies to show that anxiety disorders are related to increased levels of norepinephrine and changes in the sensitivity of norepinephrine receptors (Neumeister, Daher, & Charney, 2005). Norepinephrine is a key neurotransmitter in the activation of the sympathetic nervous system for fight-or-flight responses.

Personality: Neuroticism and Behavioral Inhibition

Two closely related personality traits, neuroticism and behavioral inhibition, both appear to predict the onset of anxiety disorders. Neuroticism is a personality trait defined by the tendency to experience frequent or intense negative affect. In studies involving more than 10,000 participants, neuroticism predicted the onset of both anxiety disorders and depression (Ormel, Jeronimus, et al., 2013). People with high neuroticism levels appear to be about twice as likely to develop an anxiety disorder compared to those with low levels (Zinbarg, Mineka, et al., 2016).

Some infants show **behavioral inhibition**, a tendency to become agitated and cry when faced with novel toys, people, or other stimuli. This trait, which has been described in infants as young as 4 months old, may set the stage for the later development of anxiety disorders. One study followed infants from 14 months through 7 years; 45% of those who showed elevated behavioral inhibition levels at 14 months showed symptoms of anxiety at age 7, compared with only 15% of those who had shown low behavioral inhibition levels (Kagan & Snidman, 1999). Behavioral inhibition is a particularly strong predictor of social anxiety disorder: Infants who showed elevated behavioral inhibition were 3.79 times as likely as those with low behavioral inhibition to develop social anxiety disorder by adolescence (Chronis-Tuscano, Degnan, et al., 2009). Multiple studies show that behavioral inhibition is a powerful predictor of the onset of anxiety disorders (Clauss & Blackford, 2012).

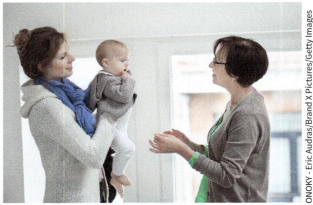

ONOKY - Eric Audras/Brand X Pictures/Getty Images

Infants and toddlers showing behavioral inhibition—high anxiety about novel situations and people—are at greater risk of developing anxiety disorders during their lifetime.

Cognitive Influences

Researchers have focused on several separate cognitive influences on anxiety disorders. Here, we concentrate on four cognitive styles: sustained negative beliefs about the future, a perceived lack of control, intolerance of uncertainty, and attention to threat.

Sustained Negative Beliefs About the Future

People with anxiety disorders often report believing that bad things are likely to happen. For example, people with panic disorder might believe that they will die when their heart begins to pound, whereas people with social anxiety disorder might believe that they will suffer humiliating rejection if they blush. As pointed out by David Clark and colleagues (Clark, Salkovskis, et al., 1999), the key issue is not why people think so negatively initially but, rather, how these beliefs are sustained. For example, by the time a person survives 100 panic attacks, you might expect the belief "this attack means I am about to die" would fade. One reason these beliefs might be sustained is that people think and act in ways that maintain these beliefs. That is, to protect against feared consequences, they engage in **safety behaviors**. For example, people who fear they will die from a fast heart rate stop all physical activity the minute they feel their heart race. They come to believe that only their safety behaviors have kept them alive. Hence, safety behaviors allow a person to maintain overly negative cognitions.

Perceived Lack of Control

People who report experiencing little sense of control over their surroundings are at risk for a broad range of anxiety disorders (Mineka & Zinbarg, 2006). Childhood experiences such as traumatic events, punitive and restrictive parenting, or abuse may promote a belief that life is not controllable. Beyond childhood experiences, more recent life events can threaten the sense of control over one's life. Indeed, about half of people with anxiety disorders report a history of childhood physical or sexual abuse (Cougle, Timpano, et al., 2010), and more than 70% of people report a severe life event before the onset of an anxiety disorder (Finlay-Jones, 1989). Other life experiences may shape the sense of control over the feared stimulus. For example, people who are used to dogs and feel comfortable about controlling dogs' behavior are much less likely to develop a phobia after a dog bite. On the whole, the degree to which a person experiences control over the environment can influence whether an anxiety disorder develops.

Animal studies have illustrated that a lack of control over the environment can promote anxiety. For example, Insel, Scanlan, et al. (1988) randomly assigned monkeys to one of two conditions. One group of monkeys grew up with the ability to choose whether and when they would receive treats. A second group of monkeys had no control over whether and when they received treats but received the same number of treats. In the third year of life, monkeys who had grown up without control behaved in ways that looked anxious when facing new situations and interacting with other monkeys; monkeys who had grown up with control showed less anxiety. In sum, animal and human studies both point toward the importance of perceived lack of control in the development of anxiety disorders.

Intolerance of Uncertainty

People who have a hard time accepting ambiguity— that is, who find it intolerable to think that something bad *might* happen in the future—are more likely to develop anxiety disorders (Dugas, Marchand, & Ladouceur, 2005). This intolerance of uncertainty, though, predicts not just anxiety disorders but also major depressive disorder and obsessive-compulsive disorder (Gentes & Ruscio, 2011; McEvoy & Mahoney, 2012).

Attention to Threat

A large body of research indicates that people with anxiety disorders pay more attention to negative cues in their environment than do people without anxiety disorders (Valadez, Pine, et al., 2022). To test attention to threatening stimuli, researchers have used a wide range of computerized measures. For example, researchers measure how quickly participants can find a threatening stimulus in a computer display of many objects, or they use gaze tracking to measure how quickly and how long people look toward threatening versus nonthreatening stimuli (Dennis-Tiwary, Roy, et al., 2019). In a meta-analysis of 172 studies, each of the specific anxiety disorders was associated with heightened attention to threatening stimuli (Bar-Haim, Lamy, et al., 2007). For example, people with social anxiety disorder have been found to selectively attend to negative faces (Bantin, Stevens, et al., 2016), whereas people with snake phobias selectively attend to cues related to snakes (Öhman, Flykt, & Esteves, 2001). This heightened attention to threatening stimuli seems to happen very quickly—before people are even consciously aware of the stimuli (Staugaard, 2010). Once a threatening object captures their attention, anxious people have a difficult time pulling their attention away from that object; they tend to stay focused on a threatening object longer than others do (Cisler & Koster, 2010). In sum, anxiety disorders are associated with selective attention to signs of threat.

Putting It All Together: Integrating Biological, Behavioral, and Social Influences

Perhaps not surprisingly, the various influences on the anxiety disorders interact in important ways. As noted in the start of this section, fear conditioning and slowed extinction of conditioned fear are core to anxiety disorders, and many of the other risk factors have important influences on conditioning processes. For example, the heightened amygdala activity shown in anxiety disorders plays a major role in fear conditioning and extinction. Childhood adversity and neuroticism are both tied to heightened amygdala activation when viewing threatening stimuli and to slowed extinction of conditioned fears (Canli, 2008; Scharfenort, Menz, & Lonsdorf, 2016). Anxiety disorders, then, provide a good example of the need to consider biology and psychosocial influences together to explain the development of psychological disorders.

Quick Summary

Many influences set the stage for anxiety disorders generally, rather than for a specific anxiety disorder. Behavioral models of anxiety disorders build from Mowrer's two-factor model (classical conditioning followed by operant conditioning). These models have been extended to propose that the classical conditioning may be driven by direct exposure to an event, observation of someone else experiencing an event (modeling), or verbal instruction. It also appears that people with anxiety disorders are slower to extinguish classically conditioned fears, and are particularly sensitive to unpredictable threats.

Genes increase risk for anxiety disorders. Neurobiological research on anxiety focuses on brain structures such as the amygdala and medial prefrontal cortex and on the connectivity of these structures. Anxiety disorders also appear to involve poor functioning of the GABA, norepinephrine, and serotonin systems. The personality traits of behavioral inhibition and neuroticism are both related to the development of anxiety disorders. From the cognitive perspective, anxiety disorders are associated with negative expectations about the future, beliefs that life is uncontrollable, intolerance of uncertainty, and a bias to attend to negative stimuli. Amygdala hyper-reactivity, adversity, and neuroticism all contribute to the propensity to sustain fear conditioning in those with anxiety disorders.

6.4 Check Your Knowledge

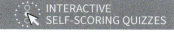 INTERACTIVE
SELF-SCORING QUIZZES

(Answers are at the end of the chapter.)
Choose the best answer for each item.

1. Research suggests that genes can explain _____% of the variance in anxiety disorders.

   a. 0–20

   b. 20–40

   c. 50–60

   d. 60–80

Answer the following question.

2. What is the definition of neuroticism?

Circle all that apply.

3. Cognitive variables found to correlate with anxiety disorders include:

   a. low self-esteem

   b. attention to signs of threat

   c. hopelessness

   d. lack of perceived control

4. A key structure related to anxiety disorders is the:

   a. cerebellum

   b. amygdala

   c. occipital cortex

   d. inferior colliculi

5. The first step in Mowrer's two-factor model involves _____ conditioning.

   a. operant

   b. predictive

   c. classical

   d. instrumental

6. Findings from the NPU task show that people with anxiety disorders are particularly reactive to _____ types of stimuli. (Fill in the blank).

Influences on Specific Anxiety Disorders

So far, we have discussed influences that might set the stage for development of anxiety disorders in general. Here, we turn to the question of how each of the specific anxiety disorders arises. That is, why does one person develop a specific phobia while another person develops generalized anxiety disorder? As we focus on the specific disorders, think about how the general influences on anxiety disorders might relate to and combine with the more specific influences described next.

Agoraphobia was only recognized as a distinct disorder in the DSM-5, and so less research is available on this diagnosis. As with other anxiety disorders, risk of agoraphobia appears to be related to genetic vulnerability and life events (Wittchen et al., 2010). As less is known about the unique influences that shape agoraphobia as compared to other anxiety disorders, we do not discuss agoraphobia in this section.

Specific Phobias

The dominant model of phobias is the two-factor model of behavioral conditioning described earlier. Here, we elaborate on how this model can be applied to understanding phobias. We'll describe some of the research evidence, as well as several refinements of the model.

In the behavioral model, specific phobias are seen as a conditioned response that develops after a threatening experience and is sustained by avoidant behavior. In one of the first illustrations of the classical conditioning part of this model, John Watson and his graduate student Rosalie Rayner published a case report in 1920 in which they demonstrated creating an intense fear of a rat (a phobia) in an infant, Little Albert, using classical conditioning. Little Albert was initially unafraid of the rat, but after repeatedly seeing the rat while a very loud noise was made, he began to cry when he saw the rat. Although this type of experiment would not be approved by modern ethics boards, the experiment provided important evidence that intense fears could be conditioned (Watson & Rayner, 1920).

As already mentioned, behavioral theory suggests that phobias *could* be conditioned by direct trauma, modeling, or verbal instruction. But do most people with a phobia report one of these types of conditioning experiences? In one study, 1937 people were asked whether they had these types of conditioning experiences before the onset of their phobias (Kendler, Myers, & Prescott, 2002). Although conditioning experiences were common, about half of the people in the

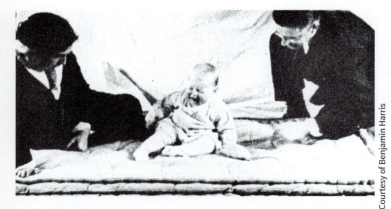

Little Albert, shown here with Rayner and Watson, was classically conditioned to develop a fear of a white rat (Watson & Rayner, 1920).

Courtesy of Benjamin Harris

study could not remember any such experiences. Obviously, if many phobias start without a conditioning experience, this is a big problem for the behavioral model. But proponents of the behavioral model argue that people may forget conditioning experiences (Mineka & Öhman, 2002a). Because of memory gaps, simple surveys asking whether people remember a conditioning experience do not provide accurate evidence about the behavioral model.

Even among those who have had a threatening experience, many do not develop a phobia. How might we understand this? To begin, the risk factors we have described, such as genetic vulnerability, neuroticism, negative cognitive styles, and propensity toward fear conditioning, probably operate as vulnerability factors that shape whether or not a phobia will develop in the context of a conditioning experience (Mineka & Sutton, 2006).

It also is believed that only certain kinds of stimuli and experiences will contribute to development of a phobia. Mowrer's original two-factor model suggests that people could be conditioned to be afraid of all types of stimuli. But people with phobias tend to fear certain types of stimuli. Typically, people do not develop phobias of flowers, lambs, or lamp shades! But phobias of insects or other animals, natural environments, and blood are common. As many as half of women report a fear of snakes; moreover, many different types of animals also fear snakes (Öhman & Mineka, 2003). Researchers have suggested that during the evolution of our species, people learned to react strongly to stimuli that could be life-threatening, such as heights, snakes, and angry humans (Seligman, 1971). That is, evolution may have biologically "prepared" us to learn fear of certain stimuli very quickly and automatically; hence, this type of learning is called **prepared learning**. In support of this idea of evolution shaping fears, researchers have shown that monkeys can be conditioned to fear snakes and crocodiles but not flowers and rabbits (Cook & Mineka, 1989).

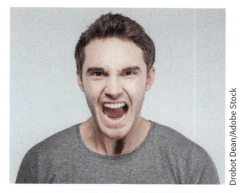

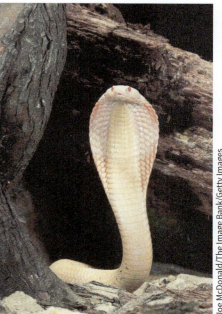

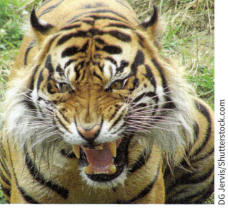

The prepared learning model suggests that we have evolved to pay special attention to signs of danger, including angry people, threatening animals, and dangerous natural environments.

Social Anxiety Disorder

In this section, we review behavioral and cognitive influences on social anxiety disorder. The trait of behavioral inhibition may also be important in the development of social anxiety disorder.

Behavioral Conditioning of Social Anxiety Disorder
As with specific phobias, behavioral perspectives on social anxiety disorder are based on the two-factor conditioning model. That is, a person could have a negative social experience (directly, through modeling, or through verbal instruction) and become classically conditioned to fear similar situations, which the person then avoids. The next step involves operant conditioning: Avoidance behavior is reinforced because it reduces the fear the person experiences. There are few opportunities for the conditioned fear to be extinguished because the person tends to avoid social situations. Even when the person interacts with others, they may show avoidant behavior in smaller ways that have been labeled as safety behaviors. Examples of safety behaviors in social anxiety disorder include avoiding eye contact, disengaging from conversation, and standing apart from others. Although these behaviors are used to avoid negative feedback, they create other problems. Other people tend to disapprove of these types of avoidant behaviors, which then intensifies the problem. (Think about how you might respond if you were trying to talk to someone who looked at the floor, failed to answer your questions, and left the room in the middle of the conversation.)

Social Cognitive Influences: Too Much Focus on Negative Self-Evaluations, Internal Cues, and Social Hierarchy
Theory focuses on several different ways in which cognitive processes might intensify social anxiety (Clark & Wells, 1995). First, people with social anxiety disorders appear to have unrealistically harsh views of their social behaviors and overly negative beliefs about the consequences of their social behaviors—for example, they may believe that others will reject them if they blush or pause while speaking. Second, they attend more to how they are doing in social situations

and their own internal sensations than other people do. Instead of attending to their conversation partner, they are often thinking about how they are performing and how others might perceive them (e.g., "He must think I'm an idiot") (Zanov & Davison, 2010). Of course, good conversation requires a focus on the other person, so too much thinking about anxiety and performance can foster social awkwardness. The resultant anxiety interferes with the ability to perform well socially, creating a vicious circle.

The evidence is clear that people with social anxiety disorder are overly negative in evaluating their social performance, even when they are not socially awkward, and they form powerful visual images of being rejected (Hirsch, Meeten, et al., 2016). For example, in one study, researchers assessed blushing in people with and without social anxiety disorder. Participants were asked to estimate how much they would blush during different tasks, such as singing a children's song. Then they were asked to engage in these different tasks. Participants with social anxiety disorder overestimated how much they would blush (Gerlach, Wilhelm, et al., 2001). Similarly, one research team asked people with social anxiety disorder to rate videos of their performance in giving a short speech. Socially anxious people rated their speeches more negatively than objective raters did, whereas people who were not socially anxious were not harsh in rating their own performance (Ashbaugh, Antony, et al., 2005). The evidence is clear that people with social anxiety disorder are unfairly harsh in their self-evaluations. Harsh self-evaluations also predict increases in social anxiety over time (Miers, Blöte, et al., 2014; Trzaskowski, Zavos, et al., 2012).

Evidence also indicates that people with social anxiety disorder attend more to internal cues than to external (social) cues. For example, people with social anxiety disorder appear to spend more time than other people do monitoring for signs of their own anxiety. In one study, researchers gave participants a chance to watch their own heart rate displayed on a computer screen or to view faces. Many of the faces were threatening. People diagnosed with social anxiety disorder attended more closely to their own heart rate than did the people who were not diagnosed with social anxiety disorder (Pineles & Mineka, 2005). Hence, rather than keeping their eye on potential external threats, people with this disorder tend to be busy monitoring their own anxiety levels.

Too much focus on internal cues could influence interactions in several ways. For example, the socially anxious person might not pay enough attention to others, who then would perceive the person as not interested in them. Paying close attention to others during social interaction certainly helps generate verbal responses. It also fosters reciprocal nonverbal behaviors (e.g., smiling back when someone smiles at us), which tends to promote rapport. People with social anxiety disorder show less reciprocal nonverbal behaviors (Asher, Kauffmann, & Aderka, 2020).

Theory also suggests that social anxiety is related to too much concern about social rank or hierarchy (Mineka & Öhman, 2022b; Trower & Gilbert, 1989). Even as children, most people can identify who is a leader in a social group, and they automatically show respect to leaders. When people fail to show expected submissiveness toward leaders, conflicts can be triggered. According to theory, because they worry more than other people do about social hierarchies, those with social anxiety disorder are expected to display more submissive behavior (Weeks, Heimberg, & Heuer, 2011). Consistent with this idea, people with higher social anxiety show more submissive behavior than others do, whether this submissiveness is rated by the person with social anxiety (Cain, Pincus, & Holtforth, 2010), an observer (Walters & Hope, 1998), or peers (Dijk, van Emmerik, & Grasman, 2018). For example, in social interactions, people with social anxiety are more likely to sit with slumped, closed body postures (Weeks, Heimberg, & Heuer, 2011) and to talk in a high-pitched voice (Gilboa-Schechtman, Galili, et al., 2014; Weeks, Srivastav, et al., 2016) and are less likely to interrupt others who are speaking (Natale, Entin, & Jaffe, 1979).

Putting It All Together: Genetic, Behavioral, and Cognitive Influences

How might all these risk variables fit together when we consider a person with social anxiety disorder, like Maureen in the **Clinical Case** presented earlier in this chapter? Maureen is likely to have inherited some tendency to be anxious when faced with new people. As she grew up, her anxiety may have interfered with her chances to acquire social skills and to gain self-confidence. This could intensify the fear that she is inferior to others. Her fear of other people's opinions and her own negative thoughts about her social

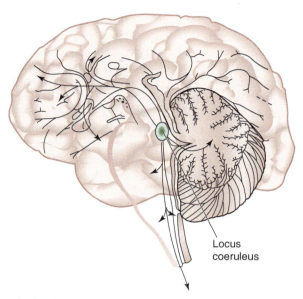

Locus
coeruleus

FIGURE 6.3 The locus coeruleus is the major source of norepinephrine. Surges in norepinephrine lead to a number of physiological shifts, including faster heart rate.

Source: From J. H. Martin, *Neuroanatomy text and atlas*, 4th ed. (1996), copyright McGraw Hill Education LLC with permission.

abilities created a vicious circle in which her intolerable anxiety led her to avoid social situations, and then the avoidance led to increased anxiety. Even when she is in social situations, her focus on her performance and anxiety levels may interfere with being fully engaged in the interaction.

Panic Disorder

In this section, we look at current thinking about the neurobiological, behavioral, and cognitive influences on panic disorder. As you will see, all these perspectives focus on how people respond to somatic (bodily) changes like increased heart rate.

Neurobiological Correlates
We have seen that a brain circuit involved in processing fear appears to play an important role in many of the anxiety disorders. Now we will see that another brain region that is involved in fear processing is especially important in panic disorder: This region is the **locus coeruleus** (see **Figure 6.3**). The locus coeruleus is the major source of the neurotransmitter norepinephrine in the brain. Surges in norepinephrine are a natural response to stress, and when these surges occur, they are associated with increased activity of the sympathetic nervous system, reflected in a faster heart rate and other psychophysiological responses that support the fight-or-flight response. People with panic disorder show a more dramatic biological response to drugs that trigger releases of norepinephrine (Neumeister, Daher, & Charney, 2005). Drugs that increase activity in the locus coeruleus can trigger panic attacks, and some imaging research is consistent with a role of norepinephrine in panic disorder as well (Bandelow, Baldwin, et al., 2017).

Behavioral Influences: Classical Conditioning
The behavioral model of panic disorder focuses on classical conditioning. This model draws from an interesting pattern— panic attacks are often triggered by internal bodily sensations of arousal. Theory suggests that panic attacks are classically conditioned responses to either the situations that trigger anxiety or the internal bodily sensations of arousal (Bouton, Mineka, & Barlow, 2001). Classical conditioning of panic attacks in response to bodily sensations has been called **interoceptive conditioning** of fear: A person experiences somatic signs of anxiety, like hyperventilation,

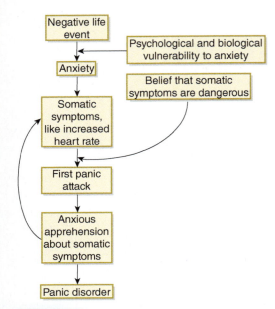

FIGURE 6.4 Interoceptive conditioning. After the first panic attack, the person is classically conditioned to fear somatic symptoms.

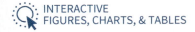

INTERACTIVE FIGURES, CHARTS, & TABLES

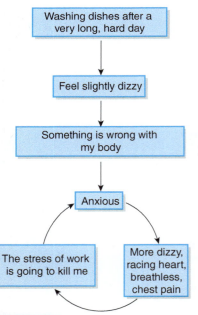

FIGURE 6.5 An example of catastrophic misinterpretation of bodily cues.

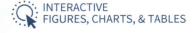

INTERACTIVE FIGURES, CHARTS, & TABLES

which are followed by the person's first panic attack; because the person then associates those somatic changes with a panic attack, panic attacks become a conditioned response to the somatic changes (see **Figure 6.4**).

Research on phenomena other than panic disorder provides ample evidence that interoceptive conditioning can happen. For example, multiple studies indicate that people quickly develop conditioned responses to cues that signal obstruction of oxygen into the lungs. From an evolutionary perspective, it makes sense that people rapidly learn to recognize cues that could signal poor oxygen flow or other key body changes. Intriguingly, these conditioned responses to interoceptive stimuli are slower to extinguish than are those to nonbodily stimuli (Van Diest, 2019), which could help explain how panic symptoms related to interoceptive conditioning could be so persistent across time.

Cognitive Influences

Cognitive perspectives on panic disorder focus on catastrophic misinterpretations of somatic changes (Clark, 1996). According to this model, panic attacks develop when a person interprets bodily sensations as signs of impending doom (see **Figure 6.5**). For example, the person may interpret the sensation of an increase in heart rate as a sign of an impending heart attack. Obviously, such thoughts will increase the person's anxiety, which produces more physical sensations, creating a vicious circle.

The evidence that this type of cognition can contribute to panic attacks is quite strong. To understand the evidence, it is important to know that panic attacks can be experimentally induced in the laboratory. For more than 75 years, research has focused on triggering panic attacks experimentally. These studies suggest that an array of influences, including more than a dozen different medications, create physiological sensations that can trigger panic attacks among people with a history of panic attacks (Swain, Koszycki, et al., 2003). Even drugs that have opposite physiological effects can set off panic attacks (Lindemann & Finesinger, 1938). Exercise alone, simple relaxation, or the physical sensations caused by an illness such as inner-ear disease also can induce panic attacks (Asmundson, Larsen, & Stein, 1998). Another commonly used procedure involves exposing people to air with high levels of carbon dioxide; in response to the diminished oxygen, breathing rate increases, and for some people this induces panic. In short, many different bodily sensations can trigger panic attacks (Barlow, 2004). Cognitive researchers have focused on how to differentiate the people who do and do not develop a panic attack in these experimental studies. People who develop panic attacks after being exposed to these agents seem to differ from those who do not develop panic attacks on only one characteristic—the extent to which they are frightened by the bodily changes (Margraf, Ehlers, & Roth, 1986).

To show the role of cognition as a predictor of panic attacks, researchers in one study experimentally manipulated carbon dioxide levels. Before breathing the carbon dioxide–enriched air, some people were given a full explanation of the physical sensations they were likely to experience, and others were given no explanation. After breathing the air, those who had received a full explanation reported that they had fewer catastrophic interpretations of their bodily sensations, and they were much less likely to have a panic attack than those who did not receive an explanation (Rapee, Mattick, & Murrell, 1986). Catastrophic interpretations of bodily sensations, then, seem to be important in triggering panic attacks.

The propensity toward catastrophic interpretations can be detected before panic disorder develops, most commonly using the Bodily Concerns subscale of the **Anxiety Sensitivity Index**, which measures the extent to which people respond fearfully to their bodily sensations and other signals of anxiety (Telch, Shermis, & Lucas, 1989). Sample items from this subscale include "Unusual body sensations scare me" and "When I notice that my heart is beating rapidly, I worry that I might have a heart attack." Scores on the Bodily Concerns subscale of this index are higher among those with anxiety disorders (Naragon-Gainey, 2010), predict the onset of panic attacks and anxiety disorders over time (Schmidt, Zvolensky, & Maner, 2006), and in twin studies, are related to the genetic risk for anxiety disorders (Brown, Waszczuk, et al., 2014).

Taken together, a large literature now supports that anxiety sensitivity is an influence on anxiety disorders (Taylor, 2020).

Many experimental studies test how high scores on the Anxiety Sensitivity Index might contribute to symptoms of panic disorder. In one study, college students with no history of panic attacks were divided into high and low scorers on the Anxiety Sensitivity Index (Telch & Harrington, 2011). Researchers then used the carbon dioxide manipulation described earlier to see who would develop panic attacks. As in the study by Rapee and colleagues, half of the participants were told that carbon dioxide would produce arousal symptoms, and half were not. With the higher level of carbon dioxide, panic attacks were most common among people who feared their bodily sensations, particularly if they were not warned that carbon dioxide would trigger arousal. This result is exactly what the model predicts: Unexplained physiological arousal in someone who is fearful of such sensations leads to panic attacks.

Generalized Anxiety Disorder

Generalized anxiety disorder (GAD) tends to co-occur with other anxiety disorders. Because the comorbidity is so high, researchers believe that many of the influences on anxiety disorders in general are important for understanding GAD. GAD, though, seems to differ from the other anxiety disorders in a few important ways. People who meet diagnostic criteria for GAD are much more likely to experience episodes of major depressive disorder (MDD) than those with other anxiety disorders are. This suggests that some of the influences involved in MDD are also likely to be important in GAD. Here, however, we focus on a specific model of GAD.

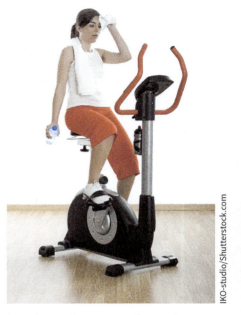

Experiments demonstrate that panic attacks can be triggered by a variety of agents that change bodily sensations, including drugs and even exercise.

Worry is the core feature of GAD. Worry is associated with negative affect and with modest increases in psychophysiological arousal. Just as you might expect, when instructed to worry, participants with and without GAD report distress and show small increases in psychophysiological arousal (Stapinski, Abbott, & Rapee, 2010). Worry is such an unpleasant experience that one might ask why anyone would worry a lot.

The **contrast avoidance model** may help explain why some people worry more than others do (Newman & Llera, 2011). Core to this model is the finding that people diagnosed with GAD find it highly aversive to experience rapid shifts in emotions. According to this theory, to ward off sudden shifts in emotion, people with GAD find it preferable to sustain a chronic state of worry and distress: A worrier confronted with a stressor has less room for a large shift in mood and psychophysiological arousal.

Several types of research indicate that worry can reduce the intensity of shifts in negative emotions. When people with GAD are presented with a laboratory stressor, they show less of an increase in mood and psychophysiological arousal than do those without GAD (McTeague & Lang, 2012). Indeed, when people with and without GAD were assigned to a worry condition, all experienced an increase in psychophysiological indicators of negative emotion as compared to a control group assigned to relaxation. The advantage, though, was clear in the next phase of the experiment, when the participants were asked to watch a frightening video clip. Compared to the relaxation control group, those who had been assigned to worry did not show as much increase in psychophysiological signs of arousal during the video clip (Kim & Newman, 2022). The point isn't that worry makes one happier or calmer during stress, but that the negative emotions are less volatile. This same profile has been shown in a study of worry in daily life: People who were worried before a stressor showed a less dramatic shift in negative mood after that stressor (Baik & Newman, 2023). Taken together, these findings suggest that worry could help a person sustain more stability in their emotional state, even if it is an uncomfortable one!

Intriguingly, worry reduces emotional volatility in a similar way for people with higher and lower GAD symptoms (Baik & Newman, 2023; Kim & Newman, 2022). The key difference for those with GAD, though, is that they find emotional volatility very aversive. Accordingly, people with GAD place greater value on these emotional effects of worry than others do (Kim & Newman, 2022; Newman, Rackoff, et al., 2023). New work suggests that people with major depressive disorder and other anxiety disorders also find emotional volatility very aversive, which could help explain why people with these disorders also tend to worry and ruminate (Newman et al., 2023).

Quick Summary

In addition to variables that increase the overall risk of developing a range of anxiety disorders, researchers have identified risk variables related to specific anxiety disorders.

Specific phobias are believed to reflect conditioning in response to a traumatic event. Many people report that they experienced traumatic conditioning experiences before developing specific phobias, but many people don't, perhaps because the conditioning experience has been forgotten. Prepared learning refers to the fact that people are more likely to fear stimuli that are evolutionarily significant.

Social anxiety disorder appears to be related to conditioning and behavioral inhibition. Cognitive influences on social anxiety disorder include self-critical evaluations of social performance, tendencies to focus on internal thoughts and sensations, and an overconcern about violating social dominance hierarchies.

Neurobiological research demonstrates that panic attacks are related to high activity in the locus coeruleus. Behavioral models emphasize the possibility that people could become classically conditioned to experience panic attacks in response to external situations or to internal somatic signs of arousal. Conditioning to somatic signs is called interoceptive conditioning. Cognitive perspectives focus on catastrophic misinterpretations of somatic symptoms, which can be measured with the Anxiety Sensitivity Index.

One cognitive model of GAD, the contrast avoidance model, suggests that worry might protect people from sudden increases in negative moods by sustaining a more chronically negative mood.

6.5 Check Your Knowledge

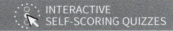
INTERACTIVE SELF-SCORING QUIZZES

(Answers are at the end of the chapter.)
Match the model to the disorder.

a. anxiety sensitivity

b. prepared learning

c. avoidance of powerful changes in negative emotions

d. too much of a focus on one's own flaws

1. Panic disorder
2. GAD
3. Specific phobias
4. Social anxiety disorder

Treatments of Anxiety Disorders

Most people who seek treatment for anxiety disorders will only visit a family doctor. In 2019, more than 6% of people living in the United States filled at least one prescription for anti-anxiety medications (Express Scripts, 2020). Although medication is the most commonly offered treatment for anxiety, a psychological treatment called exposure treatment provides as much or more relief from anxiety symptoms as medications do (Carl, Witcraft, et al., 2020; Cuijpers, Sijbrandij, et al., 2013). Because of the risk of relapse when medications are discontinued, psychological treatments are considered the preferred treatment approach for most anxiety disorders.

As with other psychological disorders, individuals from racial and ethnic minority backgrounds are less likely to seek care for anxiety disorders than are White non-Latino individuals. Some of this may be due to higher stigma, but practical barriers such as access to transportation also can impeded treatment-seeking. Programs that have provided more orientation to treatment, psychoeducation to reduce stigma, and support with transportation and pragmatic barriers have been found to be helpful for individuals with minority backgrounds (Hazlett-Stevens, 2020).

Commonalities Across Psychological Treatments

Effective psychological treatments for anxiety disorders share a common focus: exposure. That is, people must face what they deem too terrifying to face. Therapists from varying perspectives all agree that we must face up to the source of our fear or, as an ancient Chinese proverb puts it, "Go straight to the heart of danger, for there you will find safety." Even psychoanalysts, who believe that the unconscious sources of anxiety are buried in the past, eventually encourage confronting the source of fears (Zane, 1984).

Exposure is a core component of cognitive behavioral therapy (CBT). In a typical approach to exposure treatment, the therapist and the client make a list of triggers—situations and activities that might elicit anxiety or fear—and they create an "exposure hierarchy," a graded list of the difficulty of these triggers. Early sessions involve exposure to the less challenging triggers, and gradually, as the client learns that exposure will extinguish anxiety, the more challenging triggers are faced.

Dozens of randomized controlled studies have compared CBT to a control form of psychotherapy, and findings from those studies indicate that CBT works better than control treatments for the anxiety disorders (Hofmann & Smits, 2008). The odds of a treatment response are about three times larger for patients enrolled in CBT as compared to those who receive a placebo treatment (Carpenter, Andrews, et al., 2018). Nonetheless, there is room for improvement. Even though most patients show some decline in anxiety levels, only about half of patients achieve full remission (Springer, Levy, & Tolin, 2018). The benefits of CBT endure when follow-up assessments are conducted 6 months after treatment (Hollon, Stewart, & Strunk, 2006), but in the years after treatment, many people experience some return of their anxiety symptoms. Although much of the research has been conducted with samples of majority individuals, CBT has also been shown to be helpful for Latino clients (Chavira, Golinelli, et al., 2014).

The behavioral view of exposure is that it works by extinguishing the fear response. Consistent with the behavioral view, researchers have shown that people who show more rapid extinction of conditioned fears also show a better response to exposure treatment (Pittig, Treanor, et al., 2018). In one test of this idea, researchers recruited people with speech anxiety, conditioned them to fear a picture by pairing it repeatedly with a loud scream, and then examined their ability to extinguish this conditioned fear. In the next phase of the study, the researchers followed participants to see how they responded to exposure therapy. Participants who had shown better extinction of the conditioned fear response gained more symptom relief during exposure therapy (Ball, Knapp, et al., 2017). This suggests that people who more rapidly extinguish fear responses do better in exposure-based treatment.

A good deal of work has focused on how extinction works at a neurobiological level, and this information can be used to refine exposure treatment (Vervliet, Craske, & Hermans, 2013). Results of such studies suggest that extinction does not work like an eraser. Let's take dog phobia as an example. Extinction will not erase the underlying fear of dogs altogether—the conditioned fear still resides deep inside the brain, and it can resurface over time or in certain contexts. Rather, extinction involves learning new associations to stimuli related to dogs. These newly learned associations inhibit activation of the fear. Thus, extinction involves learning, not forgetting.

This idea of extinction as learning helps explain some of the key principles that are important in relapse prevention (Craske, Sandman, & Stein, 2022). First, exposure should include as many features of the feared object as possible. For example, exposure for a person with a spider phobia might include exposure to different spiders, but also a focus on different features of those spiders, such as the hairy legs and the beady eyes. Second, exposure should be conducted in as many different contexts as possible (Bouton & Waddell, 2007). As an example, it might be important to expose a person to a spider in an office and outside in nature. An elevator phobic might be urged to ride elevators in many different buildings. Repetition and mental rehearsal can be used to help consolidate the new memory. The client can be coached to attend carefully throughout the exposure and to avoid using safety behaviors. That is, good exposure treatment involves learning new responses to as many features of the feared object as possible, in as many contexts as possible.

A cognitive view of exposure treatment also has been proposed. According to this view, exposure helps people correct their mistaken beliefs that they are unable to cope with the stimulus. In this view, exposure relieves symptoms by allowing people to realize that, contrary to their beliefs, they can tolerate feared situations without loss of control (Foa & Meadows, 1997). Cognitive approaches to treatment of anxiety disorders typically focus on challenging

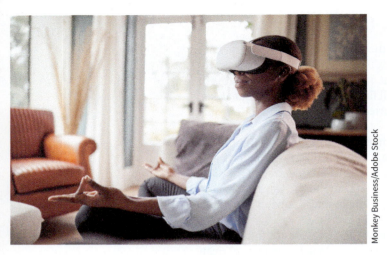

Virtual reality technology is sometimes used to facilitate exposure to feared stimuli.

Monkey Business/Adobe Stock

people's beliefs about (1) the likelihood of negative outcomes if they face an anxiety-provoking object or situation and (2) their ability to cope with the anxiety. Thus, cognitive treatments typically involve exposure in order to help people learn that they can cope with these situations. Because both behavioral and cognitive treatments involve exposure and learning to cope differently with fears, it is not surprising that most studies suggest that adding a cognitive therapy component to exposure therapy for anxiety disorders does not bolster results (Deacon & Abramowitz, 2004). Some very specific cognitive techniques, however, seem to help when added to exposure treatment, and we will discuss these as we review how treatment can be tailored for the specific anxiety disorders.

Virtual reality is sometimes used to simulate feared situations such as flying, heights, and even social interactions. Findings of randomized controlled trials indicate that exposure to these simulated situations appears to be as effective as **in vivo (real-life) exposure** (Carl, Stein, et al., 2019).

In addition to virtual reality, internet-based CBT programs appear to achieve large effects compared to control conditions, and significant benefits are shown when clients are reassessed 9 months or more after they finish the program (Andrews, Basu, et al., 2018). Such programs can help fill an important gap, as many people with anxiety disorders do not seek psychotherapy. These programs seem to work best when at least some human contact is provided. For example, therapists might conduct the initial screening to ensure that a person is enrolled in the right type of program, they might help a person develop an appropriate exposure hierarchy, or they might review homework assignments (Marks & Cavanagh, 2009). Even with this type of support, these programs substantially reduce the amount of professional contact time required to provide exposure treatment.

Although exposure treatment is considered primary, several treatments have been developed to help people take a more reflective, less reactive stance toward their intense anxiety and other emotions. These treatments include components such as mindfulness meditation and skills to promote acceptance of emotions. Most typically, these are used in combination with other CBT techniques, such as exposure treatment. Although few randomized trials are available, mindfulness meditation and acceptance treatments appear to be more powerful in reducing anxiety symptoms than are placebos and have fared as well as CBT in the treatment of mixed anxiety disorders and GAD (Hofmann & Gómez, 2017; Roemer, Williston, et al., 2013). The Unified Protocol incorporates many of these different approaches—exposure treatment, mindful emotion awareness, and identifying and reducing emotion avoidance, along with a module on improving cognitive flexibility (Barlow, Farchione, et al., 2017). The Unified Protocol was designed to be helpful in treating depressive, anxiety, and other internalizing disorders that involve emotion-related problems. Across a number of randomized controlled trials, the Unified Protocol has been shown to be more efficacious than control conditions in reducing anxious and depressive symptoms (Carlucci et al., 2021), and in one trial, it was shown to be as helpful as approaches designed to address specific anxiety disorders (Eustis, Gallagher, et al., 2020), which we turn to next.

Psychological Treatments of Specific Anxiety Disorders

Exposure treatment is used with all anxiety disorders, but next we consider how this psychotherapy can be tailored to specific anxiety disorders. Researchers have adapted exposure treatment to address the more specific content of specific anxiety disorders, and they have considered the best length and format of treatment for each of the specific anxiety disorders.

Psychological Treatment of Phobias
Many different types of exposure treatments have been developed for phobias. Exposure treatments often include in vivo (real-life) exposure to feared objects. For phobias involving fear of animals, injections, or dental work,

very brief treatments lasting only a couple of hours have been found to be highly effective (Wolitzky-Taylor, Horowitz, et al., 2008).

Psychological Treatment of Social Anxiety Disorder

CBT for social anxiety has shown efficacy compared with wait-list controls and supportive treatment (Mayo-Wilson, Dias, et al., 2014). CBT appears to be more cost-effective than medications for the treatment of social anxiety (Mavranezouli, Mayo-Wilson, et al., 2015).

As with other anxiety disorders, exposure is a core aspect of CBT for social anxiety. To provide a graded hierarchy of exposure, such treatments often begin with role playing or practicing with the therapist or in small therapy groups before undergoing exposure in more public social situations. Social skills training, in which a therapist might model effective social behavior, can help people with social anxiety disorder who may not know what to do or say in social situations. Remember that safety behaviors, like avoiding eye contact, are believed to interfere with the extinction of social anxiety. Consistent with this idea, the effects of exposure treatment seem to be enhanced when people with social anxiety disorder are taught to stop using safety behaviors (Kim, 2005). That is, not only are people asked to engage in social activities, but they are asked to make direct eye contact, to engage in conversation, and to be fully present while doing so. Doing so leads to immediate gains in how they are perceived by others and enhances outcomes of exposure treatment (Alden, Buhr, et al., 2018; Taylor & Alden, 2011).

David Clark (1997) has developed a version of cognitive therapy for social anxiety disorder that expands on other treatments in a couple of ways. The therapist helps people learn not to focus their attention internally. The therapist also helps them combat their very negative images of how others will react to them. This cognitive therapy has been shown to be more effective than either antidepressant medication or exposure treatment plus relaxation (Clark, Ehlers, et al., 2003, 2006). In one study, people who had received cognitive therapy for social anxiety continued to show positive outcomes 5 years later (Mortberg, Clark, & Bejerot, 2011).

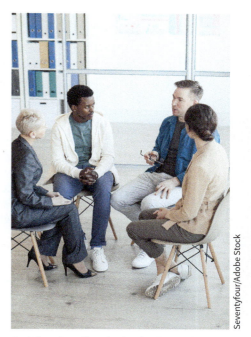

Social anxiety disorder is often treated in groups, which provide exposure to social threats and provide opportunities to practice new skills.

Psychological Treatment of Panic Disorder

Like behavioral treatments for other anxiety disorders, CBT for panic disorder focuses on exposure. Because people with panic disorder tend to overreact to bodily sensations (Craske & Barlow, 2014), the exposure sessions involve deliberately eliciting the bodily sensations associated with panic. For example, a person whose panic attacks begin with hyperventilation is asked to breathe rapidly for 3 minutes. Some examples of techniques that can be used to provoke body sensations in this type of exposure therapy are shown in Table 6.5. When sensations such as dizziness, dry mouth, lightheadedness, increased heart rate, and other somatic signs of panic begin, the person experiences them under safe conditions; in addition, the person practices coping tactics for dealing with somatic symptoms (e.g., breathing from the diaphragm to reduce hyperventilation). With practice and encouragement from the therapist, the person learns to stop seeing physical sensations as signals of loss of control and to see them instead as intrinsically harmless and controllable sensations. The person's ability to create these physical sensations and then cope with them makes them seem more predictable and less frightening (Clark, 1996).

In cognitive treatment for panic disorder (Clark, 1996), the therapist helps the person identify and challenge the thoughts that make the physical sensations threatening (see Figure 6.5

TABLE 6.5	Techniques for Provoking Somatic Symptoms During Exposure Treatment for Panic Disorder
Technique	**Body Sensation**
Rapid deep breathing for 90 seconds	Shortness of breath, sense of unreality
Attempt to swallow quickly five times in a row	Throat tightness, lump in throat
Run in place	Chest tightness, shortness of breath
Spin in chair	Dizziness

Source: Based on Abramowitz, J. S., & Braddock, A. E. (2008). *Psychological treatment of hypochondriasis and health anxiety: A biopsychosocial approach.* Hogrefe & Huber.

for an example of one patient's thoughts). For example, if a person with panic disorder imagines that they will collapse, the therapist might help the person examine the evidence for this belief and develop a different image of the consequences of a panic attack. This treatment has been shown to work well in at least seven studies and appears to be a helpful supplement to exposure treatment (Clark et al., 1999).

Psychological Treatment of Agoraphobia

CBT for agoraphobia also focuses on systematic exposure to feared situations. The person with agoraphobia may be coached to gradually tackle leaving home, then driving a couple of miles from home, then sitting in a movie theater for 5 minutes, and then staying for the full duration of a movie in a crowded theater. Exposure treatment of agoraphobia can be enhanced by involving the patient's partner (Cerny, Barlow, et al., 1987). The partner without agoraphobia is taught that recovery rests upon exposure. Many partners will have sheltered the patients from facing their fears, and through treatment, partners learn to foster exposure rather than avoidance.

Psychological Treatment of Generalized Anxiety Disorder

Multiple behavioral and cognitive treatment strategies for GAD have been developed. The most widely used behavioral technique involves relaxation training to promote calmness. Relaxation techniques can involve relaxing muscle groups one by one or generating calming mental images. With practice, clients typically learn to relax rapidly. Studies suggest that relaxation training is more effective than nondirective treatment or no treatment. Broader forms of CBT have also been developed, which include strategies to help improve problem solving and to address the thought patterns that contribute to GAD. One form of cognitive therapy includes strategies to help people tolerate uncertainty, as people with anxiety disorders seem to be distressed by uncertainty (Dugas, Brillon, et al., 2010). Other cognitive behavioral strategies used to target worry include asking people to worry only during scheduled times, asking people to test whether worry "works" by keeping a diary of the outcomes of worrying, helping people focus their thoughts on the present moment instead of worrying, and helping people address core fears (Borkovec, Alcaine, & Behar, 2004). A small number of studies indicate that broader CBT treatment is more helpful than is relaxation treatment alone (Cuijpers, Sijbrandij, et al., 2014).

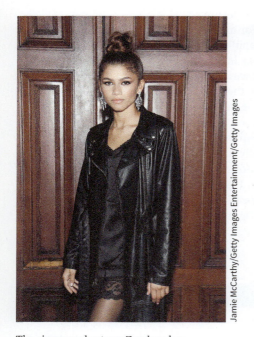

The singer and actress Zendaya has described social anxiety that led her to temporarily avoid singing engagements (*Bustle* magazine, 2019, https://www.bustle.com/p/zendaya-says-euphoria-gave-her-anxiety-every-week-that-it-aired-19202013).

Jamie McCarthy/Getty Images Entertainment/Getty Images

Quick Summary

Exposure treatment is the most validated psychological treatment for anxiety disorders. Cognitive treatments supplement exposure with interventions to challenge negative beliefs about what will happen when a person faces fears.

For specific phobias, exposure treatments can work quite quickly. For social anxiety disorder, cognitive strategies, such as teaching a person to focus less on internal thoughts and sensations, are a helpful addition to exposure treatment. The most effective treatments for panic disorder include exposure to somatic sensations, along with cognitive techniques to challenge catastrophic misinterpretations of those symptoms. Exposure treatment for agoraphobia may be enhanced by including partners. CBT for GAD can include relaxation training, strategies to help a person tolerate uncertainty and face core fears, and specific tools to combat tendencies to worry.

Medications That Reduce Anxiety

Drugs that reduce anxiety are referred to as **anxiolytics** (the suffix -*lytic* comes from a Greek word meaning "to loosen or dissolve"). Selective serotonin reuptake inhibitors (SSRIs) and serotonin-norepinephrine reuptake inhibitors (SNRIs) have both been found to be efficacious in reducing anxiety symptoms in many randomized controlled trials (Bandelow, 2020). On average, people who take SSRIs and SNRIs show large declines in their level of anxiety symptoms.

Another form of anxiolytic, **benzodiazepines** (e.g., Valium and Xanax) are commonly prescribed but are no longer recommended as a first-line treatment for two main reasons. First, people may experience severe withdrawal symptoms when they try to stop using benzodiazepines—that is, they can be addictive. Second, benzodiazepines also can have significant cognitive and motor side effects, such as memory lapses and drowsiness (Baldwin, Aitchison, et al., 2013; Rapoport, Lanctot, et al., 2009).

Antidepressants tend to have fewer side effects than benzodiazepines, and those side effects tend to become less severe in the first couple weeks of treatment (Bandelow, 2020). Some people, however, do experience side effects from SSRIs and SNRIs, including gastrointestinal distress, restlessness, insomnia, headache, and diminished sexual functioning (Bandelow, 2020). Many people stop taking anxiolytic medications because of the side effects. This is of concern as many people relapse once they stop taking medications (Wilson & Stein, 2019).

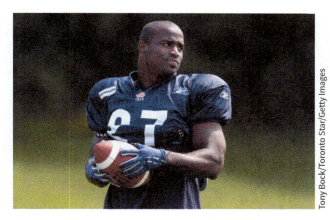

Ricky Williams, the Heisman Trophy winner who became a star for his incredible skills as a running back, obtained relief of his social anxiety symptoms from antidepressant treatment.

Tony Bock/Toronto Star/Getty Images

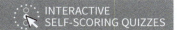

6.6 Check Your Knowledge

INTERACTIVE
SELF-SCORING QUIZZES

(Answers are at the end of the chapter.)
Answer the following questions.

1. What strategy is most commonly used in CBT for anxiety disorders?

2. List two reasons psychological treatment is a better option than medication for anxiety disorders.

3. List two reasons antidepressant medications are preferred over benzodiazepines for the treatment of most anxiety disorders.

Summary

INTERACTIVE
SELF-SCORING QUIZZES

Chapter 6 Practice Quiz

Emotions of Anxiety and Fear

- Anxiety is defined as apprehension over an anticipated problem.

- In contrast, fear is defined as a reaction to immediate danger.

- Fear can involve arousal, or sympathetic nervous system activity, and anxiety can also involve lower levels of arousal.

- Anxiety and fear are both adaptive. Anxiety helps us plan for future threats, and fear helps us respond to current threats.

Clinical Descriptions of Anxiety Disorders

- As a group, anxiety disorders are the most common type of psychological disorder.

- The five major DSM-5-TR anxiety disorders are specific phobia, social anxiety disorder, panic disorder, agoraphobia, and generalized anxiety disorder. Anxiety is common to all the anxiety disorders, and fear is common in anxiety disorders other than generalized anxiety disorder.

- Phobias are intense, unreasonable fears that interfere with functioning. Specific phobias commonly include fears of animals; natural environments such as heights; blood, injury, or injections; and situations such as crossing bridges or flying.

- Social anxiety disorder is defined by intense fear of possible social scrutiny.

- Panic disorder is defined by recurrent attacks of intense fear that occur out of the blue. Panic attacks alone are not sufficient for the diagnosis; a person must be worried about the potential of having another attack.

- Agoraphobia is defined by fear and avoidance of being in situations where escaping or getting help would be difficult if anxiety symptoms were to occur.

- The key feature of generalized anxiety disorder is worry that lasts at least 6 months.

Gender and Cultural Influences on Anxiety Disorders

- Anxiety disorders are much more common among women than men.

- The focus of anxiety, the prevalence of anxiety disorders, and the specific symptoms expressed may be shaped by culture.

Common Influences Across Anxiety Disorders

- Mowrer's two-factor model suggests that anxiety disorders are related to two types of conditioning. The first stage involves classical conditioning, in which a formerly innocuous object is paired with a feared object. This can occur through direct exposure, modeling, or verbal instruction. The second stage involves operant conditioning, in which avoidance is reinforced because it reduces anxiety, and so the person does not gain the chance to have the fears extinguished. Many people do not develop an anxiety disorder after a major threat, though, and this is a challenge to the Mowrer model. The model has been extended to include the idea that those with anxiety disorders may be particularly slow to extinguish classically conditioned fears; they also may be particularly responsive to unpredictable threats compared with other people. Many of the other risk factors may increase the propensity to develop and sustain conditioned fears.

- Genes increase risk for a broad range of anxiety disorders, and they account for about 50–60% of the variance in whether a person develops an anxiety disorder. Beyond this general risk for anxiety disorders, there may be more specific heritability for certain anxiety disorders. In addition to genetic diatheses, other biological factors involved in a range of anxiety disorders include disturbances in the activity in the amygdala and medial prefrontal cortex, poor functioning of the serotonin and GABA neurotransmitter systems, and increased norepinephrine activity.

- Cognitive influences include sustained negative beliefs about the future, lack of perceived control, intolerance of uncertainty, and heightened attention to threatening stimuli.

- Personality influences include behavioral inhibition and neuroticism.

Influences on Specific Anxiety Disorders

- Behavioral models of specific phobias build on the two-factor model of conditioning. The prepared learning model suggests that people may more easily develop fears of objects with evolutionary significance. Because not all people with negative experiences develop phobias, vulnerability factors must be important.

- The behavioral model of social anxiety disorder expands the two-factor conditioning model to consider the role of safety behaviors. Other key influences include behavioral inhibition and cognitive variables such as excessively critical self-evaluations, a focus on internal sensations rather than social cues, and an overconcern with social hierarchy.

- Neurobiological models of panic disorder have focused on the locus coeruleus, the brain region responsible for norepinephrine

release. Behavioral theories of panic attacks have posited that the attacks are classically conditioned to internal bodily sensations (interoceptive conditioning). Cognitive theories suggest that such sensations are more frightening due to catastrophic misinterpretation of somatic cues.

- The contrast avoidance model of GAD suggests that worry helps people avoid intense changes in negative emotions.

Treatments of Anxiety Disorders

- Behavior therapists focus on exposure to what is feared. For some anxiety disorders, cognitive components are also helpful in therapy.

- Exposure treatment for specific phobias tends to work quickly and well.

- Adding cognitive components to exposure treatment may help for social anxiety disorder.

- Treatment for panic disorder often involves exposure to physiological changes.

- Treatment for agoraphobia may be enhanced by including partners in the treatment process.

- Relaxation and cognitive behavioral approaches are helpful for GAD.

- Antidepressants and benzodiazepines are the most commonly prescribed medications for anxiety disorders. Benzodiazepines can be addictive.

- Discontinuing medications usually leads to relapse, and the effects of medications in providing relief from anxiety are not generally as strong as those of cognitive behavioral therapy.

Answers to Check Your Knowledge Questions

6.1 1. True; 2. False; 3. True; 4. An absence of anxiety is a problem because people are less likely to prepare adequately for threat, a little anxiety is adaptive, and a lot of anxiety is detrimental.

6.2 1. a; 2. c; 3. d; 4. b; 5. 28%; 6. worry.

6.3 1. 2 to 1; 2. the United States and European countries; 3. False.

6.4 1. c. 50–60; 2. A personality trait characterized by a tendency to experience frequent and intense negative affect; 3 b. attention to signs of threat, d. lack of perceived control; 4. b; 5. c. classical; 6. unpredictable.

6.5 1. a; 2. c; 3. b; 4. d.

6.6 1. Exposure, sometimes supplemented with cognitive approaches; 2. Although the efficacies of psychotherapy and medications are similar, medications have significant side effects, and relapse is common once medications are discontinued; 3. Side effects are more severe with benzodiazepines compared with antidepressant medications; there is a risk of addiction with benzodiazepines.

Key Terms

agoraphobia   158
anxiety   152
anxiety disorders   151
Anxiety Sensitivity Index   172
anxiolytics   178
behavioral inhibition   165
benzodiazepines   178
contrast avoidance model   173
depersonalization   157

derealization   157
fear   152
fear circuit   164
generalized anxiety disorder (GAD)   158
in vivo exposure   176
interoceptive conditioning   171
locus coeruleus   171
medial prefrontal cortex   164
Mowrer's two-factor model   162

neutral predictable unpredictable (NPU)
   threat task   163
panic attack   157
panic disorder   157
prepared learning   169
safety behaviors   166
social anxiety disorder   156
specific phobia   154

Obsessive-Compulsive-Related and Trauma-Related Disorders

LEARNING GOALS

1. Explain the symptoms and epidemiology of obsessive-compulsive and related disorders.

2. Describe the commonalities in the causes of obsessive-compulsive and related disorders, as well as the influences that shape the expression of the specific disorders within this cluster.

3. Discuss the medication and psychological treatments for obsessive-compulsive and related disorders.

4. Define the symptoms and outcomes of the trauma-related disorders: acute stress disorder and posttraumatic stress disorder.

5. Summarize how the nature and severity of trauma, as well as biological and psychological influences, contribute to whether trauma-related disorders develop.

6. Describe the medication and psychological treatments for trauma-related disorders.

Clinical Case

Jacob

Jacob was a 28-year-old graduate student when he sought treatment. Shortly after starting graduate school 2 years earlier, Jacob had begun to experience intrusive images of running over animals with his car. Although he knew that he had not done so, the images were so vivid that he could not get them out of his mind. Several times a week, he would be so disturbed by the idea that he might have hit an animal that he would feel compelled to turn his car around and drive his route again, looking for any signs of wounded or dead animals. If he spotted a wounded or dead animal, he would pull off the road and inspect his car for any signs that he might have been the person who hit the animal. Sometimes, when he finished his second trip, he would become concerned that he might have missed a wounded or dead animal,

and he would feel the need to drive the route again. This often made him late for work or appointments, but if he didn't get the chance to look for wounded or dead animals, he would ruminate about the possibility of injured animals throughout the day. He also felt compelled to engage in elaborate bathing rituals, to solve math problems again and again in his head, to chew his food a certain number of times, to flip his light switch on and off three times before he left his bedroom each morning, and to tap his right elbow three times at the top of the hour. He knew these compulsive behaviors didn't make sense, but he still felt terrible anxiety if he didn't engage in them. The images occupied his mind and the behavioral rituals absorbed his time, such that his progress in graduate school had slowed to a crawl. He sought treatment after his advisor raised concerns about the slow progress of his thesis research.

In this chapter, we examine obsessive-compulsive and related disorders, and then we turn to trauma-related disorders. Obsessive-compulsive and related disorders are defined by repetitive thoughts and behaviors that are so extreme that they interfere with everyday life. Trauma-related disorders include posttraumatic stress disorder and acute stress disorder, two conditions that are triggered by exposure to severely traumatic events.

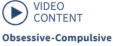

VIDEO CONTENT

Obsessive-Compulsive Disorders

As we will discuss, many people with obsessive-compulsive and related disorders, as well as those with trauma-related disorders, report feeling anxious, and they often experience anxiety disorders as well. Many of the influences on anxiety disorders contribute to these disorders, and the treatment approaches overlap a good deal as well. Nonetheless, these disorders have some causes distinct from those of anxiety disorders. As you read this chapter, consider the parallels with the anxiety disorders described in Chapter 6.

We will begin by reviewing the clinical features of obsessive-compulsive and related disorders, and then we will discuss research on their epidemiology and causes before turning to an overview of treatment approaches. Finally, we will discuss the symptoms, causes, and treatment of trauma-related disorders.

Clinical Descriptions and Epidemiology of Obsessive-Compulsive and Related Disorders

We will focus on three disorders in this section: obsessive-compulsive disorder (OCD), body dysmorphic disorder (BDD), and hoarding disorder (see **Table 7.1**). OCD, the prototypical disorder of this cluster, is defined by repetitive thoughts and urges (obsessions), as well as an irresistible need to engage in repetitive behaviors or mental acts (compulsions). BDD and hoarding disorder share the symptoms of repetitive thoughts and behaviors. People with BDD spend hours a day thinking about their appearance and engage in compulsive behaviors designed to address concerns about their appearance. People with hoarding disorder spend a good deal of their time repetitively thinking about their current and potential future possessions. They also engage in intensive efforts to acquire new objects, and these efforts can resemble the compulsions observed in OCD. For the people with all three conditions, the repetitive thoughts and behaviors feel unstoppable and consume a considerable amount of time. Thus, these three disorders share the quality of repetitive thought as well as irresistible urges to engage repetitively in some behavior or mental act. It is not surprising, then, that there is overlap in the causes and treatment of these three conditions, which will be discussed later in this chapter.

Despite the overlap, the focus of thought and behavior takes a different form across the three conditions. Likewise, there are important distinctions in the causes and treatment of these three disorders (Abramowitz, 2018). We will begin by reviewing the clinical features of obsessive-compulsive and related disorders, and then we will discuss research on their epidemiology and causes before turning to an overview of treatment approaches.

TABLE 7.1 Diagnoses of Obsessive-Compulsive and Related Disorders	INTERACTIVE FIGURES, CHARTS, & TABLES

Diagnoses	Key Features
Obsessive-compulsive disorder (OCD)	Repetitive, intrusive, uncontrollable thoughts, images or urges (obsessions)
	Repetitive behaviors or mental acts that a person feels compelled to perform (compulsions)
Body dysmorphic disorder (BDD)	Preoccupation with imagined flaws in one's appearance
	Excessive repetitive behaviors or acts regarding appearance (e.g., checking appearance, seeking reassurance)
Hoarding disorder	Acquisition of an excessive number of objects
	Inability to part with those objects

Obsessive-Compulsive Disorder

The diagnosis of **obsessive-compulsive disorder (OCD)** is based on the presence of obsessions or compulsions. Most people with OCD experience both obsessions and compulsions but having either is sufficient for diagnosis. Although many think that the chief distinction here is of thoughts (obsessions) versus behaviors (compulsions), they are mistaken. Let's consider the technical definitions of obsessions and compulsions.

Obsessions are intrusive and persistently recurring thoughts, images, or impulses that are uncontrollable (i.e., the person cannot stop the thoughts) and that often appear irrational to the person experiencing them. With a moment's reflection, most of you can likely think of a time when you had a repetitive thought. At least 80% of people briefly experience intrusive thoughts from time to time—for example, a terrible song or image gets stuck in one's head. And most of us also have thoughts now and then about behaving in ways that would be embarrassing or dangerous—thoughts about grabbing money or engaging in violence or inexplicable urges to do something dangerous like jump from a high ledge (Rachman & DeSilva, 1978). But few of us have thoughts or urges that are persistent and intrusive enough to qualify as obsessions. Like Jacob's images of animals (see the **Clinical Case of Jacob**) or David Adam's thoughts about HIV (see **Read More About It 7.1**), the obsessions of most people with OCD have such force and frequency that they interfere with normal activities. Typically, obsessions last for hours of every day for a person with OCD.

Like David Adam's thoughts, obsessions often involve fear of contamination from germs or disease. Although most of us would like to avoid germs and disease, cues that are remotely related to disease can trigger the fears of a person with OCD. Some with contamination fears describe the need to change clothes and shower after being in a room with someone who has coughed, and then to wash the clothes as well as any part of their home that the contaminated clothes might have touched. The famous mathematician Gödel was so obsessed with the idea that tainted food could poison him that he would eat only food that his wife had first tasted. When she was unable to taste his food due to illness, he starved to death (Adam, 2014).

To understand how contamination could spread so drastically from an initial threatening stimulus, researchers asked people with OCD to consider the building where the research was taking place and to identify the most contaminated object in the building. Most chose a trash can or a toilet. In this regard, the people with OCD were like people with anxiety disorders and those with no disorder. With each participant, the researcher then removed a pencil from a new box of 12 pencils and rubbed the pencil against the contaminated object. The researcher then rubbed a second pencil against the first pencil, and then rubbed a third pencil against the second pencil, and so on, through the 12 pencils. Participants were asked to rate the contamination level for each of the 12 pencils. Those without OCD generally rated the sixth pencil as free of contamination. Those with OCD rated even the 12th pencil as highly contaminated (Tolin, Worhunsky, & Maltby, 2004).

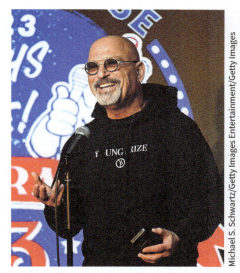

Howie Mandel describes his struggle with OCD in his book *Here's the Deal: Don't Touch Me*. Deeply afraid of germs, he has been unable to shake hands with people, touch a glass, or use a handrail without feeling the intense urge to clean. At age 6, he had trouble learning to tie his shoes because he was afraid to touch his dirty shoelaces.

Michael S. Schwartz/Getty Images Entertainment/Getty Images

Defining Symptoms of Obsessive-Compulsive Disorder (OCD)

- Obsessions and/or compulsions

Obsessions are defined by

1. Recurrent, intrusive, persistent, unwanted thoughts, urges, or images
2. The attempt to ignore, suppress, or neutralize such thoughts, urges, or images

Compulsions are defined by

1. Repetitive behaviors or mental acts that a person feels driven to perform in response to an obsession or according to rigid rules

2. The behaviors or acts are performed to reduce distress or prevent a dreaded event
3. The behaviors or acts are excessive or unlikely to prevent the dreaded event

- The thoughts or activities are time-consuming (e.g., at least 1 hour per day) or cause clinically significant distress or impairment

Read More About It 7.1

The Man Who Couldn't Stop: OCD and the True Story of a Life Lost in Thought

David Adam, an esteemed science journalist, turned his writing skills to the topic of his own struggle with and recovery from obsessive-compulsive disorder in his book, *The Man Who Couldn't Stop: OCD and the True Story of a Life Lost in Thought* (2014). His obsessions began with a fear that he could have been infected with HIV. He knew the fear was irrational—he hadn't had sex before the fear started—but even repeated testing wouldn't shake the thought. He tried to argue himself out of the thought, telling himself, "Don't be daft." But it didn't work. "I couldn't move past the idea, or the cramps of panic it caused ... I had lost the power over my own fate. As I tried to brush away the thought, the snow-flake, it squirmed from my mental grasp and settled. Quickly it was joined by another, then another, then another" (p. 29). Once these obsessional thoughts took hold, no amount of reassurance seemed to quell them. David took to calling the National AIDS Hotline so compulsively and so often that the six staff members could recognize his voice. "Every night HIV was the last thing I thought about before I went to sleep. And it was the first thing I thought of every morning. And it was pretty much all I thought of in between. I have few memories from that time of anything else. I lost interest in the stuff that had seemed important just a few months previously" (pp. 58–59).

Despite the ongoing distress and intrusion of his obsessions, Adam had many successes. He did well in school, formed close relationships, became a reporter and editor for the journal *Nature*, and won awards for his writing. It wasn't until his obsessions began to influence his relationship with his daughter that he sought treatment—19 years after his obsessions had begun. Once he sought treatment, a combination of exposure and response prevention therapy, group therapy, and antidepressant medication finally gave him relief.

His compelling book weaves together personal experiences, examples from other case histories, and succinct summaries of major findings in the field. As a science writer, Adam provides clarity on the key findings and major gaps in the science of OCD.

Source: Adam, D. (2014). *The man who couldn't stop: OCD and the true story of a life lost in thought.* Farrar, Straus and Giroux.

Beyond contamination, other frequent foci of obsessions include sex and morality, violence, religion, symmetry/order, and responsibility for harm. We provide some examples of each of these in **Table 7.2**. Obsessions are extremely uncomfortable to experience, and those with OCD will often go to great lengths to avoid situations that might trigger their obsessions (Abramowitz & Jacoby, 2015).

Compulsions can take the form of behaviors or mental acts, but in either case the person feels driven to perform them repetitively and excessively to reduce the anxiety caused by obsessive thoughts (Abramowitz & Jacoby, 2015). Jacob's need to revisit his route, described in the **Clinical Case**, fits this definition. Samuel Johnson, one of the most famous authors of the 18th century, suffered from multiple compulsions. For example, he felt compelled "to touch every post in a street or step exactly in the center of every paving stone. If he perceived one of these acts to be inaccurate, his friends were obliged to wait, dumbfounded, while he went back to fix it" (Stephen, 1900, cited in Szechtman & Woody, 2004). Like Samuel Johnson, many people with OCD feel compelled to repeat a ritual if they did not execute it with precision or did not get it "just right." The sheer frequency with which those with OCD repeat their compulsions can be staggering. See **Table 7.3** for commonly reported compulsions.

We often hear people described as compulsive gamblers or compulsive eaters. Even though people may report irresistible urges to gamble and eat, these behaviors are not considered

TABLE 7.2   Common Foci of Obsessions in OCD

Foci of Obsession	Example
Contamination	What if the public toilet I used had the coronavirus on it?
Responsibility for harm	What if I dropped my baby down the stairs by mistake?
Sex and morality	What if I could not resist the impulse to touch a stranger's breasts?
Violence	What if my husband was stabbed on his way to work today?
Religion	Inappropriate, disturbing sexual images of deities
Symmetry or order	The feeling that books, dishes, or other objects must be perfectly arranged on a shelf

Source: Adapted from Abramowitz and Jacoby (2015).

TABLE 7.3 Common Compulsive Rituals for Those with OCD

Foci of Compulsion	Example
Decontamination	Showering for hours a day, wiping down all objects upon entering the house, or asking visitors to wash before they enter the house
Checking	Returning seven or eight times in a row to see that lights, stove burners, or faucets are turned off, windows fastened, and doors locked
Repeating routine activities	Touching a body part or repeating a word again and again
Ordering/arranging	Sorting all books and cereal boxes into alphabetical order
Mental rituals	Counting, solving a math problem, or repeating a phrase in one's mind until anxiety is relieved

VIDEO CONTENT

Case Study: Obsessive-Compulsive Disorder
Pause and Ponder

compulsions because they are often experienced as pleasurable. Rather than being motivated by pleasure, compulsions are motivated by the feeling that something dire will happen if the act is not performed. A person who experiences obsessions about contamination is likely to feel intense distress if prevented from engaging in cleaning rituals, even though the person may recognize that the cleaning rituals are not warranted.

People with OCD tend to experience high levels of distress and self-doubt, and their distress is worsened as the symptoms of OCD interfere with occupational and relationship outcomes (Ruscio, Stein, et al., 2010). More than 10% of people with OCD have made a suicide attempt (Fernandez de la Cruz, Rydell, et al., 2016), OCD relates to premature mortality from suicide as well as from medical conditions (Meier, Mattheisen, et al., 2016).

Obsessions and compulsions are observed across cultures (Nicolini, Salin-Pascual, et al., 2017), but the social environment can shape the severity and content of OCD symptoms. For example, in cultures where people consider uncleanliness sinful, washing compulsions are more common (Clark & González, 2014). Data from the COVID-19 pandemic also showed the importance of social context. Among those with OCD who had contamination-related obsessions, COVID often triggered intense fear and distress. Many people who had no history of OCD at the start of the pandemic developed new obsessive fears about disease and contamination as the pandemic developed (Guzick, McCabe, & Storch, 2021). Taken together, research suggests that it is important to consider the cultural and social contexts that may shape OCD symptoms.

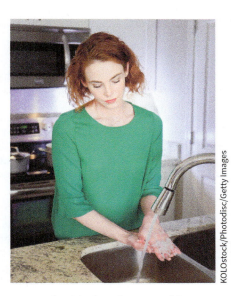

For people with obsessive-compulsive disorder (OCD), extreme fears of contamination can trigger abnormally frequent hand washing.

Body Dysmorphic Disorder

People with **body dysmorphic disorder (BDD)** are preoccupied with one or more imagined or exaggerated defects in their appearance. Although people with BDD may appear attractive to others, they perceive themselves as ugly or even "monstrous" in their appearance (Phillips, 2006). Women tend to worry about perceived flaws in their skin, hair, facial features, hips, breasts, or legs, whereas men are more likely to worry about their height, penis size, body hair, small size, or insufficient muscularity (Perugi, Akiskal, et al., 1997). Most people with BDD worry about multiple aspects of their appearance.

In a somewhat obsessional manner, people with BDD find it very hard to stop thinking about their concerns. As one woman wrote, "It's always in the back of my mind. I can't push it away. It's always there, taunting and haunting me" (Phillips, 2005, p. 69). On average, people with BDD think about their appearance for 3 to 8 hours per day (Phillips, Wilhelm, et al., 2010). Like people with OCD, people with BDD feel compelled to engage in behaviors to reduce the distress associated with these obsessional thoughts. The most common compulsive behaviors for those with BDD include checking their appearance in the mirror, comparing their appearance to that of other people, asking others for reassurance about their appearance, and using strategies to change their appearance or camouflage disliked body areas (grooming, tanning, exercising, changing clothes, and applying makeup)

(Phillips, Wilhelm, et al., 2010). While many spend several hours a day checking their appearance, some try to avoid reminders of their perceived flaws by avoiding mirrors, reflective surfaces, or bright lights (Phillips, 2005). Although most of us do things to feel better about our appearance, people with this disorder spend an inordinate amount of time and energy on these endeavors.

The symptoms are extremely distressing. About a third of clients with BDD have little insight into their overly harsh views, and so they are convinced that others will see their flaws as grotesque (Phillips, Pinto, et al., 2012). As many as a fifth of them endure plastic surgery, and many withstand multiple surgeries (Phillips, 2005). Unfortunately, plastic surgery does little to allay their concerns, such that many want to sue or hurt their physicians after the surgery (Bowyer, Krebs, et al., 2016). Among people with BDD, at least a third report some history of suicidal ideation, and about 20% have attempted suicide (Buhlmann, Glaesmer, et al., 2010; Krebs, de la Cruz, et al., 2022).

Clinical Case

Paul

After years of living with anxiety and shame over his appearance, Paul sought psychotherapy at age 33. He had first become "horrified" by his appearance during puberty, when he noticed that he was not developing the square jaw lines that many of his male friends had begun to show. For the past several years, his shame had been focused on his nose, which he perceived as being too thin. He had sought surgery, but the surgeon refused to operate on his seemingly flawless nose. Over the past two decades, his preoccupation with his appearance had often interfered with socializing and altogether prevented dating. Even when he did venture out, he had to check his appearance repeatedly throughout the evening. Sometimes he was unable to go to work in his position as a physical therapist because he was overwhelmed by his anxiety. When he did go to work, he worried that his clients were too distracted by his physical flaws to attend to his instructions.

Drawn with permission from Wilhelm, Buhlmann, et al. (2010).

As was the case for Paul (see the **Clinical Case**), preoccupation with appearance can interfere with occupational and social functioning. To cope with the intense shame they feel about their appearance, people with BDD may avoid contact with others. In one survey, about a third reported missing work or avoiding school in the past month because of concerns about their appearance (Phillips, 2005), and many take long breaks from work or interpersonal interactions to check their appearance or cope with the anxiety of being viewed by others. In another survey, about 40% of people with the disorder reported being unable to work, and some even become housebound (Didie, Menard, et al., 2008).

Defining Symptoms of Body Dysmorphic Disorder (BDD)

- Preoccupation with one or more perceived defects in appearance
- Others find the perceived defect(s) slight or unobservable
- Performance of repetitive behaviors or mental acts (e.g., mirror checking, seeking reassurance, or excessive grooming) in response to the appearance concerns
- Preoccupation is not restricted to weight or body fat concerns

---

Case reports from around the world suggest that, among those who develop BDD, the symptoms and outcomes are similar across cultures (Phillips, 2005). The body part that becomes a focus of concern sometimes differs by culture, though. For example, eyelid concerns are more common in Japan than in Western countries. In addition, Japanese patients with BDD appear more concerned about offending others than are Western patients (Suzuki, Takei, et al., 2003).

Hoarding Disorder

Collecting is a hobby for about a third of people in the United States (Frost & Steketee, 2010), and almost all children go through a phase of collecting objects, but these hobbies are distinctly different from hoarding. What distinguishes the common fascination with collections

Clinical Case

Dena

Dena was referred for treatment after animal care officials received reports from neighbors. A home inspection revealed over 100 animals living in her 3-acre yard and inside her house, many of them suffering from malnutrition and disease. When interviewed, she reported that she was running a rescue mission for animals and that she was "just a little behind" due to financial stress.

When the therapist visited her home, it became clear that her collections extended far beyond her animals. The rooms of her small home were so crowded that two of the doors to the outside had become unreachable. Heaps of clothes mixed with miscellaneous furniture parts brimmed to the ceiling of her living room. In the kitchen, a collection of theater memorabilia crowded out access to the stove and refrigerator. The dining room was covered

with assorted items—bags of trash, piles of bills, stacks of old newspapers, and several sets of china she had purchased "at a bargain" at yard sales.

When the therapist offered to help Dena organize and neaten her home, Dena became enraged. She said that she had only allowed the therapist to visit to help her broker an arrangement with the animal control authorities and that she did not want to hear any comments about her home. She described years of fighting with her family over her housekeeping, and she said she had done everything in her power to escape from their uptight expectations. She denied needing the stove, stating that she wasn't about to start cooking hot meals as a single woman living alone. After the initial unsuccessful home visit, she refused any further contact with the therapist.

Defining Symptoms of Hoarding Disorder

- Persistent difficulty discarding or parting with possessions, regardless of their actual value
- Perceived need to save items
- Distress associated with discarding items
- The accumulation of possessions clutters active living spaces to the extent that their intended use is compromised unless others intervene

from the clinical disorder of hoarding? Undoubtedly, the desire to acquire and save objects varies along a continuum (Timpano, Broman-Fulks, et al., 2013). For people with **hoarding disorder**, the need to acquire is excessive, but the bigger problem is that they abhor parting with their objects, even when others cannot perceive any potential value in them. People with hoarding disorder feel extremely attached to their possessions, feel intense distress at the prospect of discarding their possessions, and are very resistant to efforts to get rid of them. Most typically, as illustrated in the **Clinical Case of Dena**, the person acquires a huge range of different kinds of objects—they may gather collections of clothes, tools, or antiques along with old containers and bottle caps, leading to intense clutter.

Many people who hoard are unaware of the severity of their behavior (Steketee & Frost, 2015), but to those surrounding them, the consequences of hoarding are clear and sometimes severe. For those who do have insight, the difficulties of controlling one's home environment can have profound effects on self-esteem (Frost & Steketee, 2010). The accrual of objects can interfere with the ability to use the kitchen or bathroom of the home or to have safe access to exits. Consequently, poor hygiene, exposure to dirt, and difficulties with cooking can contribute to poor physical health, such as respiratory problems. Many family members sever relationships, unable to understand the attachment to the objects. About three-quarters of people with hoarding disorder engage in excessive buying (Frost, Tolin, et al., 2009), and many are unable to work (Tolin, Frost, et al., 2008), making poverty all too common among people with this condition (Samuels, Bienvenu, et al., 2007). The degree of clutter is a core facet of impairment (Timpano, Bainter, et al., 2020). As clutter levels escalate, health officials often become involved to address safety and health concerns. An estimated 10% of people with hoarding disorder are threatened with eviction at some point in their lives (Tolin et al., 2008). For some, the money spent on acquiring possessions leads to

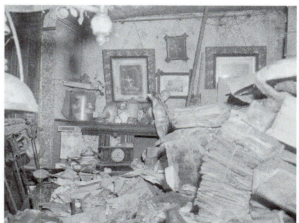

Hoarding captured the attention of the public in 1947, when the Collyer brothers were found dead, surrounded by 140 tons of objects, ranging from grand pianos to antique sculptures to a human skeleton, piled from floor to ceiling in their New York City brownstone.

Bettmann/Getty Images

homelessness (Rodriguez, Herman, et al., 2022). The lack of insight creates a challenge in conducting research on hoarding because those willing to sign up for research often are more insightful and have less cluttered homes than those with hoarding disorder served by community agencies (Woody, Lenkic, et al., 2020).

Some people with hoarding disorder—much more often women than men—engage in animal hoarding (Patronek & Nathanson, 2009). People who engage in animal hoarding sometimes think of themselves as animal rescuers, but those who witness the problem perceive it differently, as the accumulating number of animals often outstrips the person's ability to provide adequate care, shelter, and food. Animal hoarding is more associated with squalor than are other forms of hoarding. When animals are hoarded, animal protection agencies sometimes become involved.

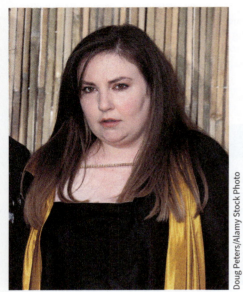

Lena Dunham has described her childhood experiences of OCD and anxiety (Dunham, 2014). Many people with OCD experience comorbid anxiety.

Doug Peters/Alamy Stock Photo

Prevalence and Comorbidity of Obsessive-Compulsive and Related Disorders

Although most of us have had a repetitive thought, have worried about our appearance, and have gone through a phase of collecting, these symptoms lead to the genuine distress or impairment required for a diagnosis in only a small proportion of people. Lifetime prevalence estimates are about 1.3% for OCD (Fawcett, Power, & Fawcett, 2020) and 3% for BDD (Schieber, Kollei, et al., 2015). Because hoarding often takes place in secret, behind closed doors, and people who engage in it may lack insight, it is hard to estimate the prevalence of this behavior. The estimated prevalence of hoarding disorder is at least 1.5% (Nordsletten, Reichenberg, et al., 2013). OCD and BDD are both slightly more common among women than men (Fawcett, Power, & Fawcett, 2020; Hartman & Buhlmann, 2017). Hoarding is equally common among men and women (Postlewaite et al., 2019).

OCD and hoarding disorder most commonly begin in childhood or early adolescence (Grisham, Frost, et al., 2006; Taylor, 2011), and BDD typically begins in adolescence. Once present, each of these disorders tends to be chronic (Eisen, Sibrava, et al., 2013; Phillips, Menard, et al., 2013). Hoarding disorder often worsens over time, because parents and lack of income can constrain the acquisition of objects earlier in life.

OCD, BDD, and hoarding disorder often co-occur. For example, about a third of people with BDD and up to a quarter of people with hoarding disorder meet the diagnostic criteria for OCD during their lifetime. About one-third of people with OCD experience at least some symptoms of hoarding (Mancebo, Eisen, et al., 2011; Weaton & Van Meter, 2015).

In addition to being comorbid, all three of the syndromes tend to co-occur with depression and anxiety disorders (Brakoulias, Starcevic, et al., 2011) and to some extent with substance use disorders (Frost, Steketee, & Tolin, 2011; Gustad & Phillips, 2003; Ruscio et al., 2010). OCD in particular is related to very high rates of comorbid anxiety disorders, with as many as three-quarters of those with OCD experiencing an anxiety disorder during their lifetime (Ruscio, Stein, et al., 2010).

Quick Summary

The obsessive-compulsive and related disorders include obsessive-compulsive disorder (OCD), body dysmorphic disorder (BDD), and hoarding disorder. OCD is defined by obsessions and/or compulsions. BDD is defined by a preoccupation with one or more imagined defects in appearance and by intensive behavioral attempts to cope with the imagined defect(s). Hoarding disorder is defined by excessive acquisition of objects and severe difficulties in discarding objects, even when they are objectively without value.

Lifetime prevalence estimates are 1.3% for OCD, 3% for BDD, and 1.5% for hoarding disorder.

People with BDD and those with hoarding disorder often have a history of OCD, and many with OCD have some history of hoarding symptoms. Obsessive-compulsive and related disorders tend to co-occur with anxiety disorders and major depressive disorder and to some extent with substance use disorders.

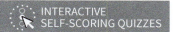
(Answers are at the end of the chapter.)
Answer the following questions.

1. Describe the most typical course of obsessive-compulsive and related disorders over time.

2. What is the chief difference between obsessions and compulsions?

Causes of the Obsessive-Compulsive and Related Disorders

There is a moderate genetic contribution to OCD, hoarding, and BDD. Heritability is estimated to be between 0.40 and 0.50 for each of these disorders (Monzani, Rijsdijk, et al., 2014).

OCD, BDD, and hoarding disorder have some overlap in genetic and neurobiological risk factors. For example, in a study of over 5,000 twins, OCD, BDD, and hoarding disorder appeared to have some shared genetic vulnerability (Monzani et al., 2014).

In regard to neurobiology, research has determined that OCD, BDD, and hoarding disorder all involve the **cortico-striatal-thalamic-cortical (CSTC) loop** and related brain regions. Brain-imaging studies indicate that three regions of the CSTC loop are unusually active in people with OCD (see **Figure 7.1**): the **orbitofrontal cortex** (an area of the medial prefrontal cortex located just above the eyes), the **caudate nucleus** (part of the basal ganglia), and the anterior cingulate cortex (Menzies, Chamberlain, et al., 2008). When people with OCD are shown objects that tend to provoke symptoms (such as a soiled glove for a person who fears contamination), brain activity in these three areas increases (Yu, Zhou, et al., 2022). The functional connectivity, or synchronization of activity, between these regions when a person is viewing objects that tend to provoke symptoms also appears to differentiate those with OCD from controls (Yu, Zhou, et al., 2022). Successful treatment, whether through cognitive behavioral therapy, antidepressant medication, or brain stimulation, changes activity in the CSTC loop (Goodman, Storch, & Sheth, 2021).

These same fronto-striatal regions are implicated in BDD and hoarding. When people with BDD observe pictures of their own face, hyperactivity of the orbitofrontal cortex and the caudate nucleus is observed (Feusner, Phillips, & Stein, 2010). When people with hoarding symptoms are faced with decisions about whether to keep or discard their possessions, such as old mail, they are more likely than a control group to exhibit hyperactivity in the orbitofrontal cortex (Tolin, Kiehl, et al., 2009) and the anterior cingulate cortex (Tolin, Stevens, et al., 2012).

While these genetic and neurobiological influences may set the stage for developing these disorders, why might one person develop OCD and another develop BDD? In addition to the overlapping brain regions, each disorder has been tied to additional brain regions. For example, BDD has been tied to more engagement of regions of the brain involved in visual processing, which could relate to patients' intense responses to viewing their bodies

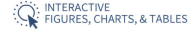
INTERACTIVE
FIGURES, CHARTS, & TABLES

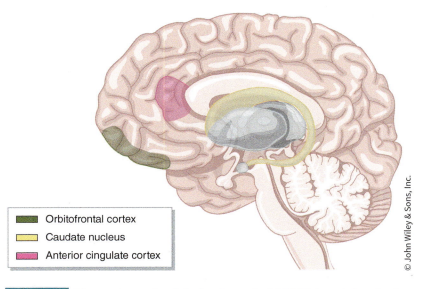

© John Wiley & Sons, Inc.

■ Orbitofrontal cortex
■ Caudate nucleus
■ Anterior cingulate cortex

FIGURE 7.1 The cortico-striatal-thalamic-cortical (CSTC) loop is involved in the obsessive-compulsive and related disorders, and includes the orbitofrontal cortex, the caudate nucleus, the anterior cingulate cortex, and the thalamus.

(Grace, Labuschagne, et al., 2017). Research suggests that psychological processes also might promote one disorder more than another. As you will learn, some of the psychological models overlap conceptually with findings from brain-imaging research.

Causes of Obsessive-Compulsive Disorder

In moderation, many of the thoughts and behaviors that disrupt the days of those with OCD, such as checking, cleaning, or reconsidering a thought, have adaptive value. Cleaning, for example, can help reduce the risk of contamination and germs. When the coronavirus caused a pandemic, international health authorities urged people to wash their hands repeatedly, highlighting the adaptive benefits of a focus on contamination. From an evolutionary perspective, having at least one person in each social group who checks everything multiple times could reap huge benefits for the group. The question, though, is why these thoughts and behaviors become so persistent, often in inappropriate contexts, as to cause real distress or impairment. Here, we consider a behavioral model of how a person might be particularly likely to develop strong conditioned associations that drive him or her to keep repeating compulsions, and then we discuss two cognitive models.

Behavioral Model
The goal of behavior theory is to understand why a person with OCD continues to show the behaviors or thoughts used to ward off an initial threat well after that threat is gone. Studies of the ability to extinguish fears once they are conditioned may help explain this. That is, when researchers pair an unconditioned stimulus (such as a neutral picture) with a conditioned stimulus (such as a shock), most people quickly develop behavioral and psychophysiological fear responses to the neutral picture. For people with OCD, those responses may be harder to override when the picture is no longer paired with shock (Cooper & Dunsmoor, 2021).

In one innovative study of conditioning, researchers conducted a two-phase experiment (Gillan, Morein-Zamir, et al., 2014). In the first phase, they created a threat by placing electrodes on participants' wrists and then teaching participants that they would receive a shock (an unconditioned stimulus) when a certain shape (the conditioned stimulus) appeared on the computer screen. To avoid the shock, participants had to press a foot pedal (the conditioned response). In this first phase, participants with and without OCD learned equally well to press the foot pedal to avoid shock. In the key second phase of the study, researchers unhooked the wrist electrodes so that participants could know that the threat of shock was gone. Even though they knew the threat had been removed and showed little psychophysiological response to the stimulus, many people with OCD either pressed the foot pedal or felt a strong urge to press the foot pedal when the conditioned stimulus (the shape) appeared on the screen. In contrast, people without OCD quit pressing the foot pedal, and most didn't have an urge to press the foot pedal. For those with OCD, previously functional responses for reducing threat were difficult to reverse after the threat was gone.

Cognitive Models
There are two different approaches to understanding cognition in OCD. Both models consider how people respond to threats, but the models are very different. First, we consider how the doubt, repetitive thoughts, and checking behaviors that people with OCD experience could be related to problems in trusting the evidence needed to make decisions and to feel confident that threats have been addressed. Second, we consider the idea that the way people with OCD interpret and respond to threat-related thoughts could contribute to obsessions.

Difficulties Using Evidence to Make Decisions
Faced with a threat, how do we know when we have done enough to feel safe? Throughout our daily lives, we have to make assumptions that the stove is truly off, that our hands are clean enough, and that other possible threats are addressed, even though the evidence is not always clear. For many people, a little evidence about the world allows them to feel safe without constantly verifying everything. For those with OCD, though, the evidence does not override the sense that things are not quite right. To address that doubt, some people feel compelled to check whether the stove is off, to wash their hands, or to engage in other compulsive behaviors again and again.

To test this idea of difficulty relying on evidence, several groups have asked people with OCD to complete tasks in which they must learn about visual or auditory stimuli, and then make decisions. For example, in the dot movement task, participants are asked to view a computer screen on which many dots are moving in the same direction, but the task is challenging because some dots are moving in random directions. Asked to decide which direction most of the dots are moving, those with OCD are slower to make a decision (Solway, Lin, & Vinaik, 2020). They also check more when asked to make perceptual decisions—for example, they review stimuli more times before making a decision (Strauss, Fradkin, et al., 2020). These findings, then, fit with the idea that those with OCD have trouble trusting their conclusions about the evidence on these tasks.

In a computational psychiatry approach, researchers created mathematical models of the multiple processes guiding how people take in and use evidence presented in laboratory tasks. These mathematical models show that people with OCD may particularly doubt evidence when the context changes—a phenomenon labeled as **transition uncertainty** (Fradkin, Adams, et al., 2020). To illustrate this, consider that we usually assume that once we turn off the stove, it remains off even when there are transitions such as leaving the room or turning off the light. According to the transition uncertainty model, people with OCD feel less confident in the adequacy of their actions (like turning off the stove or washing their hands) during small transitions, which could lead them to doubt their decisions (yielding more repetitive thoughts akin to obsessions) in those moments. To address these doubts, the person with OCD might seek comfort from repeatedly using compulsive behaviors, like turning off the stove again and again.

A Cognitive Model of Obsessions   A second cognitive model focuses on obsessions. This model suggests that people with OCD may try harder to suppress their obsessions than other people do and, in the process, may make the situation worse (Salkovskis, 1996). Several types of evidence support this model.

Several researchers have shown that people with OCD tend to believe that (1) thinking about something is as morally wrong as engaging in the action or (2) thinking about an event can make it more likely to occur. These types of beliefs have been labeled as **thought–action fusion**. People with OCD also tend to feel especially responsible for preventing harm. You can imagine how these types of thoughts lead to alarm when a negative thought or image intrudes (Clark & González, 2014). Because those with OCD tend to have these dysfunctional beliefs, the initial intrusive thought is distressing.

To rid themselves of these uncomfortable thoughts, people with OCD are more likely to attempt **thought suppression** (Amir, Cashman, & Foa, 1997). Unfortunately, it is hard to suppress thoughts. Consider the findings of one study in which researchers asked people to suppress a thought (Wegner, Schneider, et al., 1987). College students in an experimental group were asked not to think about a white bear, and a control group was asked to think about a white bear. Both groups were told to ring a bell every time they thought about a white bear. Attempts to avoid thinking about the white bear did not work—students in the experimental group thought about the bear more than once a minute when trying not to do so (more than the control group did). Beyond that, there was a rebound effect—after students tried to suppress thoughts about the bear for 5 minutes, they thought about the bear much more often during the next 5 minutes than the control group did. Trying to suppress a thought had the paradoxical effect of inducing preoccupation with it. Indeed, in one experimental study, suppressing thoughts even briefly led to more intrusions of that thought over the next four days (Trinder & Salkovskis, 1994). Across many studies, thought suppression appears most likely to fail when working memory is limited, as it would likely be when people were feeling preoccupied and worried (Wang, Hagger, & Chatzisarantis, 2020). Obviously, thought suppression is not a very good way to control obsessions when one is distressed.

According to this theory, the problem with OCD is not the initial intrusive thought but the response to that thought. To study this, one group of researchers assessed a group of people highly prone to intrusive disturbing thoughts—parents with 1-month-old babies. As expected, almost all parents reported thoughts of terrible events that could befall their baby (e.g., "What if I drop the baby?"). To test the idea that OCD might relate to thought–action fusion, researchers asked parents whether they believed that having thoughts or images could make an event more likely to occur. Those who endorsed such beliefs showed greater increases in OCD symptoms by the time their baby was 3 to 4 months old (Abramowitz, Nelson, et al., 2007). These findings illustrate that the presence of a disturbing, intrusive thought does not matter nearly as much as how people respond to that thought—consistent with thought–action fusion theory.

Causes of Body Dysmorphic Disorder

Why would Paul (see the earlier **Clinical Case**) look in the mirror, see a nose that others see as perfectly reasonable, and respond with horror? Many with BDD report vivid memories of appearance-related teasing (Osman, Cooper, et al., 2004), and many report that appearance-related teasing triggered the onset of their symptoms (Weingarden, Curley, et al., 2017). Many other people, though, experience teasing and do not develop BDD, so other vulnerabilities are clearly involved.

Cognitive models of BDD focus on what happens when people with this syndrome look at their body. People with BDD can accurately see and process their physical features without distortion. However, people with BDD are unusually detail-oriented when processing visual scenes, and this influences how they look at facial features (Lang, Kerr-Gaffney et al., 2021). Instead of considering the whole, they examine one feature at a time, which makes it more likely that they will become engrossed in considering a small flaw. Indeed, when researchers used eye-tracking measures as participants looked at photos of their own and others' faces, those with BDD spent more time than did those without BDD viewing unattractive features of their own face and others' faces (Greenberg, Reuman, et al., 2014). They also tend to be perfectionistic (Schieber, Kollei, et al., 2013) and to consider attractiveness vastly more important than do control participants (Lambrou, Veale, & Wilson, 2011). Indeed, many people with BDD believe that their self-worth is exclusively dependent on their appearance (Veale, 2004).

Causes of Hoarding Disorder

In considering hoarding, many take an evolutionary perspective (Zohar & Felz, 2001). Imagine you were a prehistoric cave dweller with no access to grocery stores to replenish food reserves and no clothing stores to provide warm clothes when the weather got cold. In that situation, it would be adaptive to store any resources you could find. The question, though, is how these basic instincts become so uncontrollable for some people. Several cognitive and behavioral influences might be involved, including poor organizational abilities, unusual beliefs about possessions, and avoidance behaviors (Timpano, Muroff, & Steketee, 2016). Let's review how each of these factors might lead to excessive acquisition as well as difficulty getting rid of objects.

People with hoarding disorder show problems sorting and categorizing objects. For example, when asked to sort objects into categories in laboratory studies, many people with hoarding disorder are slow, generate more categories than others do, and find the process highly anxiety-provoking (Wincze, Steketee, & Frost, 2007). They struggle even more when the objects to sort are personally valuable to them (Stumpf, de Souza, et al., 2022). The difficulty categorizing objects creates real life challenges in determining how to clean and organize possessions. For example, when a therapist asked one client to describe a mountain of printed material covering her dining room table, the client responded "stuff from last year" (Franklin, Budzyn, & Freeman, 2019). Many patients find it excruciatingly hard to sort through their objects and figure out what to discard, even with a supportive therapist present (Frost & Steketee, 2010). They often spend hours per day churning through their possessions without being able to discard a single object.

Beyond these organizational difficulties, the cognitive model focuses on the unusual beliefs that people with hoarding disorder hold about their possessions. First, they are able to find the potential in each of their objects. For example, a stray cap to a pen could make a good game piece, and junk mail might have some important information to offer (Frost & Steketee, 2010). People with hoarding disorder also demonstrate an extreme emotional attachment to their possessions. They report feeling comforted by their objects, feeling frightened by the idea of losing an object, seeing the objects as core to their sense of self and identity, and holding a deep sense of responsibility for taking care of those objects (Timpano, Muroff, & Steketee,

2016). Many feel grief when forced to part with an object (Frost, Steketee, & Tolin, 2012). These attachments may be even stronger when animals are involved. People who hoard animals often describe their animals as their closest confidants (Patronek & Nathanson, 2009). These beliefs about the importance of each and every object interfere with any attempt to tackle the clutter.

In the face of the anxiety of all these decisions, avoidance is common. Many with hoarding disorder find organizing their clutter so overwhelming that they delay tackling the chaos. This avoidance maintains the clutter.

Quick Summary

OCD, BDD, and hoarding disorder are moderately heritable. There is some overlap in the heritability of these disorders.

Obsessive-compulsive and related disorders appear related to dysfunction of the cortico-striatal-thalamic-cortical (CSTC) loop. OCD is characterized by high activity in the orbitofrontal cortex, the caudate nucleus, and the anterior cingulate cortex in response to symptom-provoking stimuli and by atypical connectivity of these neural regions. People with BDD show heightened activity of the orbitofrontal cortex and the caudate nucleus when viewing pictures of their own face. People with hoarding disorder show heightened activity in the orbitofrontal cortex and the anterior cingulate cortex when making decisions about possessions. Beyond these commonalities, BDD is related to greater activity in visual processing regions.

Cognitive behavioral models help explain why one might develop a specific disorder in the cluster of obsessive-compulsive and related disorders. A behavioral model of OCD suggests that people sustain conditioned responses long after the contingencies that conditioned the initial behavior have shifted. One cognitive model suggests that people with OCD have difficulty relying on evidence, and some research suggests that this problem may worsen when the environment changes (transition uncertainty). According to a second cognitive model, thought suppression may exacerbate tendencies toward obsessions, and thought–action fusion may increase the likelihood of thought suppression.

The cognitive model of BDD focuses on a detail-oriented analytic style and tendencies to overvalue the role of appearance in self-worth.

Cognitive behavioral models of hoarding disorder focus on poor organizational abilities (difficulties with categorization), unusual beliefs about possessions, and avoidance behaviors.

7.2 Check Your Knowledge

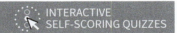 INTERACTIVE SELF-SCORING QUIZZES

(Answers are at the end of the chapter.)
Answer the following questions.

1. How heritable are the obsessive-compulsive and related disorders?
2. List four reasons to consider OCD, BDD, and hoarding as related conditions.

Treatment of the Obsessive-Compulsive and Related Disorders

Treatments that work for OCD, BDD, and hoarding disorder are somewhat similar. Each of these disorders responds to antidepressant medications. The major psychological approach for each of these disorders is exposure and response prevention, although this treatment is tailored a good deal for each of the conditions. Even though good treatments are available, many people do not receive state-of-the-art care. For BDD and hoarding disorder, problems with insight and shame often interfere with treatment seeking. As is all too common with many disorders, individuals from ethnic minority groups are less likely than others to receive treatment for OCD (de la Cruz, Llorens, et al., 2015).

Medications

Antidepressants are the medications most commonly used for obsessive-compulsive and related disorders. Although they were developed to treat depression, randomized controlled trials support their effectiveness in the treatment of OCD (Pittenger, 2023). Although selective serotonin reuptake inhibitors (SSRIs) and the tricyclic antidepressant clomipramine (Anafranil) have both been approved by the FDA for the treatment of OCD, SSRIs are recommended over other classes of antidepressants, as they have fewer side effects (Pittenger, 2023). SSRIs may require more time (up to 12 weeks) and higher doses to treat OCD than to treat depression (Pittenger, 2023), and most people with OCD continue to experience at least mild symptoms after antidepressant treatment.

Very little research has been conducted on medication treatment of BDD and hoarding disorder. Three randomized controlled trials support the efficacy of antidepressants in BDD (Castle, Beilharz, et al., 2021). As with OCD, higher doses of antidepressants may be required to treat BDD as compared with depression.

Results of two small nonrandomized trials suggest that the symptoms of hoarding disorder decrease with antidepressant treatment (Saxena, 2015), but no randomized controlled trials of medications are available for hoarding disorder. Some research focuses on hoarding symptoms among patients with OCD. Among patients with OCD, hoarding symptoms predict a poorer response to treatment; in a meta-analysis of 14 studies, patients with hoarding symptoms and OCD were about half as likely to respond to medication treatment as were those with OCD alone (Bloch, Bartley, et al., 2014).

Psychological Treatment

The most widely used psychological treatment for obsessive-compulsive and related disorders is **exposure and response prevention (ERP)**. Victor Meyer (1966) developed this approach to address the compulsive rituals of OCD by tailoring the exposure treatment discussed in Chapter 6. We'll describe this cognitive behavioral treatment for OCD and then discuss how it has been adapted for BDD and hoarding disorder.

Obsessive-Compulsive Disorder
Many with OCD hold an almost magical belief that their compulsive behavior will prevent awful things from happening. In the exposure component of ERP, clients expose themselves to situations that elicit obsessions and related anxiety. At the same time, for the response-prevention component of ERP, clients refrain from performing any compulsive ritual during the exposure. For instance, a client might be asked to touch a dirty dish and then refrain from hand washing. In addition to refraining from the overt compulsive behavior, such as hand washing, the client must also refrain from compulsive thoughts, such as covertly counting to 10. The reasoning behind the approach goes like this:

1. Not performing the ritual exposes the person to the full force of the anxiety provoked by the stimulus.
2. The exposure promotes the extinction of the conditioned response (the anxiety).
3. Facing the feared stimulus helps a person develop new, more positive thoughts in response to the stimulus.

The exposure component of ERP uses a hierarchical approach like that discussed in Chapter 6, in which a client begins with exposure to less threatening stimuli and progresses to sessions focused on more threatening stimuli. For example, clients with a focus on contamination might start by being in a dirty room and progress to placing their hands on a sticky, grimy floor. Throughout the exposure sessions, the therapist guides the client to avoid engaging in compulsions. Often, the therapist guides exposure to feared stimuli in the home (Franklin & Foa, 2014). Family members of those with OCD often have

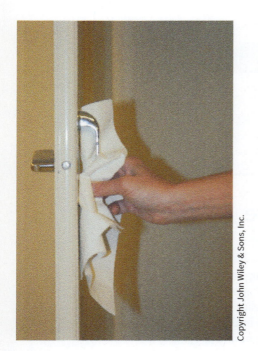

Exposure treatment for OCD involves confronting one's worst fears, such as contamination by dirty objects.

Copyright John Wiley & Sons, Inc.

developed accommodations to help their loved one avoid triggers, for example, engaging in elaborate rituals to help the family member avoid contamination-related fears. Therapists help family members avoid these accommodations, so that the person with OCD will have more exposure to the stimuli they fear (Merlo, Lehmkuhl, et al., 2009). Typically, ERP involves refraining from performing rituals during therapy sessions lasting up to 90 minutes as well as during home practice between sessions. Acute treatment typically requires up to 20 sessions. Researchers have varied in whether they conducted sessions daily, twice a week, or weekly (Ponniah, Magiati, & Hollon, 2013), and early data showed positive results with an intensive 4-day program of ERP (Hansen, Kvale, et al., 2019). Clients are often offered booster sessions in the first 6 months after acute treatment (Abramovitch, Elliott, et al., 2014).

Randomized clinical trials indicate that, in the treatment of OCD, ERP is more powerful than control conditions such as anxiety management and relaxation treatment and as powerful as antidepressants (Abramovitch, Elliott, et al., 2014; Romanelli, Wu, et al., 2014). It is effective for children and adolescents as well as adults (Franklin & Foa, 2011). About 69–75% of people who receive this treatment show significant improvement (Abramowitz & Jacoby, 2015), although mild symptoms often persist. Researchers have found excellent outcomes for ERP offered by community therapists who do not specialize in OCD (Franklin & Foa, 2011). Although some people make gains using internet-based CBT (Flygare, Lundström, et al., 2022), at least brief contact with a therapist produces better outcomes for these programs (Andersson, Mataix-Cols, & Rück, 2017).

Although the evidence to support ERP is strong, it is a demanding therapy for the clients—refraining from performing a ritual is extremely unpleasant for people with OCD. (To get some idea of how unpleasant, try delaying for a minute or two before scratching an itch.) About a third of people diagnosed with OCD are not willing to begin ERP, and among those who do enroll, about a third drop out (Abramovitch, Elliott, et al., 2014), and those in non-Western countries may be less comfortable seeking help. The challenging nature of this treatment may help explain why so few therapists offer it. In a survey of licensed psychologists, therapists were found to be more likely to offer relaxation training (which appears to be fairly ineffective) than ERP to their OCD clients (Foa & McLean, 2016).

Cognitive approaches to OCD focus on challenging people's beliefs about what will happen if they do not engage in rituals (Clark, 2006). For example, a therapist might help the client reconsider thought–action fusion and inflated perceptions of responsibility. Eventually, to help test such beliefs, these approaches will use exposure at least briefly. Most studies suggest that cognitive approaches perform as well as ERP (Reid, Laws, et al., 2021).

Body Dysmorphic Disorder   The basic principles of ERP are tailored in several ways to address the symptoms of BDD. For example, to provide exposure to the most feared activities, therapists might ask clients to interact with people who could be critical of their looks. For response prevention, therapists might ask clients to avoid activities they use to reassure themselves about their appearance, such as looking in mirrors. As illustrated in the **Clinical Case of Paul**, these behavioral techniques are supplemented with strategies to address the cognitive features of the disorder, such as excessively critical evaluations of physical features and the belief that self-worth depends on appearance.

Multiple trials have shown that ERP produces a major decrease in BDD symptoms compared with control conditions and that effects are maintained in the months after treatment ends (Harrison, Fernández de la Cruz, et al., 2016; Weingarden, Hoeppner, et al., 2021). Early evidence indicates that an internet-based version of ERP can be helpful for BDD, with about half of those treated showing a reduction in symptoms that was sustained at a 2-year follow-up (Enander, LjÓtsson, et al., 2019). Caution is warranted, though, because many people continue to experience at least mild symptoms after treatment (Harrison et al., 2016), whether it is offered in person or online.

Hoarding Disorder   To treat hoarding disorder, the exposure element of ERP focuses on the most feared situation for people with this disorder—getting rid of their objects (Steketee & Frost, 2003). The response-prevention element of ERP centers on halting the rituals that people with hoarding disorder engage in to reduce their anxiety, such as counting or

Returning to Clinical Case

CBT Treatment for Paul

Paul and his therapist agreed to work together using CBT. To begin, they reviewed childhood and current influences on Paul's symptoms. Paul described his parents' extremely high standards for appearance, along with his father's obsessive and perfectionistic style. Throughout his life, Paul had felt he could not live up to their standards.

He and the therapist then identified several cognitions (thoughts) that triggered anxiety, such as "Any flaw means I'm ugly" and "I know my client is thinking about how ugly my nose is." The therapist asked Paul to record his most negative thoughts each day and taught him ways to evaluate whether these thoughts might be overly harsh. Paul began to consider alternative ways of thinking.

As Paul's thinking became more positive, the therapist began to target his avoidant behaviors. Paul tended to avoid social events, bright lights, and even eye contact with others. Treatment consisted of exposure, in which the therapist gradually coached Paul to make eye contact, to engage in social activities, and to talk with others under bright light.

While Paul reduced his avoidant behaviors, the therapist introduced response prevention. Paul had been using rituals to try to reduce his anxiety, including engaging in facial exercises, studying others' noses, and surfing plastic surgery websites. The therapist helped him understand that the rituals did not actually relieve his anxiety. As response prevention, Paul was asked to stop conducting the rituals and to monitor his mood and anxiety as he did so.

After five sessions of treatment, Paul's therapist introduced perceptual retraining. When people with BDD look in the mirror, they focus on small details of their worst feature, and they are overly evaluative. As daily homework, the therapist asked Paul to spend time looking in the mirror but focusing on the whole of his appearance. She also asked him to describe his nose using nonevaluative, objective language. The intense anxiety he initially experienced when completing this exercise had diminished within a week. Soon, he was able to appreciate some of his features that he had previously ignored—for example, he noticed that he had nice eyes.

People with BDD often focus excessive attention on their own appearance. The therapist guided Paul to refocus his attention on people and events outside himself. For example, when Paul dined with a friend, she coached him to attend to the sound of his friend's voice, the flavor of the food, and the content of their conversation.

As Paul made gains, the therapist began to work on the more difficult and core aspects of cognitions—his deeply held beliefs about the meaning of his appearance. Paul described feeling that his physical flaws made him unlovable. The therapist helped him begin to consider his many positive qualities.

The tenth and final session consisted of reviewing the skills he had learned and discussing the strategies he would use if symptoms returned. Over the course of treatment, Paul's symptoms remitted so greatly that by the last session he was no longer distressed about his nose.

Drawn with permission from Wilhelm, Buhlmann, et al. (2010).

---

sorting their possessions. As with other exposure treatments, the client and the therapist work through a hierarchy, tackling increasingly difficult challenges as therapy progresses.

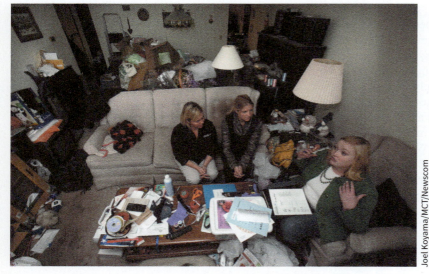

Despite the evidence that efforts to remove possessions too rapidly tend to fail, the TV show *Hoarders* featured many people who were faced with ridding themselves of objects under dire threat of eviction or other contingencies and so were forced to discard their collections immediately.

Despite the shared features with treatment for OCD, treatment for hoarding must be tailored in many ways to be efficacious. As illustrated in the Clinical Case of Dena, many people with hoarding disorder don't recognize the gravity of their symptoms. Therapy cannot begin to address the hoarding symptoms until the person develops insight. To facilitate insight, therapists use motivational strategies to help clients consider reasons to change. Once people decide to change, therapists help them make decisions about their objects and may provide tools and strategies to help them organize and remove their clutter (e.g., designating one cabinet for canned goods, one bin for paper to be discarded). Therapists often supplement their office sessions with in-home visits to assess the degree of hoarding and to conduct in vivo exercises on decluttering (Tolin, Frost, et al., 2015). Outcomes are better when clients are not rushed into quickly discarding their objects (Abramowitz, Franklin, et al., 2003).

Findings from three randomized controlled trials provide support for individual and group versions of ERP (Tolin, Frost, et al., 2021). Peer-led groups supplemented with structured readings also appear helpful (Mathews, Mackin, et al., 2018). Despite the evidence that ERP is helpful, hoarding is very difficult to treat—about half of patients continue to show clinically significant hoarding symptoms after treatment (Lin, Bacala, et al., 2023; Tolin et al., 2021). In many cities, case managers coordinate with other agencies to avoid evictions and to improve safety for those with hoarding disorder (Lin et al., 2023).

Hoarding symptoms can profoundly damage family relationships. Relatives usually try various approaches to help clear the clutter, only to become more and more distressed as those attempts fail (Drury, Ajmi, et al., 2014). Many resort to coercive strategies, like removing the hoarder's possessions while the person is away—strategies that typically create mistrust and animosity. Family approaches to treatment of hoarding begin by building rapport around these difficult issues (Tompkins & Hartl, 2013). Rather than aiming for a total absence of clutter, therapists urge family members to identify the aspects of clutter that are most dangerous—for example, lack of access to an emergency exit—to help set priorities with the person with hoarding disorder. Support groups and online communities for family members of those with hoarding disorder (e.g., Children of Hoarders) have become increasingly common.

Brain Stimulation for Treatment-Resistant OCD

About 10% of those with OCD will not respond to multiple pharmacological treatments. For those patients, two treatments involving brain stimulation have been approved by the FDA: deep transcranial magnetic stimulation (dTMS) and deep brain stimulation (DBS). dTMS involves magnetic stimulation applied to the scalp, whereas in DBS, electrodes are typically implanted into one of several regions in the basal ganglia. About half of patients treated with either form of stimulation attain significant relief within a couple months of treatment (Carmi, Tendler, et al., 2019; Freire, Cabrera-Abreu, & Milev, 2020). DBS has a chance of severe side effects from electrode implantation, and so is considered only after a board carefully reviews the case history to verify severe OCD that has failed to respond to standard treatments (Abramovitch, Elliott, et al., 2014). Despite the risks, the gains from DBS, along with those from dTMS, provide support for neurobiological models of OCD (Goodman, Storch, & Sheth, 2021).

Quick Summary

Antidepressants are the most supported medication treatment for obsessive-compulsive and related disorders.

The major psychological treatment approach for obsessive-compulsive and related disorders is exposure and response prevention (ERP). ERP for hoarding disorder often involves motivational strategies to enhance insight and willingness to consider change.

Deep transcranial magnetic stimulation (dTMS) and deep brain stimulation (DBS) are FDA-approved for treatment-resistant OCD.

7.3 Check Your Knowledge

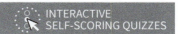
INTERACTIVE
SELF-SCORING QUIZZES

(Answers are at the end of the chapter.)
Answer the following questions.

1. What class of medication is most recommended for the treatment of obsessive-compulsive and related disorders?

2. Describe the foci of the response-prevention component of ERP for OCD, BDD, and hoarding disorder.

Clinical Description and Epidemiology of Posttraumatic Stress Disorder and Acute Stress Disorder

Trauma-related disorders are diagnosed only when a person develops symptoms after a traumatic event, such as the symptoms Ashley developed after being raped. Trauma-related diagnoses rest on the idea that horrific life experiences can trigger serious psychological symptoms. The DSM-5-TR also provides criteria for prolonged grief disorder, another syndrome related to extreme stress. These diagnoses contrast with all other major DSM diagnoses, which are defined entirely by symptom profiles. No other major DSM diagnosis places emphasis squarely on the cause.

We will begin with a focus on posttraumatic stress disorder. Then, we will more briefly discuss the DSM diagnosis for acute stress disorder.

Posttraumatic stress disorder (PTSD) entails an extreme response to a severe stressor. Although people have known for decades that the stresses of combat can have powerful adverse effects on soldiers, the aftermath of the Vietnam War spurred the development of this diagnosis.

The estimates of how many vary widely, but far too many people have experienced traumas. In large-scale studies, more than two-thirds of people report at least one serious trauma during their lifetime (Liu, Petukhova, et al., 2017). Whereas men are more likely to experience military trauma, accidental injury, serious illness, or physical assault, women are more likely to experience childhood maltreatment, sexual assault, or intimate partner violence (Kimerling, Weitlauf, & Street, 2021). An estimated one in every six women in the United States will be raped during her lifetime (Tjaden & Thoennes, 2006). All too often, the traumas experienced by women are chronic or repeated (Kimerling, Weitlauf, & Street, 2021). Transgender individuals are at particularly high risk of experiencing trauma (Stoltzer, 2009). Children are at high risk of trauma exposure compared to adults (Gunaratnam & Alisic, 2017) and are at higher risk for developing PTSD after trauma exposure (Copeland & McGinnis, 2021). Trauma rates are also higher among those with same-sex partners, and among ethnic and racial minority groups (Roberts, Austin, et al., 2010).

Exposure to trauma, however, is only one aspect of this diagnosis. Despite the very high rates of trauma in the population, it is estimated that about 5.6% of the worldwide

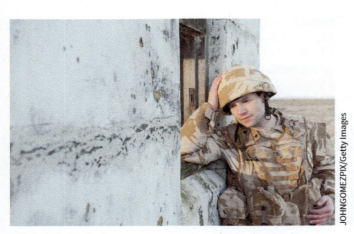

JOHNGOMEZPIX/Getty Images

Military trauma is the most common type of trauma preceding PTSD for men.

Clinical Case

Ashley

Ashley, a 20-year-old college student, sought help at the college counseling center. Three months earlier, she had been raped by a man whom she had met at a party. She sought help when the ongoing terror and associated symptoms led her to fail her classes for the semester. Since the rape, she had felt as though she were on constant alert, scanning the environment for the man who had assaulted her. When she would see anyone who looked even remotely like her attacker, her heart would pound, her knees would shake, and she would feel overwhelmed by terror. She avoided social events because the thought of interacting with men frightened her. Most nights, she would toss and turn for at least an hour

before falling asleep, and then intense nightmares related to the event would wake her. Her sleep loss often left her too exhausted to attend class, and even when she did attend class, she felt unable to concentrate. As she developed a newly cynical attitude toward people, she withdrew from most of her friends. She lost her motivation to be a part of campus life, and she stopped attending the club meetings that had been important to her before the trauma. Although she tried hard to stop thinking about the event, she faced almost daily reminders, as sexual assaults were frequently discussed in school newspapers and among her peers. Each time she was reminded of the event, she would feel overwhelmed.

population meets diagnostic criteria for PTSD (Koenen, Ratanatharathorn, et al., 2017). In addition to trauma, the diagnosis of PTSD requires that a set of symptoms be present. The diagnostic criteria for PTSD involve four symptom clusters:

- *Intrusively reexperiencing* the traumatic event. Like Ashley (see the **Clinical Case**), many people with PTSD have dreams or nightmares with themes related to the trauma night after night. Others are haunted by painfully vivid and intrusive memories. At times, the memories are so vivid that the person can feel as though they are reliving the event (Ashbaugh et al., 2017). Small sensory reminders of the event can bring on a wave of psychophysiological arousal (Orr, Metzger, et al., 2003). For example, a veteran may tremble when he hears the sound of a helicopter, which reminds him of the battlefield; for months after the event, a woman who was raped in one area of a campus may find that her heart pounds whenever she nears that area.

- *Avoidance* of stimuli associated with the event. Most people with PTSD strive to avoid thinking about the event, and some try to avoid all reminders of the event. Although most say they try to avoid remembering and reliving the event, avoidance usually fails; most people with PTSD remember the event all too often (Rubin, Berntsen, & Bohni, 2008).

- Other signs of *negative mood and thought* that developed after the trauma. Many people with PTSD feel detached from friends and activities and find that nothing in life brings joy. As they wrestle with questions of blame about the event, many come to believe that they are bad, and others develop the belief that all people are untrustworthy.

- Symptoms of *increased arousal and reactivity*. The person with PTSD often feels continuously on guard, monitoring the environment for danger. This heightened arousal can manifest in jumpiness when startled, aggressive outbursts over small events, and trouble falling asleep or sleeping through the night.

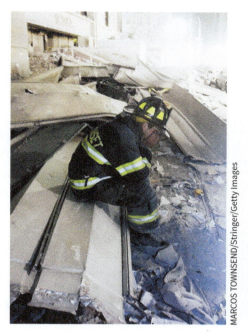

Rescue workers, such as this firefighter, could be vulnerable to PTSD.

The symptoms of PTSD may develop soon after the trauma, but sometimes the full syndrome does not develop until years after the initial event. Once PTSD develops, symptoms can be relatively chronic. Without treatment, about half of people still continue to experience diagnosable symptoms several years later (Morina, Wicherts, et al., 2014; Perkonigg, Pfister, et al., 2005). Even 40 years after the Vietnam War, some veterans who served in the war zone still met diagnostic criteria for PTSD (Marmar, Schlenger, et al., 2015).

PTSD is tied to a broad range of social and other difficulties. Many with PTSD describe feeling less satisfied in their relationships, and marital dissatisfaction and divorce are common (Bovin, Wells, et al., 2014). Unemployment is common as well (Bovin, Wells, et al., 2014). PTSD also is related to elevated rates of suicidal thoughts, suicide attempts, and incidents of nonsuicidal self-injury (Nock, Hwang, et al., 2009; Weierich & Nock, 2008). People with PTSD also show high rates of medical illness (Scott, Lim, et al., 2016). In a study of 15,288 army veterans followed for 30 years after their military service, PTSD predicted an elevated risk of early death from medical illness, accidents, and suicides (Boscarino, 2006).

It has been argued that prolonged exposure to trauma, such as repeated childhood abuse, might lead to a broader range of symptoms than those covered by the DSM criteria for PTSD. Some have proposed that this syndrome be referred to as *complex PTSD* (Herman, 1992). Authors differ in the symptom profiles they link to prolonged trauma, but most write about negative emotions, relationship disturbances, and negative self-concept (Cloitre, Courtois, et al., 2011). What does the research suggest about the effects of prolonged trauma? A comprehensive review suggests that prolonged trauma exposure can lead to more severe PTSD symptoms but does not result in a distinct subtype with unique symptomatology (Resick, Bovin, et al., 2012). Given this, the DSM-5-TR does not include a diagnosis or a specifier for complex PTSD. The ICD-11 includes a subtype of complex PTSD and also uses slightly different PTSD criteria than the DSM-5-TR does.

Like PTSD, **acute stress disorder (ASD)** is considered as a diagnosis when symptoms occur after a trauma. The symptoms of ASD are similar to those of PTSD, but the duration is shorter; this diagnosis is applicable only when the symptoms last for 3 days to 1 month. To allow

DSM-5 Defining Symptoms of Posttraumatic Stress Disorder

A. Exposure to actual or threatened death, serious injury, or sexual violence, in one or more of the following ways: experiencing the event personally, witnessing the event in person, learning that a violent or accidental death or threat of death occurred to a close other, or experiencing repeated or extreme exposure to aversive details of the event(s) other than through the media

B. At least one of the following recurrent **intrusion** symptoms:

- Intrusive distressing memories of the trauma(s) or, in children, repetitive play regarding the trauma themes
- Distressing dreams related to the event(s)
- Dissociative reactions (e.g., flashbacks) in which the individual feels or acts as if the trauma(s) were recurring or, in children, reenactment of trauma during play
- Intense or prolonged distress or physiological reactivity in response to reminders of the trauma(s)

C. At least one of the following **avoidance** symptoms:

- Avoids internal reminders of the trauma(s)
- Avoids external reminders of the trauma(s)
- In children younger than 7, attempts to avoid reminders of the trauma

D. At least two of the following persistent **negative alterations in cognitions and mood** began after the event:

- Inability to remember an important aspect of the trauma(s)
- Exaggerated negative beliefs or expectations about one's self, others, or the world
- Excessive blame of self or others about the trauma(s)

- Negative emotional state or, in children younger than 7, more frequent negative emotions
- Markedly diminished interest or participation in significant activities, or in children younger than 7, constricted play
- Feeling of detachment or estrangement from others or, in children younger than 7, social withdrawal
- Inability to experience positive emotions, or in children younger than 7, less expression of positive emotions

E. At least two of the following recurrent changes in **arousal and reactivity:**

- Irritable or aggressive behavior with little provocation
- Reckless or self-destructive behavior
- Hypervigilance
- Exaggerated startle response
- Poor concentration
- Sleep disturbance

F. The symptoms began or worsened after the trauma(s) and continued for at least 1 month

G. Among children younger than 7:

- Diagnosis requires criteria A, B, E, and F but only one symptom from either criteria C or D
- Inability to recall important parts of the trauma, exaggerated negative beliefs or expectations, excessive blame, and reckless or self-destructive behavior are not included as symptoms to consider

---

better identification of the people who are developing symptoms after a trauma, the ASD criteria are broader than the PTSD criteria. That is, ASD diagnostic criteria do not specify that symptoms from each category (e.g., intrusion symptoms, avoidance symptoms) must be present.

There is concern that the ASD diagnosis could stigmatize very common short-term reactions to serious traumas (Harvey & Bryant, 2002). For example, in the month after a rape, more than 90% of women report significant symptoms (Rothbaum, Foa, et al., 1992), and in the month after an assault, more than half of people show clinically significant symptoms (Riggs, Rothbaum, & Foa, 1995).

Despite this concern about the ASD diagnosis, it may be useful in encouraging providers to identify people who could use more support after a trauma. In a recent study of over 2,000 people who presented to emergency departments after a motor vehicle accident, the severity of trauma-related psychological symptoms in the first several days after the accident predicted the severity of symptoms 8 weeks later (Beaudoin, An, et al., 2023). When we consider treatments, we will describe evidence that treating ASD may help prevent the development of PTSD. Because less is known about ASD, we will focus on PTSD as we discuss epidemiology and causes.

PTSD is usually comorbid with other conditions. In one study of a representative community sample, researchers conducted diagnostic assessments repeatedly from age 3 until age 26. Among people who had developed PTSD by age 26, almost all (93%) had been diagnosed with another psychological disorder before age 21. Two-thirds of those with PTSD at age 26 had experienced another anxiety disorder by age 21. The other common comorbid disorders are major depressive disorder, substance use disorder, conduct disorder, and personality disorders (Koenen, Moffitt, et al., 2007; Pietrzak, Goldstein, et al., 2011). PTSD is also related to an increased risk of cardiovascular disease (Edmondson & von Känel, 2017).

Among people exposed to a trauma, women are 1.5 to 2 times as likely as men to develop PTSD, consistent with the gender ratio observed for anxiety disorders. Some argue that this is due to differential life circumstances that women face. For example, women are much more likely than men to be sexually assaulted during childhood and adulthood (Tolin & Foa, 2006). In studies that control for a history of sexual abuse and assault, men and women have comparable rates of PTSD (Tolin & Foa, 2006).

Culture and country of origin may shape the risk for PTSD in several ways. In the findings of the World Mental Health Survey, which used comparable diagnostic interviews with more than 70,000 persons, the prevalence of PTSD varied dramatically across the 24 countries studied. The prevalence of PTSD in the previous year in the United States and Northern Ireland was more than double that of other countries (Karam, Friedman, et al., 2014). Some cultural groups may be exposed to higher rates of trauma and consequently manifest higher rates of PTSD. In Northern Ireland, where civil conflict has been longstanding, events related to that strife are the primary form of trauma preceding PTSD (Atwoli, Stein, et al., 2015). Minority populations in the United States experience high rates of exposure to childhood trauma and to war-related service, and this contributes to the elevated rates of PTSD observed in Black individuals (Roberts, Gilman, et al., 2011). Nonetheless, even when trauma exposure is controlled for, rates of PTSD are high in the United States and Northern Ireland, and so trauma exposure alone cannot explain these cross-national differences (Koenen, Ratanatharathorn, et al., 2017). Refugees, and particularly those from regions with high levels of torture, genocide, and politically motivated sexual abuse, are at elevated risk of PTSD (Silove & Klein, 2021). Culture also may shape the types of symptoms observed in PTSD. *Ataque de nervios*, originally identified in Puerto Rico, involves physical symptoms and fears of going crazy in the aftermath of severe stress and thus is similar to PTSD.

VIDEO CONTENT

Case Study: PTSD Pause and Ponder

Quick Summary

Posttraumatic stress disorder (PTSD) and acute stress disorder (ASD) are both severe reactions to trauma. The symptoms of PTSD and ASD are similar, but ASD can be diagnosed only if symptoms have lasted less than 1 month. Most people who develop PTSD have a history of other psychological disorders, and two-thirds have a history of anxiety disorders.

7.4 Check Your Knowledge

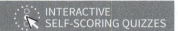
INTERACTIVE SELF-SCORING QUIZZES

(Answers are at the end of the chapter.)
Answer the following questions.

1. What is the major difference in the diagnostic criteria for PTSD and ASD?
2. Describe the four clusters of symptoms considered in the diagnosis of PTSD.
3. What is the major concern about the ASD diagnosis?

Etiology of Posttraumatic Stress Disorder

Would any of us break if exposed to severe enough life circumstances? Are some people so resilient that they could withstand whatever horrors life directs at them? Who is most likely to be haunted in the months and years after a terrible event? Consider these questions as we review the etiology of PTSD.

Earlier, we mentioned that two-thirds of people who develop PTSD have a history of an anxiety disorder. Not surprisingly, then, many of the influences on PTSD overlap with the influences on anxiety disorders described in Chapter 6 (see Table 6.4). For example, PTSD appears related to genetic risk for anxiety disorders (Smoller, 2016), childhood exposure to trauma (McLaughlin, Koenen, et al., 2017), greater activation in the amygdala and diminished activation of regions of the medial prefrontal cortex in response to cues of threat (Averill, Averill, et al., 2021), and greater emotional reactivity to cues of threat (DiGangi, Gomez, et al., 2013).

Also in parallel with anxiety disorders, Mowrer's two-factor model of conditioning has been applied to PTSD (Keane, Zimering, & Caddell, 1985). In this model, the initial fear in PTSD is assumed to arise from classical conditioning. For example, a man may come to fear walking in the neighborhood (the conditioned stimulus) where he was assaulted (the unconditioned stimulus). Like those with anxiety disorders, those with PTSD show elevated tendencies to develop and sustain conditioned fears (Hayes, VanElzakker, & Shin, 2012). This classically conditioned fear is so intense that the man avoids the neighborhood as much as possible. Operant conditioning then contributes to the maintenance of this avoidance behavior; the avoidance is reinforced by the reduction in fear that comes from not being in the presence of the conditioned stimulus. This avoidant behavior interferes with chances for the fear to extinguish.

Keeping these parallels in mind, in this section we focus on factors that are uniquely associated with PTSD. We begin by describing evidence that certain kinds of traumas may be more likely than other types to trigger PTSD. Even among people who experience serious traumas, though, not everyone develops PTSD. Thus, a great deal of research has been conducted on neurobiological and coping variables related to PTSD.

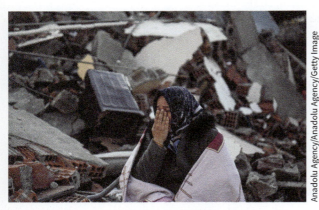

People who have experienced natural disasters, such as the Turkish earthquake in 2023, are at risk for PTSD, but their risk may not be as high as that of people who experience traumas caused by humans, such as assaults.

Anadolu Agency/Anadolu Agency/Getty Image

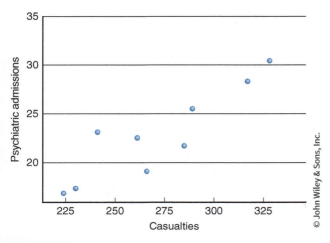

© John Wiley & Sons, Inc.

FIGURE 7.2 **Percentage of Canadian soldiers admitted for psychiatric care as a function of the number of casualties in their battalion during World War II.**

Nature of the Trauma: The Severity and Type of Trauma Matter

The severity of the trauma influences whether or not a person will develop PTSD. Consider the case of people exposed to war. Findings of the World Mental Health Survey, described earlier, indicate that simply living in a country at war does not increase the risk of PTSD, perhaps because many in these countries do not witness the violence; in contrast, those who directly witness atrocities are at a fourfold higher risk than the general population of developing PTSD (Liu et al., 2017). Among soldiers serving in Afghanistan or Iraq, the U.S. Veterans Administration estimates that rates of PTSD among those with a second tour of duty are double what they are for those with one tour of duty. About 20% of American fighters wounded in Vietnam developed PTSD, in contrast to 50% of those who were prisoners of war there (Engdahl, Dikel, et al., 1997). During Operation Desert Storm (in the 1990–1991 conflict following the Iraqi invasion of Kuwait), among those assigned to collect, tag, and bury scattered body parts of the dead, 65% developed PTSD (Sutker, Uddo, et al., 1994). As shown in **Figure 7.2**, the number of World War II soldiers in a battalion who were admitted for psychiatric care was closely related to how many casualties occurred in the battalion (Jones & Wessely, 2001). During World War II, doctors estimated that 98% of men with 60 days of continuous combat would develop psychiatric problems (Grossman, 1995). The severity of trauma also seems to matter outside of military contexts. For example, rates of PTSD are higher among persons who have been raped as compared to those who have experienced other assaultive violence (Liu et al., 2017).

Beyond severity, the nature of the trauma matters. Traumas caused by humans are more likely to cause PTSD than are natural disasters (Charuvastra & Cloitre, 2008). For example, rapes, combat experience, abuse, and assault all are associated with higher risk than are natural disasters (McMillan & Asmundson, 2016). Perhaps these events are more distressing because they challenge ideas about humans as benevolent. Consistent with the importance of events that shake the ability to trust others, intimate partner violence is related to particularly high risk of PTSD (Blanco, Hoertel, et al., 2018).

Neurobiology: The Hippocampus

Earlier, we noted that PTSD, like the anxiety disorders discussed in Chapter 6, appears related to dysregulation of the amygdala and prefrontal cortex. Also like the anxiety disorders, PTSD is tied to greater activation of the locus coeruleus and the related release of norepinephrine, which could help explain hyperreactivity to threat-related stimuli (Arnsten, 2015). In addition to these regions tied to anxiety disorders, PTSD appears uniquely related to functioning of the hippocampus, a brain region shown in **Figure 7.3** (Patel, Spreng, et al., 2012). The hippocampus plays a central role in our ability to locate autobiographical memories in space, time,

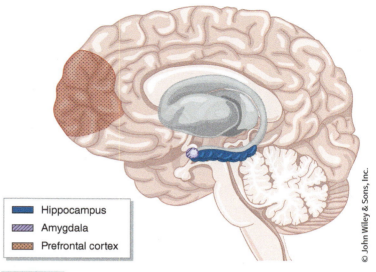

FIGURE 7.3 **People with PTSD show heightened activation of the hippocampus when completing various tasks.**

and context. Compared to those without PTSD, people with PTSD show diminished activation of the hippocampus during cognitive tasks and during tasks involving emotion regulation. In one study, researchers recruited people who were being treated at emergency rooms for a trauma. Within 2 months of the trauma, the researchers gathered fMRI data as the participants completed a cognitive task. Across two samples, blunted activation of the hippocampus during the cognitive tasks predicted the onset of PTSD symptoms within 3 to 6 months after the trauma (van Rooij, Stevens, et al., 2018). In another study, blunted activation of the hippocampus predicted the onset of PTSD only among people who also showed high levels of psychophysiological arousal in the first 2 weeks after a trauma (Tanriverdi, Gregory, et al., 2022). People with PTSD also show a smaller hippocampus than do people with a trauma history who do not have PTSD (Logue, van Rooij, et al., 2018).

Biologically based difficulties in placing memories in context could set the stage for PTSD. People with PTSD can experience fear when they have any reminder of their trauma, even out of context. For example, a soldier who witnessed bombs dropping from a plane may be frightened by all planes after he returns from the war. For those with PTSD, the cues that one is in a safe environment do not work; the fear remains as intense as it did in the moment of the trauma. Changes in the function of the hippocampus might increase the risk that a person will experience fear even in safe contexts (Liberzon, 2018).

A growing body of research examines how PTSD relates to functional connectivity, or the coordination among multiple brain regions. In PTSD, the functional connectivity of multiple networks appears to be disrupted, including the salience network involved in detecting and responding to emotionally relevant stimuli, the central executive network involved in regulation of emotions, and the default mode network involved in introspection and processing of self-relevant memories (Averill et al., 2021).

Coping

Several types of studies suggest that people who cope with a trauma by trying to avoid thinking about it are more likely than others to develop PTSD. Much of the work on avoidance coping focuses on symptoms of **dissociation**, such as feeling removed from one's body or emotions or being unable to remember the event. (We discuss dissociation in more detail in Chapter 8.) Dissociation may allow the person to avoid confronting memories of the trauma. People who have symptoms of dissociation during and immediately after the trauma are more likely to develop PTSD (Breh & Seidler, 2007). In one study, researchers interviewed women within 2 weeks of a rape about dissociation during the rape (e.g., "Did you feel numb?" and "Did you have moments of losing track of what was going on?"). Women with high levels of

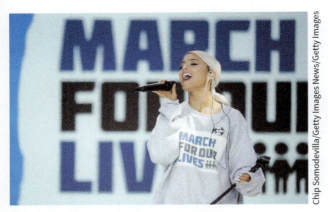

Ariana Grande developed PTSD symptoms after the Manchester Arena was bombed at the end of her performance, killing 23 people and injuring 500 others (Hattersley, G., August 14, 2018, *British Vogue*. **https://www.vogue.co.uk/article/ariana-grande-british-vogue-interview**)

dissociation were much more likely to develop PTSD symptoms than were women with low levels of dissociation. Many studies have now shown that dissociation shortly after trauma is related to a higher risk of developing PTSD over time (Carlson, Dalenberg, & McDade-Montez, 2012). Dissociation levels are usually at their highest in the weeks after the trauma and then dissipate over time. PTSD symptoms usually decline as dissociation fades (Carlson, Dalenberg, & McDade-Montez, 2012).

To encourage clinicians to consider these coping patterns, DSM-5-TR includes a dissociative symptom specifier to denote when persistent or recurrent symptoms of dissociation are present for those with PTSD. About 15% of people diagnosed with PTSD meet the criteria for this specifier (Stein, Koenen, et al., 2013).

Other protective factors may help a person cope with severe traumas more adaptively. Factors that are particularly important include strong social support (Brewin, Andrews, & Valentine, 2000) and cognitive ability (DiGangi et al., 2013). For example, veterans returning from war who report a stronger sense of social support are less likely to develop PTSD (Vogt, Smith, et al., 2011). Having better intellectual ability to make sense of horrifying events—and more friends and family members to assist in that process—helps people avoid symptoms after traumatic events.

A surprisingly high proportion of people cope quite well with trauma. For some, trauma awakens an increased appreciation of life, renews a focus on life priorities, and provides an opportunity to understand one's strengths in overcoming adversity (Bonanno, 2004).

Quick Summary

Some of the influences on anxiety disorders are involved in the development of PTSD, including genetic vulnerability, amygdala hyperactivity, heightened activity of the locus coeruleus and release of norepinephrine, diminished activity of the medial prefrontal cortex, childhood trauma exposure, and reactivity to threat. In addition, Mowrer's two-factor model of conditioning has been applied to PTSD.

Influences more specific to PTSD have been identified as well. The likelihood that a person will develop PTSD depends on the severity of the trauma. Traumas caused by humans are more likely to precede PTSD than are those involving natural disasters. People with PTSD tend to show blunted activation of the hippocampus when completing a broad range of tasks, as well as different patterns of connectivity of the salience network, the central executive network, and the default mode network. After exposure to trauma, people who rely on dissociative coping (i.e., who avoid thinking about the trauma) are more likely to develop PTSD than people who rely on other strategies. Higher cognitive ability and stronger social support can protect against the development of PTSD.

7.5 Check Your Knowledge

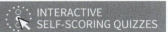
INTERACTIVE SELF-SCORING QUIZZES

(Answers are at the end of the chapter.)
Answer the following questions.

1. List major risk factors that contribute specifically to PTSD (as opposed to increasing general risk for anxiety disorders).
2. Describe the types of dissociation that are most relevant to PTSD.

Treatment of Posttraumatic Stress Disorder and Acute Stress Disorder

A good deal of work has focused on using medication and psychological treatments to treat PTSD, and some work focuses on whether treating ASD can help prevent PTSD. As we consider the treatments available for PTSD, it is important to consider that as many as 40% of those who experience PTSD do not seek treatment (Goldstein, Smith, et al., 2016) and even among those who seek treatment, many will not receive empirically supported treatments (Gavloski et al., 2021). Among those with PTSD being treated in research studies, about 15% withdraw before the treatment begins, and another quarter of patients withdraw once the treatment begins (Fernandez, Salem, et al., 2015).

Medication Treatment of PTSD

The FDA has approved two antidepressants for treatment of PTSD: paroxetine (Paxil) and sertraline (Zoloft)—both of which are selective serotonin reuptake inhibitors (SSRIs). Randomized controlled trials support the idea that these and other antidepressants (such as Venlafaxine) provide more relief from PTSD symptoms than do placebos (Davis, Pilkinston, et al., 2021), but many patients relapse after medications are discontinued. Although benzodiazapines are often prescribed for PTSD, evidence from randomized controlled trials does not support this approach, and most treatment guidelines recommend against their use (Davis et al., 2021).

Psychological Treatment of PTSD

Psychological treatments are more powerful than medications for the treatment of PTSD (Ruglass, Smith, et al., 2019). As in the psychological treatment of anxiety disorders discussed in Chapter 6, exposure treatment is the primary psychological approach to treating PTSD. In the treatment of PTSD, no approach has gained more supportive evidence than prolonged exposure treatment (Cusack, Jonas, et al., 2016). Randomized controlled trials suggest that prolonged exposure treatment provides more relief from the symptoms of PTSD than do medication, supportive unstructured psychotherapy, or relaxation therapy (Peterson, Foa, & Riggs, 2019). Prolonged exposure treatment has been found to be helpful across a broad range of cultural groups and treatment settings (Foa, Gillihan, & Bryant, 2013), and the benefits of prolonged exposure have been found to persist over a 5-year period (Foa & McLean, 2016). There is room for improvement, though, in considering how to strengthen treatment outcomes, as many clients, and particularly military clients, either withdraw from treatment or sustain some level of symptoms even after treatment (Steenkamp, Litz, & Marmar, 2020). Overall, more than a third of clients will drop out of exposure treatments (Imel, Laska, et al., 2013).

Prolonged exposure involves psychoeducation about the nature of PTSD, breathing exercises to help promote relaxation, exposure, and techniques to challenge negative beliefs about the trauma and its meaning. Exposure therapy involves facing the worst memories of the trauma, most typically by working through an exposure hierarchy from less intense fears to the most intense fears. Typically, prolonged exposure treatment involves 8 to 15 ninety-minute sessions, held once or twice per week (Foa & McLean, 2016). One goal of treatment is to extinguish the fear response, particularly the overgeneralized fear response; another goal is to challenge the idea that the person cannot cope with the anxiety and fear generated by those stimuli. As clients learn that they can deal with their anxiety, they are able to reduce their avoidance responses.

Where possible, the person is exposed directly to reminders of the trauma in vivo—for example, by returning to the scene of the event. Often, it may not be feasible or safe to return to the scene of a horrible trauma, and therapists use **imaginal exposure**—that is, the person deliberately remembers the event. Virtual reality technology can also help provide exposure (Botella, Serrano, & Baños, 2015), although it remains costly to develop stimuli relevant to the different types of traumas (Ruzek, 2021). Exposure therapy is hard for both the client and the therapist because it requires such intense focus on traumatizing events. For example, therapists might ask women who have developed PTSD after rape to recall the worst moments of the attack in vivid detail.

After a trauma, many people struggle with negative thoughts—that the world is dangerous, that they were to blame for the horrible event, or that they are not competent to cope with the dangers of the world. Within prolonged exposure treatment, as a client discusses the trauma, the therapist helps the person to develop a more positive narrative about theirability to cope with the trauma and its effects. Not surprisingly, then, negative cognitive beliefs about self-blame and the meaning of the trauma tend to change in prolonged exposure treatment (Cooper, Zoellner, et al., 2017).

Several cognitive treatments designed to directly focus on these types of negative thoughts have received support in randomized controlled trials (Cusack et al., 2016; Ehlers & Clark, 2008; Kulkarni, Barrad, & Cloitre, 2014). Benefits have been shown internationally, for example, among survivors of a terrorist attack in southern Thailand (Bryant et al., 2011). Cognitive processing therapy (CPT) was developed to help victims of rape and childhood sexual abuse dispute tendencies toward self-blame. The treatment is usually offered in 12 to 18 sessions. CPT has also received empirical support in civilian and military samples (Williams, Galovski, & Resick, 2019) and appears particularly helpful in reducing guilt (Resick, Nishith, & Griffin, 2003) and dissociation (Resick, Suvak, et al., 2012). Beneficial effects of CPT have been observed 5 to 10 years after initial treatment (Williams, Galovski, & Resick, 2019). Benefits of CPT also have been shown across countries, including among sexual assault survivors in the Democratic Republic of Congo (Bass, Annan, et al., 2013).

Eye movement desensitization and reprocessing (EMDR) is a variant of exposure treatment (Shapiro, 1999). As with prolonged exposure treatment, clients in EMDR are instructed to recall a trauma-related scene, and they are also asked to review and challenge negative thoughts related to that scene. EMDR is distinct, though, in that, as the trauma and related cognitions are discussed, the therapist moves his, her or their fingers back and forth in front of the client's eyes and asks the client to visually track the fingers. Multiple randomized controlled trials indicate that EMDR is as helpful as various forms of CBT in the short term (De Jongh, Amann, et al., 2019), although the randomized controlled trials are not of as good quality as those available for prolonged exposure (Cusack et al., 2016) and findings have not been as positive in military samples (Galovski et al., 2021). There is mixed evidence about whether the eye movement component of this treatment is helpful (Galovski et al., 2021).

Even with the clear evidence that exposure treatment (with or without additional cognitive, emotion regulation, or eye movement components) is superior to other types of treatment, many psychologists do not provide exposure treatment for their clients with PTSD (Becker, Zayfert, & Anderson, 2004). To address this lack of dissemination, over 1,500 therapists at the Veterans Affairs Medical Center (VAMC) were taught how to administer either exposure treatment or cognitive processing therapy for PTSD (Karlin & Cross, 2014). Clients offered these treatments achieved more than double the level of symptom reduction observed among clients before the training occurred (Karlin, Ruzek, et al., 2010). Sadly, in the years after the training, less than 10% of veterans with PTSD have been receiving a full dose of these interventions; therapists in the VAMC system report not having the time available to provide this type of care (Chard, Ricksecker, et al., 2012; Shiner, D'Avolio, et al., 2013).

In light of the lack of availability of these effective psychological treatments, a natural question is whether telehealth, online intervention, or apps could make treatments more accessible for people. As one example, an online clinic for anxiety and depression was able to offer assessment, information, and referral to more than 25,000 people within a 30-month period (Titov, Dear, et al., 2017). Within online treatments, support from a therapist consistently predicts better outcomes. As one example, Interapy is an online intervention for PTSD in which clients complete written exercises to facilitate exposure and cognitive reappraisal each week, and then a therapist provides feedback on the exercises. Across seven randomized controlled trials, those who took part in therapy showed more reduction in PTSD symptoms than did those assigned to a waitlist control condition. Internet-based therapy, though, tends to have higher rates of patient drop-out (Fernandez et al., 2015), and it is not yet clear if internet-based therapy offers as much benefit as face-to-face exposure treatment (Ruzek,

2021). Nonetheless, online interventions offer the potential for intervention where in-person treatment may not be readily available, such as in post-disaster or war-traumatized populations. Beyond internet-based therapy, telehealth treatment provides as much benefit as does in-person treatment for PTSD, which also opens the possibility of better care for people living in areas without specialty PTSD clinics (Galovski et al., 2021). Unfortunately, despite the rapid proliferation of apps, multiple trials have indicated that mobile apps for PTSD do not provide the long-term relief from symptoms observed with standard individual treatment (Ruzek, 2021). Nonetheless, websites and online communities can provide social support, supportive tools to supplement treatment, and information for those recovering from traumatic experiences (**http://maketheconnection.net**).

Psychological Treatment of Acute Stress Disorder

Is it possible to prevent the development of PTSD by offering treatment to people who have developed ASD? Cognitive behavioral therapy (exposure treatment) appears to do so. Multiple studies indicate that risk of PTSD is reduced among those who received exposure therapy, as compared with those who were assigned to a control condition. There is little evidence, though, that it is helpful to offer psychological treatment for those who have not developed ASD symptoms (Roberts, Kitchner, et al., 2019).

The positive effects of early exposure treatment appear to last for years. Researchers examined the long-term effect of treatment among adolescents who survived a devastating earthquake. Even 5 years after the earthquake, adolescents who had received cognitive behavioral intervention reported less severe PTSD symptoms than did those who had not received treatment (Goenjian, Walling, et al., 2005). Unfortunately, not all approaches to prevention work as well as exposure treatment (see **Focus on Discovery 7.1**).

Focus on Discovery 7.1

Critical Incident Stress Debriefing

Critical incident stress debriefing (CISD) involves immediate treatment of trauma victims, usually within the first week of the traumatic event (Mitchell, 1983). Unlike CBT, CISD is usually limited to one long group session and is given regardless of whether the person has developed symptoms. Therapists encourage people to remember the details of the trauma and to express their feelings as fully as they can. Therapists who practice this approach often visit disaster sites immediately after events, sometimes invited by local authorities; they offer therapy both to victims and to their families.

CISD is highly controversial. A review of six studies, all of which involved randomly assigning clients to receive CISD or no treatment, found that those who received CISD tended to fare worse than those who received no treatment (Litz, Gray, et al., 2002). No one is certain why harmful effects occur, but remember that many people who experience a trauma do not develop PTSD. Many experts are dubious about the idea of providing therapy for people who have not developed a disorder. Some researchers object to CISD because a person's natural coping strategies may work better than those recommended by someone else (Bonanno, 2004).

7.6 Check Your Knowledge

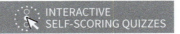

INTERACTIVE
SELF-SCORING QUIZZES

(Answers are at the end of the chapter.)
Answer the following questions.

1. In conducting exposure treatment for PTSD, _____ exposure is sometimes used because in vivo exposure cannot be carried out for experiences as horrific as war and rape.

2. Cognitive therapy, when added to exposure for PTSD, is particularly helpful in addressing (choose the answer that best fits):
   a. suicidal tendencies
   b. risk of relapse
   c. insomnia
   d. guilt

3. Describe the findings on internet-based psychotherapy for PTSD.

Summary

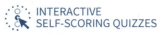

INTERACTIVE
SELF-SCORING QUIZZES

Chapter 7 Practice Quiz

Obsessive-Compulsive and Related Disorders

- People with obsessive-compulsive disorder (OCD) have intrusive, unwanted thoughts and feel compelled to engage in rituals to avoid overwhelming anxiety. People with body dysmorphic disorder (BDD) experience persistent highly self-critical thoughts that they have a flawed appearance, and they engage in intensive efforts to cope with their appearance. Hoarding disorder is characterized by the tendency to acquire an excessive number of objects and extreme difficulty in ridding oneself of those objects.

- OCD, BDD, and hoarding disorder are each moderately heritable. There is some shared genetic risk across these three disorders.

- OCD has been linked to activity in the cortico-striatal-thalamic-cortical (CSTC) loop during tasks that provoke symptoms. The CSTC includes the orbitofrontal cortex, the caduate nucleus, the thalamus and the anterior cingulate cortex. People with BDD also show hyperactivity in regions of the orbitofrontal cortex and the caudate nucleus when viewing photos of themselves. Hoarding disorder involves hyperactivity in the orbitofrontal cortex and the anterior cingulate cortex during symptom-provoking tasks. In addition to the brain regions that overlap across the OCD-related disorders, BDD has also been tied to more engagement of regions involved in visual processing.

- Tendencies toward repetitive thoughts and behaviors in OCD may be related to a tendency for conditioned responses to be sustained even after the threat is removed. People with OCD also appear to have difficulty trusting evidence needed to make decisions, particularly during transitions. Obsessions may be intensified by attempts to suppress unwanted thoughts, in part because people with OCD tend to believe that thinking about something is as bad as doing it, a tendency referred to as thought–action fusion.

- The cognitive model relates BDD to a detail-oriented analytic style and an overvaluing of the importance of appearance to self-worth.

- Cognitive behavioral influences on hoarding include poor organizational abilities, unusual beliefs about the importance of possessions and responsibility for those possessions, and avoidance behaviors.

- ERP, a well-validated approach for the treatment of OCD, involves exposure, along with strategies to prevent engaging in compulsive behaviors. ERP has been adapted for the treatment of BDD and hoarding. For the treatment of BDD, ERP is supplemented with cognitive strategies to challenge people's overly negative views of their appearance, their excessive focus on their appearance, and their belief that self-worth depends on their appearance. For hoarding disorder, therapists supplement ERP with strategies to increase insight and motivation.

- Antidepressants are the medications most commonly used for OCD, BDD, and hoarding disorder. These medications have received strong support for OCD, but little research is available concerning medication treatment for BDD or hoarding disorder.

Trauma-Related Disorders

- Posttraumatic stress disorder (PTSD) is diagnosed only after a traumatic event. It is marked by symptoms of reexperiencing the trauma, avoidance of reminders of the trauma, negative alterations in cognitions and mood, and hyper-arousal. Acute stress disorder (ASD) is defined by similar symptoms with a duration of less than 1 month. PTSD is highly comorbid with other psychological disorders, and about two-thirds of people who develop PTSD have a history of other anxiety disorders.

- Many of the influences on anxiety disorders are related to the development of PTSD, such as genetic vulnerability, hyperactivity of the amygdala and diminished function of the medial prefrontal cortex, heightened activity of the locus coeruleus and norepinephrine system, childhood trauma exposure, reactivity to negative stimuli, and behavioral conditioning. Research and theory on the causes that are specific to PTSD focus on the severity and nature of the traumatic event, as well as on hippocampal activity; functional connectivity of the salience network, the central executive network, and the default mode network; dissociation; and other factors that may enhance the ability to cope with stress, such as social support and intelligence.

- Antidepressants (SSRIs) are the medication approach best supported for treating PTSD.

- Psychological treatment of PTSD involves exposure. Exposure treatment for ASD can reduce the risk that PTSD will develop. Supplements to exposure treatment for PTSD include a more direct focus on cognition and eye movements.

Answers to Check Your Knowledge Questions

7.1. 1. chronic: 2. Obsessions involve a repetitive and intrusive thought, urge, or image; compulsions involve either a thought or a behavior that the person feels the need to engage in to ward off threats or the anxiety associated with obsessions.

7.2. 1. Heritability ranges from 0.40 to 0.50; 2. (a) All share symptoms of uncontrollable repetitive thoughts and behavior; (b) the syndromes often co-occur; (c) the genetic vulnerability for these conditions overlaps; (d) regions of the cortico-striatal-thalamic-cortical (CSTC) loop are involved in all three syndromes.

7.3. 1. antidepressants (more specifically, selective serotonin reuptake inhibitors [SSRIs]); 2. In OCD, the focus of response prevention is on compulsions; in BDD, the focus is on behaviors designed to seek reassurance or relieve anxiety about one's appearance, such as checking one's appearance in the mirror; in hoarding disorder, rituals like counting and sorting possessions are the focus.

7.4. 1. The ASD diagnosis can be considered when symptoms have lasted less than 1 month, whereas the PTSD diagnosis can be considered when symptoms have lasted at least 1 month; 2. intrusion symptoms, avoidance symptoms, negative alterations in cognition and mood, and changes in arousal and reactivity; 3. Brief symptoms may be normative after severe trauma.

7.5. 1. any two of the following: blunted activation of the hippocampus when completing a wide range of tasks; disrupted connectivity of the salience network, the central executive network, and the default mode network; avoidant coping strategies that prevent one from processing the trauma, such as dissociation; low cognitive function; poor social support; 2. People with PTSD often report feeling removed from their body or emotions or being unable to remember the traumatic event, either at the time of the trauma or after the trauma.

7.6. 1. imaginal: 2. d. guilt; 3. Internet-based CBT appears helpful, but it is not clear if it is as helpful as treatment offered in-person and drop-out rates are high. Gains are larger when there is some contact with a therapist.

Key Terms

Dissociative Disorders and Somatic Symptom and Related Disorders

---

LEARNING GOALS

1. Summarize the symptoms and epidemiology of the three major dissociative disorders.

2. Discuss the current debate regarding the causes of dissociative identity disorder.

3. Describe the available treatments for dissociative identity disorder.

4. Define the symptoms of the somatic symptom and related disorders.

5. Explain the causes of the somatic symptom and related disorders.

6. Describe the dissociative treatments for somatic symptom and related disorders.

Clinical Case

Gina

In December 1965, a woman named Gina Rinaldi sought therapy with Dr. Robert Jeans. Gina, single and 31 years old, lived with another single woman and was working successfully as a writer at a large educational publishing firm. Her friends saw her as efficient, businesslike, and productive but had observed that she was becoming forgetful and sometimes acted out of character. Gina reported that she had been sleepwalking since her early teens; her present roommate had told her that she sometimes screamed in her sleep.

The youngest of nine siblings, Gina described her 74-year-old mother as the most domineering woman she had ever known. She reported that as a child she had been a fearful and obedient daughter. At age 28, she had her first romantic relationship, with a former Jesuit priest, although it was not physical in nature. Then she became involved with T.C., a married man who assured her he would get a divorce and marry her. She indicated that she had been faithful to him since the start of their relationship. She became discouraged about their relationship when he did not come through with his promised divorce and stopped seeing Gina regularly.

After several sessions with Gina, Dr. Jeans noticed a second personality emerging. Mary Sunshine, as Gina and Dr. Jeans came to call her, was quite different from Gina. She seemed more childlike, more traditionally feminine, ebullient, and seductive. Gina felt that she walked like a coal miner, but Mary certainly did not. Some concrete incidents indicated Mary's existence. Sometimes while cleaning her home, Gina found cups that had had hot chocolate in them—neither Gina nor her roommate liked hot chocolate. She even discovered herself ordering a sewing machine on the telephone although she disliked sewing; some weeks later, she arrived at her therapy session wearing a new dress that Mary had sewn. At work, people were finding Gina more pleasant, and her colleagues took to consulting her on how to encourage people to work better with one another. All these phenomena were entirely alien to Gina. Jeans and Gina came to realize that sometimes Gina transformed into Mary.

More and more often, Jeans witnessed Gina turning into Mary in the consulting room. T.C. accompanied Gina to a session during which her posture and demeanor became more relaxed, her tone of voice warmer. Then Mary and Gina started having conversations with each other in front of Jeans.

A year after the start of therapy, a synthesis of Gina and Mary began to emerge. At first, it seemed that Gina had taken over entirely, but then Dr. Jeans noticed that Gina was not as serious as before, particularly about "getting the job done"—that is, working extremely hard on the therapy. Dr. Jeans encouraged Gina to talk with Mary. The following is that conversation:

I was lying in bed trying to go to sleep. Someone started to cry about T.C. I was sure that it was Mary. I started to talk to her. The person told me that she didn't have a name. Later she said that Mary called her Evelyn. I was suspicious at first that it was Mary pretending to be Evelyn. I changed my mind, however, because the person I talked to had too much sense to be Mary. She said that she realized that T.C. was unreliable but she still loved

him and was very lonely. She agreed that it would be best to find a reliable man. She told me that she comes out once a day for a very short time to get used to the world. She promised that she will come out to see you [Dr. Jeans] sometime when she is stronger.

(Jeans, 1976, pp. 254–255)

Throughout that month, Evelyn appeared more and more often, and Dr. Jeans felt that his patient was improving rapidly. Within a few months, she seemed to be Evelyn all the time; soon thereafter, this woman married a physician. Years later, she had shown no recurrences of the other personalities.

Drawn from Jeans, 1976.

In this chapter, we discuss the dissociative disorders and the somatic symptom and related disorders. We cover these disorders together because both types are hypothesized to be triggered by stressful experiences yet do not involve direct expressions of anxiety. In the dissociative disorders, the person experiences disruptions of consciousness—a gap in self-awareness, memory, and identity. In the somatic symptom and related disorders, the person complains of bodily symptoms that suggest a physical dysfunction, sometimes dramatic in nature. For some of these disorders, no physiological basis can be found; for others, the psychological reaction to the symptoms appears excessive.

In addition to both being related to stress, dissociative disorders and somatic symptom and related disorders are often comorbid. Patients with dissociative disorders often meet the criteria for somatic symptom and related disorders, and those with somatic symptom and related disorders are somewhat more likely than those in the general population to meet the diagnostic criteria for dissociative disorders (Akyüz, Gökalp, et al., 2017; Brown, Cardena, et al., 2007; Dell, 2006). Functional neurological symptom disorder, one of the somatic symptom-related disorders, is particularly likely to be comorbid with dissociative disorders.

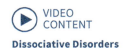

VIDEO CONTENT

Dissociative Disorders

Clinical Descriptions and Epidemiology of the Dissociative Disorders

The DSM-5-TR includes three major **dissociative disorders**: depersonalization/derealization disorder, dissociative amnesia, and dissociative identity disorder (formerly known as multiple personality disorder). **Table 8.1** summarizes the key clinical features of the dissociative disorders. **Dissociation**, the core feature of each dissociative disorder, involves some aspect

TABLE 8.1   **Diagnoses of Dissociative Disorders**

INTERACTIVE FIGURES, CHARTS, & TABLES

Diagnosis	Description
Depersonalization/derealization disorder	Experience of detachment from the self and reality
Dissociative amnesia	Lack of conscious access to memory, typically of a stressful experience. The fugue subtype involves traveling or wandering coupled with loss of memory of one's identity or past.
Dissociative identity disorder	At least two distinct personality states that act independently of each other

of emotion, memory, or experience being inaccessible consciously. Because dissociation is such a broad term, let's consider some of the different types of experience it encompasses.

Some types of dissociation are common. Many of you have probably had the experience of studying so hard for a test that you lost track of time and might not even have noticed people coming and going from the room where you were studying. Some of you may have missed a turn on the road home when thinking about a problem. These types of dissociative experiences are usually a harmless sign that one is so focused on some aspect of experience that other aspects of experience are lost from awareness.

In contrast to these common dissociative experiences, dissociative disorders are defined by more severe types of dissociation. Depersonalization/derealization disorder involves a form of dissociation characterized by detachment, in which a person feels removed from the sense of self and surroundings. The person may feel "spaced out," numb, or as though in a dream (Holmes, Brown, et al., 2005). Dissociative amnesia and dissociative identity disorder involve a more dramatic form of dissociation, in which a person cannot access important aspects of memory. In dissociative identity disorder, the gaps in memory are so extensive that the person loses the sense of a unified identity.

What causes dissociation? Both psychodynamic and behavioral theorists consider pathological dissociation to be an avoidance response that protects the person from consciously experiencing stressful events. Consistent with the idea that this is a coping response, people undergoing very intense stressors, such as advanced military survival training, often report brief moments of mild dissociation (Morgan, Hazlett, et al., 2001), and dissociation is more common when people are distressed (Buchnik-Daniely, Vannikov-Lugassi, et al., 2021) and among those who are experiencing symptoms of mood disorders (Ellickson-Larew, Stasik-O'Brien, et al., 2020). In addition to distress, sleep problems are common among people who experience dissociative disorders (Arora, Alhelali, & Grey, 2020), and naturalistic and experimentally induced sleep disruptions have been shown to trigger dissociation (Barton, Kyle, et al., 2018). Dissociation is more common when people are sleepy and after they have unusually vivid dreams (Buchnik-Daniely et al., 2021; Vannikov-Lugassi & Soffer-Dudek, 2018). Some work indicates that trauma and sleep could jointly contribute to dissociation. In one study of preschoolers, abuse led to sleep disturbance, and the sleep disturbance then predicted parental report of child dissociation (Hébert, Langevin, et al., 2016). Dissociation is also a common short-term effect of ketamine (Wodarczyk, Cubala, et al., 2021).

Researchers know less about dissociative disorders than about other disorders, and considerable controversy surrounds the etiological models for these disorders, as well as the identification of the best treatments. Even evaluating whether a person is experiencing these symptoms can be difficult. Many who endorse persistent dissociative symptoms describe unusual symptoms that are so rare as to be considered improbable (e.g., "When I hear voices I feel as though my teeth are leaving my body"), suggesting that they may be exaggerating their symptoms or experiencing genuine confusion about their experiences (Merckelbach, Boskovic, et al., 2017). To some, this controversy may seem daunting. We find the process of discovery to be fascinating, as researchers strive to untangle this complex puzzle.

Depersonalization/Derealization Disorder

Depersonalization/derealization disorder involves a disconcerting and disruptive sense of detachment from one's self or surroundings. Depersonalization is defined by a sense of being detached from one's self (e.g., being an observer outside one's body). Derealization is defined by a sense of detachment from one's surroundings, such that the surroundings seem unreal. People with this disorder may have the impression that they are outside their body, viewing themselves from a distance or looking at the world through a fog. They often report feeling physically and emotionally numb. Although more than a third of college students report that they have experienced at least fleeting moments of depersonalization or derealization in the past year (Hunter, Sierra, & David, 2004), these mild and intermittent symptoms are rarely of concern. A diagnosis of depersonalization/derealization disorder is considered only when the symptoms are persistent or recurrent. Unlike the other dissociative disorders, this disorder involves no disturbance of memory.

The following quote, drawn from a 1953 medical textbook, captures some of the experience of this disorder:

> *The world appears strange, peculiar, foreign, dream-like. Objects appear at times strangely diminished in size, at times flat. Sounds appear to come from a distance. ... The emotions likewise undergo marked alteration. Patients complain that they are capable of experiencing neither pain nor pleasure; love and hate have perished with them. They experience a fundamental change in their personality, and the climax is reached with their complaints that they have become strangers to themselves. It is as though they were dead, lifeless, mere automatons.*

> **(Schilder, 1953, pp. 304–305)**

Defining Symptoms of Depersonalization/Derealization Disorder

- **Depersonalization**: Experiences of detachment from one's mental processes or body, or
- **Derealization**: Experiences of unreality of surroundings or detachment from surroundings

- Symptoms are persistent or recurrent
- The symptoms are not explained by psychosis or other psychological or medical conditions

---

The symptoms of depersonalization and derealization are usually triggered by stress. Depersonalization/derealization disorder usually begins in adolescence, and it can start either abruptly or gradually. Most people who experience depersonalization also experience derealization, and the course is similar for both symptoms. Symptoms are often continuously present for years (Simeon, 2009). Comorbid personality disorders are frequently present, and during their lifetime, about 90% of people with this disorder will experience anxiety disorders or depression (Simeon, Knutelska, et al., 2003). As in the **Clinical Case of Mrs. A.**, childhood trauma is often reported (Michal, Adler, et al., 2016).

Clinical Case

Mrs. A.

> *Mrs. A was a 43-year-old woman who lived with her mother and son and worked in a clerical job. She had experienced symptoms of depersonalization several times per year for as long as she could remember. "It's as if the real me is taken out and put on a shelf or stored somewhere inside of me. Whatever makes me me is not there. It is like*
>
> *an opaque curtain ... like going through the motions. ..." She had found these symptoms to be extremely distressing. She had experienced panic attacks for 1 year when she was 35. She described a childhood trauma history that included nightly sexual abuse by her mother from her earliest memory to age 10.*
>
> **(Simeon, Gross, et al., 1997, p. 1109)**

The DSM diagnostic criteria for depersonalization/derealization disorder specify that the symptoms can co-occur with other disorders but should not be entirely explained by those disorders. It is important to rule out disorders that commonly involve these symptoms, including schizophrenia, acute stress disorder, posttraumatic stress disorder, and borderline personality disorder. Depersonalization is also relatively common during panic attacks and during marijuana, ketamine, or hallucinogen intoxication (Lynn, Berg, et al., 2018).

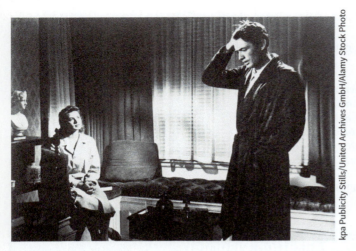

In *Spellbound*, Gregory Peck played a man with amnesia. Dissociative amnesia is typically triggered by a stressful event, as it was in the film.

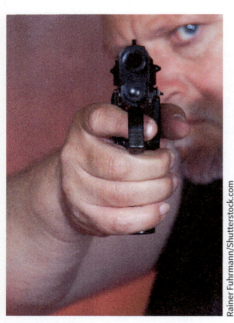

In moments of severe stress, people tend to focus on the most central element of the threat. After a hold-up, the person who was attacked may remember details of the gun but be unable to recall less threatening aspects of the situation, such as the clothes and appearance of the attacker.

Dissociative Amnesia

A person with **dissociative amnesia** is unable to recall important personal information, usually information about some traumatic experience. The holes in memory are too extensive to be ordinary forgetfulness and are not the effects of drugs or head injury. The episode of amnesia may last as briefly as several hours or as long as several years. The amnesia usually disappears as suddenly as it began, with complete recovery of memory and only a small chance of recurrence.

The DSM diagnostic criteria specify that the memory loss of amnesia typically involves information about a traumatic event or events, such as combat or childhood maltreatment, or events during a period of stress. Despite the diagnostic criteria, not all dissociative amnesias immediately follow trauma (Hacking, 1998). In addition, dissociative amnesia is rare even among people who have experienced intense trauma, such as imprisonment in a concentration camp (Merckelbach, Dekkers, et al., 2003). Whether or not the amnesia is triggered by a stressor, during the period of amnesia the person's behavior is otherwise unremarkable, except that the memory loss may cause some disorientation. Procedural memory remains intact—the person remembers how to answer the phone, ride a bike, and execute other complex actions, even though they are unable to remember specific events.

In the **dissociative fugue subtype** of dissociative amnesia (from the Latin *fugere*, "to flee"), the memory loss is more extensive. The person typically disappears from home and work. Some people wander away from home in a bewildered manner. Others take on a new name, a new home, a new job, and even a new set of personality characteristics. The person may even succeed in establishing a fairly complex social life. More often, however, the new life does not crystallize to this extent, and the fugue is more like the experience of Hannah Upp (see the **Clinical Case**)—of relatively brief duration, consisting of limited but apparently purposeful travel during which social contacts are minimal or absent. As with other forms of amnesia, recovery is usually complete, although it takes varying amounts of time; after recovery, people are fully able to remember the details of their life and experiences, except for those events that took place during the fugue.

Dissociative amnesia raises fundamental questions about how memory works under stress. Psychodynamic theory suggests that in dissociative amnesia traumatic events are repressed. Repression, as initially defined by Freud, involved suppressing unacceptably painful memories from consciousness. Many cognitive scientists, though, have questioned how repression could happen (Patihis, Ho, et al., 2021) because study after study shows that stress usually enhances rather than impairs encoding of memories for the negative event (Shields, Sazma, et al., 2017). Memory for traumatic events tends to be accurate and detailed even years later among survivors of plane crashes, natural disasters, and serious injuries (Goldfarb, Goodman, et al., 2019; McKinnon, Palombo, et al., 2015). Among a sample of veterans, those with the most severe war experiences were most likely to provide consistent descriptions of combat memories over time (Krinsley, Gallagher, et al., 2003). Norepinephrine, a neurotransmitter associated with heightened arousal, enhances memory consolidation and retrieval (Sara, 2009).

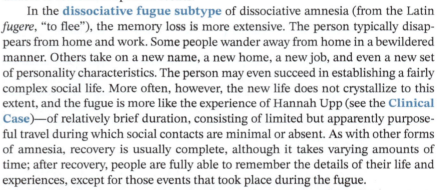

Defining Symptoms of Dissociative Amnesia

- Inability to remember important autobiographical information, usually of a traumatic or stressful nature, that is too extensive to be ordinary forgetfulness

- Specify with dissociative fugue if the amnesia is associated with bewildered or apparently purposeful wandering

Clinical Case

Hannah

In 2008, Hannah Upp's family and friends mounted an intensive search for her through media and internet outlets after she had been missing for 4 days. As reported in *The New York Times* (Marx & Ddiziulis, 2009), Hannah, a 23-year-old Spanish language teacher living in New York City, had gone for a run on the last day before the new school year began, leaving behind her ID and wallet. Almost 3 weeks later, she was rescued floating in the water about a mile southwest of Manhattan. She was suffering from dehydration and hypothermia, and she had large blisters on her heels. She had no memory of the events that had occurred during those 3 weeks, and it is believed she suffered from an episode of dissociative amnesia with dissociative fugue. When interviewed, Hannah could not identify any stressful trigger that would have provoked the episode—although her job was demanding, she loved teaching, and she was doing well in her pursuit of a master's degree. Extensive neurological tests suggested no biological explanation. Some of the events from those 3 weeks could be retraced from public video footage and reports from people who had seen her wandering around on Riverside Drive, entering an Apple store, and attending a local gym. She appears to have suffered a relapse in

2013, when she disappeared again for 2 days (Marx, 2017). In 2017, she disappeared again and had not been found by 2018 (Aviv, 2018).

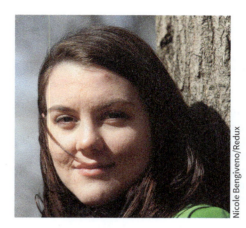

It is believed that Hannah Upp's 3-week disappearance from home and work in 2008 could have resulted from an episode of dissociative amnesia, with dissociative fugue.

The nature of attention and memory, however, does change during periods of intense stress. People under stress tend to focus on the most important features of the threatening situation and stop paying attention to peripheral features (Shields, Hunter, & Yonelinas, 2022).

Given that the usual response to trauma is enhanced memory of the central features of the threat, how can we explain the stress-related memory loss of dissociative amnesia? One answer might be that dissociative amnesia involves unusual ways of responding to stress. For example, extremely high levels of stress hormones could interfere with memory formation (Shields, Bonner, & Moons, 2015). Some have suggested that dissociative amnesia could reflect an extreme outcome of this process. Debate continues about how to understand memory loss in the context of trauma and dissociation (see **Focus on Discovery 8.1**).

Dissociative Identity Disorder

Consider what it would be like to have dissociative identity disorder, as did Gina, the woman described at the opening of this chapter. People tell you about things you have done that are out of character and about interactions of which you have no memory. How can you explain these events?

The diagnosis of **dissociative identity disorder (DID)**, formerly labeled *multiple personality disorder*, requires that a person have a disrupted sense of identity, in which the person experiences at least two separate personality states or experiences of possession—different modes of being, thinking, feeling, and acting that exist independently of one another and that emerge at different times. Each determines the person's nature and activities when it is in command. The primary identity may be totally unaware that any other identity exists and may have no memory of what those other identities do and experience when they are in control.

In most media accounts, people with DID report two or more distinct personalities or identities. According to the DSM, people with DID vary in whether they endorse having more than one personality. More commonly, they experience dramatic shifts in their sense of self and agency, along with recurrent periods of amnesia for their experiences. Usually, the personality states are quite different from one another, even polar opposites. The person with DID is often aware of lost periods of time and frequently reports hearing the voices of the others. In some cultures, people value the experience of spirits who take control of a person's body (Seligman & Kirmayer, 2008); when experiences of possession are part of a broadly accepted spiritual or cultural practice, the diagnosis of DID is not appropriate.

Focus on Discovery 8.1

Debates About Repression: Recovered Memories of Abuse in Childhood

Clearly, abuse happens all too often and exerts important effects on well-being and psychological symptoms. Here we focus on recovered memories of childhood abuse—that is, cases in which a person had no memory of being abused as a child but then "recovered" the memory. Few issues are more hotly debated in psychology than whether these recovered memories are real. On one side, some argue that these recovered memories provide evidence for repression. On the other side are those who question how valid the memories are, casting doubt on the idea that recovered memories provide evidence of repression. This debate is highly relevant to the validity of the dissociative amnesia diagnosis, as the diagnostic criteria specify that the loss of memory in this disorder is most commonly for traumatic or stressful events.

To learn more about whether memories for highly painful events are forgotten, some researchers have studied memory for traumas. In one study, 92% of people with documented childhood abuse still reported a memory of the abuse when they were asked about it almost 15 years later (Goodman, Ghetti, et al., 2003). Those with more severe abuse memories were more likely to remember and disclose their abuse.

Even for the 8% of people with documented childhood abuse who reported that they had no memory of abuse, the lack of reported recall might reflect many processes other than repression. People might not want to disclose such distressing events to a researcher. Some people might have been too young at the time of the abuse to be able to remember the events: People were less

likely to report the memory at the 15-year follow-up if they had been younger than age 5 at the time the abuse occurred. Some of the traumas may have caused brain injury that could explain the gaps in memory. Thus, failure to describe a memory may not be the same thing as repression.

Given the debate about whether repression occurs, how should we interpret it when someone develops a new memory? Where could recovered memories come from, if not from actual experiences? Many therapists who genuinely believe that adult disorders result from abuse will suggest to their clients that they were probably abused as children, and clients who received such suggestions from their therapists were 20 times more likely than others to recover previously unremembered memories of abuse during the course of therapy (Patihis & Pendergrast, 2019). Some therapists use hypnotic age regression and guided imagery to help uncover memories (Legault & Laurence, 2007). Unfortunately, techniques such as hypnosis may actually create false memories (Lynn, Lock, et al., 2003). Guided imagery, in which a person closes their eyes and tries to imagine an event occurring, tends to increase confidence that events of a false memory occurred. With three rounds of guided imagery, 30% of participants developed a false memory of committing a crime that led to police contact, and another 43% reported having an image of the event (Shaw & Porter, 2015; Wade, Garry, & Pezdek, 2018).

To examine the validity of memories recovered in therapy, one group of researchers studied three groups: persons who had continuous memories of childhood sexual abuse, those who had recovered memories without a therapist, and those who had recovered memories within the context of therapy. Striking differences emerged. Whereas about half of the continuous memories

---

DID is rarely diagnosed until adulthood, but after their diagnosis, patients often will recall symptoms dating back to childhood. This disorder is more severe and extensive than the other dissociative disorders (Mueller-Pfeiffer, Rufibach, et al., 2012). DID is much more common in women than in men. Other diagnoses are often present, including posttraumatic stress disorder, major depressive disorder, and somatic symptom disorder (American Psychiatric Association, 2013). More than half of those diagnosed with DID meet diagnostic criteria for borderline personality disorder, and other personality disorders are common as well (Lynn et al., 2018). DID is commonly accompanied by other symptoms such as headaches, hallucinations, suicide attempts, and self-injurious behavior, as well as by other dissociative symptoms such as amnesia and depersonalization. The DSM also indicates that clinicians should consider whether patients may be intentionally fabricating symptoms.

VIDEO CONTENT

Case Study: Dissociative Identity Disorder Pause and Ponder

The inclusion of DID as a diagnosis in DSM is controversial. For example, in a survey of psychiatrists, two-thirds reported reservations about the presence of DID in the DSM (Pope, Oliva, et al., 1999). Students and the public often ask, "Does DID exist?" Clinicians can describe DID reliably; it "exists" in this sense. As we will discuss later, though, controversy swirls about the reasons these symptoms occur.

Defining Symptoms of Dissociative Identity Disorder

- Disruption of identity characterized by two or more distinct personality states or an experience of possession. These disruptions lead to discontinuities in the sense of self or agency, as reflected in altered cognition, behavior, affect, perceptions, consciousness, memories, or sensory-motor functioning. This disruption may be observed by others or reported by the patient.

- Recurrent gaps in memory for events or important personal information that are beyond ordinary forgetting

- In children, symptoms are not better explained by an imaginary playmate or by fantasy play

The Epidemiology of Dissociative Disorders: Increases Over Time

We do not know how common dissociative disorders are. The most well-validated interview to assess dissociative disorders is the Structured Clinical Interview for Dissociative Disorders—Revised (SCID-D-R) (Steinberg, 1994). In one community sample of 658 adults in upper New York State who were assessed with a version of this interview, 0.8% of people endorsed diagnostic criteria for depersonalization/derealization disorder, 1.8% endorsed dissociative amnesia, and 1.5% endorsed dissociative identity disorder (Johnson, Cohen, et al., 2006).

These figures are quite high comparatively—prevalence was earlier thought to be about one in a million. Although descriptions of anxiety, depression, and psychosis have abounded in literature since ancient times, there were almost no identified reports of DID or dissociative amnesia before 1800 (Pope, Poliakoff, et al., 2006). Reports of DID increased markedly in the 1970s, particularly in the United States and Canada (Boysen & VanBergen, 2013) and to a smaller extent in countries such as Japan (Uchinuma & Sekine, 2000).

What caused the ballooning rates of the DID diagnosis over time? It is possible that more people began to experience symptoms of DID. But there are other possible explanations for the surge. The case of Eve White, popularized in the book and film adaptation of *The Three Faces of Eve*, provided a highly detailed report of DID in 1957. The popular 1973 book *Sybil* presented a dramatic case of a woman with 16 personalities (Schreiber, 1973). The book sold more than 6 million copies in the first 4 years in print, and more than a fifth of all Americans watched a TV adaptation broadcast in 1976 (Nathan, 2011). A series of other case reports were published in the 1970s as well. DSM-III, which appeared in 1980, defined the diagnosis of DID for the first time (Putnam, 1996). The diagnostic criteria and growing literature may have increased detection and recognition of symptoms. Some critics hypothesize that the heightened professional and media attention to this diagnosis led some therapists to suggest strongly to clients that they had DID, sometimes using hypnosis to probe for other personalities.

As with DID, diagnoses of dissociative fugue may vary with cultural and professional attention to the condition. The first documented case of dissociative fugue appeared in the medical literature in 1887 in France and described Albert Dadas, who traveled during his fugue states from France to Algeria, Moscow, and Constantinople (Hacking, 1998). The case received widespread attention at medical conferences, and a small epidemic of fugue cases were reported throughout Europe in the years that followed (Hacking, 1998). In the United States in the same year, newspapers covered the case of Ansel Bourne, a preacher who left his home in Rhode Island, changed his name to Albert Brown, and opened a store in Pennsylvania selling stationery and candy. After 2 months in Pennsylvania, he visited his landlord to ask where he was (Aviv, 2018).

Quick Summary

Dissociative disorders are defined on the basis of disruptions in consciousness, in which memories, self-awareness, or other aspects of cognition become inaccessible to the conscious mind. In depersonalization/derealization disorder, the person's perception of the self and surroundings is altered such that the person may feel detached from their body or may perceive the world as seeming unreal. Dissociative amnesia is defined by inability to recall important personal experience(s), usually of a traumatic nature. In the fugue subtype of dissociative amnesia, the person not only is unable to recall important information but also leaves home and wanders without regard to work or social obligations. The person with dissociative identity disorder has two or more distinct personality states, each with unique memories, behavior patterns, and relationships.

The epidemiology of the dissociative disorders is not well researched. The number of diagnosed cases of DID surged during the 1970s, and some attribute this to the increased media and professional attention to the syndrome.

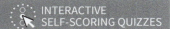

8.1 Check Your Knowledge

(Answers are at the end of the chapter.)
Answer the following questions.

1. What is the key feature of the fugue subtype of dissociative amnesia?
2. What is the key feature of dissociative identity disorder?
3. Describe historical changes in rates of DID.

Causes of Dissociative Disorders

There is considerably less research on dissociative disorders compared to other psychological syndromes. Few studies have tested the models of causes in people who had been formally diagnosed with dissociative disorders. Instead, many of the available studies have relied on a self-report scale called the Dissociative Experiences Survey that has been shown to have low reliability and easily misinterpreted items (Trujillo, Brown, et al., 2022). Because so little is known about dissociative amnesia, we will focus on the causes of depersonalization/derealization disorder and DID.

Causes of Depersonalization/Derealization Disorder

Some research findings indicate that some experiences of depersonalization/derealization may relate to problems in the way that the brain integrates information from different sensory and bodily sources (Lynn et al., 2018). In a small PET study, eight patients with depersonalization/derealization disorder showed atypical activity in regions involved in integrating information from sensory cortex areas (e.g., visual, auditory, and somatosensory) and bodily cues (Simeon, Guralnick, et al., 2000). Other research has shown that brief symptoms of depersonalization and derealization can be induced in individuals who do not have depersonalization/derealization disorder by providing mismatched or unexpected sensory experiences. For example, asking participants to wear goggles that distort visual information about where a person is being touched can produce temporary experiences of depersonalization and derealization (Jáuregui Renaud, 2015; Lickel, Nelson, et al., 2008). Among those with depersonalization/derealization disorder, brain regions that are involved in processing bodily cues related to emotion experience, such as the anterior cingulate cortex, appear to be underactive when viewing emotionally evocative images, which could contribute to the sense of feeling affectively numb (Medford, 2012). Taken together, depersonalization/derealization symptoms may be triggered when neural signals from various bodily or sensory cues are mismatched (Lynn et al., 2018).

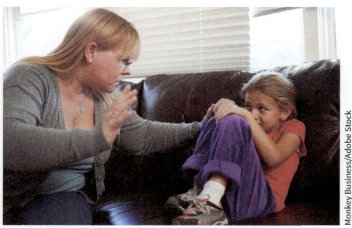

Monkey Business/Adobe Stock

According to the posttraumatic model, physical or sexual abuse in childhood is regarded as a major factor in the development of dissociative disorders.

Causes of Dissociative Identity Disorder

There are two major theories regarding the causes of DID: the **posttraumatic model** and the **sociocognitive model**. Both models focus on why some people develop DID. As we will discuss, considerable debate has arisen between the proponents of these two approaches.

The Posttraumatic Model   It is widely acknowledged that child abuse has profoundly negative effects (Curran, Adamson, et al., 2016). The posttraumatic model proposes that some people are particularly likely to use dissociation to cope with trauma and that dissociation is the key reason people develop alternate personalities after trauma (Gleaves, 1996). Research supports two important tenets of this model (Dalenberg, Brand, et al., 2012). First, children who are abused are at risk for developing dissociative symptoms. Second, children who dissociate are more likely to develop psychological symptoms after the trauma (Ensink, Berthelot, et al., 2017).

There is debate, though, about whether these childhood experiences shape DID symptoms in adulthood. On the one hand, most patients in therapy for DID report severe childhood abuse (Dalenberg et al., 2012). Patients, though, may be biased in their judgments about whether to describe early childhood experiences as abuse. A few studies have considered whether objective evaluations of childhood abuse (for example, from child protection agencies) predict tendencies to dissociate in adulthood. Those studies have yielded mixed findings about whether childhood abuse predicts tendencies for adults to dissociate (Lynn et al., 2018).

The Sociocognitive Model

According to the sociocognitive model, people who have been abused seek explanations for their symptoms and distress, and their alternate personality states appear in response to suggestions by therapists, exposure to media reports of DID, or other cultural influences (Lilienfeld, Lynn, et al., 1999). Proponents of this model note that the prevalence of DID surged when media and professionals began to place more emphasis on the diagnosis. This model, then, implies that DID could be iatrogenic (created within treatment) in that the person often learns to role-play these symptoms within treatment. This does not mean, however, that DID is conceptualized as conscious deception; the issue is not whether DID is real but how it develops.

Many of the treatment manuals for DID recommend therapeutic techniques that reinforce clients' identification of alternate personality states, such as interviewing clients about their identities after administering hypnosis or sodium pentothal (Nathan, 2011). The reinforcement and suggestive techniques might promote false memories and DID symptoms in vulnerable people (Lilienfeld et al., 1999), such as those who are more suggestible (Wieder, Brown, et al., 2022). The famous case of Sybil is now widely cited as an example of how a therapist might elicit and reinforce stories of alternate personalities. It has been claimed that in Sybil's case, the alternate personalities were created by a therapist who gave substance to Sybil's different emotional states by giving them names, and who helped Sybil elaborate on her early childhood experiences while administering sodium pentothal, a drug that has been shown to contribute to false memories (Borch-Jacobsen, 1997; Nathan, 2011). As another example of troubling therapeutic techniques, the Clinical Case of Elizabeth provides an extreme example of a therapist who unwittingly encouraged her client to adopt a diagnosis of DID when it wasn't justified by the symptoms. All the symptoms Elizabeth described are common experiences; indeed, none of the symptoms listed are actual diagnostic criteria for DID.

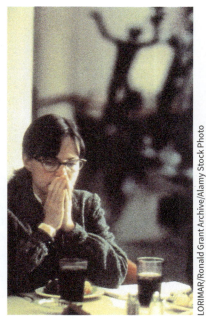

In the film version of *Sybil*, about a famous case of dissociative identity disorder, the title role was played by Sally Field. A later review of case notes suggested that "Sybil's personalities had not popped up spontaneously but were provoked over many years of rogue treatment." (Nathan, D. 2011).

LORIMAR/Ronald Grant Archive/Alamy Stock Photo

Clinical Case

Elizabeth

An Example of Unwarranted Diagnosis of DID

The book *Creating Hysteria: Women and Multiple Personality Disorder* (Acocella, 1999) provides a personal account of a person who received a false diagnosis of DID. Elizabeth Carlson, a 35-year-old married woman, was referred to a psychiatrist after being hospitalized for severe depression. Elizabeth reported that soon after treatment began, her psychiatrist suggested to her that perhaps her problem was the elusive, often undiagnosed condition of multiple personality disorder (MPD, now referred to as DID). Her psychiatrist reviewed

... certain telltale signs of MPD. Did Carlson ever "zone out" while driving and arrive at her

destination without remembering how she got there? Why yes, Carlson said. Well, that was an alter [an alternate personality] taking over the driving and then vanishing again, leaving her, the "host" personality, to account for the blackout. Did Carlson ever have internal arguments—for example, telling herself, "Turn right" and then "No, turn left"? Yes, Carlson replied, that happened sometimes. Well, that was the alters fighting with each other inside her head. Carlson was amazed and embarrassed. All these years, she had done these things, never realizing that they were symptoms of a severe mental disorder.

(Acocella, 1999, p. 1)

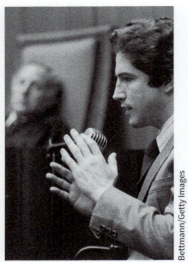

Ken Bianchi, a serial killer known as the Hillside strangler, unsuccessfully attempted an insanity defense, claiming that he suffered from DID. The jury decided that he was faking the symptoms of DID.

We will never have experimental evidence for the sociocognitive model, since it would be unethical to intentionally reinforce dissociative symptoms. Given this reality, what kinds of evidence have researchers raised in support of the sociocognitive model?

DID Symptoms Can Be Role-Played Across 20 studies, researchers have shown that people can role-play the symptoms of DID (Boysen & VanBergen, 2014). When instructed to generate a second personality, many participants can even produce responses on personality tests that differ considerably from their initial profile. These findings indicate that people can adeptly role-play DID. This evidence has been criticized, though—people can mimic having a broken leg (and many other symptoms), but this does not cast doubt on the reality of broken legs.

Some Therapists Reinforce DID Symptoms in Their Clients Therapists who diagnose more people with DID tend to use hypnosis, to urge clients to try to unbury unremembered abuse experiences, or to name alternate personality states (Powell & Gee, 2000). Consistent with the idea that treatment evokes the DID symptoms, most patients are unaware of having alternate personality states until after they begin treatment, and as treatment progresses, they report a rapid increase in the number of personalities they can identify.

Alternate Personalities Share Memories, Even When They Report Amnesia One of the defining features of DID is the inability to recall information experienced by one personality when a different personality is present. One way to test whether personalities share memory is to use implicit tests of memory (Huntjen, Postma, et al., 2003). In tests of **explicit memory**, researchers might ask a person to remember words. In tests of **implicit memory**, researchers determine if the word lists have subtler effects on performance. For example, if people are first shown a word list that included the word lullaby, they might be quicker on a second task to identify *lullaby* as a word that fills in the puzzle l_l_a_y. People with DID were taught an initial word list and were then asked to complete the implicit memory test when they returned to the second session in a different personality state. Twenty-one of the participants diagnosed with DID claimed at the second testing session that they had no memory of the first session. On tests of implicit memory, however, these 21 people performed comparably to people without DID. That is, memories were transferred between personalities. Many, but not all, studies replicate this finding (Boysen & VanBergen, 2013). Implicit memory tests also show transfer of autobiographical memories between personality states (Marsh, Dorahy, et al., 2018). People with DID demonstrate more shared memories than they tend to acknowledge.

Quick Summary

Little research is available concerning the causes of the dissociative disorders. Depersonalization/derealization disorder is related to difficulties in integrating somatic sensations from different channels. DID is related to severe abuse, but considerable debate exists about the other causes of this disorder. The posttraumatic model suggests that DID is the result of using dissociation as a coping strategy to deal with the abuse. The sociocognitive model suggests that DID occurs when social influences, including therapist suggestions, lead vulnerable patients to believe in the alternate personality states, such that the patients begin to play a role. Proponents of the sociocognitive model note the dramatic shifts in diagnosis over time, the use of suggestive techniques among therapists who frequently diagnose DID, the increases in number of personalities recognized after treatment begins, and the evidence that people can role-play symptoms of DID and that personalities share more information than they acknowledge.

8.2 Check Your Knowledge

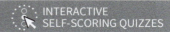
INTERACTIVE
SELF-SCORING QUIZZES

(Answers are at the end of the chapter.)
True or false?

1. Most patients with DID report childhood abuse.
2. List the major sources of evidence for the sociocognitive model of DID.

Treatment of Dissociative Disorders

No treatments for the dissociative disorders are well validated. No randomized controlled trials have assessed psychological treatment. Medications have not been shown to relieve the symptoms of dissociative disorders (Lynn, Polizzi, et al., 2022).

In the absence of strong evidence, expert clinicians agree on several principles in the treatment of dissociative identity disorder (International Society for the Study of Dissociation, 2011). These include the importance of an empathic and gentle stance. The goal of treatment should be to convince the person that splitting into different personalities is no longer necessary to deal with traumas. In addition, as DID is conceptualized as a means of escaping from severe stress, therapists can help teach the person more effective ways to cope with stress and to regulate emotions (Mohajerin, Lynn, et al., 2020). Psychoeducation can help a person to understand why dissociation occurs and to begin to identify the triggers for dissociative responses in day-to-day life (Brand, Myrick, et al., 2012). Often, people with DID are hospitalized to help them avoid self-harm and to offer more intensive treatment.

Psychodynamic treatment is probably used more for DID and the other dissociative disorders than for any other psychological disorder. The goal of this treatment is to overcome repressions (MacGregor, 1996), as DID is believed to arise from traumatic events that the person is trying to block from consciousness. Unfortunately, some psychodynamic practitioners use hypnosis as a means of helping patients diagnosed with dissociative disorders to gain access to repressed material (International Society for the Study of Dissociation, 2011). Typically, the person is hypnotized and encouraged to go back in their mind to traumatic events in childhood—a technique called *age regression*. The hope is that accessing these traumatic memories will allow the person to realize that childhood threats are no longer present and that adult life need not be governed by these ghosts from the past (Grinker & Spiegel, 1944). Using hypnosis to promote age regression and recovered memories, though, can exacerbate DID symptoms (Lilienfeld, 2007). More than 100 patients have sued therapists for harm caused by treatment of DID (Hanson, 1998). Hypnotic techniques have become less popular as the problems have received more attention.

Quick Summary

There are no randomized controlled trials of psychological treatments for the dissociative disorders. No medications have been shown to reduce symptoms of dissociative disorders.

In the safe, supportive context of therapy, patients with DID are encouraged to learn new strategies for coping with emotions, so as to gain better control over tendencies to rely on dissociation. Hypnosis and age regression techniques to recover memories are contraindicated for DID.

8.3 Check Your Knowledge

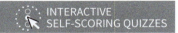 INTERACTIVE
SELF-SCORING QUIZZES

(Answers are at the end of the chapter.)
Answer the following questions.

1. How many randomized controlled trials are available to assess the efficacy of psychological treatments of DID?

2. Which medications reduce DID symptoms?

3. Which types of interventions for DID appear to be harmful?

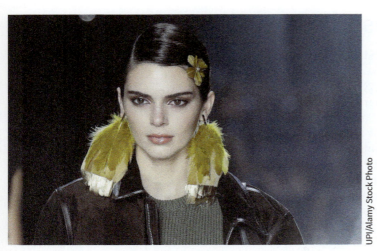

In a 2018 interview on *Keeping up with the Kardashians*, Kendall Jenner described her experiences of health anxiety.

Clinical Description of Somatic Symptom and Related Disorders

Somatic symptom and related disorders are defined by excessive concerns about physical symptoms or health. As shown in **Table 8.2**, the DSM-5-TR includes three major disorders in this category: somatic symptom disorder, illness anxiety disorder, and functional neurological symptom disorder. Many of us use the term *hypochondriasis* to describe chronic worries about developing a serious medical illness. Although hypochondriasis is not a DSM-5-TR diagnosis, both somatic symptom disorder and illness anxiety disorder overlap to some degree with hypochondriasis in that they involve high levels of distress and energy expenditure about a health concern. In somatic symptom disorder, the distress revolves around a somatic symptom that exists, whereas in illness anxiety disorder, the distress is about the potential for a medical illness in the absence of significant somatic symptoms. Functional neurological symptom disorder involves neurological symptoms that are medically unexplained (labeled as *functional neurological disorder* in medical literature). Table 8.2 also lists a fourth somatic symptom-related disorder, factitious disorder, and a disorder to be ruled out in considering the somatic symptom and related disorders, malingering. We discuss these two disorders in **Focus on Discovery 8.2**.

People with somatic symptom and related disorders tend to seek frequent medical treatment, typically leading to thousands of dollars per year in medical expense. They often visit several different physicians for a given health concern and try many different medications; they may even seek surgery. Although people with these disorders seek medical care frequently, they are often dissatisfied when doctors cannot provide a medical explanation or cure. They often describe their physicians as incompetent and uncaring (Persing, Stuart, et al., 2000). Despite their negative assessment of the medical profession, they will often continue extensive treatment seeking, visiting new doctors and demanding new tests. Many patients become unable to work because of the severity of their concerns (van der Leeuw, Gerrits, et al., 2015). For patients for whom pain is a concern, dependency on painkillers is a risk.

Although there is no doubt that the outcomes are troubling, there are important criticisms of the diagnostic criteria for somatic symptom and related disorders:

- Up to 80% of the general population report having had a somatic symptom in the past week that led to some concern or impairment (Hiller, Rief, & Brähler, 2006). The threshold for when to diagnose somatic symptom and related disorders, then, can be very subjective.

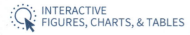
INTERACTIVE FIGURES, CHARTS, & TABLES

TABLE 8.2   **Diagnoses of Somatic Symptom and Related Disorders, and Malingering**

Diagnosis	Description
Somatic symptom disorder	Excessive thought, distress, and behavior related to somatic symptoms
Illness anxiety disorder	Unwarranted fears about a serious illness in the absence of any significant somatic symptoms
Functional neurological symptom disorder	Neurological symptom(s) that cannot be explained by medical disease or culturally sanctioned behavior
Factitious disorder	Falsification of psychological or physical symptoms, without evidence of gains from those symptoms
Malingering	Intentionally faking psychological or somatic symptoms to gain from those symptoms

- Patients often find the diagnosis of somatic symptom and related disorders stigmatizing. This may interfere with applying diagnoses of these disorders in clinical practice.

Because these disorders are defined differently than they were in DSM-IV-TR (where they were labeled *somatoform disorders*), we don't have data on the epidemiology or course of somatic symptom and related disorders. When the fears about a serious disease are accompanied by somatic symptoms, the appropriate DSM-5-TR diagnosis is somatic symptom disorder. Because so few people with intense fears about their health are free of somatic symptoms, somatic symptom disorder is estimated to be three times as common as illness anxiety disorder (Bailer, Kerstner, et al., 2016).

Somatic symptom related disorders tend to develop by early adulthood (Carson & Lehn, 2016; Herzog, et al., 2018) and tend to have a chronic course. In longitudinal studies, less than half of those with somatic symptom or related disorders achieve full remission within a 5-year period (olde Hartman, Borghuis, et al., 2009), although the severity of symptoms may wax and wane. Somatic symptom and related disorders tend to co-occur with anxiety disorders, mood disorders, and personality disorders (American Psychiatric Association, 2013).

Symptoms of these disorders may begin or intensify after some conflict or stress. To an outside observer, it may seem that the person is using the health concern to avoid some unpleasant activity or to get attention and sympathy. People with somatic symptom and related disorders have no sense of this, however; they experience their symptoms as completely medical. Their distress over their symptoms is authentic.

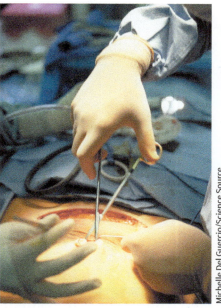

People with somatic symptom disorder may undergo unnecessary surgeries in hopes of finding a cure for their medical symptoms.

Clinical Description of Somatic Symptom Disorder

The key feature of **somatic symptom disorder** is excessive anxiety, energy, or behavior focused on somatic symptoms that persists for at least 6 months. The person with this disorder is typically quite worried about their health and tends to perceive even small physical concerns as a sign of looming disease. Tormented by a broad range of somatic symptoms that were not solved by visiting 20 different doctors (Campbell & Matthews, 2005), for 6 years Charles Darwin completed a log of his bodily complaints, which was dominated by ratings of his flatulence and other gastrointestinal complaints. Although his symptoms were likely genuine, his extensive notes signal that he was spending too much energy monitoring his health (Dillon, 2010). As illustrated by the **Clinical Case of Maria**, some might experience a multitude of symptoms from many different body systems. Others experience pain as the major concern.

Clinical Case

Maria

Maria was 32 when her physician referred her to a psychologist after seeing her 23 times in 6 months for a range of complaints— general aches and pains, bouts of nausea, fatigue, irregular menstruation, and dizziness. Various tests, including complete blood workups, X-rays, and spinal taps, had not revealed any pathology.

On meeting her therapist, Maria let him know that she was a reluctant client: "I'm here only because I trust my doctor, and she urged me to come. I'm physically sick and don't see how a psychologist is going to help." But when the therapist asked Maria to describe the history of her physical problems, she quickly warmed to the task.

According to Maria, she had always been sick. As a child, she had had episodes of high fever, frequent respiratory infections, convulsions, and her first two operations—an appendectomy

and a tonsillectomy. During her 20s, Maria had gone from one physician to another. She had experienced unbearable periods of vomiting. She had seen several gynecologists for her menstrual irregularity and for pain during intercourse. She had been referred to neurologists for her headaches, dizziness, and fainting spells, and they had performed EEGs, spinal taps, and a CT scan. Other physicians had ordered EKGs for her chest pains. Maria seemed genuinely distressed by her health problems, and doctors responding to her desperate pleas for a cure had performed rectal and gallbladder surgery.

When the interview shifted away from Maria's medical history, it became clear that she was anxious in many situations, particularly those in which she feared others might evaluate her. Indeed, some of her physical symptoms were typical of those experienced by people diagnosed with anxiety disorders.

Somatic symptom disorder can be diagnosed regardless of whether symptoms can be explained medically. It is nearly impossible to determine whether some symptoms are biologically caused. Doctors often disagree on whether a symptom has a medical cause (Rief & Broadbent, 2007). Indeed, when asked about their physical symptoms, people receiving primary care report that two-thirds of their symptoms have not received a medical explanation (Steinbrecher, Koerber, et al., 2011). Some people might have a condition that defies diagnosis because of limits in medical knowledge and technology. As technology has improved, the medical profession now understands some conditions that were historically difficult to explain. One example is complex regional pain syndrome; it was previously believed to be caused by psychological factors, but animal and human research now indicates that these symptoms result from inflammation secondary to autoimmune disorder (Cooper & Clark, 2013). Many common syndromes remain a focus of research because their causes are not well understood, including irritable bowel syndrome, fibromyalgia, chronic fatigue, nonulcer dyspepsia, and some forms of chronic pain (Cooper & Clark, 2013). The presence of these syndromes is not a reason to diagnose somatic symptom disorder. When psychological factors exert a negative effect on medical symptoms, an alternative DSM diagnosis, labeled *psychological factors affecting other medical conditions*, may be appropriately considered.

Defining Symptoms of Somatic Symptom Disorder

- At least one somatic symptom that is distressing or disrupts daily life
- Excessive thoughts, distress, and behavior related to somatic symptom(s) or health concerns, as indicated by at least one of the following:

1. health-related anxiety

2. disproportionate and persistent concerns about the seriousness of symptoms

3. excessive time and energy devoted to health concerns

- Duration of at least 6 months, although somatic symptoms do not have to be continuously present during that time
- Specify if predominant pain

Clinical Description of Illness Anxiety Disorder

VIDEO CONTENT

Case Study: Illness Anxiety Disorder
Pause and Ponder

The main feature of **illness anxiety disorder** is a preoccupation with fears of having a serious disease despite having no significant somatic symptoms, accompanied by excessive care seeking or maladaptive avoidance behaviors, that persists for at least 6 months. People with this disorder are easily alarmed about their health, and they tend to worry about the possibility of cancer, heart attacks, AIDS, and strokes (Rachman, 2012). They may be haunted by powerful visual images of becoming ill or dying (Muse, McManus, et al., 2010). They may react with anxiety when they hear about illnesses in their friends or in the broader community. Their fears are not easily calmed.

Defining Symptoms of Illness Anxiety Disorder

- Preoccupation with and anxiety about having or acquiring a serious disease
- Excessive illness behavior (e.g., checking for signs of illness, seeking reassurance) or maladaptive avoidance (e.g., avoiding medical care)

- No more than mild somatic symptoms are present, or anxiety is disproportionate to medical conditions
- Preoccupation lasts at least 6 months, although the specific illness feared may change during that time

Clinical Description of Functional Neurological Symptom Disorder

In **functional neurological symptom disorder**, the person suddenly develops neurological symptoms, such as blindness, seizures, or paralysis. The symptoms suggest an illness related to neurological damage, but medical tests indicate that the bodily organs and nervous system are fine. People may experience partial or complete paralysis of arms or legs; seizures; coordination disturbances; a sensation of prickling, tingling, or creeping on the skin; insensitivity to pain; or anesthesia—the loss of sensation. Vision may be seriously impaired; the person may become partially or completely blind or have tunnel vision, in which the visual field is constricted as it would be if the person were peering through a tube. *Aphonia*, loss of voice other than for whispered speech, can also occur. Many people with functional neurological symptom disorder do not connect their symptoms with their stressful situations. Sigmund Freud thought that anxiety and psychological conflict were converted into physical symptoms (see the **Clinical Case of Anna O.**, an influential case for Freud's theory).

When a patient reports a neurological symptom, the clinician must be careful to assess whether that symptom has a true neurological basis. Some symptoms that might seem medically implausible have been shown to have a biological basis. Consider, for instance, the classic example of "glove anesthesia," in which the person experiences little or no sensation in the part of the hand and lower arm that would be covered by a glove. For years, this was considered a textbook illustration of anatomical nonsense because the nerves run continuously from the hand up the arm. Yet, now it appears that carpal tunnel syndrome, a recognized medical condition, can produce symptoms like those of glove anesthesia. Nerves in the wrist run through a tunnel formed by the wrist bones and membranes. Swelling in this tunnel can pinch the nerves, leading to tingling, numbness, and pain in the hand. Beyond the symptoms of glove anesthesia, other symptoms that would intuitively seem difficult to explain medically, such as the perception of a burning sensation when touching a cold object, have clear medical explanations (in this case, ciguatera, a disease caused by eating certain reef fish).

It is estimated that genuinely physical problems are misdiagnosed as functional neurological symptom disorder about 4% of the time (Stone, Smyth, et al., 2005). Some tests can help clinicians make an accurate diagnosis. Nonepileptic seizure disorder, a common form of functional neurological symptom disorder, is defined by seizure-like events that occur at the same time that a normal EEG pattern is recorded (Stone, LaFrance, et al., 2010). Arm tremors might disappear when the person is asked to move the arm rhythmically. Leg weakness might not be consistent when tested with resistance (Stone et al., 2010). Tunnel vision, another functional neurological symptom, is incompatible with the biology of the visual system. To enhance the reliability of diagnoses, the DSM-5-TR provides guidance to clinicians about how to assess whether symptoms might be medically unexplained.

Defining Symptoms of Functional Neurological Symptom Disorder

- One or more symptoms affecting voluntary motor or sensory function
- The clinical findings are incompatible with any recognized medical disorder
- Symptoms cause significant distress or functional impairment or warrant medical evaluation

---

Clinical Case

Anna O.

As described in a case report, Anna O. was sitting at the bedside of her seriously ill father when she dropped off into a waking dream. She saw a black snake come toward her sick father to bite him. She tried to ward it off, but her arm had gone to sleep. When she looked at her hand, her fingers seemed to turn into little snakes with death's heads. The next day, when a bent branch caused her to recall her waking dream of the snake, her right arm became rigidly extended. After that, whenever some object revived her hallucination, her arm responded in the same way—with rigid extension. Later, her symptoms extended to paralysis and anesthesia of her entire right side.

Drawn from Breuer and Freud (1982).

Some, but not all, people with functional neurological symptom disorder seem motivated to appear ill. When relevant neurological abilities are tested (e.g., visual tests for a person with functional neurological symptom disorder involving blindness), some with functional neurological symptom disorders perform more poorly than what would be achieved by chance and show evidence of little effort on the tests related to their deficit (Drane, Williamson, et al., 2006). Some with these disorders endorse multiple implausible and rare neurological symptoms (Benge, Wisdom, et al., 2012; Peck, Schroeder, et al., 2013). Some report a symptom, such as a tremor, much more continuously than is observed with objective measures, such as wristbands that monitor motion (Parees, Saifee, et al., 2012). Many people with functional neurological symptom disorder, though, show no signs that they are amplifying their symptoms. When present, any amplification of symptoms may be outside conscious awareness. See **Focus on Discovery 8.2** for diagnoses to be considered when a person appears to be consciously producing symptoms.

Focus on Discovery 8.2

Malingering and Factitious Disorder

In evaluating somatic symptoms, clinicians must rule out factitious disorder and malingering. Both can involve somatic symptoms. In **malingering**, a person intentionally fakes a symptom to avoid a responsibility, such as work or military duty, or to achieve some reward, such as an insurance settlement. This contrasts with factitious disorder, where the sole goal is to adopt the patient role.

To distinguish between malingering and functional neurological symptom disorder, clinicians try to determine whether the symptoms have been adopted consciously or unconsciously; in malingering, the symptoms are under voluntary control, which is not thought to be the case in functional neurological symptom disorder. Insurance companies often go to great lengths to show that a person is faking symptoms and can function well outside of doctors' offices. When such detective work fails, though, it is often difficult, if not impossible, to know whether the behavior is consciously or unconsciously motivated.

In **factitious disorder**, people intentionally produce symptoms to assume the role of a patient. Most of the symptoms are physical, but some people produce psychological symptoms as well. They may make up symptoms—for example, reporting acute pain. Some will take extraordinary measures to make themselves ill. They may injure themselves, take damaging medications, or inject themselves with toxins.

In one of the most severe examples of factitious disorder reported, a woman named Miss Scott described being hospitalized at more than 600 hospitals and having 42 operations, nearly all of which were not needed (Grady, 1999). Some days she would leave one hospital and be admitted to a different hospital by nightfall. One doctor who examined the scars on her abdomen reported that "she looked as if she had lost a duel with Zorro." When asked about her treatment seeking, she reported, "To begin with, it was just something I did when I needed someone to care about me. Then it became something I had to do. It was as if something took me over. I just had to be in the hospital. I had to."

She had grown up as an abused, lonely child, and one of her early positive memories was the care she received from a nurse after having her appendix removed. After that experience, she once walked into her local hospital feigning a stomachache, hoping that someone would care about her experience. She spent several days there appreciating the attention that she received. Over the course of the next year, she began to seek care at a series of different hospitals. "Soon she was spending all her time hitchhiking from town to town, trying to get into the hospital (Grady, 1999, p. D5). For Miss Scott, being a patient became her chief way of gaining support and nurturance.

Factitious disorder may also be diagnosed in a parent who creates physical illness in a child; in this case, it is called *factitious disorder imposed on another,* or *Munchausen syndrome by proxy.* In one extreme case, a 7-year-old girl was hospitalized more than 300 times and experienced 40 surgeries at a cost of over $2 million. Her mother, Kathleen Bush, had caused her illnesses by administering drugs and even contaminating her feeding tube with fecal material (Toufexis, Blackman, & Drummond, 1996). The motivation in a case such as this appears to be a need to be regarded as an excellent parent who is tireless in attending to the child's needs.

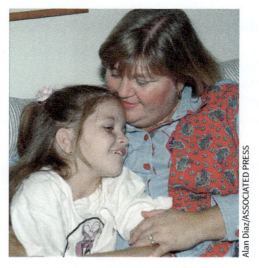

Kathleen Bush was charged with child abuse and fraud for deliberately causing her child's illnesses.

Defining Symptoms of Factitious Disorder

- Fabrication or induction of physical or psychological symptoms, injury, or disease

- Deceptive behavior is present in the absence of obvious external rewards

- In factitious disorder imposed on self, the person presents themself to others as ill, impaired, or injured

- In factitious disorder imposed on another, the person fabricates or induces symptoms in another person and then presents that person to others as ill, impaired, or injured

The onset of functional neurological symptom disorder is usually rapid, with symptoms developing in less than 1 day (Carson & Lehn, 2016). Many patients with functional neurological symptoms disorder experience work-related disability (Carson & Lehn, 2016). An episode may end abruptly, but about 40% show symptoms when reassessed 5 years later (Gelauff, Stone, et al., 2013). Although there are no community-based studies using diagnostic interviews, the prevalence of functional neurological symptom disorder is estimated to be less than 1% in the community but more common among patients visiting neurology clinics, where as many as 10% of patients have symptoms that have no medical explanation (Carson & Lehn, 2016). More women than men are given the diagnosis (Carson & Lehn, 2016). Patients with functional neurological symptom disorder are highly likely to meet the criteria for another somatic symptom disorder (Brown, et al., 2007).

Quick Summary

The common feature of somatic symptom and related disorders is the excessive focus on physical symptoms. The nature of the concern, however, varies by disorder. The major somatic symptom and related disorders in the DSM-5-TR are somatic symptom disorder, illness anxiety disorder, and functional neurological symptom disorder. Somatic symptom disorder is defined by excessive anxiety, worry, or behavior focused on somatic symptoms. Illness anxiety disorder is defined by fears of a severe disease in the absence of significant somatic symptoms. Functional neurological symptom disorder is defined by sensory and motor dysfunctions that cannot be explained by medical tests. These disorders may arise suddenly in stressful situations. Somatic symptom and related disorders often develop by early adulthood.

8.4 Check Your Knowledge

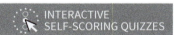 INTERACTIVE SELF-SCORING QUIZZES

(Answers are at the end of the chapter.)
Match the case description to the disorder. Assume that the symptoms cause significant distress or impairment.

a. somatic symptom disorder

b. illness anxiety disorder

c. functional neurological symptom disorder

1. Paula, a 24-year-old librarian, sought psychological help on the advice of her brother because of deep fears about her health. In daily phone calls with her brother, Paula would describe worries that she had cancer or a brain tumor. She had no somatic symptoms or signs of these conditions, but every time she saw an internet report, a TV program, or a newspaper article on some new serious condition, she became worried she might have it. She had seen doctors frequently for years, but when they identified no disease, she became annoyed with them, criticized the insensitivity of their medical tests, and sought a new consultant.

2. John's surgeon referred him for psychological treatment because he seemed excessively nervous about his health. In the past 5 years, John, now 35 years old, had sought a stunning array of medical treatments and tests for stomach distress, itching, frequent urination, and any number of other complaints. He had received 10 MRIs and too many X-rays to count and had seen 15 different specialists.

Each test had been negative. He genuinely seemed to experience physical symptoms, and there was no indication that he stood to gain from a medical diagnosis.

3. Thomas's ophthalmologist referred him for psychological treatment. Thomas reported that 2 weeks before, he had suddenly developed tunnel vision. Medical tests failed to reveal any reason for his tunnel vision, and there was no sign he was faking symptoms.

Causes of Somatic Symptom and Related Disorders

The major features of somatic symptom disorder and illness anxiety disorder include excessive attention to somatic symptoms and disproportionate anxiety about one's health. Neurobiological and cognitive behavioral models have focused on understanding these two tendencies, and we describe those models here. After discussing that research, we consider models of functional neurological symptom disorder.

Neurobiological Factors That Increase Awareness of and Distress Over Somatic Symptoms

Everyone experiences occasional somatic symptoms. For example, we may feel muscle pain after a tough workout, small signs of an impending cold, or a faster heart rate as we exercise. In understanding somatic symptom and related disorders, then, the key issue is not whether people have some bodily sensation but rather why some people are more focused on and distressed by these sensations. Health anxiety does appear to be moderately heritable (Taylor & Asmundson, 2012). How might the vulnerability to health anxiety unfold?

Neurobiological models of somatic symptom and related disorders focus on brain regions activated by unpleasant body sensations. Pain and uncomfortable physical sensations, such as heat, increase activity in two regions of the brain: the rostral anterior insula and the anterior cingulate cortex (ACC) (Price, Craggs, et al., 2009). These regions have strong connections with the somatosensory cortex, a region of the brain involved with processing bodily sensations (see **Figure 8.1**). Heightened activity in these regions is related to greater propensity for

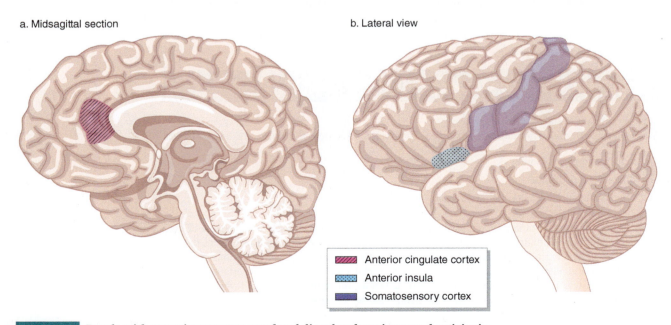

a. Midsagittal section   b. Lateral view

	Anterior cingulate cortex
	Anterior insula
	Somatosensory cortex

FIGURE 8.1 People with somatic symptom or related disorders have increased activity in brain regions implicated in evaluating the unpleasantness of body sensations: the rostral anterior insula, the anterior cingulate cortex, and the somatosensory cortex. The anterior cingulate cortex is also involved in depression and anxiety.

somatic symptoms (Landgrebe, Barta, et al., 2008) and more intense pain ratings in response to a standardized stimulus (Mayer, Berman, et al., 2005). Some people, then, may have hyperactivity in brain regions that are involved in evaluating the unpleasantness of body sensations (Bourke, Langford, & White, 2015). This would help explain why they are more vulnerable to experiencing somatic symptoms and pain.

Pain and somatic symptoms can be increased by anxiety, depression, and stress hormones, and those with somatic symptom or related disorders show elevated rates of trauma, anxiety, and depression (Rief & Martin, 2014). Depression and anxiety also directly relate to activity in specific regions of the ACC (Shackman, Salomons, et al., 2011; Wiech & Tracey, 2009). Even brief experiences of emotional pain, such as remembering a relationship breakup, can activate the ACC and the anterior insula. The involvement of these regions in experiences of physical and emotional pain may help explain why distress and depression can intensify experiences of pain (Villemure & Bushnell, 2009).

In an interesting study, researchers investigated whether learning to control ACC activity using real-time functional magnetic resonance imaging (fMRI) feedback could help reduce pain (deCharms, Maeda, et al., 2005). In this study, healthy individuals with no somatic symptom or related disorder completed brain-scanning sessions in which they viewed graphs showing the changing level of activity in key regions of the ACC as they were exposed to uncomfortable sensations (a heat bar was attached to their hand, and pulses of 116–120° heat were sent to the bar). They were told various strategies for manipulating activity in their ACC, such as attending toward or away from the heat, changing their thoughts about their heat (e.g., to consider it as neutral rather than tissue-damaging), and trying to think of it as high or low intensity. Within three sessions, most individuals did learn to control the activity in their ACC. The more people learned to control their ACC, the more they could reduce their experiences of pain. The fMRI feedback training was more powerful in reducing pain than control conditions of false fMRI feedback or no fMRI feedback. In a second study, ACC feedback training was found to be helpful for people who suffered from chronic pain. These findings, then, support the idea that the ACC is important in experiences of pain.

Cognitive Behavioral Factors That Increase Awareness of and Distress Over Somatic Symptoms

Like the neurobiological models of somatic symptom and related disorders, cognitive behavioral models focus on the mechanisms that could contribute to the excessive focus on and anxiety over health concerns. **Figure 8.2** illustrates one model of how these cognitive and behavioral influences could fit together. The orange boxes are relevant to understanding how a person might initially develop a somatic symptom. The blue boxes are relevant to understanding reactions to a somatic symptom. As shown in the blue boxes, once a somatic symptom develops, two cognitive variables are important: attention to body sensations and interpretation of those sensations. The purple boxes show some of the troubling outcomes of the health anxiety.

People with health worries tend to be overly focused on their somatic symptoms, particularly when they are in a negative mood (Shi, Taylor, et al., 2022). Once they attend to those somatic symptoms, they tend to interpret their physical symptoms in the worst possible way (Du, Witthöft, et al., 2022). They may interpret small physical symptoms as a sign of impending catastrophe. For example, one person might interpret a red blotch on the skin as a sign of cancer (Marcus, Gurley, et al., 2007). Another person might overestimate the odds that a symptom is a sign of a disease (Rief, Buhlmann, et al., 2006). The exact form of the cognitive bias may vary, but once these negative thoughts begin, the resultant elevations of anxiety may exacerbate somatic symptoms and distress over those symptoms. Not only are catastrophic thoughts about somatic symptoms

INTERACTIVE
FIGURES, CHARTS, & TABLES

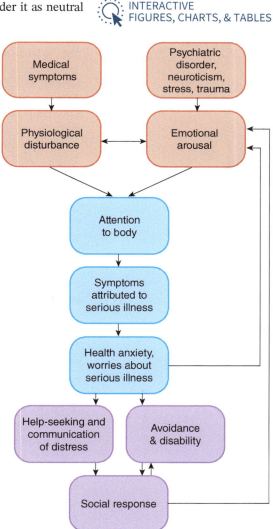

FIGURE 8.2 **Mechanisms involved in somatic symptom and related disorders (Looper & Kirmayer, 2002).**

elevated among those with somatic symptom or related disorders (Witthöft, Gropalis, & Weck, 2018), but they predict more severe pain and fatigue among those with medical conditions (Rief & Martin, 2014).

In Chapters 6 and 7, we described similar cognitive processes as part of panic disorder and obsessive-compulsive disorder. That is, people with panic disorder are likely to overreact to physiological symptoms. In panic disorder, the person often believes that the symptoms are a sign of an immediate threat (e.g., a heart attack), whereas in somatic symptom disorder, the person believes that the symptoms are a sign of an underlying long-term disease (e.g., cancer or AIDS). As we saw in Chapter 7, the obsessions that torment those with obsessive-compulsive disorder can involve fears of disease and contamination. Unlike the person with health worries, the person with obsessions sees those worries about disease as unwarranted.

A growing body of experimental research shows how negative thoughts might even trigger the onset of some somatic symptoms. In one example of this work, researchers randomly assigned participants to watch a TV documentary about the effects of exposure to Wi-Fi signals on somatic symptoms or to watch a control film (Witthoft & Rubin, 2013). After the films, experimenters falsely stated that they would be exposing all participants to a new type of Wi-Fi signal for 15 minutes; in actuality, no Wi-Fi signals were emitted during that time. Those who had seen the documentary reported significant increases in physical symptoms (including GI, head, and skin-tingling symptoms) after the sham Wi-Fi signal exposure, particularly if they were more anxious at baseline. Those who saw the control film did not report these symptoms. This is exactly what a theory would predict—beliefs predicted physical symptoms even when there was no medical explanation for those symptoms. These findings illustrate that worrying about possible symptoms can make them more likely to occur, and the effect of those worries may be particularly strong for those who are already anxious.

A fear of impending illness is likely to have behavioral consequences. The person may assume the role of being sick and avoid work, exercise, and social activities (Martin & Jacobi, 2006), and these avoidant behaviors in turn can intensify poor health. Some people are reinforced for disengagement from these key roles. For example, people receive disability payments based on how much symptoms interfere with their daily activities.

Beyond avoidance, many with health anxiety engage in "safety behaviors." As we discussed in Chapter 7, people use safety behaviors to try to reduce immediate anxiety. For health anxiety, safety behaviors involve seeking reassurance from doctors, family members, and the internet or taking other steps to protect health (e.g., conducting self-exams, disinfecting household surfaces). Safety behaviors may help quell anxiety briefly, and reassurance seeking can elicit attention or sympathy. Nonetheless, safety behaviors are believed to be counterproductive for several reasons. Some people may come to believe that they have warded off serious health problems only because they engaged in safety behaviors. Also, some safety behaviors prevent focused exposure to the initial somatic symptom and thus prevent the person from extinguishing their fear of that symptom. At the same time, safety behaviors may keep the person focused on potential health problems, and so may intensify distress (Brown, Skelly, & Chew-Graham, 2020).

In an experiment designed to test whether safety behaviors intensify health anxiety, researchers randomly assigned undergraduates to a control condition or an experimental condition for 1 week. Those in the control condition were asked to monitor their use of health safety behaviors each day. Those in the experimental condition were asked to engage in health safety behaviors as many times per day as they could. To foster these behaviors, they were given diagrams of how to conduct breast or testicular self-exams, bottles of hand sanitizer to be carried at all times, disinfectant wipes to clean their office and home, tongue depressors to check their throats each day, and instructions for avoiding contamination. The experimental manipulation worked: People in the experimental group engaged in an average of 116 safety behaviors during the week, compared with an average of 26 for the control participants. More importantly, after 1 week of engaging in safety behaviors, the experimental group developed a set of new symptoms. They reported anxiety about their health, worries that they could have a serious illness, and a lack of willingness to approach a potentially contaminated object (e.g., a dirty tissue) in a lab task. The control group showed none of these changes. Taken together, the findings indicate that health safety behaviors can intensify health anxiety (at least until participants were debriefed). Of course, it would be unethical to conduct this experiment in a clinical population, and so caution is warranted in interpreting how well these effects generalize to those with diagnosable disorders (Olatunji, Etzel, et al., 2011).

Many different behavioral and cognitive influences can maintain and intensify health anxiety. We'll return to a number of these influences when we discuss cognitive behavior therapy for health anxiety.

Causes of Functional Neurological Symptom Disorder

We mentioned earlier that stress is a potential trigger of the somatic symptom and related disorders. To evaluate this idea, researchers have tested whether functional neurological symptom disorder might be triggered by overwhelming stress and by difficulty coping with the resultant emotions. Although those with functional neurological symptom disorder report major life stressors in the month before onset, as well as childhood neglect and abuse, more often than other psychiatric patients do, not all people with functional neurological symptom disorder report a history of these adversities (Ludwig, Pasman, et al., 2018). Moreover, findings are inconsistent on the coping and emotion profiles of those with functional neurological symptom disorder (Roberts & Reuber, 2014). In this section, then, we focus on the idea that functional neurological symptom disorder symptoms can be produced unconsciously. Then we consider sociocultural influences.

Psychodynamic and Neuroscience Perspectives on the Unconscious in Functional Neurological Symptom Disorder
Functional neurological symptom disorder occupies a central place in psychodynamic theories because the symptoms provide a clear example of the role of the unconscious. Consider trying to diagnose a woman who says that she awoke one morning with a paralyzed left arm. Assume that a series of neurological tests reveals no neurological disorder. Perhaps she has decided to fake paralysis to achieve some end—this would be an example of malingering (see Focus on Discovery 8.2). But what if you believe her? You would almost have to conclude that unconscious processes were operating, making her unable to move her arm despite the absence of any physical cause. Psychodynamic theory suggests that the physical symptom is a response to an unconscious psychological conflict.

Neuroscience supports the idea that much of our perceptual processing may operate outside our conscious awareness. Take as an example unexplained blindness. The vision system relies on a set of brain regions. If these regions are not coordinated in an overarching conscious fashion, the brain may process some visual input in such a way that the person can do well on certain visual tests yet still lack a conscious sense of "seeing" certain types of stimuli. In one case study, a person with functional neurological symptom of blindness showed activity in brain regions involved with processing low levels of visual stimuli (such as lines and squares) but showed diminished activity in higher-level visual cortex regions involved in integrating visual inputs into a consolidated whole (such as a house) (Becker, Scheele, et al., 2013). If people were not processing visual inputs at a higher level, they could truthfully claim that they could not see, even when tests suggested that they could.

The idea of neural processing outside consciousness has been applied to medically inexplicable tremors, one form of functional neurological symptom disorder. If a person were actually initiating the tremor but the brain's monitoring system was not processing this fact, the person could experience the tremor as involuntary (Brown, 2016). Consistent with this idea, some people with medically unexplained tremors show diminished activation of association cortices involved in conscious monitoring of motor movements (Hallett, 2016). Intriguingly, several studies suggest differential connectivity of the amygdala with these motor control regions and with regions involved in processing physical sensations. This is consistent with the idea that emotion could contribute to these motoric issues (Jungilligens, Paredes-Echeverri, et al., 2022). Although these few small studies provide illustrations that brain systems involved in awareness could be involved, neuroimaging findings remain mixed, and no central neural process has emerged that could explain the lack of conscious awareness or the influence of emotions on that awareness across patients with different symptoms of DID (Aybek & Vuilleumier, 2016).

Social and Cultural Influences on Functional Neurological Symptom Disorder
Social and cultural factors shape the symptoms of functional neurological symptom disorder. For example, symptoms of functional neurological symptom disorder are more common among people from rural areas and people of lower socioeconomic status

(Binzer & Kullgren, 1996). The influence of social factors is also supported by the many documented cases of "mass hysteria," in which a group of people with close contact, such as schoolmates or coworkers, develop inexplicable medical symptoms that would likely warrant a diagnosis of functional neurological symptom disorder. Consider the outbreak of seizure-type symptoms (a relatively common functional neurological symptom) in a cotton-processing facility, described in 1787: "A girl ... put a mouse into the breast of another girl who had great dread of mice. She was immediately thrown into a fit and continued in it with the most violent convulsions for 24 hours. On the following day, three more girls were seized in the same manner, and the day after, six more." Within 3 days, 24 girls were affected (Dr. St. Clare, 1787, *Gentleman's Magazine,* p. 268). Incidents like this one suggest that social factors, including modeling, shape how functional neurological symptoms disorder unfold.

Quick Summary

Health anxiety appears to be moderately heritable. Neurobiological models suggest that some people may have a propensity toward hyperactivity in those regions of the brain involved in processing the unpleasantness of somatic sensations, including the anterior cingulate cortex and the rostral anterior insula. These brain regions are also implicated in negative emotions and depression. Cognitive behavioral models focus on attention to and interpretation of somatic symptoms. Behavioral responses to health concerns can include disengagement and isolation, as well as excessive safety and help-seeking behaviors.

Psychodynamic theories of functional neurological symptom disorder focus on the idea that people can be unaware (unconscious) of their perceptions or their own control of a motor symptom like tremor. Social influences on functional neurological symptom disorder seem important, particularly given that sometimes cases cluster within small groups of coworkers or schoolmates.

8.5 Check Your Knowledge

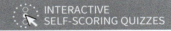
INTERACTIVE
SELF-SCORING QUIZZES

(Answers are at the end of the chapter.)
True or false?

1. The psychodynamic model of functional neurological symptom disorder emphasizes failures of conscious awareness.
2. Somatic symptom disorder involves hyperactivation of the cerebellum.

Treatment of Somatic Symptom and Related Disorders

One of the major obstacles to treatment is that most people with somatic symptom and related disorders want medical care, not mental health care (Lehn, Gelauff, et al., 2016). Indeed, most do not receive psychological or psychiatric treatment in the first 10 years after symptom onset (Herzog, Shedden-Mora, et al., 2018). Patients may resent a mental health referral from their physician because they interpret such a referral as a sign that the doctor thinks the illness is "all in their head." It is not a good idea for a provider to try to convince a patient that psychological factors are causing the symptoms. Most somatic and pain concerns have both physical and psychological components, and so it is unwise for the physician to debate the source of these symptoms with the patient. For many patients, a gentle reminder of the mind–body connection will enhance their willingness to consider psychological treatment. With this caution as a backdrop, we will consider interventions for those with the intense health anxiety of somatic symptom disorder and illness anxiety, and then we will look at novel evidence for cognitive behavioral treatment of functional neurological symptom disorders.

Somatic Symptom Disorder and Illness Anxiety Disorder

Because most people with somatic symptom and related disorders seek treatment from general practitioners, one approach has been to teach primary care teams how to tailor care for people with these disorders. The goal is to establish a strong doctor–patient relationship that bolsters the patient's sense of trust and comfort, so that the patient will feel reassured about their health. In one study, researchers randomly assigned patients with distressing and medically unexplained gastrointestinal symptoms to receive standard care or high levels of warmth, attention, and reassurance from doctors. Those who received high levels of support showed more improvement in symptoms and quality of life over the next 6 weeks than those who received standard care (Kaptchuk, Kelley, et al., 2008).

Another healthcare system intervention involves alerting physicians when a patient is an intensive user of healthcare services so as to minimize the use of diagnostic tests and medications. This type of intervention with physicians can reduce the unnecessary provision of costly healthcare services (Konnopka, Schaefert, et al., 2012).

Cognitive behavior therapy (CBT) makes use of many different techniques to help people with somatic symptom and related disorders. As illustrated by the Clinical Case of Louis, these techniques include helping people (1) identify and change the emotions that trigger somatic concerns, (2) change cognitions regarding their somatic symptoms, and (3) change

Clinical Case

Louis

Louis, a 66-year-old man, was referred to a psychiatrist by his cardiologist because of health anxiety. Although Louis acknowledged years of depressive and anxiety symptoms, he reported being much more concerned about his potential for heart problems. Several years before, he had developed intermittent symptoms of heart palpitations and chest pressure. Despite extensive medical test results within the normal range, he continued to seek additional tests. He had gathered a thick file of articles on cardiovascular conditions, had adopted a highly restrictive diet, and had stopped all activities that might be too exciting and therefore challenging to his heart, such as travel and sex. He had even retired early from running his restaurant. By the time he sought treatment, he was measuring his blood pressure four times a day using two machines so that he could average the readings, and he was keeping extensive logs of his blood pressure readings.

Before treatment could begin, Louis had to understand that the way he was thinking about his physical symptoms was intensifying those physical symptoms as well as creating emotional distress. His therapist taught him a model of symptom amplification, in which initial physical symptoms are exacerbated by negative thoughts and emotions. The therapist used statements such as "A headache you believe is due to a brain tumor hurts much more than a headache you believe is due to eye strain." Once Louis understood that his thoughts and behavior might be increasing his medical concerns, treatment focused on four goals. First, the therapist coached Louis to identify one doctor with whom to routinely discuss health concerns and to stop seeking multiple medical opinions. Second, the therapist taught Louis to reduce the time spent engaging in illness-related safety behaviors, such as logging his blood pressure. His therapist showed him that these behaviors were actually increasing his anxiety rather than providing relief. Third, the therapist taught Louis to challenge the negative and pessimistic thoughts he had in response to his symptoms. For example, the therapist and Louis identified ways in which he tended to catastrophize harmless physical sensations by viewing them as

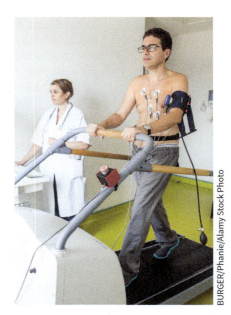

BURGER/Phanie/Alamy Stock Photo

People with health anxiety are not easily reassured that they are well, even when extensive medical tests indicate no problems.

evidence of heart disease. Louis began to consider more benign reasons for his physical symptoms. Finally, Louis was encouraged to build other aspects of his life to diminish the focus on physical symptoms, and in response, he began to consult for restaurants. Taken together, these interventions helped Louis reduce his anxiety, diminish his focus on and concern about his health, and begin to lead a more enjoyable life.

Adapted from Barsky, 2006.

behaviors so as to improve social interactions (Looper & Kirmayer, 2002). Family interventions are also often provided. Let's review each of these techniques.

As we discussed earlier, the negative emotions that accompany anxiety and depressive disorders often trigger physiological symptoms and intensify the distress about those somatic symptoms. It should be no surprise that treating anxiety and depression often reduces somatic symptoms and that providers use many of the medication and psychological interventions that we discussed in Chapters 5 and 6 (Payne & Blanchard, 1995).

Therapists also use many different cognitive strategies to treat somatic symptom and related disorders. Some involve training people to pay less attention to their body. Alternatively, cognitive strategies might help people identify and challenge negative thoughts about their health (Warwick & Salkovskis, 2001). The person who struggles with thoughts such as "I cannot cope with this pain" might be taught to make more positive self-statements, such as "I've been able to manage bouts of pain on other days, and I'll get through this one as well" (Christensen, Frostholm, et al., 2015). Mindfulness can also help clients disengage from a focus on their symptoms; clients who were taught to engage in daily mindfulness practice reported less health anxiety than participants who received standard medical care (McManus, Surawy, et al., 2012).

Behavioral techniques might help people reduce safety behaviors, resume healthy activities, and rebuild a lifestyle damaged by too much focus on illness-related concerns (Warwick & Salkovskis, 2001). Maria, the woman described earlier in a **Clinical Case**, revealed that she was extremely anxious about her shaky marriage and about situations in which other people might judge her. Couples therapy, assertiveness training, and social skills training—for example, coaching Maria in effective ways to approach and talk to people—could help her improve her social interactions. In general, behavioral and couples work can encourage patients to re-engage in satisfying activities and improve relationships.

Behavioral and family approaches could also help change Maria's reliance on playing the role of a sick person (Warwick & Salkovskis, 2001). If Maria's family members have adjusted to her illness by reinforcing her avoidance of responsibilities, family therapy might involve teaching family members about operant conditioning so that they reduce the amount of attention (reinforcement) they give to her somatic symptoms.

CBT is more efficacious in reducing health concerns, depression, and anxiety than is standard medical care or psychodynamic treatment of somatic symptom and related disorders (Olatunji, Kauffman, et al., 2014), and benefits are sustained 8 years after treatment (Tyrer, Wang, et al., 2021). In one study, CBT was as effective as antidepressant treatment in reducing illness anxiety symptoms (Greeven, van Balkom, et al., 2007). CBT interventions do more to reduce the *distress* about somatic symptoms than they do to reduce the actual somatic symptoms (van Dessel, den Boeft, et al., 2014).

Internet-based treatment can be helpful, particularly when it involves some brief guidance from a clinician (Axelsson, Andersson, et al., 2020; Newby, Smith, et al., 2018). Improvements associated with internet-based CBT have been shown to be sustained at follow-up assessments (Newby et al., 2018).

When the focus of somatic symptom disorder is on pain, several techniques can be helpful. Low-dose antidepressants, CBT, hypnosis, and a variant of CBT called acceptance and commitment therapy (ACT) have all been found to be helpful in randomized controlled trials (Ehde, Dillworth, & Turner, 2014; Fishbain, Cutler, et al., 2000; Jensen & Patterson, 2014; Veehof, Oskam, et al., 2011). In ACT, the therapist encourages the client to adopt a more accepting attitude toward pain, suffering, and moments of depression and anxiety and to consider these as a natural part of life (McCracken & Vowles, 2014). Although pain is harder to treat than is health anxiety (Rief & Martin, 2014), these treatments are preferred over opioid medications, which are highly addictive (Streltzer & Johansen, 2006).

Functional Neurological Symptom Disorder

Four randomized controlled trials indicate beneficial effects of CBT for specific forms of functional neurological symptom disorder. In one trial, researchers randomly assigned 61 individuals who had medically unexplained gait disorders, such as limping or foot dragging, to immediate treatment or a wait-list control (Jordbru, Smedstad, et al., 2014). As a first step in treatment, therapists explained to patients and their family members that medical tests had not revealed an explanation for gait disturbance but disconnections in the interface of the nervous system and the body are common. Patients were then hospitalized for 3 weeks so that they could take part in daily physical training. The CBT had two major components. First, patients were reinforced for taking part in the training. Second, to avoid reinforcing functional neurological symptoms, the treatment team ignored ongoing signs of gait disturbance. Patients showed large increases in their mobility, independence, and quality of life during the CBT intervention, and those gains were present 1 year later. In the other two trials, researchers found that outpatient CBT was more helpful than standard medical care or supportive therapy in reducing the rate of nonepileptic seizures, although some benefits are less clear at the 1-year follow-up (Fobian, Long, & Szaflarski, 2020; Goldstein, Robinson, et al., 2022; LaFrance, Baird, et al., 2014). CBT is often combined with physical therapy techniques (Nielsen, Stone, et al., 2015).

8.6 Check Your Knowledge

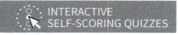
INTERACTIVE
SELF-SCORING QUIZZES

(Answers are at the end of the chapter.)
Answer the following questions.

1. Describe outcomes that have been shown to be improved by using CBT with somatic symptom and related disorders.

2. Describe treatments to reduce pain in somatic symptom and related disorders.

Summary

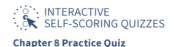
INTERACTIVE
SELF-SCORING QUIZZES
Chapter 8 Practice Quiz

Dissociative Disorders

- Dissociative disorders are defined by disruptions in the conscious awareness of experience, memory, or identity.

- The key symptom of dissociative disorders is dissociation. Mild dissociation can be triggered in the general population by stress, sleep disruption, and some drugs.

- As described in **Table 8.1**, the DSM-5-TR dissociative disorders include depersonalization/derealization disorder, dissociative amnesia, and dissociative identity disorder.

- Little is known about the causes of dissociative amnesia.

- Depersonalization/derealization disorder is believed to be related to difficulties integrating somatic and sensory information.

- Most of the writing about the causes of dissociative disorders focuses on dissociative identity disorder. People with dissociative identity disorder (DID) often retrospectively report severe physical or sexual abuse during childhood, but prospective research does not suggest that early adversity predicts the onset of DID. One model, the posttraumatic model, suggests that extensive reliance on dissociation to fend off overwhelming feelings arising from abuse puts people at risk for developing dissociative identity disorder. The sociocognitive model, though, proposes that these symptoms are elicited by treatment. Proponents of the sociocognitive model point out that some therapists use strategies that suggest such symptoms to people and that most people do not recognize the presence of alternate personalities until after they see a therapist. Although one of the defining features of DID is the lack of shared memories among alternative personality states, evidence suggests that the alternate personalities may share more memories than they report. Also, symptoms of DID can be role-played effectively.

- Regardless of theoretical orientation, clinicians focus their treatment efforts on helping clients cope with anxiety, face fears more directly, and operate in a manner that integrates their memory and consciousness.

- Psychodynamic treatment is perhaps the most commonly used treatment for dissociative disorders, but some of the techniques involved, such as hypnosis and age regression, may make symptoms worse.

Somatic Symptom and Related Disorders

- Somatic symptom and related disorders share a common focus on physical symptoms. As shown in Table 8.2, the major somatic symptom and related disorders include somatic symptom disorder, illness anxiety disorder, and functional neurological symptom disorder.

- Health anxiety is moderately heritable.

- Neurobiological models suggest that key brain regions involved in processing the unpleasantness of bodily sensations may be hyperactive among people with somatic symptom and related disorders. These regions include the anterior cingulate cortex and the rostral anterior insula. Cognitive variables are also important: Some people are overly attentive to physical concerns and make overly negative interpretations of symptoms and their implications. Avoidance may lead to health declines, and behavioral reinforcement may maintain help-seeking behavior. Safety behaviors may prolong and intensify health anxiety.

- Brain-imaging findings are consistent with the psychodynamic idea that people with functional neurological symptom disorder may not be conscious of their perceptions (in the case of functional blindness) or their control of movements (in the case of functional movement symptoms). Sociocultural influences also appear important in functional neurological symptom disorder.

- People with somatic symptom and related disorders often resent being referred for mental health care. Programs in which primary care physicians are encouraged to address these symptoms by providing warmth and reassurance while limiting medical tests have been shown to be helpful. Cognitive behavioral treatments of somatic symptoms, which are efficacious approaches to addressing the distress over such symptoms, try to relieve depressive and anxious symptoms, to reduce the excessive attention to bodily cues, to address the overly negative interpretations of physical symptoms, and to reinforce behavior that is not consistent with the sick role. Meditation may also help patients reduce their health focus and anxiety. When pain is a primary concern in somatic symptom disorder, CBT, hypnosis, ACT, and low doses of antidepressant medication may be helpful. Small trials indicate that CBT may also be helpful for functional neurological symptom disorder.

Answers to Check Your Knowledge Questions

8.1 1. Assumption of a new identity or bewildered wandering; 2. Disruption of identity characterized by distinct personality states or experience(s) of possession; 3. Before 1800, very few cases were recorded. There was a marked increase with media attention, and diagnostic criteria were introduced in the 1970s.

8.2 1. True; 2. Base rates of the disorder increased with media attention to the disorder; the therapists who treat the most DID cases rely on techniques like hypnosis, which could produce distinct personality states; most clients are unaware of alternate personality states until after they receive psychotherapy; DID can be role-played; most people with DID do appear to share memories among alternate personalities when sophisticated memory tests are used.

8.3 1. 0; 2. None; 3. age regression and hypnosis.

8.4 1. b; 2. a; 3. c.

8.5 1. True; 2. False.

8.6 1. Diminished health anxiety, lower anxiety and depression, slightly decreased pain and somatic symptoms in somatic symptom and related disorders, improved gait disturbance and lowered rate of nonepileptic seizures in functional neurological symptoms disorder; 2. CBT, hypnosis, ACT, and low-dose antidepressants

Key Terms

depersonalization 213
depersonalization/derealization
  disorder 212
derealization 213
dissociation 211
dissociative amnesia 214
dissociative disorders 211

dissociative fugue subtype 214
dissociative identity disorder (DID) 215
explicit memory 220
factitious disorder 226
functional neurological symptom
  disorder 224
iatrogenic 219

illness anxiety disorder 224
implicit memory 220
malingering 226
posttraumatic model (of DID) 218
sociocognitive model (of DID) 218
somatic symptom and related disorders 222
somatic symptom disorder 223

Schizophrenia

LEARNING GOALS

1. Describe the clinical symptoms of schizophrenia, including positive, negative, and disorganized symptoms.

2. Differentiate the genetic influences, both behavioral and molecular, in the cause of schizophrenia.

3. Understand the psychological influences in schizophrenia, including sociocultural, familial, and developmental influences.

4. Distinguish the medication treatments and psychological treatments for schizophrenia.

Clinical Case

A Woman with Schizophrenia

All of a sudden things weren't going so well. I began to lose control of my life and, most of all, myself. I couldn't concentrate on my schoolwork, I couldn't sleep, and when I did sleep, I had dreams about dying. I was afraid to go to class, imagined that people were talking about me, and on top of that I heard voices. I called my mother in Pittsburgh and asked for her advice. She told me to move off campus into an apartment with my sister.

After I moved in with my sister, things got worse. I was afraid to go outside, and when I looked out of the window, it seemed that everyone outside was yelling, "Kill her, kill her." My sister forced me to go to school. I would go out of the house until I knew she had gone to work; then I would return home. Things continued to get worse. I imagined that I had a foul body odor, and I sometimes took up to 6 showers a day. I recall going to the grocery store one day, and I imagined that the people in the store were saying, "Get saved, Jesus is the answer." Things worsened—I couldn't remember a thing. I had a notebook full of reminders telling me what to do on that particular day. I couldn't remember my schoolwork, and I would study from 6:00 p.m. until 4:00 a.m. but never had

the courage to go to class on the following day. I tried to tell my sister about it, but she didn't understand. She suggested that I see a psychiatrist, but I was afraid to go out of the house to see him.

One day I decided that I couldn't take this trauma anymore, so I took an overdose of 35 Darvon pills. At the same moment, a voice inside me said, "What did you do that for? Now you won't go to heaven." At that instant, I realized that I didn't really want to die. I wanted to live, and I was afraid. I got on the phone and called the psychiatrist whom my sister had recommended. I told him I had taken an overdose of Darvon and that I was afraid. He told me to take a taxi to the hospital. When I arrived at the hospital, I began vomiting, but I didn't pass out. Somehow, I just couldn't accept the fact that I was really going to see a psychiatrist. I thought that psychiatrists were only for crazy people, and I definitely didn't think I was crazy. As a result, I did not admit myself right away. As a matter of fact, I left the hospital and ended up meeting my sister on the way home. She told me to turn right back around because I was definitely going to be admitted. We then called my mother, and she said she would fly down the following day.

Quoted in O'Neal, 1984, pp. 109–110.

Clinical Descriptions and Epidemiology of Schizophrenia

The young woman described in the preceding Clinical Case was diagnosed with schizophrenia. Schizophrenia is a disorder characterized by disordered thinking, in which ideas are not logically related; faulty perception and attention; a lack of emotional expressiveness; and disturbances in behavior, such as a disheveled appearance. People with schizophrenia may withdraw from other people and from everyday reality, often into a life of odd beliefs (delusions) and hallucinations. Given that schizophrenia is associated with such widespread disruptions in a person's life, it has been difficult to uncover the causes of the disorder and develop effective methods to treat it. Unfortunately, schizophrenia is one of the most stigmatized of psychological disorders. For example, an analysis of nearly 2,000 tweets using #schizophrenia or #schizophrenic found that the tweets were used in a sarcastic, inappropriate, or derogatory way more often than tweets using #diabetes or #diabetic (Josephs, Tandon, et al., 2015). We still have a long way to go before we fully understand the multiple factors that trigger schizophrenia, develop treatments that are both effective and free of unpleasant side effects, and reduce misinformation and stigma about the disorder.

The symptoms of schizophrenia invade every aspect of a person: the way someone thinks, feels, and behaves. Not surprisingly, then, these symptoms can interfere with maintaining a job, living independently, and having close relationships with other people. They can also provoke ridicule and persecution. Substance use rates are high among people with schizophrenia (Hartz, Pato, et al., 2014), perhaps reflecting shared genetic vulnerability between substance use disorder and schizophrenia (Hartz, Horton, et al., 2017) or an attempt to achieve some relief from the symptoms (Blanchard, Squires, et al., 1999). Moreover, the suicide rate among people with schizophrenia is high. Indeed, they are 12 times more likely to die of suicide than people in the general population. People with schizophrenia are also more likely to die from any cause than people in the general population (Laursen, Nordentoft, & Mortensen, 2014; Olfson, Gerhard, et al., 2015), and their mortality rates are as high as or higher than the rates for people who smoke (Chesney, Goodwin, & Fazel, 2014).

The lifetime prevalence of schizophrenia is around 1%, and it affects men slightly more often than women (Kirkbride, Fearon, et al., 2006; Walker, Kestler, et al., 2004). Schizophrenia is diagnosed more frequently among some groups, such as Black and Latino Americans (Barr, Bigdeli, & Meyers, 2022; Schwartz & Blankenship, 2014), though this may reflect a bias among those making the diagnosis (Schwartz, Docherty, et al., 2019) and experiences of discrimination, trauma, and structural racism (DeVylder, Munson, et al., 2023). Indeed, several studies have found that Black or Latino people in the United States report more psychotic experiences than White people (Anglin, 2023), and such racial disparities are driven in part by experiences of discrimination and racism (Anglin, Ereshefsky, et al., 2021). Schizophrenia rarely begins in childhood; it usually appears in late adolescence or early adulthood and usually somewhat earlier in men than in women. However, psychotic-like experiences can occur in childhood, and experiencing these is associated with a great risk of developing schizophrenia as we discuss later in the chapter. These psychotic-like experiences in childhood are higher among Black and Latino children compared to White children, although these experiences are also strongly related to experiences of discrimination (Karcher, Klaunig, et al., 2022). People with schizophrenia typically have several acute episodes of their symptoms and less severe symptoms between episodes.

The range of symptoms in the diagnosis of schizophrenia is extensive, although people with the disorder typically have only some of these symptoms at any given time

Defining Symptoms of Schizophrenia

For a diagnosis of schizophrenia, a person has to have at least two symptoms, and one of these should be delusions, hallucinations, or disorganized speech:

- delusions
- hallucinations

- disorganized speech
- disorganized (or catatonic) behavior
- negative symptoms (diminished motivation or emotional expression)

TABLE 9.1   Summary of the Major Symptom Domains in Schizophrenia

Positive Symptoms	Negative Symptoms	Disorganized Symptoms
Delusions, hallucinations	Avolition, alogia, anhedonia, blunted affect, asociality	Disorganized behavior, disorganized speech

(see the Defining Symptoms box). Schizophrenia symptoms are often described in three broad domains: positive, negative, and disorganized. **Table 9.1** shows the symptoms that comprise these domains.

When assessing the symptoms of schizophrenia, it is important to consider a person's culture. Beliefs, experiences, and behaviors vary from culture to culture, and what may seem to be a symptom in one culture may be a common behavior or practice in another culture (Maietta, Paul, & Allen, 2020).

Positive Symptoms

Positive symptoms comprise excesses and distortions and include hallucinations and delusions. For the most part, acute episodes of schizophrenia are characterized by positive symptoms. These symptoms are also referred to as *psychotic symptoms*.

Delusions   No doubt all of us at one time or another have been concerned because we believed that others thought ill of us. Some of the time this belief may be justified. After all, who is universally loved? Consider, though, the anguish you would feel if you were firmly convinced that many people did not like you—indeed, that they disliked you so much that they were plotting against you. Imagine that your persecutors have hacked your phone in order to listen in on your most private conversations and gather evidence in a plot to discredit you. Those around you, including your loved ones, are unable to reassure you that people are not spying on you. Even your closest friends are gradually joining forces with your tormentors. Anxious and angry, you begin taking counteractions against your persecutors. When you meet people for the first time, you question them at great length to determine whether they are part of the plot against you.

Such **delusions**, which are beliefs contrary to reality and firmly held despite disconfirming evidence, are common positive symptoms of schizophrenia. Delusions may take several forms, as shown in **Table 9.2**.

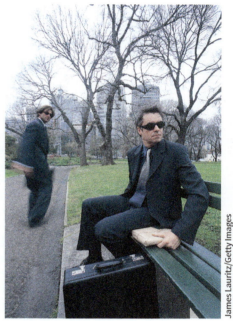

Believing that others are taking special notice is a common paranoid delusion.

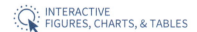
INTERACTIVE FIGURES, CHARTS, & TABLES

TABLE 9.2   Descriptions of Delusions in Schizophrenia

Delusion	Definition	Example
Thought insertion	A person may believe that thoughts that are not their own have been placed in their mind by an external source.	A woman may believe that the government has inserted a computer chip in her brain so that thoughts can be inserted into her head.
Thought broadcasting	A person may believe that their thoughts are broadcast or transmitted, so others know what they are thinking.	When walking down the street, a man may look suspiciously at passersby, thinking that they are able to hear what he is thinking even though he is not saying anything out loud.
Delusion of reference	A person may incorporate unimportant events within a delusional framework and read personal significance into the trivial activities of others.	A man might think that overheard segments of conversations are about him, that the frequent appearance of the same person on a street where he customarily walks means that he is being watched, and that what he sees on TV somehow refers to him.
Delusion of control	A person may believe that an external force controls their feelings or behaviors.	A person may believe that their behavior is being controlled by the signals emitted from cell phone towers.
Grandiose delusion	A person may have an exaggerated sense of their own importance, power, knowledge, or identity.	A woman may believe that she can cause the wind to change direction just by moving her hands.
Persecutory delusion	A person may believe that others are going out of their way to harm, harass, discredit, or conspire against them.	A man may think someone is poisoning his food in order to harm him.

Hallucinations

Hallucinations are sensory experiences in the absence of any relevant stimulation from the environment. They are more often auditory than visual.

Some people with schizophrenia report hearing their own thoughts spoken by another voice. Other people hear voices arguing, and still others hear voices commenting on their behavior. Many people with schizophrenia experience their hallucinations as frightening or annoying. In one study of nearly 200 people with schizophrenia, those whose hallucinations were longer, louder, more frequent, and experienced in the third person found the hallucinations unpleasant. Hallucinations that were believed to come from a known person were experienced more positively (Copolov, Mackinnon, & Trauer, 2004).

Meta-analyses of neuroimaging studies have examined what happens in the brain during auditory hallucinations. These studies have found greater activity in Broca's area (an area of the frontal cortex that supports our ability to produce speech) and in Wernicke's area (an area of the temporal cortex that supports our ability to understand speech) when people with schizophrenia report hearing voices (Jardri, Pouchet, et al., 2011; Zmigrod, Garrison, et al., 2016). These data suggest that there is a problem in the connections between the frontal lobe areas that enable the production of speech and the temporal lobe areas that enable the understanding of speech (Ford, Mathalon, et al., 2002).

Negative Symptoms

The **negative symptoms** of schizophrenia consist of deficits in motivation, pleasure, social closeness, and emotion expression (Kirkpatrick, Fenton, et al., 2006). These symptoms tend to endure beyond an acute episode and have profound effects on the lives of people with schizophrenia. They are also important prognostically; the presence of many negative symptoms is a strong predictor of a poor quality of life (e.g., occupational impairment, few friends) (Degnan, Berry, et al., 2018; Fervaha, Foussias, et al., 2014; Mahmood, Keller, et al., 2019).

Avolition

Apathy, or **avolition**, refers to diminished motivation and a seeming absence of interest or persistence in what are usually routine activities, including work or school, hobbies, or social activities. For example, people with avolition may not be motivated to go to a movie or hang out with friends. They may have difficulty persisting at work, school, or household chores. One study examined the types of motivation deficits in schizophrenia by interviewing people with and without schizophrenia four times a day for 7 days about their daily goals using ecological momentary assessment (EMA; see Chapter 3). The researchers found that people with schizophrenia were less motivated than people without schizophrenia by goals associated with autonomy (self-expression), gaining new knowledge or skills, or praise but were more motivated by goals that had to do with reducing boredom (Gard, Sanchez, et al., 2014). People with schizophrenia were equally motivated, however, by goals that had to do with interacting with others and with avoiding criticism. Thus, it appears that people with schizophrenia may have trouble with motivation for certain life areas but not for others.

Asociality

Some people with schizophrenia have impairments in social relationships, referred to as **asociality**. They may have few friends, poor social skills, and very little interest in being with other people. They may not desire close relationships with family, friends, or romantic partners. Instead, they may wish to spend much of their time alone. When around others, people with this symptom may interact only superficially and briefly and may appear aloof or indifferent to the social interaction.

Anhedonia

A loss of interest in or a reported lessening of the experience of pleasure is called **anhedonia**. Anhedonia can interfere with day-to-day functioning in people with schizophrenia even more than the positive symptoms (Abplanalp, Braff, et al., 2022). There are two types of pleasure experiences in the anhedonia construct. The first, called **consummatory pleasure**, refers to the amount of pleasure experienced in the moment or in the presence of something pleasurable. For example, the amount of pleasure you experience as you are eating a good meal is known as consummatory pleasure. The second type of pleasure, called **anticipatory pleasure**, refers to the amount of expected or anticipated pleasure from future events or activities. For example, the amount of pleasure you expect to feel after graduating from college is anticipatory pleasure. People with schizophrenia appear to have a deficit in anticipatory pleasure but not consummatory pleasure (Gard, Kring, et al., 2007; Kring & Elis, 2013). That is, when asked about expected future situations or activities that are pleasurable for most people (e.g., good food, recreational activities, social interactions) on an anhedonia questionnaire, people with schizophrenia report that they derive less pleasure from these sorts of activities than do people without schizophrenia. However, when presented with actual pleasant activities, such as amusing films or tasty beverages, people with schizophrenia report experiencing as much pleasure as do people without schizophrenia. Thus, the anhedonia deficit in schizophrenia appears to be in anticipating pleasure, not experiencing pleasure in the presence of pleasurable things. Notably, anticipatory pleasure is also observed in depression (Hallford & Sharma, 2019).

Blunted Affect

Blunted affect refers to a lack of outward expression of emotion. A person with this symptom may stare vacantly, the muscles of the face motionless, the eyes lifeless. When spoken to, the person may answer in a flat and toneless voice and not look at their conversational partner.

The concept of blunted affect refers only to the outward expression of emotion, not to the person's inner experience, which is not impoverished at all. Over 20 different studies have shown that people with schizophrenia are much less facially expressive than are people without schizophrenia; this is true both in daily life and in laboratory studies when emotionally evocative stimuli (films, pictures, foods) are presented. However, people with schizophrenia report experiencing the same amount of or *even more* emotion than people without schizophrenia (Kring & Elis, 2013).

Alogia

Alogia refers to a significant reduction in the amount of speech. Simply put, people with this symptom do not talk much. A person may answer a question with one or two words and is not likely to elaborate on an answer with additional detail. For example, if you ask a person with alogia to describe a happy life experience, the person might respond "getting married" and then fail to elaborate, even when asked for additional information.

Although we have just described five different negative symptoms, research suggests that these symptoms can be understood more simply as representing two domains (Blanchard, Bradshaw, et al., 2017). The first domain, involving motivation, emotional experience, and sociality, is sometimes referred to as the *motivation and pleasure domain*. The second domain, involving outward expression of emotion and vocalization, is referred to as the *expression domain*.

Disorganized Symptoms

Disorganized symptoms include disorganized speech and disorganized behavior.

Disorganized Speech

Also known as *formal thought disorder*, **disorganized speech** refers to problems in organizing ideas and in speaking so that a listener can understand. The following excerpt illustrates the incoherence sometimes found in the conversation of people with schizophrenia as an interviewer tries to ask John, a person with schizophrenia, several questions (Neale & Oltmanns, 1980).

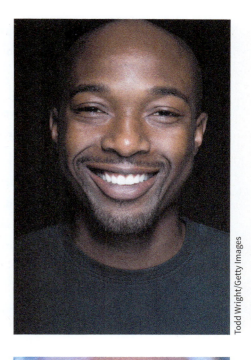

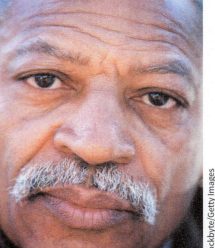

People with schizophrenia who have blunted affect may not outwardly show happiness, but they will feel it as strongly as people who smile.

Interviewer:	Have you been nervous or tense lately?
John:	No, I got a head of lettuce.
Interviewer:	You got a head of lettuce? I don't understand.
John:	Well, it's just a head of lettuce.

Interviewer:	Tell me about lettuce. What do you mean?
John:	Well ... lettuce is a transformation of a dead cougar that suffered a relapse on the lion's toe. And he swallowed the lion and something happened. The ... see, the ... Gloria and Tommy, they're two heads and they're not whales. But they escaped with herds of vomit, and things like that.
Interviewer:	What does all that mean?
John:	Well, you see, I have to leave the hospital. I'm supposed to have an operation on my legs, you know. And it comes to be pretty sickly that I don't want to keep my legs. That's why I wish I could have an operation.
Interviewer:	You want to have your legs taken off?
John:	It's possible, you know.
Interviewer:	Why would you want to do that?
John:	I didn't have any legs to begin with. So I would imagine that if I was a fast runner, I'd be scared to be a wife, because I had a splinter inside of my head of lettuce. (Neale & Oltmanns, 1980, pp. 103–104)

Although John may make repeated references to central ideas or themes, the images and fragments of thought are not connected; it is difficult to understand what he is trying to tell the interviewer.

Speech may also be disorganized by what are called **loose associations (derailment)**, in which case the person may be more successful in communicating with a listener but has difficulty sticking to one topic. Steve Lopez, a reporter for the *Los Angeles Times*, befriended a man with schizophrenia named Nathaniel in the L.A. area who was a gifted musician (and also homeless). Lopez wrote about their friendship in the book *The Soloist* (Lopez, 2008). Nathaniel often exhibited loose associations. For example, in response to a question about Beethoven, Nathaniel replied:

> *Cleveland doesn't have the Beethoven statue. That's a military-oriented city, occupied, preoccupied, with all the military figures of American history, the great soldiers and generals, but you don't see the musicians on parade, although you do have Severance Hall, Cleveland Music School Settlement, Ohio University Bobcats, Buckeyes of Ohio State. All the great soldiers are there from the United States Military, World War Two, Korean War, whereas in Los Angeles you have the LAPD, Los Angeles County Jail, Los Angeles Times, Mr. Steve Lopez. That's an army, right?*
>
> **(Quoted in Lopez, 2008, pp. 23–24)**

As this quote illustrates, a person with this symptom seems to drift off on a train of associations evoked by an idea from the past.

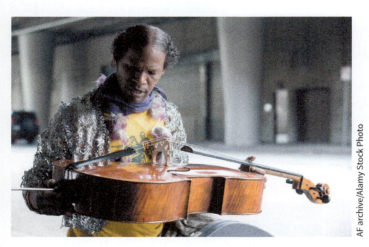

Jamie Foxx played Nathaniel in the movie version of *The Soloist* (2009).

AF archive/Alamy Stock Photo

Disorganized Behavior   People with the symptom of **disorganized behavior** may go into inexplicable bouts of agitation, dress in unusual clothes, act in a silly manner, or wander with no particular destination. They seem to lose the ability to organize their behavior and make it conform to community standards. They also have difficulty performing the tasks of everyday living.

In DSM-5-TR, one manifestation of disorganized behavior is called **catatonia**. People with this symptom may gesture repeatedly, using peculiar and sometimes complex sequences of finger, hand, and arm movements, which often seem to be purposeful. Some people manifest an unusual increase in their overall level of activity, including much excitement, flailing of the limbs, and great expenditure of energy similar to that seen in mania. At the other end of the spectrum is immobility: People adopt unusual postures and maintain them for very long periods of time.

Focus on Discovery 9.1

History of the Concept of Schizophrenia

Two European psychiatrists, Emil Kraepelin and Eugen Bleuler, initially formulated the concept of schizophrenia. Kraepelin first described *dementia praecox*, his term for what we now call schizophrenia, in 1898. The term *dementia praecox* reflected what he believed to be that core—an early-onset (praecox) and a progressive, inevitable intellectual deterioration (dementia). The dementia in dementia praecox is not the same as the dementias we discuss in the chapter on neurocognitive disorders (Chapter 14). Kraepelin's term referred to a general "mental enfeeblement."

Bleuler broke with Kraepelin's description on two major points: He believed that the disorder did not necessarily have an early onset, and he believed that it did not inevitably progress toward dementia. Thus, the label "dementia praecox" was no longer appropriate, and in 1908 Bleuler proposed his own term, *schizophrenia*, from the Greek words *schizein* ("to split") and *phren* ("mind"), capturing what he viewed as the essential nature of the condition.

Bleuler used a metaphor—the "breaking of associative threads"—to describe the essential features of schizophrenia. For Bleuler, associative threads joined not only words but also thoughts. Thus, goal-directed, efficient thinking and communication were possible only when these hypothetical structures were intact. The notion that associative threads were disrupted in people with schizophrenia could then be used to account for the range of other symptoms.

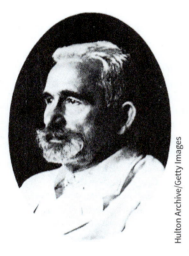

Hulton Archive/Getty Images

Emil Kraepelin (1856–1926), a German psychiatrist, articulated descriptions of schizophrenia (then called dementia praecox) that have proved remarkably durable in light of contemporary research.

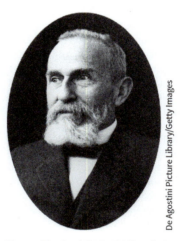

De Agostini Picture Library/Getty Images

Eugen Bleuler (1857–1939), a Swiss psychiatrist, contributed to our conceptions of schizophrenia and coined the term.

Catatonia is seldom seen today in people with schizophrenia, perhaps because medications work effectively on these disturbed movements or postures. See **Focus on Discovery 9.1** for more details on the history of schizophrenia and its symptoms.

 VIDEO CONTENT

Case Study: Schizophrenia Pause and Ponder

Other Schizophrenia Spectrum Disorders

Schizophrenia is part of the DSM-5-TR chapter entitled "Schizophrenia Spectrum and Other Psychotic Disorders." Two other psychotic disorders appearing in this chapter are **schizophreniform disorder** and **brief psychotic disorder**. The symptoms of schizophreniform disorder are the same as those of schizophrenia but last only 1 to 6 months. For a diagnosis of schizophrenia, symptoms have to last for at least 6 months. Brief psychotic disorder lasts from 1 day to 1 month and is often brought on by extreme stress.

Schizoaffective disorder comprises a mixture of symptoms of schizophrenia and mood disorders. The DSM-5-TR requires either a depressive or a manic episode rather than simply mood disorder symptoms. This can be a difficult diagnosis to make. We describe this diagnostic difficulty in **Read More About It 9.1**.

A person with **delusional disorder** is troubled by persistent delusions. These can be delusions of persecution or jealousy, such as the unfounded conviction that a spouse or lover is unfaithful. Other delusions seen in this disorder include grandiose delusions,

Read More About It 9.1

The Collected Schizophrenias

The author Esmé Weijun Wang writes beautifully about her journey with schizoaffective disorder in her collection of essays entitled *The Collected Schizophrenias*, published in 2019. It took 8 years from the time that she first experienced symptoms (hallucinations) for her to receive this diagnosis. She was first diagnosed with bipolar disorder based on her manic symptoms. But the psychotic symptoms she also experiences, which include hallucinations and delusions, led to the new diagnosis of schizoaffective disorder, bipolar type.

What's in a name? Having the incorrect diagnosis can mean receiving the wrong treatment. In Wang's case, she first received Depakote, an anticonvulsant medication that is also mood stabilizing and used for treating bipolar disorder (see Chapter 5). This medication, like most medications for psychological disorders, has unpleasant side effects that go along with any benefits. She first took this medication before and during her time in college, though she reports that she did not receive a clinically effective dose (perhaps to minimize the likelihood of the medication damaging her liver). Later, she received a first-generation antipsychotic medication called haloperidol, or Haldol (see Table 9.6); this medication is more often prescribed for psychotic disorders such as schizophrenia and schizoaffective disorder.

In an essay called "High Functioning," she describes her experience talking to two different groups: One was a group of people with severe mental illness, and another was a group of mental health professionals. She describes how she tried to show that she was doing well even though she had a diagnosis of schizoaffective disorder by inserting certain "signifiers" into her talk (such as mentioning that she had attended a prestigious university) and by wearing her wedding ring. These were meant to signal: I am OK; I am smart; I am just like other people. She expands on distinctions between "high-functioning" people with psychological disorders and those who have a harder time with such problems. She is able to work; she has achieved a great deal. Yet, she is cognizant that others do not fare as well and that others would view her differently if she had not been so successful. In short, she recognizes that stigma is unfortunately alive and well.

Even though she attended a prestigious university (actually more than one), she does not mince words when it comes to her experience with receiving treatment and accommodation for her disorder in the context of her undergraduate education. She was hospitalized twice during her first three semesters in college; the university asked her to take a medical leave and then would not accept her back on campus. Simply put, the college would not provide mental health accommodations. Although Wang's college experience took place nearly two decades ago, providing appropriate and sufficient mental health care is something many colleges and universities still struggle to achieve.

Wang describes her awareness of her developing psychotic symptoms with clarity, vivid imagery, and honesty:

> *... I am aware enough to know something's wrong. Something is wrong, then it is completely wrong. After the prodromal phase, I settle into a way of being that is almost intolerable. The moment of shifting from one phase to the other is usually sharp and clear; I turn my head and in a single moment realized that my coworkers have been replaced by robots, or glance at my sewing table as the thought settles over me, fine and gray as soot, that I am dead. In this way I have become, and have remained, delusional for months at a time, which feels like breaking through a thin barrier to another world that sways and bucks and won't throw me back through again no matter how many pills I swallow or how much I struggle to return.*

The collection of essays discusses many aspects of mental health and conveys what it is like to have a serious psychological disorder and at the same time achieve a great deal. It is both inspiring and realistic.

---

delusions of erotomania (believing that one is loved by some other person, usually a complete stranger with a higher social status), and somatic delusions (e.g., delusions about body functions).

The DSM-5 added a new category to the "Conditions for Further Study" part of Section III called *attenuated psychosis syndrome*. We discuss this disorder in more detail in **Focus on Discovery 9.2**.

Quick Summary

Schizophrenia affects men slightly more often than women and typically begins in late adolescence or early adulthood. Symptoms can be distinguished as positive, negative, and disorganized. Positive symptoms include hallucinations and delusions; negative symptoms include avolition, alogia, blunted affect, anhedonia, and asociality. Together, the negative symptoms represent two domains: motivation/pleasure and expression. Disorganized symptoms include disorganized speech and disorganized behavior. Other schizophrenia spectrum disorders include schizophreniform disorder and brief psychotic disorder, which differ from schizophrenia in duration. Schizoaffective disorder involves symptoms of both schizophrenia and either a depressive or a manic episode. Delusional disorder involves delusions but no other symptoms of schizophrenia.

9.1 Check Your Knowledge

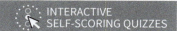
INTERACTIVE
SELF-SCORING QUIZZES

(Answers are at the end of the chapter.)
List the symptom that each clinical vignette describes.

1. Charlie enjoyed going to the movies. They particularly liked to see horror movies because they made them feel really scared. Their sister was surprised to learn this because when they went to the movies with Charlie, they didn't gasp out loud or show fear on their face.

2. Marlene was convinced that Christian Bale was sending them messages. In the movie *The Dark Knight*, their battles with the Joker were a signal that they were prepared to fight for them to be together. That they signed autographs at the movie opening also told Marlene that they were trying to get in touch with them.

3. Sophia didn't want to go out to dinner with her family. She reasoned that these dinners were always the same food and conversation, and it just didn't sound like fun. Later in the week, her mother mentioned that Sophia was not doing much around the house. Sophia said that nothing she could think of to do would be fun.

4. Jevon was talking with the doctor about the side effects of their medication. He talked about having dry mouth and then immediately began talking about cottonmouth snakes and jungle safaris and how hiking was good for your health, but that Joe Biden was in better shape than Donald Trump.

Focus on Discovery 9.2

Attenuated Psychosis Syndrome

When DSM-5 first considered adding to the chapter "Schizophrenia Spectrum and Other Psychotic Disorders" a new disorder called attenuated psychosis syndrome (APS), the proposal generated a good deal of discussion and debate in the field. Ultimately, APS was placed in Section III of DSM-5, which covers conditions in need of further research before being included in the DSM.

The idea for APS came from research over the past two decades that has sought to identify young people who are at risk for developing schizophrenia. These types of studies are called clinical high-risk studies, and the starting point for these prospective, longitudinal studies is the reliable identification of youth who present with mild positive symptoms that might later develop into schizophrenia (Miller, McGlashan, et al., 2002). Such people have been referred to as prodromal; the word *prodrome* refers to the early signs of a disease. Young people who show these mild symptoms differ from young people who do not in several domains, including their everyday functioning and their rate of conversion to schizophrenia spectrum disorders (Woods, Addington, et al., 2009). Between 10% and 30% of people meeting prodromal criteria develop a schizophrenia spectrum disorder, compared with only 0.2% of the general population (Carpenter & van Os, 2011; Yung, Woods, et al., 2012). The duration of the prodromal period, at least among those identified as being clinical high risk, is just under 2 years (Powers, Addington, et al., 2020).

What were some of the arguments in favor of adding this new category to DSM-5? First, identifying APS may help people get treatment when otherwise they would go unnoticed by mental health professionals. Unfortunately, under the current health insurance system in the United States, people often cannot get treatment unless they have an official diagnosis. Second, the hope is that the identification and treatment of people with APS might prevent them from developing schizophrenia or other schizophrenia spectrum disorders.

However, there were also several arguments against adding this new category (Yung et al., 2012). First, the category itself does not yet have enough reliability and validity to support its inclusion in the DSM. Second, there is a high level of comorbidity with prodromal symptoms: Over 60% of young people with the prodromal symptoms have a history of depression, raising the possibility that APS is really part of a mood disorder, not a schizophrenia spectrum disorder. Third, there is concern that applying a new diagnostic label, particularly to young people, might be stigmatizing or lead to discrimination. Because not all people with APS will develop schizophrenia, it may unnecessarily alarm young people and their families. Finally, although providing treatment for people with distressing or disabling attenuated positive symptoms is a laudable goal, the treatment may too closely resemble that for schizophrenia, further blurring the line between the two conditions. Indeed, there is not yet an effective treatment for APS (Carpenter & van Os, 2011).

Causes of Schizophrenia

What can explain the scattering and disconnection of thoughts, delusions, hallucinations, and diminished motivation and emotion expression of people with schizophrenia? As we will see, many influences contribute to the cause of this complex disorder. Longitudinal studies are beginning to help sort out the ways in which these influences unfold over the course of development. What appears to be happening is that genetic, neural, and social influences (e.g., early adversity) bidirectionally influence one another over the course of development to produce the symptoms of schizophrenia (Cannon, 2015; Murray, Bhavasar, et al., 2017).

Genetic Influences

A good deal of research supports the idea that schizophrenia has a genetic component, as we discuss in the following sections on behavior genetics and molecular genetics research. The evidence is somewhat more convincing from behavior genetics studies, largely because they have been well replicated (see Chapter 4 for a discussion of the importance of replication). The heritability estimate for schizophrenia based on behavior genetics studies is between 0.77 and 0.81 (Smoller, Andreassen, et al., 2019; Sullivan, Kendler, & Neale, 2003). Like nearly all disorders we discuss in this text, schizophrenia is genetically heterogeneous—that is, genetic influences may vary from person to person.

Behavior Genetics Research   Behavior genetics studies (described in Chapter 4) support the idea that genetic factors play a role in schizophrenia. Many of these studies were conducted when the definition of schizophrenia was considerably broader than it is now. However, behavior genetics investigators collected extensive descriptive data on their samples, allowing the results to be reanalyzed later using new diagnostic criteria.

Family Studies   Table 9.3 presents a summary of the risk for schizophrenia in various relatives of people with schizophrenia. (In evaluating the figures, keep in mind that the risk for schizophrenia in the general population is a little less than 1%.) Quite clearly, relatives of people with schizophrenia are at higher risk, and the risk increases as the genetic relationship between the person with schizophrenia and the relative becomes closer.

A family study examined over 2 million people from Denmark from the Danish Civil Registration System (Gottesman, Laursen, et al., 2010). This system records all inpatient and outpatient admissions for health-related issues, including psychological disorders. The researchers examined the cumulative incidence of schizophrenia and bipolar disorder among people with one, two, or no biological parents who had been admitted for treatment for schizophrenia or bipolar disorder. They also examined the incidence of these disorders among children who had one parent admitted for schizophrenia and one parent admitted for bipolar disorder. The findings are presented in Table 9.4. As you might expect, the incidence of schizophrenia was highest for children who had two parents admitted for schizophrenia. For people who had one parent admitted for schizophrenia and one parent admitted for bipolar disorder, the incidence of schizophrenia was higher than for those people who had just one parent admitted for schizophrenia. These findings suggest that there may be some shared genetic vulnerability between schizophrenia and bipolar disorder; molecular genetics studies, which we turn to shortly, also suggest such a link.

TABLE 9.3   **Summary of Major Family and Twin Studies of the Genetics of Schizophrenia**

Relation to Person with Schizophrenia	Percentage with Schizophrenia
Spouse	1.00
Grandchildren	2.84
Nieces/nephews	2.65
Children	9.35
Siblings	7.30
DZ twins	12.08
MZ twins	44.30

Source: Gottesman, McGuffin, & Farmer (1987).

TABLE 9.4	Summary of the Findings of the Family Study by Gottesman and Colleagues (2010)
Psychopathology in Parents	**Incidence of Schizophrenia**
Both parents with schizophrenia	27.3%
One parent with schizophrenia	7.0%
No parent with schizophrenia	0.86%
One parent with schizophrenia and one parent with bipolar disorder	15.6%

A different type of family study is called a **familial high-risk study**. This type of study begins with one or two biological parents with schizophrenia and follows their children longitudinally to identify how many of them develop schizophrenia and what types of childhood neurobiological and behavioral factors may predict the disorder's onset (Mednick & Schulsinger, 1968).

A meta-analysis of 33 familial high-risk studies that included offspring of parents with schizophrenia, bipolar disorder, or major depressive disorder found that the risk of developing schizophrenia was highest for the offspring of a parent with schizophrenia. Furthermore, compared with the offspring of parents with no psychological disorders, the offspring having a parent with schizophrenia were at nearly two times greater risk of developing any severe psychological disorder (Rasic, Hajek, et al., 2014). Thus, having a parent with schizophrenia is associated with a greater risk of developing not only schizophrenia, but other disorders as well.

Family studies show that genes likely play a role in schizophrenia, but of course the relatives of a person with schizophrenia share not only genes but also common experiences. We present a book about a very interesting family in **Read More About It 9.2**; therefore, the influence of the environment cannot be discounted in explaining the higher risks among relatives.

Twin and Adoption Studies   As Table 9.3 shows, although the risk for identical (MZ) twins of people with schizophrenia (44.3%) is greater than that for fraternal (DZ) twins of people with schizophrenia (12.08%), it is still much less than 100%. A meta-analysis of 12 twin studies concluded that the studies provided evidence of high heritability but also evidence for small but significant environmental contributions (Sullivan, Kendler, & Neale, 2003). The less-than-100% concordance in MZ twins is important: If genetic transmission alone accounted for schizophrenia and one identical twin had schizophrenia, the other twin would also have schizophrenia.

As with family studies, of course, there is a critical problem in interpreting the results of twin studies. Common shared (e.g., child-rearing practices) and nonshared (e.g., peer relationships) environmental factors rather than common genetic factors could account for some portion of the increased risk.

Studying children whose biological mothers had schizophrenia but who were reared from early infancy by adoptive parents without schizophrenia is another useful behavior genetics research method. Such studies eliminate the possible effects of being reared in an environment where a parent has schizophrenia.

A large study of adopted offspring of mothers with schizophrenia found that the risk for developing schizophrenia or a related diagnosis for the 164 adoptees who had a biological mother with schizophrenia was 8.1%; the risk for the 197 control adoptees who did not have a biological parent with schizophrenia was significantly lower, at 2.3% (Tienari, Wynne, et al., 2000).

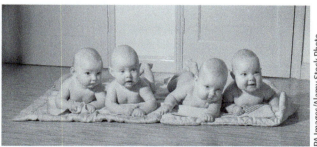

PA Images/Alamy Stock Photo

Behavior genetics studies focus often on twins and more rarely on triplets or quadruplets. In one rare case, all of the "Genain" quadruplet girls (not their real name and not pictured), born in 1930, developed schizophrenia. Two of the still surviving sisters were evaluated at age 81, and both were still taking antipsychotic medications (Mirsky, Bieliauskas, et al., 2013). As of 2022, only one of the quadruplets was still living. Sadly, all four girls experienced severe maltreatment as children, and thus, the interaction of genes, brain injury at birth, and early trauma likely contributed to the development of schizophrenia (Farley, 2023).

Read More About It 9.2

Hidden Valley Road: Inside the Mind of an American Family

In 2020, author Robert Kolker published *Hidden Valley Road: Inside the Mind of an American Family*. This book tells the story of the Galvin family and their experiences with schizophrenia. Don and Mimi Galvin had 12 children between 1945 and 1965. There were 10 boys and 2 girls; the youngest two children were the girls.

A remarkable 6 of the 10 Galvin boys were believed to have had schizophrenia. The eldest son, Donald, began experiencing symptoms in high school, but he did not receive a diagnosis until he was in college in the mid-1960s. The second son, Jim, exhibited what we would today call disorganized behavior and was first hospitalized in the late 1960s. The fourth son, Brian, was taking antipsychotic medications at the time he died by suicide (medical records were not available to determine if a diagnosis of schizophrenia had been given). Two other sons also had schizophrenia—Joseph, the seventh son, who had been quiet and withdrawn, was diagnosed at age 26, and Matthew, the ninth son, who had strong delusions, was diagnosed around age 18. The tenth son, Peter, was diagnosed at the youngest age; he was just 14. Peter was hospitalized more frequently than his brothers and at one point was taking eight different medications. Upon discharge from the hospital, he would usually stop taking his medications and would be rehospitalized. His diagnosis changed over the years; ultimately, bipolar disorder with psychotic features appeared to be the more accurate diagnosis for him.

In the 1960s and 1970s, the family did not discuss the sons' experiences with mental illness, working instead to put on a façade of a remarkably large family doing well in America. The stigma associated with mental illness no doubt contributed to the silence (Read More About It 1.1 in Chapter 1 focuses on books on stigma and mental illness by Steve Hinshaw). But shame also likely played a role. After all, the theorizing of Fromm-Reichman was prominent, and mothers were often singled out for blame in causing schizophrenia in their children. Mimi, the family matriarch, was told repeatedly that the illness befalling her sons was her doing, even as her husband, the father of the children, did his best to keep as far from home as possible during the years the children were growing up.

Kolker's engrossing book tells the story of the boys who were ill as well as that of the other family members. It is a mesmerizing account of the impact of schizophrenia on a family and the family's efforts to do the best they can. The period of time during which the Galvin children grew up was a time of great change in psychopathology research. Medications for schizophrenia were not identified until the late 1950s. Behavior genetics research produced many findings in the 1960s. A gradual decrease in the number of hospital beds for people with schizophrenia and other serious disorders started in the 1960s and continues today. Fortunately for the Galvin boys, they were able to have short hospital stays to help stabilize their symptoms. Yet, they were not always offered effective treatments, and this created a good deal of turmoil in the Galvin house on Hidden Valley Road, for those with and without schizophrenia, for many years.

How could so many of the Galvin children develop schizophrenia? In the 1960s and 1970s, genetics researchers who studied the presence of schizophrenia in more than one family member (in so-called *multiplex families*) struggled to get the field to accept the approach. Some in the field countered that twin and adoption studies were better suited to determining genetic and environmental contributions. Molecular genetics researchers focused on identifying candidate genes and genetic mutations. What the decades of research in behavior and molecular genetics have made clear, however, is that the genetic vulnerability to schizophrenia varies a great deal from person to person. The field has finally, more than 50 years later, come to value the importance of studying multiplex families. Using findings of genetic mutations from GWAS, researchers can now better pinpoint what particular mutation(s) may be passed along in families like the Galvins. The Galvin children, and now their children, have participated in genetics research since the 1970s. Mimi, the family matriarch, spearheaded the effort after realizing that she was not to blame and that her family could help other families. Most of the children continue to participate in research. Sadly, two of the ill brothers (Jim and Joseph) died in their 50s, likely from complications brought on by medication side effects.

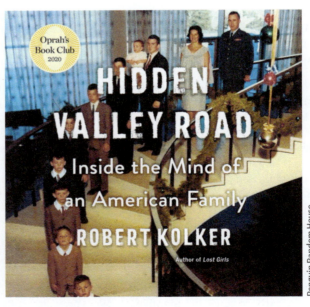

The Galvin family had 12 children (10 boys, 2 girls). Six of the boys were diagnosed with schizophrenia, although the diagnosis was later changed for one of them.

Molecular Genetics Research   Finding that schizophrenia can be influenced by genes is in many ways just the starting point for research. Understanding exactly what constitutes the genetic influence is the challenge faced by molecular genetics researchers. As with nearly all disorders we cover in this book, vulnerability for schizophrenia is not transmitted by a single gene. Furthermore, research has found that there are multiple common genes associated with schizophrenia and other disorders (Anttila, Bulik-Sullivan, et al., 2018; Cross-Disorder Group of the Psychiatric Genomics Consortium, 2013; Lam, Chen, et al., 2019), suggesting that the genetic vulnerability is not likely even specific to schizophrenia. As we discussed in Chapter 2, recent evidence from genetics research suggests that genetic vulnerability increases risk for psychopathology in general more than for specific disorders, including schizophrenia.

Recall from Chapter 2 that the GWAS technique allows researchers to identify rare mutations, such as CNVs (copy number variations), in genes rather than just known gene loci (locations). Mutations are changes in a gene that occur randomly and for unknown reasons. A CNV refers to an abnormality (a deletion or a duplication) in a copy of one or more sections of DNA in a gene (see Chapter 2). Across two different samples of people, one GWAS found that over 50 rare CNV mutations were three times more common among people with schizophrenia than among people without schizophrenia (Walsh, McClellan, et al., 2008). Some of the identified gene mutations are known to be associated with other presumed risk factors in the cause of schizophrenia, including the neurotransmitter glutamate and proteins that promote the proper placement of neurons in the brain during brain development. However, even though the identified mutations were more common in people with schizophrenia than in people without schizophrenia, they were identified in only about 20% of the people with schizophrenia.

CNV deletions such as 22q11.21, 15q13.3, and 1q21 (see **Figure 9.1** for how to decode these strings of letters and numbers) have been identified in reviews of GWAS on schizophrenia, and these studies meet the stringent replication requirements of modern-day genetics research (Rees, Walters, et al., 2014; Sullivan, Agrawal, et al., 2018; Tang & Gur, 2017). Consistent with evidence that genetic vulnerability is common across different disorders, many CNVs observed in schizophrenia are also observed in other disorders, including autism spectrum disorder and intellectual disability, suggesting that these CNVs are not specific to schizophrenia (Fromer, Pocklington, et al., 2013).

GWAS of the sequence of genes have also been conducted. These studies seek to identify single nucleotide polymorphisms (SNPs; see Chapter 2) that are associated with schizophrenia. SNP studies, like the familial high-risk and CNV studies, suggest that there may be a common genetic vulnerability for schizophrenia and bipolar disorder (Smeland, Bahrami, et al., 2020; Sullivan, Daly, & O'Donovan, 2012) and other disorders, such as autism spectrum disorder, depression, and ADHD (Anttila et al., 2018; Lam et al., 2019).

Two key methodological requirements for any GWAS are (1) very large sample sizes and (2) replication and rigorous statistical tests (see Chapter 4 for more on these topics). When one is looking at the entire human genome—over 20,000 genes—and then comparing groups of people with and without a psychological disorder, the odds of finding a difference between groups by chance alone are large unless the sample size is very big. To address the sample size challenge, the Psychiatric Genomics Consortium (PGC) formed in 2007. The PGC includes over 800 researchers from around the world who work together by combining individual samples into very large samples for GWAS.

In 2014, the Schizophrenia Working Group of the PGC conducted a GWAS with over 36,000 people with schizophrenia and over 110,00 people without schizophrenia. They

What do all the letters and numbers mean?

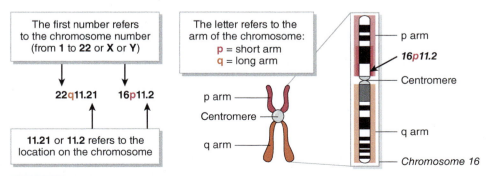

FIGURE 9.1 Decoding the language of genes.

identified 108 different genetic loci containing SNPs that were associated with schizophrenia (Ripke, Neale, et al., 2014). The statistical tests were very rigorous, and the researchers conducted replication studies within this very large sample. In 2022, this group, along with other collaborators from around the world, conducted an even larger GWAS with over 76,000 people with schizophrenia and over 240,000 without schizophrenia (Trubetskoy, Pardiñas, et al., 2022). They replicated the findings from 2014 and found even more loci associated with schizophrenia in this larger sample. That so many different locations were found supports the finding that schizophrenia is polygenic (involves many genes).

We can make three important points about GWAS findings:

1. Observed mutations are rare—CNVs account for less than 1% of genetic variance (Schwab & Wildenauer, 2013), and SNPs account for less than 25% of genetic variance (Ripke, Sanders, et al., 2011);

2. Only some people with these rare mutations have schizophrenia; and

3. The mutations are not specific to schizophrenia.

Does the fact that the genetic mutations are so rare mean that these researchers are on the wrong track in identifying genetic vulnerability to schizophrenia? Not necessarily. These findings confirm the genetic heterogeneity of schizophrenia and the idea that people with the same disorder (schizophrenia) may not necessarily have the same genetic factors contributing to the disorder. Current genetics research supports the idea that the genetic vulnerability to schizophrenia may be made up of many rare mutations.

The Role of Neurotransmitters

A great deal of research over the past decades has been devoted to evaluating different neurotransmitters to see what role they might play in the cause of schizophrenia. It has been challenging to pinpoint the ways in which neurotransmitters are involved in schizophrenia. This is in part because most neurotransmitter discoveries were based on finding out, quite serendipitously, that a medication alleviated the symptoms. Researchers then worked backward to identify how the medication was influencing neurotransmitters. Translating the way a medication works into the cause of schizophrenia, however, has not yielded solid evidence for neurotransmitters as causes, as we illustrate next with the story of the dopamine theory.

Dopamine Theory The theory that schizophrenia is related to excess activity of the neurotransmitter dopamine is based principally on the knowledge that drugs effective in treating schizophrenia reduce dopamine activity. Researchers have noted that antipsychotic drugs, in addition to being useful in treating some symptoms of schizophrenia, produce side effects resembling the symptoms of Parkinson's disease. Parkinson's disease is caused in part by low levels of dopamine in a particular area of the brain. Antipsychotic drugs fit into and thereby block a type of postsynaptic dopamine receptor called the D2 receptor (Seeman, 2013). Based on this knowledge about the action of the drugs that help people with schizophrenia, it was natural to conjecture that schizophrenia resulted from excess activity in dopamine.

However, as other studies progressed, this assumption turned out to be too simple to account for schizophrenia's wide range of symptoms (Scull, 2022). For example, an excess of dopamine activity appears to be related mainly to positive and disorganization symptoms, and antipsychotic medications help these symptoms by blocking dopamine receptors (Yilmaz, Zai, et al., 2012), thereby lowering dopamine activity. Evidence linking dopamine to the negative symptoms is less robust, with most research indicating a link between dopamine and avolition and anhedonia. Specifically, research in animals and people without schizophrenia has shown that dopamine in the brain region called the striatum is important for reward, anticipation, and motivation. In people with schizophrenia, anticipatory pleasure motivational deficits have been linked to problems in this brain region (Kring & Barch, 2014; Robison, Thakkar, & Diwadkar, 2020).

Later revisions to the theory suggest that interactions between stress and other parts of the brain, including the hippocampus and HPA axis (see Chapter 2), may trigger the excess release of dopamine (Howes & Kapur, 2009; Howes, McCutcheon, & Stone, 2015; Walker, Mittal, & Tessner, 2008). Because schizophrenia is a disorder with widespread symptoms covering perception, emotion, cognition, and social behavior, no single neurotransmitter can account for all of them. Thus, schizophrenia researchers cast a broader neurotransmitter net, moving away from an emphasis on dopamine.

Other Neurotransmitters   Research on other neurotransmitters has also not led to strong evidence for causal influences in schizophrenia. Instead, much of the research has shown how medications used to treat schizophrenia impact other neurotransmitters. As we discuss later, some drugs used in treating schizophrenia implicate serotonin because they block the serotonin receptor 5HT2 as well as dopamine D2 receptors.

Glutamate is another neurotransmitter that has been studied in schizophrenia (Javitt & Kantrowitz, 2022). Low levels of glutamate have been found in the cerebrospinal fluid of people with schizophrenia, and postmortem studies have revealed low levels of the enzyme needed to produce glutamate (Weickert, Fung, et al., 2013). The drugs PCP and ketamine can induce both positive and negative symptoms in people without schizophrenia by interfering with NMDA receptors that are part of the glutamate system. Brain-imaging studies have found evidence for decreased NMDA receptor activity (Pilowsky, Bressan, et al., 2006) and lower levels of glutamate (Marsman, van den Heuvel, et al., 2013) in the prefrontal cortex. Additional evidence suggests that cognitive deficits in schizophrenia supported by the prefrontal cortex, as well as symptoms of disorganization, may be connected to deficits involving NMDA (Howes, McCutcheon, & Stone, 2015; MacDonald & Chafee, 2006). Even if glutamate plays a role, medications targeting glutamate have thus far been only modestly effective (Egerton, Grace, et al., 2020).

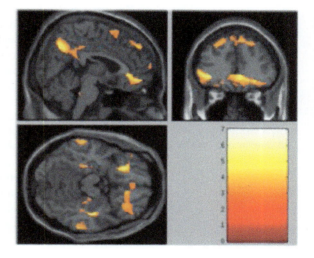

Brain Structure and Function   Because schizophrenia affects so many domains (thought, emotion, and behavior), it makes sense that a single brain region cannot account for all of schizophrenia's symptoms. Among the most well-replicated findings of brain abnormalities in schizophrenia are enlargement of the ventricles, reduced cortical thickness and other dysfunction in the prefrontal cortex and temporal cortex, as well as surrounding brain regions. Research has also identified problems in how different areas of the brain are connected to one another (Crossley, Mechelli, et al., 2016).

Enlarged Ventricles   As discussed in Chapter 2, the brain has four ventricles, which are spaces in the brain filled with cerebrospinal fluid. Having larger fluid-filled spaces implies a loss of brain cells. Meta-analyses of several neuroimaging studies have revealed that some people with schizophrenia, even very early in the course of the illness and across the course of the illness, have enlarged ventricles (Mendrek & Mancini-Marïe, 2016).

Further evidence concerning enlarged ventricles comes from a meta-analysis of 69 studies that included over 2,000 people with schizophrenia who had never taken antipsychotic medication (Haijma, Van Haren, et al., 2013). This is important because it helps to rule out the possibility that enlarged ventricles or other overall brain size reductions may be due to the side effects of medications.

Problems in the Cortex and Subcortical Regions of the Brain   The prefrontal cortex is known to play a role in behaviors such as speech, memory encoding, decision making, emotion, and goal-directed behavior, which are disrupted in schizophrenia. Brain imaging studies have shown reductions in gray matter and overall volume (size) in the prefrontal cortex (Goodkind, Eikhoff, et al., 2015; Guo, Ragland, & Carter, 2019; Gupta, Calhoun, et al., 2015; Ohtani, Levitt, et al., 2014; Ragland, Laird, et al., 2009) even in people early in the course of the

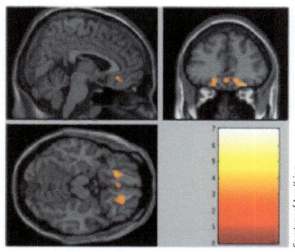

fMRI is used to assess brain function. These pictures show brain activation from an fMRI study that involved maintaining a pleasant emotional experience over a 12-second delay. The control group (top panel) showed greater activation in areas of the frontal cortex than did the group with schizophrenia (bottom panel).

Courtesy of Ann Kring

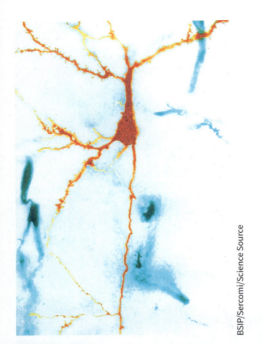

BSIP/Sercomi/Science Source

FIGURE 9.2 **Micrograph of a neuron showing dendrites. The bumps on the dendrites are dendritic spines, which receive inputs from other neurons. Having fewer dendritic spines may impair connections among neurons and may be a factor in schizophrenia.**

illness (Cannon, Chung, et al., 2015; Sun, Phillips, et al., 2009). In addition, a large meta-analysis has confirmed that the cortex of people with schizophrenia is thinner, particularly in the frontal and temporal regions (van Erp, Walton, et al., 2018). Unfortunately, antipsychotic medications may contribute to some of these issues (Ho, Andreasen, et al., 2011; Torres, Portela-Oliveira, et al., 2013).

People with schizophrenia perform more poorly than people without schizophrenia on neuropsychological tests designed to tap functions supported by the prefrontal region, including working memory, or the ability to hold bits of information in memory (Lesh, Niendam, et al., 2012), and there is some evidence that performance on some of these tests declines from before disorder onset to when people are in their late 30s (Meier, Caspi, et al., 2014).

Despite the reduced volume of the gray matter in the prefrontal cortex, the number of neurons in this area does not appear to be reduced. More detailed studies indicate that what is lost is called a *dendritic spine* (Cannon, 2015; Glausier & Lewis, 2013; McGlashan & Hoffman, 2000; Moyer, Shelton, & Sweet, 2015). Dendritic spines are small projections on the shafts of dendrites where nerve impulses are received from other neurons at the synapse (see **Figure 9.2**). The loss of these dendritic spines means that communication among neurons (i.e., functioning of the synapses) is disrupted, resulting in what some have termed a "disconnection syndrome." One possible result of the failure of neural systems to communicate could be the speech and behavioral disorganization seen in schizophrenia. Research has also linked these abnormalities in dendritic spines with CNVs identified in schizophrenia, discussed in the earlier section on genetic influences (Copf, 2016; Penzes, Cahill, et al., 2011).

Research has found that people with schizophrenia have structural and functional abnormalities in the temporal cortex, including areas such as the temporal gyrus, hippocampus, parts of the insula, fusiform gyrus, amygdala, and cingulate cortex. For example, research shows a reduction in cortical gray matter in temporal as well as frontal brain regions (Gupta et al., 2015) and reduced volume in the insula (Sheffield, Huang, et al., 2021), basal ganglia (e.g., the caudate nucleus), hippocampus, and amygdala (Glahn, Laird, et al., 2008; Mathew, Gardin, et al., 2014). A meta-analysis of MRI studies conducted with over 2,000 people with schizophrenia concluded that the volume of the hippocampus was significantly reduced compared to that of people without schizophrenia (van Erp, Hibar, et al., 2016). This large meta-analysis also found smaller volumes in other subcortical brain regions, including the amygdala, thalamus, and basal ganglia.

An additional interesting piece of evidence regarding the hippocampus comes from a meta-analysis of nine studies assessing the brain volume of more than 400 first-degree relatives of people with schizophrenia and more than 600 first-degree relatives of people without schizophrenia (Boos, Aleman, et al., 2007). Relatives of people with schizophrenia had smaller hippocampal volumes than relatives of people without schizophrenia. These findings suggest that reduced hippocampal volume in people with schizophrenia may reflect a combination of genetic and environmental factors.

What makes these findings about the hippocampus all the more intriguing is the fact that the hypothalamic-pituitary-adrenal (HPA) axis is closely connected to this area of the brain. Chronic stress is associated with reductions in hippocampal volume in other disorders, such as posttraumatic stress disorder (see Chapter 7). Although people with schizophrenia do not necessarily experience more stress than people without schizophrenia, they may be more reactive to stress. Other evidence indicates that the HPA axis is disrupted in schizophrenia, particularly very early in the course of the disorder (Walker, Mittal, & Tessner, 2008; Walker, Trotman, et al., 2013). Taken together, stress reactivity and a disrupted HPA axis likely contribute to the reductions in hippocampal volume observed in people with schizophrenia (Walker, Mittal, & Tessner, 2008).

Connectivity in the Brain

As we discussed in Chapter 2, current neuroimaging methods measure how different areas of the brain are connected to each other. A meta-analysis of over 50 studies found less connectivity within and between brain networks in schizophrenia, further demonstrating the widespread brain dysfunction in schizophrenia (Dong, Wang, et al., 2018). Brain connectivity research in schizophrenia has also revealed that there is less connectivity between brain networks, including the frontoparietal and default-mode networks, and this diminished connectivity is correlated with poor performance on cognitive tests (Unschuld, Buchholz, et al., 2014) and negative symptoms (Brady, Gonsalvez, et al., 2019). Research has also found diminished connectivity among healthy relatives of people with schizophrenia, suggesting that diminished connectivity might be part of the genetic vulnerability for schizophrenia (Collin, Kahn, et al., 2014; Unschuld et al., 2014).

Brain-imaging studies using fMRI can demonstrate that symptoms or behaviors are correlated with brain activity, but they cannot easily demonstrate causation. Brain stimulation methods, such as rTMS, can come closer to demonstrating causation. Recall from Chapter 3 that rTMS allows researchers to stimulate particular areas of the brain to see the resulting impact on behavior. In one study, researchers stimulated parts of the brain in a prefrontal cortex network and showed that doing so increased brain connectivity and decreased negative symptoms (Brady et al., 2019). This finding suggests that interventions that increase connectivity in these regions, whether through rTMS, medication, or psychosocial treatments, may reduce negative symptoms. Other studies of brain connectivity in schizophrenia have found measures of connectivity to be helpful in predicting who will respond well to antipsychotic medication treatment. In one study, researchers found that greater connectivity between the striatum, an area of the brain rich in dopamine, and other areas of the brain predicted a greater reduction in symptoms early in the course of a hospital stay (Sarpal, Argyelan, et al., 2016).

Environmental Factors Influencing the Developing Brain

Several different environmental factors have been studied as possible contributing factors to schizophrenia (van Os, Kenis, & Rutten, 2010). A possible cause of some of the observed brain abnormalities in schizophrenia is damage during gestation or birth. Many studies have shown high rates of delivery complications in people with schizophrenia (Davies, Segre, et al., 2020); such complications could have resulted in a reduced supply of oxygen to the brain, resulting in loss of cortical gray matter (Cannon, van Erp, et al., 2002). These obstetrical complications do not raise the risk for schizophrenia in everyone who experiences them. Rather, the risk for schizophrenia is increased in those who experience complications and have a genetic vulnerability (Mittall, Ellman, & Cannon, 2008; Paquin, Lapierre, et al., 2021).

Additional research suggests that maternal infections during pregnancy are associated with greater risk of the children developing schizophrenia when they become adults (Brown & Derkits, 2010). For example, one study found that maternal exposure to the parasite *Toxoplasma gondii* was associated with a nearly 2.5 times greater risk of schizophrenia among the mothers' children when they became adults (Brown, Schaefer, et al., 2005; Pedersen, Stevens, et al., 2011). This is a common parasite, carried by many people with no ill effects. Stress during pregnancy has also been shown to increase the risk of offspring developing schizophrenia (Fineberg, Ellman, et al., 2016).

If, as the findings we have just reviewed suggest, the development of the brains of people with schizophrenia go awry very early, why does the disorder begin many years later, in adolescence or early adulthood? The prefrontal cortex is a brain structure that matures late, typically in adolescence or early adulthood. Thus, a problem in this area, even one that begins early in the course of development, may not show itself in the person's behavior until the period of development when the prefrontal cortex begins to play a larger role in behavior (Weinberger, 1987). Notably, dopamine activity peaks in adolescence, which may further set the stage for the onset of schizophrenia symptoms (Walker, Mittal, & Tessner, 2008). Adolescence is also typically a developmental period that is fraught with stress. Recall from our discussion in Chapter 2 that stress activates the HPA axis, causing cortisol to be secreted. Research has demonstrated that cortisol increases dopamine activity, perhaps increasing the likelihood of developing schizophrenia symptoms (Pruessner, Cullen, et al., 2017).

Another proposed explanation is that the development of symptoms in adolescence could reflect a loss of synapses due to excessive pruning, the elimination of synaptic connections (Cannon, 2015). Pruning is a normal part of brain development that occurs at different rates in different areas of the brain. It is mostly complete in sensory areas by about age 2 but continues in the prefrontal cortex until mid-adolescence. If too extensive, pruning may result in the loss of necessary communication among neurons (McGlashan & Hoffman, 2000; Sekar, Bialas, et al., 2016).

An additional environmental factor that has been studied as a risk factor for schizophrenia among adolescents is cannabis (marijuana) use. Among people already diagnosed with schizophrenia, cannabis use is associated with a worsening of symptoms (Foti, Kotov, et al., 2010). But does cannabis use contribute to the onset of schizophrenia? A longitudinal study examining the prospective relationship between cannabis use in adolescence and the onset of schizophrenia in adolescence or adulthood indicated that the risk of developing schizophrenia symptoms was greater among those who used cannabis than among those who did not (Arseneault, Cannon, et al., 2002), and meta-analyses of both cross-sectional and longitudinal studies show that cannabis use is associated with increased risk for schizophrenia or psychosis symptoms (Hasan, Keller, et al., 2020; Marconi, Di Forti, et al., 2016; Moore, Zammit, et al., 2007). Furthermore, more frequent use, higher-potency cannabis, and using more over time are associated with greater risk (Di Forti, Sallis, et al., 2013; Kelley, Wan, et al., 2016). However, recall from Chapter 4 that correlation does not mean causation. Other studies suggest that the linkage between cannabis use and risk of developing schizophrenia is observed only among those who are genetically vulnerable to schizophrenia (Aas, Melle, et al., 2018).

Psychological Influences

People with schizophrenia do not appear to experience more stress in daily life than people without schizophrenia (Phillips, Francey, et al., 2007; Walker, Mittal, & Tessner, 2008). However, people with the disorder appear to be very reactive to the stressors we all encounter in daily living. In one study, people with psychotic disorders (92% with schizophrenia), their first-degree relatives, and people without any psychiatric disorder participated in a 6-day ecological momentary assessment study in which they recorded stress and mood several times each day. Daily life stress predicted greater decreases in positive moods in both people with schizophrenia and their relatives compared with controls. Stress also predicted greater increases in negative moods in the people with schizophrenia compared with both relatives and controls (Myin-Germeys, van Os, et al., 2001). Thus, people with schizophrenia were particularly vulnerable to daily stress. Research also shows that, as with many of the disorders we have discussed in this book, increases in life stress increase the likelihood of a relapse (Walker, Mittal, & Tessner, 2008).

Additional research on psychological influences in the development and relapse of schizophrenia has focused on sociocultural factors, the family, and developmental factors.

Sociocultural Influences: Poverty, Trauma, Urbanicity, and Migration

Four sociocultural influences that have been associated with schizophrenia are poverty (socioeconomic status), trauma, urbanicity (living in cities), and migration (moving from one country to another). These three variables can be related to one another, but each appears to be independently associated with a higher risk of developing schizophrenia.

For many years, we have known that the highest rates of schizophrenia are found in people with the highest poverty levels (Hollingshead & Redlich, 1958; Kohn, 1968). The correlation between poverty and schizophrenia is consistent but difficult to interpret in causal terms. Does the stress associated with poverty—such as low education, limited opportunities, and stigma from others of high status—contribute to the development of schizophrenia? Or is it the case that during the course of their developing illness, people with schizophrenia drift into low income neighborhoods because their illness impairs their earning power and they cannot afford to live elsewhere? Though it is difficult to sort out these two possibilities, the bulk of the evidence supports the notion that people with schizophrenia drift into poor neighborhoods as a consequence of the illness (Dohrenwend, Levav, et al., 1992).

As we discussed in Chapter 2, trauma or maltreatment in childhood, whether in the form of physical abuse, sexual abuse, or neglect, is a risk factor for nearly all psychological disorders (Caspi & Moffitt, 2018). This is true for schizophrenia. In a comprehensive review of the literature, Gibson and colleagues (2016) present evidence that childhood maltreatment, as well as other traumatic life events, increases the risk for schizophrenia and psychotic disorders.

Note, however, that although trauma interacts with genetic vulnerability and neurobiological factors to increase the risk, experiencing trauma does not necessarily mean someone will develop schizophrenia or any other disorder.

Another sociocultural influence that has been linked with schizophrenia is urbanicity. That is, the likelihood of developing schizophrenia is higher for people living in urban areas (i.e., densely populated cities) than for those in rural areas. A meta-analysis of 20 studies found that risk for developing schizophrenia was nearly three times higher among people living in urban areas than among those living in rural areas (March, Hatch, et al., 2008). These effects were not the result of drift to urban areas in adolescence or adulthood (just prior to the onset of schizophrenia) but rather showed that people born and raised in urban areas had a greater risk of developing schizophrenia in adulthood. A separate recent meta-analysis confirmed these findings: The more the urbanicity, the greater the incidence of schizophrenia (Vassos, Pedersen, et al., 2012).

What about living in densely populated cities might increase the risk for developing schizophrenia? The answer to this question is not fully known, but researchers have speculated that living in such areas may be more stressful or that exposure to infection or other environmental toxins may be more likely than in less densely populated areas (Tost, Champagne, & Meyer-Lindenberg, 2015). Additional research finds that the relationship between urbanicity and schizophrenia in the United States may have to do with poverty or air pollution. That is, in the United States, the link between urbanicity and schizophrenia was explained in part by higher air pollution and higher poverty (Bakolis, Mammoud, et al., 2021; Saxena & Dodell-Feder, 2022).

A final sociocultural influence that is associated with a greater risk of developing schizophrenia is migration. In this context, *migration* refers to people who were born in one country and moved to another (first-generation migrant) or a person whose parents (one or both) were born in a different country (second-generation migrant). A meta-analysis of 18 studies found that the risk for developing schizophrenia was three times higher among first-generation migrants and four times higher among second-generation migrants than among people who did not migrate to a different country (Cantor-Graae & Seleten, 2005). The risk was particularly high for people of color, which may reflect a bias in diagnostic practices, exposure to greater stress, less access to treatment, or, more likely, some combination of these factors (Kirkbride, Barker, et al., 2008).

As with genetic and neuroscience influences, environmental, psychological, and sociocultural influences do not work on their own. Rather, they are related to one another and these in turn influence the developing brain and gene expression (Anglin, 2023; Anglin, et al., 2021).

Developmental Factors   What are people who develop schizophrenia like before their symptoms begin? Studies have found that adults with schizophrenia scored lower on IQ and other cognitive tests as children than did adults without schizophrenia (Woodberry, Giuliano, & Seidman, 2008). In one very clever study, Elaine Walker and colleagues analyzed the home movies of children who later developed schizophrenia. The movies were made as part of typical family life and were made before the onset of schizophrenia (Walker, Davis, & Savoie, 1994; Walker, Grimes, et al., 1993). Compared with their siblings who did not later develop schizophrenia, the children who developed schizophrenia as young adults showed poorer motor skills and more expressions of negative emotions.

As intriguing as these findings are, these studies were not necessarily designed with the intention of predicting the development of schizophrenia from childhood behavior. Rather, they began with an adult sample of people with schizophrenia and then looked back at records and data collected from their childhoods to see if there were characteristics that distinguished them as young children.

Prospective studies begin with a sample of people with schizophrenia or at risk for developing it and follow them forward in time. One prospective study identified childhood characteristics that were associated with the development of schizophrenia in early adulthood (Reichenberg, Avshalom, et al., 2010). In this study, a large sample of people from Dunedin, New Zealand, were assessed several times between the ages of 7 and 32. IQ tests were administered at ages 7, 9, 11, and 13; diagnostic

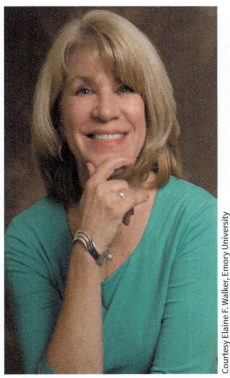

Elaine Walker has conducted many studies on the development of schizophrenia.

Courtesy Elaine F. Walker, Emory University

assessments were conducted at ages 21, 26, and 32. The researchers found that lower scores on the IQ test in childhood predicted the onset of schizophrenia in young adulthood, even after they controlled for low socioeconomic status (which is associated with lower IQ scores; see Chapter 3). Thus, children who developed schizophrenia as adults had signs of a cognitive deficit at age 7 that remained stable through adolescence.

Another prospective study assessed several cognitive abilities in a sample of over 100 people when they were first diagnosed with schizophrenia and then again 10 years later (Zanelli, Mollan, et al., 2019). Researchers found that IQ scores continued to decline over the 10-year period. Performance on other neuropsychological tests (see Chapter 3) assessing verbal learning and memory also declined. However, performance on other tests, including tests of executive functioning, processing speed, and visuospatial skills, did not decline. These findings suggest that although it can be helpful to intervene early for some cognitive skills, receiving a diagnosis of schizophrenia does not mean that a person will have an inevitable and widespread decline in cognitive functioning.

Another type of prospective study is a **clinical high-risk study**. As we noted earlier, a clinical high-risk study identifies people with early, attenuated signs of schizophrenia, most often milder forms of hallucinations, delusions, or disorganization that nonetheless cause impairment (see Focus on Discovery 9.2). One such study followed people ages 14 to 30 in Australia who were referred to a mental health clinic in the mid-1990s (Yung, McGorry, et al., 1995). None of the participants had schizophrenia when they entered the study, but many later exhibited varying degrees of schizophrenia symptoms, and some, but not all, had a biological relative with a psychotic disorder. These participants were deemed to be at "ultra-high risk" of developing schizophrenia or psychotic disorders. Over about the next 10 years, 41 of the original 104 participants developed some type of psychotic disorder (Yung, Phillips, et al., 2004).

A similar longitudinal study, the North American Prodrome Longitudinal Study (NAPLS), and its follow-ups (NAPLS-2, NAPLS-3) were carried out at eight different centers in the United States and Canada. Participants were identified as clinical high risk based on the Structured Interview for Prodromal Syndromes (see Focus on Discovery 9.2). In the NAPLS study, 82 of the 291 clinical high-risk (CHR) participants who also had a family history of schizophrenia (familial high risk, or FHR) developed schizophrenia or some type of psychotic disorder (Cannon, Cadenhead, et al., 2008). The researchers identified several factors that predicted a greater likelihood of developing a psychotic disorder, including having a biological relative with schizophrenia, a recent decline in functioning, high levels of positive symptoms, and high levels of social impairment. Other findings from the NAPLS sample are that social and academic difficulties in childhood predicted conversion to a psychotic disorder (Tarbox, Addington, et al., 2013).

The NAPLS-2 and NAPLS-3 studies were larger than the first study and built on its findings (Addington, Cadenhead, et al., 2012; Addington, Liu, et al., 2020). In NAPLS-2, impaired cognition—particularly attention and working memory, which are associated with the prefrontal cortex—was found to be impaired among those identified as clinical high-risk (Seidman, Shapiro, et al., 2016). The researchers developed a risk calculator to help determine who among those at high risk would go on to develop schizophrenia (Cannon, Yu, et al., 2016). Based on clinical symptoms, cognitive functioning, and other individual characteristics, the risk calculator identifies people at high risk who develop schizophrenia with about the same accuracy as risk calculators that predict who will develop cardiovascular disease. The risk calculator has been used successfully in other samples that were not part of NAPLS (Carrion, Cornblatt, et al., 2016; Osborne & Mittal, 2019), and it has also predicted a positive response to family treatment (Worthington, Miklowitz, et al., 2020).

Quick Summary

Given the complexity of the disorder, several causal factors likely contribute to schizophrenia. The genetic evidence is strong, with much of it coming from family, twin, and adoption studies. Familial high-risk studies have found that children with a biological parent with schizophrenia are more likely to develop adult psychopathology, including schizophrenia, and have difficulties with attention and motor control, among other things. Molecular genetics studies include candidate gene studies and GWAS.

GWAS have pointed to rare mutations, including copy number variations (CNVs) and single nucleotide polymorphisms (SNPs) that are associated with genetic vulnerability to schizophrenia, though some of these findings are not specific to schizophrenia.

Neurotransmitters have been studied schizophrenia, and we know that medications used to treat schizophrenia influence neurotransmitters including dopamine, serotonin, and glutamate. However, there is no solid evidence that these neurotransmitters cause schizophrenia. Many different brain areas have been implicated in schizophrenia. One of the most widely replicated findings involves enlarged ventricles. Other research supports the role of the prefrontal cortex, the temporal cortex, and subcortical brain areas such as the hippocampus. Brain networks and limited connectivity between brain regions are also disrupted in schizophrenia.

Environmental factors, such as obstetric complications and prenatal infections, may impact the developing brain and increase the risk of schizophrenia. Cannabis use among adolescents has been associated with greater risk of schizophrenia, particularly among those who are genetically vulnerable to the disorder.

Research has examined the role of sociocultural risk factors, including poverty, trauma, urbanicity, and migration. This work supports the idea that people with schizophrenia may drift into poverty as the illness develops, but that being born and raised in a densely populated urban area is a distinct risk factor. Furthermore, people who were born in one country but move to another are at greater risk for schizophrenia, particularly if they are people of color.

Developmental studies that look back at the childhood records of adults with schizophrenia have found that adults with schizophrenia scored lower on cognitive tests, including an IQ test. Other studies found that adults who later developed schizophrenia expressed more negative emotion and had poor motor skills as children. A prospective study confirmed that lower IQ in childhood is a predictor of the later onset of schizophrenia and that the IQ deficits are stable across childhood. Clinical high-risk studies identify people who are showing early signs of schizophrenia.

9.2 Check Your Knowledge

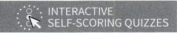
INTERACTIVE
SELF-SCORING QUIZZES

(Answers are at the end of the chapter.)
Answer the following questions.

1. What types of studies do not do a very good job of evaluating genetic and environmental effects in schizophrenia?
2. _____ genetic studies find rare mutations in schizophrenia and other psychological disorders, including _____ and _____.
3. Some studies showing that the _____ area of the brain is disrupted in schizophrenia also show that people with schizophrenia do poorly on tasks that rely on this area, such as planning and problem solving.
4. What are four sociocultural risk factors for schizophrenia?

Treatment of Schizophrenia

Treatments for schizophrenia may include a combination of short-term hospital stays (during the acute phases of the illness), medication, and psychosocial treatments.

Medications

The most common type of medication used to treat schizophrenia is collectively called **antipsychotic drugs** (also referred to as *neuroleptics* because they produce side effects similar to the symptoms of a neurological disease). **Focus on Discovery 9.3** presents a brief history of the development of these drugs. As we will see, medications have their own drawbacks.

The most recent clinical practice guideline from the American Psychiatric Association calls for treatment of schizophrenia with an antipsychotic medication and close, careful

Focus on Discovery 9.3

Stumbling Toward a Cure: The Development of Antipsychotic Medications

One of the more frequently prescribed antipsychotic drugs, phenothiazine, was first produced by a German chemist in the late 19th century. But it was not until the discovery of the antihistamines, which are derived from phenothiazine, in the 1940s that phenothiazines received much attention.

Reaching beyond the use of antihistamines to treat the common cold and asthma, the French surgeon Henri Laborit pioneered their use to reduce surgical shock. He noticed that they made his patients somewhat sleepy and less fearful about the impending operation. Laborit's work encouraged pharmaceutical companies to reexamine antihistamines in light of their tranquilizing effects. Shortly thereafter, the French chemist Paul Charpentier prepared a new phenothiazine derivative, which he called chlorpromazine. This drug proved very effective in calming people with schizophrenia. Phenothiazines derive their therapeutic properties by blocking dopamine receptors in the brain, thus reducing the influence of dopamine on thought, emotion, and behavior.

Chlorpromazine (trade name Thorazine) was first used therapeutically in the United States in 1954 and rapidly became the preferred treatment for schizophrenia. By 1970, more than 85% of all people in treatment were receiving chlorpromazine or another phenothiazine.

monitoring for side effects. This guideline also recommends nonmedication treatments, which we discuss later. The practice guideline recommends continued treatment with antipsychotic medications even if symptoms have been reduced (American Psychiatric Association [APA], 2020). That is, people who respond positively to the antipsychotics are typically kept on so-called maintenance doses of the drug, just enough to continue the therapeutic effect.

The commonly reported side effects of all antipsychotics include sedation, dizziness, blurred vision, restlessness, and sexual dysfunction. In addition, some particularly disturbing side effects, termed *extrapyramidal side effects*, resemble the symptoms of Parkinson's disease. People taking antipsychotics may develop tremors of the fingers, a shuffling gait, and drooling. Other side effects can include dystonia, a state of muscular rigidity, and dyskinesia, an abnormal motion of voluntary and involuntary muscles, producing chewing movements as well as other movements of the lips, fingers, and legs. Another side effect is akathisia, an inability to remain still; some people on antipsychotics pace constantly and fidget.

In a rare muscular disturbance called *tardive dyskinesia*, the mouth muscles involuntarily make sucking, lip-smacking, and chin-wagging motions. In more severe cases, the whole body can be subject to involuntary motor movements.

We present examples and descriptions of side effects in Table 9.5. Because of these serious side effects, treatment providers must closely and continuously assess for these and adjust dosages or medication types accordingly.

First-Generation Antipsychotic Drugs and Their Side Effects
The first-generation antipsychotic drugs are those broad classes of medications that were the first to be discovered. See Table 9.6 for a summary of major drugs used to treat schizophrenia. These drugs can reduce the positive and disorganization symptoms of schizophrenia but have little or no effect on the negative symptoms. Despite the enthusiasm with which these drugs are prescribed, they are not a cure. About 30% of people with schizophrenia do not respond favorably to the first-generation antipsychotics, about half the people who take any antipsychotic drug quit after 1 year, and up to three-quarters quit before 2 years because the side effects are so unpleasant (Lieberman, Stroup, et al., 2005).

Second-Generation Antipsychotic Drugs and Their Side Effects
In the decades following the introduction of the first-generation antipsychotic drugs, there was little interest in developing new drugs to treat schizophrenia. Nevertheless, it was clear that the existing drugs did not help everyone, and they produced troubling side effects.

Drug companies thus began to search for other drugs that might be more effective than first-generation antipsychotics. These drugs are referred to as the second-generation antipsychotic drugs because their mechanism of action is not like that of the first-generation antipsychotic medications. Examples are shown in Table 9.6. Although the hope was that these newer drugs would be more effective and have fewer side effects, two decades of research have failed to demonstrate a strong advantage for second-generation drugs. And sadly, they have their own unpleasant side effects.

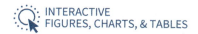
INTERACTIVE
FIGURES, CHARTS, & TABLES

TABLE 9.5   **Side Effects Associated with First- and Second-Generation Antipsychotic Drugs**

Side Effect	First-Generation Drugs	Second-Generation Drugs
Extrapyramidal signs	✓	✓
Drowsiness/sedation/fatigue	✓	✓
Blurred vision	✓	✓
Weight gain		✓
Restlessness	✓	
Dizziness		✓
Sexual dysfunction	✓	
Dry mouth	✓	
Tachycardia		✓
Constipation	✓	✓
Nausea		✓
Insomnia		✓
Headache		✓
Urinary incontinence		✓

TABLE 9.6   **Summary of Major Drugs Used in Treating Schizophrenia**

Drug Category	Generic Name	Trade Name
First-generation drugs	chlorpromazine	Thorazine
	fluphenazine	Prolixin
	haloperidol	Haldol
	thiothixene	Navane
	trifluoperazine	Stelazine
Second-generation drugs	clozapine	Clozaril
	aripiprazole	Abilify
	olanzapine	Zyprexa
	risperidone	Risperdal
	ziprasidone	Geodon
	quetiapine	Seroquel

In a landmark randomized controlled clinical trial (called Clinical Antipsychotic Trials of Intervention Effectiveness, or CATIE), researchers compared four second-generation drugs (olanzapine, risperidone, ziprasidone, and quetiapine) and one first-generation drug (perphenazine) with one another (Lieberman et al., 2005). Close to 1,500 people from all over the United States were in the study. What set this study apart from other studies was that it was not sponsored by one of the drug companies that make the drugs. Among the many findings from this study, three stand out. First, the second-generation drugs were not more effective than the older, first-generation drugs. Second, the second-generation drugs did not produce fewer unpleasant side effects. And third, nearly three-quarters of the people stopped taking the medications before the 18 months of the study design had ended.

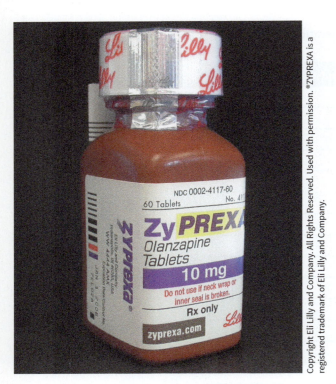

Second-generation antipsychotic drugs such as olanzapine may have different side effects than first-generation antipsychotic drugs, but they still have side effects.

These results have been confirmed in later meta-analyses of randomized controlled trials. In a large meta-analysis of over 400 studies with over 50,000 people compared the efficacy and side effect profiles of 32 different first- and second-generation medications (Huhn, Nikolakopoulou, et al., 2019). All but six of the drugs did a better job than a placebo of reducing symptoms, and there was little difference between the drugs in terms of how effective they were at reducing symptoms. The greatest effect was on positive and disorganization symptoms. Medications, whether first or second generation, are not very effective for negative symptoms (Fusar-Poli, Papanastasiou, et al., 2015). The side-effect profiles of the first- and second-generation medications were different, but all had unpleasant side effects.

One of the most common side effects of the second-generation antipsychotics is weight gain (Huhn et al., 2019; Wu, Siafis, et al., 2022). In addition to being unpleasant, weight gain is associated with other serious health problems, such as increased cholesterol levels and increases in blood glucose, collectively referred to as "metabolic syndrome" which can cause cardiovascular disease and type 2 diabetes (Correll, Solmi, et al., 2017; Pillinger, McCutcheon, et al., 2020; Vancampfort, Stubbs, et al., 2015). For example, clozapine and olanzapine have been related to the development of type 2 diabetes (Leslie & Rosenheck, 2004). By 2007, the drug company that produces olanzapine, Eli Lilly, had settled more than 25,000 lawsuits, paying out over $1.2 billion to people taking the drug. The company was sued for failing to adequately warn people of these serious side effects. The drug's label now contains warnings about possible side effects, including weight gain and elevated blood sugar and cholesterol levels.

Another disturbing aspect of the second-generation antipsychotic medications is that Black people do not tend to receive them. At least three different studies have found that Black people were more likely to be prescribed first-generation than second-generation antipsychotic medications (Kreyenbuhl, Zito, et al., 2003; Robinson, Schooler, et al., 2014; Valenti, Narendran, & Pristach, 2003). This is unfortunate for many reasons, but particularly because Black people may experience more side effects than White people in response to the first-generation medications (Frackiewicz, Sramek, et al., 1997). More broadly, these results echo the findings of the Surgeon General's supplement to the landmark report on mental health in 2001, which elucidated several disparities in mental health treatment among members of racial and ethnic minority groups (U.S. Department of Health and Human Services, 2001).

At this point in time, antipsychotic drugs are the most commonly used treatment for schizophrenia. A review of 60 years' worth of clinical trials with these drugs found that just over half of the people with schizophrenia had a minimally better response to the drug than to a placebo, but only 23% had a good response (Leucht, Leucht, et al., 2017). Thus, even though these drugs work better than a placebo, they do not work well for many people. Furthermore, the mixed success of second-generation antipsychotic drugs has stimulated a continuing effort to find new and more effective drug therapies for schizophrenia. A newer drug called Lumateperone appears to be effective based on three clinical trials. It works on multiple neurotransmitter systems (dopamine, glutamate, and serotonin) and may have fewer side effects (Kane, Durgam, et al., 2021). Even if the side effects are less, however, the need for additional effective treatments for schizophrenia remains.

Other Biological Treatments   Newer treatments capitalize on developments in brain stimulation methods such as tDCS (transcranial direct current stimulation; see Chapter 3). Treatment with tDCS involves placing a small device on the head that contains electrodes that apply a weak current (2 milliamps or mA) for several minutes. A person receives between 5 and 15 sessions over days or weeks that are about 20 minutes each. This noninvasive brain stimulation is targeted to the frontal and temporal cortex.

Small meta-analyses of randomized controlled clinical trials using tDCS found that this method of stimulating the frontal/temporal regions of the brain reduced the severity of auditory hallucinations and this effect lasted for at least 3 months post-treatment (Yang, Fang, et al., 2019). tDCS also helped to alleviate negative symptoms, though the reason why this was effective is a topic of further investigation (Cheng, Louie, et al., 2020).

Psychological Treatments

The limits of antipsychotic medications have spurred efforts to develop psychosocial treatments that can be used in addition to the medications. Indeed, the current APA practice guideline for schizophrenia (APA, 2020) and the current treatment recommendations compiled by the schizophrenia Patient Outcomes Research Team (PORT) include psychosocial interventions in addition to medications (Kreyenbuhl, Buchanan, et al., 2010). Both sets of recommendations are based on extensive reviews of treatment research recommendations and include different types of psychosocial treatments. Several psychosocial interventions, including skills training, cognitive behavior therapy, and family-based treatments, have a solid evidence base to support their use as an adjunctive treatment to medications (Dixon, Dickerson, et al., 2010; McDonagh, Dana, et al., 2022). In addition, several psychological treatments have been adapted for different cultural groups (Paul, Maietta, & Allen, 2020).

See **Read More About It 9.3** for another example of a successful combination treatment approach.

Social Skills Training   Social skills training is
designed to teach people with schizophrenia how to successfully manage a wide variety of interpersonal situations—discussing their medications with their psychiatrist, ordering meals in a restaurant, filling out job applications, interviewing for jobs, saying no to drug dealers on the street, reading bus schedules. Most of us take these skills for granted and give little thought to them in our daily lives, but people with schizophrenia cannot consider them a given—they need to work hard to acquire or reacquire such skills (Heinssen, Liberman, & Kopelowicz, 2000; Liberman, Eckman, et al., 2000). Social skills training typically involves role-playing and other group exercises to practice skills, both in a therapy group and in actual social situations.

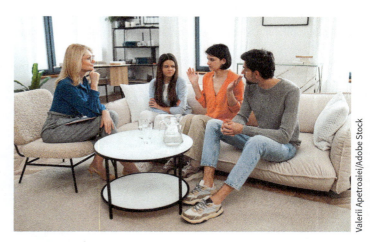

Family therapy can help educate people with schizophrenia and their families about schizophrenia and reduce expressed emotion.

Research has shown that social skills training can help people with schizophrenia achieve fewer relapses, better social functioning, and a higher quality of life (Almerie, Okba al Marhi, et al., 2015; Kopelowicz, Liberman, & Zarate, 2006; Kurtz & Mueser, 2008). Social skills training is usually a component of treatments for schizophrenia that go beyond the use of medications alone, including family therapies for lowering expressed emotion, which we discuss next. Social skills training that included family therapy was found to be more effective than treatment as usual (medication plus a 20-minute monthly meeting with a psychiatrist) in a randomized controlled trial conducted in Mexico (Valencia, Racon, et al., 2007). There is some evidence that social skills training may also be effective in reducing negative symptoms (Elis, Caponigro, & Kring, 2013).

Family Therapies   Many people with schizophrenia
live with their families. Although families do not cause schizophrenia, they can have an impact on recovery and relapse. In a pioneering study conducted in London, researchers interviewed families of people with schizophrenia and rated three characteristics—critical comments,

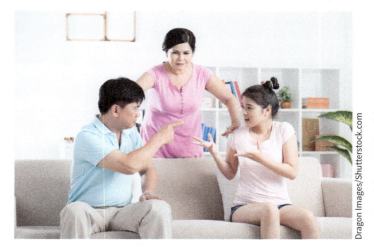

Expressed emotion, which includes hostility, critical comments, and emotional overinvolvement, has been linked with relapse in schizophrenia.

Read More About It 9.3

The Center Cannot Hold: My Journey Through Madness

A heartening example of one woman's struggles with and triumphs over schizophrenia is found in the 2007 book *The Center Cannot Hold: My Journey Through Madness*. This book was written by Elyn Saks, an endowed professor of law at the University of Southern California, who also happens to have schizophrenia (Saks, 2007). In the book, she describes her lifelong experience with this illness. Prior to the publication of the book, only a few of Professor Saks's close friends even knew that she had schizophrenia. Why did she keep it a secret? Certainly, stigma is part of the reason. As we have discussed throughout this book, stigma toward people with psychological disorders is very much alive in the 21st century and can have seriously negative consequences for people with disorders such as schizophrenia.

What makes Saks's life story particularly encouraging is that she has achieved exceptional professional and personal success in her life despite having such a serious psychological disorder. She grew up in a loving and supportive family; earned a bachelor's degree from Vanderbilt University, graduating as her class valedictorian; received a prestigious Marshall fellowship to study philosophy at Oxford in the United Kingdom; graduated from Yale Law School as editor of the prestigious *Yale Law Review*; and is a tenured professor of law at a major university. How did she do it?

She believes that a combination of treatments (including psychoanalysis and medications), social support from family and friends, hard work, and acknowledgment of the seriousness of her illness have all helped her cope with schizophrenia and its sometimes unpredictable and frightening symptoms. Although psychoanalysis does not have a good deal of empirical support for its efficacy with schizophrenia, it was and remains a central part of Saks's treatment regimen. Thus, even though some treatments may not be effective for a group of people, they can nonetheless be beneficial for individuals. One characteristic that appears to have been helpful for Saks, from her early days in psychoanalysis as a Marshall scholar at Oxford University until the present, has been her ability to "be psychotic" when she is with her psychoanalyst. So much of her energy was spent trying to hide her symptoms and keep them from interfering with her life; psychoanalysis became a safe place

for her to bring these symptoms more fully out into the open. The different analysts she has had over the years were also among the chief proponents of adding antipsychotic medication to her treatment, something that Professor Saks resisted for many years. Having the unwavering support of close friends and her husband has also been a tremendous help, particularly during her more symptomatic periods. Her loved ones would not turn and run the other way when she was psychotic. Instead, they would support her and help her get additional treatment if it was needed.

Saks still experiences symptoms, sometimes every day. Her symptoms include paranoid delusions, which she describes as very frightening (e.g., believing that her thoughts have killed people). She also experiences disorganization symptoms, which she eloquently describes in the book:

> *Consciousness gradually loses its coherence. One's center gives way. The center cannot hold. The "me" becomes a haze, and the solid center from which one experiences reality breaks up like a bad radio signal. There is no longer a sturdy vantage point from which to look out, take things in, assess what's happening. No core holds things together, providing the lens through which to see the world, to make judgments and comprehend risk.*
>
> (Saks, 2007, p. 13)

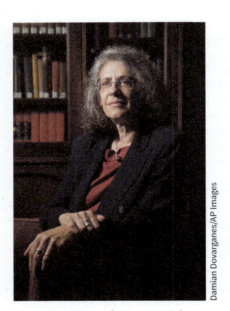

Damian Dovarganes/AP Images

Elyn Saks, a law professor at USC, has schizophrenia.

Even though she still experiences symptoms, she has come to terms with the fact that schizophrenia is a part of her life. Would she prefer not to have the illness? Sure. But she recognizes that she has a wonderful life filled with friends, loved ones, and meaningful work. She is not defined by her illness, and she importantly notes that "the humanity we all share is more important than the mental illness we may not" (Saks, 2007, p. 336). Her life is an inspiration to all, not just those with psychological disorders. Her story reminds us that life is difficult, more so for some than for others, but that it can be lived—and lived to the fullest.

hostility, and emotional overinvolvement (Brown, Bone, et al., 1966). Combining these three characteristics make up what is called **expressed emotion (EE)**. Families in the original study were divided into two groups: those revealing a great deal of expressed emotion (high-EE families) and those revealing little (low-EE families). At the end of the follow-up period, only 10% of the people returning to low-EE homes had relapsed, but 58% of the people returning to high-EE homes had gone back to the hospital. This research, which has since been replicated (Butzlaff & Hooley, 1998), indicates that the home environment of people with schizophrenia can influence how soon they relapse.

EE has been observed in different cultures, but the components that are linked to relapse differ. For example, emotional overinvolvement may be more common in European American caregivers compared to Mexican American caregivers (Aguilera, Lopez, et al., 2010; Lopez, Garcia, et al., 2009). In addition, the relationship between emotional overinvolvement and relapse in European and Asian countries is not as robust as it is in North American countries (Singh, Harley, & Suhail, 2013). The different findings may be attributed either to emotional overinvolvement being measured differently across countries and cultures or to emotional overinvolvement being more harmful in some cultures and countries than in others. This issue needs to be sorted out in future research.

Following from EE research, a few family therapies have been developed. These therapies may differ in length, setting, and specific techniques, but they have several features in common:

- **Education about schizophrenia—specifically about the genetic or neurobiological factors that predispose some people to the illness, the cognitive problems associated with schizophrenia, the symptoms of schizophrenia, and the signs of impending relapse.** Knowing, for example, that neurobiology has a lot to do with having schizophrenia and that the illness involves problems in thinking clearly and rationally may help family members be more accepting and understanding of their relative's actions.

- **Information about antipsychotic medication.** Therapists impress on both the family and the ill relative the pros and cons of taking antipsychotic medication. When they become better informed about the intended effects and the side effects of the medication, they are in a better position to take responsibility for monitoring response to medication and for seeking medical consultation rather than discontinuing the medication if adverse side effects occur.

- **Blame avoidance and reduction.** Therapists encourage family members to blame neither themselves nor their relative for the illness and for the difficulties all may have in coping with it.

- **Communication and problem-solving skills within the family.** Therapists focus on teaching the family ways to express both positive and negative feelings in a constructive, empathic, nondemanding manner rather than in a finger-pointing, critical, or overprotective manner. They also focus on making personal conflicts less stressful by teaching family members ways to work together to solve everyday problems.

- **Social network expansion.** Therapists encourage people with schizophrenia and their families to expand their social contacts, especially their support networks.

- **Hope.** Therapists instill hope that things can improve, including the hope that the person with schizophrenia may not have to return to the hospital.

Therapists use various techniques to implement these strategies. Examples include identifying stressors that could trigger relapse and training families in communication skills and problem solving (Penn & Mueser, 1996). Family therapy and family psychoeducation are effective at reducing relapse (McFarlane, 2016; Pharoah, Mari, et al., 2010; Rodolico, Bighelli, et al., 2022) and improving symptoms and functioning (Mueser, Deavers, et al., 2013). Compared with medication alone, family therapy plus medication has lowered relapse, particularly in studies in which the treatment lasted for at least 9 months (Hogarty, Anderson, et al., 1986, 1991; Kopelowicz, Liberman, & Zarate, 2002).

Psychoeducation

As we discussed in Chapter 5 in the context of bipolar disorder, psychoeducation is an approach that seeks to educate people about their illness, including the symptoms of the disorder, the expected time course of symptoms, the biological and psychological triggers for symptoms, and treatment strategies. A meta-analysis of 44 studies of psychoeducation in schizophrenia found that, in combination with medication, it was effective in reducing relapse and rehospitalization and increasing medication compliance (Xia, Merinder, & Belgamwar, 2011).

Cognitive Behavior Therapy At one time, researchers assumed that it was futile to try to alter the cognitive distortions, including delusions, of people with schizophrenia. Now, however, a growing body of evidence has demonstrated that some people with schizophrenia can in fact benefit from the use of cognitive behavior therapy (CBT) (Garety, Fowler, & Kuipers, 2000; Wykes, Steel, et al., 2008). The use of CBT in schizophrenia is often referred to as CBTp, where "p" stands for *psychosis* to make it clear that the therapy has been adapted for people with psychosis, such as those with schizophrenia.

People with schizophrenia can be encouraged to test out their delusional beliefs in much the same way as people without schizophrenia test out their beliefs. Through collaborative discussions (and in the context of other modes of treatment, including antipsychotic drugs), some people with schizophrenia have been helped to attach a nonpsychotic meaning to paranoid symptoms and thereby reduce their intensity and aversive nature (Beck & Rector, 2005; Turkington, Kingdon, & Weiden, 2006). Researchers have found that CBT can also reduce negative symptoms by, for example, challenging belief structures tied to low expectations for success (avolition) and low expectations for pleasure (anticipatory pleasure deficit in anhedonia) (Grant, Huh, et al., 2012; Wykes et al., 2008).

Results from meta-analyses of over 50 studies of more than 2,000 people with schizophrenia across eight countries have found small to moderate effect sizes for positive symptoms, negative symptoms, mood, and general life functioning (Jauhar, McKenna, et al., 2014; Wykes et al., 2008). CBT is currently the most effective treatment for these symptoms (Elis, Caponigro, & Kring, 2013). CBT has been used as an adjunctive treatment for schizophrenia in Great Britain for many years, and the results have been positive, even in community settings (Sensky, Turkington, et al., 2000; Turkington, Kingdon, & Turner, 2002; Wykes et al., 2008).

A newer therapy for schizophrenia combines two effective treatments: social skills training and cognitive behavior therapy (Granholm, McQuaid, & Holden, 2016). Termed *cognitive-behavioral social skills training* (CBSST), this treatment focuses on reducing symptoms and improving functioning. Randomized controlled clinical trials have shown it to be effective (Granholm, Holden, et al., 2014; Granholm, McQuaid, et al., 2005), and it has also shown promise among people early in the course of the disorder (Herman, Shireen, et al., 2016). CBSST is a group therapy, and it lasts longer than some other treatments, but the length of treatment has been shown to be associated with better outcomes. It may well take longer to work on complex symptoms and skills. How long? CBSST typically lasts for 6 to 9 months, which may well be a good investment in time.

Another type of combined treatment that has shown promise for young people early in the course of schizophrenia is called NAVIGATE (Mueser, Penn, et al., 2015). This treatment involves medication, family psychoeducation, individual therapy, and help with employment and education. In a large randomized controlled clinical trial called the Recovery After an Initial Schizophrenia Episode Early Treatment Program (RAISE-ETP), researchers found that this combined treatment was more effective than standard community care. This was particularly true for people who got into treatment sooner. That is, the longer psychosis was left untreated, the worse the outcome for participants (Kane, Robinson, et al., 2016). A later analysis of the data found that Black and White participants similarly benefited from NAVIGATE with one exception. There was less improvement in positive symptoms for Black participants compared to White participants, largely due to symptoms of suspiciousness and paranoia (Nagendra, Weiss, et al., 2023). It is likely that these symptoms reflect more than symptoms but also adaptive responses to experiences of racism (Anglin, 2023; Nagendra et al., 2023).

We emphasize two important conclusions from this study that are true for any treatment for schizophrenia: (1) Combined and comprehensive treatments in community settings are important to develop and implement for people with schizophrenia, and (2) the earlier treatment begins, the better.

Community-Based Care As we discussed in Chapter 1 and will return to in Chapter 16, the zeal to discharge people with schizophrenia from hospitals and provide treatment in the community did not match the needs of all people with the disorder. Some people did and still do need treatment in a hospital, even if for a short time. Unfortunately, it is difficult to receive such treatment today because of the cost and limited availability of hospital beds for people with schizophrenia and other psychological disorders.

The need in the United States for effective community treatment cannot be underestimated (Torrey, 2014). People with schizophrenia almost always need follow-up community-based services, and these services are scarce. Indeed, today a large percentage of unhoused people in the United States have a psychological disorder, many with schizophrenia. Social Security disability benefits are available to those with schizophrenia, but if they do not have an address, they often do not receive all the benefits to which they are entitled. Although good community treatment programs are available, there simply are not enough of them.

9.3 Check Your Knowledge

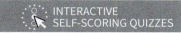 INTERACTIVE SELF-SCORING QUIZZES

(Answers are at the end of the chapter.)
True or false?

1. First-generation antipsychotics include medications like Haldol or prolixin; second-generation antipsychotics include clozapine and olanzapine.

2. Second-generation antipsychotics produce more motor side effects than first-generation antipsychotics.

3. Cognitive behavior therapy, but not family therapy, is effective for schizophrenia, if given along with medications.

4. Name the three components of expressed emotion.

Summary

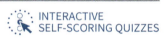 INTERACTIVE SELF-SCORING QUIZZES

Chapter 9 Practice Quiz

Clinical Description of Schizophrenia

- The symptoms of schizophrenia involve several areas, including thought, perception, and attention; motor behavior; and emotion. Symptoms are typically divided into positive, negative, and disorganized categories. Positive symptoms include excesses and distortions, such as delusions and hallucinations. Negative symptoms are behavioral deficits, which include avolition, asociality, anhedonia, blunted affect, and alogia. Disorganized symptoms include disorganized speech and behavior. Schizophrenia is diagnosed more frequently in Black and Latino people, though this may be due to bias among those making the diagnosis and experiences of discrimination, trauma, and structural racism.

- Other schizophrenia spectrum disorders in the DSM-5-TR include schizophreniform disorder, brief psychotic disorder, schizoaffective disorder, and delusional disorder.

Causes of Schizophrenia

- The evidence for genetic vulnerability to schizophrenia is relatively strong. Family and twin studies suggest a genetic component; adoption studies show a strong relationship between having a parent with schizophrenia and the likelihood of developing the disorder, typically in early adulthood. Familial high-risk studies have longitudinally studied the offspring of a parent with schizophrenia to determine if problems in childhood might predict the onset of the disorder. Genome-wide association studies (GWAS) have found rare genetic mutations called copy number variations (CNVs) and single nucleotide polymorphisms (SNPs) to be associated with schizophrenia.

- Neurotransmitters, including dopamine, serotonin, and glutamate have been studied in schizophrenia, though the causal evidence for these neurotransmitters is not solid. Medications that work on dopamine and serotonin can be effective in treating schizophrenia, but this does not mean that problems in the neurotransmitters caused the disorder.

- The brains of some people with schizophrenia have enlarged ventricles as well as problems with the prefrontal cortex, the temporal cortex, subcortical regions, and connectivity between brain regions. Some of these structural abnormalities could result from maternal viral infection during the first trimester of pregnancy or from damage sustained during a difficult birth. The combination of brain development during adolescence, stress, and the activity of the HPA axis is important for understanding why symptoms typically emerge during late adolescence, even if a brain disturbance has been in place since gestation. Cannabis use in adolescence has been linked to a higher risk for developing schizophrenia, primarily for those who are genetically vulnerable to schizophrenia.

- Four sociocultural factors that have been associated with schizophrenia are poverty, trauma, urbanicity, and migration.

- Developmental studies have identified problems in childhood that existed prior to the onset of schizophrenia. Because these studies were not designed to predict schizophrenia, however, it is difficult to interpret the findings. Clinical high-risk studies have identified young people with mild symptoms who are at high risk for developing schizophrenia spectrum disorders.

Treatment of Schizophrenia

- Antipsychotic drugs are widely used to treat schizophrenia. The first-generation drugs are somewhat effective, but they can also produce serious side effects. Second-generation antipsychotic drugs are as effective as the first-generation drugs, but they have their own set of side effects. Drugs alone are not a completely effective treatment, though, as people with schizophrenia may need support in dealing with the challenges of everyday life. Brain stimulation methods, such as tDCS, show promise.

- Several psychological interventions are effective at reducing symptoms and improving overall functioning. Family therapy, social skills training, psychoeducation, and cognitive behavior therapy are examples of helpful psychological treatments. Family therapy and social skill straining are valuable in preventing relapse. Community-based care is needed but not as widely available.

Answers to Check Your Knowledge Questions

9.1. 1. blunted affect; 2. delusion (delusion of reference); 3. anhedonia (anticipatory pleasure deficit); 4. disorganized thinking or derailment

9.2. 1. family and twin; 2. molecular; CNVs; SNPs; 3. prefrontal; 4. poverty, trauma, urbanicity, migration

9.3. 1. True; 2. False; 3. False; 4. hostility, critical comments, emotional overinvolvement

Key Terms

alogia   241
anhedonia   240
anticipatory pleasure   240
antipsychotic drugs   257
asociality   240
avolition   240
blunted affect   241
brief psychotic disorder   243
catatonia   242

clinical high-risk study   256
consummatory pleasure   240
delusional disorder   243
delusions   239
disorganized behavior   242
disorganized speech   241
disorganized symptoms   241
expressed emotion (EE)   262
familial high-risk study   247

hallucinations   240
loose associations (derailment)   242
negative symptoms   240
positive symptoms   239
schizoaffective disorder   243
schizophrenia   238
schizophreniform disorder   243
second-generation antipsychotic drugs   258
social skills training   261

Substance Use Disorders

LEARNING GOALS

1. Describe substance use disorder and its symptoms.

2. Describe the epidemiology and symptoms associated with alcohol, tobacco, and marijuana use disorders.

3. Describe the epidemiology and symptoms associated with opioid, stimulant, and other drug use disorders.

4. Understand the major causal influences for substance use disorders, including genetic,

neurobiological, psychological, and sociocultural influences.

5. Describe the approaches to treating substance use disorders, including psychological treatments, medications, and drug substitution treatments.

For centuries, people have used various substances in the hope of reducing pain or negative emotion, increasing positive emotion, or altering states of consciousness. The United States is a drug culture. Americans use drugs to wake up (coffee or tea), to stay alert throughout the day (soft drinks), to relax (alcohol), and to reduce pain (aspirin). The widespread availability and frequent use of drugs set the stage for the potential abuse of drugs, the topic of this chapter. Many authors have poignantly described their struggles with alcohol and drugs, such as Leslie Jamison, who wrote the searing and personal 2018 book *The Recovering: Intoxication and Its Aftermath*.

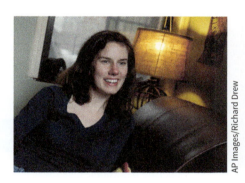

Author Leslie Jamison wrote a best-selling book, *The Recovering: Intoxication and its Aftermath*, which describes her years-long journey with alcohol use and abuse. (Jamison, 2018).

Overview: Substance Use by the Numbers

How common is substance use? In 2018, nearly 32 million people over the age of 12 in the United States reported having used an illicit drug in the past month (Substance Abuse and Mental Health Services Administration [SAMHSA], 2022). Marijuana was the most frequently used, with 36.4 million people over the age of 12 reporting using it in the past month. Alcohol remains the most used substance, with more than 133.1 million Americans over the age of 12 reporting alcohol use of some kind, and 60 million Americans reported at least one episode of binge drinking (defined as having five or more drinks for men and four or more drinks for women in a short period of time) in the last 30 days (SAMHSA, 2022).

Recent data on the frequency of use of several drugs, legal and illegal, in the United States are presented in **Table 10.1**. These figures do not represent the frequency of substance use disorders but simply indicate the pervasiveness of drug and alcohol use in the United States. Across the world, men use substances more frequently than women, but the gap between men and women is narrowing (McHugh, Votaw, et al., 2018). There are also important differences in use depending upon culture, race, and ethnicity, which we will present throughout the chapter.

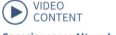

VIDEO CONTENT

Consciousness Altered: Drugs

TABLE 10.1	Number of People in the United States Who Reported Use in Past Year (2021)
Substance	**Number of People**
Alcohol	179.3 million
Cigarettes	57.4 million
Marijuana	52.5 million
Pain medications (misuse)	8.7 million
Hallucinogens	7.4 million
Cocaine	4.8 million
Inhalants	2.2 million
Methamphetamine	2.5 million
Heroin	1.1 million

Source: SAMHSA (2022). Numbers include people age 12 and older.

Using a substance is not the same thing as having a substance use disorder. DSM-5-TR includes **substance use disorder** for many specific substances, such as alcohol, opioids, and tobacco. See the box for descriptions of the defining symptoms of a substance use disorder. In 2021, 46.3 million people in the United States had a substance use disorder in the past year. Of this large number of people, most (29.5 million) had alcohol use disorder. Another 24 million had a drug use disorder, and 7.3 million met the DSM-5-TR criteria for both drug and alcohol use disorders (SAMHSA, 2022).

Defining Symptoms for Substance Use Disorder

- A person has trouble meeting obligations
- A person keeps using a substance even if it is dangerous to do so
- A person has ongoing relationship problems linked to use of the substance
- A person keeps using even though doing so causes problems in a person's life
- Tolerance

- Withdrawal
- A person takes more of the substance than originally intended
- Efforts to reduce or control substance use do not work
- A person spends a lot of time trying to get the substance
- A person gives up or reduces social events, hobbies, and/or work
- A person experiences strong craving to use the substance

Two symptoms that often are part of a substance use disorder are tolerance and withdrawal. **Tolerance** is indicated by either (1) larger doses of the substance being needed to produce the desired effect or (2) the effects of the drug becoming markedly less if the usual amount is taken. **Withdrawal** refers to the negative physical and psychological effects that develop when a person stops taking the substance or reduces the amount. Substance withdrawal symptoms can include muscle pains and twitching, sweating, vomiting, diarrhea, and insomnia.

Beginning with DSM-5, a nonsubstance category was added to the chapter "Substance-Related and Addictive Disorders": Gambling disorder. We discuss this disorder in **Focus on Discovery 10.1**. The term *addiction* is not in the DSM, but it is a term we are all familiar with. It typically refers to a severe substance use disorder.

Focus on Discovery 10.1

Is Gambling the Same as Other Substance Use Disorders?

DSM-5 added a nonsubstance condition—gambling disorder—in the chapter "Substance-Related and Addictive Disorders." Although the name is new and the disorder is now explicitly considered alongside substance use disorders, the disorder itself is not new to the DSM. Pathological gambling disorder was first included in the DSM in 1980.

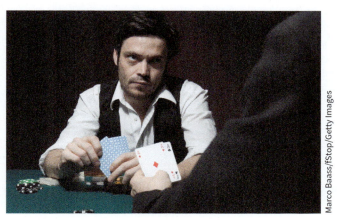

Marco Baass/fStop/Getty Images

Although gambling may look like fun, for many people it gets out of control, as in gambling disorder.

Some mental health professionals worry that including gambling disorder as an addictive disorder may create a "slippery slope" such that other types of behavioral "addictions" (shopping? exercise? sex?) will soon be added. In fact, internet gaming disorder is included in the DSM-5-TR Appendix as a condition in need of further study, and it was added as a full diagnostic category in ICD-11. Research on problematic gaming is under way, and some findings suggest it can be impairing, particularly in the case of role-playing games such as massively multiplayer online role-playing games (MMORGPs) (King, Delfabbro, et al., 2019). Internet gaming disorder may well make it into the next revision of the DSM.

What are some of the similarities and differences between substance use disorders/addictions and behavioral addictions like gambling disorder? One difference is that gambling does not involve putting some type of substance into the body, and thus, it is difficult to determine whether someone with gambling disorder can have withdrawal symptoms. Tolerance, however, is something that may be relevant to both types of addictive disorders. Other similarities include the consequences of the behavior. Whether people are gambling or ingesting a substance, there are significant consequences for work, school, and relationships.

Defining Symptoms for Gambling Disorder

1. Gambling often occurs when a person feels negative emotions
2. Efforts to stop or reduce gambling cause negative emotions
3. Having to ask other people to fix financial consequences of gambling
4. A person keeps gambling even though it causes relationship, job, or school problems
5. A person keeps gambling to try to recoup losses
6. A person lies to others about gambling
7. Gambling with more money is needed to get the desired good feelings
8. Efforts to reduce or control gambling do not work
9. A person spends a lot of time thinking about and planning gambling

Do people with gambling disorder participate in some types of gambling more often than those without a gambling disorder? It turns out that the answer to this question is no. Playing the lottery is the most common type of gambling for all people, whether they have a problem with gambling or not. However, those with gambling disorder are likely to have participated in a wider variety of gambling activities (e.g., sports betting, casino gambling, internet gambling, slot machines) than people who do not have problems with gambling (Kessler, Hwang, et al., 2008). Indeed, one of the characteristics that may put a person at higher risk for moving from social or recreational gambling to developing a gambling disorder is the frequency with which the person gambles.

What distinguishes professional gamblers from people with gambling disorder? After all, professional gamblers gamble even more than people with gambling disorder (Weinstock, Massura, & Petry, 2013). One study compared 22 professional gamblers with 13 people in the now-obsolete pathological gambling disorder category and found some interesting similarities and several key differences. Card games were the most frequent type of gambling among both groups, and both groups gambled at a pretty high frequency. However, professional gamblers won more money (about $125,000) than those with gambling disorder. In fact, people with gambling disorder had no income from their gambling. In addition, people with gambling disorder reported more stressful life events, a lower quality of life, more impulsivity, and more comorbid psychological disorders than professional gamblers.

Drug and alcohol use disorders are among the most stigmatized of disorders. Terms such as *addict* and *alcoholic* are tossed about carelessly, as if these words captured the essence of people, not the disorder from which they suffer. Historically, drug and alcohol problems have been viewed as moral lapses rather than as conditions in need of treatment. Unfortunately, such attitudes persist today. True, people make decisions about whether to try alcohol or drugs, but the ways in which these decisions and the substances involved interact with an individual's neurobiology, social setting, culture, and other environmental factors, all conspire to create a substance use disorder. Thus, it is a mistake to consider substance use disorders as somehow being solely the result of moral failing or personal choice.

Clinical Descriptions: Alcohol, Tobacco, and Cannabis Use Disorders

Clinical Case

Alice

Alice was 54 and living alone when her family finally persuaded her to check into an alcohol rehabilitation clinic. She had taken a bad fall while drunk, and it may have been this event that got her to admit that something was wrong. Her drinking had been out of control for several years. She began each day with a drink, continued drinking through the morning, and was totally intoxicated by the afternoon. She seldom had any memory for events after noon of any day. Since early adulthood, she had drunk regularly, but rarely during the day and never to the point of drunkenness. The sudden death of her husband in an automobile accident 2 years earlier had triggered a quick increase in her drinking, and within 6 months she had slipped into a pattern of severe alcohol use. She had little desire to go out of her house and had cut back on social activities with family and friends. Repeated efforts by her family to get her to curtail her intake of alcohol had only led to angry confrontations.

We turn now to an overview of some of the major substance use disorders: Those involving alcohol, tobacco, marijuana, opioids, stimulants, and hallucinogens.

Alcohol Use Disorder

Alcohol use disorder is the most common substance use disorder. People who develop tolerance or withdrawal generally have severe alcohol use disorder. Withdrawal symptoms for alcohol use disorder may be rather dramatic because the body has become accustomed to alcohol. Specifically, a person may experience feeling anxious, depressed, weak, restless, and unable to sleep. They may have muscle tremors, especially of the fingers, face, eyelids, lips, and tongue; and pulse, blood pressure, and temperature may be elevated.

In relatively rare cases, a person who has been drinking heavily for several years may also experience **delirium tremens (DTs)** when the level of alcohol in the blood drops suddenly. The person becomes delirious as well as tremulous and has hallucinations that are primarily visual but may be tactile as well. Unpleasant and very active creatures—snakes, cockroaches, spiders, and the like—may appear to be crawling up the wall or over the person's body or to be filling the room. Feverish, disoriented, and terrified, the person may claw frantically at their skin to get rid of the creatures.

Alcohol use disorder is associated with other drug use (Grant, Goldstein, et al., 2015). It is estimated, for example, that 80–85% of people who abuse alcohol are smokers. This very high comorbidity may occur because alcohol and nicotine are cross-tolerant; that is, nicotine can induce tolerance for the rewarding effects of alcohol, and vice versa. Thus, consumption of both drugs may be increased to maintain their rewarding effects (Rose, Brauer, et al., 2004). Evidence from animal studies suggests that this may happen because nicotine influences the way alcohol works in the brain's dopamine pathways associated with reward (Doyon, Dong, et al., 2013), a topic we turn to later in this chapter.

Prevalence of Alcohol Use Disorder   Results from the annual survey conducted by SAMHSA indicate that 29.5 million people in the United States age 12 or older met criteria for alcohol use disorder in 2021—more than the total population of the states of North Carolina, Michigan, and Virginia combined.

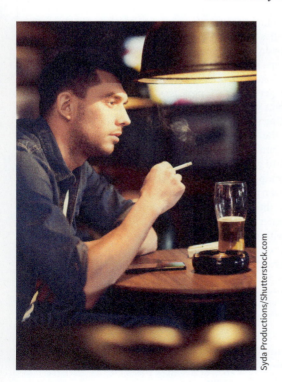

Alcohol and nicotine are a frequent combination, although most people who smoke and drink in social situations do not have problems with these substances.

Syda Productions/Shutterstock.com

TABLE 10.2	**Prevalence of Alcohol Use Disorder by Sex Assigned at Birth, Race, and Ethnicity (2021)**
Group	**Percentage**
Women	9.1
Men	12.1
Black or African American	10.1
Native American or Alaska Native	15.6
White	11.0
Hispanic or Latino	10.3
Asian	6.0
Multiracial	14.7

Source: SAMHSA (2022).
Data are percentages of people in the United States ages 12 or older.

The prevalence of alcohol use disorder varies by sex assigned at birth, race, and education level, as is shown in Table 10.2. Historically, men have had more problems with alcohol than women, but this sex difference has shrunk in the past few decades. In an analysis of studies from 1948 to 2014, researchers found that among those born in the early to mid-20th century, men were three times as likely to have alcohol problems as women. However, among those born after 1991, men were only 1.2 times as likely as women to have alcohol problems (Slade, Chapman, et al., 2016).

Short-Term Effects of Alcohol   After being swallowed and reaching the stomach, alcohol begins to be metabolized by enzymes. Most of it goes into the small intestine and from there it is absorbed into the blood. It is then broken down, primarily in the liver, which can metabolize about 1 ounce of 100-proof (50% alcohol) liquor per hour.

Figure 10.1 shows mean blood alcohol levels based on a person's weight and amount of alcohol consumption. Importantly, however, the effects of alcohol vary with its concentration in the bloodstream. Levels in the bloodstream depend on the amount ingested in a particular period of time, how much food is in the stomach (food retains the alcohol and reduces its absorption rate), the weight and body fat of the person drinking, and the efficiency of the liver. Two ounces of alcohol will thus have a different effect on a 180-pound man who has just eaten than on a 110-pound woman with an empty stomach. However, women achieve higher blood alcohol concentrations even after adjustment for differences in body weight, due to differences between men and women in body water content and in the enzyme that breaks down alcohol (alcohol dehydrogenase) (McHugh et al., 2018).

It is also important to consider this question: What counts as a drink? A 12-ounce glass of beer, a 5-ounce glass of wine, and 1.5 ounces of "hard liquor" (like a shot of tequila) are all considered one drink. The size of the drink is not what matters. Rather, it is the alcohol content of the beverage (http://rethinkingdrinking.niaaa.nih.gov).

Alcohol produces its effects through its interactions with several neurotransmitters. It stimulates gamma-aminobutyric acid (GABA) receptors, which may partially account for its ability to reduce tension. (GABA is a major inhibitory neurotransmitter; the benzodiazepines, such as Xanax, have an effect on GABA receptors similar to that of alcohol.) Alcohol also acts on serotonin and dopamine, which may contribute to its ability to produce pleasurable effects. Finally, alcohol inhibits glutamate receptors, which may influence the cognitive effects of alcohol intoxication, such as slowed thinking and memory loss.

A novel study examined the effects of alcohol on both the brain and behavior. Participants were given different doses of alcohol while in an fMRI scanner performing a simulated driving test (Calhoun, Pekar, & Pearlson, 2004). The low dose (0.04 blood alcohol content) led to just a small impairment in motor functioning, but the high dose (0.08 blood alcohol content) led to more significant motor impairment that interfered with driving ability. Furthermore, the effects of alcohol in the brain were in areas associated with monitoring errors and making

Blood Alcohol Concentration Calculator

# OF DRINKS CONSUMED/SEX		WEIGHT							
		100	120	140	160	180	200	220	240
1	Male	.04	.04	.03	.03	.02	.02	.02	.02
	Female	.05	.04	.04	.03	.03	.03	.02	.02
2	Male	.09	.07	.06	.05	.05	.04	.04	.04
	Female	.10	.08	.07	.06	.06	.05	.05	.04
3	Male	.13	.11	.09	.08	.07	.07	.06	.05
	Female	.15	.13	.11	.10	.08	.08	.07	.06
4	Male	.17	.15	.13	.11	.10	.09	.08	.07
	Female	.20	.17	.15	.13	.11	.10	.09	.09
5	Male	.22	.18	.16	.14	.12	.11	.10	.09
	Female	.25	.21	.18	.16	.14	.13	.12	.11
6	Male	.26	.22	.19	.16	.15	.13	.12	.11
	Female	.30	.26	.22	.19	.17	.15	.14	.13
7	Male	.30	.25	.22	.19	.17	.15	.14	.13
	Female	.36	.30	.26	.22	.20	.18	.16	.15
8	Male	.35	.29	.25	.22	.19	.17	.16	.15
	Female	.41	.33	.29	.26	.23	.20	.18	.16
9	Male	.39	.35	.28	.25	.22	.20	.18	.16
	Female	.46	.38	.33	.29	.26	.23	.21	.19
10	Male	.39	.35	.28	.25	.22	.20	.18	.16
	Female	.51	.42	.36	.32	.28	.25	.23	.21
11	Male	.48	.40	.34	.30	.26	.24	.22	.20
	Female	.56	.46	.40	.35	.31	.27	.25	.23
12	Male	.53	.43	.37	.32	.29	.26	.24	.21
	Female	.61	.50	.43	.37	.33	.30	.28	.25
13	Male	.57	.47	.40	.35	.31	.29	.26	.23
	Female	.66	.55	.47	.40	.36	.32	.30	.27
14	Male	.62	.50	.43	.37	.34	.31	.28	.25
	Female	.71	.59	.51	.43	.39	.35	.32	.29
15	Male	.66	.54	.47	.40	.36	.34	.30	.27
	Female	.76	.63	.55	.46	.42	.37	.35	.32

© John Wiley & Sons, Inc.

FIGURE 10.1 Blood alcohol concentration (BAC) calculator. Note that values are estimates. An actual BAC will vary depending on metabolism and amount of food in the stomach.

decisions (the anterior cingulate cortex and orbitofrontal cortex). Based on this finding, the researchers suggested that people at the legal limit of alcohol may make poor decisions about driving and may not realize they are making mistakes.

Long-Term Effects of Prolonged Alcohol Abuse Prolonged consumption of alcohol adversely affects every tissue and organ of the body. For example, alcohol impairs the digestion of food and absorption of vitamins. In older people who have chronically abused alcohol, a deficiency of B-complex vitamins can cause a severe loss of memory for both recent and long-past events.

Prolonged alcohol use plus reduction in the intake of proteins contributes to the development of cirrhosis of the liver, a disease in which some liver cells become engorged with fat and protein, which impede their functioning. Some cells die, triggering an inflammatory process, and when scar tissue develops, blood flow is obstructed.

Heavy alcohol consumption by a woman during pregnancy is associated with a range of problems in the developing fetus—broadly, fetal alcohol spectrum disorders, including **fetal alcohol syndrome (FAS)**, partial FAS, and alcohol-related neurodevelopmental disorder (Lange, Probst, et al., 2017). Between 1% and 5% of children in the United States may have a fetal alcohol spectrum disorder (May, Chambers, et al., 2018). The most serious and rare of these

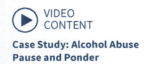

VIDEO CONTENT

Case Study: Alcohol Abuse Pause and Ponder

disorders is FAS, accounting for less than 20% of fetal alcohol spectrum disorders (May et al., 2018). FAS is a leading known cause of intellectual disability among children. The growth of the fetus is slowed, and cranial, facial, and limb anomalies can be produced. Even moderate drinking can produce undesirable, if less severe, effects on the fetus, leading the National Institute on Alcohol Abuse and Alcoholism to counsel total abstention during pregnancy as the safest course.

There has long been debate about whether alcohol in moderation might have some positive health benefits. For example, light to moderate drinking has been related to lower risk of coronary heart disease for some people (Griswold, Fullman, et al., 2018; Zhao, Stockwell, et al., 2017). Other evidence, however, suggests that even moderate drinking can have ill effects on health. For example, a prospective study with more than 500 people in the United Kingdom found that greater alcohol consumption predicted less gray matter density, particularly in the hippocampus, 30 years later (Topiwala, Allan, et al., 2017). Recall from Chapter 2 that gray matter refers to the neural tissue that constitutes the cortex and the hippocampus, areas of the brain that support memory. Other studies have found that the so-called protective effects of light to moderate alcohol consumption on cardiovascular health are likely accounted for by the overall better health (e.g., lower BMI, more exercise, better diet) of those who are light to moderate drinkers (Biddinger, Emdin, et al., 2022). A large meta-analysis published in 2023 that included over 100 studies with nearly 5 million people found no evidence for lower mortality from any cause for light and moderate drinkers (Zhao, Stockwell, et al., 2023). In short, it appears that there are no clear health benefits for light to moderate drinking.

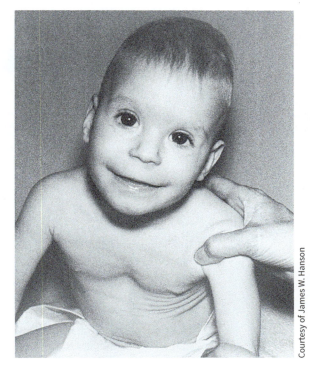

Heavy drinking during pregnancy can cause fetal alcohol syndrome. Children with this disorder can have facial abnormalities and intellectual developmental disorder.

Tobacco Use Disorder

Nicotine is the addicting agent in tobacco. The neural pathways that become activated stimulate the dopamine neurons in the mesolimbic area that seem to be involved in producing the reinforcing effects of most drugs (Stein, Pankiewicz, et al., 1998).

Prevalence and Health Consequences of Smoking
The threats to health posed by smoking have been documented convincingly by the Surgeon General of the United States since the 1960s. Although more than 20 million Americans died from smoking between 1964 and 2014, another 45 million quit smoking, which no doubt saved many lives. Unfortunately, the declines in smoking have not affected everyone equally. Smoking among people with a college degree declined by 83%, but it declined by only 39% among people with less than a high school degree. Worldwide, the number of people who smoke declined by about a third from 1990 to 2015 (Reitsma, Fullman, et al., 2017). Although these trends are encouraging, smoking remains the single most preventable cause of premature death in the United States, as well as in other parts of the world.

Among the other medical problems associated with—and almost certainly caused or exacerbated by—long-term cigarette smoking are emphysema; cancers of the larynx, esophagus, pancreas, bladder, cervix, and stomach; complications during pregnancy; sudden infant death syndrome; periodontitis; and a number of cardiovascular disorders (U.S. Department of Health and Human Services [USDHHS], 2014). The most probable harmful components in the smoke from burning tobacco are nicotine, carbon monoxide, and tar, which consists primarily of certain hydrocarbons, many of which are known carcinogens. Results from a longitudinal study with close to 300,000 people found that people who smoked as little as one cigarette per day were more likely to die from any cause than people who never smoked (Inoue-Choi, Liao, et al., 2017).

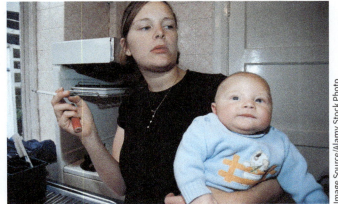

Children of mothers who smoke are at increased risk for respiratory infections, bronchitis, and inner-ear infections.

TABLE 10.3	Use of Any Tobacco Product or Nicotine Vaping in 2021 by Sex Assigned at Birth, Race, and Ethnicity	
Group		**Percentage**
Women		17.8
Men		26.4
Black or African American		23.6
Native American or Alaska Native		36.1
White		24.6
Hispanic or Latino		14.9
Asian		9.3
Multiracial		29.7

Source: SAMHSA (2022).
Data are percentages of people in the United States ages 12 and older who used any tobacco product (cigarettes, smokeless tobacco, cigars, pipe tobacco) or nicotine vaping—during the past month in year 2021.

In 2021, 66.8 million people in the United States had used a tobacco product (cigarette, cigar, smokeless tobacco, pipe) in the past year, with 52.44 million of these people smoking cigarettes (SAMHSA, 2022). The number of people who used any tobacco product or nicotine vaping in 2021 is nontrivial, as shown in Table 10.3. Encouragingly, tobacco use among people ages 18–25 has continued to decline between 2015 and 2021. Smoking is more prevalent among people with lower incomes (Dwyer-Lindgren, Mokdad, et al., 2014), likely adding to the disparity in health between those with high and low incomes in the United States.

Research has demonstrated the significance of race in nicotine addiction as well as the intricate interplay among behavioral, social, and neurobiological factors. It has been known for years that Black cigarette smokers are less likely to quit and are more likely, if they continue to smoke, to get lung cancer. Why? It turns out that they retain nicotine in their blood longer than do White smokers; that is, they metabolize it more slowly (Mustonen, Spencer, et al., 2005). The type of cigarette smoked also matters. Black people are more likely to smoke menthol cigarettes, largely due to extensive advertising of these types of cigarettes to this community beginning in the 1950s and continuing today (Kreslake, Wayne, & Connolly, 2008; Moreland-Russell, Harris, et al., 2013; USDHHS, 2014). Research shows that people who smoke menthol inhale more deeply and hold in the smoke for a longer time, thus providing more opportunity for deleterious effects (Celebucki,

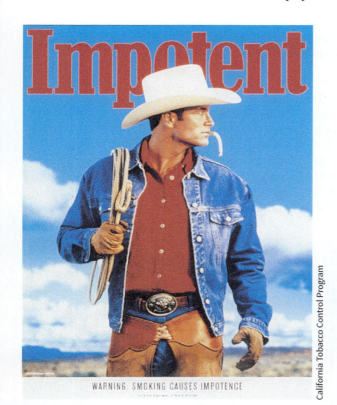

California Tobacco Control Program

WARNING: SMOKING CAUSES IMPOTENCE

California's Tobacco Education Media Campaign parodies tobacco ads to illustrate the health risks associated with smoking and to attack pro-tobacco influences (see more at http://tobaccofreeca.com/resources/).

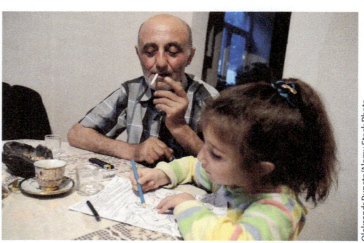

Oleksandr Rupeta/Alamy Stock Photo

Parental smoking greatly increases the chances that children will begin to smoke.

Wayne, et al., 2005). Given the additional health concerns associated with menthol cigarettes, the Food and Drug Administration (FDA) proposed a rule to remove them from the market in 2022. It will likely take a few years for this to go into effect.

Health Consequences of Secondhand Smoke

As we have known for many years, the health hazards of smoking are not restricted to those who smoke. The smoke coming from the burning end of a cigarette, called **secondhand smoke** or environmental tobacco smoke (ETS), contains higher concentrations of ammonia, carbon monoxide, nicotine, and tar than does the smoke inhaled by the smoker. In 2014, the Surgeon General updated the report detailing the health hazards of secondhand smoke. The National Institutes of Health has classified ETS as a known carcinogen, indicating that evidence has established a cause–effect relationship between ETS and cancer. The effects of ETS include the following:

- Nonsmokers can suffer lung damage, possibly permanent, from extended exposure to cigarette smoke. Those living with smokers are at greatest risk. Precancerous lung abnormalities have been observed in those living with smokers, and they are at greater-than-average risk for developing cardiovascular disease and lung cancer.
- Babies of women exposed to secondhand smoke during pregnancy are more likely to be born prematurely, to have low birth weights, and to have birth defects.
- Children of smokers are more likely to have upper respiratory infections, asthma, bronchitis, and inner-ear infections than are their peers whose parents do not smoke.

The Surgeon General has stated that the best way of preventing exposure to secondhand smoke is to promote smoke-free environments, since there is really no safe level of exposure to secondhand smoke (USDHHS, 2014). As of 2023, 23 states[1] plus the District of Columbia had received an A grade from the American Lung Association for their strong smoke-free-air laws, which ban smoking in nearly all public places, including restaurants and bars (https://www.lung.org/research/sotc/state-grades/state-rankings).

E-Cigarettes and Vaping

Electronic cigarettes, or e-cigarettes, sometimes look like cigarettes, but they are made of plastic or metal and are filled with liquid nicotine that is mixed with other chemicals. They are battery-operated and work by heating up the nicotine liquid concoction so that users can inhale and then exhale the vapor. The term *vaping* has come to mean smoking an e-cigarette. Often, e-cigarettes are not called cigarettes at all, but are instead called vape pipes, vaping pens, hookah pens, or e-hookahs. Although it is true that these devices do not always contain nicotine (many were sold with flavored water vapor until 2020 when the FDA placed restrictions on flavored cartridges), they can all be used to deliver liquid nicotine. They also contain other ingredients that are used to heat and convert nicotine to vapor but are not always listed on packages, and the health impact of these ingredients is not yet fully known (National Academies of Sciences, Engineering, and Medicine, 2018; Talih, Balhas, et al., 2015; Varlet, Farsalinos, et al., 2015).

Vaping among high school students doubled between 2017 and 2019 (Miech, Johnston, et al., 2019). However, vaping among high school students decreased during the COVID-19 pandemic and has remained at lower levels through 2022 (Miech, Johnston, et al., 2023). The declines are promising but not well understood. It could be that the COVID-19 pandemic disrupted access to vaping materials or that distance from peers during school closures contributed to less use. Nevertheless, e-cigarettes have been more frequently used than cigarettes among young people since 2014 (Gentzke, Wang, et al., 2022). In 2021, over 60% of

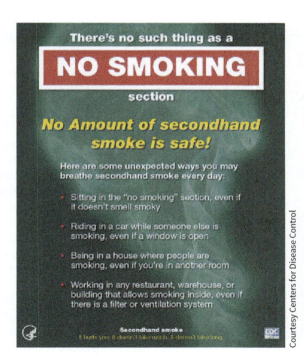

The Surgeon General's report from 2006 noted that no amount of secondhand smoke is safe.

---

[1]Arizona, California, Delaware, Hawaii, Illinois, Iowa, Kansas, Maine, Maryland, Massachusetts, Minnesota, Montana, Nebraska, North Dakota, New Jersey, New York, Ohio, Oregon, Rhode Island, Utah, Vermont, Washington, and Wisconsin

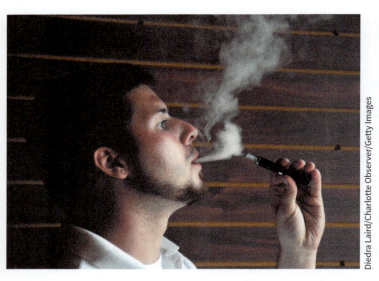

E-cigarettes are more popular among high school students, even though we do not yet know about the safety of these products.

adolescents ages 12–17 who reported using tobacco products did so exclusively by vaping. By contrast, under a third of young adults age 18–25 who used tobacco did so by vaping (SAMHSA, 2022). Longitudinal studies show that among young people, those who vape are more likely to take up smoking old-fashioned tobacco cigarettes and use alcohol and marijuana (Hershberger, Argyriou, & Cyders, 2020; Miech, Patrick, et al., 2017; Park, Livingston, et al., 2020).

The FDA first published regulations for vaping and e-cigarettes in 2016. These regulations treat e-cigarettes like any other regulated tobacco product, thus making it illegal to sell them to children under the age of 18, requiring warning labels about nicotine's addictive properties, and calling for scientific evidence to support any claims about their safety relative to other tobacco products. As of 2020, vaping products must first be approved the FDA Center for Tobacco Products; it will no longer approve flavored cartridges for vaping products.

Some argue that e-cigarettes are safer alternatives to cigarettes containing tar and other carcinogens and that they may assist people who want to quit smoking and dissuade others from trying actual cigarettes. In 2018, the National Academies of Sciences, Engineering, and Medicine published a comprehensive report that reviewed the evidence on the health effects of e-cigarettes (National Academies of Sciences, Engineering, and Medicine, 2018). A few key findings of this report are as follows:

- E-cigarettes were less toxic than traditional combustible cigarettes;
- E-cigarettes can be helpful tools for smoking cessation, but only for adults;
- Young people, who use e-cigarettes more than adults, are *more* likely to transition to smoking cigarettes; and
- Secondhand aerosols from e-cigarettes contain nicotine and other chemicals that can impact others in the surrounding area.

Cannabis Use Disorder

The dried and crushed leaves and flowering tops of the hemp plant, *Cannabis sativa* are commonly referred to as **marijuana**. It is most often smoked, but it may be chewed, prepared as a tea, or eaten in baked goods (referred to as edibles). In DSM-5-TR, *cannabis use disorder* is the category name that includes marijuana.

Synthetic cannabis contains artificially created chemicals similar to those contained in cannabis. These chemicals are typically sprayed onto inert plant materials and placed in small packages and sold under names such as Spice or K2. Synthetic marijuana was made illegal in 2011, and use among high school students declined from 11% to less than 2% from 2011 to 2022 (Miech, et al., 2023).

Prevalence of Cannabis Use
Although it is considered an illicit (illegal) drug by SAMHSA, cannabis is legal for all uses in 22 states and the District of Columbia. All but five states have deemed it legal for medicinal use and/or have decriminalized it (i.e., people are not prosecuted for possessing a small amount). In 2021, 36.4 million people reported using marijuana in the past month, and it was the most commonly used drug across all age groups (SAMHSA, 2022). (See **Figure 10.2** for data on usage in the past year from 2012 to 2021.) Vaping of marijuana among high school students increased dramatically in 2019, showing the largest 1-year increase for any drug in 45 years (Miech, Johnston, et al., 2020). This increase may reflect that fact that possession of cannabis by adults is currently legal for all uses in 22 states (Alaska, Arizona, California, Colorado, Connecticut, Delaware, Illinois, Maine, Maryland, Massachusetts, Michigan, Minnesota, Missouri, Montana, Nevada, New Jersey, New Mexico,

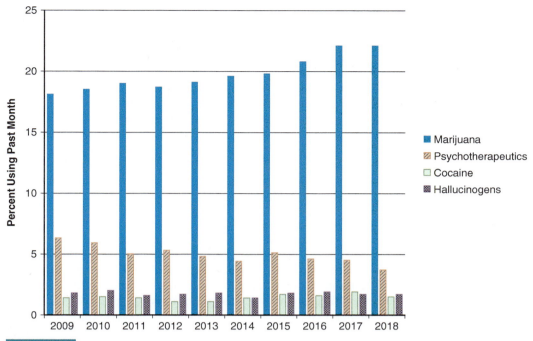

FIGURE 10.2   **Trends in drug use among people ages 18–25 (SAMHSA, 2022).**

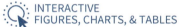
INTERACTIVE
FIGURES, CHARTS, & TABLES

Note: Psychotherapeutics refers to the misuse of pain relievers, tranquilizers, stimulants, or sedatives; it does not include over-the-counter medications. Data collection in 2020 during the COVID-19 pandemic was not as complete as in other years.

New York, Oregon, Rhode Island, Vermont, and Washington) and the District of Columbia. It is approved for medical use in many more states, a topic we return to later.

Effects of Cannabis   As with most other drugs, legal or not, cannabis use has its risks. Generally, the more we learn about a drug, the less benign it turns out to be, at least for some people, and cannabis is no exception (see **Focus on Discovery 10.2**).

Focus on Discovery 10.2

Is Marijuana a Gateway Drug?

The so-called gateway hypothesis of marijuana use has been around for a long time. According to this perspective, marijuana is dangerous not only in itself but also because it is a first step for young people on the path to developing problems with other drugs, such as heroin.

Is there evidence that marijuana is indeed a gateway to more serious substance use? Overall, the answer to this question is no. Most young people who use marijuana do *not* go on to use such drugs as heroin and cocaine (Hall & Lynskey, 2005; National Academies of Sciences, Engineering, and Medicine, 2017). So, if by *gateway* we mean that escalation to a more serious drug is inevitable, then marijuana is not a gateway drug. However, we do know that many, but far from all, of those who use heroin and cocaine began their drug experimentation with marijuana. And some evidence suggests that users of marijuana are more likely than nonusers to experiment later with heroin and cocaine (Kandel & Kandel, 2015; Miller & Volk, 1996).

Has legalization of marijuana changed patterns of use? Thus far, the data show that there is more marijuana use in states that have legalized marijuana. However, there appears to be less use of other drugs and alcohol in these states (Alley, Kerr, & Bae, 2020; Anderson & Rees, 2021; Bae & Kerr, 2020; Zellers, Ross, et al., 2023).

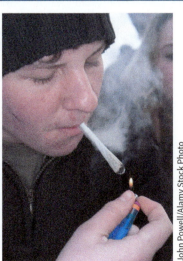

John Powell/Alamy Stock Photo

Most people who use marijuana do not go on to use other drugs, but many drug users do begin their drug use with marijuana.

Cannabinoids are the active chemicals in cannabis. The major cannabinoid in marijuana is delta-9-tetrahydrocannabinol (delta-9-THC or THC). The amount of THC in marijuana is variable, but marijuana is much more potent now than it was 30 years ago (ElSohly, Chandra, et al., 2020). A second cannabinoid in cannabis is cannabidiol, better known as CBD. The main difference between the two cannabinoids is that THC is associated with feeling high and CBD is not. Delta-8—tetrahydrocannabinol is less abundant in the cannabis sativa plant, but it can be manufactured from CBD. Delta-8-THC levels are particularly elevated in edibles, and the FDA has released warning statements about this and the potential for ill effects among children (https://www.fda.gov/food/alerts-advisories-safety-information/fda-warns-consumers-about-accidental-ingestion-children-food-products-containing-thc). In addition to greater potency, users smoke more now than in the past. For example, a "blunt" contains more cannabis than a joint. Edibles (e.g., brownies, gummies) are even more potent and were not as readily available before cannabis was legalized in many states.

Psychological Effects   The intoxicating effects of cannabis, like those of most drugs, depend in part on the potency and size of the dose. Smokers of marijuana find that it makes them feel relaxed and sociable. Large doses can bring rapid shifts in emotion, dull attention, fragmented thoughts, impair memory, and give the sense that time is moving more slowly. Extremely heavy doses have sometimes induced hallucinations and other effects similar to those of hallucinogens, including extreme panic, sometimes arising from the belief that a frightening experience will never end. Dosage can be difficult to regulate because it may take up to half an hour after smoking marijuana for its effects to appear; many users thus get much higher than they intended.

Accumulated scientific evidence indicates that cannabis can interfere with cognitive functioning in areas such as attention, planning, decision making, working memory, and problem solving (Broyd, van Hell, et al., 2016; Crean, Crane, & Mason, 2011). Does chronic use of cannabis affect cognitive functioning, even when the person is not using the drug? Unfortunately, not many well-controlled studies have been conducted to address this question. One large longitudinal study of people from New Zealand assessed marijuana use at five time points from the ages of 18 to 38. Neuropsychological functioning was assessed at age 13, prior to initiation of marijuana use, and again at age 38. The researchers found that those people who persistently met the criteria for what would now be called severe cannabis use disorder had reductions in IQ points and poorer performance on tests assessing working memory and processing than people who had never used marijuana or did so less persistently (Meier, Caspi, et al., 2012). This was particularly true for those who began using marijuana chronically as adolescents. Those people in the study who used marijuana, but not regularly, showed no decline in IQ or impairment on the neuropsychological tests. An additional follow-up study of participants at age 45 found similar results (Meier, Caspi, et al., 2022). Long-term cannabis users (weekly use) performed more poorly on cognitive tests compared to long-term users of tobacco or alcohol.

Studies have demonstrated that being high on marijuana can impair complex psychomotor skills necessary for driving (Rogeberg & Elvik, 2016). Poor performance after smoking one or two marijuana cigarettes containing 2% THC can persist for up to 8 hours after a person believes they are no longer high. This creates the danger that people will drive when they are not functioning adequately.

Physical Consequences   The short-term effects of cannabis include bloodshot and itchy eyes, dry mouth and throat, increased appetite, reduced pressure within the eye, and somewhat raised blood pressure.

We know that the long-term use of marijuana can impair lung structure and function (Martinasek, McGrogan, & Maysonet, 2016). Even though marijuana users smoke far fewer cigarettes than do tobacco smokers, most inhale marijuana smoke more deeply and retain it in their lungs for much longer periods of time. Since marijuana has some of the same carcinogens found in tobacco, it too has harmful effects.

How does cannabis affect the brain? Researchers have identified two cannabinoid brain receptors, called CB1 and CB2 (Matsuda, Lolait, et al., 1990; Munro, Thomas, & Abu-Shaar, 1993). CB1 receptors are found throughout the body and the brain, with a particularly high number in the hippocampus, an important region of the brain for learning and memory. Researchers have found that the cognitive problems associated with marijuana use are linked to the effects of marijuana on these receptors in the hippocampus (Ranganathan & D'Souza, 2006). The longitudinal study in New Zealand described earlier found that long-term cannabis use (using cannabis weekly) was associated with lower hippocampus volume (size) at age 45 than noncannabis users (Meier et al., 2022).

An fMRI study of people who did and did not regularly use cannabis found that regular users showed different patterns of connectivity (see Chapter 2) between the amygdala and frontal cortex while attempting to regulate negative emotions (Zimmermann, Walz, et al., 2017). These findings might help explain some of the psychological effects associated with marijuana use, including changes in emotion and attentional capabilities.

Cannabis users can develop tolerance, and withdrawal symptoms such as restlessness, depression, anxiety, tension, stomach pains, and insomnia can occur if marijuana use is discontinued (Hasin, Keyes, et al., 2008).

Therapeutic Effects and Legalization

The potential benefits of cannabis were confirmed over 20 years ago (Institute of Medicine, 1999) and have been reaffirmed since (National Academies of Sciences, Engineering, and Medicine, 2017). These include reduction in the nausea and loss of appetite that accompany chemotherapy for some people with cancer and alleviation of glaucoma, chronic pain, muscle spasms, and discomfort for those with AIDS. There is also limited evidence that cannabinoids can help ease the symptoms of Tourette's syndrome, social anxiety, dementia, or sleep disorders (National Academies of Sciences, Engineering, and Medicine, 2017).

California was the first state to pass a law legalizing medical use of marijuana in 1996. Since then, all but 12 states have approved the use of marijuana for medical purposes.[2] These state laws are currently in conflict with a federal law that makes any marijuana use illegal. Thus, state officials in these states will not prosecute people for using medical marijuana, even though federal officials may do so.

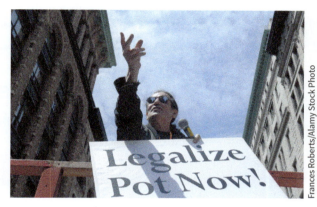

Demonstrator advocates the legalization of marijuana.

Quick Summary

Alcohol and drug use is common in the United States. DSM-5-TR lists substance use disorders for alcohol and many other substances.

Withdrawal from alcohol can involve hallucinations and delirium tremens (DT). People who use alcohol or have severe alcohol use disorder may use other drugs as well, particularly nicotine. Alcohol use is particularly high among college students; men are more likely to drink alcohol than women, though this difference continues to shrink, and differences in alcohol use disorder by race and ethnicity have been observed. Light to moderate drinking does not appear to have any health benefits, but it can cause problems during pregnancy.

Smoking remains widespread, though it has been on the decline. Cigarette smoking causes several illnesses, including several cancers, heart disease, and other lung diseases. The ill effects of tobacco are greater for Black people. Secondhand smoke, also called environmental tobacco smoke (ETS), is linked to many serious health problems. E-cigarettes rapidly became popular among young people, though there use appears to have decreased slightly since the COVID-19 pandemic. The ill effects of the nicotine in these products are the same as those for cigarettes; additional studies suggest that there may be negative effects on health from the aerosol products used in vape pipes.

Cannabis makes people feel relaxed and sociable, but it can interfere with cognitive functioning. In addition, smoking marijuana has been linked to lung-related problems. It remains the most prevalently used drug, particularly among younger people. Users can develop tolerance to and suffer withdrawal symptoms from cannabis. Marijuana also has therapeutic benefits, particularly for those experiencing the side effects of chemotherapy and for those with AIDS, glaucoma, chronic pain, and muscle spasms.

---

[2] Six states (Georgia, Indiana, Iowa, Tennessee, Texas, and Wisconsin) permit CBD oil only for medicinal purposes.

10.1 Check Your Knowledge

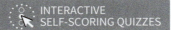
INTERACTIVE
SELF-SCORING QUIZZES

(Answers are at the end of the chapter.)
True or false?

1. Symptoms of a substance use disorder include tolerance and withdrawal.
2. Research suggests that nicotine can enhance the rewarding properties of alcohol.
3. Even moderate drinking by pregnant women can cause learning and attention problems in their children.

Answer the following questions or fill in the blank.

4. List three types of cancer that are caused by smoking.
5. Cannabis can have _____ effects on learning and memory.
6. List three of the therapeutic benefits of marijuana.
7. Describe two similarities and two differences between e-cigarettes and cigarettes.

Clinical Descriptions: Opioid, Stimulant, and Other Drug Use Disorders

Clinical Case

Brandon

Brandon played middle linebacker on his high school football team in a small town in Ohio. Impressed by his speed, agility, and strength, his coaches were talking about college scholarships. During his junior year, Brandon injured his knee. He had surgery and was up and around the day after. He was prescribed Vicodin for pain, and this helped him recover with less pain and get the most out of his physical therapy. Brandon noticed that not only was the medication helpful for his pain, it also helped him "even out" and feel better all around. He found that taking an extra pill here and there was beneficial. With the pills, he would not get so upset by his girlfriend Brianna's complaints about him taking more and more pills or his parents' nagging about doing housework. At spring practice, he felt invincible. No matter how hard the hit, he could take it.

By summer, he was having a hard time getting by without pain pills. When he tried to stop, he felt awful, as if he had the flu. He would sweat and have the chills, even shake. He couldn't eat, and this was bad for bulking up for the season. Even though his doctor continued to provide him with new prescriptions, the supply that should have lasted a month was gone in a few days. He could buy more from a guy downtown, but he was running out of money. The pills cost $5

each, and he needed as many as 20 a day. He wondered if he had a problem, but he thought football was a contact sport and pain went with it. Other guys on the team were taking stuff too. Plus, his senior year was coming up and recruiters were going to be at the games.

The guy who sold him pain pills told him he could sell him heroin for a lot less than the Norco he was now taking. He thought heroin was for losers and guys who shot up in the low-income parts of the city. The guy gave him a small bag for free and told him he could sniff it and not shoot it. It lasted for 3 days. He reasoned he would take it just until the season was over, and then he would stop for good.

Brianna was furious with him when she found out he was taking heroin, and she threatened to tell his parents. Brandon pleaded with her not to and said that he would stop. He quit taking it, but again felt horrible—the worst flu ever. He decided to drive downtown and get another bag, just to help him slowly stop.

The police found Brandon slumped over the front seat of his car. They tried reviving him with Narcan, but it was too late. He was pronounced dead at the scene. An autopsy revealed that he had fentanyl—a synthetic opioid—in his system. Brandon thought he was buying heroin, but his dealer had likely substituted fentanyl without telling him. Brandon was 17 years old.

Opioids

The **opioids** include opium, morphine, **heroin**, and codeine. Misuse of these drugs has exploded in the past 25 years. In moderate doses, they can relieve pain, which is of tremendous relief to many people. Unfortunately, prescription pain medications have become among the most abused of the drugs we discuss. In 2021, over 8.7 million people misused prescription pain medications (SAMHSA, 2022). DSM-5-TR categorizes the misuse of such drugs as *opioid use disorder*. In 2021, over 5.5 million people met criteria for opioid use disorder (SAMHSA, 2022), and although this is a high number, some evidence suggests that the prevalence rates have decreased or plateaued since 2016 (Keyes, Rutherford, et al., 2022). We discuss two recent books on the severe problems associated with opioid use in **Read More About It 10.1**.

Read More About It 10.1

Dopesick: Dealers, Doctors, and the Drug Company That Addicted America

In 2018, Beth Macy published *Dopesick: Dealers, Doctors, and the Drug Company That Addicted America*. This book is the culmination of years of reporting that Macy did, beginning in Roanoke, Virginia. She tells the story of people who battled with opioid addiction, some successfully and some not, throughout that state. She tells the stories of people who became addicted following a legitimate prescription for pain medication, as well as the stories of young people who began taking a family member's pain medicine to get high, only to then move on to heroin and then fentanyl. The allure of these drugs is clear, as one young person told her:

> *It was like shooting Jesus up into your arm. ... it's like this white explosion of light in your head. You're floating on a cloud. You don't yet know that the first time is the best. After that, you're just chasing that first high.*
>
> **(Macy, 2018, p. 136)**

Many young people in their teens and twenties died. Others went to prison. Still others went to rehab, only to relapse again and again.

Macy also tells the stories of dealers, those who began selling to their friends in suburban high schools behind a school building and in shopping centers and moved on to larger endeavors. She tells the story of the head of one of the largest drug rings in the region and the many law enforcement professionals who eventually caught and incarcerated him, only to find new rings sprouting up as quickly as new peas in a vegetable garden.

She tells the stories of doctors, nuns, and volunteers who spent countless hours counseling, cajoling, and taking care of those in the grip of prescription pain medicine, heroin, or fentanyl, as well as consoling family members in the seemingly unending ocean of grief after losing a son, a daughter, a parent, or a spouse to an overdose death.

She tells the story of the drug companies who make these medications, focusing mostly on Purdue Pharma, which created OxyContin, aggressively marketed it, downplayed its addictive potential, remade its formula in response to public and official outcries, and ultimately paid millions of dollars in fines and to families whose lives were ravaged by the company's product.

This clear-eyed and sobering look at the havoc created by a confluence of poverty, pain, greed, and desperation is not an altogether uplifting story. But it is essential reading for understanding how opioids came to grip this country so fiercely, and it may help us move purposefully and effectively toward solutions and prevention efforts before we lose more young people due to the misuse of opioids. Perhaps most hopefully, the book emphasizes the effectiveness of medication-assisted treatment and behavioral interventions, leading readers toward the clear conclusion that we must invest more in the treatment and support of people who struggle with opioid addiction.

In 2022, Beth Macy published a follow-up book called *Raising Lazarus: Hope, Justice, and the Future of America's Overdose Crisis*. In this book, she focuses on the frontline workers who are trying to treat those who have opioid use disorder. She also traces the story of the Sackler family, the owners of the company (Purdue Pharma) that created OxyContin.

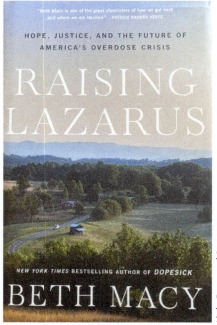

There are many different pain medications that can be legally prescribed, including **hydrocodone** and **oxycodone**. Hydrocodone is most often combined with other drugs, such as acetaminophen (the active agent in Tylenol), to create prescription pain medicines such as Vicodin, Zydone, and Lortab. Oxycodone is found in medicines such as Percodan, Tylox, and OxyContin. Vicodin is one of the most commonly abused drugs containing hydrocodone, and OxyContin is one of the most commonly abused drugs containing oxycodone. Fentanyl is another prescription pain medicine that has become a serious and deadly drug of abuse since 2015. In

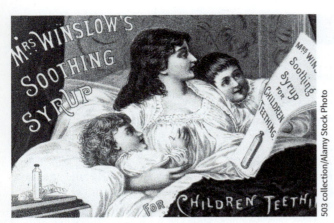

Heroin was synthesized from opium in 1874 and was soon added to a variety of medicines that could be purchased without prescription. This ad shows a teething remedy containing heroin. It probably worked.

fact, overdose deaths from opioids have been increasing since the turn of the century, and the most recent "wave" of deaths, beginning around 2013, is largely due to fentanyl and other synthetic opioids (Jalal, Buchanich, et al., 2018; Kiang, Basu, et al., 2019). Synthetic opioids like fentanyl are opioids that are made (synthesized) in a laboratory. The first wave of opioid deaths, starting in the 1990s, was driven mostly by prescription pain medicines; the second wave, beginning around 2010 was driven by heroin. The third wave which is still continuing is driven by fentanyl. In short, opioid overdose deaths continue to rise in a troubling way. During the COVID-19 pandemic, yearly overdose deaths from any drug reached 100,000 in 12 months, and that number has continued to grow in 2021 and 2022. Most of these deaths are due to synthetic opioid overdoses (National Center for Health Statistics, 2023; Spencer, Warner, & Chisewski, 2023).

Prevalence of Opioid Use and Its Consequences About 1.1 million people over age 12 in the United States reported using heroin in 2021 (SAMHSA, 2022). Slightly more men than women use heroin, but both use heroin most often after first taking prescription pain medicines (Cicero, Ellis, et al., 2014), as the **Clinical Case of Brandon** illustrates.

Prescription pain medicines used for nonprescribed purposes are the most commonly abused opioids. Nearly two million people met the criteria for opioid use disorder based on misuse of prescription pain medicines (SAMHSA, 2022). Although more women than men used prescription pain medicines in 2018, slightly more men than women *misused* or abused them. Misuse is substantially higher among White Americans than among any other ethnic or racial group (SAMHSA, 2022). **Table 10.4** lists some of the common pain medications.

Pharmaceutical companies encouraged use of prescription pain medicines, arguing that the risk of addiction was very low (Macy, 2018; Quinones, 2015). Once it became clear that addiction was not as rare as these companies promised in their sales materials, lawsuits were filed. Pharmaceutical companies then began to change their practices. For example, medicines such as OxyContin and Opana came in a pill format, with a polymer coating that made the pill easy to dissolve or crush into a form that could then be injected or snorted. Companies replaced the polymer-coated pills with a newly developed extended-release formula that is not as susceptible to crushing for injection.

With greater awareness and regulation of the misuse of prescription pain medications, overdose deaths from prescription pain medications have begun to decline. Unfortunately, overdose deaths from synthetic opioids, including fentanyl, have risen dramatically since 2015 (Centers for Disease Control and Prevention [CDC], 2018; Spencer, Warner, & Chisewski, 2023). The number of fentanyl overdose deaths more than tripled between 2015 and 2021 (Spencer, Warner, & Chisewski, 2023). By contrast, oxycodone overdose deaths decreased by 21% during the same period.

TABLE 10.4 **Types of Prescription Pain Medications**

Category	Commonly Prescribed Examples
Oxycodone	OxyContin, Percocet, Percodan
Hydrocodone	Vicodin, Lortab, Norco
Morphine	Avinza, MS Contin
Fentanyl	Actiq, Fentora
Tramadol	Ultram, Ultracet
Oxymorphone	Opana
Hydromorphone	Dilaudid, Exalgo
Buprenorphine*	Suboxone
Methadone*	

*Buprenorphine and methadone are also used to treat opioid addiction.

Psychological and Physical Effects

Opioids produce euphoria, drowsiness, and sometimes a lack of coordination. Heroin and OxyContin also produce a "rush," a feeling of warm, suffusing ecstasy immediately after an intravenous injection. The user sheds worry and fear and has great self-confidence for 4 to 6 hours. However, the user then experiences a severe letdown, bordering on stupor.

Opioids produce their effects by stimulating neural receptors of the body's own opioid system (the body naturally produces opioids, called *endorphins* and *enkephalins*). Heroin, for example, is converted into morphine in the brain and then binds to opioid receptors, which are located throughout the brain. Some evidence suggests that a link between these receptors and the dopamine system is responsible for opioids' pleasurable effects. However, evidence from animal studies suggests that opioids may achieve their pleasurable effects via their action in the area of the brain called the *nucleus accumbens* (Wade, Kallupi, et al., 2017).

Clinical Case

James

James was a 27-year-old man who had been addicted to heroin for 7 years. He first tried heroin during his time in the Marine Corps. Unable to control his habit, he was dishonorably discharged from the Marines a year later. He lived with his family for a short time, but after stealing money and valuables to support his habit, he was asked to leave the house. He then began living on the street, panhandling for money to support his habit. He also donated blood platelets when he was physically able. Over the years, James lost a tremendous amount of weight and became quite malnourished. He was over 6 feet tall, but he weighed only 150 pounds. Food wasn't a priority on most days, though he was usually able to gather a meal of scraps from the local diner. James tried to get into several rehabilitation programs, but they required that he remain free of heroin for at least a week before he could be admitted. James was able to resist for a day or two, but then withdrawal symptoms would begin, making it too painful to continue without the drug. A friend from the streets, formerly addicted to heroin, had recently helped James get to a methadone clinic. James tried methadone for a few weeks but was unable to tolerate the long waits outside the clinic each morning and the shame of being stared at by people passing on their way to work. Still, having been free of heroin for over a week, James gained admittance to a residential treatment program. One of the physicians at the program prescribed a newly approved medication called Suboxone that eased the discomfort of heroin withdrawal while replacing the cravings for heroin. James no longer needed to go to the methadone clinic, and he was getting job training at the treatment program. He was hopeful that he would shake his habit for good.

Opioids users develop tolerance and show withdrawal symptoms. Withdrawal from heroin, sometimes called "dopesick," may begin within 8 hours of the last injection in users who have built up high tolerance. During the next few hours after withdrawal begins, the person typically experiences muscle pain, sneezing, and sweating; becomes tearful; and yawns a great deal. The symptoms resemble those of influenza. Within 36 hours, the withdrawal symptoms become more severe. There may be uncontrollable muscle twitching, cramps, chills alternating with excessive flushing and sweating, and a rise in heart rate and blood pressure. The person is unable to sleep, vomits, and has diarrhea. These symptoms typically persist for about 72 hours and then diminish gradually over a 5- to 10-day period.

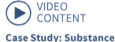

VIDEO CONTENT

Case Study: Substance Dependence Pause and Ponder

Stimulants

Stimulants act on the brain and the sympathetic nervous system to increase alertness and motor activity. Amphetamines are synthetic stimulants; cocaine is a natural stimulant extracted from the coca leaf. **Focus on Discovery 10.3** discusses a less risky and more prevalently used stimulant: caffeine. In DSM-5-TR, misuse of stimulants is called stimulant use disorder.

Amphetamines

Amphetamines such as Dexedrine and Adderall produce their effects by causing the release of norepinephrine and dopamine and blocking the reuptake of these neurotransmitters. **Amphetamines** are taken orally or intravenously. Amphetamines can heighten wakefulness, inhibit intestinal functions, and suppress appetite—hence, their use in dieting. They can quicken the heart rate and constrict blood vessels. A person becomes alert, euphoric, and outgoing and feels boundless energy and self-confidence. Larger doses can make a person nervous, agitated, and confused; other symptoms include palpitations, headaches, dizziness, and sleeplessness. Sometimes heavy users become extremely suspicious and hostile, to the extent that they can be dangerous to others.

Focus on Discovery 10.3

Our Tastiest Addiction—Caffeine

What may be the world's most popular drug is seldom viewed as a drug at all, and yet, it has strong effects. People can develop tolerance and experience withdrawal symptoms if they stop taking it (Hughes, Higgins, et al., 1991). Users and nonusers joke about it, and most readers of this book have probably had some this very day. We are, of course, referring to caffeine, a substance found in coffee, tea, cocoa, cola and other soft drinks, some cold remedies, and some diet pills.

A "grande" (16 ounces) cup of coffee from Starbucks contains 300 milligrams of caffeine. As little as 150 milligrams of caffeine can affect most people within half an hour. Metabolism, body temperature, and blood pressure all increase; urine production goes up; there may be hand tremors; appetite can diminish; and, most familiar of all, sleepiness is warded off. Extremely large doses of caffeine can cause headache, diarrhea, nervousness, severe agitation, and even convulsions and death. Death, though, is very rare unless a person takes a very large amount of caffeine in a very short period of time, because the drug is eliminated by the kidneys without much accumulation. Unfortunately, this is just what happened to a 16-year-old high school student in 2017. He consumed coffee, a soft drink, and an energy drink in 2 hours or less and subsequently died from cardiac arrest, probably caused by a heart arrhythmia triggered by the excessive caffeine. His heart was healthy; the caffeine was just too much for it.

Although it has long been recognized that drinkers of very large amounts of caffeinated coffee daily can experience withdrawal symptoms when consumption ceases, people who drink no more than two cups of coffee a day can suffer from headaches, fatigue, and anxiety if caffeine is withdrawn from their daily diet (Ferré, 2008), and these symptoms can interfere with social and occupational functioning. These findings are important because two-thirds of Americans have at least one cup of coffee a day, and coffee drinkers report having close to three cups a day according to a 2015 Gallup poll (Saad, 2015). And although parents may prohibit coffee, they often allow their children to have caffeine-laden soft drinks, energy drinks, or hot chocolate and to eat chocolate. Thus, our addiction to caffeine can begin to develop as early as 6 months of age, the form of it changing as we move from childhood to adulthood.

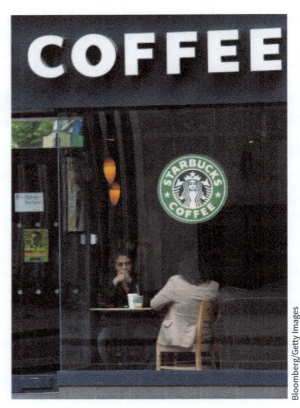

The caffeine found in coffee, tea, and soft drinks is probably the world's favorite drug.

Tolerance to amphetamines develops rapidly, so more and more of the drug is required to produce the stimulating effect. One study has demonstrated tolerance after just 6 days of repeated use (Comer, Hart, et al., 2001).

Methamphetamine   The most commonly abused stimulant drug is an amphetamine derivative called methamphetamine. Most methamphetamine comes from illicit sources. In 2021, over 2.5 million people ages 12 or older reported having used methamphetamine in the past year (SAMHSA, 2022).

Men are more likely to abuse methamphetamine than women; in contrast, few sex differences occur in the abuse of other amphetamines. Methamphetamine is used (and manufactured) in small towns in the United States as much as, if not more than, in big cities. The loss of manufacturing jobs in rural towns, along with consolidation of the American food business into a few big conglomerates instead of many smaller family farms, may have contributed to a rise in methamphetamine use (Macy, 2018; Redding, 2009).

Like other amphetamines, methamphetamine can be taken orally, intravenously, or intranasally (i.e., by snorting). In a clear crystal form, the drug is often referred to as "crystal meth" or "ice." Craving for methamphetamine is particularly strong, often lasting several years after use is discontinued. Craving is also a reliable predictor of later use (Hartz, Frederick-Osborne, & Galloway, 2001). As with other amphetamines, users of methamphetamine get an immediate high, or rush, that can last for hours. This includes feelings of euphoria as well as changes to the body, such as increases in blood flow to the heart and other organs and an increase in body temperature. The high eventually levels off (the "shoulder"), and then it comes crashing down ("tweaking"). Not only do the good feelings crash, but the person becomes very agitated. Physiological dependence on methamphetamine often includes both tolerance and withdrawal. Overdoses from methamphetamine can happen and are often fatal. Between 2015 and 2021, the number of methamphetamine overdose deaths more than quadrupled (Spencer, Warner, & Chisewski, 2023).

Several animal and human studies have indicated that chronic use of methamphetamine causes damage to the brain, affecting both the dopamine and the serotonin systems (Ashok, Mizuno, et al., 2017; Frost & Cadet, 2000). Neuroimaging studies of humans have found that methamphetamine use is associated with reductions in brain volume (size) in areas in the temporal and frontal cortices (Chen, Hsu, et al., 2019; Hall, Alhassoon, et al., 2015; Mackey & Paulus, 2013). For example, one study of chronic meth users found damage to the hippocampus (see **Figure 10.3**). The volume of the hippocampus was smaller among chronic meth users, which correlated with poorer performance on a memory test (Thompson, Hayashi, et al., 2004).

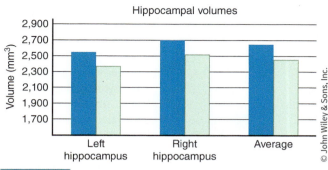

FIGURE 10.3 Results from an fMRI study showing that those who abused methamphetamine (green bars) had smaller hippocampal volume (size) than those in the control group (blue bars) who did not abuse methamphetamine.

© John Wiley & Sons, Inc.

Clinical Case

Anton

Anton, a 37-year-old man, had just been arrested for a parole violation: stealing a package of string cheese from a convenience store. He was also found to be under the influence of methamphetamine. Two months earlier, he had been released from prison after serving time for petty theft and for purchasing methamphetamine. He was determined to remain out of prison, but his cravings for meth were so intense that he was unable to abide by the terms of his parole. He had been using meth since he was 26 years old and had been arrested numerous times for drug-related offenses, including prostitution (to get money to support his habit).

Meta-analyses of brain-imaging studies indicate that areas of the brain impacted by methamphetamine use are areas associated with reward and decision making, such as the insula, areas of the frontal and temporal cortex, and the striatum (Ersche, Williams, et al., 2013; Hall et al., 2015). One study found that lower activation in these regions during a decision-making task predicted relapse to methamphetamine use 1 year after treatment (Paulus, Tapert, & Schuckit, 2005). Although it may seem obvious that poor decision making might put one at higher risk for relapse, it is less clear whether the methamphetamine damaged these areas or whether these areas were damaged before methamphetamine use began.

A caveat should be noted here. One difficulty with conducting these types of studies is finding participants who use only the drug of interest (in this case, methamphetamine) so that any observed effects can be linked exclusively to that drug. It is difficult to find meth users who have not at some point used other substances, particularly alcohol and nicotine. For example, in one of the studies described earlier, the meth users did not differ from the control group in alcohol consumption, but they did smoke more (Thompson et al., 2004). Nevertheless, it seems clear that the deleterious effects of methamphetamine are many and serious.

Cocaine   The drug **cocaine** comes from the leaves of the coca shrub. A form of cocaine called **crack** was developed in the mid-1980s; it comes in a rock-crystal form that is then heated, melted, and smoked. The name *crack* comes from the crackling sound the rock makes when being heated.

In 2021, 4.76 million people over the age of 12 reported using cocaine in the past year, about the same number and percentage (1.7% of people age 12 and older) as in 2015 (SAMHSA, 2022). The use of crack has also remained steady at just under a million in 2021 or 0.4% of people ages 12 and older (SAMHSA, 2022). Men use cocaine and crack more often than women do.

Cocaine can be sniffed (snorted), smoked in pipes or cigarettes, swallowed, or even injected into the veins; some heroin users mix the two drugs. Cocaine acts rapidly on the brain, blocking

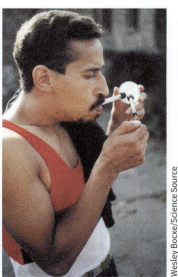

Crack cocaine is in rock-crystal form and "crackles" when heated.

Wesley Bocxe/Science Source

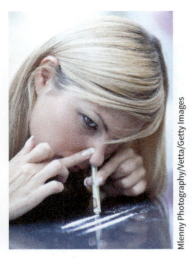

Cocaine can be smoked, swallowed, injected, or snorted, as shown here.

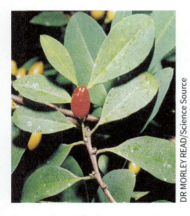

A coca plant. The leaves contain about 1% cocaine.

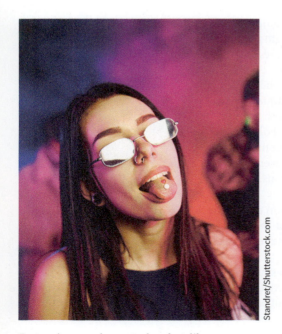

Ecstasy is a popular party drug but, like many drugs, is not free of ill effects.

the reuptake of dopamine in mesolimbic areas. Cocaine yields pleasurable states because dopamine left in the synapse facilitates neural transmission. Self-reports of pleasure induced by cocaine are related to the extent to which the drug has blocked dopamine reuptake (Volkow, Wang, et al., 1997). Cocaine can produce feelings of self-confidence, well-being, and stamina. An overdose may bring on chills, nausea, and insomnia, as well as strong paranoid feelings and terrifying hallucinations of insects crawling beneath the skin. Chronic use can lead to heightened irritability, impaired social relationships, paranoid thinking, and disturbances in eating and sleeping. Some, but not all, users develop tolerance to cocaine, requiring a larger dose to achieve the same effect. Stopping cocaine use appears to cause severe withdrawal symptoms.

Cocaine is a vasoconstrictor, causing the blood vessels to narrow. As users take larger and larger doses of the purer forms of cocaine, they are often rushed to emergency rooms and may die of an overdose, often from a heart attack. Cocaine also increases a person's risk for stroke and causes cognitive impairments, such as difficulty paying attention and remembering.

Hallucinogens, Ecstasy, and PCP

LSD and Other Hallucinogens

Hallucinogens include drugs such as LSD, psilocybin, Ecstasy, and mescaline. The term **hallucinogen** refers to the main effect of such drugs: hallucinations. Unlike the hallucinations in schizophrenia, however, these hallucinations are usually recognized by the person as being caused by the drug. The DSM-5-TR diagnosis that includes these substances is called *other hallucinogen use disorder*. In 2021, 7.4 million people over the age of 12 used some type of hallucinogen.

LSD (lysergic acid diethylamide) was very popular in the 1960s, but regular use generally declined over the next 50 years. However, the number of people using LSD increased to 403,000 in 2018, up from 352,000 in 2015 (SAMHSA, 2022). In 2019, LSD use among high school students was at its highest level since 2000 (Miech et al., 2020). There is no evidence of withdrawal symptoms, but tolerance appears to develop rapidly (Halberstadt, 2015).

Hallucinogens appear to exert their effects via the serotonin system and the 5-HT$_{2A}$ receptor (Halberstadt, 2015). In addition to producing hallucinations, LSD can alter a person's sense of time (it seems to go slowly). A person using LSD may have sharp mood swings, but can also experience an expanded consciousness such that they seem to appreciate sights and sounds as never before. These effects take place within 30 minutes of taking LSD and can last for up to 12 hours (Schmid, Enzler, et al., 2015).

Some users feel anxious after taking LSD, in part because the perceptual experiences and hallucinations can provoke fears that the user is "going crazy." The anxiety usually subsides as the drug is metabolized. Paradoxically, LSD has shown modest success for reducing anxiety in people diagnosed with life-threatening illnesses (Gasser, Holstein, et al., 2014).

Flashbacks are recurrences of perceptual experiences after the physiological effects of the drug have worn off. In DSM-5-TR, the diagnostic category *hallucinogen persisting perception disorder* involves re-experiences of flashbacks and other perceptual symptoms that occurred during hallucinogen use, even though the drug is no longer used.

Psilocybin has gained in popularity over the past several years, and research has intensified into using this hallucinogen to produce positive benefits for mental health and end-of-life experiences (Nutt, Erritzoe, & Carhart-Harris, 2020; Pollan, 2018; Rucker, Iliff, & Nutt, 2018). In 2020, Oregon decriminalized the use of psilocybin and approved it for medical use, and many other states are considering similar measures. Statistical modeling of state and local legislative initiatives suggests that a majority of U.S. states will legalize psychedelics in the next 10 to 15 years (Siegel, Daily, et al., 2023).

MDMA (Ecstasy)

The hallucinogen-like substance **Ecstasy** is made from compounds from both the hallucinogen and the amphetamine families, including **MDMA** (methylenedioxymethamphetamine).

Ecstasy began as a popular drug on college campuses and in clubs, though it is now used among over 2% of high school students (Miech et al., 2023). In 2021, 2.1% of people age 18 or older reported using Ecstasy during the past year (SAMHSA, 2022). **Focus on Discovery 10.4** discusses the use and effects of another club drug: nitrous oxide. MDMA can be taken in pill form but is often mixed with other substances (e.g., caffeine) or drugs (e.g., LSD, ketamine, talcum powder), making the effects vary dramatically. A purer powder version of Ecstasy is referred to as "Molly." Whether it is actually purer requires a leap of faith, as powder can also be mixed with other substances.

Clinical Case

Tamara

Tamara tried Ecstasy (X) for the first time when she was a freshman in college. She went to her first rave, and a friend gave her a pill she thought was a Sweet Tart. Within a short period of time, she began to feel almost magical, as if she were seeing everything around her in a new light. She felt incredibly close to her friends and even to men and women she had just met. Hugging and close dancing were intensely pleasurable in a completely new way. A few days after the party, she asked her friend about the "Sweet Tart" and found out how she could obtain more. But the next time she tried X, she was unable to achieve the same pleasurable feelings. Instead, she felt more subdued, even anxious. After several more times using X, she noticed that despite her enthusiasm and even craving for the effects, instead she felt a little depressed and anxious, even several days after taking the drug.

Ecstasy acts primarily by contributing to both the release and the subsequent reuptake of serotonin (Liechti, Baumann, et al., 2000; Morgan, 2000).

Users report that Ecstasy enhances intimacy and insight, improves interpersonal relationships, elevates positive emotion and self-confidence, and promotes aesthetic awareness. It can also cause muscle tension, rapid eye movements, jaw clenching, nausea, faintness, chills or sweating, anxiety, depression, depersonalization, and confusion. Like psilocybin, MDMA is being assessed to see if it might relieve mental distress. For example, a randomized controlled clinical trial found that MDMA in combination with therapy (MDMA-assisted psychotherapy) was safer and more effective than a placebo for people with PTSD (Mitchell, Bogenshutz, et al., 2021).

PCP   Abuse of **PCP** (phencyclidine), often called *angel dust*, is coded as *phencyclidine use disorder* in DSM-5-TR and is in the section on hallucinogen-related disorders. Abuse of ketamine is also classified as phencyclidine use disorder in DSM-5-TR. As with most drugs, more men than women use PCP and ketamine.

Focus on Discovery 10.4

Nitrous Oxide—Not a Laughing Matter

Nitrous oxide is a colorless gas that has been available since the 19th century. Within seconds, it induces lightheadedness and a state of euphoria in most people; for some, important insights seem to flood the mind. Many people find otherwise mundane events and thoughts irresistibly funny, hence the nickname *laughing gas*.

Many people have received nitrous oxide at a dentist's office to facilitate relaxation and otherwise make a potentially uncomfortable and intimidating dental procedure more palatable. A major advantage of nitrous oxide over other analgesics and relaxants is that a person can return to a normal waking state within minutes of again breathing enriched oxygen or normal air.

Nitrous oxide fits in the broader category of inhalants and has been used recreationally since it first became available, although it has been illegal for many years in most states except as administered by appropriate health professionals. As with the other drugs examined in this chapter, illegality has not prevented unsupervised use. It is one of the most commonly used inhalants among teens and young adults (along with sniffing glue, gasoline, and paint). Sometimes called "hippie crack" or "whippets," nitrous oxide balloons are often used along with Ecstasy and other drugs at parties with bright laser lights and loud dance music (i.e., at raves).

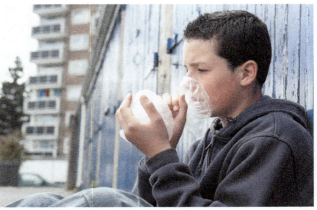

Nitrous oxide is no laughing matter.

PCP generally causes serious negative reactions, including severe paranoia and violence. Coma and death are also possible. PCP affects multiple neurotransmitters in the brain, and chronic use is associated with a variety of neuropsychological deficits. People who abuse PCP are likely to have used other drugs either before or concurrently with PCP, so it is difficult to sort out whether neuropsychological impairments are due solely to PCP, to other drugs, or to the combination.

Quick Summary

Opioids include heroin and other pain medications such as hydrocodone and oxycodone. Abuse of prescription pain medications rose dramatically in the 1990s, and overdoses are common. Overdose deaths due to synthetic opioids such as fentanyl are still increasing and is a severe problem. Initial effects of opioids include euphoria; later, users experience a letdown. Withdrawal is extremely unpleasant for opioids, often referred to as "dopesick." Amphetamines are stimulants that produce wakefulness, alertness, and euphoria. Men and women use these equally. Tolerance develops quickly. Methamphetamine is a synthesized amphetamine; its use increased dramatically in the 1990s but has leveled off in recent years. Methamphetamine can damage the brain, including the hippocampus. Cocaine can increase sexual desire, feelings of well-being, and alertness, but chronic use is associated with problems in relationships, paranoia, and trouble sleeping, among other things.

LSD was a popular hallucinogen in the 1960s, often thought of as a mind-expanding drug. Other such mind-expanding drugs include psilocybin and MDMA (Ecstasy). A so-called purer form of Ecstasy called Molly is used, but its purity cannot be ascertained. The therapeutic benefits of hallucinogens are being tested and early results are promising. Although these drugs do not typically elicit withdrawal symptoms, tolerance can develop. PCP can cause severe paranoia and violence.

10.2 Check Your Knowledge

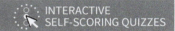 INTERACTIVE SELF-SCORING QUIZZES

(Answers are at the end of the chapter.)
True or false?

1. Withdrawal from heroin begins slowly, days after use has been discontinued.
2. The opioid crisis began with fentanyl in the 1990s and now mostly involves prescription pain medications.
3. Methamphetamine is a less potent form of amphetamine and so is less likely to be associated with brain impairment.
4. MDMA (Ecstasy) contains compounds associated with hallucinogens and amphetamines.

Causes of Substance Use Disorders

As with all the other disorders we have discussed in this book, several factors contribute to the cause of substance use disorders. Indeed, substance use disorders are caused by a complex interaction of psychological and sociocultural factors (e.g., deciding to first use a substance) with the brain (that becomes sensitized after repeated substance use) and genes (Ray & Grodin, 2021). One of the key questions about the cause of substance use disorders is why some people develop a disorder after substance use and others do not. In the following sections, we discuss genetic, neurobiological, psychological, and sociocultural influences associated with substance use disorders. Keep in mind that these influences are likely to be differently related to different substances. Genetic factors, for example, may play a role in alcohol use disorder but may be less important in hallucinogen use disorder.

Genetic Influences

Much research has addressed the possibility that there is a genetic contribution to drug and alcohol use disorders. Heritability estimates range from 0.40 to 0.60, suggesting that genes do play a role in such disorders. Like most all disorders discussed in the book, multiple genes are involved (Deak & Johnson, 2021; Gelernter & Polimanti, 2021), and there is commonality in the genetic susceptibility across substance use disorders according to large GWAS results (Hatoum, Colbert, et al., 2023). Evidence from twin studies suggests genetic involvement in alcohol use disorder (McGue, Pickens, & Svikis, 1992), smoking (Li, Cheng, et al., 2003), heavy use of marijuana (Kendler & Prescott, 1998), and drug use disorders in general (Tsuang, Lyons, et al., 1998).

Of course, genes do their work via the environment, and research has uncovered gene–environment relationships in alcohol and drug use disorders (Kendler, Chen, et al., 2012; Kendler, Ohlsson, et al., 2019). In a Swedish study of close to a million people, those who had a family history of alcohol problems were more likely to develop alcohol use disorder following a divorce, suggesting a gene–environment interaction (Kendler, Lönn, et al., 2016). Among adolescents, peers appear to be particularly important environmental variables. For example, a large twin study in Finland found that heritability for alcohol problems among adolescents was higher among those teens who had many peers who drank than among those who had a smaller number of peers who drank (Dick, Pagan, et al., 2007). The environmental factor in this case was peer-group drinking behavior. Another study found that heritability for both alcohol and smoking among adolescents was higher for those teens whose best friend smoked and drank (Harden, Hill, et al., 2008). In this case, the environmental factor was best-friend behavior. Another study found that heritability for smoking was greater for teens who went to schools where the "popular crowd" smoked than for students at schools where such students did not smoke (Boardman, Saint Onge, et al., 2008).

Genetics may also play a protective role in alcohol use. For example, some Asian people may have a low rate of alcohol problems because of physiological intolerance caused by an inherited deficiency in the enzymes involved in alcohol metabolism, called *alcohol dehydrogenases* (ADH). Mutations in genes called *ADH2* and *ADH3* code proteins that make up the ADH enzymes, and these genes have been linked with alcohol use disorders generally as well as among some Asian populations specifically (Edenberg, Xuie, et al., 2006; Sher, Grekin, & Williams, 2005). About three-quarters of Asian people experience unpleasant effects such as flushing (blood flow to the face) from small quantities of alcohol, which may protect them from developing tolerance to or withdrawal from alcohol. Similarly, genes that code for aldehyde dehydrogenase (ADLH), another substance that metabolizes alcohol have been identified in GWAS as genetic influences for alcohol use disorder (Edenberg, Gelernter, & Agrawal, 2019).

Research has also emerged on the mechanism through which genetics plays a role in smoking and alcohol.

A gene called *CYP2A6* codes for an enzyme that metabolizes nicotine may contribute to nicotine use disorder (Furberg, Kim, et al., 2010). Slower nicotine metabolism means that nicotine stays in the brain longer. Evidence suggests that variants of this gene are linked to more smoking per day (Murphy, 2017); people who metabolize nicotine more quickly are likely to smoke more. In addition, a prospective study of smokers found that *CYP2A6* was associated with a greater risk of developing lung cancer even after controlling for other variables, such as amount of smoking (Park, Murphy, et al., 2017). One of the largest GWAS to date identified several SNPs in the region of the *CYP2A6* gene (Buchwald, Chenowith, et al., 2020). Other evidence has found that people who show reduced activity of the *CYP2A6* gene smoke fewer cigarettes and are less likely to become dependent on nicotine or develop lung cancer (Audrain-McGovern & Tercyak, 2011; Johani, Majid, et al., 2020). This is an interesting example of a gene polymorphism serving a protective function.

The role of genes in marijuana use has also been studied. In a GWAS with over 32,000 people, four different genes were associated with marijuana use, but none of the SNPs reached statistical significance at the genome-wide level, even with this large sample (Stringer, Minica, et al., 2016). As we have seen, finding the set of genes associated with any psychological disorder remains a very big challenge.

Neurobiological Influences

You may have noticed that in our discussions of specific drugs the neurotransmitter dopamine has almost always been mentioned. This is not surprising given that dopamine pathways in the brain are linked to pleasure and reward. Drug use typically results in rewarding or pleasurable feelings, and it is via the dopamine system that these feelings are produced. Research with both humans and animals shows that nearly all drugs, including alcohol, stimulate the dopamine pathways in the brain (see **Figure 10.4**), particularly the mesolimbic pathway

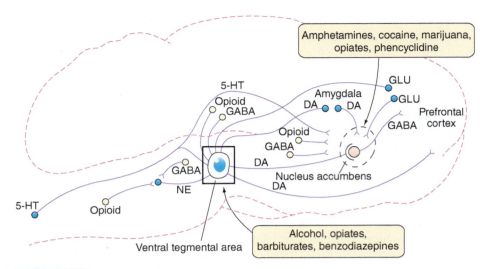

FIGURE 10.4 Reward pathways in the brain that are affected by different drugs. DA = dopamine; GABA = gamma-aminobutyric acid; GLU = glutamate; 5-HT = serotonin; NE = norepinephrine.

(Koob & Le Moal, 2008; Volkow & Boyle, 2018). Researchers have wondered, then, whether problems in the dopamine pathways in the brain might somehow account for why certain people develop substance use disorders.

It is difficult to determine whether problems in the dopamine system increase the vulnerability of some people to developing a substance use disorder, sometimes called the "vulnerability model," or whether problems in the dopamine system are the consequence of taking substances, the "toxic effect model." For drugs such as cocaine and opioids, current research supports both views (Bechara, Berridge, et al., 2019).

Although people take drugs to feel good, they also take them to feel less bad. This is particularly true for people who struggle with substances such as alcohol, methamphetamine, or heroin, whose withdrawal symptoms are excruciatingly unpleasant. In other words, people continue to take drugs to avoid the bad feelings associated with withdrawal. Moreover, they may be particularly sensitive to stress just after stopping use of a substance, and exposure to stress may then trigger a return to use (Kaye, Bradford, et al., 2017). A substantial body of research with animals supports this motivation for drug-taking behavior (Koob & Le Moal, 2008). Newer research supports this motivation in humans as well. For example, one study found that people with alcohol use disorder who had recently stopped drinking exhibited larger physiological responses to unpredictable stress than did people who did not have alcohol use disorder (Moberg, Bradford, et al., 2017). This research helps to explain why relapse is so common.

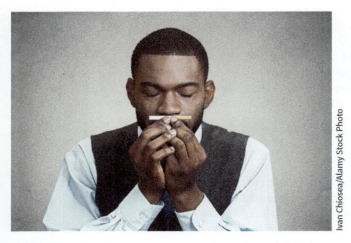

Craving, or wanting, a substance is an important component of substance use disorders.

Investigators have proposed a neurobiological theory to explain cravings, referred to as the *incentive-sensitization theory,* which considers both the craving for drugs ("wanting") and the pleasure that comes with taking the drugs ("liking") (Robinson & Berridge, 1993, 2003). According to this theory, the dopamine system, which is linked to pleasure, or liking, becomes supersensitive not just to the direct effects of drugs but also to the cues associated with drugs (e.g., needles, spoons, rolling paper). This sensitivity to cues induces craving, or wanting, and people go to extreme lengths to seek out and obtain drugs. Over time, the liking for drugs decreases, but the wanting remains very intense. These investigators argue that the transition from liking to powerful wanting, accomplished by the drug' effects on brain pathways involving dopamine, is what maintains the addiction.

Many researchers have studied the neurobiology of cravings. A number of laboratory studies have shown that cues for a particular drug can elicit responses not altogether unlike those associated with actual use of the drug. For example, compared with people not dependent on cocaine, those who were dependent on cocaine exhibited more changes in physiological arousal, increases in cravings and "high" feelings, and increases in negative emotions in response to cues of cocaine (which consisted of audio and video recordings of people preparing to inject or snort cocaine) (e.g., Robbins, Ehrman, et al., 2000). Brain-imaging studies have shown that cues for a drug, such as a needle or a cigarette, activate the reward and pleasure areas of the brain implicated in drug use. One study of smokers found that anticipating smoking by looking at a cigarette prior to a stressful task lessened physiological and self-reported stress responses more than actually smoking prior to the task (Bradford, Curtin, & Piper, 2015). A meta-analysis of over 200 studies that prospectively assessed exposure to cues or reports of craving with subsequent substance use or relapse found that such exposure or craving more than doubled the likelihood of drug use or relapse, suggesting the powerful role of cues and cravings as causal influences (Vafale & Kober, 2022).

What about the psychology of craving? Do people with stronger cravings for a substance actually use it more, even when they are trying to quit? The answer appears to be yes. In a longitudinal study of heavy drinkers, the more participants reported wanting (craving) and liking samples of alcohol (carefully presented to reduce expectancies about alcohol) at a baseline assessment, the more alcohol use disorder symptoms they had 6 years later (King, McNamara, et al., 2014).

An experience-sampling study (see Chapter 3) of people who were trying to quit smoking showed that more craving was associated with more smoking (Berkman, Falk, & Lieberman, 2011). People who had just started a smoking-cessation program were given text messages 8 times a day for 21 consecutive days. At each text prompt, they reported how many cigarettes they had smoked, how much they were craving a cigarette, and how they were feeling. Reports of more craving predicted a greater likelihood of smoking when the participants received their next text. These investigators also used fMRI to examine participants' brain activation during a task called the "go/no-go task." In this task, people are presented with onscreen letters one at a time and are instructed to press a button when they see certain letters (e.g., L, V, T, N; the "go" part) but refrain from pressing the button when they see another letter (X; the "no-go" part). There are many more "go" trials than "no-go" trials, and thus, it is challenging to keep from pressing the button during a "no-go" trial because people get into the habit of pressing the button many times in a row on the "go" trials. Areas of the brain that showed greater activation during "no-go" trials than during "go" trials included the basal ganglia, inferofrontal gyrus, and premotor areas. People who showed greater activation in these areas during the task were better able to inhibit their button pressing; their brain was therefore likely doing a better job of providing support for inhibiting a response when needed. In addition, greater activation in these brain regions was associated with less linkage between craving and smoking. That is, people who showed greater brain activation when inhibiting a button press were less likely to act on their cravings and begin to smoke again.

Valuing the Short Term over the Long Term

A related psychological and neurobiological model emphasizes the distinction between the values people place on short-term (immediate) versus long-term (delayed) rewards. People with a substance use disorder often value the immediate, even impulsive, pleasure and reward that come from taking a drug more than they do a delayed reward, such as a monthly paycheck from work.

Laboratory experiments to assess whether people value immediate or delayed rewards typically present people with choices of monetary rewards that are immediate but small (e.g., $1 now) or delayed but larger (e.g., $10 in a day). The extent to which people opt for the smaller, immediate reward can be calculated mathematically and is referred to as *delay discounting*. In other words, researchers can compute the extent to which people discount the value of larger, delayed rewards. People who substance use disorders include substances such as opioids, nicotine, heroin, and cocaine, discount delayed rewards more steeply than do people without these disorders (Bickel, Koffarnus, et al., 2014). One longitudinal study found that the extent of delay discounting predicted smoking initiation in adolescents that continued into early adulthood (Audrain-McGovern, Rodriguez, et al., 2009).

At the level of the brain, valuing immediate and delayed rewards recruits different brain regions. Researchers have hypothesized that these brain regions compete with one another when people are faced with a decision about whether to take a drug. In fMRI studies, valuing the delayed reward is associated with activation of the prefrontal cortex; valuing the immediate reward is associated with activation in the amygdala and the nucleus accumbens (Bechara, 2005; Bechara et al., 2019; Bickel, Miller, et al., 2007).

Risky Decision Making

Another psychological and neurobiological theory on substance use disorders involves decision making. Specifically, people with drug or alcohol use disorders are prone to make *risky* decisions when it comes to substance use or drug-seeking behavior (Chen, Yang, et al., 2020). What may contribute to the making of such risky decisions are difficulties with tolerating risks, whether they are known risks (e.g., "If I take this drug, I know I will be late for work") or ambiguous risks (e.g., "If I take this drug, I might get caught by my boss").

In a study of people currently in treatment for opioid use disorder, researchers found that people who had low tolerance for ambiguous risks, but not for known risks, were more likely to begin using opioids again during the course of a 7-month treatment program (Konova, Lopez-Guzman, et al., 2020). The researchers were able to prospectively predict who was at risk for such a relapse by using a computer game that assesses tolerance for known versus ambiguous financial risks.

Brain regions that support risky decision making are similar to those identified as being involved in delay discounting, but there are also distinct regions linked with decision making. Specifically, a meta-analysis of fMRI studies found that risky decision making is associated with activation in brain regions including the orbitofrontal cortex, parietal cortex, and rostral parts of the anterior cingulate cortex. Tolerance for ambiguity is associated with the dorsolateral prefrontal cortex, parietal cortex, and dorsal parts of the anterior cingulate cortex (Krain, Wilson, et al., 2006).

Psychological Influences

In this section, we look at three other types of psychological influences that may contribute to the cause of substance use disorders. First, we consider the effects of drugs (particularly alcohol and nicotine) on emotion regulation; we examine the situations in which a tension-reducing effect occurs and the role of cognition in this process. Second, we consider people's expectancies about the effects of substances on behavior, including beliefs about the prevalence with which a drug is used and about the health risks associated with using that drug. Third, we consider personality traits that may make some people more likely to use drugs heavily.

Emotion Regulation

It is generally assumed that one of the main psychological motives for using drugs is to alter emotion—that is, drug use is reinforced because it enhances positive feelings or diminishes negative ones (Sayette, 2017). For example, most people believe that stress or negative emotion (e.g., because of a bad day at work) leads to increased alcohol consumption.

Unfortunately, people with substance use disorders may be less successful than people without substance use disorders in regulating negative emotion, at least when it comes to recruiting brain regions and networks that support regulation, such as the prefrontal cortex (Wilcox, Pommy, & Adinoff, 2016). Whether this is a cause or consequence of substance use is not entirely clear, but most brain-imaging studies that have examined emotion regulation have done so following at least 2 weeks of abstinence.

Subsequent research has examined why substances appear to reduce negative emotion in some situations but not others. Three factors appear to be important: uncertainty, unpredictability, and distraction. Laboratory studies have demonstrated that alcohol reduces self-reported and physiological indicators of negative emotion, particularly when there is uncertainty (e.g.,

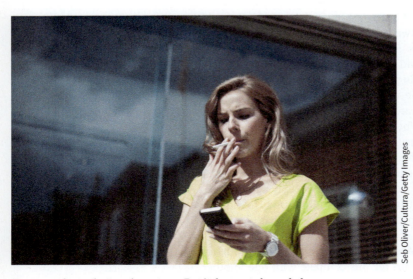

Seb Oliver/Cultura/Getty Images

Some people smoke to reduce stress. But it does not always help.

having arrived home late after having drinks with friends, will you argue with your spouse?) or uncontrollability (e.g., my car won't start) about a negative event (Bradford, Shapiro, & Curtin, 2013; Bradford, Shireman, et al., 2022).

Other studies have found that emotion effects are more likely to occur when distractions are present (Fairbairn & Sayette, 2013; Josephs & Steele, 1990; Steele & Josephs, 1988). Alcohol narrows our attention to the most immediately available cues, resulting in "alcohol myopia" (Steele & Josephs, 1990). In other words, an intoxicated person has less cognitive capacity and tends to use that capacity to focus on the immediate situation, which may be a distraction from negative emotion, and thus, negative emotions may decrease.

Research has also documented the added benefits of distraction for relieving anxiety with nicotine. Specifically, smokers who smoked during a distracting activity experienced a reduction in anxiety, whereas smokers who smoked without a distracting activity did not experience lessened anxiety (Kassel & Shiffman, 1997; Kassel & Unrod, 2000). However, alcohol and nicotine may increase negative emotion when no distractions are present. For example, a person drinking alone may focus all of their limited cognitive capacity on unpleasant thoughts, begin brooding, and become increasingly tense and anxious, a situation reflected in the expression "crying in one's beer."

Another reason people may opt to use substances is to increase positive emotion in social situations. Sayette and colleagues (Fairbairn & Sayette, 2014) have proposed that people may turn to alcohol as an emotion regulation tool in social situations because it can help them damp down thoughts of being rejected ("I must sound so stupid to these people") and focus instead on the pleasures of being around others ("This is so much fun laughing together!").

In one study, participants were placed in groups of three unacquainted people to do assigned tasks and talk about whatever they wished. Some of these small groups were given alcohol to drink (cranberry juice and vodka); others were given cranberry juice. Other groups were told they were drinking alcohol but were actually given nonalcoholic beverages (tonic and cranberry juice with vodka on the outside of the glass for smell). The researchers found that the participants in the groups that drank alcohol smiled and bonded more than those in the other two groups (Sayette, Creswell, et al., 2012). In this study, the effects of alcohol were stronger than the expectations about alcohol. As we discuss in the next section, however, simply expecting to receive alcohol can have a profound impact on behavior.

Expectancies About Alcohol and Drug Effects

If substances don't always reduce negative emotion or increase positive emotion, why do so many people who drink or take drugs believe that it helps them unwind? Expectation may play a role here—that is, people may drink not because it actually reduces negative emotion but because they expect it to do so. In support of this idea, studies have shown that people who expect alcohol to reduce stress and anxiety are more likely to be frequent users (Sher, Walitzer, et al., 1991; Tran, Haaga, & Chambless, 1997). Furthermore, the expectation that drinking will reduce anxiety increases drinking, which in turn makes the positive expectancies even stronger (Sher, Wood, et al., 1996; Smith, Goldman, et al., 1995). More broadly, expectancies about alcohol and its effects, particularly social effects (e.g., people are more friendly, people are mean), develop in childhood, as early as age 4 (Voogt, Beusink, et al., 2017). Throughout development and particularly after first exposure to alcohol, expectancies about alcohol become more positive (Smit, Voogt, et al., 2018). Alcohol expectancies also prospectively predict alcohol use and problem drinking among adolescents, and thus addressing these expectations can be an important focus of prevention programs (Smit et al., 2018).

Other research has shown that expectancies about a drug's effects—for example, the belief that a drug will increase sexual responsiveness—predict increased drug use in general (Stacy, Newcomb, & Bentler, 1991). Similarly, people who believe (falsely) that alcohol will make them seem more socially skilled are likely to drink more heavily than those who accurately perceive that alcohol can interfere with social interactions. In now-classic experiments demonstrating the power of expectancies, participants who believe they are consuming a quantity

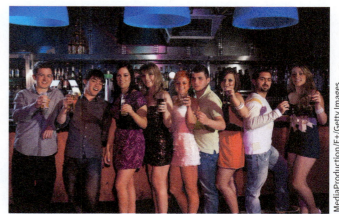

Expectations about alcohol influence whether people will drink.

of alcohol when they are actually consuming an alcohol-free beverage subsequently become more aggressive (Lang, Goeckner, et al., 1975). Alcohol consumption is associated with increased aggression, but expectancies about alcohol's effects can also play a role (Bushman & Cooper, 1990; Ito, Miller, & Pollock, 1996). Thus, as we have seen in other contexts, cognitions can have a powerful effect on behavior.

The extent to which a person expects a drug to be harmful and the perceived prevalence of use by others are also factors related to use. In general, the greater the perceived risk of a drug, the less likely it is to be used. For example, the illegal drug most commonly used by high school students is marijuana; it is also the drug with the lowest perceived risk of harm in this age group (Miech et al., 2020).

Personality Factors   Personality factors that appear to be important in predicting the later onset of substance use disorders include high levels of negative affect, sometimes called *negative emotionality* or *neuroticism*; a persistent desire for arousal, along with increased positive affect; and constraint, which refers to cautious behavior, harm avoidance, and conservative moral standards. One longitudinal study found that 18-year-olds who were low in constraint but high in negative emotionality were more likely to develop a substance use disorder as young adults (Krueger, 1999).

Another prospective longitudinal study investigated whether personality factors could predict the onset of substance use disorders in over 1,000 male and female adolescents at age 17 and then again at age 20 (Elkins, King, et al., 2006). Low constraint and high negative emotionality predicted the onset of alcohol, nicotine, and illicit drug use disorders for both men and women.

A large meta-analysis of both cross-sectional and prospective studies assessing personality traits and psychopathology, including substance use disorders, found strong associations with low levels of agreeableness and conscientiousness and with high levels of disinhibition (i.e., low constraint), as well as moderate associations with neuroticism (Kotov, Gamez, et al., 2010).

Sociocultural Influences

Sociocultural influences play a widely varying role in substance use disorders. People's interest in and access to drugs are influenced by peers, the media, and cultural norms about acceptable behavior.

At the broadest level, we can look at great cross-national variation in substance consumption. Some research suggests that there are commonalities in substance use across countries. For example, a cross-national study of alcohol and drug use among high school students in 36 countries found that alcohol was the substance most commonly used across countries, despite great variation in the proportions of students who consumed alcohol, ranging from 32% in Zimbabwe to 99% in Wales (Smart & Ogburne, 2000). In all but two of the countries studied, marijuana was the next most commonly used drug. In those countries where marijuana was used most often (with more than 15% of high school students having ever used marijuana), there were also higher rates of use of amphetamines, Ecstasy, and cocaine.

Despite the commonalities across countries, other research has documented cross-national differences in alcohol consumption. For example, a cross-national study found that in some countries (e.g., Argentina, Australia, France, and Norway), 80% or more of the population drank alcohol. In other countries (e.g., Algeria, China, India, and Saudi Arabia), less than 20% of the population drank alcohol (Griswold et al., 2018).

The social setting in which a person operates can also affect substance use (Dimoff & Sayette, 2017; Fairbairn & Sayette, 2014). For example, studies showed that having friends who smoke predicts smoking. In longitudinal studies, peer-group identification in the 7th grade predicted smoking in the 8th grade (Sussman, Dent, et al., 1994) and increased drug use over a 3-year period (Chassin, Curran, et al., 1996). Peer influences are

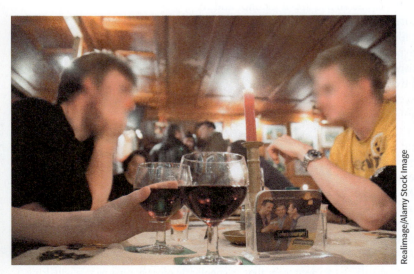

Realimage/Alamy Stock Image

Alcohol use disorder is more prevalent in countries in which alcohol use is heavy.

also important in promoting the use of alcohol (Deutsch, Chernyavskiy, et al., 2015; Hussong, Hicks, et al., 2001; Kelly, Chan, et al., 2012), e-cigarettes (Pentz, Shin, et al., 2015), and other drugs (Chan, Kelly, et al., 2017).

These findings support the idea that social networks influence a person's drug and alcohol behavior. However, other evidence indicates that people who are inclined to develop substance use disorders may select social networks that conform to their own drinking or drug use patterns. Thus, we have two broad explanations for how the social environment is related to substance use disorders: a social influence model and a social selection model. A longitudinal study of over 1,200 adults, designed to test which model better accounted for drinking behavior, found support for both models (Bullers, Cooper, & Russell, 2001). A person's social network predicted individual drinking, but individual drinking also predicted subsequent social network drinking. In fact, the social selection effects were stronger, indicating that people often choose social networks with drinking patterns like their own. No doubt the selected networks then support or reinforce their drinking.

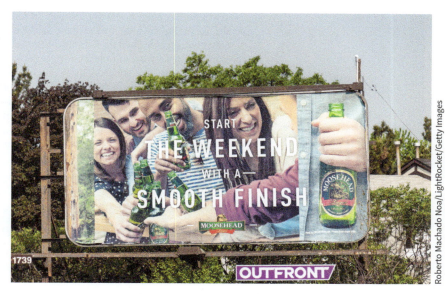

Advertising is one variable that affects expectancies about drug or alcohol use.

Another variable to be considered is the influence of the media. Television commercials associate beer with attractive men and women having a good time. Billboards equate cigarettes with excitement, relaxation, and being in style. A review of studies found that tobacco billboards were more than twice as common in primarily Black neighborhoods than they were in primarily White neighborhoods (Primack, Bost, et al., 2007).

Does advertising change substance use patterns among young people? Some evidence indicates that it does. A review of 12 studies across the world of young people who were exposed to alcohol marketing were more likely to start drinking alcohol and experience episodes of binge drinking (Jernigen, Noel, et al., 2016). In a longitudinal study of nonsmoking adolescents, those who had a favorite cigarette ad were twice as likely to begin smoking subsequently or to be willing to do so (Pierce, Choi, et al., 1998). A longitudinal study in Germany found that adolescents who were exposed to ads for e-cigarettes were more likely to try them (Hansen, Hanewinkel, & Morgenstern, 2020). On the flip side, advertising about the ill effects of smoking is associated with a lower likelihood of becoming a smoker (Emery, Kim, et al., 2012).

As part of the 1998 settlement of a class-action suit brought by 46 states that charged U.S. tobacco companies with manipulating nicotine levels to keep smokers addicted, several companies agreed to stop advertising and marketing efforts aimed at children. Despite these promises by tobacco companies, an analysis of internal documents of several of these companies (made public thanks to the lawsuit) by researchers at the Harvard School of Public Health revealed that they were still targeting their advertising toward young people (Kreslake, Wayne, Alpert, et al., 2008). The tobacco companies' own research had found that cigarettes with mild menthol appealed more to young people, and thus, they made efforts to market these milder menthol brands to young people. In 2017 and 2018, over half of adolescent smokers chose menthol cigarettes (Azagba, King, et al., 2020). Adolescents who begin smoking menthol cigarettes are more likely to continue smoking than those who do not begin with menthol cigarettes (Nonnemaker, Hersey, et al., 2013).

Quick Summary

Several etiological factors have been proposed with respect to substance use disorders. Genetic factors play a role in both alcohol and nicotine use disorders. The ability to tolerate alcohol or metabolize nicotine may be what is heritable. Several studies have shown how genes interact with the environment to cause smoking and alcohol use disorders. The most studied neurobiological influences are brain systems associated with dopamine pathways—the major reward pathways in the brain. The incentive-sensitization theory describes brain pathways involved in liking and wanting (i.e., craving) drugs. People with substance use problems value immediate rewards more than delayed rewards.

Psychological influences have also been evaluated, and there is support for the idea that emotion regulation plays a role, but only under certain circumstances, such as when distractions are present. Expectancies about the effects of drugs, such as reducing tension and increasing social skills, have been shown to predict drug and alcohol use. Expectancies are powerful: The greater the perceived risk of a drug, the less likely it is to be used. Studies of personality factors further help us understand why some people may be more prone than others to abuse drugs and alcohol.

Sociocultural influences play a role, including the culture, availability of a substance, family factors, social settings and networks, and advertising. Support exists for both a social influence model and a social selection model.

10.3 Check Your Knowledge

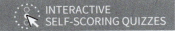 INTERACTIVE SELF-SCORING QUIZZES

(Answers are at the end of the chapter.)
Select the best answer to each question.

1. Which of the following is *not* one of the sociocultural factors implicated in the cause of substance use disorders?
   a. the media
   b. cultural norms
   c. availability of a substance
   d. peers

2. Which of the following statements best captures the link between wanting, liking, and drinking, according to a large prospective study?
   a. Wanting, but not liking, predicted more drinking among heavy drinkers.
   b. Wanting predicted more drinking for heavy drinkers; liking predicted more drinking for light drinkers.
   c. Wanting and liking predicted more drinking among heavy drinkers.
   d. Sedation predicted less drinking for all types of drinkers.

3. Genetics research on substance use indicates that:
   a. genetic factors are the same for many drugs
   b. additional studies need to be done to determine heritability
   c. the *CYP2A6* gene may contribute to nicotine use disorder
   d. twin studies show that the environment is not important

---

Treatment of Substance Use Disorders

The chronicity of addiction is really a kind of fatalism writ large. If an addict knows in his heart he is going to use again, why not today? But if a thin reed of hope appears, the possibility that it will not always be so, things change. You live another day and then get up and do it again. Hope is oxygen to someone who is suffocating on despair.

(Carr, 2008)

The challenges in treating people with substance use disorders are great, as illustrated by the preceding quote. Substance use disorders are typically chronic, and relapse occurs often. In view of these challenges, the field is continually working to develop new and effective treatments, many of which we review in this section. The author of the quote, David Carr, was formerly addicted to cocaine, crack, and alcohol. He wrote about his experiences in a beautiful memoir while working as a media columnist for *The New York Times*. For him, residential treatment was successful.

Many who work with those with alcohol or drug use disorders suggest that the first step to successful treatment is admitting there is a problem. To a certain extent, this makes sense.

Why would someone get treatment for something that is not deemed a problem? Unfortunately, several treatment programs require people not only to admit a problem but also to demonstrate their commitment to treatment by stopping their use of alcohol or drugs before beginning treatment. This requirement can exclude many who desire and need treatment. For example, James, who was featured in a **Clinical Case** earlier in the chapter, might not have been admitted to a residential program had he not been free of heroin for a week before trying to gain admission. Imagine if people with lung cancer were told they had to demonstrate their commitment to treatment by stopping smoking before the cancer could be treated.

Most treatments for substance use disorders are psychological. The FDA has approved medication treatments for three substance use disorders: alcohol, tobacco, and opioids (Volkow, 2020). There are currently no effective medications for cocaine use disorder (Chan, Kondo, et al., 2019). Regrettably, many who need treatment for substance use disorders do not receive it. In 2021, over 40 million people needed treatment for a substance use problem (SAMHSA, 2022). Unfortunately, 91% of those needing treatment did not get it (SAMHSA, 2022). The Surgeon General's report on addiction published in 2016 reported that only 1 out of 10 people who needed it received treatment (USDHHS, 2016b). We must do better.

For either an alcohol or a drug use disorder, relapse prevention is a cognitive behavioral treatment that is useful as a stand-alone treatment or in addition to other treatments (Brandon, Vidrine, & Litvin, 2007; Hendershot, Witkiewitz, & Marlatt, 2011). Unfortunately, relapse is the norm when it comes to any substance use disorder. The relapse prevention approach developed by Marlatt and colleagues (Marlatt & Gordon, 1985; Witkiewitz & Marlatt, 2004) emphasizes that relapse should be regarded as a learning experience rather than as a sign that all is lost. Broadly, the goal is to help people avoid relapsing into problematic drinking or drug use.

Treatment of Alcohol Use Disorder

Treatment for alcohol problems can be done in a special treatment facility ("rehab"), but most often it takes place on an outpatient basis, either with a mental health professional or in a self-help group such as Alcoholics Anonymous. As with all substance use problems, there are many more people who need treatment for alcohol problems than receive it.

Inpatient Hospital Treatment
Often, the first step in treatment for substance use disorders is called **detoxification**, or *detox* for short. Withdrawal from substances, including alcohol, can be difficult, both physically and psychologically. Although detox does not have to occur in a hospital, it can be less unpleasant in such a supervised setting. Alice, the woman described in an earlier **Clinical Case**, would likely need hospital treatment, at least for detox.

Inpatient treatment is much more expensive than outpatient treatment, and most people receive outpatient treatment. In 2021, over 1.5 million people received treatment for alcohol use disorders at an outpatient facility, and over 1.4 million received treatment in an inpatient rehabilitation or hospital setting (SAMHSA, 2022).

Alcoholics Anonymous
The largest and most widely known self-help group in the world is Alcoholics Anonymous (AA), founded in 1935 by two men with alcohol problems. It has over 100,000 chapters and a membership numbering more than 2 million people around the world. In 2021, over 1.2 million people who received treatment for alcohol use disorders did so through a self-help program like AA (SAMHSA, 2022).

Each AA chapter runs regular and frequent meetings at which attendees announce that they are alcoholics and give testimonials relating the stories of their problems with alcohol and how their lives have improved with the help of AA. The group provides emotional support, understanding, and close counseling as well as a social network. Members are urged to call on one another around the clock when they need companionship and encouragement not to relapse. Programs modeled after AA are available for other substances; examples are Narcotics Anonymous, Cocaine Anonymous, and Marijuana Anonymous.

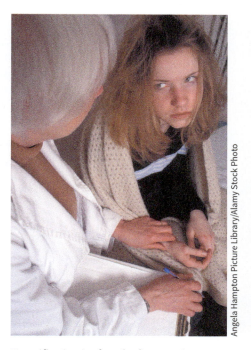

Detoxification is often the first step in treatment for alcohol use disorder.

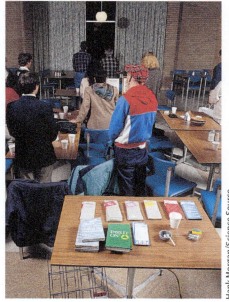

Alcoholics Anonymous is the largest self-help group in the world. At the regular meetings, attendees announce their addiction and receive advice and support from others.

TABLE 10.5   **The 12 Steps of Alcoholics Anonymous**

1. We admitted we were powerless over alcohol—that our lives had become unmanageable.

2. Came to believe that a power greater than ourselves could restore us to sanity.

3. Made a decision to turn our will and our lives over to the care of God as we understood Him.

4. Made a searching and fearless moral inventory of ourselves.

5. Admitted to God, to ourselves, and to another human being the exact nature of our wrongs.

6. Were entirely ready to have God remove all these defects of character.

7. Humbly asked Him to remove our shortcomings.

8. Made a list of all persons we had harmed and became willing to make amends to them all.

9. Made direct amends to such people wherever possible, except when to do so would injure them or others.

10. Continued to take personal inventory and, when we were wrong, promptly admitted it.

11. Sought through prayer and meditation to improve our conscious contact with God as we understood Him, praying only for knowledge of His will for us and the power to carry that out.

12. Having had a spiritual awakening as the result of these steps, we tried to carry this message to alcoholics and to practice these principles in all our affairs.

Source: The Twelve Steps are reprinted with permission of Alcoholics Anonymous World Services, Inc. ("A.A.W.S."). Permission to reprint the Twelve Steps does not mean that A.A.W.S. has reviewed or approved the contents of this publication, or that A.A. necessarily agrees with the views expressed herein. A.A. is a program of recovery from alcoholism only—use of the Twelve Steps in connection with programs and activities which are patterned after A.A., but which address other problems, or in any other non-A.A., does not imply otherwise.

The AA program tries to instill in each member the belief that alcohol use disorder is a disease that can never be cured, and that continuing vigilance is necessary to resist taking even a single drink, lest uncontrollable drinking begin all over again. AA's principles, which include some spiritual aspects, are outlined in the 12 steps, shown in Table 10.5. Even if the person has not consumed any alcohol for 15 years or more, the designation "alcoholic" is still necessary according to the tenets of AA, since the person always has the disorder, even if it is currently under control.

The largest evaluation of whether AA is effective included 27 studies (21 of these were randomized or semi-randomized controlled trials) with over 10,000 participants (Kelly, Humphreys, & Ferri, 2020). This review showed that AA, when led by peers or professionals who followed the treatment manual, was more effective than other treatments, such as cognitive behavior therapy or motivational interviewing, and was effective for helping people remain abstinent for up to 3 years. The primary goal of AA is complete abstinence, so this is good news. Other treatments may not have abstinence as the primary treatment goal, as we discuss later.

All of this sounds like good news for people participating in AA. However, AA has very high dropout rates, and the dropouts are not always factored into the results of studies (Dodes & Dodes, 2014). In the large review by Kelly and colleagues (2020), a third of the studies had 20% or more of the participants drop out. Unfortunately, dropping out (also referred to as *attrition*) was also high in other treatments.

Couples Therapy   Behaviorally oriented couples therapy has been found to achieve some reduction in problem drinking as well as some improvement in couples' distress generally (McCrady, Epstein, et al., 2009; McCrady, Wilson, et al., 2016; O'Farrell & Clements, 2012). It appears to be effective for straight, gay, and lesbian couples (Fals-Stewart, O'Farrell, & Lam, 2009). This treatment combines the skills covered in individual cognitive behavior therapy with a focus on the couple's relationship and dealing with alcohol-related stressors together as a couple. A meta-analysis of 12 studies found that behaviorally oriented couples therapy was more effective than individual treatment approaches (Powers, Vedel, & Emmelkamp, 2008).

Motivational Interventions   As we noted earlier, heavy drinking is particularly common among college students. One team of investigators designed a brief intervention to try to curb heavy drinking in college (Carey, Carey, et al., 2006). The intervention had two parts: (1) a comprehensive assessment of drinking in the past 3 months, and (2) a brief motivational treatment that included individualized feedback about a person's drinking in relation to community and national averages, education about the effects of alcohol, and tips for reducing harm and moderating drinking. Results from the study showed that the TLFB alone decreased drinking behavior, but that the combination of the TLFB and motivational intervention was associated with a longer-lasting reduction in drinking behavior, up to 1 year after the interview and intervention.

Moderation in Drinking

At least since the advent of Alcoholics Anonymous, the popular belief has been that people with alcohol use disorder must abstain completely if they are to be successfully treated, for they presumably have no control over drinking once they take that first drink. This continues to be the belief of AA, but as noted earlier, many people drop out of that program.

A different treatment approach that emphasizes moderation in drinking instead of total abstinence was developed by Mark and Linda Sobell and is called *guided self-change* (Sobell & Sobell, 1993, 2005). The basic assumption is that people have the potential to exercise more control over their drinking than they typically believe and that heightened awareness of the costs of drinking to excess, as well as of the benefits of cutting down, can help. For example, getting a person to delay 20 minutes before taking a second or third drink can help them reflect on the costs versus the benefits of drinking to excess. Evidence supports the effectiveness of this approach in helping people moderate their intake and otherwise improve their lives (Sobell & Sobell, 1993). A randomized controlled clinical trial demonstrated that guided self-change was just as effective as individual or group treatment (Sobell, Sobell, & Agrawal, 2009). A randomized controlled clinical trial with adolescents found that this approach reduced alcohol (and drug) use and that the effects continued at the 3-month follow-up (Wagner, Hospital et al., 2014).

Medications

Disulfiram, or Antabuse, is a medication that discourages drinking by causing violent vomiting after one drinks alcohol. As you can imagine, adherence to an Antabuse regimen is difficult, and the person using this treatment must already be strongly committed to change. In a large multicenter study, Antabuse was not shown to have any benefit, and dropout rates were as high as 80% (Fuller, 1988).

The opiate antagonist naltrexone blocks the activity of endorphins that are stimulated by alcohol, thus reducing the craving for it. Evidence is mixed regarding whether this drug is more effective than a placebo in reducing drinking when it is the only treatment offered (Krystal, Cramer, et al., 2001; Lobmaier, Kunøe, et al., 2011). But it does appear to add to overall treatment effectiveness when combined with cognitive behavior therapy (Pettinati, Oslin, et al., 2010; Streeton & Whelan, 2001). In addition, it may help to dampen cravings for alcohol (Helstrom, Blow, et al., 2016).

The drug acamprosate has been shown to be somewhat effective. Meta-analyses have found acamprosate more effective than a placebo in reducing drinking and cravings (Donoghue, Elzerbi, et al., 2015; Rösner, Hackl-Herrwerth, et al., 2010). A meta-analysis comparing the effectiveness of acamprosate and naltrexone found them to be equally effective (Kranzler & van Kirk, 2001). Researchers believe that acamprosate impacts the glutamate system and thereby reduces the cravings associated with withdrawal.

Antabuse is used to treat alcohol use disorder.

Courtesy of Teva Pharmaceuticals

Quick Summary

Inpatient hospital treatment for alcohol use disorder is not as common today as it was in earlier years, primarily due to the cost. Detoxification from severe alcohol use disorder often takes place in hospitals, but other treatments are more commonly done in outpatient settings.

Alcoholics Anonymous is the program most commonly used for treatment of alcohol use disorder. This group-based self-help treatment instills the notion that alcohol use disorder is always with you and abstinence is the only suitable outcome. Uncontrolled studies suggest that AA is effective, but randomized controlled trials do not. There is some evidence that couples therapy is an effective treatment. The guided self-change approach emphasizes moderation over drinking, the costs of drinking to excess, and the benefits of abstaining.

Medications for alcohol use disorder treatment include Antabuse, naltrexone, and acamprosate. Antabuse is not an effective treatment in the long run because noncompliance is common. Some evidence suggests that other medications are effective on their own, but they seem more beneficial in combination with other treatments.

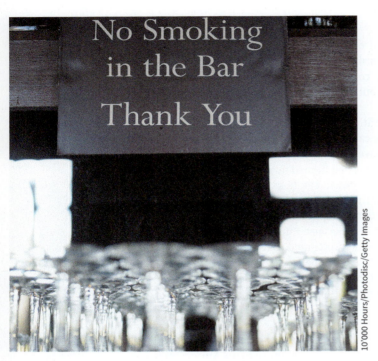

Laws that have banned smoking in many places have probably increased the quit rate.

10'000 Hours/Photodisc/Getty Images

Treatments for Smoking

The numerous laws that currently prohibit smoking in almost all public places are part of a social context that provides incentives and support to stop smoking. In addition, people are more likely to quit smoking if other people around them quit. A longitudinal study of over 12,000 people demonstrated that if people in one's social network (e.g., spouses, siblings, friends, or co-workers) quit smoking, the odds that a person will quit smoking are much greater (Christakis & Fowler, 2008). For example, if a person's spouse stopped smoking, their chances of continuing to smoke decreased by nearly 70%. In short, peer pressure to quit smoking appears to be as effective as peer pressure to start smoking.

Some smokers who want to quit attend smoking clinics or consult with professionals for specialized smoking-reduction programs. Even so, it is estimated that only about half of those who go through smoking-cessation programs succeed in abstaining by the time the program is over; and only a very small percentage of those who have succeeded in the short term remain nonsmokers after a year (Brandon, Vidrine, & Litvin, 2007).

Psychological Treatments
Probably the most widespread psychological treatment consists of a physician telling a person to stop smoking. Each year, millions of smokers are given this advice—because of hypertension, heart disease, lung disease, or diabetes or on general grounds of preserving or improving health. In addition, healthcare providers can also direct smokers to a quitline—a phone number that provides support for smoking cessation—or other digital interventions (e.g., website, social media, text line) to help with quitting (Baker & McCarthy, 2021).

Recent efforts have begun to target cravings for cigarettes. Overcoming the urge to smoke when it arises is extremely difficult. In a clever approach, researchers presented pleasant olfactory cues (i.e., smells) to people when they craved a cigarette (Sayette, Marchetti, et al., 2019). They found that these smells (e.g., chocolate, cumin, peppermint, lemon, apple) damped down the craving for as long as 5 minutes. That may not seem like very long, but it may well be enough to get over the immediate and urgent craving for a cigarette.

Should people quit smoking abruptly or gradually? For some people, quitting abruptly is too difficult even though it is one of the most common approaches to quitting (Caraballo, Shafer, et al., 2017). Gradually reducing the number of cigarettes smoked is also commonly used, leading up to a "target quit day," appears to be more effective than stopping all at once (Lindson-Hawley, Aveyard, & Hughes, 2012).

One of the most commonly used psychological treatments for smoking cessation is a treatment that teaches skills and coping (Baker & McCarthy, 2021). This type of intervention can emphasize relapse prevention skills that help a person identify cues that trigger the urge or craving to smoke and then coping skills to resist these urges. This type of treatment has been shown to be effective in smoking cessation and relapse prevention (Baker & McCarthy, 2021; Livingston-Banks, Norris, et al., 2019).

Much effort has been directed at getting young people to stop smoking. One school-based program called Project EX appears to work and to maintain the benefits up to 1 year post-treatment. The treatment includes training in coping skills and a psychoeducational component about the harmful effects of smoking. This program, translated and adapted for each culture, has been found to be effective in the United States (Sussman, Miyano, et al., 2007), China (Zheng, Sussman, et al., 2004), Spain (Espada, Gonzálvez, et al., 2015), Korea (Yu, Galimov, et al., 2019), Thailand (Chansatitporn, Charoenca, et al., 2016), and Russia (Idrisov, Sun, et al., 2013). Cognitive behavioral approaches that focus on problem-solving and coping skills have also shown promise (Curry, Mermelstein, & Sporer, 2009).

Nicotine Replacement Treatments and Medications

Nicotine replacement therapy (NRT) substitutes a different delivery system for nicotine (in the form of gum, lozenges, mouth sprays, inhalers, patches, or e-cigarettes) to allay cravings while dosages are gradually reduced, with the goal of eliminating reliance on nicotine. Although NRT is often intended to alleviate withdrawal symptoms, the severity of withdrawal is only minimally related to success in stopping smoking (Ferguson, Shiffman, & Gwaltney, 2006).

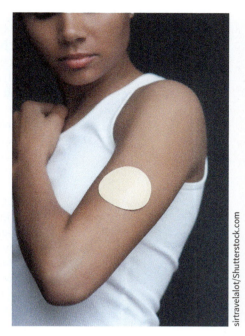

Nicotine patches are available over the counter to help quit smoking and relieve withdrawal symptoms.

The nicotine in nicotine gum, available over the counter, is absorbed much more slowly and steadily than that in tobacco. Nevertheless, gum, lozenges, and sprays are considered faster-acting NRT compared to the patch (discussed next). These faster-acting methods deliver an amount of nicotine equivalent to one cigarette an hour and can cause cardiovascular changes, such as increased blood pressure, that can be dangerous to people with cardiovascular diseases. Even if people do not manage to completely wean themselves from using a faster-acting method such as gum, some experts believe that prolonged, continued use of the gum is healthier than obtaining nicotine by smoking because the carcinogens are avoided (de Wit & Zacny, 2000).

Nicotine patches, also available over the counter, consist of a polyethylene patch, taped to the arm, that slowly and steadily releases the drug into the bloodstream transdermally (through the skin); the drug is then carried to the brain. An advantage of the patch over nicotine gum is that the person need only apply one patch each day and need not remove it until applying the next patch, making compliance easier. Even still, adherence remains a problem, with one study finding that only 40% of people used the patch daily as directed (Schlam, Cook, et al., 2018). Treatment can be effective after 8 weeks of use for most smokers (Stead, Perera, et al., 2012), with the dosage tapering down as treatment progresses. Some evidence suggests that a longer course of treatment may increase the likelihood of smoking cessation success (Baker & McCarthy, 2021).

Evidence suggests that the nicotine patch is superior to the placebo patch in terms of both abstinence and craving (Cahill, Stevens, et al., 2013). In addition, the nicotine patch is effective for men and women (Smith, Kasza, et al., 2015). Two large meta-analyses of over 200 studies of all types of nicotine replacement treatments (patch, gum, nasal spray, inhaler, tablets) found that NRT was more effective than a placebo in smoking cessation (Cahill, et al., 2013; Stead et al., 2012). Combination treatments that include a faster-acting method and the patch appear to be the most effective (Theodoulou, Chepkin, et al., 2023). People who begin to stop smoking after wearing the patch but before dedicated cessation efforts begin are more likely to remain abstinent from smoking at the end of NRT (Rose, Herskovic, et al., 2009). However, NRT is not a panacea. Abstinence rates are less than 50% at 12-month follow-ups (Baker, Piper, et al., 2016; Cahill et al., 2013). The manufacturers state that the patch is to be used only as part of a psychological smoking-cessation program and then for not more than 3 months at a time.

There is continued debate about whether e-cigarettes are an effective form of NRT. A recent meta-analysis of 61 studies, including 34 randomized controlled clinical trials, found moderate-certainty evidence that people assigned to e-cigarettes with nicotine were more likely to quit than those assigned to other NRT or to e-cigarettes without nicotine (Hartmann-Boyce, McRobbie, et al., 2021). The authors noted additional randomized controlled trials are needed to more fully investigate whether e-cigarettes are effective.

Two medications are effective in reducing smoking: the antidepressant bupropion (trade name Wellbutrin) and varenicline (trade name Chantix). NRT plus bupropion is not more effective than NRT alone, but it may be more effective than bupropion alone (Cahill et al., 2013; Stead et al., 2012). Varenicline is effective alone or in combination with behavioral treatment or NRT (Baker et al., 2016; Cahill, Stead, & Lancaster, 2007; Tonstad, Tonnesen, et al., 2006), and it is effective for both men and women (Smith et al., 2015). One randomized trial found that bupropion combined with varenicline was more effective than varenicline alone (Rose & Behm, 2014).

Treatment of Drug Use Disorders

Central to the treatment of people who use drugs such as opioids and cocaine is detoxification—withdrawal from the drug itself. Opioid withdrawal reactions range from relatively mild bouts of anxiety, nausea, and restlessness for several days to more severe and frightening bouts of delirium and panic. The cravings for the substance often remain even after the substance has been removed through detoxification.

Psychological Treatments

Cognitive behavior therapy has been shown to be effective in treating alcohol and some drug use disorders (Carroll & Weiss, 2017; Magill & Ray, 2009; Magill, Ray, et al., 2019). With CBT, people learn how to avoid high-risk situations (e.g., being around people using the drug), recognize the lure of the drug for them, and develop alternatives to using the drug (e.g., recreational activities with nonusers). People also learn strategies for coping with the craving and for resisting the tendency to regard a slip as a catastrophe.

An iteration of CBT is computer-based training for CBT, or CBT4CBT. One study found that CBT4CBT was more effective than standard substance abuse counseling in helping people remain abstinent from cocaine (Carroll, Kiluk, et al., 2014) for up to 6 months after treatment. An additional study of people with a broad range of drug or alcohol use disorders also found CBT4CBT to be more effective than clinician-led CBT at the 6-month follow-up (Kiluk, Nich, et al., 2018). Participants in CBT4CBT were also less likely to drop out of treatment. A meta-analysis of various forms of computer-based (or tech) CBT found that this treatment is effective, particularly for alcohol use disorder (Kiluk, Ray, et al., 2019).

Contingency management involves teaching people with drug use disorders and those close to them to reinforce behaviors inconsistent with drug use—for example, taking the drug methadone (discussed later in the chapter) and avoiding situations associated with drug use in the past. This treatment is based on the belief that environmental contingencies can play an important role in encouraging or discouraging drug use. Vouchers are provided for not using a substance (verified by urine samples) and are exchangeable for things that the person would like to have more of.

Contingency management with vouchers or prizes has been shown to be helpful for cocaine, methamphetamine, nicotine, marijuana, and opioid use disorders (Bolívar, Klemperer, et al., 2021; Cahill, Hartmann-Boyce, & Perera, 2015; De Crescenzo, Ciabattini, et al., 2018; DePhilippis, Petry, et al., 2018; Dugosh, Abraham, et al., 2016; Petry, Alessi, et al., 2017). Studies of contingency management for cocaine use disorder find that it is associated with a greater likelihood of abstinence and a better quality of life (Petry, Alessi, & Hanson, 2007).

Motivational interviewing has also shown promise (McHugh, Hearon, & Otto, 2010). This treatment involves a combination of CBT techniques and techniques associated with helping people generate solutions that work for themselves. A meta-analysis of this treatment found that it was effective for both alcohol and drug use disorders (Burke, Arkowitz, & Menchola, 2003).

Self-help residential programs are another psychological approach to treating heroin and other types of drug use disorders. Daytop Village, Phoenix House, Odyssey House, and other drug-rehabilitation homes share the following features:

- Separation of people from previous social contacts, on the assumption that these relationships have been instrumental in maintaining the drug use disorder

- A comprehensive environment in which drugs are not available and continuing support is offered to ease the transition from regular drug use to a drug-free existence

- The presence of role models—people formerly with a drug use disorder who appear to be meeting life's challenges without drugs

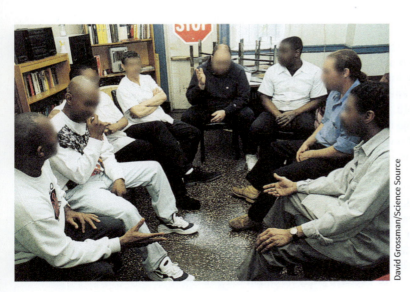

David Grossman/Science Source

Group therapy in residential settings is frequently used to treat drug use disorders.

- Direct, often intense, confrontation in group therapy, in which people are urged to accept responsibility for their problems and for their drug habits and are encouraged to take charge of their lives
- A setting in which people are respected as human beings rather than stigmatized as failures or criminals

There are several obstacles to evaluating the efficacy of residential drug-treatment programs. Because the dropout rate is high, those who remain cannot be regarded as representative of the population of people with substance use disorders; their motivation to stop using drugs is probably much stronger than that of people who don't volunteer for treatment or people who drop out. Any improvement participants in these programs make may reflect their strong motivation to quit more than the specific qualities of the treatment program.

Ninety percent of people who need treatment for substance use disorder do not get it (SAMHSA, 2022). What happens? Many people end up going to prison, some for drug use and many for crimes associated with drug use (e.g., stealing to get money to buy drugs). Yet, treating a substance use problem is substantially less costly than imprisoning someone (Florence, Zhou, et al., 2016)—and possibly more effective, too.

All states have drug courts. Though the specifics vary by state, the general idea behind them is to offer people the option of treatment instead of jail time for nonviolent drug offenses. California found that 4 out of 10 people completed the treatment program (failure to do so meant a return to jail). This number may seem low, but it is quite favorable in comparison to completion rates of other programs, particularly those to which offenders are referred by the criminal justice system (Longshore, Urada, et al., 2003, 2005; Urada, Evans, et al., 2009). The program also saved money. Prison would have cost four times what treatment cost (Longshore, Hawken, et al., 2006). The news was not all good, however. Participants who went into treatment were more likely to be rearrested for drug offenses than were people who had similar offenses before the California drug treatment diversion program was begun (Longshore et al., 2005; Urada et al., 2009).

Developing effective treatments for methamphetamine use remains a challenge. People like Anton, described in a **Clinical Case** earlier in this chapter, do not have many places to turn for treatment. The largest research effort to date is a randomized controlled clinical trial conducted across eight different sites and referred to as the Methamphetamine Treatment Project (Rawson, Martinelli-Casey, et al., 2004). This study compared a multifaceted treatment called Matrix with treatment as usual. The Matrix treatment consisted of 16 CBT group sessions, 12 family education sessions, 4 individual therapy sessions, and 4 social support group sessions. Treatment as usual (TAU) consisted of the best available treatment currently being offered at the eight outpatient clinics. This treatment varied quite a bit across the sites, with some offering individual counseling and others offering group counseling, some offering 4 weeks of treatment and others offering 16 weeks. Results of the study were somewhat supportive of the Matrix treatment. Compared to those in TAU, those people receiving Matrix stayed in treatment longer and were less likely to use methamphetamine during treatment (confirmed with urine analysis). Unfortunately, at the end of treatment and at the 6-month follow-up, people who received Matrix were no less likely to have used methamphetamine than those in TAU. The good news is that all participants were less likely to have used methamphetamine after 6 months, regardless of whether they received Matrix or TAU. Although these results are promising, additional work is clearly needed to develop effective treatments for methamphetamine problems.

Medications   Use of medications, sometimes referred to as *medication-assisted treatment* or MAT, is effective for treating opioid use disorders (Mattick, Breen, et al., 2014; Volkow, Jones, et al., 2019). Two broad types of medications are effective: (1) *Opioid substitutes* (also known as agonists) are chemically similar to the opioids and can dampen the body's craving for those drugs, and (2) *opioid antagonists* prevent the user from experiencing the high. An antagonist is a drug that dampens the activity of neurotransmitters, and an agonist is a drug that stimulates neurotransmitters. In 2019, the National Academies of Sciences, Engineering, and Medicine published a Consensus Study Report noting that, despite its effectiveness, MAT is often not provided, in part because of the stigma surrounding drug use (National Academies of Sciences, Engineering, and Medicine, 2019). As we have discussed throughout the book, stigma remains a barrier to understanding psychological disorders and to availability of treatment.

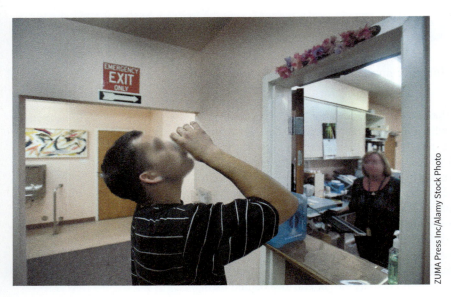

Methadone is an opioid substitute. People come to clinics each day and swallow their dose.

Opioid substitutes include methadone and buprenorphine. Since these drugs are themselves addicting, people often consider that this treatment means converting a person's dependence on one type of opioid into dependence on a different one. However, because these medications do not create the same high and they dampen the cravings, the problems associated with opioid use are diminished. Abrupt discontinuation of these medications can cause withdrawal reactions, but these reactions are less severe than those with heroin or prescription pain medications. The use of opioid substitutes is also linked with a lower risk of overdose death (Sordo, Barrio, et al., 2017).

Methadone treatment typically involves going to a drug-treatment clinic and swallowing the drug in the presence of a staff member. There is some evidence that methadone maintenance can be carried out more simply and just as effectively through weekly visits to a physician (Fiellin, O'Connor, et al., 2001). The effectiveness of methadone treatment is improved if a high (80- to 100-milligram) dose is used as opposed to the more typical 40- to 50-milligram dose (Strain, Bigelow, et al., 1999) and if it is combined with regular psychological counseling (Ball & Ross, 1991). Drug treatment experts generally believe that treatment with methadone is best conducted in the context of a supportive social interaction, not merely as a medical encounter (Lilly, Quirk, et al., 2000).

Since methadone does not provide a euphoric high, many people will return to heroin if it becomes available to them. To improve outcomes, researchers have tried adding contingency management to the usual treatment at methadone clinics. In one randomized controlled trial (Pierce, Petry, et al., 2006), people receiving methadone from a clinic could draw for prizes each time they submitted a (carefully supervised and obtained) urine sample that had no trace of illegal drugs or alcohol. Prizes ranged from praise to televisions. People who were in the contingency management group were more likely to remain drug-free than those people who received only usual care from the methadone clinic.

Unfortunately, many people drop out of methadone programs, in part because of side effects such as insomnia, constipation, excessive sweating, and diminished sexual functioning. The stigma associated with going to methadone clinics is also linked to dropout rates, as illustrated in the **Clinical Case of James** presented earlier.

One of the advantages of buprenorphine (e.g., brand name Subutex) is that it can be taken at home rather than at a clinic. Up until recently, physicians had to receive specialized training to get a waiver from the Drug Enforcement Agency (DEA) in order to prescribe it. As of December 2022, however, physicians need only register with the DEA to prescribe buprenorphine and this ought to make it easier for people to receive this treatment. Unfortunately, barriers still must be overcome. For example, many people, particularly in rural areas, must still go to a clinic daily to receive it (Andrilla, Coulthard, & Larson, 2017). In addition, minoritized groups are less likely to receive buprenorphine than Whites in the United States (Lagisetty, Ross, et al., 2019).

Buprenorphine is a partial opioid agonist, which means it does not have the same powerfully addicting properties as other opioids. Nevertheless, it can and has been abused (Macy, 2018). To help combat the potential for abuse, another type of this medication (trade name Suboxone) has been produced containing two agents: buprenorphine and naloxone (e.g., trade name Narcan). Naloxone is an opioid antagonist, which is often used to reverse opioid overdose effects in the form of a nasal spray or injection. By

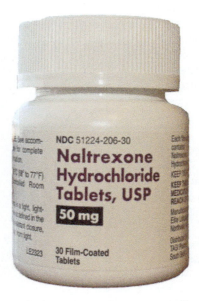

Opioid antagonists such as naltrexone or can be helpful in treating opioid.

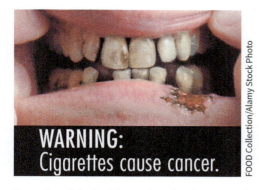
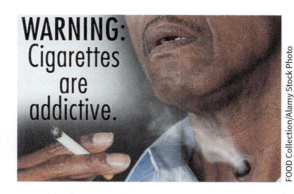

Examples of the health warnings for cigarette packages proposed by the FDA. Tobacco companies sued to prevent the graphic images from being added to packages, and a federal judge and appeals panel ruled in their favor. Antismoking groups have now sued over the FDA's delay in developing new graphic labels.

itself, it has no addicting properties. In 2023, the FDA approved naloxone nasal spray to be sold over the counter so that people could get this without a prescription. The unique combination of buprenorphine and naloxone in Suboxone does not produce an intense high, is only mildly addictive, and lasts for as long as 3 days. Suboxone is effective at relieving withdrawal symptoms (Gowing, Ali, & White, 2009), something that researchers hope will reduce the likelihood of relapse. Still, some users may miss the more euphoric high associated with heroin or pain medications and return to those deadlier opioids. Indeed, unless treatment is continued for longer than 12 weeks or coupled with behavioral counseling, relapse is likely (Weiss, Potter, et al., 2011).

The FDA has also approved two longer-acting types of buprenorphine. Specifically, an implanted version can last for up to 6 months, and an injection can be given once a month.

Another opioid antagonist used as a treatment is a drug called naltrexone (e.g., brand name Vivitrol). First, people are gradually weaned from either heroin or pain medications. Then they receive increasing dosages of naltrexone, which prevents them from experiencing any high should they later take other opioids. Naltrexone works because it has great affinity for the receptors to which opioids usually bind; its molecules occupy the receptors without stimulating them. This leaves heroin or pain medication molecules with no place to go, so these deadlier opioids do not have the usual effect. Like buprenorphine, naltrexone can be prescribed in pill form to be taken at home, and there are also implant and injection versions available. One study compared two different naltrexone treatments: the daily pill naltrexone and surgically implanted naltrexone that was slowly released into the body over 30 days. People with implanted naltrexone used opioids less and reported fewer cravings than those who received oral doses of naltrexone (Hulse, Ngo, & Tait, 2010).

Quick Summary

Psychological treatments have not been all that effective in achieving smoking cessation. Nicotine gum appears to be somewhat effective, though users may never stop chewing the gum. Nicotine patches are more effective than placebo patches, but 9 months after the treatment, abstinence differences between those who received the drug and those who received a placebo disappear. Adding bupropion or therapy to the use of nicotine patches may be effective for adults but not for adolescents. Early evidence about the effectiveness of e-cigarettes as a treatment to stop smoking is not promising, but more research needs to be done.

Detoxification, or detox, is usually the first step in treatment for drug use disorders. There is some evidence that CBT is an effective treatment for cocaine use disorder. Motivational interviewing has shown promise for the treatment of alcohol and other drug use disorders. Residential treatment homes have not been adequately evaluated for their efficacy, though they are a common way of providing treatment. Treating methamphetamine use disorder remains a challenge.

The use of heroin substitutes, such as methadone or naltrexone, is an effective treatment for heroin use disorder. Methadone can be administered only in a special clinic, and there is stigma associated with this type of treatment. A prescription drug called buprenorphine can be taken at home.

10.4 Check Your Knowledge

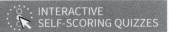
INTERACTIVE
SELF-SCORING QUIZZES

(Answers are at the end of the chapter.)

Match the treatment approach to the type of substance(s).

Substance:

  a. alcohol

  b. opioid

  c. cocaine

  d. nicotine

  e. methamphetamine

Treatment:

1. Suboxone

2. AA

3. couples therapy

4. opioid antagonist

5. antidepressant

6. NRT

7. Matrix

8. Cognitive behavior therapy

Summary

INTERACTIVE
SELF-SCORING QUIZZES

Chapter 10 Practice Quiz

Clinical Descriptions of Substance Use Disorders

- DSM-5-TR includes substance use disorder for alcohol and drug disorders. The number of symptoms present determines severity.

- Alcohol has a variety of short-term and long-term effects on individuals, ranging from poor judgment and impaired motor coordination to chronic health problems.

- Medical problems associated with long-term cigarette smoking include many cancers, emphysema, and cardiovascular disease. Moreover, the health hazards of smoking are not restricted to those who smoke, because secondhand (environmental) smoke can also cause lung damage and other problems. The 2018 report of the National Academies of Sciences, Engineering, and Medicine highlights the known hazards of nicotine in e-cigarettes.

- When used regularly, marijuana can damage the lungs and cardiovascular system and can lead to cognitive impairments. Tolerance to marijuana may develop. However, marijuana also has therapeutic effects, easing the nausea experienced by people undergoing chemotherapy and relieving the discomfort associated with AIDS, glaucoma, chronic pain, and muscle spasms.

- Opioids slow the activities of the body; in moderate doses, they are used to relieve pain and induce sleep. Addiction to prescription pain medications skyrocketed starting in the 1990s, but it has begun to lessen. Unfortunately, use of heroin persists, and use of synthetic opioids such as fentanyl has increased as have deaths from fentanyl overdose. Deaths from prescription pain medicines are also high and a severe problem.

- Stimulants, which include amphetamines and cocaine, act on the brain and the sympathetic nervous system to increase alertness and motor activity. Use of methamphetamine, a derivative of amphetamine, has declined since the 1990s but remains a problem, and use may be once again on the rise.

- Hallucinogens such as LSD and psilocybin alter or expand consciousness. Use of the hallucinogen-like drug Ecstasy is associated with positive feelings. PCP use often leads to violence.

Causes of Substance Use Disorders

- Several factors are related to the causes of substance use disorders. Genetic influences have been studied most often in the context of alcohol and tobacco use disorders.

- Neurobiological influences involving the brain's reward pathways appear to play a role in the use of some substances. Many substances are used to regulate emotion (e.g., to reduce negative or increase positive emotion), and people with certain personality traits, such as being high in negative affect or low in constraint, are especially likely to use drugs. Psychological variables, such as the expectation that the drug will yield positive effects, are also important.

- Sociocultural influences, such as cultural norms, peer influences, and media portrayal of the substance, are all related to how frequently a substance is used.

Treatment of Substance Use Disorders

- Medications are effective for a few drug use disorders. For opioid use disorders, medications lessen the high and dampen cravings. Benefits have been observed for medications such as methadone, buprenorphine, and naltrexone.

- Nicotine replacement via gum, lozenges, sprays, patches, or inhalers has met with some success in reducing cigarette smoking. E-cigarettes can also help people stop smoking.

- Psychological treatments that are effective in treating alcohol use disorder include cognitive behavior therapy, couples therapy, skills training, and contingency management. Alcoholics Anonymous is also effective, and it is a standard part of many treatment programs.

Answers to Check Your Knowledge Questions

10.1. 1. True; 2. True; 3. True; 4. lung, larynx, esophagus, pancreas, bladder, cervix, stomach; 5. short-term; 6. pain relief, glaucoma relief, reduction of nausea, increased appetite, relief from the discomfort from AIDS; 7. similarities: contain nicotine, regulated by the FDA; differences: more carcinogens in cigarettes, aerosol products in vape pipes.

10.2. 1. False; 2. False; 3. False; 4. True

10.3. 1. b. cultural norms; 2. c. wanting and liking predicted more drinking among heavy drinkers; 3. the *CYP2A6* gene may contribute to nicotine use disorder.

10.4. 1. b; 2. a; 3. a; 4. b; 5. d; 6. d; 7. e; 8. a; c.

Key Terms

amphetamines 283
caffeine 284
cocaine 285
crack 285
delirium tremens (DTs) 270
detoxification 297
Ecstasy 286
fetal alcohol syndrome (FAS) 272
flashbacks 286

hallucinogen 286
heroin 280
hydrocodone 281
LSD 286
marijuana 276
MDMA 286
methamphetamine 284
nicotine 273
opioids 280

oxycodone 281
PCP 287
psilocybin 286
secondhand smoke 275
stimulants 283
substance use disorder 268
tolerance 268
withdrawal 268

Eating Disorders

LEARNING GOALS

1. Distinguish the symptoms associated with anorexia, bulimia, and binge eating disorder, and distinguish among the different eating disorders.

2. Describe the neurobiological, sociocultural, and psychological influences implicated in the causes of eating disorders.

3. Discuss the issues surrounding the growing epidemic of obesity in the United States.

4. Describe the treatments for eating disorders and the evidence supporting their effectiveness.

Clinical Case

Lynne

Lynne, a 24-year-old White woman, was admitted to the psychiatric ward of a general hospital for treatment of anorexia nervosa. Although she didn't really think anything was wrong with her, her parents had consulted with a psychiatrist, and the three of them had confronted her with the choice to admit herself or be committed involuntarily.

At the time, Lynne stood 5 feet, 5 inches and weighed only 78 pounds. She hadn't menstruated for 3 years, and she had a variety of medical problems—hypotension, irregularities in her heartbeat, and abnormally low levels of potassium and calcium.

Lynne had experienced several episodes of dramatic weight loss, beginning at age 18 when she first left home for college. But none of the prior episodes had been this severe, and she had not sought treatment before. She had an intense fear of gaining weight, and although she had never been overweight, she felt that her buttocks and abdomen were far too large. (This belief persisted even when she weighed 78 pounds.) During the periods of weight loss, she severely restricted food intake and used laxatives heavily. She had occasionally had episodes of binge eating, typically followed by self-induced vomiting so that she would not gain any weight.

Many cultures are preoccupied with food. In the United States today, numerous apps, websites, and TV shows are devoted to food and food preparation. Grocery stores in the United States are stocked with embarrassingly huge quantities of food, and food prices in the United States remain relatively low, even following periods of inflation. Dieting to lose weight is common, and the desire of many people, especially women, to be thinner fuels a multibillion-dollar-a-year industry.

Like most of the other disorders we cover in this book, eating disorders are likely to be stigmatized. In one study, college students were presented with vignettes depicting fictional women with different disorders and were then asked to rate these fictional women on several dimensions (Wingfield, Kelly, et al., 2011). Participants rated the women depicted with eating disorders as self-destructive and responsible for their conditions. Men in the study were particularly likely to believe that eating disorders were easy to overcome. In another study (Roehrig & McLean, 2010), participants were randomly assigned to read a vignette about a woman with an eating disorder or a woman with depression. Compared with participants who read about the woman with depression, participants who read about the woman with the eating disorder viewed the woman in their vignette as more responsible, more fragile, and more likely to be trying to get attention with her disorder. These types of attitudes and beliefs are not consistent with the current research on eating disorders.

More broadly, there is stigma about body shape and weight, particularly for women. The cultural expectation for women is that they be thin, but some women are pushing back via social media. For example, the model Tess Holliday has written a book called *The Not So Subtle Art of Being a Fat Girl: Love the Skin You're In* and has posted many photos on Instagram proudly showcasing her size 22 body. Other hashtags, such as #bodyshaming and #bodyacceptance, appear on Instagram and Twitter to promote body shapes of all sizes.

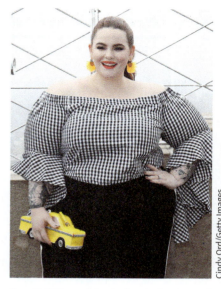

Tess Holliday celebrates her body size and is a successful model.

Clinical Descriptions and Epidemiology of Eating Disorders

We will discuss three DSM-5-TR eating disorders: anorexia nervosa, bulimia nervosa, and binge eating disorder. Although DSM-5-TR includes subtypes and specifiers for these three disorders, the validity for these categories is poor, and thus, we do not discuss them here (Smith, Ellison, et al., 2017). DSM-5-TR also includes disorders of early childhood such as pica (eating nonfood substances for extended periods), rumination disorder (repeated regurgitation of foods). Avoidant/restrictive food intake disorder (diminished interest in food based mostly on the sensory aspects of food) typically begins in childhood but may persist into adulthood.

Anorexia Nervosa

Lynne, the woman described in the chapter-opening Clinical Case, had **anorexia nervosa**. The term *anorexia* refers to loss of appetite, and *nervosa* indicates that the loss is due to emotional reasons. The term is something of a misnomer because most people with anorexia nervosa do not lose their appetite or interest in food. On the contrary, while starving themselves, most people with the disorder become preoccupied with food; they may read cookbooks constantly and prepare gourmet meals for their families.

Lynne exhibited all three features of anorexia nervosa (see Defining Symptoms of Anorexia Nervosa):

1. *Restriction of behaviors that promote healthy body weight.* This is usually taken to mean that the person weighs much less than is considered normal for that person's age and height—e.g., a **body mass index (BMI)** of less than 18.5 for an adult (see **Table 11.1**). Weight loss is typically achieved through dieting, although purging (self-induced vomiting, heavy use of laxatives or diuretics) and excessive exercise can also be part of the picture.

2. *Strong fear of gaining weight or behavior that interferes with gaining weight.* This fear is not reduced by weight loss. The person believes that there is no such thing as "too thin."

3. *Distorted body image or sense of body shape.* Even when emaciated, those with anorexia nervosa maintain that they are overweight and that certain parts of their bodies, particularly the abdomen, hips, and thighs, are too fat. To check on their body size, they typically weigh themselves frequently, measure the size of different parts of the body, and gaze critically at their reflections in mirrors. Their self-esteem is closely linked to maintaining thinness.

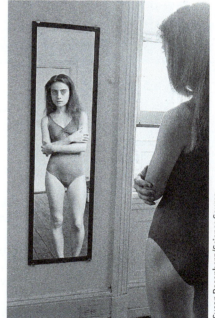

Despite being thin, women with anorexia believe that parts of their bodies are too fat, and they spend a lot of time critically examining themselves in front of mirrors.

In both DSM-5-TR and ICD-11, the severity of anorexia nervosa is based on the BMI (the lower the BMI, the higher the severity). The BMI is calculated by dividing weight in kilograms by height in meters squared and is considered a more valid estimate of body fat than many others. For women, a healthy BMI is between 20 and 25. To calculate your own BMI, see Table 11.1. The BMI is not a perfect measure. Many people have a higher or lower

TABLE 11.1   **Computing Your Body Mass Index (BMI)**

WEIGHT lbs	100	105	110	115	120	125	130	135	140	145	150	155	160	165	170	175	180	185	190	195	200	205	210	215
kgs	45.5	47.7	50.0	52.3	54.5	56.8	59.1	61.4	63.6	65.9	68.2	70.5	72.7	75.0	77.3	79.5	81.8	84.1	86.4	88.6	90.9	93.2	95.5	97.7

HEIGHT in/cm   ▨ Underweight   ▨ Healthy   ▨ Overweight   ▨ Obese   ▨ Extremely obese

HEIGHT in/cm	100	105	110	115	120	125	130	135	140	145	150	155	160	165	170	175	180	185	190	195	200	205	210	215
5'0" - 152.4	19	20	21	22	23	24	25	26	27	28	29	30	31	32	33	34	35	36	37	38	39	40	41	42
5'1" - 154.9	18	19	20	21	22	23	24	25	26	27	28	29	30	31	32	33	34	35	36	36	37	38	39	40
5'2" - 157.4	18	19	20	21	22	22	23	24	25	26	27	28	29	30	31	32	33	33	34	35	36	37	38	39
5'3" - 160.0	17	18	19	20	21	22	23	24	24	25	26	27	28	29	30	31	32	32	33	34	35	36	37	38
5'4" - 162.5	17	18	18	19	20	21	22	23	24	24	25	26	27	28	29	30	31	31	32	33	34	35	36	37
5'5" - 165.1	16	17	18	19	20	20	21	22	23	24	25	25	26	27	28	29	30	30	31	32	33	34	35	35
5'6" - 167.6	16	17	17	18	19	20	21	21	22	23	24	25	25	26	27	28	29	29	30	31	32	33	34	34
5'7" - 170.1	15	16	17	18	18	19	20	21	22	22	23	24	25	25	26	27	28	29	29	30	31	32	33	33
5'8" - 172.7	15	16	16	17	18	19	20	21	22	23	24	25	25	26	27	28	28	29	30	31	32	32	33	33
5'9" - 175.2	14	15	16	17	17	18	19	20	20	21	22	22	23	24	25	25	26	27	28	28	29	30	31	31
5'10" - 177.8	14	15	15	16	17	18	18	19	20	20	21	22	23	23	24	25	25	26	27	28	28	29	30	30
5'11" - 180.3	14	14	15	16	16	17	18	18	19	20	21	21	22	23	23	24	25	25	26	27	28	28	29	30
6'0" - 182.8	13	14	14	15	16	17	17	18	19	19	20	21	21	22	23	23	24	25	25	26	27	27	28	29
6'1" - 185.4	13	13	14	15	15	16	17	17	18	19	19	20	21	21	22	23	23	24	25	25	26	27	27	28
6'2" - 187.9	12	13	14	14	15	16	16	17	18	18	19	19	20	21	21	22	23	23	24	25	25	26	27	27
6'3" - 190.5	12	13	13	14	15	15	16	16	17	18	18	19	20	20	21	21	22	23	23	24	25	25	26	26
6'4" - 193.0	12	12	13	14	14	15	15	16	17	17	18	18	19	20	20	21	22	22	23	23	24	25	25	26

than ideal BMI for reasons that do not have to do with body fat. For example, someone who is very muscular will likely have a high BMI but will not be overweight or obese. By contrast, an elite runner may be very lean and have a low BMI but not have anorexia.

The distorted body image that accompanies anorexia nervosa has been assessed in several ways, most frequently by a questionnaire such as the Eating Disorders Inventory (Garner, Olmsted, & Polivy, 1983). Some of the items on this questionnaire are presented in Table 11.2. In another type of assessment, people with anorexia nervosa are shown line drawings of women with varying body weights and asked to pick the one closest to their own body size and the one that represents their ideal shape (see Figure 11.1). People with anorexia overestimate their own body size and choose a thin figure as their ideal. Despite this distortion in their image of their body size, people with anorexia nervosa are fairly accurate when reporting their actual weight (McCabe, McFarlane, et al., 2001), perhaps because they weigh themselves frequently.

Defining Symptoms of Anorexia Nervosa

- Restriction of food that leads to very low body weight; body weight is significantly below normal
- Strong fear of weight gain or behavior that interferes with weight gain
- Distorted body image

Anorexia nervosa typically begins in the early to middle teenage years. Estimates of lifetime prevalence of anorexia range from less than 1% to over 3% (Brown & Keel, 2023; Galmiche, Dechelotte, et al., 2019; Udo & Grilo, 2018). Anorexia nervosa is at least three times more frequent in women than in men (Hudson, Hiripi, et al., 2007; Udo & Grilo, 2018).

When anorexia nervosa does occur in men, symptoms can differ, with more of an emphasis on muscularity as well as thin or lean bodies (Murray, Nagata, et al., 2017). As we discuss more fully later in this chapter, the sex difference in the prevalence of anorexia most likely reflects the greater cultural emphasis on women's beauty, which has promoted a thin body shape as the ideal over the past several decades.

TABLE 11.2   Subscales and Illustrative Items from the Eating Disorders Inventory

Drive for thinness	I think about dieting.
	I feel extremely guilty after overeating.
	I am preoccupied with the desire to be thinner.
Bulimia	I stuff myself with food.
	I have gone on eating binges where I have felt that I could not stop.
	I have the thought of trying to vomit in order to lose weight.
Body dissatisfaction	I think that my thighs are too large.
	I think that my buttocks are too large.
	I think that my hips are too big.
Ineffectiveness	I feel inadequate.
	I have a low opinion of myself.
	I feel empty inside (emotionally).
Perfectionism	Only outstanding performance is good enough in my family.
	As a child, I tried hard to avoid disappointing my parents and teachers.
	I hate being less than best at things.
Interpersonal distrust	I have trouble expressing my emotions to others.
	I need to keep people at a certain distance (feel uncomfortable if someone tries to get too close).
Interoceptive awareness	I get confused about what emotion I am feeling.
	I don't know what's going on inside me.
	I get confused as to whether or not I am hungry.
Maturity fears	I wish that I could return to the security of childhood.
	I feel that people are happiest when they are children.
	The demands of adulthood are too great.

Note: Responses use a 6-point scale ranging from "always" to "never."
Source: From Garner, Olmsted, and Polivy (1983).

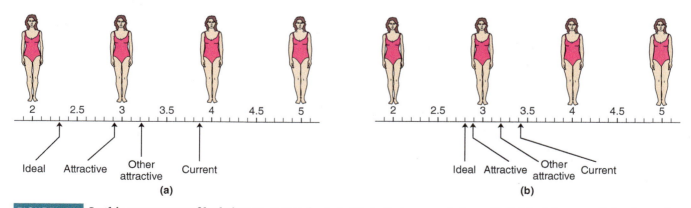

FIGURE 11.1 In this assessment of body image, respondents indicate their current shape, their ideal shape, and the shape they think is most attractive to the opposite sex. The figure rated as most attractive by members of the opposite sex is shown in both panels. Ratings of women who scored high on a measure of distorted attitudes toward eating are shown in (a); ratings of women who scored low on that measure are shown in (b). The high scorers overestimated their current size and ideally would be very thin (Zellner, Harner, & Adler, 1989).

▶ VIDEO
CONTENT

**Case Study: Anorexia
Pause and Ponder**

For both men and women, anorexia nervosa is frequently comorbid with depression, obsessive-compulsive disorder, specific phobias, social anxiety disorder, panic disorder, substance use disorders, and various personality disorders (Brown & Keel, 2023; Baker, Mitchell, et al., 2010; Hudson, Hiripi, et al., et al., 2007; Mandelli, Draghetti, et al., 2020; Root, Pinheiro, et al., 2010). Suicide rates are quite high for people with anorexia, with as many as 5% dying by suicide and 20% attempting suicide (Arcelus, Mitchell, et al., 2011; Franko & Keel, 2006).

Physical Consequences of Anorexia Nervosa
Self-starvation and use of laxatives to lose weight produce numerous undesirable consequences in people with anorexia nervosa. Blood pressure often falls, heart rate slows, kidney and gastrointestinal problems develop, bone mass declines, the skin dries out, nails become brittle, hormone levels change, and mild anemia may occur. Some people lose hair from the scalp, and they may develop *lanugo*—fine, soft hair—on their bodies. As in Lynne's case, levels of electrolytes, such as potassium and sodium, are altered. These ionized salts, present in various bodily fluids, are essential to neural transmission, and lowered levels can lead to tiredness, weakness, cardiac arrhythmias, and even sudden death.

Prognosis
From 50% to 70% of people with anorexia eventually recover or at least significantly improve (Keel & Brown, 2010). However, recovery often takes 6 or 7 years, and relapses are common before a stable pattern of eating and weight maintenance is achieved (Steinhausen, 2002). One long-term study of over 100 women with anorexia found that nearly a third had recovered 9 years after diagnosis and nearly two-thirds had recovered 22 years after diagnosis (Eddy, Tabri, et al., 2017). As we discuss later, changing people's distorted views of themselves is very difficult, particularly in cultures that value thinness.

Anorexia nervosa is a life-threatening illness; death rates are 10 times higher among people with the disorder than among the general population and twice as high as among people with other psychological disorders. Mortality rates among women with anorexia range from 3% to 5% (Crow, Peterson, et al., 2009; Keel & Brown, 2010); anorexia has a higher death rate than either bulimia nervosa or binge eating disorder (Arcelus et al., 2011). Death most often results from physical complications of the disorder—for example, congestive heart failure—and is more likely among those who struggle with the illness for many years (Franko, Keshaviah, et al., 2013; Herzog, Greenwood, et al., 2000; Steinhausen, 2002).

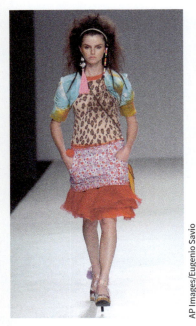

Anorexia nervosa can be a life-threatening condition. It is especially prevalent among young women who are under intense pressure to keep their weight low. Brazilian model Ana Carolina Reston died from the condition in 2006 at age 21.

AP Images/Eugenio Savio

Clinical Case

Jill

Jill was the second child born to her parents. Both she and her brother became intensely involved in athletics at an early age, Jill in gymnastics and her brother in Little League baseball. At age 4, Jill was enrolled in gymnastics school, where she excelled. By the time she was 9, her mother had decided that Jill had outgrown the coaching abilities of the local instructors and began driving her to a nationally recognized coach several times a week. Over the next few years, Jill's trophy case swelled and her aspirations for a place on the Olympic team grew. As she reached puberty,

though, her thin frame began to fill out, raising concerns about the effects of weight gain on her performance as a gymnast. She began to restrict her intake of food but found that after several days of semistarvation she would lose control and go on an eating binge. This pattern of dieting and bingeing lasted for several months, and Jill's fear of gaining weight seemed to increase during that time. At age 13, she hit on the solution of self-induced vomiting. She quickly fell into a pattern of episodes of bingeing and vomiting three or four times per week. Although she maintained this pattern in secret for a while, eventually her parents caught on and initiated treatment for her.

A new category called "other specified feeding or eating disorder (OSFED)" was added to DSM-5, and one of the manifestations of OSFED is **atypical anorexia nervosa**. Atypical anorexia nervosa includes all the symptoms of anorexia nervosa *except* for very low body weight. People with atypical anorexia may be overweight or even obese (Walsh, Hagan, & Lockwood, 2023). Although a fairly new disorder, some evidence suggests that it is increasing, particularly among young people (Agostino, Burstein, et al., 2021; Freizinger, Recto, et al., 2022). Compared to anorexia, atypical anorexia is more prevalent and has comparable health consequences and psychological comborbities (Harrop, Mensinger, et al., 2021; Wilkop, Wade, et al., 2023). A recent meta-analysis of 69 studies found that people with atypical anorexia have more eating pathology (e.g., restricting food intake) than people with anorexia (Wilkop et al., 2023), suggesting the need for treatment. Unfortunately, data show that people with atypical anorexia are less likely to receive treatment (Harrop et al., 2021).

Bulimia Nervosa

Jill's behavior illustrates the features of **bulimia nervosa**. *Bulimia* is from a Greek word meaning "ox hunger." This disorder involves episodes of rapid consumption of a large amount of food, followed by compensatory behavior such as vomiting, fasting, or excessive exercise to prevent weight gain. A *binge* has two characteristics: First, it involves eating an excessive amount of food—that is, much more than most people would eat (usually more than 1,000 calories; Forney, Holland, et al., 2015), within a short period of time (e.g., 2 hours). Second, it involves a feeling of losing control over eating—as if one couldn't stop. Bulimia nervosa is not diagnosed if the bingeing and purging occur only in the context of anorexia nervosa and its extreme weight loss. The key difference between anorexia and bulimia is weight loss: People with anorexia nervosa lose a tremendous amount of weight, whereas people with bulimia nervosa do not.

In bulimia, binges typically occur in secret; they may be triggered by stress and negative emotions, and they continue until the person is uncomfortably full. In the case of Jill, she was likely to binge after periods of stress associated with being an elite athlete. Foods that can be rapidly consumed, especially sweets such as ice cream and cake, are usually part of a binge. One study found that women with bulimia nervosa were more likely to binge while alone and during the morning or afternoon. In addition, avoiding a craved food on one day was associated with a binge episode with that food the next morning (Waters, Hill, & Waller, 2001). Other studies have shown that a binge is likely to occur after a negative social interaction—or, at least, the perception of a negative social exchange (Steiger, Gauvin, et al., 1999) or negative mood (Chami, Reichenberger, et al., 2021; Lavender, Utzinger, et al., 2016).

People report that they lose control during a binge, to the point of experiencing something akin to what happens in addiction (Lowe, Arigo, et al., 2016; Smith & Robbins, 2013), even losing awareness of their behavior. They are usually ashamed of their binges and try to conceal them.

After the binge is over, feelings of discomfort, disgust, and fear of weight gain lead to the second step of bulimia nervosa—the inappropriate compensatory behavior (also known as *purging*) to attempt to undo the caloric effects of the binge. People with bulimia most often stick their fingers down their throats to cause gagging, but after a time many can induce vomiting at will without gagging themselves. Laxative abuse and diuretic abuse (which do little to reduce body weight), as well as fasting and excessive exercise, are also used to prevent weight gain.

Like people with anorexia nervosa, people with bulimia nervosa depend heavily on maintaining normal weight to maintain self-esteem. Whereas people without eating disorders typically underreport their weight and say they are taller than they actually are, people with bulimia nervosa are more accurate in their reports (Doll & Fairburn, 1998; McCabe et al., 2001). Yet, people with bulimia nervosa are also likely to be highly dissatisfied with their bodies.

Bulimia nervosa typically begins in late adolescence or early adulthood. About 90% of people with bulimia are women; prevalence rates for men and women are thought to be about 1–2% of the population (Baker & Keel, 2023; Hudson et al., 2007; Klump, Culbert, & Sisk, 2017). Although both anorexia nervosa and bulimia nervosa among women begin in adolescence, they can persist into adulthood and middle age (Keel, Gravener, et al., 2010; Slevec & Tiggemann, 2011).

Bulimia nervosa is comorbid with other disorders, including depression, personality disorders, anxiety disorders, substance use disorders, and conduct disorder (Baker & Keel, 2023; Baker et al., 2010; Gadalla & Piran, 2007; Godart, Flament, et al., 2002; Root et al., 2010; Stice, Burton, & Shaw, 2004). Suicide rates are higher among people with bulimia nervosa than in the general population (Keel, 2018) but substantially lower than among people with anorexia (Arcelus et al., 2011; Franko & Keel, 2006).

Which comes first, bulimia nervosa or the comorbid disorders? With respect to substance use disorders, a prospective study of over 1,200 twin pairs found that bulimia symptoms surfaced before substance use disorder symptoms (Baker et al., 2010). For depression, a prospective study found that bulimia symptoms predicted the onset of depression symptoms in adolescent girls. However, the converse was also true: Depression symptoms predicted the onset of bulimia symptoms (Stice, Burton, & Shaw, 2004). Thus, it appears that each disorder increases the risk for the other.

Defining Symptoms of Bulimia Nervosa

- Repeated episodes of binge eating
- Repeated compensatory behaviors to prevent weight gain, such as vomiting
- Body shape and weight are extremely important for self-evaluation

---

Physical Consequences of Bulimia Nervosa   Bulimia nervosa, like anorexia, is a serious disorder with many unfortunate medical consequences (Mehler, 2011). For example, frequent purging can cause potassium depletion. Heavy use of laxatives induces diarrhea, which can lead to changes in electrolytes and cause irregularities in the heartbeat. Recurrent vomiting may lead to tearing of tissue in the stomach and throat and to loss of dental enamel as stomach acids eat away at the teeth, which become ragged. The salivary glands may become swollen. Death from bulimia nervosa is less common than death from anorexia nervosa (Herzog et al., 2000; Keel & Brown, 2010), but mortality rates are higher than for other disorders (Arcelus et al., 2011; Crow et al., 2009).

Prognosis   Long-term follow-ups of people with bulimia nervosa reveal that 68–75% of them recover, although about 10–20% remain fully symptomatic (Eddy et al., 2017; Keel et al., 2010; Steinhausen & Weber, 2009). Intervening soon after a diagnosis is made (i.e., within the first few years) is linked with a better prognosis (Reas, Williamson, et al., 2000).

Clinical Case

Amy

Amy, a 27-year-old Black woman, reported a lifelong struggle with her weight. She was described as "chubby" as a child, and peers often called her "fatty." She went on several diets as a child, but none of them were successful. Currently, Amy is 5 feet, 4 inches tall and weighs 212 pounds (with a BMI of 35).

Amy experienced several episodes of binge eating beginning at age 18, when she first left home for college. After being left out of a social group on campus, she retreated to her dorm room alone, where she ate two large pizzas and a bag of Doritos. After the binge, she felt very full and went to sleep. After that first binge, she found herself doing this as often as twice a week throughout college. She was not always hungry when she binged, but even though she felt extremely full, she could not stop eating. Afterward, she felt ashamed and angry at herself for having eaten so much. She gained 70 pounds during her college years.

Amy reported that she currently binges at least once a week, typically when she has had a very stressful day at work. She recently confided in a friend about her troubled eating, and her friend recommended that she seek treatment at the local university mental health clinic.

Binge Eating Disorder

Binge eating disorder was first included as a diagnosis in DSM-5. This disorder involves recurrent binges (one time per week for at least 3 months), lack of control during the bingeing episode, and distress about bingeing, as well as other characteristics such as rapid eating and eating alone. As in bulimia nervosa, binges often include sweets and other rapidly consumed foods. Binge eating disorder is distinguished from bulimia, however, by the absence of compensatory behaviors (purging, fasting, or excessive exercise) and from anorexia by the absence of weight loss.

Most people with binge eating disorder are **obese**. A person with a BMI greater than 30 is considered obese. With the current explosion in the prevalence of obesity in the United States, it is perhaps not surprising that research on binge eating disorder continues to increase (Attia, Becker, et al., 2013). Although it may seem intuitive that bingeing is associated with weight gain, this has now been confirmed in a prospective longitudinal study. Binge eating at the beginning of the study predicted a higher BMI 2 years later in a group of women in college (Rohde, Arigo, et al., 2018).

It is important to point out, however, that not all obese people meet the criteria for binge eating disorder. Indeed, only those who have binge episodes and report feeling a loss of control over their eating qualify for this diagnosis; they comprise from 2% to 25% of obese people (Wonderlich, Gordon, et al., 2009). For further discussion of obesity, see **Focus on Discovery 11.1**.

Defining Symptoms of Binge Eating Disorder

- Repeated binge eating episodes
- The binge eating episodes must include several features (e.g., eating fast, eating even if not hungry, eating past feeling full, feeling bad about eating so much)

Focus on Discovery 11.1

Obesity: A 21st-Century Epidemic

Obesity is not an eating disorder, though it is a serious public health problem, estimated to account for yearly healthcare costs of nearly $150 billion in the United States (Finkelstein, Trogdon, et al., 2009; Kim & Basu, 2016). The projected lifetime cost of treating the obesity-related health care problems of *one* 10-year-old child in the United States is $19,000; the total for all the 10-year-olds who are currently obese comes to $14 billion (Finkelstein, Graham, & Malhotra, 2014). Why are the healthcare costs so high? Obesity is linked to many health problems,

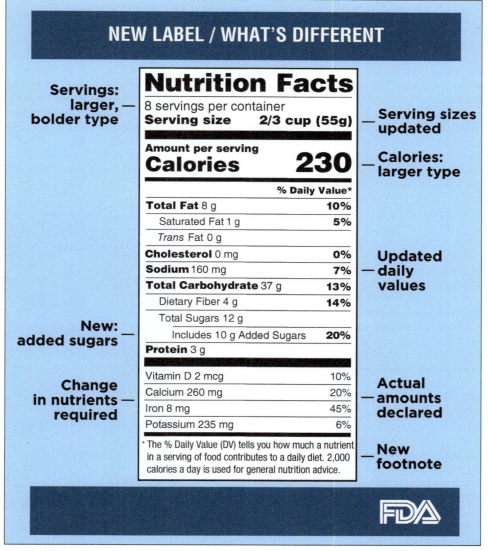

Nutrition facts labels approved in 2016 for packaged foods make it easier to see the serving size and number of calories per serving.

including diabetes, hypertension, cardiovascular disease, and several forms of cancer.

Between 2000 and 2020, the prevalence rate for obesity in the United States grew from 30% to 42% (Hales, Carroll, et al., 2020). Unfortunately, obesity is not just a problem for adults. The World Health Organization (WHO) estimated that 38 million children around the world *under the age of 5* were overweight or obese in 2019 (WHO, 2020). Rates of obesity are much higher in the United States than in many other countries. Nevertheless, obesity is also increasing in other parts of the world, from Aborigines in Australia to children in Egypt, and in Siberia and Peru (NCD Risk Factor Collaboration [NCD-RisC], 2017; Ng, Fleming, et al., 2014).

Why are so many people overweight? Several factors play a role, including the environment we live in. In the United States, the availability and amount of all food, not just fast food, have exponentially increased in the past decades. We pay far less for our food now, spending less than 10% of our income on food today compared to 25% in the 1920s (Cohen, 2014). We can buy food at any time of day or night, with most grocery stores featuring unhealthy items (with higher profit margins) more prominently than healthy items. Many of the foods that we can purchase are highly processed foods, and these are associated with weight gain and obesity (Hall, Azyuketah, et al., 2019). At the same time, many people, including children, have become more sedentary, spending more time than ever before working at a desk job, playing on a computer or smartphone, and watching TV. Furthermore, physical education programs for children in schools have been declining for decades (Critser, 2003). People eat in restaurants more than ever before (at least one-third of total calories consumed by people in the United States are consumed in restaurants, according to the Food and Drug Administration [FDA]), and portion sizes of foods, both in restaurants and in grocery stores, are larger than ever.

In fact, most people do not even know the portion sizes of most foods that are recommended by the U.S. Department of Agriculture, even though the FDA now requires packaged foods to use nutrition facts labels that prominently display serving size and number of calories. A 20-ounce bottle of soda is not one serving, but two and a half servings. The recommended serving size of cheese is 1½ ounces, about the size of a 9-volt battery.

Americans today eat an average of 2,700 calories daily compared with closer to 2,200 calories a day more than 50 years ago. The ever-increasing portion sizes, as well as the greater availability of unhealthy foods, impact the amount we eat. The limited availability and higher cost of healthy foods in low-income neighborhoods also contribute to obesity. Research has shown that low-income neighborhoods have fewer grocery stores, more fast-food restaurants, and fewer healthy food selections in their stores (Moreland, Wing, et al., 2002). And people in low-income neighborhoods may not have a means of transportation to and from grocery stores that carry more affordable, healthy food choices but are farther away.

We are all subject to the continuing impact of advertisements, especially those promoting alluring high-calorie products such as snack foods, sodas, and meals at fast-food restaurants. Showing the direct effects of TV marketing, one study provided snacks to children as they watched either a TV cartoon containing commercials for snack foods or a TV cartoon containing commercials for other products. Children randomly assigned to watch the show with the snack food commercials ate more snacks than children assigned to watch the cartoon with nonfood advertising (Harris, Bargh, & Brownell, 2009). Given the power of advertising to influence emotion and food choice, several steps have been taken to minimize the impact. For example, the FDA instituted a nationwide rule in 2018 requiring chain restaurants with more than 20 locations to post information about the calorie content of their menu items. Other regulations intended to limit food marketing, add information or warning labels, and place taxes on unhealthy foods are being implemented around the world (Roberto, 2020).

Advertisements can also serve as powerful cues about food. Cues in turn create cravings for food. Research suggests that people with obesity may be particularly sensitive to these cues and experience intense cravings for food which promotes overeating and weight gain (Boswell & Kober, 2016; Devoto, Zapparoli, et al., 2018; Morales & Berridge, 2020). Brain imaging studies have found that people who are obese show greater activation in areas of the brain associated with dopamine and reward in response to food cues, even when they are not hungry (Devoto et al., 2018).

Along with the environment, heredity plays a role in obesity. In behavioral genetics terms, 25–40% of the variance in obesity is attributed to genetics (O'Rahilly & Farooqi, 2008). Heredity could produce its effects by regulating metabolic rate, affecting the hypothalamus, or influencing the production of enzymes that make it easier to store fat and gain weight (Loos & Yeo, 2022).

Related to genetics is the role of the neural pathways associated with reward. Prospective studies have found that brain activation in areas associated with reward (e.g., striatum and nucleus accumbens) in response to tasty, high-calorie foods or cues about food (e.g., pictures of food) predict weight gain (Stice & Burger, 2019; Stice & Yokum, 2016). Indeed, a meta-analysis of 45 food cue studies found medium effect sizes (see Chapter 4) for food cues in predicting greater eating and weight gain (Boswell & Kober, 2016). Activation in these regions is linked to genes associated with the neurotransmitter dopamine, which is also part of the brain's reward system.

Studying the combination of genetic, neural, endocrine (e.g., hormones such as leptin and ghrelin), and environmental influences will lead to the clearest understanding of how obesity

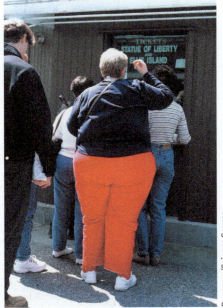

Obesity has become quite prevalent, particularly in the United States, in the past 30 years.

develops (Schwartz, Seeley, et al., 2017). In 2011, researchers published a study showing that many mammals, not just humans, have been gaining weight over the past decades (Klimentidis, Beasley, et al., 2011). The researchers examined different kinds of monkeys, as well as mice, rats, and marmosets, all of which were raised in captivity, and found that these animals have all become heavier over the decades even though they were fed highly controlled diets that have not markedly changed over the years in quantity or quality. Clearly, animals are not gaining weight based on advertising or access to fast food or even limited exercise. The researchers' findings indicate that changes in the environment, such as chemicals that disrupt the endocrine system, bacteria or other infectious agents, and stress, are influencing the obesity epidemic in humans (Schwartz et al., 2017).

Indeed, stress and its associated negative moods can induce eating in some people (Tomiyama, 2019), and research with humans and rodents shows that foods rich in fat and sugar may reduce stress in the short term, giving new meaning to the term *comfort food* (Dallman, Pecoraro, et al., 2003; Kessler, 2009; Wardle, Chida, et al., 2011). Unfortunately, prolonged stress can negatively impact the HPA axis and increase the release of cortisol (see Chapter 2), which can also promote weight gain (Tomiyama, 2019). And, even if some foods bring comfort in the short term, research shows that negative moods usually get worse after binge eating (Haedt-Matt & Keel, 2011).

The stigma associated with being overweight is also stressful. Several reality TV shows are devoted to watching obese people struggle to lose weight; one is *My 600-lb Life* that showcases the challenges of people who weigh 600 pounds or more as they try to lose weight and keep it off (a spin-off series is *My 600-lb Life: Where Are They Now*?). Obese people are now presented as entertainment: This does not seem to be an effective way to reduce stigma. Further, studies have shown that the stress linked to weight stigma is associated with weight gain (Tomiyama, 2019). This creates a vicious cycle: A person who is overweight feels shame and stress from weight stigma and may turn to comfort food, which in turn promotes weight gain, which in turn maintains or even strengthens the stigma. In children and adolescents, research shows that there is greater bullying about weight than about other characteristics (e.g., race or sexual orientation; Puhl, Latner, et al., 2016). Reducing weight stigma will no doubt help us in the fight against obesity.

Stigma can also perpetuate the idea that obesity is simply a matter of personal responsibility—the belief that if people would just eat less and exercise more, obesity would not be a problem. But the science behind self-control tells another story. Given the multitude of factors contributing to obesity, such a simple solution is not reasonable.

Evidence suggests that psychological treatments for obesity can be effective. The journal *American Psychologist* published a special issue in March 2020 entitled "Obesity: Psychosocial and Behavioral Aspects of a Modern Epidemic." Two of the articles in this issue covered behavioral treatments for obesity. The American Psychological Association (APA) recommended that treatments include the family and have at least 26 hours of contact with a professional (Guideline Development Panel for Treatment of Obesity, American Psychological Association, 2020). The earlier the treatment can begin, the better. The treatment recommendations indicate that the treatments should include three aspects: physical activity, diet change, and behavioral techniques to help make and sustain changes in diet and physical activity. In addition, participation in behavioral weight loss programs should continue for at least 1 year (Wadden, Tronieri, & Butryn, 2020). The program should cover diet changes, education about health and diet, and physical activity. These programs can be implemented in person, one-on-one or in a group, or by using a digital platform (e.g., an internet or smartphone telehealth app).

Medications that can help with weight loss became so popular in 2022 that there were severe shortages. Some of these medications were originally developed to treat Type 2 diabetes, such as Ozempic (contains semaglutide) or Mounjaro (contains tirzepatide). One semaglutide medication (Wegovy) was approved explicitly as a medication for obesity and weight loss. In addition to reducing A1C (a measure of blood sugar important for diabetes assessment), these medications also lead to weight loss. These medications mimic the action of a hormone called GLP-1 that is released after you eat and helps to reduce appetite and increase feelings of fullness. With a smaller appetite, people eat less. And feelings of fullness help keep people from overeating.

These medications are commonly injected daily into the abdomen (dubbed by some as "skinny pens") and discontinuing the medication is linked to regaining most of the weight what was lost (Wilding, Batterham, et al., 2022). Like many medications, these can have some unpleasant side effects, including nausea, vomiting, and diarrhea.

Even as we learn more about the causes of obesity, the prevalence rates continue to rise. Behavioral and medication interventions can help, but work needs to be done to halt the obesity epidemic.

Binge eating disorder is comorbid with several disorders, including mood disorders, anxiety disorders, ADHD, conduct disorder, and substance use disorders (Kessler, Berglund, et al., 2013; Lydecker & Grilo, 2022; Wonderlich et al., 2009). Risk factors for developing binge eating disorder include childhood obesity, critical comments about being overweight, weight-loss attempts in childhood, low self-concept, depression, and childhood physical or sexual abuse (Rubinstein, McGinn, et al., 2010).

Binge eating disorder is more prevalent than either anorexia nervosa or bulimia nervosa (Hudson et al., 2007; Kessler et al., 2013; Stice, Marti, & Rohde, 2013). In one study of several countries, the lifetime prevalence ranged from 0.2% to 4.7% (Kessler et al., 2013). Binge eating disorder is more common in women than men, although the sex difference is not as great as it is for anorexia or bulimia (Kessler et al., 2013). Though only a few epidemiological studies have been done, binge eating disorder appears to be equally prevalent among European, African, Asian, and Hispanic Americans (Striegel-Moore & Franco, 2008).

Physical Consequences of Binge Eating Disorder

Like the other eating disorders, binge eating disorder has physical consequences. Many of the physical consequences appear likely to be a function of the associated obesity, including increased risk of type 2 diabetes, cardiovascular problems, chronic back pain, and headaches, even after controlling for the independent effects of other comorbid disorders (Kessler et al., 2013). Research shows that people with binge eating disorder have many physical problems that are independent from co-occurring obesity, including sleep problems, anxiety, depression, irritable bowel syndrome, and, for women, early onset of menstruation (Bulik & Reichborn-Kjennerud, 2003).

Prognosis

Research suggests that 25–82% of people with binge eating disorder recover (Keel & Brown, 2010; Striegel-Moore & Franco, 2008). One epidemiological study of binge eating disorder in several countries reported a duration of just over 4 years (Kessler et al., 2013).

Quick Summary

Anorexia nervosa has three characteristics: restriction of behaviors to promote a healthy body weight, an intense fear of gaining weight, and a distorted body image. Anorexia usually begins in the early teen years and is more common in women than men. Bodily changes that can occur after severe weight loss can be serious and life threatening. As many as 70% of women with anorexia eventually recover, but it can take many years.

Bulimia nervosa involves both bingeing and compensatory behavior. Bingeing often involves sweet foods and is more likely to occur when someone is alone, after a negative social encounter, and in the morning or afternoon. One striking difference between anorexia and bulimia is weight loss: People with anorexia nervosa lose a tremendous amount of weight, whereas people with bulimia nervosa do not lose weight. Atypical anorexia nervosa, which is a manifestation of the category other specified feeding or eating disorder (OSFED), includes all the symptoms of anorexia nervosa *except* for very low body weight. Bulimia typically begins in late adolescence and is more common in women than men. Dangerous changes to the body can also occur as a result of bulimia, particularly the use of laxatives and recurrent vomiting, such as changes in electrolytes, irregularities in the heartbeat, tearing in tissues of the stomach and throat, and swelling of the salivary glands.

Binge eating disorder is characterized by several binges, and most (but not all) people who have it are obese (defined as having a BMI greater than 30). Not all obese people meet the criteria for binge eating disorder—only those who have binge episodes and report feeling a loss of control over their eating qualify. Binge eating disorder is more common than anorexia and bulimia and is more common in women than men, though the sex difference is not as great as it is for anorexia and bulimia. Recovery may take even longer than recovery for anorexia or bulimia.

11.1 Check Your Knowledge

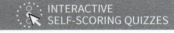
INTERACTIVE
SELF-SCORING QUIZZES

(Answers are at the end of the chapter.)
Answer the following questions.

1. All the following are symptoms of anorexia *except*:
   a. fear of gaining weight
   b. unwillingness to maintain normal weight
   c. perfectionism
   d. distorted body image

2. Which statement is true regarding binge eating disorder?
   a. It is more common in men than women.
   b. It was not an eating disorder category in DSM-IV-TR.
   c. It is synonymous with obesity.
   d. It includes binges and purges.

3. Which of the following are characteristics of both anorexia and bulimia?

   a. Both involve a good deal of weight loss.

   b. Both are more common in women than men.

   c. Both have physical side effects (e.g., menstrual irregularities).

   d. All of the above except (a) are correct.

4. List three factors that contribute to obesity.

Causes of Eating Disorders

As with other disorders, any single influence is unlikely to cause an eating disorder. Several areas of current research—genetics, neurobiology, cognitive behavioral influences, sociocultural pressures to be thin, personality, and the role of the family—suggest that eating disorders result when several influences converge in a person's life. Prospective studies identify and measure causal influences *before* the onset of an eating disorder and demonstrate that the influences predict the onset of disorder (Stice, 2016). Prospective studies can come closer to identifying causes rather than consequences of eating disorders. Unfortunately, there are currently too few of these prospective studies.

Stress and negative emotion also play a role in eating disorders as it does in all psychological disorders. The stress associated with the COVID-19 pandemic and eating disorders has been studied, and the impacts of the pandemic were substantial. A review of studies that collected data before and during the pandemic found that hospital admissions for eating disorders increased by an average of 48% during the pandemic. Over a third of the studies found that eating disorder symptoms worsened during the pandemic (Devoe, Han, et al., 2023).

Genetic Influences

Heritability estimates for anorexia range from 0.48 to 0.74, and those for bulimia from 0.55 to 0.62 (Yilmaz, Hardaway, & Bulik, 2015). Although eating disorders are less frequent among men, one study found that first-degree relatives of men with anorexia nervosa were at greater risk for having anorexia nervosa (though not bulimia) than relatives of men without anorexia (Strober, Freeman, et al., 2000). A family study (Hudson, Lalonde, et al., 2006) found that relatives of people with binge eating disorder and obesity were more likely to have binge eating disorder themselves (20%) than were relatives of people who were obese but did not have binge eating disorder (9%).

Twin studies of eating disorders also suggest a genetic influence. Most studies of both anorexia and bulimia report higher concordance rates for MZ twins than for DZ twins (Bulik, Wade, & Kendler, 2000) and show that genes account for a portion of the variance among twins with eating disorders (Wade & Bulik, 2018). On the other hand, research has shown that nonshared/unique environmental factors (see Chapter 2), such as different interactions with parents or different peer groups, also contribute to the development of eating disorders (Klump, McGue, & Iacono, 2002; Wade & Bulik, 2018). For example, a study of more than 1,200 twin pairs found that 42% of the variance in bulimia symptoms was attributable to genetic influences, but 58% of the variance was attributable to unique environmental factors (Baker et al., 2010). Research also suggests that key features of the eating disorders, such as dissatisfaction with one's body, a strong desire to be thin, binge eating, and preoccupation with weight, are heritable (Klump, McGue, & Iacono, 2002; Wade & Bulik, 2018). Additional evidence suggests that common genetic factors may account for the relationship between certain personality characteristics, such as negative emotionality and constraint, with eating disorders (Keel, 2018; Klump, McGue, & Iacono, 2002; Wade & Bulik, 2018). The largest GWAS to date included nearly 17,000 people with anorexia and over 55,000 without anorexia from around the world (Watson, Yilmaz, et al., 2019); it identified eight genetic loci. However, this study did not replicate results from a smaller GWAS (Duncan, Yilmaz, et al., 2017). Given that anorexia is a rare psychological disorder, it will be challenging to identify the multiple genes and genetic mutations that may be involved.

Neurobiological Influences

The hypothalamus is a key brain center for regulating hunger and eating. Research on animals with lesions to the lateral hypothalamus indicates that they lose weight and have no appetite (Hoebel & Teitelbaum, 1966). Thus, it is not surprising that the hypothalamus has been proposed to play a role in anorexia. The level of some hormones regulated by the hypothalamus, such as cortisol, is indeed different in people with anorexia. Rather than causing the disorder, however, these hormonal differences occur as a result of self-starvation, and levels return to normal after weight gain (Doerr, Fichter, et al., 1980; Stoving, Hangaard, et al., 1999). Furthermore, the evidence from animals with hypothalamic lesions does not parallel what we know about anorexia. These animals appear to have no hunger and to become indifferent to food, whereas people with anorexia continue to starve themselves despite being hungry and having an interest in food. Nor does the hypothalamic model account for body-image disturbance or fear of gaining weight. Thus, a dysfunctional hypothalamus does not seem a likely causal factor in anorexia nervosa.

Brain imaging studies have examined areas of the brain associated with rewards in people with and without anorexia. These studies have found that, compared to people without anorexia, people with anorexia display different patterns of activation when viewing pictures of food or tasting food (Steinglass & Walsh, 2016). One fMRI study of 21 women hospitalized with anorexia and 21 women without anorexia examined brain activity when the women made choices between two foods (Foerde, Steinglass, et al., 2015). Not surprisingly, women with anorexia chose high-fat foods less often than women without anorexia. Interestingly, however, both groups of women showed comparable brain activation in the ventral striatum, an area associated with reward, during the food choice task. Where the groups differed was in the dorsal striatum, an area of the brain linked with habitual choices and anxiety. These findings suggest that eating habits may be important in anorexia. That is, dieting or restrictive eating may become habitual, and these habits may themselves become rewarding (O'Hara, Campbell, & Schmidt, 2015; Walsh, 2013).

Researchers have also examined the role of dopamine, a neurotransmitter that is linked to reward and other pleasurable things, including food (Kaye, Wierenga, et al., 2013). For anorexia, the evidence suggests that changes to the dopamine system may be a consequence of the disorder rather than a cause (Södersten, Bergh, et al., 2016). That is, severe food restriction and weight loss may lead to problems in the dopamine system. Research has yet to identify specific vulnerabilities in the dopamine system that are present before the onset of anorexia (or any eating disorder) and might set off a bidirectional process in which the dopamine system and eating behaviors continue to influence one another (Steinglass & Foerde, 2018).

One theory about the role of dopamine in eating disorders comes from research on substance use disorders (discussed in Chapter 10). The *incentive-sensitization theory* considers both the craving ("wanting") of food and the pleasure ("liking") that comes with eating foods, particularly tasty, high-calorie foods (Berridge, Ho, et al., 2010). In this model, dopamine plays a key role in the "liking" of food and the "wanting" or anticipation of food. People who binge, whether in binge eating disorder, bulimia, or obesity, may experience excessive "wanting" or craving for tasty foods but not excessive "liking" of food (Morales & Berridge, 2020). Cravings for food can be triggered by cues in the environment, not just hunger. Cues about food (e.g., billboards, photos on food packaging) can elicit dopamine responses that in turn promote strong cravings for food that some people have a hard time resisting. You can probably remember a time when you saw an ad on TV for some food (e.g., Taco Bell tacos) or read about a food (e.g., donuts) and then found yourself wanting that very food! The theory suggests that the cues can thus create cravings, which can then promote (over)eating or bingeing. Evidence from a meta-analysis supports this theory: Cravings and food cues prospectively predict more eating and

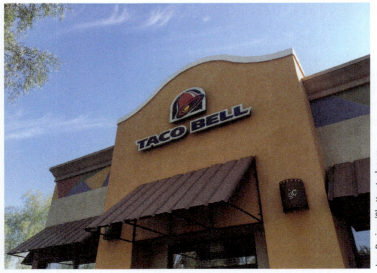

Java Designs/Shutterstock.com

Cravings can be a powerful driver of behavior, including eating.

weight gain (Boswell & Kober, 2016). Brain imaging studies have found that people who show greater activation in areas of the brain associated with dopamine and reward during the presentation of food cues are more likely to subsequently gain weight (Stice & Burger, 2019; Stice & Yokum, 2016). Research also suggests that people with binge eating disorder are particularly sensitive to cravings and cues about food (Kober & Boswell, 2018).

Finally, some research has focused on the neurotransmitter serotonin, which is related to eating and satiety (feeling full). Like research on dopamine, much of the research on serotonin suggests that changes to the serotonin system may be a consequence of an eating disorder (Culbert, Racine, & Klump, 2015; Kaye et al., 2013; Sjögren, Nielsen, et al., 2019). Researchers examining levels of serotonin metabolites have found low levels among people with anorexia and bulimia (Kaye et al., 2013; Sjögren et al., 2019). Low levels of a neurotransmitter's metabolites are one indicator that neurotransmitter activity is underactive. Antidepressant drugs can be effective treatments for some people with bulimia and binge eating disorder (treatments are discussed later in this chapter) and are known to influence serotonin, adding to evidence for the possible relevance of that neurotransmitter.

Although we can expect further neuroscience research in the future, keep in mind that much of this work focuses on brain mechanisms relevant to hunger, eating, and satiety (and a lot of the research focuses on animals) but does little to account for other key features of eating disorders, in particular the intense fear of gaining weight. Furthermore, as suggested, much of the evidence so far does not show that brain changes come before the onset of eating disorders. Brain changes may happen because of under- or overeating, not the other way around. In other words, we know that brain activity is correlated with eating disorders, not that these processes cause eating disorders.

Cognitive Behavioral and Emotion Influences

Cognitive behavioral theories of eating disorders focus on understanding the thoughts, feelings, and behaviors that contribute to distorted body image, fear of weight gain, and loss of control over eating.

Anorexia Nervosa   Cognitive behavioral theories of anorexia nervosa emphasize body-image disturbance as the motivating factor that powerfully reinforces weight loss. Many people who develop anorexia symptoms report that the onset followed a period of weight loss and dieting. Behaviors that achieve or maintain thinness are negatively reinforced by the reduction of anxiety about gaining weight as well as positively reinforced by comments from others (e.g., "Did you lose weight? You look great!"). Dieting and weight loss may also be positively reinforced by the sense of mastery or self-control they create (Fairburn, Shafran, & Cooper, 1999; Garner, Vitousek, & Pike, 1997). Body-image disturbance coupled with a low BMI increases the risk for developing anorexia (Stice & Desjardins, 2018).

Another important factor in producing a strong drive for thinness and a disturbed body image is criticism from peers and parents about being overweight (Gondoli, Corning, et al., 2011; Helfert & Warschburger, 2011). In one study supporting this conclusion,

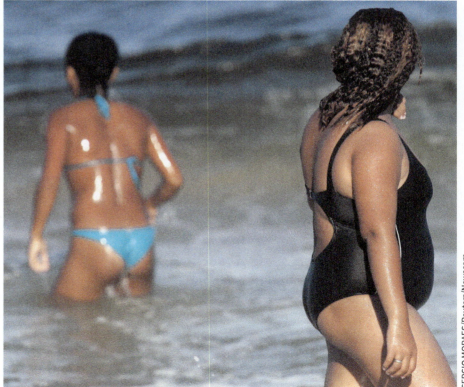

SERGIO MORAES/Reuters/Newscom

The fear of weight gain, which is so important in eating disorders, is partly based on society's negative stereotypes of overweight people.

adolescent girls ages 10 to 15 were evaluated twice, with a 3-year interval between assessments. Obesity at the first assessment was related to being teased by peers, and at the second assessment it was linked to dissatisfaction with their bodies. Dissatisfaction was in turn related to symptoms of an eating disorder (Paxton, Schutz, et al., 1999).

Research has also examined the role of emotion in anorexia nervosa. Not surprisingly, people with anorexia experience many negative emotions. Researchers have sought to understand whether negative emotions predict restricted eating (sometimes called *dietary restraint*) or whether restricted eating predicts negative emotions. That is, does a person with anorexia feel bad and then restrict eating? Or does restricting eating lead to feeling more negative emotions? The answer appears to be both. In a longitudinal study, researchers found that restricting eating in the prior month predicted more negative emotions 2 weeks later and also that experiencing more negative emotions in the prior month predicted more restricted eating 2 weeks later (Pila, Murray, et al., 2019).

Of course, people with anorexia also experience positive emotion, even though they may not distinguish among different positive emotional states all that well (Selby, Wonderlich, et al., 2013). In other words, people with anorexia may experience a positive emotion such as pride very intensely after losing weight or avoiding eating a piece of cake at a party. This emotion may in turn be indistinguishable from happiness or success, an inability referred to as *low positive emotion differentiation*. One study found that low positive emotion differentiation prospectively predicted eating disorder behaviors such as vomiting, checking weight, exercising excessively, and using laxatives in a group of 118 women with anorexia (Selby et al., 2013). Feeling stronger negative emotions also predicted these behaviors.

Bulimia Nervosa and Binge Eating Disorder

People with bulimia nervosa are thought to be overly concerned with weight gain and body appearance; indeed, they often view their self-worth in terms of their weight and shape. They may have low self-esteem, and because weight and shape are somewhat more controllable than are other features of the self, they tend to focus on weight and shape, hoping their efforts in this area will make them feel better generally. They may try to follow a very rigid pattern of restrictive eating, with strict rules regarding how much to eat, what kinds of food to eat, and when to eat. These strict rules are inevitably broken, and the lapse escalates into a binge. After the binge, feelings of shame, disgust and fear of becoming fat build up, leading to compensatory actions such as vomiting. Although purging temporarily reduces the negative feelings from having eaten too much, it also lowers the person's self-esteem, which triggers still more bingeing and purging—a vicious cycle that maintains desired body weight but has serious medical consequences (see **Figure 11.2** for a summary of this theory).

People with bulimia nervosa or binge eating disorder typically binge when they encounter stress and experience negative emotions, as has been shown in several studies. In fact, the propensity to experience negative emotions has been shown to predict the onset of eating disorders (Culbert, Racine, & Klump, 2015). Using ecological momentary assessment (EMA; see Chapter 3), investigators have shown how specific binge-and-purge events are linked to

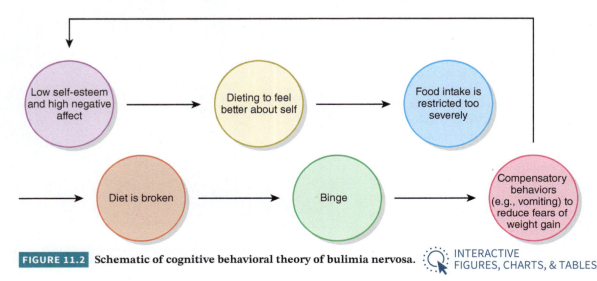

FIGURE 11.2 **Schematic of cognitive behavioral theory of bulimia nervosa.** INTERACTIVE FIGURES, CHARTS, & TABLES

changes in emotions and stress in the course of daily life (Smyth, Wonderlich, et al., 2007). A meta-analysis of 82 EMA studies found that negative emotion preceded the onset of a binge among people with bulimia and people with binge eating disorder, but the effect sizes (see Chapter 4) were stronger for binge eating disorder than for bulimia (Haedt-Matt & Keel, 2011).

An EMA study of over 100 people with binge eating disorder found that in the hours leading up to a binge, people reported increases in negative affect and guilt and decreases in positive affect. In the hours after the binge, positive affect remained stable, but negative affect and guilt decreased (Schaefer, Smith, et al., 2020). Thus, people with binge eating disorder may binge in order to reduce negative feelings, even if positive feelings do not always increase. By contrast, an EMA study of people with bulimia found that negative feelings decreased and positive feelings increased after a binge (Smyth et al., 2007), suggesting that emotional changes may differ between these two disorders.

Another EMA study found that low positive emotion differentiation prospectively predicted binge eating episodes (Mikhail, Keel, et al., 2020). One reason binges are not necessarily associated with an increase in positive feelings may be that people have difficulty distinguishing among positive feelings (e.g., happy, content, satisfied, excited, proud).

Evidence also supports the idea that stress and negative emotion are relieved by purging. That is, negative emotion levels decline and positive emotion levels increase after a purge event, suggesting that purging may be reinforced by a reduction in negative affect (Haedt-Matt & Keel, 2011; Smyth et al., 2007).

Research methods from cognitive science have been used to study how attention, memory, and problem solving are affected in people with eating disorders. Research shows that people with anorexia and bulimia focus their attention on food-related words or images more than other images (Brooks, Prince, et al., 2011). People with anorexia nervosa and people who score high on restrained eating (Polivy, Herman, & Howard, 1988) remember food words better when they are full but not when they are hungry (Brooks et al., 2011). Other studies have found that college women with eating disorder symptoms are better at paying attention to and remembering images depicting other people's body size than images depicting emotion (Treat & Viken, 2010). Thus, women with eating disorders pay greater attention not only to their own bodies, food, and weight but also to other women's bodies, food, and shapes. This tendency to (over) attend to food and body image may make it hard for women with eating disorders to change their thinking patterns. As we shall see later, cognitive behavior therapy (CBT) devotes a good bit of time to teaching people with eating disorders to alter these memory and attention processes.

Sociocultural Influences

Throughout history, the standards societies have set for the ideal body—especially the ideal female body—have varied greatly. Think of the famous nudes painted by Rubens in the 17th century: According to modern standards, these women are chubby. Over the past 60 years, the American cultural ideal for body shape has progressed steadily toward increased thinness, particularly for White women.

At the same time, the prevalence of obesity (see **Focus on Discovery 11.1**) has doubled since 1980 in 70 countries (GBD 2015 Obesity Collaborators, 2017), and the rates show no signs of declining (WHO, 2020). Currently, over two-thirds of Americans are overweight (and over 40% are obese), setting the stage for greater conflict between the cultural ideal and reality.

Dieting to lose weight is very common; in a survey of over 4,000 women ages 25 to 45, a third of the women reported spending more than half of their lifetime trying to lose weight (Reba-Harrelson, Von Holle, et al., 2009). Procedures such as liposuction (vacuuming out fat deposits just under the skin) and bariatric surgery (surgically changing the stomach so that it cannot digest as much food) are popular despite their risks (Sarwer & Heinberg, 2020). In fact, the American Academy of Pediatrics issued a recommendation that access to

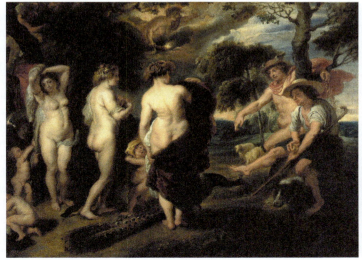

AKG London/SuperStock

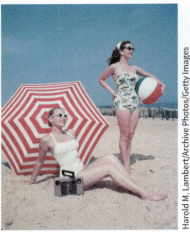
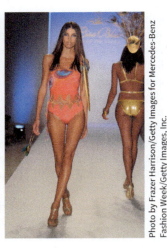

Cultural standards regarding the ideal feminine shape have changed over time. Even in the 1950s and 1960s, the feminine ideal was considerably heavier than what it became in the 1970s and is today.

bariatric surgery be increased for adolescents who are severely obese (Armstrong, Bolling, et al., 2019).

Women are more likely than men to be dieters. The onset of eating disorders is typically preceded by dieting or other concerns about weight, supporting the idea that social standards stressing the importance of thinness play a role in the development of these disorders (Rubinstein et al., 2010; Stice, 2002, 2016).

It is likely that women who either are overweight or fear becoming so are dissatisfied with their bodies. Not surprisingly, studies have found that women and adolescent girls with both a high BMI and body dissatisfaction are at higher risk for developing eating disorders (Grabe, Ward, & Hyde, 2008; Stice, 2001, 2022; Stice & Van Ryzin, 2018). Preoccupation with being thin or feeling pressure to be thin predicts an increase in body dissatisfaction among adolescent girls, which in turn predicts more dieting, eating pathology, and negative emotions (Stice, 2001, 2022); these factors were operating in the Clinical Case of Jill, presented earlier. Indeed, prospective studies indicate that body dissatisfaction, dieting, and the desire to be thin all predict the onset of bulimia (Stice, 2016).

Does the media play a role in body dissatisfaction? Overall, the evidence from meta-analyses show that the effect sizes on such influences are small. Experimental studies (see Chapter 4) have found that exposure to media portrayals of unrealistically thin models can influence reports of body dissatisfaction. In one creative experimental study, researchers randomly assigned women to one of four groups (Bury, Tiggemann, & Slater, 2017). The women viewed ads from magazines in which photos of fashion models either had or had not been digitally altered, and they either did or did not read a disclaimer noting that the ads had been digitally altered. The disclaimer said the images had been altered to enhance the appearance of the models. No matter what group participants were assigned to, they all reported lower body dissatisfaction after viewing the ads than before viewing the ads. In other words, providing the participants with knowledge that the ads were not real (i.e., the disclaimer) did not help them feel less worse about their own bodies after the experiment. In addition, the women rated all the ads as similarly realistic even if they were given a disclaimer. This study confirms how difficult it can be to reduce the influence of media. Even if we know that images have been altered, we may still view them as real and feel worse about ourselves. This is likely to continue as images produced or altered by AI (artificial intelligence) proliferate.

The sociocultural ideal of thinness is likely one vehicle through which people learn to fear weight gain or even feeling fat, and it was probably influential for both Lynne and Jill (see the earlier **Clinical Cases**). In addition to creating an undesired physical shape, being overweight has negative connotations, such as being unsuccessful and having little self-control. People who are obese are viewed by others as less smart and are stereotyped as lonely, lazy, shy, and greedy for the affection of others (Puhl, Himmelstein, & Pearl, 2020). Even more disturbing is the finding that health professionals who specialize in obesity have exhibited beliefs that obese people are lazy, stupid, or worthless (Schwartz, Chambliss, et al., 2003). Reducing the stigma associated with being overweight will be beneficial to those with eating disorders as well as those who are obese.

In much the same way as the fear of weight gain contributes to eating pathology, the celebration of extreme thinness via Twitter, Instagram, YouTube, and magazines may also play a role. Hashtags or sites that are "pro-ana" ("ana" is shorthand for *anorexia*) or "pro-mia" ("mia" is shorthand for *bulimia*) have developed a following of women and girls who seek support and encouragement for losing weight, often to a dangerously low level. So-called "ed twitter" includes images and videos with hashtags like #proana, #edtwitter,

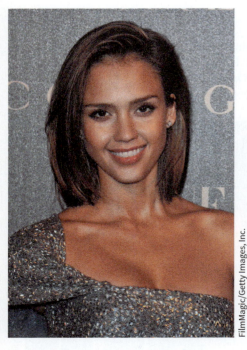

Jessica Alba has spoken openly about her eating disorder.

and #thinspo. These sites often post photos of female celebrities who are extremely thin as inspiration (hence the terms *thinspiration* and *thinspo*). Some of these women have publicly discussed their struggles with eating disorders (e.g., the actress Jessica Alba), but others have not. The low BMI that goes along with extreme thinness has been shown to prospectively predict the onset of anorexia (Stice, 2016), and therefore, sites that promote such low weight may nurture a risk factor for anorexia.

A review of the impact of these "pro–eating disorder" social media sites and websites noted that women who visited these sites were more dissatisfied with their bodies, had more eating disorder symptoms, and had experienced more prior hospitalizations for eating disorders (Rouleau & von Ranson, 2011). To distinguish causation from correlation, researchers have randomly assigned healthy women to view either pro–eating disorder, other health-related, or tourist websites (Jett, La Porte, & Wanchism, 2010), supposedly as part of a website evaluation survey. The women completed food diaries for 1 week before and 1 week after viewing these websites. Women assigned to the pro–eating disorder website condition restricted their eating more the following week than did the women assigned to the other website conditions. These results suggest that viewing pro–eating disorder websites have the potential to cause unhealthful changes in eating behavior.

Sex and Gender Influences

We have noted that eating disorders are more common in women than in men. One primary reason is likely the fact that Western cultural standards emphasize and reinforce the desirability of being thin more for women than for men. For men, magazines focus attention on the masculine ideal of normal body weight or on increased muscle mass (Halliwell, Dittmar, & Orsborn, 2007; Strother, Lemberg, et al., 2012). The risk for eating disorders appears to be especially high among groups of women who might be expected to be particularly concerned with thinness and their weight—such as dancers or gymnasts, as in the case of Jill (Bratland-Sanda & Sundgot-Borgen, 2013; Murray et al., 2017; Thompson, Petrie, & Anderson, 2017).

However, eating disorders and symptoms are more common among sexual minoritized men and women—gay, lesbian, bisexual—than heterosexual people (Kamody, Grilo, & Udo, 2020; Shepherd, Brochu, & Rodriguez-Seijas, 2022). Eating disorders in gender minoritized men and women is a newer area of research focus. Thus, noting sex differences in eating disorders between men and women without attention to sexual or gender minoritized status will not allow for a complete understanding of how men and women may or may not differ.

There is another sociocultural factor that has remained remarkably resilient to change— namely, the objectification of women's bodies. Women's bodies are often viewed through a sexual lens; in effect, women are defined by their bodies, whereas men are esteemed more for their accomplishments. According to objectification theory (Fredrickson & Roberts, 1997), the prevalence of objectification messages in Western culture (in television, advertisements, and so forth) has led some women to "self-objectify," which means that they see their own bodies through the eyes of others. Research has shown that self-objectification causes women to feel more shame about their bodies. Shame is most often elicited in situations where an individual's ideal falls short of a cultural ideal or standard. Thus, women may experience body shame when they observe a mismatch between their ideal self and the cultural (objectified) view of women. Research has also shown that both self-objectification and body shame are associated with disordered eating among racially and ethnically diverse women (Davies, Burnette, & Mazzeo, 2020; McKinley & Hyde, 1996; Noll & Fredrickson, 1998; Schaefer, Burke, et al., 2018; Tiggemann & Williams, 2012).

Do eating disorders and weight concerns go away as men and women get older? A large prospective study has followed a group of nearly 1,000 men and women since they were in college in the early 1980s. Assessments were conducted in college and then 10, 20, and 30 years later (Brown, Forney, et al., 2020; Keel, Baxter, et al., 2007). At each time point, eating disorder prevalence rates were computed and risk factors such as dieting, BMI, body image, and drive for thinness were assessed. By the 30-year follow-up assessment, the men and women were around age 50. The researchers found that after 30 years, a quarter of the women who had an eating disorder diagnosis continued to meet the diagnostic criteria at age 50. The most dramatic drop was between ages 20 and 30; after age 30, the number of women receiving a diagnosis stayed low. For men, the prevalence rates were stable since college, but there were very few men who met the diagnosis of any eating disorder (10 in college; 7 at age 50), so it

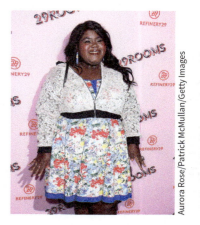

Gabourey Sidibe, Oscar-nominated actress and author of the memoir *This Is Just My Face: Try Not to Stare*, had bariatric surgery to accomplish weight loss.

Aurora Rose/Patrick McMullan/Getty Images

was hard to draw strong conclusions about the men. At age 40, women dieted less and were less concerned about their weight and body image than they had been in college, even though they weighed more. By the time women reached age 50, their eating disorder symptoms had decreased, as had the risk factors for eating disorders (concern about body image, drive for thinness, frequency of dieting). Changes in life roles—having a life partner, having a child—were also associated with decreases in eating disorder symptoms for women. By contrast, over the 30 years, men had become more concerned about their weight and were dieting more. Like women, they weighed more in their early 40s than they had when they were in college.

Cross-Cultural Studies   How much evidence there is for the presence of eating disorders across cultures depends on the disorder. Anorexia or its symptoms have been observed in several cultures and countries besides the United States—for example, in Hong Kong, China, Taiwan, England, Korea, Japan, Denmark, Nigeria, South Africa, Zimbabwe, Ethiopia, Jordan, Saudi Arabia, Kuwait, UAE, Iran, Malaysia, India, Pakistan, Australia, the Netherlands, and Egypt (Keel & Klump, 2003; Melisse, de Beurs, & van Furth, 2020; Pike & Dunne, 2015). Furthermore, cases of anorexia have been documented in cultures with very little Western cultural influence. An important caveat must be made, however. The anorexia observed in these diverse cultures does not always include the intense fear of gaining weight that is part of the DSM criteria, at least initially. Thus, intense fear of weight gain likely reflects an ideal more widely espoused in more Westernized cultures.

The variation in the clinical presentation of anorexia across cultures provides a window into the importance of culture in establishing realistic versus potentially disordered views of one's body. However, there is evidence that this cultural variation is diminishing when it comes to eating disorders. A 20-year study of eating disorders in Hong Kong found evidence of Western influence in both the prevalence and the presentation of eating disorders (Lee, Ng, et al., 2010). First, both anorexia and bulimia were twice as common in 2007 as they had been in 1987. Second, 25% more women reported body dissatisfaction and fear of fat in 2007 than in 1987. Thus, in a fairly short period of time, eating disorders in Hong Kong appear to have become more Western.

Bulimia nervosa appears to be more common in industrialized societies, such as the United States, Canada, Japan, Australia, and Europe, than in nonindustrialized nations. However, as cultures undergo social changes associated with adopting the practices of more Westernized cultures, including having access to more food, the incidence of bulimia appears to increase (Keel & Klump, 2003; Kolar, Rodriguez, et al., 2016; Lee et al., 2010; van Hoeken, Burns, & Hoek, 2016).

One study examined the prevalence rates of women seeking treatment for anorexia, bulimia, or binge eating disorder in a Kyoto, Japan, hospital across four decades, from 1963 to 2004 (Nakai, Nin, et al., 2018). Anorexia was

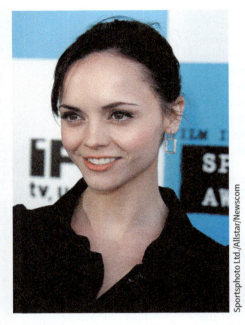
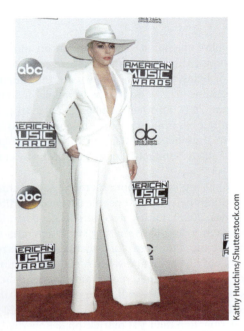

Celebrities such as Christina Ricci and Lady Gaga have publicly discussed their struggles with eating disorders.

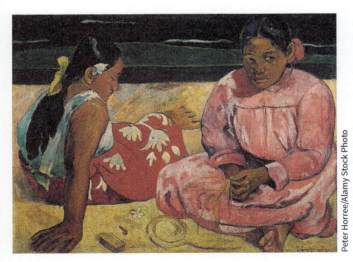

Standards of beauty vary across cultures, as Gauguin's painting of Tahitian women shows.

present in the 1960s. People seeking treatment for bulimia or binge eating disorder appeared in 1980. Rates of treatment seeking for all three disorders increased across the four decades. The researchers noted that cultural influences within Japan as well as from elsewhere (e.g., American emphasis on thinness as a beauty ideal) may have contributed to this rise.

Racial and Ethnic Differences   Some evidence indicates that anorexia nervosa is more prevalent among White women than among Black or Hispanic women (Udo & Grilo, 2018). However, for bulimia nervosa or binge eating disorder, differences in prevalence among racial and ethnic groups are minimal (Cheng, Perko, et al., 2019; Wildes, Emery, & Simons, 2001). Data from one epidemiological study of Latina women age 18 or older showed that binge eating disorder was more prevalent than bulimia nervosa but that the prevalence rates for both disorders were comparable to prevalence rates in non-Latina women (Alegria, Woo, et al., 2007). The diagnosis of bulimia was more likely for women who had lived in the United States for several years than for women who had recently immigrated to the United States, indicating that acculturation may play a role.

Current evidence suggests that there are more similarities than differences in eating disorder risk factors or features. The differences between White and Black women appear to be most pronounced in college student samples; fewer differences are observed in either high school or nonclinical community samples (Udo & Grilo, 2018; Wildes, Emery, & Simons, 2001). A meta-analysis indicated that White women and Latina women reported greater body dissatisfaction than Black women, but no other ethnic differences were reliably found (Grabe & Hyde, 2006). A more recent study found that Asian American women endorsed more thin-ideal beliefs than either White or Black women (Cheng et al., 2019).

Other Influences Contributing to the Causes of Eating Disorders

Personality Influences   We have already seen that neurobiological changes are associated with eating disorders. It is also important to keep in mind that the eating disorder itself can affect the personality. A study of semistarvation in male conscientious objectors conducted in the late 1940s supports the idea that the personality of people with eating disorders, particularly those with anorexia, is affected by their weight loss (Keys, Brozek, et al., 1950). For a period of 6 weeks, the men were given two meals a day, totaling 1,500 calories, to simulate the meals in a concentration camp. On average, the men lost 25% of their body weight. They all soon became preoccupied with food; they also reported increased fatigue, poor concentration, lack of sexual interest, irritability, moodiness, and insomnia. Four became depressed, and one developed bipolar disorder. This research shows vividly how severe restriction of food intake can have powerful effects on personality and behavior, which we need to consider when evaluating the personalities of people with anorexia and bulimia.

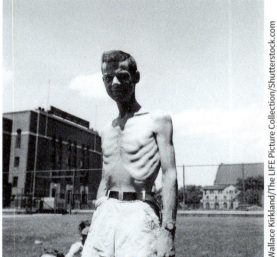

Severe food restriction can have profound effects on behavior and personality, as illustrated by the study of male conscientious objectors in the 1940s.

Wallace Kirkland/The LIFE Picture Collection/Shutterstock.com

One personality characteristic that has been studied is perfectionism. Perfectionism refers to setting high standards for oneself and being self-critical when the standards are not met (Frost, Marten, et al., 1990). Perfectionism is multifaceted and may be self-oriented (setting high standards for oneself), other-oriented (setting high standards for others), or socially oriented (trying to conform to the high standards imposed by others). In addition, perfectionism is not necessarily problematic, but when the standards are impossibly high and the self-criticism unrelenting, it can interfere with many aspects of daily life.

Reviews of many studies concluded that perfectionism, no matter how it is measured, is higher among girls with anorexia than among girls without anorexia and that perfectionism remains high even after successful treatment for anorexia (Bardone-Cone, Wonderlich, et al., 2007; Dahlenburg, Gleaves, & Hutchinson, 2019). Additional evidence from reviews and meta-analyses shows that perfectionism is correlated with binge eating disorder and bulimia

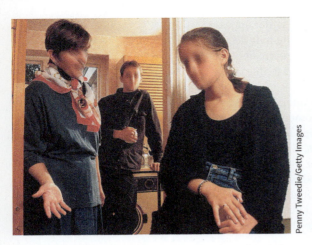

People with eating disorders consistently report that their family life was high in conflict.

nervosa (Cassin & von Ranson, 2005), and prospectively predicts the onset of eating disorder symptoms, but not necessarily eating disorders (Stice, 2016, 2022). Perfectionism combined with body dissatisfaction also predicts drive for thinness and concern about weight (Boone, Soenens, & Luyten, 2014).

In one prospective study, more than 2,000 students in a suburban Minneapolis school district completed several tests, including measures of personality characteristics and the Eating Disorders Inventory, for 3 consecutive years. During year 1 of the study, cross-sectional predictors of disordered eating included body dissatisfaction; poor interoceptive awareness, which is the extent to which people can distinguish different biological states of their bodies (see Table 11.2 for items that assess interoceptive awareness); and a propensity to experience negative emotions (Leon, Fulkerson, et al., 1995). At year 3, these same variables were found to have prospectively predicted disordered eating (Leon, Fulkerson, et al., 1999).

Characteristics of Families   Studies of the characteristics of families of people with eating disorders have yielded variable results. Some of the variation stems from the different methods used to collect the data and from the sources of the information. For example, self-reports of people with eating disorders reveal high levels of conflict in the family (Holtom-Viesel & Allan, 2014; Quiles Marcos, Quiles Sebastián, et al., 2013). Reports of parents, however, do not necessarily indicate high levels of family problems. Indeed, parent and child reports do not always agree when it comes to describing characteristics of families of people with eating disorders.

Quick Summary

Genetic influences appear to play a role in anorexia and bulimia. Both disorders tend to run in families, and twin studies support a role for genetics in the disorders and their characteristics, such as body dissatisfaction, preoccupation with thinness, and binge eating. The hypothalamus does not appear to be directly involved in eating disorders. Serotonin may play a role in bulimia and binge eating disorders, but evidence suggests that changes to the serotonin system may be a consequence of an eating disorder more than a cause. Research linking dopamine to the brain's reward system can help account for how the bingeing that is part of bulimia and binge eating disorder influences the dopamine system. Changes in serotonin and dopamine both appear to be a consequence of eating disorders rather than a cause. Neurobiological influences do not account very well for some key features of anorexia and bulimia, in particular the intense fear of gaining weight.

Cognitive behavioral and emotion influences include body dissatisfaction, preoccupation with thinness, negative emotion, and attention and memory. People are more likely to binge when under stress or experiencing negative emotions. People with eating disorders pay greater attention to words and images related to food and body image, and they tend to remember these better as well, suggesting that their attention and memory may be biased toward food and body image.

Sociocultural influences, including society's preoccupation with thinness, may play a role in eating disorders. This preoccupation is linked to dieting efforts, and dieting precedes the development of eating disorders among many people. In addition, a preoccupation with thinness, as well as exposure to media portrayals of thin women, predicts an increase in body dissatisfaction, which also precedes the development of eating disorders. The stigma associated with being overweight also contributes. Women are more likely to have eating disorders than men; the ways in which women's bodies are objectified may lead some women to see their bodies as others do (self-objectify), which in turn may increase body dissatisfaction and eating pathology. Anorexia appears to occur in many cultures, whereas bulimia appears to be more common in industrialized and Westernized societies. Anorexia may be slightly more common among White women than women of color, but there are few ethnic or racial differences in bulimia and binge eating disorder.

Research on personality characteristics finds that perfectionism may play a role in eating disorders. Troubled family relationships are fairly common among people with eating disorders, but this could be a result of the eating disorder, not necessarily a cause of it.

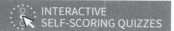

11.2 Check Your Knowledge

INTERACTIVE
SELF-SCORING QUIZZES

(Answers are at the end of the chapter.)
True or false?

1. The strongest evidence for genetic influences in eating disorders is found in twin studies.
2. Research on dopamine and serotonin shows that these neurotransmitters are disrupted prior to the onset of an eating disorder.
3. Prospective studies of personality and eating disorders indicate that the tendency to experience negative emotions is related to disordered eating.
4. Anorexia appears to be specific to Western culture; bulimia is seen all over the world and is thus not culture-specific.
5. Research on race and ethnic factors suggests that there are more similarities than differences in the risk factors and features associated with eating disorders.

Treatment of Eating Disorders

Hospitalization is frequently required to treat people with anorexia so that their ingestion of food can be gradually increased and carefully monitored. This was necessary for Lynne. Weight loss can be so severe that intravenous feeding is necessary to save the person's life. The medical complications of anorexia, such as electrolyte imbalances, also require treatment. For both anorexia and bulimia, both medications and psychological treatments have been used.

Medications

Because bulimia nervosa is often comorbid with depression, it has been treated with various antidepressants. Findings from most studies, including double-blind randomized controlled trials with placebo controls, confirm the efficacy of a variety of antidepressants in reducing purging and binge eating (McElroy, Guerdjikova, et al., 2019; Reas & Grilo, 2015).

Medications have also been used to treat anorexia nervosa, but with little success in improving weight or other core features of anorexia (Crow, 2019). Medication treatment for binge eating disorder has not been as well studied. Limited evidence suggests that antidepressant medications are not effective in reducing binges or weight loss (Peat, Berkman, et al., 2017). A randomized controlled trial compared three groups. One group received the antidepressant medication fluoxetine (Prozac). A second group received CBT plus CBT fluoxetine; the third group received CBT plus a placebo. The results indicated that CBT plus a placebo was more effective in reducing binge episodes than either condition including fluoxetine, and this remained the case at a 12-month follow-up (Grilo, Crosby, et al., 2012).

Psychological Treatment of Anorexia Nervosa

Therapy for anorexia is generally thought of as a two-tiered process. The immediate goal is to help the person gain weight so as to avoid medical complications and the possibility of death. The person is often so weak and physiological functioning so disturbed that hospital treatment is medically imperative (in addition to being needed to ensure that the patient ingests some food). The second goal of treatment— long-term maintenance of weight gain—remains a challenge for the field.

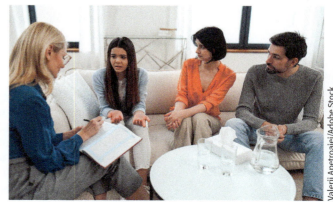

Valerii Apetroaiei/Adobe Stock

Family therapy is a main form of treatment for anorexia nervosa.

Beyond interventions aimed at immediate weight gain, psychological treatment for anorexia can involve CBT. One study that combined hospital treatment with CBT found that reductions in many anorexia symptoms persisted up to 1 year after treatment (Bowers & Ansher, 2008). Other studies have found that CBT is effective after hospitalization in reducing the risk of relapse (Pike, Walsh, et al., 2003). A randomized controlled clinical trial compared CBT to supportive psychotherapy plus education about anorexia and found that both were equally effective for women with anorexia nervosa in reducing eating disorder symptoms and depression (Touyz, Le Grange, et al., 2013). Although BMI had increased at the end of treatment and remained stable at the 12-month follow-up, the average BMIs for women in both treatment groups were still not fully back to a healthy range. Additional analyses of the results indicated that women who were older and had more severe symptoms benefited the most from CBT (Le Grange, Fitzsimmons-Craft, et al., 2014).

Family therapy is another form of psychological treatment for anorexia; it is based on the notion that interactions among members of the patient's family can play a role in treating the disorder (Le Grange & Rienecke, 2018). Results from meta-analyses indicate that family-based therapies are the most effective treatments for anorexia nervosa, particularly for weight gain and remission of symptoms (Correll, Cortese, et al., 2021; Monteleone, Pellegrino, et al., 2022). A family-based therapy (FBT) developed in England focuses on helping parents restore their daughter to a healthy weight while at the same time building up family functioning in the context of adolescent development (Lock, Le Grange, et al., 2001; Loeb, Walsh, et al., 2007). A randomized controlled clinical trial compared FBT with individual therapy and found that both treatments were equally effective at the end of 24 sessions. However, 1 year after treatment, more girls receiving FBT were in full remission (49%) than girls receiving individual therapy (23%) (Lock, Le Grange, et al., 2010). Other randomized trials of FBT found that the girls who had gained weight by session 4 were more likely to be in full remission at the end of treatment (Agras, Lock, et al., 2014; Doyle, Le Grange, et al., 2010). Thus, early weight gain may be an important predictor of a good outcome.

Psychological Treatment of Bulimia Nervosa

CBT is the best-validated and has the most evidence to support its use in the treatment of bulimia (Agras & Bohon, 2021; Fairburn, Cooper, et al., 2009; Monteleone et al., 2022), and it is the top recommended treatment in clinical practice guidelines around the world (Hilbert, Hoek, & Schmidt, 2017). In CBT, people with bulimia are encouraged to question society's standards for physical attractiveness. People with bulimia must also uncover and then change their beliefs about food, weight, and attractiveness. They must be helped to see that healthy body weight can be maintained without severe dieting and that unrealistic restriction of food intake can often trigger a binge. They are taught that all is not lost with just one bite of high-calorie food and that snacking need not trigger a binge, which will be followed by induced vomiting or taking laxatives, which in turn will lead to still lower self-esteem and depression. Altering this all-or-nothing thinking can help people begin to eat more moderately.

The overall goal of treatment for bulimia nervosa is to develop more healthy eating patterns. People with bulimia need to learn to eat three meals a day and even some snacks between meals without sliding back into bingeing and purging. Regular meals control hunger and thereby, it is hoped, the urge to eat enormous amounts of food, the effects of which are counteracted by purging. To help people with bulimia develop less extreme beliefs about themselves, the cognitive behavior therapist gently but firmly challenges such beliefs as "No one will respect me if I am a few pounds heavier than I am now" or "Eric loves me only because I weigh 112 pounds and would surely reject me if I ballooned to 120 pounds." Unrealistic demands and other cognitive distortions—such as the belief that eating a small amount of high-calorie food means that the person is an utter failure and doomed never to improve—are continually challenged. The therapist works collaboratively with the person to identify events, thoughts, and feelings that trigger an urge to binge and then to learn more adaptive ways to cope with these situations.

In the case of Jill, she and her therapist discovered that bingeing often took place after she was criticized by her coach. Therapy included the following:

- Encouraging Jill to assert herself if the criticism is unwarranted
- Desensitizing her to social evaluation and encouraging her to question society's standards for ideal weight and the pressures on women to be thin—not an easy task by any means
- Teaching her that, even if the coach's criticism is valid, it is not a catastrophe to make a mistake, and it is not necessary to be perfect

Findings from reviews and meta-analyses indicate that CBT is effective (Agras & Bohon, 2021; Monteleone et al., 2022); it often results in less frequent bingeing and purging, with reductions ranging from 70% to more than 90%. For example, one randomized controlled clinical trial compared 5 months of CBT with 2 years of psychoanalytic therapy and found that those who received CBT had far fewer bingeing and purging episodes, both at the end of 5 months and at the end of 2 years (Poulsen, Lunn, et al., 2014). Other studies have found that therapeutic gains are maintained at a 1-year follow-up (Agras, Crow, et al., 2000), nearly 6 years later (Fairburn, Norman, et al., 1995), and 10 years later (Keel, Mitchell, et al., 2002).

CBT alone is more effective than any available medication (Wilson, 2018), and a meta-analysis showed that CBT yielded better results than antidepressant medications (Monteleone et al., 2022). But are outcomes better when antidepressant medication is added to CBT? Evidence on this front is mixed. Adding antidepressant drugs may be useful in helping to alleviate the depression that often occurs with bulimia (Keel et al., 2002).

Another form of CBT, called CBT-guided self-help (CBT-gsh), has shown promise (Hilbert, Hoek, & Schmidt, 2017). In this type of treatment, people receive self-help (via a book or on the internet) on topics such as perfectionism, body image, negative thinking, and food and health. Participants meet for a small number of sessions with a therapist who helps guide them through the self-help material. This appears to be an effective treatment, based on comparison to a wait-list control group and to traditional CBT for bulimia (Agras & Bohon, 2021; Traviss-Turner, West, & Hill, 2017). In the United Kingdom, guided self-help CBT is recommended as the first-line treatment for bulimia and binge eating disorder, followed by individual CBT (National Collaborating Centre for Mental Health, 2017).

Interpersonal therapy (IPT) has also been used for bulimia, though it does not produce results as quickly as CBT (Agras & Bohon, 2021; Fairburn, Jones, et al., 1991, 1993). The two modes of intervention were equivalent at 1-year follow-up in effecting change in bingeing, purging, and maladaptive attitudes about body shape and weight (Wilson, 1995). This pattern—CBT superior to IPT immediately after treatment but IPT catching up at follow-up—was replicated (Agras et al., 2000). A small meta-analysis found that CBT had a slight advantage over IPT, but long-term follow-ups were not conducted in most of the studies included in the meta-analysis (Cuijpers, Donker, et al., 2016).

Family therapy may be effective for bulimia, though it has been studied less frequently than either CBT or IPT. Two randomized clinical trials have found that family-based therapy was effective for adolescents with bulimia with respect to decreasing bingeing and purging up to 6 and 12 months after treatment was completed (Le Grange, Crosby, et al., 2007; Le Grange, Hughes, et al., 2016). International treatment guidelines recommend family therapy for children or adolescents but CBT for adults (Hilbert, Hoek, & Schmidt, 2017).

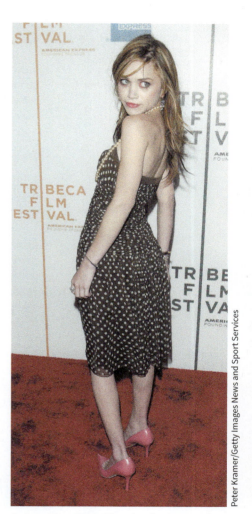

Actress Mary-Kate Olsen has been treated for an eating disorder.

Peter Kramer/Getty Images News and Sport Services

Psychological Treatment of Binge Eating Disorder

Although not as extensively studied with binge eating disorder as with bulimia nervosa, CBT has been shown to be effective for binge eating disorder in several studies (Agras & Bohon, 2021; Hilbert, Petroff, et al., 2019; Linardon, Wade, et al., 2017; Peat et al., 2017). CBT for binge eating disorder targets binges as well as emphasizing self-monitoring, self-control, and problem solving related to eating (Fairburn, 2013). Gains from CBT appear to last up to 1 year after treatment. CBT appears to be more effective than treatment with fluoxetine (Wilson, 2018). Randomized controlled clinical trials have shown that IPT is as effective as CBT and CBT-guided self-help for binge eating disorder (Wilfley, Welch, et al., 2002; Wilson, Wilfley, et al., 2010). These three treatments are more effective than behavioral weight-loss programs, which are often used to treat obesity. More specifically, CBT and IPT reduce binge eating (but not necessarily weight), whereas behavioral weight-loss programs may promote weight loss but do not curb binge eating.

One study compared three treatments for binge eating disorder: (1) therapist-led group CBT, (2) therapist-assisted group CBT, and (3) structured self-help group CBT with no therapist. Results showed that people in the therapist-led group CBT had the greatest reduction in binge eating at 6-month and 12-month follow-ups but that all groups had a greater reduction in binges than a group of people assigned to a wait-list control group (Peterson, Mitchell, et al., 2009). Fewer people dropped out of the therapist-led group as well. Thus, having a therapist lead a CBT group may help keep people in treatment and help reduce binges, but, importantly, people in the therapist-assisted and therapist-free groups also showed reductions in binges. Given that cost and/or availability may limit therapist-led treatment for some people, having options such as these available is promising.

Another form of CBT, called CBT-guided self-help (CBT-gsh), is effective for binge eating disorder (Agras & Bohon, 2021; Ghaderi, Odeberg, et al., 2018; Traviss-Turner et al., 2017). It appears be more effective for binge eating disorder than for bulimia, but additional research is needed to better understand why this may be the case. Current treatment recommendations suggest pointing to CBT-gsh if fully therapist led CBT is not available or accessible (Agras & Bohon, 2021).

Preventive Interventions for Eating Disorders

A different approach to treating eating disorders involves prevention. Intervening with children or adolescents before the onset of eating disorders may help to prevent these disorders from ever developing.

One effective prevention program is called the Body Project (Stice, Marti, et al., 2019). It is a dissonance reduction intervention, focused on de-emphasizing sociocultural influences on thinness. In an early study showing its efficacy (Stice, Marti, et al., 2008), adolescent girls were randomly assigned either to the Body Project or to a program called Healthy Weight, which targeted eating disorder risk factors. Specifically, girls in the Body Project intervention talked, wrote, and role-played with one another to challenge society's notions of beauty (i.e., the thin ideal). Girls in the Healthy Weight intervention worked together on developing healthy weight and exercise programs for themselves. Compared with girls who did not participate in a session, girls in both programs showed less negative affect, less body dissatisfaction, lower thin-ideal internalization, and lower risk of developing eating disorder symptoms 2 to 3 years after the session. The Body Project has also been successfully implemented with other high school samples and college women, with evidence suggesting that the Body Project may be more effective than Healthy Weight (Stice, Becker, & Yokum, 2013; Stice et al., 2019). A further follow-up study supported that evidence, showing that the effects last up to 4 years after the program (Stice, Rohde, et al., 2020). An online version of the Body Project (eBodyProject) is also effective (Stice, Durant, et al., 2014; Stice, Rohde, et al., 2013, 2017).

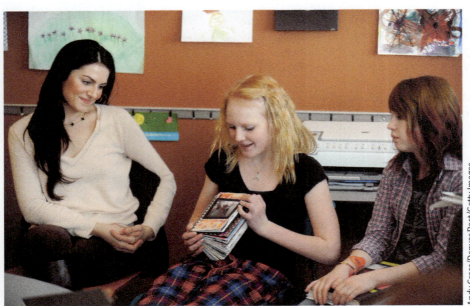

Interactive prevention programs have been effective for girls at risk of eating disorders.

Andy Cross/Denver Post/Getty Images

11.3 Check Your Knowledge

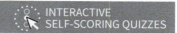

INTERACTIVE
SELF-SCORING QUIZZES

(Answers are at the end of the chapter.)
Fill in the blanks.

1. Research suggests that _____ therapy is an effective treatment for bulimia, in both the short and the long term.

2. For anorexia, _____ may be required to get the patient to gain weight. There are not many _____ that have been shown to be effective. The most common type of therapy used to treat anorexia is _____.

3. Research on prevention programs has shown that a _____ prevention program called _____ is effective up to 4 years after the intervention.

Summary

INTERACTIVE
SELF-SCORING QUIZZES

Chapter 11 Practice Quiz

Clinical Descriptions of Eating Disorders

- Three DSM-5-TR eating disorders are anorexia nervosa, bulimia nervosa, and binge eating disorder. The symptoms of anorexia nervosa include restriction of food that leads to very low body weight, strong fear of weight gain, and a distorted body image. Anorexia typically begins in adolescence, is at least three times more frequent in women than in men, and is comorbid with several other disorders. Many people recover, but it can take years. The disorder can be life-threatening.

- The symptoms of bulimia nervosa include episodes of binge eating followed by purging and a distorted body image. Like anorexia, bulimia begins in adolescence, is much more frequent in women than in men, and is comorbid with other diagnoses, such as depression. Prognosis for this disorder is somewhat more favorable than for anorexia.

- The symptoms of binge eating disorder include episodes of bingeing and a feeling of losing control over eating but no compensatory purging. People with binge eating disorder are often obese, but not all obese people have binge eating disorder.

Causes of Eating Disorders

- Evidence is consistent with possible genetic contributions to eating disorders. Serotonin, which plays a role in mediating hunger and satiety, has been examined in connection with eating disorders. Low levels of serotonin metabolites have been found in people with eating disorders, but evidence that these cause eating disorders is limited. Dopamine is involved with the rewarding aspects of eating, but the dopamine system may be altered because of eating disturbances and not cause them.

- Research on cognitive behavioral influences shows that fear of weight gain and body-image distortion make weight loss a powerful reinforcer. Among people with bulimia nervosa, negative affect and stress precipitate binges that create anxiety, which is then relieved by purging. Restricting eating exacerbates negative feelings, which in turn exacerbate more restricted eating.

- As sociocultural standards changed to favor a thinner shape as the ideal for women, the frequency of eating disorders increased. The objectification of women's bodies exerts pressure on women to see themselves through this sociocultural lens. The prevalence of eating disorders is higher in countries where the cultural pressure to be thin is strongest. White women are more likely to have anorexia than are Black or Latina women, though the prevalence rates for bulimia and binge eating disorder do not differ between ethnic and racial groups.

- Studies of personality have found that people with eating disorders are high in negative emotion and perfectionism and low in interoceptive awareness and positive emotion differentiation. Reports of people with eating disorders indicate high levels of conflict in their families.

Treatment of Eating Disorders

- The main neurobiological treatment for eating disorders is the use of antidepressant medications. Although they are somewhat effective for bulimia, they are not effective for anorexia or binge eating disorder. Dropout rates from drug-treatment programs are high, and relapse is common when people stop taking the medication. Treatment of anorexia often requires hospitalization to reduce the medical complications of the disorder. Cognitive behavioral treatment (CBT) has been shown to be somewhat effective for anorexia, and family-based treatments show promise but need further study.

- Cognitive behavioral treatment for bulimia focuses on questioning beliefs about physical attractiveness and food restriction and on developing healthy eating patterns. Outcomes are good, in both the short and the long term. Cognitive behavior therapy for binge eating disorder focuses on reducing binges, and it appears to be effective, as does CBT-guided self-help.

- Prevention programs are effective, particularly the Body Project.

Answers to Check Your Knowledge Questions

11.1　1. c. perfectionism; 2. b. It was not an eating disorder category in DSM-IV-TR.; 3. d. All of the above except (a) are correct.; 4. limited availability of healthy food; minimal awareness of recommended portion sizes; abundance and low cost of food; processed foods; genetics; marketing/advertising

11.2　1. True; 2. False; 3. True; 4. False; 5. True

11.3　1. cognitive behavior; 2. hospitalization; medications; family therapy; 3. dissonance reduction; Body Project.

Key Terms

anorexia nervosa　309
atypical anorexia nervosa　312

binge eating disorder　314
body mass index (BMI)　309

bulimia nervosa　313
obese　314

Sexual Disorders

LEARNING GOALS

1. Describe the influence of culture and gender on sexual norms and some of the research methods and issues in sexuality research.

2. Explain the symptoms of the DSM-5-TR sexual dysfunction disorders and the prevalence of sexual dysfunctions.

3. Discuss the biological and psychosocial influences on sexual dysfunctions.

4. Describe psychological and medication treatments for sexual dysfunctions.

5. Discuss the symptoms of the paraphilic disorders and the debates about these diagnoses.

6. Explain the neurobiological, social, and psychological influences on paraphilic disorders and limits in the knowledge concerning these influences.

7. Discuss common psychological and medication treatments for paraphilic disorders, the current state of evidence about treatment efficacy, and the debates about community prevention programs.

Clinical Case

Anne

Anne, a 26-year-old woman, sought treatment after beginning her first "steady" sexual relationship. She reported that she and her partner, Colin, enjoyed their sexual life together. Nonetheless, Colin had begun to express concerns because she had been unable to achieve an orgasm. She sought therapy independently to talk about this concern. In therapy, she described that she had not really enjoyed sexual activities with her former partners and that she had rarely masturbated. Anne disclosed to the therapist that her brother had raped her when she was 12 years old, an event that she had not been able to disclose to anyone in the past. The therapist provided directed masturbation exercises (described when we review treatments later in this chapter) for Anne to begin to explore and enjoy her body independently, and in sessions they discussed her abuse history and her feelings about sexuality. With the use of a vibrator, Anne began to enjoy orgasms. As her comfort with her body and sexuality increased, Anne learned to discuss her sexual preferences more openly with Colin.

Adapted from Graham (2014).

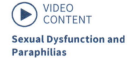

VIDEO CONTENT

Sexual Dysfunction and Paraphilias

Sexuality is one of the most personal areas of life. Each of us is a sexual being with preferences and fantasies that may surprise or even shock us from time to time. Usually, these are part of normal sexual functioning. But when our fantasies or desires begin to affect us or others in unwanted or harmful ways, they begin to qualify as abnormal.

For perspective, we begin by briefly describing norms and healthy sexual behavior. Then we consider two forms of sexual problems: sexual dysfunctions and paraphilic disorders. In the DSM, these are covered in separate chapters because they deal with such distinct problems with sexuality. Sexual dysfunctions are defined as persistent and troubling (1) disruptions in the ability to experience sexual arousal, desire, or orgasm or (2) pain associated with intercourse. Paraphilic disorders are defined as persistent and troubling attractions to unusual sexual activities or objects.

Sexual Norms and Behavior

Definitions of what is normal or desirable in human sexual behavior vary with time and place. In contemporary Western worldviews, *inhibition* of sexual expression is seen as a problem. Contrast this with the 19th- and early-20th-century view that *excess* was the culprit; in particular, excessive masturbation in childhood was widely believed to lead to sexual problems in adulthood. Von Krafft-Ebing (1902) postulated that early masturbation damaged the sexual organs and exhausted a finite reservoir of sexual energy, resulting in diminished ability to function sexually in adulthood. The general Victorian view was that sexual appetite was dangerous and therefore had to be restrained. For example, to discourage children from handling their genitals, metal mittens were promoted; to distract adults from too much sex, outdoor exercise and a bland diet were recommended. In fact, Kellogg's Corn Flakes and graham crackers were developed as foods that would lessen sexual interest. They didn't.

More recent historical changes have influenced people's attitudes and experiences of sexuality. The availability of the birth control pill contributed to a major shift in attitudes toward premarital sex and to the sexual revolution of the 1970s. The AIDS epidemic in the 1980s changed the risks associated with sexual behavior. The number of people accessing sexual content on the internet increased dramatically in the 1990s.

Like changes across generations, differences across cultures shape attitudes and beliefs about sexuality. In some cultures, sexuality is viewed as an important part of well-being and pleasure, whereas in others, sexuality is seen as relevant only for procreation (Bhugra, Popelyuk, & McMullen, 2010). The level of acceptance of same-gender sexual behavior differs by culture and across time. For example, Herdt wrote in 1984 about rituals among Sambians living in Papua New Guinea in which pubescent males engage in oral sex with older men as a way of learning about their sexuality. In other cultures, it is common to stigmatize same-gender sexual behavior. In the United States, the DSM contained a diagnosis for homosexuality as recently as 1973. More recently, though, findings from a large representative community survey, as shown in Table 12.1, indicate that many people have engaged in behavior involving same-sex partners (Herbenick, Reece, et al., 2010b) and as shown in Figure 12.1, the percentage of adults who identify as lesbian, gay, bisexual, or transgender has increased with each recent generation.

Clearly, we must keep varying cultural norms and response biases in mind as we study human sexual behavior. See Focus on Discovery 12.1 for a discussion of one of the most debated diagnoses in the DSM—gender dysphoria, a diagnosis that some argue reflects outdated cultural views.

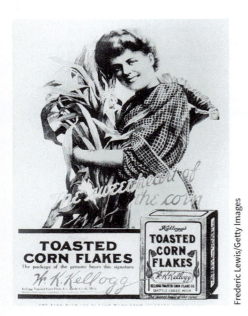

Norms about sexuality have fluctuated a great deal over time. In the early 20th century, corn flakes were promoted as part of a bland diet designed to reduce sexual desire.

Frederic Lewis/Getty Images

TABLE 12.1 Percentages of People Who Self-Report Lifetime Participation in Selected Sexual Behaviors by Gender and Age Group

Age	Masturbated Alone	Received Oral from Female	Received Oral from Male	Gave Oral to Female	Gave Oral to Male	Vaginal Intercourse	Inserted Penis into Anus	Received Penis in Anus
Males (N = 2,857)								
16–17	79	34	3	20	3	30	6	1
18–19	86	59	9	61	10	62	10	4
20–24	92	74	9	71	9	70	24	11
25–29	94	91	8	86	6	89	45	5
30–39	93	90	9	88	7	93	44	6
40–49	92	86	14	84	13	89	43	8
50–59	89	83	15	77	13	86	40	10
60–69	90	75	9	72	6	87	27	4
70+	80	58	8	62	5	88	14	5
Females (N = 2,813)								
16–17	52	7	26	9	29	32		7
18–19	66	8	62	8	61	64		20
20–24	77	17	80	14	78	86		40
25–29	85	11	88	10	89	91		46
30–39	80	16	82	14	80	89		40
40–49	78	10	86	12	83	94		41
50–59	77	8	83	7	80	94		35
60–69	72	4	79	3	73	92		30
70+	58	2	47	2	43	89		21

From Herbenick et al. (2010b).

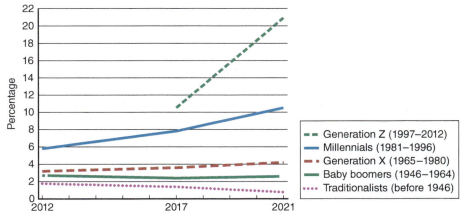

This is from an article published by Gallup News online:
Jones, J. M. (Feb 17, 2022). LGBT identification in U.S. ticks up to 7.1%. Gallup News.
https://news.gallup.com/poll/389792/lgbt-identification-ticks-up.aspx

FIGURE 12.1 Percentages of U.S. adults identifying as lesbian, gay, bisexual, or transgender by birth cohort.

Focus on Discovery 12.1

Debates About Gender Dysphoria

Gender identity refers to a person's inherent sense of being male or female, which is distinct from sexual orientation. Transgender people feel deep within themselves, usually from early childhood, that they are of the opposite sex. They are not persuaded by the presence of their genitals or by others' perceptions of their gender. A man can look at himself in a mirror, see the body of a biological man, and yet experience that body as belonging to a woman. In a large representative survey in the United States, about 1 out of every 200 adults endorsed being transgender, with higher prevalence among younger age groups (Crissman, Berger, et al., 2017). In addition to those who identify as transgender, there has been increasing recognition that gender identity is not binary—some people do not feel that they fit entirely with the sense of being male or female.

Some people who desire to change their gender identity pursue hormonal treatments to change secondary sexual characteristics and sex-reassignment surgery to alter the genitalia to be like those of the opposite sex. Surveys of hundreds of people 1 year after they have undergone such surgery indicate that about 90% of them are satisfied and do not regret the surgery (Gijs & Brewaeys, 2007). Sex-reassignment surgery is related to improvements over presurgery levels in psychological symptoms, life satisfaction, social and partner relationships, and sexual satisfaction (Monstrey, Vercruysse, & De Cuypere, 2009).

DSM-5-TR includes a diagnosis of gender dysphoria for people who experience a strong and persistent identification that differs from the sex they were assigned at birth. The DSM-5-TR diagnostic criteria for gender dysphoria specify that the conflict between their gender identity and their biological sex causes marked distress or functional impairment. Gender dysphoria is one of the most debated categories in the DSM (Vance, Cohen-Kettenis, et al., 2010). Clearly, there are many transgender people with the intense belief that their identity does not fit their sex assigned at birth. But should this be labeled as a disorder? There are several reasons to think it should not be.

- Cross-gender behavior is universal. In countless species, biologically male animals will adopt behavior, courtship rituals, and mating strategies that parallel those seen in female animals (Roughgarden, 2004). In humans, most children engage in play that violates gender roles (Zucker, 2005). It does not make sense to conceptualize such universal behavior as a disorder.

- The existence of this diagnosis implicitly contradicts the need for treatments to change a person's body to suit the person's gender identity. The diagnosis is philosophically incongruent with the positive outcomes of sex-reassignment surgery.

- Rather than promoting psychological health, diagnosing gender nonconformity might foster more stigma. Rates of victimization, including physical attacks and denial of employment attributed to transgender status, are far too common (Barboza, Dominguez, & Chance, 2016).

Research Methods in the Study of Sexuality

Research aimed at understanding normative sexual behavior has many tools available. Beyond self-report and interview-based assessments, researchers can gather physiological measurements as people watch erotic scenes (see **Figure 12.2** for the sexual anatomy of men and women). Important insights have been gained by directly measuring physiological responses to sexual stimuli, using tools such as a **penile plethysmograph** or a **vaginal plethysmograph** to measure biological arousal, defined as blood flow to the genitalia (see **Figure 12.3**).

Nonetheless, there are challenges in conducting research to understand sexual practices and attitudes. How can one be certain that participants are honest in their responses, particularly when asked about stigmatized aspects of sexuality? As we consider findings, we have to consider response biases that may differ by gender, age group, cohort, and culture.

Gender and Sexuality

Throughout this chapter, you will learn that gender shapes sexual disorders in many ways. Few topics, though, raise as much debate as gender differences in sexuality. Are reported gender differences based on cultural prohibitions regarding women's sexuality? Do they reflect gender differences in willingness to disclose sexual behavior? Are they based on biological differences? Are they tied to women's role in child-bearing?

The pioneering work of the sex therapists William H. Masters and Virginia Johnson helped launch a candid and scientific appraisal of human sexuality.

Bettmann/Getty Images

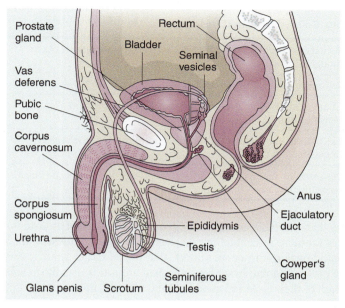

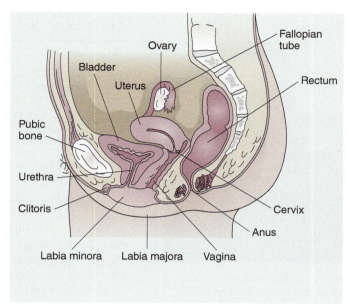

FIGURE 12.2 **The male and female sexual anatomy.**

INTERACTIVE FIGURES, CHARTS, & TABLES

On many dimensions, men and women may be more similar than stereotypes suggest. Take, for example, the commonly held idea that women, more than men, are motivated to have sex to promote relationship closeness. In a survey of more than 1,000 women, many reported that their primary motivation for having sex was sexual attraction and physical gratification (Meston & Buss, 2009). It would be an exaggeration to claim that the sole reason women are having sex is to promote relationship closeness.

Across hundreds of worldwide surveys, many gender differences in sexuality have been seen to decrease over time and to be less apparent in cultures with more empowered attitudes toward women. Nonetheless, men continue to endorse engaging in slightly more masturbation, using somewhat more pornography than women (Petersen & Hyde, 2010), and experiencing higher levels of sex drive (Frankenbach, Weber, et al., 2022). Is this gender difference genuine, or could it reflect disclosure patterns? To examine this question, researchers randomly assigned men and women to complete questionnaires about sexuality in conditions with or without a sham; in the sham condition, the researchers applied physiological sensors and said they were administering a lie detector test (Alexander & Fisher, 2003). In the conditions without the lie detector, women reported less masturbation and use of pornography than men did, just as has been found in the large surveys. In the sham condition, men's and women's levels of reported masturbation and pornography did not differ. That is, gender differences in reported sexual behavior may be biased by respondents' attempts to match cultural expectations.

Researchers have also used laboratory research, including penile and vaginal plethysmography, to understand the relationship of **sexual interest**, **subjective arousal**, and **biological arousal** for men versus women. See **Table 12.2** for definitions of these terms. Older theory, based on research in men, had suggested that sexual interest would precede subjective arousal and that biological arousal would follow this subjective arousal (Kaplan, 1974). But when researchers included women in their studies, they found that interest and subjective arousal often co-occur for women (Graham, 2010) and that women's sexual interest often follows (rather than precedes) their biological arousal (Carvalheira, Brotto, & Leal, 2010).

Placed over penis

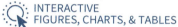

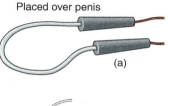

(a)

Photocell
Acrylic tube

(b)   (c)

© John Wiley & Sons, Inc.

FIGURE 12.3 **Behavioral researchers use genital devices for measuring biological sexual arousal.** These devices are sensitive indicators of blood flow into the genitalia, a key physiological process in sexual arousal. For men, the penile plethysmograph measures changes in the size of the penis. **(a)** In one version of the penile plethysmograph, a very thin rubber tube is used. As the penis enlarges with blood, the tube stretches, changing its electrical resistance. **(b)** Less commonly, a rubber sheath is inserted over the penis, and then a chamber is placed over the penis. As the penis enlarges, the volume of air displaced is measured, providing a more accurate measure of change. **(c)** For women, biological sexual arousal can be measured by a vaginal plethysmograph. This tampon-shaped apparatus can be inserted into the vagina to measure increases in blood flow. Biological arousal may not be associated with subjective arousal or desire for women.

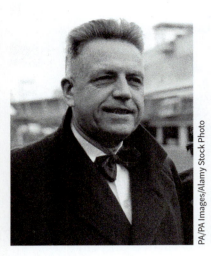

As portrayed in the movie *Kinsey*, Alfred Kinsey (shown here) shocked many people when he began to conduct interviews to understand more about norms in sexual behavior.

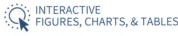
INTERACTIVE FIGURES, CHARTS, & TABLES

TABLE 12.2	Key Terms Related to Sexual Responses
Sexual interest	Sexual desire, often associated with sexually arousing fantasies or thoughts
Subjective arousal	Self-perceptions of sexual excitement
Biological arousal	Changes in blood flow to genitalia, which can be measured by penile or vaginal plethysmography
Orgasm	Ejaculation in men; contraction of the outer walls of the vagina in women
Resolution	Post-orgasm phase; for men further erection is not possible during a refractory period

Research also suggests that subjective arousal may not mirror biological arousal for women, even though it does for men. When biological arousal is measured, most women experience a rapid, automatic response to erotic stimuli that depict either gender; this differs from the normative profile in men, in whom biological arousal is usually greater when watching sexual stimuli of their preferred gender (Huberman & Chivers, 2015). But the amount of blood flow to the vagina has little correlation with women's subjective level of desire or arousal (Basson, Brotto, et al., 2005). Indeed, many women report little or no subjective arousal when biological arousal occurs (Chivers, Seto, et al., 2010). As we will discuss when we consider sexual dysfunctions, biological and subjective arousal need to be considered separately for women, even though they are highly correlated for men.

Quick Summary

Sexuality is profoundly shaped by culture and experience. Attitudes about masturbation, premarital sex, homosexuality, and gender roles in sexuality vary across time and cultures, and the attitudes prevalent for a given culture at a given time affect disclosure levels in survey research. To study sexuality, researchers sometimes gather psychophysiological data on biological arousal in laboratory settings.

Gender differences in sexuality are less pronounced in studies designed to consider reporting biases. Women are less likely to report sexual interest preceding arousal than men are, and their biological and subjective arousal are less correlated than men's.

12.1 Check Your Knowledge

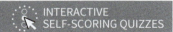
INTERACTIVE SELF-SCORING QUIZZES

(Answers are at the end of the chapter.)
Answer the following questions.

1. Describe the gender differences most often observed in current survey research on sexuality.
2. Identify three historical changes that influenced sexuality in the 20th century.

Clinical Descriptions of Sexual Dysfunctions

At its best, sexuality provides a forum for connection and shared pleasure. For better or for worse, our sexuality shapes at least part of our self-concept. Do we please the people we love, or, more simply, are we able to enjoy fulfillment from a pleasurable sexual experience?

We turn now to sexual problems that interfere with sexual enjoyment for many people at some time during their life. We begin by describing the different types of sexual dysfunctions described in DSM-5-TR. Then we discuss causes and treatments for these problems.

TABLE 12.3   **Diagnoses of Sexual Dysfunction**

Category of Dysfunction	Diagnoses in Women	Diagnoses in Men
Sexual interest, desire, and arousal	Female sexual interest/arousal disorder	Male hypoactive sexual desire disorder
		Erectile disorder
Orgasmic disorder	Female orgasmic disorder	Premature ejaculation
		Delayed ejaculation
Sexual pain	Genito-pelvic pain/penetration disorder	

TABLE 12.4   **Prevalence of Sexual Difficulties Among Sexually Active Individuals Aged 16 to 74 in the National Survey of Sexual Attitudes and Lifestyles (Mitchell et al., 2016)**

	Lacked Interest or Arousal in Sex	Difficulty Reaching Orgasm	Physical Pain During Sex	Orgasm Reached Too Quickly	Trouble Maintaining or Achieving an Erection	One or More of These Problems
Percentage reporting problems for 3 months of the past year						
Men	15	9.2	NA*	14.9	12.9	38
Women	6.5	16.3	7.4	NA	NA	23
Percentage meeting DSM-5 criteria regarding persistence and distress						
Men	0.8	0.5	NA	1.7	1.8	4.2
Women	0.6	1.9	1.9	NA	NA	3.6

*NA = not analyzed

DSM-5-TR divides **sexual dysfunctions** into three categories: those involving sexual desire, arousal, and interest; orgasmic disorders; and a disorder involving sexual pain (see **Table 12.3**). Separate diagnoses are provided for men and women. The diagnostic criteria for all sexual dysfunctions specify that dysfunction should be persistent and recurrent and should cause clinically significant distress for the affected person. A diagnosis of sexual dysfunction is not appropriate if the problem is due entirely to a medical illness (such as advanced diabetes, which can cause erectile problems in men) or to another psychological disorder (such as major depressive disorder).

One might not expect people to be willing to report problems as personal as sexual dysfunction in community surveys. But many people do report these symptoms—the prevalence of occasional symptoms of sexual dysfunction is quite high. **Table 12.4** presents data from a community survey of more than 11,000 men and women who completed questionnaires and interviews about symptoms of sexual dysfunction lasting at least 3 months in the past year. Among those who endorsed a symptom, the researchers assessed DSM-5 diagnostic criteria regarding whether the symptom had persisted for 6 months and caused distress (Mitchell, Jones, et al., 2016). As shown in the data, many people reported brief periods of symptoms in the past year, but less than 5% reported that these symptoms persisted and caused distress.

Sexual concerns that arise consequent to severe relationship distress, such as partner abuse, should not be diagnosed as sexual dysfunctions. Especially for women, sexuality has strong links with relationship satisfaction (Tiefer, Hall, & Tavris, 2002). The data shown in Table 12.4 do not consider whether problems were due to relationship concerns, and so they may overestimate prevalence rates.

Many people with one form of sexual dysfunction will report a second form of sexual dysfunction (Mitchell et al., 2016). Some of these reports may be due to a vicious cycle. For example, men who develop premature ejaculation may begin to worry about sex and then experience problems with sexual desire or sexual arousal (Wincze & Weisberg, 2015). Beyond the consequences for the individual, sexual problems in one person may lead to sexual problems in the partner (Kaya, Gunes, et al., 2015).

Disorders Involving Sexual Interest, Desire, and Arousal

The DSM-5-TR includes three disorders involving a lack of sexual interest, desire, or arousal. **Female sexual interest/arousal disorder** refers to persistent deficits in sexual interest, biological arousal, or subjective arousal. For men, the DSM-5-TR diagnoses consider sexual interest and biological arousal separately: **Male hypoactive sexual desire disorder** refers to deficient or absent sexual fantasies and urges, and **erectile disorder** refers to failure to attain or maintain an erection through completion of the sexual activity. The **Clinical Case of Robert** provides an illustration of hypoactive sexual desire disorder.

Defining Symptoms of Female Sexual Interest/Arousal Disorder

Diminished, absent, or reduced frequency of at least three of the following:

- Interest in sexual activity
- Erotic thoughts or fantasies
- Initiation of sexual activity and responsiveness to partner's attempts to initiate

- Sexual excitement/pleasure during at least 75% of sexual encounters
- Sexual interest/arousal elicited by any internal or external erotic cues
- Genital or nongenital sensations during at least 75% of sexual encounters

Defining Symptoms of Male Hypoactive Sexual Desire Disorder

- Sexual fantasies and desires, as judged by the clinician, are deficient or absent

Defining Symptoms of Erectile Disorder

On at least 75% of sexual occasions:

- Inability to attain an erection or
- Inability to maintain an erection for completion of sexual activity or

- Marked decrease in erectile rigidity that interferes with penetration or pleasure

Clinical Case

Robert

Robert, a very bright 25-year-old graduate student in physics at a leading university, sought treatment for what he called "sexual diffidence" toward his fiancée. He said he loved his fiancée very much and felt compatible with her in every conceivable way except in bed. There, try as he might, and with understanding from his fiancée, he found himself uninterested in initiating or responding to sex. He and his fiancée had attributed these problems to the academic pressures he had faced for the past 2 years, but a discussion with the therapist revealed that Robert had had little interest in sex—either with men or with women—for as far back as he could remember, even when work pressures were not present. He asserted that he found his fiancée very attractive, but as with other women he had known, he did not feel passion for her.

He had masturbated very rarely in adolescence and did not begin dating until late in college, though he had had many female acquaintances. His general approach to life, including sex, was analytical and intellectual, and he described his problems in a very unemotional and detached way to the therapist. He freely admitted that he would not have contacted a therapist at all were it not for the quietly stated wishes of his fiancée, who worried that his lack of interest in sex would interfere with their future relationship.

After a few individual sessions, the therapist asked the young man to invite his fiancée to a therapy session, which the client readily agreed to do. During a joint session, the couple appeared to be in love and looking forward to a life together, despite the woman's concern about Robert's lack of sexual interest.

Of all the sexual dysfunction diagnoses, the sexual interest and desire disorders, often colloquially referred to as "low sex drive," are the most subjective. How often should a person want sex? And with what intensity? Often, one partner will encourage the other partner to see a clinician. Female sexual interest/arousal disorder and male hypoactive desire disorder may owe their existence to the high expectations some people have about being sexual, and those high expectations may be shaped by cultural norms about how much sex a person "should" want. Among women who experienced low sexual desire in the last month, American women were more likely to report distress about the symptom than were European women (Hayes, Dennerstein, et al., 2007). Age may also influence expectations. Postmenopausal women are more likely than women in their 20s to report low levels of sexual desire and arousal, but they are less likely to be distressed by these lower levels (Hendrickx, Gijs, & Enzlin, 2015). Because ideals regarding how much sex one should have are so subjective, some object to labeling these individual differences as disorders (Segal, 2015).

DSM-5 criteria for sexual interest/arousal disorder in women include biologically or subjectively low arousal or desire. Women tend to be more concerned by a lack of subjective desire than by a lack of biological arousal (Basson, Althof, et al., 2004). Most commonly, women with this disorder report that previously exciting stimuli, such as their partner's touch or a sensual dance, no longer trigger desire (Brotto & Luria, 2014). When studies are conducted using a vaginal plethysmograph, women who experience a subjective lack of desire often have normative levels of biological response to erotic stimuli (Graham, 2010). This again highlights the distinction between biological and subjective arousal in women.

Erectile disorder is distinct from low sex drive—many with erectile disorder report frequent desires for sex. In erectile disorder, the problem is physical arousal. The prevalence of erectile disorder increases sharply with age, with as many as 50% of men aged 60 and older reporting at least occasional erectile dysfunction (Rosen, Miner, & Wincze, 2014).

Orgasmic Disorders

DSM-5-TR includes separate diagnoses for problems in achieving orgasm for women and men. **Female orgasmic disorder** refers to the persistent absence or reduced intensity of orgasm after sexual excitement. Women differ in their thresholds for orgasm. Although some women have orgasms quickly and without much clitoral stimulation, others need prolonged clitoral stimulation. Women become more likely to have orgasms as they age, perhaps because they learn more about their bodies and sexual needs over time (Wincze & Weisberg, 2015). They are also more likely to have orgasms in close relationships than they are in casual, short-term relationships (Armstrong, England, & Fogarty, 2009). For many women, enjoying a sense of emotional closeness to their partner is more important than achieving an orgasm. About two-thirds of women report that they have faked an orgasm, and most say that they did so to try to protect their partner's feelings (Muehlenhard & Shippee, 2010). Many men are unaware (or at least don't report) that their partners don't achieve orgasms (Herbenick, Reece, et al., 2010a).

Women's problems reaching orgasm are distinct from problems with sexual arousal. As in the **Clinical Case of Anne** presented at the beginning of this chapter, many women with orgasmic disorder achieve sexual arousal and enjoy sexual contact, even though they have difficulty reaching orgasm. Indeed, laboratory research has shown that arousal levels while viewing erotic stimuli do not distinguish women with orgasmic disorder from those without orgasmic disorder (Meston & Gorzalka, 1995).

DSM-5-TR includes two orgasmic disorders of men: **premature (early) ejaculation**, defined by ejaculation that occurs too quickly, and **delayed ejaculation disorder**, defined by persistent difficulty in ejaculating. Consistent with what Bill experienced in the **Clinical Case**, DSM-5 introduced the definition of "premature" as less than 1 minute after the penis is inserted. One minute was chosen based on cross-national studies showing that the median time to ejaculation is 5 minutes after penis insertion (Waldinger, Quinn, et al., 2005). Many men who seek treatment concerned about premature ejaculation are well within the norms in the duration of their erections—in their case, psychoeducation can help them set realistic expectations (Wincze & Weisberg, 2015).

Delayed ejaculation is the least common sexual dysfunction among men. Most men who seek treatment for delayed ejaculation report that it happens during intercourse but not when masturbating (Wincze & Weisberg, 2015).

Clinical Case

Bill

Bill, age 42, and Mary, his girlfriend of 18 months, sought treatment due to concerns about premature ejaculation. Both were divorced with children, and they stayed together every other weekend. Bill had a history of hypertension, hyperlipidemia, and low total testosterone levels. Bill's symptom, though, began well before these medical issues—he reported that he had never been able to maintain an erection for more than a minute after insertion. Mary was his first partner to label this as premature ejaculation, and she often worried that it was an indicator that he did not find her attractive. Mary urged him to seek treatment.

The therapist helped Bill and Mary understand that his rapid ejaculation was likely biologically based and that he had developed "performance anxiety" in response to this pattern. The therapist encouraged Bill and Mary to put a premium on pleasure and intimacy instead of controlling the timing of his ejaculation. Mary was helped to understand that, rather than a sign of lack of arousal, premature ejaculation could be viewed as a sign of intense arousal. The therapist also explained that their limited time together could be intensifying the pressure and thus encouraged them to schedule times between their weekends together to enjoy intimacy. With the pressures removed, Bill and Mary developed a more satisfying sex life.

Adapted from Wincze and Weisberg (2015).

Defining Symptoms of Female Orgasmic Disorder

On at least 75% of sexual occasions:

- Marked delay, infrequency, or absence of orgasm or

- Markedly reduced intensity of orgasmic sensation

Defining Symptoms of Premature Ejaculation

On at least 75% of partnered sexual occasions:

- Tendency to ejaculate within 1 minute of penile insertion

Defining Symptoms of Delayed Ejaculation

On at least 75% of partnered sexual occasions:

- Marked delay, infrequency, or absence of orgasm

Sexual Pain Disorder

The major symptom of **genito-pelvic pain/penetration disorder** is persistent or recurrent pain during intercourse. Although some men experience recurrent pain during sex, very few men seek treatment for it. For this reason, the DSM-5 criteria focus on women. Women with this disorder often experience vaginismus, defined by involuntary muscle spasms of the outer third of the vagina to a degree that makes intercourse impossible (Binik, 2010). A first step in diagnosing genito-pelvic/penetration disorder is ensuring that the pain is not caused by a medical problem, such as an infection, or by a lack of vaginal lubrication due to low desire or postmenopausal changes. Without adequate treatment, one study found that half of women with genito-pelvic pain disorder had sustained symptoms across a 2-year follow-up, and another quarter had a fluctuating course of remission and relapse (Reed, Harlow, et al., 2016).

Defining Symptoms of Genito-Pelvic Pain/Penetration Disorder

Persistent or recurrent difficulties with at least one of the following:

- Inability to have vaginal penetration during intercourse
- Marked vulvar, vaginal, or pelvic pain during vaginal penetration or intercourse attempts

- Marked fear or anxiety about pain or penetration
- Marked tensing of the pelvic floor muscles during attempted vaginal penetration

The symptoms are not due to severe relationship distress, partner violence, or other significant stressors.

Most women diagnosed with this disorder experience sexual arousal and can have orgasms from manual or oral stimulation that does not involve penetration. Women who experience pain when attempting sexual intercourse show normative sexual arousal to films of oral sex, but not surprisingly, their arousal is blunted when they watch a depiction of intercourse (Wouda, Hartman, et al., 1998).

Quick Summary

In DSM-5-TR, the sexual dysfunction disorders are divided as follows:

- Sexual interest, desire, and arousal disorders (female sexual interest/arousal disorder, male hypoactive sexual desire disorder and erectile disorder)
- Orgasmic disorders (female orgasmic disorder, premature ejaculation, and delayed ejaculation)
- Sexual pain disorder (genito-pelvic pain/penetration disorder)

Although more than a quarter of people report at least brief symptoms of sexual dysfunction, less than 5% report that these symptoms persist for 6 months and cause distress.

12.2 Check Your Knowledge

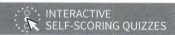
INTERACTIVE
SELF-SCORING QUIZZES

(Answers are at the end of the chapter.)
True or false?

1. A person who experiences a brief problem with sexual arousal, orgasm, or desire is highly likely to meet the diagnostic criteria for a sexual dysfunction.
2. People with one sexual dysfunction tend to have other comorbid sexual dysfunctions.

Answer the following questions.
3. In the survey conducted by Mitchell and colleagues, which sexual dysfunction symptoms did women most commonly report?
4. In the same survey, which sexual dysfunction symptoms did men most commonly report?

Causes of Sexual Dysfunctions

We now turn to research on the causes of sexual dysfunctions. **Table 12.5** summarizes key influences on sexual dysfunctions.

Biological Influences

As noted earlier, a first step in making a diagnosis of sexual dysfunction is to rule out medical disease as the cause. DSM-5-TR includes separate diagnoses for sexual dysfunctions that are caused by medical illnesses. Some have criticized this division in the diagnoses because sexual

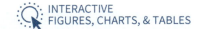

INTERACTIVE
FIGURES, CHARTS, & TABLES

TABLE 12.5   **Predictors of Sexual Dysfunction**

Domain	Predictors
Biological influences	Heavy smoking
	Heavy drinking
	Cardiovascular disease
	Diabetes
	Neurological disease
	Hormone dysfunction
	SSRI medications
	Other medical illnesses and medications
Social influences	Rape or sexual abuse
	Lack of opportunity to learn about sexuality
	Relationship difficulties
	Negative cultural attitudes toward sexuality
Psychological influences	Depression and anxiety
	Low physiological arousal/exhaustion
	Negative cognitions about sex, appearance, or sexual performance; guilt and self-blame

dysfunctions often have both biological and psychological causes. Biological causes of sexual dysfunctions can include diseases such as diabetes, multiple sclerosis, and spinal cord injury; heavy alcohol use before sex; chronic alcohol use; and heavy cigarette smoking (Wincze & Weisberg, 2015). Laboratory tests of hormone levels are a routine part of assessment of sexual dysfunctions (Buvat, Maggi, et al., 2010) because sexual dysfunctions among men can be exacerbated either by low levels of testosterone or by the high levels induced by chronic use of anabolic steroids or testosterone supplements. Certain medications, such as selective serotonin reuptake inhibitor (SSRI) antidepressant drugs (e.g., Prozac and Zoloft), have effects on sexual function, including decreased arousal and higher rates of orgasmic disorders (Kronstein, Ishida, et al., 2015).

Beyond these general biological contributions, some biological factors may be specific to certain sexual dysfunctions. Biological explanations are particularly important for erectile disorder and premature ejaculation. Erectile disorder symptoms are often related to vascular disorder, which restricts blood flow into the veins of the penis (Rastrelli, Corona, et al., 2015). SSRI treatment can blunt sexual sensitivity, and this finding has led to a focus on abnormal serotonin receptors as a major explanation of premature ejaculation (Wincze & Weisberg, 2015). For women, there is evidence that a neurologically based supersensitivity to pain could contribute to genito-pelvic pain/penetration disorder (van Lankveld, Granot, et al., 2010) and that atypically low estradiol (Cappelletti & Wallen, 2016) or testosterone levels (Davis, Worsley, et al., 2016) can contribute to low sexual desire.

Psychosocial Influences

Some sexual dysfunctions can be traced to rape, sexual abuse, or an absence of positive sexual experiences. Childhood sexual abuse is associated with diminished arousal and desire, with higher rates of genital pain, and, among men, with double the rate of premature ejaculation (Graham, Mercer, et al., 2017; Latthe, Mignini, et al., 2006; Laumann, Paik, & Rosen, 1999). See **Focus on Discovery 12.2** for a discussion of childhood sexual abuse and its repercussions. Just as traumatic experiences may play a negative role, positive experiences have important benefits—many people with sexual problems have not had opportunities to learn about their sexuality and develop sexual skills.

Focus on Discovery 12.2

The Effects of Pedophilic Disorder: Outcomes After Childhood Sexual Abuse

It is hard to estimate the prevalence of childhood sexual abuse (CSA), as researchers vary in their definitions of abuse. Nonetheless, CSA clearly happens far too often. In one major community survey, about 10% of adults reported some form of CSA, with CSA occurring three times as often to girls as to boys (Pérez-Fuentes, Olfson, et al., 2013).

A child abuser is usually not a stranger. They may be a father, an uncle, a brother, a teacher, a coach, or even a cleric. Recent lawsuits have highlighted disturbing rates of abuse from clergy, coaches, and Boy Scout pack leaders. The abuser is often an adult whom the child knows and trusts. When the abuser is someone close to the child, the child is likely to feel torn between, on the one hand, allegiance to the abuser and, on the other hand, fear, revulsion, and the knowledge that what is happening is wrong. The betrayal of trust makes the crime more abhorrent than it would be if no prior relationship existed between the abuser and the child. As with childhood incest, molestation or sexual harassment by an authority figure violates trust and respect. The child, whatever their age, cannot give meaningful consent. The power differential is just too great.

Here, we consider two central questions. How does the all-too-common experience of CSA affect psychological health during childhood and beyond? What can be done to help children heal from CSA?

Effects on the Child

After CSA, many children will develop symptoms such as depression, low self-esteem, conduct disorder, anxiety disorders, or posttraumatic stress disorder (PTSD). On the other hand, many children do not exhibit symptoms immediately after CSA. What factors contribute to how CSA affects a child? Negative outcomes are more pronounced when the CSA involves sexual intercourse (Nelson, Heath, et al., 2002) or violence (Dunn, Gilman, et al., 2012) or when the CSA starts at an earlier age (Kaplow & Widom, 2007). Outcomes are better when the child has a supportive relationship with a nonabusive parent (Widom, 2014).

In adulthood, CSA is related to higher risk of many different psychological disorders. These effects are observed in large-scale representative community samples, as well as smaller longitudinal studies in which researchers have followed abused children over time (Widom, 2014). A history of CSA is common among adults experiencing many different psychological disorders—notably, dissociative identity disorder, PTSD, eating disorders, borderline personality disorder, major depressive disorder, and substance use disorder. CSA is also tied to lower self-esteem, less life satisfaction, poorer romantic relationships, and greater risk of sexual dysfunctions during adulthood (Fergusson, McLeod, & Horwood, 2013).

An issue in interpreting these correlations, though, is that families in which abuse occurs are often experiencing a broad array of problems, such as substance use disorder in one or both parents, which may be entangled with other genetic and environmental risks for psychological disorders. As a result, it is hard to isolate whether CSA is genuinely the factor that heightens the risk for a clinical disorder—most children exposed to child abuse also experience other forms of early adversity (Green, McLaughlin, et al., 2010). Twin studies provide a way to disentangle these effects, particularly when one twin but not the other has been abused, because the twin who was not abused shares genetic and at least some environmental influences. In one study of almost 2,000 twin pairs, adults with a history of CSA had a substantially higher risk of depression, suicide, conduct disorder, alcohol use disorder, social anxiety, rape, and divorce than their nonabused twins (Nelson et al., 2002).

Dealing with the Problem

When they suspect that something is awry, parents must raise the issue with their children; unfortunately, many adults are uncomfortable doing so. Clinicians also need to be sensitive to signs of sexual abuse. The law requires healthcare professionals who suspect sexual or nonsexual child abuse to report their suspicions to the police or a child protective agency. Despite this, many crimes are not reported.

For a child, reporting sexual abuse can be extremely difficult. We tend to forget how helpless and dependent a child feels, and it is difficult even to imagine how frightening it would be to tell one's parents that one had been fondled by a brother or grandfather.

Most cases of sexual abuse do not leave any physical evidence, such as torn vaginal tissue, and there is no behavioral sign or emotional syndrome that unequivocally indicates that abuse has occurred. Therefore, the child's own report is the primary source of information about whether CSA has occurred. Leading questions, though, can produce some false reports (Larson, Cartwright, & Goodman, 2016). Great skill is required in questioning a child about possible sexual abuse to avoid biasing the youngster one way or the other.

Many children who have been abused need treatment. Trauma-related treatments typically focus on exposure to memories of the trauma through discussion in a safe and supportive therapeutic atmosphere. As with rape, it is important to change the person's attribution of responsibility from "I was bad" to "They were bad." Such treatments have been shown to help abused children find relief from their symptoms and reduce their sense of shame (Cohen, Deblinger, et al., 2004; O'Callaghan, McMullen, et al., 2013).

Relationship problems often interfere with sexual arousal and pleasure (Burri & Spector, 2011). More than half of women with symptoms of sexual dysfunction believe those symptoms are caused by relationship problems (Nicholls, 2008). For women, concerns about a partner's affection are particularly likely to lower sexual satisfaction (Nobre & Pinto-Gouveia, 2008). As one might expect, people who are angry with their partners are less likely to want sex (Beck & Bozman, 1995). Even in couples who are satisfied with other realms of the relationship, poor communication around sex can contribute to sexual dysfunction, particularly for women

(Mallory, Stanton, & Handy, 2019). For any number of reasons, including embarrassment, worry about the partner's feelings, or fear, one lover may not tell the other about preferences even if a partner is engaging in unstimulating or even aversive behaviors during sex.

Depression and anxiety increase the risk of sexual dysfunctions. People with a clinical diagnosis of a mood disorder are more than three times as likely as those without a mood disorder to report a general dissatisfaction with their sexual life, and those with anxiety disorder are more than twice as likely to report sexual dissatisfaction (Vanwesenbeeck, Have, & de Graaf, 2014). Anxiety and depression are particularly likely to be comorbid with sexual pain (Meana, Binik, et al., 1998), lack of sexual desire or arousal (Graham et al., 2017), and female orgasmic disorder (Leeners, Hengartner, et al., 2014).

Beyond the detrimental effects of depression and anxiety, several studies suggest that low general physiological arousal can interfere with sexual arousal. Meston and Gorzalka (1995) examined the role of arousal by assigning women to exercise or no-exercise conditions and then asking the women to watch erotic films. Consistent with the positive role of higher arousal, exercise facilitated sexual arousal. No wonder, then, that exhausted couples, turning to sex after a full day of work, parenting, socializing, and other roles, can encounter problems with sexuality.

Negative cognitions, including worries about pregnancy or AIDS or negative attitudes about sex, can interfere with sexual functioning (Wincze & Weisberg, 2015). Intrusive negative thoughts about their weight or appearance impinge on sexual enjoyment for many women (Pujols, Seal, & Meston, 2010). But worries about one's sexual performance can be significant problems for both men and women (Carvalho & Nobre, 2010; Rowland, Adamski, et al., 2015). Consider the fact that variability in sexual performance is common; a stressful day, a distracting context, a relationship concern, or any number of other issues may diminish sexual responsiveness. The key factor may be how people think about their diminished physical response when it happens. One theory is that people who blame themselves for decreased sexual performance will be more likely to develop recurrent sexual problems.

In a test of the role of self-blame in erectile dysfunction, researchers asked male participants to watch erotic videos (Weisberg, Brown, et al., 2001). During the videos, their sexual arousal (penile circumference) was measured using a **penile plethysmograph** (see **Figure 12.3**). Regardless of their actual arousal, the men were given false feedback that the size of their erection was smaller than that typically measured among aroused men. Men were randomly assigned to receive two different explanations for this false feedback. In the first, they were told that the films were not working for most men (external explanation). In the second, they were told that the pattern of their responses on questionnaires about sexuality might help explain the low arousal (internal explanation). After receiving this feedback, the men were asked to watch one more film. The men who were given an internal explanation reported less subjective arousal and also showed less physiological arousal during this film than those given an external explanation. These results support the idea that people who blame themselves when their body doesn't perform will experience diminished subsequent arousal. Needless to say, men in this study were carefully debriefed after the experiment!

In considering the source of negative cognitions, many patients have learned negative views of sexuality from their social and cultural surroundings (Masters & Johnson, 1970). For example, some religions and cultures discourage sexuality for the sake of pleasure, particularly outside marriage. Other cultures disapprove of sexual initiative or behavior among women, other than for the sake of procreation. Guilt about engaging in sexual behavior varies by cultural group and can inhibit sexual desire (Woo, Brotto, & Gorzalka, 2011).

Putting It All Together: Integrating Biological and Psychosocial Influences on Sexual Dysfunction

Although we have described biological and psychosocial influences separately, these influences usually interact to jointly contribute to sexual dysfunction. Take erectile dysfunction as an example. Particularly in older men, erectile dysfunction may become more likely because cardiovascular disease constricts blood flow into the penis. For a man struggling with depression or anxiety or worrying about his ability to satisfy his partner, the change in erections may be especially distressing, and that distress, in turn, can diminish arousal. Biological, social, and psychological influences can combine in numerous ways to trigger symptoms.

Quick Summary

In diagnosing sexual dysfunction, it is important to rule out potential medical and pharmacological explanations. If biological factors are the main cause of the dysfunction, separate diagnoses are applied. Key psychosocial etiological variables involved in sexual dysfunctions are sexual abuse or rape, lack of sexual knowledge, relationship problems, psychological disorders such as depression or anxiety, exhaustion, and negative cognitions and attitudes about sexuality.

12.3 Check Your Knowledge

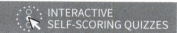 INTERACTIVE SELF-SCORING QUIZZES

(Answers are at the end of the chapter.)
Answer the following questions.

1. What proportion of women attribute their sexual dysfunction symptoms to relationship concerns?
2. How large are the effects of depression and anxiety on sexual dissatisfaction?

Treatments of Sexual Dysfunctions

Among those who experience sexual dysfunction disorders, just over a third in the United States will seek professional help (Mitchell et al., 2016). For those who do seek help, it is perhaps no surprise that therapists often draw on a rich array of strategies to help address the many different factors that can contribute to sexual dysfunction. When biological factors are contributing, a first step involves ensuring that those are addressed. A therapist may choose only one technique for a given case, but the multifaceted nature of sexual dysfunctions often requires the use of a combination of relationship and more focused sex therapy techniques, as illustrated by the **Clinical Case of Carol**.

Clinical Case

Carol

Carol, a 52-year-old woman, sought treatment for her lack of interest in sex. Carol and Darren had been married for 11 years. Although they had engaged in sex once or twice per week in the early years of their marriage, her interest in sex had waned over the past 5 years. She began to refuse Darren's requests for sex 2 years ago, and they had not had intercourse for 9 months. Indeed, Carol tried to avoid any physical contact, including holding hands, as she did not want to send the signal that she was interested in sex. She also reported that she had stopped masturbating or having sexual fantasies.

Carol was raised in a devout Catholic family and had been taught that strong sex drives were immoral for women. In college, she had been able to enjoy sex with a few partners. She also had enjoyed sex with Darren during the early years of their relationship, even though she described feeling awkward about sex and uncomfortable describing her needs to a partner. The past several years had been very stressful for her, with taking care of her ill mother and coping with budget cuts in her workplace. As is typical with aging, she had noticed more vaginal dryness, and this made sex more physically uncomfortable. Darren reported feeling rejected and angry about their lack of sex, and Carol reported that she felt guilty but that his anger only made her less interested in sex. In the context of her stress, Darren's requests for sex had begun to feel like one more demand in her life.

Carol's case illustrates how complicated sexual dysfunction can be. Carol described beliefs that sex drive is shameful, difficulty communicating about sexual needs, significant life stress, normative age-related changes in vaginal lubrication, and tension and lack of communication in her partnership. The therapist worked to address each of these concerns. To reduce the pressure and conflict around sex, the therapist banned the couple from having sex while they engaged in sensate-focus exercises (discussed later in this section). Carol's shame and negative beliefs about her sexuality were tackled using cognitive approaches. Carol and Darren were coached in communication skills to improve their relationship and their sexual communication. Carol was encouraged to use a lubricant. Combining these different approaches restored their sexual intimacy and renewed their closeness.

Adapted from Wincze and Weisberg (2015).

Throughout assessment and intervention, it is important to consider that cultural and religious background can shape a person's comfort with seeking treatment, discussing their sexuality, and their personal values concerning sexuality (Newlands, Britto, & Denning, 2020). Therapists do well to practice cultural humility and to be sensitive toward how a patient's background may have shaped their attitudes toward sexuality and treatment.

We will begin by considering interventions that are helpful across a broad range of sexual dysfunctions. Randomized controlled trials indicate that these interventions are more helpful than control treatments, and the evidence is particularly strong for female sexual interest/arousal disorder and female orgasmic disorder (Frühauf, Gerger, et al., 2013). After discussing approaches useful for addressing multiple sexual dysfunctions, we will describe interventions developed for specific sexual dysfunctions. As we discuss the treatment options, it is worth noting that with one exception we will discuss, there has been only limited success in identifying medical treatments for sexual dysfunction disorders among women (Weinberger, Houman, et al., 2019). Some have argued that the extensive focus on medical treatments fails to recognize the complex social and psychological contributions to women's sexual concerns (Kleinplatz, 2018).

Psychoeducation

For many clients, the first step of treatment is to provide good information about how common sexual dysfunction is. By providing clear information about the sources of these types of issues, therapists can normalize the concern, reduce anxiety, model effective communication about sexuality, and eliminate blame (Wincze & Weisberg, 2015). For example, many men with premature ejaculation become focused on self-blame, and simply understanding that there is a likely biological basis for these symptoms can be a relief. Beyond normalizing the symptoms, therapists often provide written materials and videos to help clients understand more about the body and sexual techniques.

Couples Therapy

Some sexual dysfunctions are embedded in a distressed relationship, and in turn, sometimes sexual difficulties create problems between partners. Troubled couples often need training in nonsexual communication skills (Wincze & Weisberg, 2015). Some therapists focus on nonsexual issues, such as difficulties with in-laws or with child rearing—either in addition to or instead of interventions directly focused on sex. For some couples, planning romantic events together is recommended to restore closeness and intimacy (Wincze & Weisberg, 2015).

Encouraging partners to communicate their sexual likes and dislikes to each other can help resolve a range of sexual dysfunctions (Wincze & Weisberg, 2015). Sexual skill and communication training is particularly warranted when sexual dysfunction is specific to a given relationship and was not a concern with previous partners.

Cognitive Interventions

Cognitive interventions are often used to challenge the self-demanding, perfectionistic thoughts that cause problems for many people with sexual dysfunctions. A therapist might try to reduce the pressure a man with erectile dysfunction feels by challenging his belief that intercourse is the only true form of sexual activity. Therapists might coach women who are hypercritical of their appearance to consider more positive ways of viewing their bodies and their sexuality. In some versions of cognitive therapy, mindfulness meditation training is provided to help foster awareness of the moment and a nonjudgemental attitude (Brotto & Basson, 2014).

Sensate Focus

To help couples refocus on the sensual pleasure of their intimacy, many therapists prescribe *sensate focus*, a technique introduced by Masters and Johnson (1970). The therapist instructs the couple not to have intercourse during sensate-focus exercises and, indeed, not even to touch each other's genitalia initially. Rather, the therapist instructs them to choose a time when both partners feel a sense of warmth and compatibility and to undress and give each other pleasure by touching each other's bodies. Therapists appoint one partner to do the first pleasuring; the partner who is "getting" is simply to enjoy being touched. The one being touched is not required to feel a sexual response and is responsible for immediately telling the partner if something becomes uncomfortable. Then the roles are switched.

The sensate-focus assignment usually promotes contact, constituting a first step toward reestablishing sexual intimacy. Most of the time, partners begin to realize that their physical encounters could be intimate and pleasurable without necessarily being a prelude to sexual intercourse. Sensate focus often helps counter the destructive tendency to think about one's performance or attractiveness during sex, and it helps a couple begin to communicate more constructively about their sexual preferences.

Treatments for Specific Sexual Dysfunctions

Therapists often use more specific techniques for female sexual interest/arousal disorder, female orgasmic disorder, genito-pelvic pain/penetration disorder, premature ejaculation, and erectile disorder, and we discuss these next. Many of these specific techniques are combined with the general treatments we already discussed.

Female Sexual Interest/Arousal Disorder   In the United States, the FDA has approved two medications for premenopausal women with low sexual desire: flibanserin (Addyi) and bremelanotide (Vyleesi). Addyi, though, shows limited efficacy compared to a placebo, and both show high rates of side effects (Rosen, Brotto, & Zucker, 2018; Simon, Kingsberg, et al., 2019).

Female Orgasmic Disorder   Directed masturbation was developed to enhance women's comfort with and enjoyment of their sexuality (LoPiccolo & Lobitz, 1972). The first step is for the woman to examine her genitals and to identify various areas with the aid of diagrams. Next, she is instructed to touch her genitals and to find areas that produce pleasure. Then she increases the intensity of masturbation using erotic fantasies. If she does not achieve orgasm, she is to use a vibrator in her masturbation. Finally, her partner joins in, first watching her masturbate, then doing for her what she has been doing for herself, and finally having intercourse in a position that allows him to stimulate her genitals manually or with a vibrator. As illustrated in the **Clinical Case of Anne** at the beginning of this chapter, directed masturbation has been shown to help treat female orgasmic disorder, particularly when women have a lifelong inability to experience orgasm, with 60–90% of that subgroup achieving orgasm posttreatment (ter Kuile, Both, & van Lankveld, 2012).

Genito-Pelvic Pain/Penetration Disorder   A woman with genito-pelvic pain/penetration disorder might first be trained in relaxation and then practice inserting her fingers or dilators into her vagina, starting with inserting smaller dilators and working up to larger ones. Such programs have been shown to help many women with sexual pain disorder (ter Kuile & Reissing, 2014).

Premature Ejaculation   SSRI antidepressants have been found to help reduce premature ejaculation. The SSRI dapoxetine (Priligy) has been approved for the treatment of premature ejaculation in 50 countries. It is taken as needed in the hour before sex (Althof, McMahon, et al., 2014).

As a behavioral treatment of premature ejaculation, the squeeze technique is often used, in which a partner is trained to squeeze the penis in the area where the head and shaft meet to rapidly reduce arousal. This technique is practiced without insertion, and then during insertion, the penis is withdrawn and the squeeze is repeated as needed. In a similar approach, men are taught to withdraw their penis as needed during intercourse to reduce arousal. Behavioral techniques are not as powerful as antidepressant medications for premature ejaculation, but they are helpful as a supplement to medication (Cooper, Martyn-St James, et al., 2015). Psychotherapy can also help men regain confidence after experiences of premature ejaculation (Althof, 2014).

Erectile Disorder   The most common intervention for erectile disorder is a phosphodi-esterase type 5 (PDE-5) inhibitor, such as sildenafil (Viagra), tadafil (Cialis), vardenafil (Levitra), or avanafil (Stendra). PDE-5 inhibitors relax smooth muscles and thereby allow blood to flow into the penis, creating an erection during sexual stimulation but not in its absence (Eardley, Donatucci, et al., 2010). Some PDE-5 inhibitors have a long half-life and can be taken daily, and others can be taken 15–30 minutes before sex (Rosen, Brotto, & Zucker, 2018). Although some men stop taking these medications due to side effects such as headaches and indigestion, most men will tolerate the side effects to gain relief from their sexual symptoms. Indeed, worldwide sales of PDE-5 inhibitors have surpassed $5 billion (Wilson, 2011).

Across 27 treatment studies, about 83% of men who took sildenafil were able to success-fully have intercourse compared with about 45% of men who took a placebo (Fink, Mac Don-ald, et al., 2002). Some men continue to experience intermittent erectile dysfunction on PDE-5 inhibitors, and so sex therapy is a helpful addition to medication treatment (Melnik, Soares, & Nasello, 2008).

Quick Summary

Key cognitive behavioral treatments for sexual dysfunction include psychoeducation, couples therapy, cognitive interventions, and sensate focus. Flibanserin (Addyi) and bremelanotide (Vyleesi) have been FDA-approved for female sexual interest/arousal disorder, directed masturbation is often used to treat female orgasmic disorder, relaxation coupled with the use of dilators is used for pain disorder, SSRIs and variants of the squeeze technique are used for premature ejaculation, and PDE-5 inhibitors such as silde-nafil (Viagra) and tadafil (Cialis) are used for erectile disorder.

12.4 Check Your Knowledge

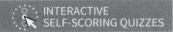
INTERACTIVE
SELF-SCORING QUIZZES

(Answers are at the end of the chapter.)
Answer the following question.

1. Describe the sensate-focus technique.

Which is the most effective treatment for each of the following?
2. Female orgasmic disorder

3. Premature ejaculation

4. Erectile disorder

True or false?
5. Sex therapists may recommend that a woman who does not achieve orgasm practice masturbation without her partner present.

Clinical Descriptions of the Paraphilic Disorders

The core feature of the **paraphilic disorders** is recurrent sexual attraction to unusual objects or activities, lasting at least 6 months. In other words, there is a deviation *(para)* in what the person is attracted to *(philia)*. DSM-5-TR differentiates the paraphilic disorders based on the source of arousal; for example, it provides one diagnostic category for people whose sexual attractions are focused on causing pain and another diagnostic category for people whose attractions are focused on children (see **Table 12.6**). Large surveys have shown that many people occasionally fantasize about some of the activities we will be describing, and some engage in these behaviors. Voyeuristic attractions may be particularly common: More than 40% of people report fantasies of watching unsuspecting people undress, have sex, or be naked

TABLE 12.6   Paraphilic Disorders Included in DSM-5-TR

Diagnosis	Object of Sexual Attraction
Fetishistic disorder	An inanimate object or nongenital body part
Transvestic disorder	Cross-dressing
Pedophilic disorder	Children
Voyeuristic disorder	Watching unsuspecting others undress or have sex
Exhibitionistic disorder	Exposing one's genitals to an unwilling stranger
Frotteuristic disorder	Sexual touching of an unsuspecting person
Sexual sadism disorder	Inflicting pain
Sexual masochism disorder	Receiving pain

(Joyal & Carpentier, 2017). About 7.7% report that they had been aroused by spying on others having sex, 7% report that they had engaged in sadomasochistic sex at least once, 3.1% report that they had been aroused by exposing their genitalia to a stranger at least once during their lifetime, and 3.1% of adult men report having had fantasies or sexual interest in children ages 13 to 15 in the past year (although a smaller percentage, 0.4%, endorsed an interest in children 12 and younger) (Holvoet, Huys, et al., 2017; Långström & Seto, 2006; Santtila, Antfolk, et al., 2015). The website fetlife.com, a social network site for people interested in sadomasochistic and fetishistic sex, lists more than 6 million members. *Fifty Shades of Gray*, a book describing a sadomasochistic relationship, was a worldwide bestseller. Some of these foci, such as sadomasochistic sex, appear to have a long history: *The Kama Sutra*, a sex manual published around 450 CE, discusses biting, marks left during sex, and love blows (Moser & Kleinplatz, 2020). Although many people are interested in or have tried these sexual activities, many fewer people report that these interests are sustained, uncontrollable, or distressing (Joyal & Carpentier, 2017).

Distress, impairment, and engagement of nonconsenting others are important boundaries between normative and problematic sexual behavior. It is important to note that some of the paraphilias do not involve nonconsenting others. When paraphilias do not involve nonconsenting others, DSM-5-TR specifies that these diagnoses can be applied if the sexual attractions cause marked distress or impairment.

Some have argued that it is inappropriate to diagnose paraphilias that involve sexual behavior with consenting adults and typically do not induce distress or impairment (Richters, De Visser, et al., 2008). Indeed, the World Health Organization removed fetishistic disorder, sexual sadism disorder, sexual masochism disorder, and transvestic disorder from their psychiatric classification system (WHO, 2018) but retained a diagnostic category for coercive sexual sadism disorder. DSM-5-TR retains labels for sexual sadism, sexual masochism, fetishistic disorder, and transvestic paraphilias, but the word *disorder* is added to the title of these diagnoses to emphasize that the clinician is to consider these diagnoses only if the sexual attractions cause marked distress or impairment or if the person engages in the sexual activities with a nonconsenting person.

Transvestic disorder and fetishistic disorder do not typically involve nonconsenting others and rarely lead to impairment; the diagnosis of these disorders rests on the presence of distress. But diagnostic criteria that rely on distress about sexual desires and behaviors are somewhat illogical. The person who cross-dresses for sexual gratification and accepts the behavior won't meet the diagnostic criteria. In contrast, the person who feels guilty and ashamed because they have internalized stigma about this behavior is diagnosable. Because fetishistic and transvestic behaviors so rarely lead to impairment or involve nonconsenting others, we do not discuss these two disorders further here.

Accurate prevalence statistics are not available for the paraphilic disorders. Research is limited by the reluctance of many people with paraphilias to reveal their proclivities. Because some people with paraphilic disorders seek nonconsenting partners or otherwise violate people's rights in offensive ways (as in the exhibitionistic and pedophilic disorders), these disorders can have legal consequences. But statistics on arrests underestimate prevalence because so many crimes go unreported and because some paraphilias (e.g., voyeuristic disorder) involve an unsuspecting victim. The data do indicate, however, that most people with paraphilic disorders are male and heterosexual; even with sexual masochism and voyeurism disorders, which occur in noticeable numbers of women, men outnumber women (Richters et al., 2008). The onset of sexual sadism disorder and sexual masochism disorder tends to occur by early adulthood (Balon, 2016; Grundmann, Krupp, et al., 2016). Many of the paraphilic interests, including fetishistic, voyeuristic, exhibitionistic, and pedophilic interests, typically emerge during adolescence. Nonetheless, the DSM-5-TR specifies that voyeuristic disorder should not be diagnosed before age 18. A person with one form of paraphilic interests is often aroused by other paraphilic stimuli—that is, tendencies to engage in exhibitionism, sexual sadism, sexual masochism, and voyeurism are correlated (Baur, Forsman, et al., 2016). Here we provide clinical descriptions of the paraphilic disorders.

Pedophilic Disorder and Incest

According to DSM-5-TR, **pedophilic disorder** (*pedes* is Greek for "child") is diagnosed when persons age 16 and older derive sexual gratification through sexual contact with prepubescent children or, in the absence of any actions, when their recurrent and intense desires for sexual contact with prepubescent children cause distress either for themselves or for others. Pedophilic disorder is diagnosed only when adults act on their sexual urges toward children or when the urges reach the frequency or intensity to be distressing to the person or those close to them. Sometimes a man with pedophilic disorder is content to stroke the child's hair, but he may also manipulate the child's genitalia, encourage the child to manipulate his, and, less often, attempt penile insertion. The molestations may be repeated over a period of weeks, months, or years.

People with pedophilic disorder generally molest children whom they know, such as neighbors or friends of the family. Most with pedophilic disorder do not engage in violence other than the sexual act, although when they do become violent, it is often a focus of lurid stories in the media. Because overt physical force is seldom used in pedophilic disorder, the child molester often denies that he is forcing himself on his victim. Despite molesters' distorted beliefs, child sexual abuse inherently involves a betrayal of trust and other serious negative consequences, as discussed earlier in **Focus on Discovery 12.2**.

Defining Symptoms of Pedophilic Disorder

- For at least 6 months, recurrent and intense sexually arousing fantasies, urges, or behaviors involving sexual contact with a prepubescent child
- Person has acted on these urges or the urges and fantasies cause marked distress or interpersonal problems

- Person is at least 16 years old and 5 years older than the child
- Person is not an older adolescent involved in ongoing sexual relationship with a 12- or 13-year-old

---

What are the demographic characteristics of people who meet the criteria for pedophilic disorder? Although some women acknowledge pedophilic interests or behavior (Fromuth & Conn, 1997), most of the people convicted of pedophilia are men. People with pedophilic disorder can be straight or gay, though most are heterosexual. Among those convicted of pedophilic offenses, about half have never been married (Seto & Eke, 2017).

Sexual arousal in response to pictures of young children can be measured by the penile plethysmograph. In large-scale studies, arousal as measured in this way discriminates those who have committed sexual offenses with children (Cantor & McPhail, 2015), and it is one of the strongest predictors of repeated sexual offenses (Hanson & Bussiere, 1998). Nonetheless, arousal in response to pictures of children is not a perfect predictor of pedophilic disorder. Many men who are conventional in their sexual interests and behavior can be sexually aroused by erotic pictures of children. In a study using both self-reports and penile plethysmography, one-quarter of men drawn from a community sample showed or reported arousal when viewing sexually provocative pictures of children (Hall, Hirschman, & Oliver, 1995). The *relative* level of interest in children versus adults may be more telling. People with pedophilic disorder show more arousal to sexual stimuli involving children than to stimuli involving adults; those without pedophilic disorder tend to show relatively more arousal to stimuli involving adults (McPhail, Hermann, et al., 2019). As you consider these findings, it is important to remember that a diagnosis of pedophilic disorder is not based on sexual interest alone.

Incest is listed as a subtype of pedophilic disorder. **Incest** refers to sexual relations between close relatives for whom marriage is forbidden. It is most common between brother and sister. The next most common form, which is considered more pathological, is between father and daughter. Fathers who abuse their daughters tend to do so after the daughter reaches puberty.

Clinical Case

William

William and Nancy sought marital therapy after Nancy learned that William had a long history of voyeurism. Nancy had been startled to walk into their guest room and find him viewing the neighbor with binoculars while masturbating. Upon confrontation, William shared with his wife that he had felt intense and uncontrollable urges to watch strangers undress since his early adolescence.

William and Nancy had been married for 20 years, and they reported that neither had ever found their sexual life very satisfying. Nancy was concerned that he rarely initiated sexual contact with her, and indeed, in an individual session, William reported that he preferred watching strangers to having sex with his wife. He had never found sex with a consenting partner as exciting as the forbidden. William had tried different strategies to gain control over his voyeuristic urges, including reading self-help books and attending a support group, with no success. He reported that he came from an extremely strict family and had been teased relentlessly by his father. Although his desire to watch strangers haunted him, he had always felt too ashamed to discuss his sexual preferences. His sexual detachment was part of a broader pattern of emotional distance and lack of disclosure with others in his life.

In therapy, William began to explore the sense of social rejection that he had experienced since early childhood. As his wife learned of his past, they achieved a stronger emotional bond, which freed them to discuss their sexuality more openly. As their sex life improved, William reported that his desire to watch others undress faded.

Adapted from Kleinplatz (2014).

The taboo against incest is virtually universal in human societies (Ford & Beach, 1951). The incest taboo makes sense according to present-day scientific knowledge. The offspring from a father–daughter or a brother–sister union have a greater probability of inheriting a pair of recessive genes, one from each parent. Many recessive genes have negative biological effects, such as serious birth defects. The incest taboo, then, has adaptive evolutionary significance.

Voyeuristic Disorder

The central feature of **voyeuristic disorder** is an intense and recurrent desire to obtain sexual gratification by watching unsuspecting others who are naked or engaged in sexual behavior. Voyeuristic fantasies are quite common in men, but as with the other paraphilic disorders, fantasies alone do not warrant a diagnosis. For some men with this disorder, voyeurism is their only means of attaining sexual arousal; for others, like William in the **Clinical Case**, it is preferred but not essential for sexual arousal. People with voyeuristic disorder achieve orgasm by masturbation, either while watching or later while remembering the scene. Sometimes the person with voyeuristic disorder fantasizes about having sexual contact with the observed person, but it remains a fantasy; they seldom contact the observed person. Most voyeurs do not find it exciting to watch someone undress for their benefit. The element of risk and the threat of discovery are important.

Defining Symptoms of Voyeuristic Disorder

- For at least 6 months, recurrent and intense sexually arousing fantasies, urges, or behaviors involving the observation of unsuspecting other who is naked, disrobing, or engaged in sexual activity

- Person has acted on these urges with a nonconsenting person, or the urges and fantasies cause marked distress or interpersonal problems
- At least 18 years of age

Exhibitionistic Disorder

The focus of sexual desire in **exhibitionistic disorder** is on exposing one's genitals to an unwilling stranger, sometimes a child. As with voyeuristic disorder, there is seldom an attempt to have other contact with the stranger. Many exhibitionists masturbate during the exposure. In most cases, there is a desire to shock or embarrass the observer. In one study, people diagnosed with exhibitionistic disorder reported that they had been arrested for only 1 out of every 150 incidents (Abel, Becker, et al., 1987).

Defining Symptoms of Exhibitionistic Disorder

- For at least 6 months, recurrent, intense, and sexually arousing fantasies, urges, or behaviors involving showing one's genitals to an unsuspecting person

- Person has acted on these urges toward a nonconsenting person, or the urges and fantasies cause clinically significant distress or interpersonal problems

Frotteuristic Disorder

The focus of sexual desire and urges in **frotteuristic disorder** is on touching an unsuspecting person. The person with this disorder may rub his penis against a woman's thighs or buttocks or fondle her breasts or genitals. These attacks typically occur in places such as a crowded bus or sidewalk that provide an easy means of escape. Most men who engage in frotteurism report doing so dozens of times (Abel et al., 1987).

Defining Symptoms of Frotteuristic Disorder

- For at least 6 months, recurrent and intense and sexually arousing fantasies, urges, or behaviors involving touching or rubbing against a nonconsenting person

- Person has acted on these urges with a nonconsenting person, or the urges and fantasies cause clinically significant distress or problems

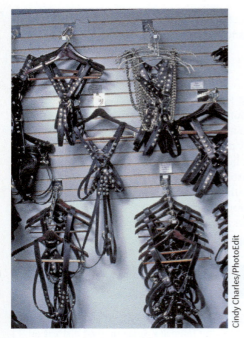

Many people experiment with sadomasochism. Paraphilias are not diagnosed unless the sexual interests cause marked distress or impairment.

Sexual Sadism and Masochism Disorders

The focus of desire in **sexual sadism disorder** is on inflicting pain or psychological suffering (such as humiliation) on another, and the focus of desire in **sexual masochism disorder** is on being subjected to pain or humiliation. Sexual sadism and masochism can span a wide range of activities. Examples include physical bondage, blindfolding, spanking, whipping, electric shocks, cutting, humiliation (e.g., being urinated or defecated on, being forced to wear a collar and bark like a dog, or being put on display naked), and taking the role of an enslaved person and submitting to orders and commands. Most sadists establish relationships with masochists to derive mutual sexual gratification. Although many alternate between dominant and submissive roles, masochists outnumber sadists.

Sadistic and masochistic sexual behaviors have become more accepted over time. In many cities, clubs cater to members seeking sadomasochistic partnerships. Most people who engage in sadomasochistic behaviors are comfortable with their sexual practices and would not meet the diagnostic criteria requiring that the desires lead to distress or impairment. Sadomasochistic sexual behaviors are not usually related to maladaptive personality traits, impairment, or distress and are rarely a focus of treatment. In an unpublished review of over 500 million visits to psychiatrists, gynecologists, urologists, and other physicians, no doctor recorded a diagnosis of sexual sadism disorder or sexual masochism disorder (Narrow, 2008, cited in Krueger, 2010a).

Given the absence of evidence for distress or treatment seeking, there was debate about whether these diagnoses should be retained in DSM-5 (Krueger, 2010b; Wismeijer & van Assen, 2013). These diagnostic labels were retained because some sadistic and masochistic practices can be dangerous. One particularly dangerous

Defining Symptoms of Sexual Sadism Disorder

- For at least 6 months, recurrent, intense, and sexually arousing fantasies, urges, or behaviors involving the physical or psychological suffering of another person

- Causes marked distress or impairment in functioning or the person has acted on these urges with a nonconsenting person

Defining Symptoms of Sexual Masochism Disorder

- For at least 6 months, recurrent, intense, and sexually arousing fantasies, urges, or behaviors involving the act of being humiliated, beaten, bound, or made to suffer

- Causes marked distress or impairment in functioning

form of masochism, called *asphyxiophilia*, can result in death or brain damage; it involves sexual arousal by restricting breathing, which can be achieved using a noose or a plastic bag or by chest compression.

Quick Summary

Paraphilic disorders are defined as sexual attraction to an unusual sexual object or activity that lasts at least 6 months and causes significant distress or impairment or involves sexual actions toward a nonconsenting person. The DSM-5-TR diagnostic criteria for paraphilic disorders are distinguished based on the object of sexual attraction. The major DSM-5-TR diagnoses of paraphilias include pedophilic disorder, voyeuristic disorder, exhibitionistic disorder, frotteuristic disorder, sexual sadism disorder, sexual masochism disorder, fetishistic disorder, and transvestic disorder. (The last two diagnoses are not discussed in this book.) Researchers do not know the prevalence of these disorders.

12.5 Check Your Knowledge

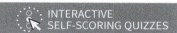 INTERACTIVE SELF-SCORING QUIZZES

(Answers are at the end of the chapter.)
Choose the diagnostic category that best fits each vignette. If the problem described is not diagnosable, state so.

1. Joe can obtain sexual arousal only by rubbing their body against strangers. They usually choose to engage in this behavior in a crowded bus.

2. Sam and Terry enjoy a good sexual relationship. They have mutually satisfying sex at least weekly. Occasionally, Terry likes to be tied down before sex but can enjoy sex without bondage as well. Most of their sex life involves no hint of pain or bondage.

3. Matt feels aroused only when they cause pain to someone as part of engaging in sex. Most of the time, they indulge in these activities at a sadomasochism club. They have not been able to sustain a relationship with any of the women they have met in clubs. They are deeply distressed by their inability to enjoy other forms of sexuality.

4. Barry is a 40-year-old single man who has never had a sustained romantic or sexual relationship. Several times a week, Barry parks their car, masturbates, and then finds a way to lure a woman to their car, usually by asking for directions. Barry is unable to have an orgasm unless the woman notices their erection. Barry has been arrested three times for this behavior.

Causes of the Paraphilic Disorders

Given that many people have interests in sexual sadism, masochism, or exhibitionism, why do some of these interests become difficult to control for some people, such that they reach a diagnosable level? As we consider possible causes of the paraphilic disorders, including neurobiological influences, early abuse, and psychological influences, keep in mind that there are many gaps in knowledge. Some research focuses on understanding paraphilic interests that do not lead to distress or impairment; this research indicates, for example, that people with paraphilic interests tend not to have histories of childhood sexual abuse or psychological traits that would indicate risk (Långström & Seto, 2006; Richters et al., 2008). Such work does not tell us, though, why some people become unable to control their paraphilic interests and develop a paraphilic disorder. Because many people do not want to talk about their paraphilic disorders, researchers have few opportunities to understand their causes. Indeed, almost all studies rely on samples of less than 25 people with paraphilic disorders (Kafka, 2010). Beyond the problem of small sample sizes, most of the available research focuses on men who are arrested for their sexual behavior; little is known about those whose sexual behavior does not lead to arrest. Hence, much of this literature is most relevant for understanding sexual offenders, who represent a severe subset of those with paraphilic disorders.

Neurobiological Influences

Because the vast majority of people with paraphilic disorders include men, there has been speculation that androgens (hormones like testosterone) play a role. Androgens regulate sexual desire, and sexual desire appears atypically high among some sexual offenders with paraphilic disorders. Nonetheless, men with paraphilic disorders do not appear to have high levels of testosterone or other androgens (Thibaut, De La Barra, et al., 2010).

Childhood Sexual Abuse

Childhood sexual abuse is relevant in understanding the most severe forms of paraphilic disorder. That is, across multiple studies, about 40–66% of adult sexual offenders reported a history of sexual abuse; rates are substantially higher than the rates among those charged with nonsexual offenses or among those in the general population (Jespersen, Lalumiere, & Seto, 2009; Levenson & Grady, 2016). This suggests that sexual abuse is tied to sexual offending. Nonetheless, sexual abuse cannot be the whole story—large-scale follow-up studies of boys with confirmed sexual abuse have shown that fewer than 5% were charged with any type of sexual offense as adults (Ogloff, Cutajar, et al., 2012; Salter, McMillan, et al., 2003).

Psychological Influences

Some people with paraphilic disorders report that their sexual behaviors are more likely to happen in the context of negative moods, suggesting that sexual activity is being used to escape from negative affect. Relatedly, people with paraphilic disorders tend to show longer-term problems with emotion regulation (Ward & Beech, 2006).

For the paraphilias that involve sexual behaviors directed toward nonconsenting others, succumbing to the sexual urge can be thought of as an impulsive act, in which the person loses control over their behavior. Alcohol decreases the ability to inhibit impulses, and accordingly, many incidents of pedophilic disorder, voyeuristic disorder, and exhibitionistic disorder occur in the context of alcohol use. People with paraphilic disorders involving nonconsenting others also tend to show heightened impulsivity (Moser & Kleinplatz, 2020; Ward & Beech, 2006).

In addition to a loss of control, men who engage in paraphilic behaviors that involve nonconsenting women or children may have hostile attitudes and a lack of empathy toward their sexual targets (Babchishin, Hanson, & VanZuylen, 2015). See **Focus on Discovery 12.3** for a discussion of rape.

A separate line of work focuses on pedophilia. Because most of the available research on pedophilia focuses only on men, we will focus our discussion on the causes of pedophilia among men. It is increasingly well recognized that many men who are sexually attracted to children do not engage in sexual behavior toward children (Seto & Eke, 2017). This raises the question of why some can restrain these impulses. In one study, researchers compared empathy levels in three groups: men who engaged in pedophilic behavior, men who were sexually attracted to children yet did not act on those attractions, and controls who endorsed neither attractions nor behaviors with children. To study empathy, the researchers asked participants to view pictures of adults and children and to judge the emotion expressions. While the men who had engaged in pedophilic behavior were poor in judging the children's emotion expressions, those who had resisted acting on their sexual attractions were better than average in judging the children's emotion expressions. The authors concluded that the ability to infer another person's emotional state could help protect against acting on pedophilic urges (Schuler, Mohnke, et al., 2019).

Focus on Discovery 12.3

Rape

Rape is one of the most disturbing of human behaviors. It is typically defined as "attempted or completed vaginal, anal, or oral intercourse obtained through force, through the threat of force, or when the victim is incapacitated and unable to give consent" (Abbey & McAuslan, 2004). The rapist is usually known to the victim.

Many more women than men are raped: In the United States, an estimated 19.3% of women and 1.7% of men have been raped during their lifetime. For three-quarters of women who are raped, the rape occurs before the age of 25 (Zinzow & Thompson, 2015).

Coercive sexual behavior, in which a person is pressured to engage in sexual contact, is even more common than rape. It has been extremely difficult to estimate just how common coercive behavior is; more than a dozen scales have been used to ask about such behavior, and the results from different scales vary widely—from 6.7% to more than 60% of respondents saying they have experienced it (Anderson, Silver, et al., 2019). Even estimates of 6.7% are troublingly high.

The high rates of rape and coercive sexual behavior have led many to suggest that sexual violence reflects a social and cultural problem (Gavey & Senn, 2014). This has led to policy efforts to provide education about the negative outcomes of rape and coercive sexual behavior and to strengthen laws and response systems (DeMatteo, Galloway, et al., 2015).

Even if it is the case that this behavior must be viewed in a social context, it is only natural to ask questions about rapists. Who are the men who perpetrate these acts? Can treatment reduce the risk of recidivism?

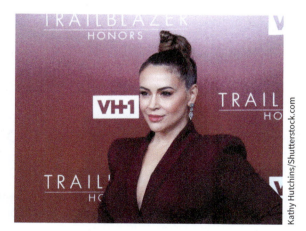

Alyssa Milano used the Twitter hashtag "#MeToo" to encourage people to respond and showcase the magnitude of the problem of sexual violence. Capturing public attention, the hashtag was used 12 million times in the first 24 hours (CBS, 2017), and the MeToo movement brought considerable attention to the troubling prevalence of sexual coercion worldwide.

Understanding the Causes of Rape

Sexually aggressive men tend to show antisocial and impulsive personality traits, unusually high hostility toward women, and

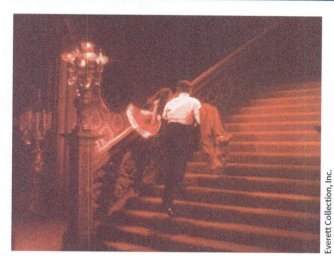

This famous scene from the movie *Gone with the Wind* illustrates one of the myths about rape—that despite initial resistance, women like to be "taken."

distorted beliefs about sexual coercion (e.g., "women mean yes when they say no" or tendencies to place blame on the victim) (Trottier, Benbouriche, & Bonneville, 2019; Zinzow & Thompson, 2015). It is also likely that there are different subgroups of rapists: Some show more sadistic traits, some show more hypersexuality, and others show more impulsive traits (Krstic, Neumann, et al., 2017).

Data suggest that exposure to violence may increase the likelihood of rape. That is, rapists are more likely than nonrapists to have been the victim of sexual and physical abuse (Knight & Sims-Knight, 2011). Even watching violence against women in films can lead men to view violence as more acceptable. At least eight experiments have been conducted in which men were asked to watch videos that contained sexual activities either with or without violence. After watching the videos that contained violence, men were significantly more likely to report that violence toward women was acceptable (Allen, D'Alessio, & Brezgel, 1995). This research suggests that rape may be encouraged by pornography that depicts violent sexual relations, and more broadly, it highlights the importance of social influences.

Treatment for Rapists

Treatment programs for rapists rely on the general approaches we describe for paraphilic disorders: motivational strategies, cognitive behavioral techniques, and pharmacological treatments. As with the research on treatment for paraphilic disorders, the evidence regarding the effectiveness of these approaches is remarkably slim—only 24 rapists were followed in the best available randomized controlled trial (Marques, Wiederanders, et al., 2005). Outcomes of that study suggested that 20% of rapists assigned to cognitive behavioral treatment committed an offense during the 5-year follow-up period, compared with 29% in the no-treatment group. Although this may seem like a small gain from treatment, any gain is important with such a difficult problem.

Other evidence suggests neurocognitive problems associated with pedophilia. On average, men with pedophilic disorder have a slightly lower IQ and higher rates of neurocognitive problems than the general population (Cantor, Blanchard, et al., 2005; Suchy, Eastvold, et al., 2014). Men with pedophilia also show minor physical anomalies related to atypical prenatal development more often than those with other paraphilic sexual behaviors do (Dyshniku, Murray, et al., 2015).

There may be more than one psychological pathway to pedophilia (Knight & King, 2012). Some people with pedophilic disorder show an intense preoccupation with sex, a sense of emotional compatibility with children, and a specific sexual preference for children (Konrad, Kuhle, et al., 2018). Others with this disorder demonstrate more general tendencies toward elevated impulsivity and psychopathy (Mann, Hanson, & Thornton, 2010).

Quick Summary

Neurobiological theory of paraphilic disorders has focused on excessively high testosterone levels, but the theory has not received support. Sexual offenders report higher rates of being sexually abused than do other offenders, but very few children who are abused grow up to engage in sexual offenses against others.

Alcohol use and negative affect are often immediate triggers of inappropriate sexual behaviors. When paraphilic behavior is directed at nonconsenting others, impulsivity, hostility, and lack of empathy may be involved.

Among those with pedophilia, neurocognitive deficits, lower IQ, and signs of atypical prenatal development are sometimes observed. Empathy toward children may relate to less likelihood of acting on pedophilic urges. There may be more than one pathway toward pedophilia: Some men are sexually preoccupied with children and experience a sense of emotional compatibility with children; other men have a profile of more general impulsive, psychopathic traits.

12.6 Check Your Knowledge

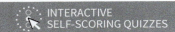 INTERACTIVE SELF-SCORING QUIZZES

(Answers are at the end of the chapter.)
Answer the following questions.

1. Describe the major problems with the research findings on the prevalence and causes of paraphilic disorders.
2. What types of factors might contribute to the loss of control over sexual urges for those with paraphilic disorders?

Treatments and Community Prevention for the Paraphilic Disorders

We now describe motivational, cognitive behavioral, hormone, and SSRI treatments for the paraphilic disorders. After we discuss treatment approaches, we will turn to a discussion of issues in addressing the legal and public ramifications of sexual offending.

We know very little about the effectiveness of the treatments used for paraphilic disorders. First, most of the available research on treatment focuses on men who have been charged with sexual offenses, so we know little about treatment of those in the community. Second, only very small amounts of long-term treatment data are available. Third, because many researchers consider it unethical to withhold treatment when the consequences of sexual offenses are so severe, most studies have not randomly assigned people into control groups— very few randomized controlled trials (RCTs) are available. Indeed, no RCTs are available to consider the efficacy of SSRIs for paraphilic disorders (Balon, 2016). Little long-term outcome data are available for behavioral treatments designed to change sexual arousal to atypical objects or activities (Ware, McIvor, & Fernandez, 2021).

What do the findings of the available RCTs indicate about treatment of paraphilic disorders? In the largest available RCT of cognitive behavior therapy (CBT) for adults, no significant effects were observed on legal recidivism (Marques et al., 2005). In contrast, two studies have shown benefits of offering intensive individual and family therapy for juvenile offenders (Schmucker & Lösel, 2015). More research is needed overall, as there are very few randomized controlled trials testing the efficacy of psychotherapy. Across six available RCTs, hormone agents reduce arousal to paraphilic stimuli, as measured using penile plethysmography (Thibaut et al., 2010), but only very small amounts of data are available on whether medications reduce sexual offending (Khan, Ferriter, et al., 2015). Findings of the studies of hormone agents are difficult to interpret due to issues such as high drop-out rates (Khan et al., 2015).

Strategies to Enhance Motivation

Sex offenders often lack the motivation to change their illegal behavior. They may deny their problem or minimize the seriousness of their problem. Many refuse to take part in treatment, and even among those who begin treatment, many will drop out. To enhance motivation for treatment, a therapist can bolster the client's hope that they can gain control over their urges through treatment. The therapist can help the client focus on reasons for change, including the potential legal and other consequences of continued engagement in the same sexual behavior (Miller & Rollnick, 1991).

Cognitive Behavioral Treatment

In the earliest years of behavioral treatment, paraphilic disorders were narrowly viewed as attractions to inappropriate objects and activities. Looking to behavioral psychology for ways to reduce these attractions, researchers fixed on aversion therapy. Thus, a person with a pedophilic disorder would be given a shock on the hands or a drug that produces nausea when looking at a photograph of a nude child, and so on. In the form of aversion therapy called *satiation*, men are coached to pair their paraphilic fantasies with another aversive stimulus: masturbating for 55 minutes after orgasm (Kaplan & Krueger, 2012). In covert sensitization, people would be asked to imagine negative consequences of their inappropriate sexual behavior. Over time, as the difficulty of changing arousal patterns became clearer, therapists began to use a broader array of techniques to help patients avoid acting on problematic urges.

Cognitive interventions are often used to counter the distorted thinking of people with paraphilic disorders. For example, an exhibitionist might claim that the girls he exposes himself to are too young to be harmed by it. The therapist would counter this distortion by pointing out that the younger the victim, the worse the harm will be (Kaplan & Krueger, 2012).

Many other techniques have become common (Balon, 2016; Kaplan & Krueger, 2012). Therapists often offer social skills training and teach sexual impulse control strategies such as distraction. As warranted, they might focus on early abuse experiences. Training in empathy toward others is another common technique; teaching the sex offender to consider how their behavior would affect someone else may lessen the tendency to engage in such activities. Relapse prevention, modeled after the work on substance abuse described in Chapter 10, is also an important component of many broader treatment programs. A therapist who uses relapse prevention techniques would help a person identify situations and emotions that might trigger symptomatic behavior.

Biological Treatments

Several medications have been used to treat paraphilic disorders, particularly among adult sex offenders. These medications are considered supplements to psychological treatment (Thibaut, Cosyns, et al., 2020). Among men, sexual drive and functioning are regulated by androgens (such as testosterone). Hence, hormonal agents that reduce androgens have been used to treat paraphilic disorders; these agents include medroxyprogesterone acetate (MPA, trade name Depo-Provera) and cyproterone acetate (CPA) (Khan et al., 2015). In addition to the weak evidence for the efficacy of hormonal agents, another concern is ethical issues raised by their long-term use, which is associated with several negative side effects, including feminization, infertility, osteoporosis, diabetes, and depression. Informed consent concerning these risks must be obtained, and many patients will not agree to use these drugs long term (Balon, 2016). Besides drugs that influence hormones, SSRI antidepressants are commonly used, despite the absence of evidence supporting the effectiveness of this approach.

Prevention

All too often, treatment for paraphilias takes place only once an individual is charged with a crime. In 2004, major initiatives began to identify and provide intervention for men who experienced sexual attractions to children, through community outreach in several countries. As part of the Dunkelfeld Project, media advertisements were launched with the message "You are not guilty because of your sexual desire, but you are responsible for your sexual behavior. There is help! Don't become an offender!" More than 11,000 men contacted the Dunkelfeld center. More than 1,000 were treated, and many of those traveled more than a hundred miles to take part in assessments. For those living near the center, a 1-year treatment is offered, including cognitive behavior therapy and the option to consider medication (Beier, 2018). Among the first 53 men who took part in the treatment program, changes were apparent from before to after treatment in cognitions about victims and in perceived ability to regulate sexual urges; nonetheless, these changes were not significantly better than the changes observed among those assigned to a wait-list control (Mokros & Banse, 2019), and of 25 who had engaged in child sexual abuse before treatment, 5 continued to engage in these sexual behaviors (Beier, Grundmann, et al., 2015). Findings based on the fuller sample will be important in evaluating the success of this program more fully.

In many countries, this type of face-to-face treatment would be difficult to offer because therapists are mandated to report sexual abuse to authorities; with such laws, some patients might not be willing to disclose their sexual behaviors. Anonymous treatment online is now offered internationally to help prevent sexual abuse of children (https://troubled-desire.com/en/). The large number of individuals who sign up for these online programs suggests a need for such interventions, but there is little data on their effectiveness (Stephens, Elchuk, et al., 2022).

Balancing Efforts to Protect the Public Against the Civil Liberties of Those with Paraphilias

Most people are frightened by sexual offenses, so balancing the protection of the public against the civil liberties of sexual offenders is not easy. Issues arise in multiple aspects of the legal process, including how diagnoses of paraphilic disorders can influence institutionalization, as well as with laws concerning the public's "right to know" when a sex offender is released.

In the United States, it is generally unconstitutional to detain a person on the basis of their potential for *future* crimes. Nonetheless, the Supreme Court has ruled that a person deemed at high risk for a sex crime can be detained if the risk is related to a psychological disorder that diminishes the person's ability to control their sexual behavior. The diagnosis of a paraphilic disorder, then, has significant implications for civil liberties: Receipt of a paraphilic diagnosis can lead to placement in a psychiatric facility after a prison term is completed. In this context, it has been argued that particular care should be taken to ensure the validity of these diagnoses (Wakefield, 2011).

Legal statutes referred to as Megan's Law allow police to publicize the whereabouts of registered sex offenders if they are considered a potential danger. Citizens can use computerized police records to determine whether sex offenders are living in their neighborhood. Megan's Law and related statutes arose from public outrage at the brutal murder of a 2nd grader in New Jersey who was kidnapped while walking home from school. The person convicted of this crime had been convicted twice for child sexual abuse. The hope behind these laws is that they will protect against repeat offenses; however, findings have been mixed about whether they are successful in reducing sexual crimes. One unintended consequence of these laws is that some people have committed violent crimes toward sex offenders in their neighborhoods (Younglove & Vitello, 2003). Not surprisingly, civil liberties groups are challenging these laws. Navigating the tension between protecting the public and civil liberties for offenders is not easy.

12.7 Check Your Knowledge

(Answers are at the end of the chapter.)
Answer the following questions.

1. The most common biological treatments to reduce sexual desire and paraphilic behaviors are:
   a. surgical castration
   b. hormonal agents and antidepressants
   c. antianxiety medications
   d. None of the above are used to reduce sexual desire and paraphilic behaviors.
2. Name four cognitive behavioral strategies used in the treatment of paraphilic disorders.
3. Describe the evidence base for the psychological and biological treatments of paraphilic disorders.

Summary

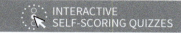
Chapter 12 Practice Quiz

Sexual Norms and Behavior

- Sexual behaviors and attitudes are heavily influenced by culture, so any discussion of disorders in sexuality must be sensitive to the ideas that norms are likely to change across time and place and that those norms will influence people's reports in surveys.
- Gender differences in sexual behavior are less apparent when researchers use research methods designed to reduce bias in reporting. Nonetheless, for women, desire may not precede biological arousal, and biological and subjective arousal may not be correlated.

Sexual Dysfunctions

- DSM-5-TR includes sexual dysfunction diagnoses relevant to arousal and desire (female sexual interest/arousal disorder, male hypoactive sexual desire disorder, and erectile disorder), to orgasm (female orgasmic disorder, premature ejaculation, and delayed ejaculation), and to pain (genito-pelvic pain/penetration disorder). Many people experience brief sexual symptoms, but these are not diagnosable unless they are recurrent, cause either distress or impairment, and are not explained by severe relationship distress or by medical conditions.
- Research on sexual dysfunctions is difficult to conduct, as survey responses may be limited by willingness to disclose problems, and data from laboratory measures may be difficult to gather. Researchers have identified many different variables that contribute to sexual dysfunctions, including biological variables, previous sexual experiences, relationship issues, psychological disorders, low arousal, and cognitions (e.g., self-blame).
- Many effective cognitive behavioral interventions for sexual dysfunctions are available. Strategies include psychoeducation, couples therapy, cognitive interventions, sensate focus, and techniques to address more specific dysfunctions, such as

directed masturbation for female orgasmic disorder, relaxation and use of dilators for genito-pelvic pain/penetration disorder, SSRIs and squeeze techniques for premature ejaculation, and PDE-5 inhibitors for erectile disorder.

Paraphilic Disorders

- The paraphilic disorders are defined by attractions and urges toward unusual sexual objects or behaviors that are persistent and lead to distress or impairment. The major DSM-5-TR paraphilic disorders are pedophilic disorder, voyeuristic disorder, exhibitionistic disorder, frotteuristic disorder, sexual sadism disorder, sexual masochism disorder, fetishistic disorder, and transvestic disorder. (We do not discuss the last two disorders.)
- Exposure to childhood sexual abuse may be a risk factor for paraphilic disorders. Negative affect and emotion dysregulation appear involved. Alcohol use may increase the odds of acting on sexual urges. Impulsivity, hostility, and lack of empathy appear relevant when sexual behaviors are directed toward nonconsenting others.
- Stronger ability to read children's emotional expressions is related to less likelihood of acting on pedophilic urges. Pedophilic disorder has been related to neurocognitive deficits and lower IQ. Some men with pedophilic disorder are obsessed with sex and strongly attracted to children both emotionally and sexually; other men with pedophilic disorder act out of more general impulsive and antisocial traits.
- The research evidence regarding treatments for paraphilic disorders is limited. Treatment approaches must begin by engaging and motivating the person, which is often difficult to do. Early cognitive behavioral approaches focused on aversion therapy. Cognitive techniques are used to challenge distorted beliefs about the consequences of sexual behaviors. Over time,

cognitive behavioral therapists have begun to use techniques to improve social skills, help people control impulses, increase empathy for potential victims, and identify potential high-risk situations for the return of symptoms. Very few randomized controlled trials have tested the efficacy of psychological interventions for paraphilic disorders, and the findings of the available trials are mixed. Hormonal agents that reduce testosterone levels have been found to reduce sexual arousal to the paraphilic object, but because of the side effects, there are ethical issues involved in the long-term use of these medications.

SSRI antidepressants are commonly prescribed to reduce the sexual drive of men with paraphilic disorders, but no RCTs are available.

- Community outreach efforts attempt to prevent pedophilic behavior among men who are attracted to children.
- A diagnosis of paraphilic disorder has relevance for whether a person can be detained in a psychiatric facility to prevent possible future crimes. Laws allow the public to access information about where sexual offenders live, but some offenders have been victimized when such information became public.

Answers to Check Your Knowledge Questions

12.1 1. Men report a higher frequency of masturbation and more use of pornography than do women; 2. the availability of the birth control pill in the 1970s, the AIDS epidemic in the 1980s, and the availability of sexual content on the internet in the 1990s.

12.2 1. False; 2. True; 3. difficulty reaching orgasm; 4. lack of interest or arousal.

12.3 1. more than half; 2. Depression is associated with more than a threefold increase in risk of sexual dissatisfaction and anxiety with more than a twofold increase.

12.4 1. The clients are instructed not to have intercourse. They are to focus on sensual touching, excluding genitals initially. They are to take turns pleasuring each other and receiving; 2. directed masturbation; 3. SSRIs (specifically dapoxetine); 4. PDE-5 inhibitors; 5. True.

12.5 1. frotteuristic disorder; 2. not diagnosable, as there is no evidence of distress or impairment; 3. sexual sadism disorder; 4. exhibitionistic disorder.

12.6 1. small samples, often consisting of sexual offenders; discomfort of many to disclose these symptoms; and few studies; 2. alcohol use and impulsivity

12.7 1. b. hormonal agents and antidepressants; 2. any four of the following: aversion therapy, satiation, covert sensitization, cognitive interventions to address maladaptive beliefs, social skills training, sexual impulse control training, therapy focused on early abuse, empathy training, relapse prevention; 3. The largest RCT for CBT showed little effect on repeat offending; hormonal agents reduce sexual desire toward deviant objects; no RCT is available for SSRIs; available trials typically focus on sexual offenders; and only small amounts of long-term data are available.

Key Terms

biological arousal 339
delayed ejaculation disorder 343
erectile disorder 342
exhibitionistic disorder 356
female orgasmic disorder 343
female sexual interest/arousal disorder 342
frotteuristic disorder 356
genito-pelvic pain/penetration disorder 344

incest 355
male hypoactive sexual desire disorder 342
orgasm 340
paraphilic disorders 352
pedophilic disorder 354
penile plethysmograph 338
premature (early) ejaculation 343
sexual dysfunctions 341

sexual interest 339
sexual masochism disorder 356
sexual sadism disorder 356
subjective arousal 339
vaginal plethysmograph 338
voyeuristic disorder 355

Disorders of Childhood

LEARNING GOALS

1. Describe the issues in the diagnosis of psychopathology in children.

2. Discuss the description, causes, and treatments for externalizing problems, including ADHD and conduct disorder.

3. Discuss the description, causes, and treatments for internalizing problems, including depression and anxiety disorders.

4. Understand the description, causes, and treatments for intellectual disability.

5. Describe the symptoms, causes, and treatments for autism spectrum disorder.

Clinical Case

Eric

"Eric. Eric? Eric!" His teacher's voice and the laughter of his classmates roused the boy from his daydreaming. Glancing at the book of the girl sitting next to him, he noticed that the class was pages ahead of him. He was supposed to be answering a question about the Declaration of Independence, but he had been lost in thought, wondering about what seats he and his father would have for the baseball game they'd be attending that evening. A tall, lanky 12-year-old, Eric had just begun 7th grade. His history teacher had already warned him about being late to class and not paying attention, but Eric just couldn't seem to get from one class to the next without stopping for a drink of water or to investigate an altercation between classmates. In class, he was rarely prepared to answer when the teacher called on him, and he usually forgot to write down the homework assignment. He already had a reputation among his peers as an "airhead."

Eric's relief at the sound of the bell was quickly replaced by anxiety as he reached the field for baseball tryouts. Despite his speed and physical strength, Eric was always picked last for sports teams. During tryouts, the boys were assigned into two teams. His team was up to bat first, and Eric sat down to wait his turn. Absorbed in studying a pile of pebbles at his feet, he failed to notice his team's third out and missed the change of innings. The other team had already come in from the outfield before Eric

noticed that his team was out in the field—too late to avoid the irate yells of the coach to take his place at third base. Resolved to watch for his chance to field the ball, Eric nonetheless found himself without his glove on when a sharply hit ball rocketed his way; he had taken it off to toss it in the air in the middle of the pitch.

At home, Eric's father told him he had to finish his homework before they could go to the Giants game. He had only one page of math problems and was determined to finish them quickly. Thirty minutes later, his father emerged from the shower to find Eric building an elaborate Lego structure on the floor of his room; the math homework was only half done. In exasperation, Eric's father left for the game without him.

At bedtime, frustrated and discouraged, Eric was unable to sleep. He often lay awake for what seemed like hours, reviewing the disappointments of the day and berating himself for his failures. On this night, he ruminated about his lack of friends, the frustration of his teachers, and his parents' exhortations to pay attention and "get it together." Feeling hopeless about doing better, despite his daily resolve, Eric often found his thoughts turning to suicide. Tonight, he reviewed his fantasy of wandering out into the street in front of a passing car. Although Eric had never acted on his suicidal thoughts, he frequently replayed in his mind his parents' sorrow and remorse, his classmates' irritation with him, and the concern of his teachers.

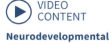
VIDEO
CONTENT

Neurodevelopmental Disorders

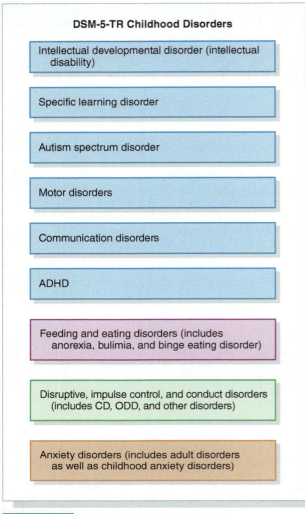

FIGURE 13.1   DSM-5-TR childhood disorders.

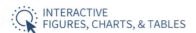

INTERACTIVE
FIGURES, CHARTS, & TABLES

Childhood disorders, like adult disorders, involve a combination of genetic, neurobiological, behavioral, cognitive, and social influences in their causes and treatment. The number of children diagnosed with and treated for different psychological disorders has dramatically increased in the past three decades, but not without controversy (as discussed in Focus on Discovery 13.2 later in this chapter).

In this chapter, we discuss several of the disorders that are most likely to arise in childhood and adolescence. We consider first disorders involving inattention, impulsivity, and disruptive behavior, followed by depression and anxiety disorders. Finally, we discuss disorders involving problems in the acquisition of cognitive, language, or social skills. These include specific learning disorder, intellectual disability, and autism spectrum disorder (ASD).

Classification and Diagnosis of Childhood Disorders

Before making a diagnosis of a disorder in a child, clinicians must first consider what is typical for a particular age. Children who lie on the floor kicking and screaming when they don't get their way are assessed differently at age 2 than at age 7. The field of **developmental psychopathology** focuses on the disorders of childhood within the context of development over the life span, enabling us to identify behaviors that are considered appropriate at one stage but not at another. Childhood disorders included in DSM-5-TR are shown in **Figure 13.1**.

The more prevalent childhood disorders are often divided into two broad domains: externalizing disorders and internalizing disorders. **Externalizing disorders** are characterized by more outward-directed behaviors, such as aggressiveness, noncompliance, overactivity, and impulsiveness; the category includes attention-deficit/hyperactivity disorder, conduct disorder, and oppositional defiant disorder. **Internalizing disorders** are characterized by more inward-focused experiences and behaviors, such as depression, social withdrawal, and anxiety; the category includes childhood anxiety and mood disorders. Children and adolescents may exhibit symptoms from both domains, as was evident in the **Clinical Case of Eric**.

Focus on Discovery 13.1 discusses the possible role of culture in the prevalence of childhood disorders.

Externalizing Disorders: ADHD and Conduct Disorder

Attention-Deficit/Hyperactivity Disorder

The term *hyperactive* is familiar to most people, especially parents and teachers. The child who is constantly in motion—tapping fingers, jiggling legs, poking others for no apparent reason, talking out of turn, and fidgeting—is often called hyperactive. Often, these children have difficulty concentrating on the task at hand for an appropriate period of time. When such problems are severe and persistent enough, these children may meet the criteria for diagnosis of **attention-deficit/hyperactivity disorder (ADHD)**.

Focus on Discovery 13.1

The Role of Culture in Internalizing and Externalizing Behaviors

The values of a culture may play a role in whether a certain pattern of child behavior develops or is considered a problem. Studies have found that internalizing and externalizing problems are observed in children around the world (e.g., Rescorla, Achenbach, et al., 2011); there are more differences between the prevalences of the two types within a culture or society than there are among societies.

One study found that in Thailand, the children who were more commonly referred to mental health clinics for treatment were those with internalizing behavior problems such as fearfulness, whereas in the United States, the children referred for treatment were those with externalizing behavior problems such as aggressiveness

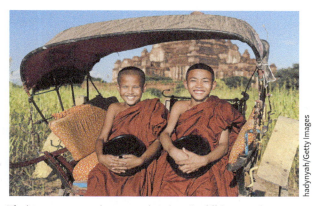

Thai teenagers serving as novices in a Buddhist temple. Buddhist culture may contribute to the relatively low prevalence of externalizing disorders in Thailand.

and hyperactivity (Weisz, Suwanlert, et al., 1987). The researchers attributed these differences to the fact that Buddhism, which disapproves of and discourages aggression, is widely practiced in Thailand. In other words, cultural sanctions against acting out in aggressive ways may have kept those behaviors from developing in Thailand at the rate they do in the United States. One of the issues in this study was that the researchers used only assessment measures that were based on norms from U.S. samples, leaving open the possibility that behavior differences between the two cultures were missed because they were not validly assessed for both cultures (see Chapter 3 for more discussion of culture and assessment).

Indeed, follow-up studies suggest that the behavior problems described in the same terms may not really be the same across Thai and U.S. cultures (Weisz, Weiss, et al., 2003, 2006). These studies compared specific behavior problems (e.g., somatic complaints, aggressive behavior) and the broad categories of internalizing and externalizing behaviors, using U.S. and Thai assessment measures. Internalizing and externalizing behaviors were the same in Thai and U.S. children, but more specific problems within those categories were not. Among boys, somatic complaints were seen consistently across cultures, but shyness was seen less consistently. Among girls, shyness was seen consistently across cultures, but verbal aggressive behavior was not.

These studies point to the importance of studying psychopathology across cultures. It is dangerous to assume that the measures we develop to assess psychological disorders in the United States will work as well in other cultures. As Weisz and colleagues point out, our theories about the causes of psychological disorders should take into account cultural variation in factors such as parenting practices, beliefs, and values and the ways in which parents report on their child's behavior problems. This remains an urgent and important challenge for our field.

Clinical Descriptions, Prevalence, and Prognosis of ADHD

Clinical Descriptions   What distinguishes the typical range of hyperactive behaviors from a diagnosable disorder? When these behaviors are extreme for a given developmental period, persistent across different situations, and linked to significant impairments in functioning, the diagnosis of ADHD may be appropriate (Hinshaw & Scheffler, 2014).

Many children with ADHD struggle to get along with peers and to establish friendships (Blachman & Hinshaw, 2002), perhaps because their behavior can be aggressive and intrusive and perhaps also because of the stigma associated with ADHD (Mikami, Miller, & Lerner, 2019). Although these children are usually friendly and talkative, they often miss subtle social cues—failing to notice, for example, when other children are tiring of their constant jiggling. Unfortunately, children with ADHD often overestimate their ability to navigate social situations with peers (Hoza, Murray-Close, et al., 2010). A longitudinal study of children with and without ADHD who were followed up every year for 6 years found that poor social skills, aggressive behavior, and self-overestimation of performance in social situations all predicted problems with peers up to 6 years later. The researchers also found "vicious cycles" in the areas of poor social skills, aggressive behavior, and overestimation of one's social abilities, which predicted a decline in these abilities at the next follow-up, which in turn predicted greater problems with peers at the next follow-up (Murray-Close, Hoza, et al., 2010). Another longitudinal study of over 2,000 children assessed at ages 5, 7, 10, and 12 found that increases in ADHD symptoms predicted future increases in social isolation.

In another study, children were asked to exchange instant messages (IMs) with other children in what appeared to be an online chat room (Mikami, Huang-Pollack, et al., 2007). In reality, the children were interacting with four computer-simulated peers in the chat room, and all children got the same IMs from the simulated peers. The researchers evaluated the participants' messages and their reported experiences of the chat room elicited during subsequent interviews. Children with ADHD were more likely to send IMs that were hostile and off the topic than were children without ADHD, and children's chat room experiences were related to other measures of social skills difficulties, suggesting that the ability to interact even when the interaction is not face to face is impaired among children with ADHD.

Defining Symptoms of Attention-Deficit/Hyperactivity Disorder

ADHD involves symptoms of inattention and/or hyperactivity-impulsivity that interfere with school, work, or relationships. These symptoms and behaviors don't fit with what is expected at a particular age or developmental level:

A. Manifestations of inattention could include making careless mistakes, not listening well, not following instructions, being easily distracted, or being forgetful in daily activities

B. Manifestations of hyperactivity-impulsivity could include fidgeting, running about inappropriately (in adults, restlessness), acting as if "driven by a motor," interrupting or intruding, or nonstop talking

ADHD in DSM-5-TR and Comorbidities   In DSM-5-TR, symptoms must begin before age 12 and take place in two or more settings (e.g., home, school, after-school care, work). For children, six symptoms are needed for the diagnosis to be made; for adults, five symptoms are needed. DSM-5-TR includes three specifiers to indicate which symptoms predominate:

1. Predominantly inattentive presentation: children whose problems are primarily those of poor attention

2. Predominantly hyperactive-impulsive presentation: children whose difficulties result primarily from hyperactive/impulsive behavior

3. Combined presentation: children who have both sets of problems

Most children with ADHD meet the criteria for the combined specifier. Children with the predominantly inattentive specifier have more difficulties with focused attention.

ADHD and conduct disorder (discussed later in this chapter) frequently co-occur and have some features in common (Beauchaine, Hinshaw, & Pang, 2010). There are some differences, however. ADHD is associated more with off-task behavior in school, cognitive and achievement deficits, and a better long-term prognosis.

Substance use disorders, particularly those involving nicotine or illegal substances, co-occur with ADHD (Howard, Kennedy, et al., 2020; Lee, Humphreys, et al., 2011). Internalizing disorders, such as anxiety and depression, also frequently co-occur with ADHD (Hechtman, Swanson, et al., 2016). A longitudinal study of girls with ADHD found that young women who had experienced childhood maltreatment were more likely than those who had not been maltreated as children to experience internalizing disorders, as well as to attempt suicide and engage in self-harm (Guendelman, Owens, et al., 2016). In addition, about 15–30% of children with ADHD have a learning disorder (DuPaul, Gormley, & Laracy, 2013).

Prevalence   The prevalence of ADHD is between 7% to 11% (Merikangas, He, et al., 2010; Noordermeer & Oosterlaan, 2023). Results of a recent meta-analysis

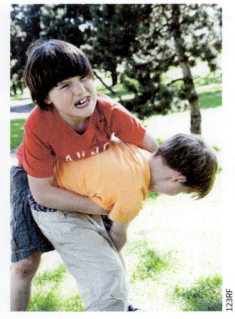

Aggression is not uncommon among boys with ADHD, and it contributes to their being rejected by peers.

indicate that the prevalence of ADHD is higher in Black youth than White youth (Cénat, Blaiss-Rochette, et al., 2021).

A nationally representative study conducted by the Centers for Disease Control and Prevention (CDC) reported a prevalence rate of 11% in 2011 (Visser, Danielson, et al., 2014). By contrast, a study from one large health care system in California reported a prevalence rate of just over 3% (Getahun, Jacobsen, et al., 2013). Why the difference in rates? Several explanations are possible, suggesting that the increase is due to factors other than an actual increase in the disorder. For example, most children receive a diagnosis after a brief visit with a pediatrician, but correct diagnoses require careful and thorough assessments (Hinshaw & Scheffler, 2014). Thus, many children may be getting the diagnosis when it is not warranted. In addition, DSM-5 changed the criteria such that symptoms must appear before age 12 compared to before age 7 in DSM-IV; it is likely that more children now meet the DSM-5 criteria who may have been excluded from DSM-IV.

Sex Differences   Evidence indicates that ADHD is two to three times more common in boys than in girls (Kessler, Avenevoli, et al., 2012; Merikangas et al., 2010), and for years ADHD studies focused mostly on boys. Two groups of researchers have conducted large and long-term prospective studies of ADHD in girls that have greatly increased our understanding of the development course of ADHD in girls and young women. Here are some of the key findings about girls and young women with ADHD (Biederman & Faraone, 2004; Biederman, Petty, et al., 2010; Hinshaw, 2002; Hinshaw, Carte, et al., 2002; Hinshaw, Owens, et al., 2006, 2012; Owens & Hinshaw, 2019; Owens, Zalecki, et al., 2017).

For example, girls with ADHD were more likely to have internalizing symptoms (anxiety, depression) than were girls without ADHD, and this remained true 16 years after initial diagnosis. Girls with ADHD exhibited several neuropsychological deficits, particularly in executive functioning (e.g., planning, solving problems), more often than girls without ADHD. However, boys and girls with ADHD show the same level of impairment in executive functioning (Loyer Carbonneau, Demers, et al., 2021). In addition, girls with ADHD are less likely to exhibit hyperactivity than boys with ADHD (Loyer Carbonneau et al., 2021).

By early adulthood, girls with ADHD preferred online social interactions (e.g., Facebook) over actual interactions, but the quality of their online Facebook interactions was not as rich (e.g., fewer friends, less support from friends; Mikami, Szwedo, et al., 2015).

Young women with ADHD were more likely than young women without ADHD to have an unplanned pregnancy, due to greater rates of risky sexual behavior in adolescence, which were in turn predicted by lower academic achievement and greater substance use in earlier adolescence.

ADHD in Adulthood   At one time, it was thought that ADHD simply went away as children entered adolescence. However, this belief has been challenged by numerous longitudinal studies (Barkley, Fischer, et al., 2002; Lee, Lahey, et al., 2008; Owens et al., 2017). Although some people show reduced severity of symptoms in adolescence and early adulthood, 65–80% of children with ADHD still have symptoms associated with impairments in adolescence (Biederman, Monuteaux, et al., 2006; Hinshaw et al., 2006; Lahey, Lee, et al., 2016). **Table 13.1** provides a sample of behaviors that are found more often among adolescents with ADHD than among adolescents without it (Barkley, DuPaul, & McMurray, 1990). Many children with ADHD do not appear to take a "hit" with respect to academic achievement, however—many studies indicate that their achievement is within the average range for both adolescent boys (Lee et al., 2008) and girls (Hinshaw et al., 2006).

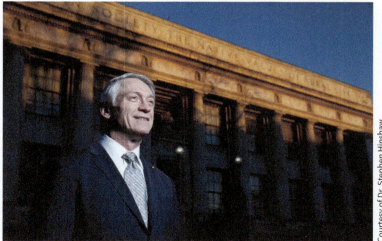

Stephen Hinshaw, a renowned developmental psychopathology researcher and expert on mental illness stigma, is conducting one of the largest ongoing studies of girls with ADHD.

Courtesy of Dr. Stephen Hinshaw

TABLE 13.1 Behaviors in Adolescents with and Without ADHD

Behavior	Percentage of Adolescents Who Show This Behavior	
	With ADHD	Without ADHD
Blurts out answers	65.0	10.6
Is easily distracted	82.1	15.2
Doesn't complete task before moving to another	77.2	16.7
Doesn't sustain attention	79.7	16.7
Doesn't follow instructions	83.7	12.1
Doesn't listen to others well	80.5	15.2
Engages in physically dangerous activities	37.4	3.0
Fidgets	73.2	10.6
Finds it hard to play quietly	39.8	7.6
Gets out of seat often	60.2	3.0
Interrupts others	65.9	10.6
Loses things needed for tasks	62.6	12.1
Talks a lot	43.9	6.1

Source: Adapted from Barkley, DuPaul, & McMurray (1990).

In early adulthood, more than half of those who were diagnosed with ADHD as children continue to exhibit symptoms associated with impairment in several domains (Cheung, Rijdijk, et al., 2015; Faraone, Biederman, & Mick, 2005; Hechtman et al., 2016; Owens et al., 2017). For example, in a large prospective study of girls with ADHD, 57% of girls diagnosed with ADHD at ages 6–12 continued to meet the diagnostic criteria 16 years later, and 74% of the girls continued to exhibit ADHD symptoms. Unfortunately, the young women who continued to meet ADHD diagnostic criteria in their mid-20s exhibited difficulties with work, educational achievement, and social functioning (Owens et al., 2017). Another prospective study of over 350 adults who were diagnosed with ADHD as children found that by age 30, these people were doing worse financially (i.e., earning less and more likely to be financially dependent upon their parents) than a comparable group who did not receive an ADHD diagnosis in childhood. This difference in financial functioning at age 30 was found even if the adults were not currently experiencing symptoms (Pelham, Page, et al., 2020).

Causes of ADHD

Genetic Influences
Substantial evidence indicates that genetics plays a role in ADHD (Faraone & Larsson, 2019; Thapar, 2018). Adoption studies (Sprich, Biederman, et al., 2000) and twin studies (Burt, 2009a; Larsson, Chang, et al., 2014) indicate that ADHD has a genetic component, with heritability estimates as high as 0.70–0.80 (Thapar, 2018). As with nearly all the disorders we cover in the book, many genes contribute to ADHD, making the search for them all the more difficult. In addition, several of these genes are not specific to ADHD, and thus the set of genes or genetic mutations that contribute to ADHD vulnerability may also be part of the genetic vulnerability for other psychological disorders (Andersson, Tuvblad, et al., 2020; Demontis, Walters, et al., 2019; Faraone & Larsson, 2019; Hamshere, Langley, et al., 2013).

Brain and Environmental Influences
Studies show that brain structure, function, and connectivity differ in children with and without ADHD, particularly in areas of the brain linked to the neurotransmitter dopamine. A large meta-analysis of structural brain imaging studies found that children with ADHD had

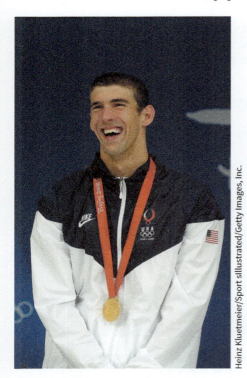

Michael Phelps won more Olympic medals (28) than any other athlete in history. He won his medals (23 gold, 3 silver, and 2 bronze) in swimming. He also struggled with ADHD as a child.

Heinz Kluetmeier/Sport sIllustrated/Getty Images, Inc.

smaller volumes (sizes) of the amygdala, hippocampus, nucleus accumbens, caudate nucleus, and putamen (Hoogman, Bralten, et al., 2017). A meta-analysis of 55 functional brain-imaging studies found that children with ADHD exhibited less activation in frontal areas of the brain (Cortese, Kelly, et al., 2012). Moreover, children with ADHD perform poorly on neuropsychological tests that rely on the frontal lobes, such as selective attention (i.e., selecting to focus on one thing and not another; Mueller, Hong, et al., 2017), working memory (i.e., how much can be held in the mind at any given time while doing a task; Fair, Bathula, et al., 2012), and inhibition of behavioral responses (Faraone, Asherson, et al., 2015; Barkley, 1997). This evidence provides support for the theory that a deficit in the frontal cortex may be related to the disorder (Matthews, Nigg, & Fair, 2014; Nigg & Casey, 2005).

Perinatal and Prenatal Factors   Perinatal and prenatal complications are also risk factors for ADHD, such as fetal distress, pregnancy complications, or a mother's high blood pressure during pregnancy (Noordermeer & Oosterlaan, 2023). Low birth weight is another predictor of the development of ADHD (Franz, Bolat, et al., 2018).

Environmental Toxins   Research has found that elements of the diet, particularly additives, may influence ADHD symptoms for a subset of children. Two meta-analyses reported small effect sizes for artificial food coloring on hyperactive behavior among children with ADHD (Nigg, Lewis, et al., 2012; Schnab & Trinh, 2004).

Some evidence suggests that higher blood levels of lead may be associated to a small degree with symptoms of ADHD (Nigg, Elmore, et al., 2016; Nilsen & Tulve, 2020). Given the unfortunate frequency with which children are exposed to low levels of lead, investigators continue to examine how lead exposure might play a role, perhaps by influencing other cognitive abilities.

Nicotine—specifically, maternal smoking—may play a role in the development of ADHD. A review of 24 studies examining the association between maternal smoking and ADHD found that exposure to tobacco in utero was associated with ADHD symptoms (Linnet, Dalsgaard, et al., 2003). However, an interesting study distinguishes correlation from causation. Thapar and colleagues (2009) examined ADHD symptoms in the offspring of two groups of mothers who were regular smokers when pregnant. One group of smoking mothers delivered babies that were not genetically related to them (e.g., a surrogate mother delivering a genetically unrelated baby for another family); the other group of mothers delivered babies that were genetically related to them. The researchers reasoned that if maternal smoking during pregnancy was an important factor in ADHD, smoking ought to be related to ADHD symptoms in the offspring from both groups of mothers. By contrast, if genetic factors were important, then the association between smoking and ADHD symptoms ought to be higher in the offspring of genetically related mothers. They found that ADHD symptoms were related to maternal smoking in both groups, but the association was significantly higher in the group of children whose genetically related mothers smoked during pregnancy. These findings suggest that smoking might not be a causal factor by itself but that it is related to other genetic factors or maternal behavior and psychopathology that might increase the risk of ADHD (Faraone, Banaschewski, et al., 2021).

Family Factors in ADHD   Family factors such as parenting practices may contribute to maintenance or exacerbation of symptoms and to consequences of ADHD; however, there is little evidence to suggest that families cause ADHD (Hinshaw, 2018; Sellers, Harold, et al., 2019). The relationship between parenting and child behavior is bidirectional. For example, parents of children with ADHD may try to manage problem behaviors by issuing more commands; these children may in turn be less compliant, thus escalating negative interactions between parents and children (Wells, Epstein, et al., 2000).

It is also important to consider parents' own histories of ADHD. As noted earlier, ADHD appears to have a substantial genetic component. Thus, it is not surprising that many parents of children with ADHD have ADHD themselves. In one study that examined couples' parenting practices with their ADHD children, fathers who had a diagnosis of ADHD were found to be less effective parents, suggesting that parental psychopathology may make parenting more difficult (Arnold, O'Leary, & Edwards, 1997).

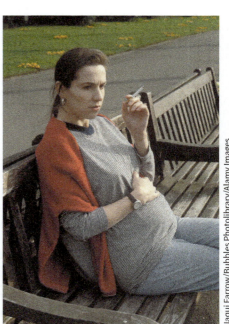

Children born to mothers who smoked cigarettes during pregnancy have an increased risk for ADHD.

Jaqui Farrow/Bubbles Photolibrary/Alamy Images

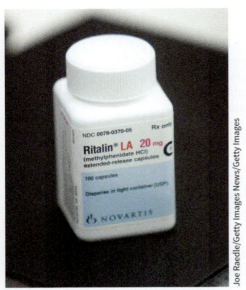

Ritalin is a commonly prescribed and effective drug treatment for ADHD.

Joe Raedle/Getty Images News/Getty Images

Treatment of ADHD

ADHD is typically treated with medication and with behavioral therapies based on operant conditioning principles.

Stimulant Medications

Stimulant medications, such as methylphenidate (Ritalin), have been prescribed for ADHD since the early 1960s. Other medications used to treat ADHD include Adderall, Concerta, and Strattera. In 2022, 15% of seniors in high school reported ever having used prescribed medication for ADHD (Miech, Johnston, et al., 2023). The prescription of these medications often continues into adolescence and adulthood because of accumulating evidence that the symptoms of ADHD do not usually disappear with the passage of time. During the pandemic, prescribed and nonprescribed use of medications for ADHD increased (McCabe, Shulenberg, et al., 2023; Miech et al., 2023). In October 2022, the U.S. Food and Drug Administration announced a shortage of Adderall (https://www.fda.gov/drugs/drug-safety-and-availability/fda-announces-shortage-adderall).

The drugs used to treat ADHD reduce disruptive behavior and impulsivity and improve ability to focus attention (Hinshaw & Scheffler, 2014). A large meta-analysis of randomized controlled trials found that stimulants were more effective than placebos (Catalá-López, Hutton, et al., 2017).

The Multimodal Treatment of ADHD (MTA) study is an influential and well-designed randomized controlled trial of treatments for ADHD. Conducted at six different sites for 14 months with nearly 600 children with ADHD, the study compared standard community-based care with three other treatments: (1) medication alone, (2) medication plus intensive behavioral treatment involving both parents and teachers, and (3) intensive behavioral treatment alone. Over the 14-month period, children receiving medication alone had fewer ADHD symptoms than children receiving intensive behavioral treatment alone. The combined treatment was slightly superior to the medication alone and had the advantage of not requiring as high a dosage of Ritalin to reduce ADHD symptoms. In addition, the combined treatment yielded improved functioning in areas such as social skills more than did medication alone. The medication alone and the combined treatment were superior to community-based care, although behavioral treatment alone was not (MTA Cooperative Group, 1999a, 1999b).

Despite the initially promising findings from the MTA study, additional follow-ups of this study have not been quite as encouraging, at least where medication is concerned (Hinshaw & Arnold, 2015). Importantly, all the children maintained the gains made during the 14-month treatment, even as they all returned to receiving standard community care, and this was true at the 3-, 6-, and 8-year follow-ups. However, children in the medication alone group or the combined treatment group were no longer doing better than children who received intensive behavioral treatment or standard community care at the 3-year follow-up (Jensen, Arnold, et al., 2007) or the 6- and 8-year follow-ups (Molina, Hinshaw, et al., 2009). In other words, the relatively superior effects of medication that were observed in the combined treatment and medication alone groups did not persist beyond the study, at least for some of the children (Swanson, Hinshaw, et al., 2007).

Does this mean that medication does not work? Not necessarily. The MTA study demonstrated that carefully prescribed and managed stimulant medication is effective for children with ADHD. However, medication as it is administered in the community may not offer any benefits above and beyond other forms of treatment, according to these MTA follow-up studies.

These findings are important in light of the side effects that stimulant medication can have, such as transient loss of appetite, changes in weight, stomach pain, reduction in height, and sleep problems (Catalá-López et al., 2017; Greenhill, Swanson, et al., 2020). In 2006 and again in 2011, the FDA recommended but did not mandate that a "black box" warning, the strongest possible safety warning the FDA can issue for medications, about cardiovascular risks (e.g., heart attack) be added to the packaging of stimulant medications.

Psychological Treatment

Other treatments for ADHD involve parent training and changes in classroom management (Chronis, Jones, & Raggi, 2006; Hinshaw, 2018). These programs have demonstrated at least short-term success in improving both social and academic behavior. In these treatments, children's behavior is monitored at home and in school, and they are reinforced for behaving appropriately—for example, for remaining in their seats and working on assignments. Point systems and daily report cards (DRCs) are typical components of these programs. Children earn points or stars for behaving in certain ways; the children can then spend their earnings for rewards. The DRCs also allow parents to see how their child is doing in school. The focus of these programs is on improving academic work, completing household tasks, or learning specific social skills rather than on reducing ADHD symptoms. Parent-training programs are also effective, although it is unclear whether they improve children's behavior more than treatment with medication does (MTA Cooperative Group, 1999a, 1999b).

Findings from the MTA study indicate that intensive behavioral therapies can be very helpful to children with ADHD. In that study, some of the children participated in an intensive 8-week summer program that included several validated behavioral treatments. At the end of the summer program, children receiving the combined treatment had very few more significant improvements than children receiving the intensive behavioral treatment alone (Arnold, Elliott, et al., 2003; Pelham, Gnagy, et al., 2000). This finding suggests that intensive behavioral therapy may be as effective as Ritalin combined with less intensive behavioral therapy.

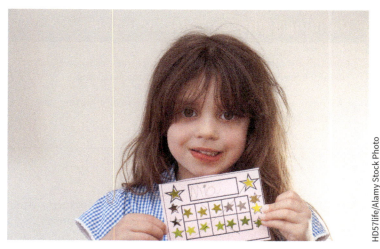

Point systems and star charts, which are common in classrooms, are particularly useful in the treatment of ADHD.

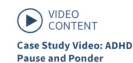

VIDEO CONTENT

Case Study Video: ADHD Pause and Ponder

Conduct Disorder

Before discussing the externalizing disorder known as conduct disorder, we will briefly discuss two other related disorders. These three disorders are in the DSM-5-TR chapter called "Disruptive, Impulse-Control, and Conduct Disorders."

Intermittent explosive disorder (IED) involves recurrent verbal or physical aggressive outbursts that are far out of proportion to the circumstances. What distinguishes IED from conduct disorder is that the aggression is impulsive and not preplanned toward other people (American Psychiatric Association, 2013). For example, a child with IED may have an aggressive outburst after not getting their way but would not plan aggressive retaliation.

Another DSM disorder, *oppositional defiant disorder* (ODD), is diagnosed if a child does not meet the criteria for conduct disorder—most especially, extreme physical aggressiveness—but exhibits such behaviors as losing his or her temper, arguing with adults, repeatedly refusing to comply with requests from adults, deliberately doing things to annoy others, and being angry, spiteful, touchy, or vindictive. The prevalence rate of ODD is around 8% (Kessler et al., 2012).

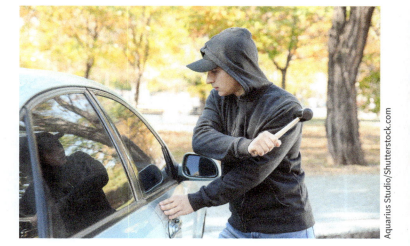

Conduct disorder is diagnosed among those who are aggressive, steal, lie, and vandalize property.

ODD and ADHD frequently occur together, but ODD is different from ADHD in that the defiant behavior is not thought to arise from attentional deficits or impulsiveness. One manifestation of difference is that children with ODD are more deliberate in their unruly behavior than children with ADHD. Although conduct disorder is three to four times more common among boys than among girls, research suggests that boys are only slightly more likely to have ODD, and some studies find no difference in prevalence rates for ODD between boys and girls (Loeber, Burke, et al., 2000; Merikangas et al., 2010).

Clinical Description, Prevalence, and Prognosis of Conduct Disorder   Perhaps more than any other childhood disorder, **conduct disorder** is defined by the impact of the child's behavior on people and surroundings.

Defining Symptoms of Conduct Disorder

Conduct disorder involves a pattern of repeated destructive and harmful behavior that can take different forms, including:

A. Aggressive behavior (e.g., bullying, physically hurting animals or people)

B. Destroying property (e.g., vandalizing a building, setting a fire)

C. Lying or stealing (e.g., shoplifting, breaking into a house and stealing items, lying about behavior)

D. Breaking rules (e.g., skipping school, missing curfew)

Clinical Descriptions   Conduct disorder involves aggressive behaviors (e.g., physical cruelty to people or animals), serious rule violations (e.g., truancy), property destruction, and deceitfulness. Often the behavior is marked by callousness, viciousness, and lack of remorse.

DSM-5-TR includes a "limited prosocial emotions" diagnostic specifier for children who have what are referred to as callous and unemotional traits. These traits are characteristics such as shallow emotions and a lack of feelings of remorse, empathy, and guilt. A longitudinal study found that children with high levels of conduct problems and high levels of callous and unemotional traits had more problems with symptoms, peers, and families than did children with conduct problems but low levels of callous and unemotional traits (Fontaine, McCrory, et al., 2011). A comprehensive review of callous and unemotional traits in children and adolescence revealed that these traits are associated with a more severe course, more cognitive deficits, more antisocial behavior, poorer response to treatment, and perhaps distinct etiologies (Frick, Ray, et al., 2014).

Comorbidities and Longitudinal Course   Many children with conduct disorder display other problems, such as substance abuse and internalizing disorders. Some research suggests that conduct disorder precedes substance use problems (Nock, Kazdin, et al., 2006), but other findings suggest that conduct disorder and substance use occur concomitantly, with the two conditions exacerbating each other (Loeber et al., 2000).

Anxiety and depression are common among children with conduct disorder, with comorbidity estimates varying from 15% to 45% (Loeber & Keenan, 1994; Loeber et al., 2000). Evidence suggests that conduct disorder precedes depression and most anxiety disorders, with the exceptions of specific phobias and social anxiety, which appear to precede conduct disorder (Nock et al., 2006).

How early does conduct disorder begin? Studies estimate that as many as 7% of preschool children exhibit the symptoms of conduct disorder (Egger & Angold, 2006). One longitudinal study assessed a group of preschool children at age 3 and again at age 6 (Rolon-Arroyo, Arnold, & Harvey, 2013). Parents were interviewed using diagnostic interviews at the two time points. The researchers found that conduct disorder symptoms at age 3 predicted conduct disorder symptoms at age 6, even when symptoms of ADHD and ODD were controlled for. These findings suggest that assessing conduct disorder early is important because these symptoms are not just manifestations of typical disruptive behaviors related to development.

Moffitt (1993) theorized that two different courses of conduct problems should be distinguished. Some people seem to show a life-course-persistent pattern of antisocial behavior, beginning to show conduct problems by age 3 and continuing to commit serious transgressions into adulthood. Other conduct problems are adolescence-limited—the people have typical childhoods, engage in high levels of antisocial behavior during adolescence, and have typical and nonproblematic adulthoods. Moffitt proposed that the adolescence-limited pattern of antisocial behavior is the result of a maturity gap between the adolescent's physical

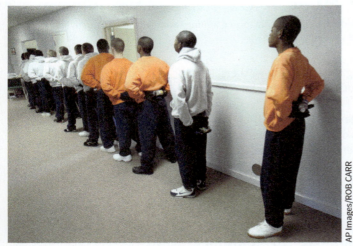

AP Images/ROB CARR

Children with the life-course-persistent type of conduct disorder continue to have trouble with the law into their mid-20s and beyond

maturation and their opportunity to assume adult responsibilities and obtain the rewards usually accorded such behavior.

Cumulative evidence supports this distinction across cultures (Hinshaw & Lee, 2003). The original sample from which Moffitt and colleagues made the life-course-persistent and adolescence-limited distinction was a sample of over 1,000 people from Dunedin, New Zealand, who were assessed every 2 or 3 years from age 3 to age 32. Both boys and girls with the life-course-persistent form of conduct disorder had an early onset of antisocial behavior that persisted through adolescence and into adulthood (Moffitt, 2007).

Those who were classified as life-course-persistent continued to have the most severe problems, including psychopathology, poorer physical health, lower socioeconomic status, lower levels of education, partner and child abuse, and violent behavior, at age 32; this was true for both men and women (Odgers, Moffitt, et al., 2008).

Interestingly, those classified as adolescence-limited, who were expected to "grow out" of their aggressive and antisocial behavior, continued to have troubles with substance use, impulsivity, crime, and overall mental health in their mid-20s (Moffitt, Caspi, et al., 2002). By age 32, women with the adolescent-onset type of conduct problems were not having difficulties with violent behavior, but men still were. However, both men and women continued to have substance use problems, economic problems, and physical health problems (Odgers et al., 2008).

Prevalence   Estimates suggest that conduct disorder is fairly common, with prevalence rates between 5% and 6% (Kessler et al., 2012; Merikangas et al., 2010). Like ADHD, conduct disorder is more common in boys than in girls. The adolescence-limited type is more common than the life-course-persistent type for boys and girls (Moore, Silberg, et al., 2017; Odgers et al., 2008).

Prognosis   The prognosis for children diagnosed with conduct disorder is mixed. Research results show that men and women with the life-course-persistent type of conduct disorder will likely continue to have all sorts of problems in adulthood, including violent and antisocial behavior. However, conduct disorder in childhood does not inevitably lead to antisocial behavior in adulthood. For example, a longitudinal study indicated that about half of boys with conduct disorder did not fully meet the criteria for the diagnosis at a later assessment (1 to 4 years later), although almost all of them continued to demonstrate some conduct problems (Lahey, Loeber, et al., 2005).

Causes of Conduct Disorder

Multiple influences are involved in the causes of conduct disorder, including genetic, neurobiological, psychological, and social factors that interact in a complex manner (**Figure 13.2**). The evidence favors causes that include heritable temperamental characteristics that interact with other neurobiological difficulties (e.g., neuropsychological deficits) and with a host of environmental factors (e.g., parenting, school performance, peer influences) (Beauchaine & McNulty, 2013; Hinshaw & Lee, 2003).

Genetic Influences

Heritability plays a part in conduct disorder, but some of the genetic influences are shared with other disorders, including ADHD and depression, and some of the genetic influences are specific to conduct disorder or antisocial behavior (Lahey, Van Hulle, et al., 2011; Lahey & Waldman, 2012; Rhee & Waldman, 2002). Like other disorders discussed in this text, we know that single genes are not likely to tell the genetic story for any psychological disorder and that genes do their work via the environment (Hyde & Dotterer, 2022; Taylor & Kim-Cohen, 2007).

Distinguishing types of conduct problems may help to clarify findings on the heritability of conduct disorder (Burt, 2012). Evidence from twin studies indicates that aggressive behavior (e.g., cruelty to animals, fighting, destroying property) is more heritable than other rule-breaking behavior (e.g., stealing, running away, truancy) (Burt, 2009b; Burt, Klump, et al., 2016). In a study of twins ages 6–10, Burt and colleagues found that the genetic influence of rule-breaking behavior varied depending on

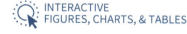
INTERACTIVE FIGURES, CHARTS, & TABLES

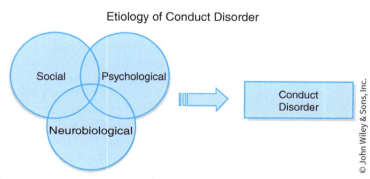

FIGURE 13.2 Neurobiological, psychological, and social influences all play a role in conduct disorder.

© John Wiley & Sons, Inc.

the wealth of the neighborhood (Burt et al., 2016). Specifically, genetics played more of a role in rule-breaking behavior for twins raised in wealthier neighborhoods than for twins raised in low-income neighborhoods. This finding reveals an important gene–environment interaction and underscores the impact that poverty can have on childhood misconduct.

Other evidence indicates that the combination of conduct problems and callous and unemotional traits is more highly heritable than conduct problems alone (Moore, Blair, et al., 2019). A clever longitudinal adoption study examined the development of callous and unemotional traits in very young children (Hyde, Waller, et al., 2016). In this study, callous and unemotional behaviors were measured in over 500 adopted children at age 18 months and again at 27 months. The researchers also measured antisocial behaviors in biological mothers and adoptive mothers. Children of biological mothers who had exhibited severe antisocial behavior were more likely to exhibit callous and unemotional behaviors, but not if the adoptive mother gave a lot of positive reinforcement. In other words, parenting of the adoptive mother appeared to exert a buffer against the genetic propensity passed down from the biological mother. The same thing was found in a twin study where lower heritability of callous and unemotional traits was observed in families with more parental warmth (Tomlinson, Hyde, et al., 2022).

Finally, evidence suggests that the age when antisocial and aggressive behavior problems begin is related to heritability. For example, aggressive and antisocial behaviors that begin in childhood, as in the case of Moffitt's life-course-persistent type, are more heritable than similar behaviors that begin in adolescence (Burt & Neiderhiser, 2009; Taylor, Iacono, & McGue, 2000).

Neurobiological Influences   Neuroimaging studies of children with conduct disorder have revealed deficits in regions of the brain that support emotion, particularly empathetic responses. For example, children with callous and unemotional traits have difficulty perceiving distress (fear, sadness, or pain) and happiness on the faces of others but do not have trouble perceiving anger (Marsh & Blair, 2008). In addition, these children show reduced activation in brain regions associated with emotion and reward, such as the amygdala, ventral striatum, and prefrontal cortex (Alegria, Radua, & Rubia, 2016; Blair, 2013; Cardinale, Breeden, et al., 2018). Children with callous and unemotional traits also do not learn to associate their behavior with reward or punishment as easily as do other children, and this difficulty is associated with dysfunction in brain regions associated with emotion (e.g., amygdala) and reward (e.g., ventral striatum) (Blair, 2013).

Psychological Influences   An important part of typical child development is the growth of social emotions and moral awareness—the acquisition of a sense of what is right and wrong and the ability, even desire, to abide by rules and norms. Most people refrain from hurting others not only because it is illegal but also because it would make them feel guilty. Children with conduct disorder, particularly those with callous and unemotional traits, seem to be deficient in this moral awareness, lacking remorse for their wrongdoing (Blair, 2013; Frick et al., 2014; Waller, Wagner, et al., 2020). In adulthood, these traits figure prominently in antisocial personality disorder and psychopathy (discussed in Chapter 15), and are considered a risk factor for adult APD and psychopathy (Hyde & Dotterer, 2022).

The relationship between parenting and callous, unemotional traits appears to be bidirectional. Parenting can contribute to the exacerbation of callous and unemotional traits (Waller & Hyde, 2018). In twin studies, researchers have disentangled heritability from parenting. Specifically, they examined a group of MZ (identical) twins and found differences in callous and unemotional traits, aggressive behavior, and rule breaking between twins that were associated with differential parenting. That is, the twin who received harsher parenting was more likely than the other twin to exhibit callous and unemotional traits as well as aggressive behavior and rule breaking (Burt, Clark, et al., 2021; Waller, Hyde, et al., 2018). These finding suggest that callous and unemotional traits may develop, in part, from nonshared environmental factors (see Chapter 2) like parenting.

Callous and unemotional traits can also contribute to decreases in parental warmth. Results from a large longitudinal study showed callous and unemotional traits predicted a lessening in parental warmth over time (Vaughan, Frick, et al., 2022). Adolescents with these traits are less likely to show warmth toward others, including parents, and over time, this may influence how parents respond to their children. Unfortunately, this study also found that more parental warmth did not lead to reductions in these traits over time.

The work of Kenneth Dodge and colleagues provides a social-cognitive perspective on aggressive behavior (and, by extension, conduct disorder). In one of his early studies (Dodge & Frame, 1982), Dodge found that the social information processing of aggressive children had a hostile bias; these children interpreted ambiguous acts, such as being bumped in line, as evidence of hostile intent. Such perceptions may lead these children to retaliate aggressively for actions that may not have been intended as provocative. This can create a vicious cycle: Their peers, remembering these aggressive behaviors, may tend to be aggressive more often in return, further angering the already aggressive children (see **Figure 13.3**).

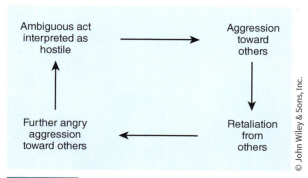

FIGURE 13.3 **Dodge's cognitive theory of aggression. The interpretation of ambiguous acts as hostile is part of a vicious cycle that includes aggression toward and from others.**

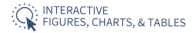
INTERACTIVE
FIGURES, CHARTS, & TABLES

Peer Influences   Investigations of how peers influence aggressive and antisocial behavior in children have focused on two broad areas: (1) acceptance or rejection by peers and (2) affiliation with delinquent peers. Studies have shown that being rejected by peers is causally related to aggressive behavior, particularly in combination with ADHD (Hinshaw & Scheffler, 2014). Other studies have shown that being rejected by peers as early as 1st grade can predict later aggressive behavior, even after prior levels of aggressive behavior are controlled for (Coie & Dodge, 1998; Miller-Johnson, Coie, et al., 2002). Additional longitudinal evidence suggests that children who are more prone to react negatively to situations are in turn more likely to be rejected by peers and subsequently more likely to engage in antisocial behavior (Buil, van Lier, et al., 2017).

Associating with other delinquent peers also increases the likelihood of delinquent behavior (Forgatch, Patterson, et al., 2009), perhaps due to modeling or even to being coerced by peers (Dishion, Kim, & Tien, 2015). Do children with conduct disorder choose to associate with like-minded peers, thus continuing their path of antisocial behavior (a social selection view), or does simply being around delinquent peers help initiate antisocial behavior (a social influence view)? Studies examining gene–environment interactions have shed light on this question, and the answer appears to be that both views are correct (Burt, 2022). That is, we know that genetic influences are at play in conduct disorder, and these influences in turn play a role in encouraging children with conduct disorder to select more deviant peers to associate with. However, environmental influences, particularly neighborhood (e.g., socioeconomic disadvantage, exposure to violence in the neighborhood) and family (e.g., parental monitoring) factors, play a role in whether children associate with deviant peers, and this in turn influences and exacerbates conduct disorder (Jennings, Perez, & Reingle Gonzales, 2018; Kendler, Jacobson, et al., 2008).

Treatment of Conduct Disorder

The treatment of conduct disorder appears to be most effective when it addresses the multiple systems involved in the life of a child (family, peers, school, and neighborhood).

Family Interventions   Some of the most promising approaches to treating conduct disorder involve intervening with the parents and family of the child. In addition, evidence suggests that intervening early, if even just briefly, can make an impact. An intervention called the *family checkup* (FCU) has been shown to have positive effects in preventing conduct problems and aggression in children. FCU involves three meetings to get to know, assess, and provide feedback to parents regarding their children and parenting practices. In the first randomized controlled trial (Shaw, Dishion, et al., 2006), FCU was offered to families with toddlers who were at high risk of developing conduct problems (based on the presence of conduct or substance abuse problems in parents or early signs of conduct problems in the child). This brief, three-session intervention was associated with less disruptive behavior than was no treatment, even 2 years after the intervention. Additional trials (Dishion, Shaw, et al., 2008) have confirmed the effectiveness of the FCU, showing that the preventive intervention is associated with less aggressive behavior and conduct problems in the early years of school (Dishion, Brennan, et al., 2014).

Gerald Patterson and colleagues developed a very successful behavioral program called **parent management training (PMT)**, in which parents are taught to modify their responses to their children so that prosocial rather than antisocial behavior is consistently

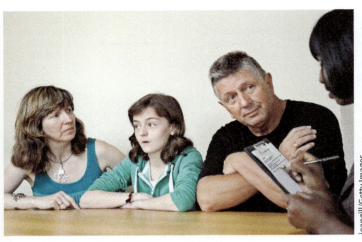

Parent management training can be effective in treating conduct disorder.

rewarded. Parents are taught to use techniques such as positive reinforcement when the child exhibits positive behaviors and time-out and loss of privileges for aggressive or antisocial behaviors.

This treatment has been modified by others, but, in general, it is the most efficacious intervention for children with conduct disorder and oppositional defiant disorder. Both parents' and teachers' reports of children's behavior and direct observation of behavior at home and at school support the program's effectiveness (Kazdin, 2005; Patterson, 1982). PMT has been shown to alter parent–child interactions, which in turn is associated with a decrease in antisocial and aggressive behavior (Dishion & Andrews, 1995). PMT has been adapted for families in many different cultures and countries (Dishion, Forgatch, et al., 2016), and it has been adapted to focus on callous and unemotional traits (Fleming, Neo, et al., 2022).

Multisystemic Treatment　Another treatment for conduct disorder is **multisystemic treatment (MST)** (Henggeler, Schoenwald, et al., 2009). MST involves delivering intensive and comprehensive therapy services in the community, targeting the adolescent, the family, the school, and, in some cases, the peer group (**Figure 13.4**). The treatment is based on the view that conduct problems are influenced by multiple factors within the family as well as interactions between the family and other social systems.

The strategies used by MST therapists are varied, incorporating behavioral, cognitive, family-systems, and case-management techniques. The therapy's uniqueness lies in emphasizing individual and family strengths, identifying the social context for the conduct problems, using present-focused and action-oriented interventions, and using interventions that require daily or weekly efforts by family members. Treatment is provided in homes, schools, or local recreational centers to maximize the chances that improvement will carry through into the regular daily lives of children and their families. MST has been shown to be effective in several studies around the world (Curtis, Ronan, & Borduin, 2004; Henggeler, 2011).

INTERACTIVE
FIGURES, CHARTS, & TABLES

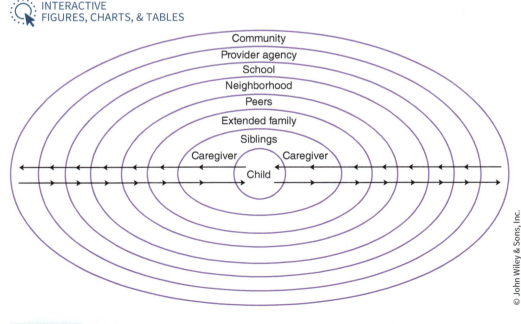

FIGURE 13.4　In multisystemic treatment (MST), many different factors are considered in developing a child's treatment, including family, school, community, and peers.

Prevention Programs   It would be ideal if we could prevent conduct disorder from ever developing. Can this be done? One study followed a group of children until they were age 25 and involved a prevention program called Fast Track. Findings of the Conduct Problems Prevention Research Group (CPPRG), the group of researchers who developed, implemented, and evaluated Fast Track, showed impressive reductions in later psychopathology (Conduct Problems Prevention Research Group, 2020).

The study evaluated 10,000 kindergarten children from four low-income, high-crime regions in the United States, and nearly 900 children who were exhibiting conduct problems were randomly assigned to either the Fast Track intervention or a control intervention. The Fast Track intervention was designed to help children academically, socially, and behaviorally, focusing on areas that are problematic in conduct disorder, including peer relationships, aggressive and disruptive behavior, social information processing, and parent–child relationships. The intervention was delivered over the course of 10 years in groups and at individual families' homes, with a more intensive treatment in years 1 to 5 and a less intensive treatment in years 6 to 10.

Results from the study showed that children who received the Fast Track intervention benefited. Some of the benefits lasted for many years. For example, at the 9th-grade and 12th-grade assessments, the children who had had the most severe problem behaviors at the baseline assessment in kindergarten and who had received Fast Track exhibited fewer delinquent behaviors and were less likely to have a diagnosis of conduct disorder or any externalizing disorder than children in the control group (CPPRG, 2010a, 2010b, 2011). The impact of Fast Track on reducing behavior problems was due, in part, to a decrease in the hostile attribution bias discussed earlier (Dodge & Godwin, 2013). By age 25, a full 8 years after the intervention ended, the young adults who had received the Fast Track intervention were less likely to have externalizing or internalizing psychopathology, substance use problems, or antisocial personality disorder. In addition, those young people were less likely to have been involved in violent crimes (Dodge, Bierman, et al., 2015). By age 34, women, but not men, who participated in Fast Track as girls were less likely to have depression or substance use problems (Rothenberg, Lansford, et al., 2023). These are indeed impressive results, and they suggest that intensive preventive interventions can make a positive impact in reducing later conduct disorder and antisocial behavior among children at risk (Dodge, 2020).

Quick Summary

ADHD and conduct disorder are referred to as externalizing disorders. They appear across cultures, although there are also differences in the manifestation of externalizing symptoms in different cultures. Both disorders are more common in boys than girls. A number of factors work together to cause attention-deficit/hyperactivity disorder (ADHD) and conduct disorder. Genetic factors play a particularly important role in ADHD but are also implicated in conduct disorder. Other risk factors for ADHD include low birth weight and maternal smoking. Family and peer variables are also important factors to consider, especially their interactions with genetic and neurobiological vulnerabilities. The most effective treatment for ADHD is a combination of stimulant medication and behavioral therapy. For conduct disorder, family-based treatments, such as parent management training (PMT), are effective, as are treatments that include multiple points for intervention, as in multisystemic treatment (MST). Prevention approaches, such as Fast Track, can also be helpful.

13.1 Check Your Knowledge

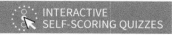
INTERACTIVE
SELF-SCORING QUIZZES

(Answers are at the end of the chapter.)
True or false?

1. The two broad categories of childhood psychopathology are internalizing disorders and externalizing disorders.

2. Young adult women who continue to meet the diagnostic criteria for ADHD are more likely to have internalizing and externalizing psychopathology than are young adult women without ADHD.

3. Dopamine has been investigated in ADHD, with respect to both genes and the brain.

4. The most effective treatment for ADHD is behavioral treatment without medication.

Answer the following questions.

5. Moffitt and colleagues have provided a good deal of evidence for two types of conduct disorder. The _____ type is associated with an early age of onset and continued problems into adolescence and adulthood. The adolescent-onset type begins in the teenage years and is hypothesized to remit by adulthood, though a recent follow-up study has not supported the idea that this type remits.

6. What are three problems that can co-occur with conduct disorder?

7. One successful treatment for conduct disorder that involves the family is called _____.

Internalizing Disorders: Depression and Anxiety Disorders

The internalizing disorders, which include depression and anxiety disorders, first begin in childhood or adolescence but are quite common in adults as well. Much richer descriptions of these disorders are presented in Chapter 5 (mood disorders) and Chapters 6 and 7 (anxiety disorders, obsessive-compulsive disorder, and trauma-related disorders). Here, we describe the ways in which the symptoms, causes, and treatments of these disorders are different for children than for adults. We present the lifetime prevalence rates of these disorders in Table 13.2 (Merikangas et al., 2010).

Depression

Clinical Descriptions, Prevalence, and Comorbidities of Depression in Childhood and Adolescence
There are both similarities and differences in the symptomatology of children and adults with major depressive disorder. Children and adolescents ages 7–17 and adults show the following symptoms: depressed mood, inability to experience pleasure, fatigue, concentration problems, and suicidal ideation. Children and adolescents differ from adults in showing more guilt but lower rates of early-morning wakefulness, early-morning depression, loss of appetite, and weight loss. As in adults, depression in children is recurrent. Longitudinal studies have demonstrated that both children and adolescents with major depression are likely to continue to exhibit significant depressive symptoms when assessed even 4 to 8 years later (Garber, Kelly, & Martin, 2002; Lewinsohn, Rohde, et al., 2000).

Prevalence rates for depression and anxiety are higher among racially minoritized youth (Anderson & Mayes, 2010), but there is also evidence to indicate that commonly used

TABLE 13.2	Lifetime Prevalence Rates of Mood and Anxiety Disorders in Adolescents	
Disorder	**Lifetime Prevalence Rate**
Depression (or dysthymia)	11.7%
Bipolar disorder (I or II)	2.9%
Specific phobia	19.3%
Social anxiety disorder	9.1%
Separation anxiety disorder	7.6%
Generalized anxiety disorder	2.2%
Posttraumatic stress disorder	5.0%

Source: Merikangas et al. (2010).

assessment measures, at least for depression, do not work the same across different race and ethnic groups (Vaughn-Coaxum, Mair, & Weisz, 2016). This suggests that the differences in prevalence rates may reflect a bias in our diagnostic and assessment tools.

The prevalence among adolescent girls (15.9%) is almost twice that among adolescent boys (7.7%), the same ratio as for adult depression (Merikangas et al., 2010). Interestingly, the sex difference does not occur before age 12 (Hankin, Abramson, et al., 1998). Unfortunately, the overall prevalence rates for depression have been increasing for over a decade; the COVID-19 pandemic exacerbated this trend. Between 2010 and 2017, depression rates in adolescents between the ages of 12 and 17 increased by 63%, with much of this increase found in girls (Twenge, Cooper, et al., 2019). Depression occurs in 2–3% of school-age children under age 12 (Costello, Erkanli, & Angold, 2006). In 2021, the U.S. Surgeon General issued an advisory called "Protecting Youth Mental Health" to underscore the importance of these increases and to provide a road map for making positive changes (https://www.hhs.gov/sites/default/files/surgeon-general-youth-mental-health-advisory.pdf).

As with adults, depression is comorbid with anxiety in children, particularly adolescents (Cummings, Caporino, & Kendall, 2014). There is evidence that comorbidity between depression and anxiety in adolescence may be caused in part by shared genetic vulnerabilities (Waszczuk, Zavos, et al., 2014).

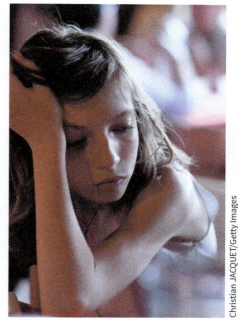

Many of the symptoms of childhood depression are the same as those of adult depression, including sad mood.

Causes of Depression in Childhood and Adolescence

What causes a young person to become depressed? As with adults, evidence suggests that genetic factors play a role (Kopala-Sibley & Klein, 2017). Indeed, the results of genetic studies with adults (see Chapter 5) also apply to children and adolescents because genetic influences are present from birth, though they may not be expressed right away. A child with a depressed parent has as much as four times the risk of developing depression as a child without a depressed parent (Hammen & Brennan, 2001). Of course, having a depressed parent confers risk via both genes and environment.

What about screen time and use of social media? In a large meta-analysis of over 225 studies published between 2006 and 2018, social media use was associated with depression and anxiety (Hancock, Liu, et al., 2022). However, correlation and causation are not the same. Can the increase in depression in the last 15 years be attributed in part to the concomitant increase in the use of smartphones and social media? Although it is certainly true that children and adolescents have increased their use of technology, the latest evidence suggests that time spent using smartphones and social media is not strongly causally linked with psychological disorders or symptoms such as depression (Odgers & Jensen, 2020). A few small experimental studies that randomly assigned college students to more or less social media (Facebook) time found that those who spent less time reported less depression (Twenge, 2020). On the other hand, a large EMA study (see Chapter 3) of over 2,000 children (ages 11–15) found that there was no increase in reported symptoms of anxiety and depression on days when digital technology was used more frequently (Jensen, George, et al., 2019). It seems, then, that the number of hours spent using smartphones and social media is not strongly causally linked to mental health in youth. Nevertheless, it may be that technology use heightens symptoms for those who are already at risk for depression and anxiety (Odgers, 2018; Prinstein, Nesi, & Telzer, 2020).

As with adults, other types of early adversity, interpersonal stress, and other negative life events also play a role (Garber, 2006; Hammen, 2009). For example, one study found that early adversity (e.g., financial hardship, maternal depression, chronic illness as a child) predicted depression from age 15 through age 20, particularly among adolescents who had experienced a number of negative life events by age 15 (Hazel, Hamman, et al., 2008). Results from the Youth Emotion Project found that interpersonal stress and the personality trait neuroticism predicted the onset of depression in adolescents across a 5-year period (Mineka, Williams, et al., 2020).

As we learned in Chapters 2 and 5, our bodies respond to stress via the HPA axis and the release of cortisol. Additional results from the Youth Emotion Project indicate that cortisol levels upon awakening prospectively predicted the onset of a major depressive episode up to 2.5 years later (Vrshek-Schallhorn, Doane, et al., 2013). These results are consistent with findings in adults. Together, the evidence from the different studies reviewed here suggests that genes, stressful life events, cortisol, and the brain are all important considerations in depression in adolescence.

Consistent with both Beck's theory and the hopelessness theory of depression (see Chapter 5), cognitive distortions and negative attributions are associated with depression in children and adolescents in ways similar to how they are associated in adults (Cole, Zelkowitz, et al., 2019; Garber, Kelly, & Martin, 2002; Lewinsohn et al., 2000). Negative thoughts and hopelessness also predict slower recovery from depression among adolescents (Rhode, Seeley, et al., 2006).

This is a key question in the study of children with depression: When do children develop stable attributional styles? That is, can young children have a stable way of thinking about themselves in the midst of such profound cognitive development? A longitudinal study examined the development of attributional style in children (Cole, Ciesla, et al., 2008). Specifically, the researchers prospectively studied three groups of children for 4 years each. At year 1 of the study, the three groups were (1) children in 2nd grade, (2) children in 4th grade, and (3) children in 6th grade. These three groups were followed yearly until the children were in grades 5, 7, and 9, respectively. The researchers found that attributional style didn't appear to be stable until children were early adolescents. In addition, attributional style did not interact with negative life events to predict depression for young children. Thus, results of this study suggest that attributional style becomes stable by early adolescence and serves as a cognitive diathesis for depression by the middle school years.

Treatment of Childhood and Adolescent Depression   Cognitive behavior therapy (CBT) and interpersonal therapy (see Chapter 2) are effective treatments for depression in adolescents, according to the results of a large meta-analysis of 55 studies (Eckshtain, Kuppens, et al., 2020). Importantly, these treatments were equally effective across all race and ethnic groups.

Antidepressant medications are only modestly strongly effective for children. Results from a large randomized controlled trial called the Treatment for Adolescents with Depression Study (TADS) provide some support for the efficacy of antidepressants. In TADS, adolescents were randomized to receive Prozac, cognitive behavioral therapy (CBT), or both. Results indicated that the treatment consisting of both CBT and Prozac was the most effective through 12 weeks and that Prozac had modest advantages compared to CBT (March, Silva, et al., 2004), a pattern that remained true after 36 weeks (TADS team, 2007). A meta-analysis of 27 randomized controlled trials of antidepressant medication treatment for depression and anxiety disorders in children found that the medications were most effective for anxiety disorders other than obsessive-compulsive disorder (OCD) and less effective for OCD and depression (Bridge, Iyengar, et al., 2007). Similarly, another meta-analysis of antidepressant use in children found a very small effect size for the efficacy of these medications in treating childhood depression (Feeney, Hock, et al., 2022).

Despite their modest effectiveness, antidepressant prescriptions for adolescents have risen by over 40% since 2017 (Schwartz, 2022). In addition, however, several concerns have been raised about antidepressants (see **Focus on Discovery 13.2**). The side effects experienced by some children taking antidepressants include diarrhea, nausea, sleep problems, and agitation (Barber, 2008). More importantly, concerns with respect to suicidality prompted a series of hearings in the United States and the United Kingdom about the safety of antidepressants for children. In the meta-analysis by Bridge and colleagues (2007), the researchers looked at suicidality rates in the studies of depression. The risk of suicidal ideation was 3% for those children taking antidepressants and 2% for those taking a placebo. It is important to note that this analysis shows that children taking medication were at risk for suicidal ideation, not that medication caused the suicide thoughts or attempts. No children or adolescents lost their lives to suicide in any of the 27 studies reviewed.

How long do the treatment effects studied last? A naturalistic follow-up of just under half the adolescents in TADS found that, although most participants (96%) had recovered 2 years after the study, close to half of those who had recovered by the end of treatment had a recurrent episode of depression 5 years later (Curry, Silva, et al., 2011). Girls were more likely to have a recurrence than boys, as were adolescents who had a comorbid anxiety disorder. However, the rate of recurrence did not differ depending on the kind of treatment the adolescents

Focus on Discovery 13.2

Controversies in the Diagnosis and Treatment of Children with Psychopathology

The number of children diagnosed with psychological disorders continues to rise, sometimes dramatically, as does the number of children taking psychoactive medications. Here we briefly discuss some of the controversies and current evidence accumulated to address these issues.

Emotion Difficulties in Children: How Many Diagnoses Do We Need?

For years, professionals have struggled to distinguish problems with emotions and emotion regulation in children. DSM-5-TR includes several disorders that include problems with emotion regulation, including ADHD, ODD, bipolar disorder, and disruptive mood dysregulation disorder (DMDD). DMDD was added to help distinguish episodic irritability seen in childhood bipolar disorder from more chronic irritability. But the diagnosis of DMDD is not without controversy. In addition, it can often be challenging to distinguish bipolar disorder from ADHD in children, and there is even evidence of shared genetic vulnerability between the two (Hosang, Lichtenstein, et al., 2019). Do we have too many or too few disorders involving emotion problems in children?

The DSM-5 added DMDD in the hope that this diagnosis would help clinicians distinguish episodic irritability that is part of bipolar disorder from severe and chronic irritability. DMDD is distinguished by severe temper outbursts that happen many times a week and in two different settings for at least a year. By contrast, irritability in bipolar disorder needs to last for just a week and can happen in just one setting.

Unfortunately, there is not yet much evidence to support the DMDD diagnosis. The reliability of the diagnosis was quite low in the DSM-5 field trials (Regier, Narrow, et al., 2013), and recall from Chapter 3 that the question of validity cannot be addressed without first establishing reliability. Perhaps not surprisingly, given the problems with reliability, prevalence rates vary widely, from 1% to over 30% (Copeland, Angold, et al., 2013; Dougherty, Smith, et al., 2016; Freeman, Youngstrom, et al., 2016; Margulies, Weintraub, et al., 2012). The evidence on whether the DMDD symptoms are stable across time is also mixed (Dougherty et al., 2016; Mayes, Mathiowetz, et al., 2015). Other difficulties with diagnosing DMDD include the high comorbidity with other disorders, including depression, ODD, and ADHD (Copeland et al., 2013; Mayes, Waxmonsky, et al., 2016). In short, the inclusion of DMDD in DSM-5 remains controversial.

Antidepressant Medications

Can antidepressant medications increase the likelihood of suicide in adolescents? Findings from the Treatment of Adolescent Depression Study (TADS) indicated that the most effective treatment was a combination of Prozac and cognitive behavioral therapy (CBT) (March et al., 2004). However, the authors also reported that six adolescents taking Prozac attempted suicide (1.5% of the sample), whereas only one receiving cognitive behavioral therapy attempted suicide. The participants in the study were randomly assigned to treatment conditions, so it is less likely that the adolescents taking Prozac were more seriously ill or suicidal than the ones receiving CBT.

Antidepressants can take as long as 3–4 weeks to start working, and one analysis of adolescent suicide attempts and antidepressant use found that the risk for suicide was highest in the first 3–4 weeks of treatment. Thus, it could be the case that the medications did not have sufficient time to begin working in the adolescents who attempted suicide. It may also be true that the combined treatment in TADS was most effective because CBT began working earlier in the course of treatment.

Nevertheless, findings from the TADS study prompted the FDA to mandate a "black-box" warning to accompany information sent to physicians on the use of antidepressants with adolescents. This is the strongest safety warning the FDA can issue with medications. In the United Kingdom, the equivalent regulatory agency, the Medicines and Healthcare Products Regulatory Agency (MHRA), also recommended warnings for antidepressant labels. The 2014 UK guidelines for treating depression in young people suggest that the risks associated with antidepressants outweigh the benefits (https://www.gov.uk/government/publications/ssris-and-snris-use-and-safety/selective-serotonin-reuptake-inhibitors-ssris-and-serotonin-and-noradrenaline-reuptake-inhibitors-snris-use-and-safety). Following the instituting of the warnings, the number of prescriptions for antidepressants declined initially (Kurian, Ray, et al., 2007), but it has once again risen (Sarginson, Webb, et al., 2017).

Stimulant Medications

The number of children taking stimulant medications has risen dramatically since they were introduced in the 1960s (Hinshaw, 2018). Does the use of stimulant medications lead to increases in illicit drug use among children? Evidence from longitudinal studies suggests that the answer to this question is no. In one study, two groups of children with ADHD were studied for 13 years (Barkley, Fischer, et al., 2003). One group of children had been treated with stimulant medication for 3½ years on average, and the other group had never received stimulant medication. At follow-up in young adulthood, those who had taken stimulant medication were not more likely to have used illicit drugs than those who had not been treated, with one exception—those who had taken stimulant medication were at greater risk for having tried cocaine. However, after controlling for the severity of conduct disorder symptoms, the relationship between stimulant medication use and trying cocaine disappeared. This suggests that having severe conduct disorder symptoms accounts for the link between stimulant medication and trying cocaine, not the use of stimulant medication per se.

Another study followed up children 8 years after they participated in the MTA study (discussed earlier in this chapter), when they were in middle to late adolescence (Molina, Hinshaw, et al., 2013). The children with ADHD, regardless of treatment type, were more likely to have used alcohol, tobacco, marijuana, and other drugs in adolescence than were the children without ADHD. However, there was no relationship between stimulant medication use and later drug use. Neither the total amount of medication taken, the dosage of medication, initial MTA treatment group (medication alone or combined treatment), nor continued use of medication after the MTA study was associated with later drug or alcohol use. Thus, children with ADHD are at a higher risk for substance use, but it is not because they have taken stimulant medication.

Autism Spectrum Disorder: Diagnosis and Causes

The number of cases of autism spectrum disorder (ASD) has increased dramatically since the turn of the century. As reported by the Centers for Disease Control and Prevention (CDC), the prevalence rate of ASD in the United States rose

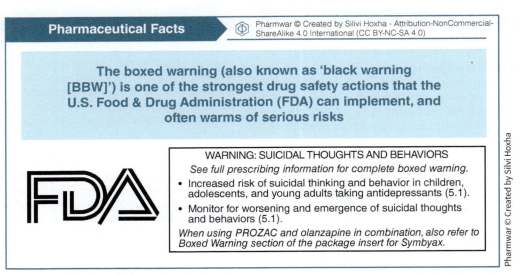

The FDA now requires that black-box warnings be included with antidepressants used with adolescents.

from 1 in 150 children to 1 in 36 children between 2000 and 2020 (Maenner, Warren, et al., 2023; https://www.cdc.gov/ncbddd/autism/data.html). Why has there been such an increase? Are there that many more children with autism, or have mental health professionals gotten better at making a diagnosis?

Both appear to be true. The diagnostic criteria have broadened between DSM-III and DSM-5-TR, and more children meet the criteria for a diagnosis of ASD under the broader criteria than they did under the narrower criteria (Gernsbacher, Dawson, & Goldsmith, 2005). The method that the CDC uses for defining ASD to compute prevalence rates changed in 2018, but it does not appear to account for the higher rates (Maenner, Graves, et al., 2021). Additionally, there is greater public awareness of ASD, and this may spur families to seek out mental health professionals for a formal psychological assessment. Indeed, the delay in or lack of language acquisition has become a widely recognized warning sign among parents and mental health professionals that ASD may be a possibility. In addition, public schools are mandated by law to provide services for children with ASD, and this may have helped families to seek a formal diagnosis.

Although the rise in autism diagnoses may be accounted for in part by better diagnosis, awareness, and mandated services, most experts agree that there are indeed more cases today than there were 20 years ago.

One thing that is not responsible for an increase in ASD is vaccines. Based largely on celebrity proclamations, parents became particularly worried that vaccines routinely given to toddlers might cause ASD. The MMR vaccine (for measles, mumps, and rubella) is given to children at about the same age when autism signs and symptoms begin to appear. A related concern was that the product used to preserve these vaccines—a substance called thimerosal, which contains mercury—could be responsible for autism.

There is no evidence, however, linking autism with either the MMR vaccine or thimerosal (Institute of Medicine, 2004; Wessel, 2017). A meta-analysis including more than 1.2 million children found no link between autism and the vaccine (Taylor, Swerdfeger, & Eslick, 2014).

Vaccines have not been stored in thimerosal for many years, and even those vaccines that were stored in thimerosal contained very small amounts of mercury. By 2001, all but the smallest trace of thimerosal had been removed from childhood vaccines. If thimerosal was causing autism, the decline in its use in vaccines should have corresponded to a decrease in the number of new cases of autism. However, results of a study of ASD across 12 years found no such association (Schecter & Grether, 2008). In fact, the number of new cases of autism increased.

received during TADS. In other words, the modest benefits of Prozac over cognitive behavior therapy observed in TADS did not seem to protect this group of adolescents from having a future episode of depression 5 years later. The **Clinical Case of Sharon** illustrates CBT techniques with an adolescent.

Prevention of Depression in Childhood and Adolescence
Professional groups including the U.S. Preventive Services Task Force (USPSTF) and the Guidelines for Adolescent Depression in Primary Care (GLAD-PC) recommend annual screening for depression in adolescents beginning at age 12 (USPSTF, 2022a, 2022b; Zuckerbrot, Cheung, et al., 2018).

Research has also focused on how to prevent the onset of depression in adolescents and children. Selective prevention programs target youth based on family risk factors (e.g., parents with depression), environmental factors (e.g., poverty), or personal factors (e.g., hopelessness). Universal programs target large groups, typically in schools, and seek to

Clinical Case

Sharon

When initially seen, Sharon was extremely sad, experienced recurrent suicidal ideation, and displayed numerous other signs of depression. ... [After being] placed on antidepressant medication ... she was introduced to a cognitive behavioral approach to depression. ... She was able to understand how her mood was affected by her thoughts and behavior and was able to engage in behavioral planning to increase the occurrence of pleasurable and mastery-oriented events. Sharon manifested extremely high standards for evaluating her performance in several areas, and it became clear that her parents also subscribed to these standards, so family therapy sessions were held to encourage Sharon and her parents to reevaluate their standards.

Sharon had difficulty with the notion of changing her standards and noted that when she was not depressed, she valued her perfectionism. At that point she resisted the therapy because she perceived it as trying to change something she valued in herself. With this in mind, we began to explore and identify those situations or domains in which her perfectionism worked for her and when and how it might work against her. She became increasingly comfortable with this perspective and decided she wanted to continue to set high standards regarding her performance in mathematical course work (which was a clear area of strength), but she did not need to be so demanding of herself regarding art or physical education.

Adapted from Braswell & Kendall, 1988, p. 194.

provide education and information about depression. Results of meta-analyses indicate that selective prevention programs are more effective than universal programs in preventing depression symptoms among adolescents (Garber, Brunwasser, et al., 2016; Werner-Seidler, Spanos, et al., 2021).

For example, one large randomized control clinical trial of a selective prevention program for at-risk adolescents randomly assigned adolescents to either a group CBT intervention that focused on problem-solving skills and changing negative thoughts or a usual care group (i.e., any mental health care they sought out on their own). The incidence of depression episodes was lower for adolescents in the CBT group than for those in the usual care group; therefore, the treatment may have had an effective preventative effect (Garber, Clarke, et al., 2009). Results from follow-ups at 33 months and 75 months indicated that the effects held: Those who received the prevention program had fewer depression episodes than those in the usual care group (Brent, Brunwasser, et al., 2015; Beardslee, Brent, et al., 2013).

Anxiety

Just about every child experiences fears and worries as part of the typical course of development. Common fears, most of which the child outgrows, include fear of the dark and of imaginary creatures and fear of being separated from parents. For fears and worries to be considered as disorders, children's functioning must be impaired; unlike adults, however, children need not regard their fear as excessive or unreasonable, because children sometimes are unable to make such judgments.

Not only do children experience, as do adults, the aversiveness of being anxious—simply put, anxiety doesn't feel good—but their anxiety may also work against their acquisition of skills appropriate to various stages of their development. For example, a child who is painfully anxious around others and finds interacting with peers virtually intolerable may have difficulty learning important social skills.

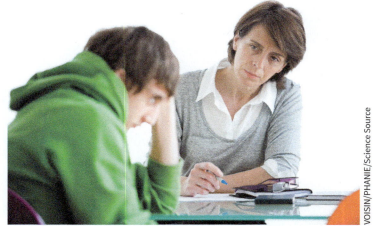

Clinical Descriptions and Prevalence of Anxiety in Childhood and Adolescence

About 9% of children and adolescents are diagnosed as having an anxiety disorder (Bitsko, Claussen, et al., 2022). See Table 13.2 for the prevalence rates of the individual anxiety disorders.

Anxiety disorders in childhood and adolescence can interfere with other aspects of development.

VOISIN/PHANIE/Science Source

Defining Symptoms of Separation Anxiety Disorder

- Experiencing a great deal of distress when separated from a parent or caregiver
- Experiencing intense worry that something bad will happen to a parent (or a person to whom a child is closely attached)
- Refusing to go to school or showing a great bit of trepidation about going to school, called *school refusal* by mental health professionals

- Refusing to sleep away from home (e.g., at a sleepover or at a relative's house) or showing trepidation about doing so
- Having bad dreams or nightmares about being separated
- Experiencing a great deal of physical problems (e.g., headache, stomachache) when separated

Separation anxiety disorder is characterized by constant worry that some harm will befall the children's parents or the children themselves when they are away from their parents. When at home, such children shadow one or both of their parents. Since the beginning of school is often the first circumstance that requires lengthy and frequent separations of children from their parents, separation anxiety is often first observed when children begin school. Separation anxiety disorder is associated with the development of other internalizing and externalizing disorders at later ages, and this is true in several countries around the world (Silove, Alonso, et al., 2015).

Children and adolescents also suffer from social anxiety disorder. Most classrooms include at least one or two children who are extremely quiet and shy. Often these children will play only with family members or familiar peers, avoiding strangers both young and old. Their social anxiety may prevent them from acquiring skills and participating in a variety of activities enjoyed by most of their peers, for they avoid playgrounds and stay out of games played by other children. Extremely shy children may refuse to speak at all in unfamiliar social circumstances, a condition called *selective mutism*.

Children who are exposed to traumas, such as chronic abuse, community violence, or natural disasters, may experience symptoms of posttraumatic stress disorder (PTSD) similar to those experienced by adults. For children older than 6, these symptoms are organized into the same four broad categories used for adults: (1) intrusively reexperiencing the traumatic event, as in nightmares, flashbacks, or intrusive thoughts; (2) avoiding trauma-related situations or information and experiencing a general numbing of responses, as in feelings of detachment or anhedonia; (3) negative changes in cognitions or mood related to the traumatic event; and (4) increased arousal and reactivity, which can include irritability, sleep problems, and hypervigilance.

DSM-5 added distinct symptoms for PTSD in children age 6 and younger. The symptoms for these younger children fall into the same four broad categories just described, but they are presented in ways that are more developmentally appropriate for younger children. For example, extreme temper tantrums are an example of an increased reactivity symptom; intrusive thoughts about the trauma may be experienced as reenactment play. In addition, some of the symptom descriptors that don't apply to young children have been removed from these criteria. For example, holding negative beliefs about oneself is part of the negative changes in cognitions or mood symptoms cluster that does not apply to very young children.

OCD is found among children and adolescents, with prevalence estimates ranging from less than 1% to 4% (Rapee, Schniering, & Hudson, 2009). The symptoms in childhood are similar to symptoms in adulthood; both obsessions and compulsions are involved. The most common obsessions in childhood involve dirt or contamination as well as

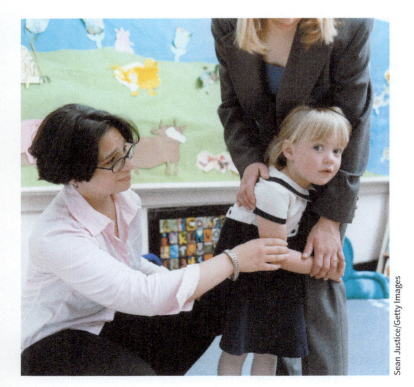

Sean Justice/Getty Images

Separation anxiety disorder involves an intense fear of being away from parents or other attachment figures.

aggression; recurrent thoughts about sex or religion become more common in adolescence (Turner, 2006). In children, OCD is more common in boys than girls, but by adulthood, OCD is slightly more common in women than men.

Causes of Anxiety Disorders in Childhood and Adolescence   As with adults, genetics plays a role in anxiety among children, with heritability estimates ranging from 29% to 50% in one study (Lau, Gregory, et al., 2007). However, genes do their work via the environment. For example, genetics plays a role in separation anxiety in the context of more negative life events experienced by a child (Lau et al., 2007). Furthermore, shared environment factors (see Chapter 2) also play a significant part in childhood anxiety disorders (Burt, 2014).

Parenting practices have a small role in childhood anxiety. Specifically, parental control and overprotectiveness, more than parental rejection, are associated with childhood anxiety. However, parental control accounted for only 4% of the variance in childhood anxiety according to a meta-analysis of 47 studies (McLeod, Weisz, & Wood, 2007). Other meta-analyses similarly found significant effects for parental practices, including abuse, conflict between parents, warmth, and overinvolvement, but these factors accounted for only 2–4% of the variance in childhood anxiety generally (Yap & Jorm, 2015) or PTSD specifically (Williamson, Creswell, et al., 2017).

Another factor studied in childhood anxiety is the role of being bullied. Prospective studies have found that children who had been bullied in childhood or early adolescence were more likely to develop an anxiety disorder or depression in early adulthood (Copeland, Wolke, et al., 2013; Stapinski, Bowes, et al., 2014). A meta-analysis of over 600 studies found that childhood maltreatment of any kind (physical abuse, sexual abuse, emotional abuse, neglect, or exposure to intimate partner violence) is a risk factor for anxiety and depression in children (Gardner, Thomas, & Erskine, 2019).

Other causes of social anxiety in children are generally similar to those for adults (Spence & Rapee, 2016). For example, research has shown that children with anxiety disorders overestimate danger in social situations and underestimate their ability to cope with social challenges (Boegels & Zigterman, 2000; Miers, Blöte, et al., 2009). The anxiety created by these thoughts then interferes with social interactions, causing the children to avoid social situations (Wong & Rapee, 2016) and thus not get much practice with social skills. In adolescence, peer relationships are important (Spence & Rapee, 2016). One longitudinal study found that adolescents who perceived that their peers did not accept them were more likely to be socially anxious (Teachman & Allen, 2007). Other research points to behavioral inhibition as an important risk factor for developing social anxiety (also discussed in Chapter 6). Children who had high levels of behavioral inhibition at age 4 were 10 times as likely as children with lower levels to have social anxiety disorder by age 9 (Essex, Klein, et al., 2010).

Causes of PTSD are similar for children and adults. For both, there must be exposure to a trauma, either experienced or witnessed. Like adults, children who have a propensity to experience anxiety may be at more risk for developing PTSD after exposure to trauma. Specific risk factors for children may include high levels of family stress, low levels of social support, low socioeconomic status of the family, poor family functioning, and past experiences with trauma (Trickey, Siddaway, et al., 2012).

Treatment of Anxiety in Childhood and Adolescence   In 2022, the U.S. Preventive Service Task Force recommended screening for anxiety in children and adolescents ages 8–18. Given how common and troubling anxiety can be, intervening early can help young people.

Evidence from a meta-analysis of 48 randomized controlled trials indicates that cognitive behavior therapy can be helpful to many children with anxiety disorders (Reynolds, Wilson, et al., 2012). There is also evidence to suggest that the earlier a child receives treatment, the more likely the treatment effects are to last (Ginsburg, Becker-Haimes, et al., 2018).

General Treatments for Anxiety   One of the more widely used treatments is a type of CBT called Coping Cat (Kendall, Aschenbrand, & Hudson, 2003). This treatment focuses on confrontation of fears, development of new ways to think about fears, exposure to feared situations, and relapse prevention. Parents are also included in a couple of sessions. Data from randomized controlled clinical trials have shown this treatment to be effective in the short term (Kendall, Flannery-Schroeder, et al., 1997), 7 years later (Kendall, Safford, et al., 2004), and 19 years later (Benjamin, Harrison, et al., 2013). Coping Cat is recommended by the Children and Young People's Improving Access to Psychological Therapies Program in the United Kingdom as a treatment for social anxiety, GAD, and separation anxiety disorder (Oldham-Cooper & Loades, 2017).

A large randomized controlled trial compared the Coping Cat treatment alone; the medication sertraline (Zoloft) alone; and a combination of the two for children with separation anxiety, general anxiety, and social anxiety and found that the combined treatment was more effective than either Coping Cat or medication alone (Walkup, Albano, et al., 2008). Perhaps not surprisingly, given the characteristics of the Coping Cat treatment, follow-up analyses indicated that improvements in children's coping ability seemed to drive the change in both the Coping Cat alone and the combined treatment groups (Kendall, Cummings, et al., 2016). Two- and 3-year follow-up studies of these children found that children assigned to the Coping Cat treatment alone or medication alone continued to get better; that is, either of these two conditions was as effective in reducing anxiety as the combined treatment (Piacentini, Bennett, et al., 2014). Thus, the combined treatment appears to provide the most immediate improvement, but over time the Coping Cat treatment (or medication alone) yielded the same benefits.

Another randomized controlled trial compared individual CBT, family CBT, and family psychoeducation for the treatment of childhood anxiety. Both individual and family CBT included the Coping Cat workbook, and both were more effective than family psychoeducation at reducing anxiety (Kendall, Hudson, et al., 2008); also, the effects persisted after 1 year and 7 years (Benjamin et al., 2013). Family CBT was more effective than individual CBT when both parents had an anxiety disorder. This study points to the importance of considering not only the child's anxiety but also levels of parental anxiety when deciding on a treatment for childhood anxiety.

A new family-based intervention called SPACE (Supportive Parenting for Anxious Childhood Emotions) shows promise. This treatment focuses entirely on parents and not the child with anxiety. The treatment involves psychoeducation but also efforts to teach parents how to bolster coping skills and confidence in children and alter the accommodations they make to a child's anxiety. For example, if a child reports being afraid to sleep alone, parents are given tools to boost the child's confidence about sleeping alone and asked to use these tools rather than letting the child sleep with them. In one randomized controlled clinical trial, SPACE was found to be as effective as CBT (not the Coping Cat version), suggesting that this may be a promising additional approach to treating childhood anxiety (Lebowitz, Marin, et al., 2020).

Psychological treatments are also effective for adolescents. Results from a meta-analysis covering 50 years of psychotherapy research found a medium effect size across all the studies (Weisz, Kuppens, et al., 2017). The analysis included studies of behavioral treatments (including CBT), nonbehavioral treatments (e.g., psychodynamic), and family-focused interventions. Importantly, these treatments were just as effective for ethnic minority adolescents.

Treatments for Specific Anxiety Disorders   Behavior therapy and group cognitive behavior therapy have been found to be effective for social anxiety disorder in children (Davis, May, & Whiting, 2011). CBT is recommended as the first-line treatment for mild to moderate OCD, according to the American Association of Child and Adolescent Psychiatry (AACP) (Geller & March, 2012), and it is effective in children and adolescents, with effect sizes larger than those for medication (Freeman, Sapyta, et al., 2014; Watson & Rees, 2008).

For severe OCD, the AACP guidelines recommend medication plus CBT. In the Pediatric OCD Treatment Studies, a combination of CBT and sertraline (Zoloft) was more effective than CBT alone for children and adolescents with severe OCD (Franklin, Sapyta, et al., 2011; Pediatric OCD Treatment Study [POTS] Team, 2004).

Only a few studies have evaluated the efficacy of treatment of PTSD among children and adolescents, but the available research suggests that cognitive behavioral treatments, whether individual or group, are effective (Davis, May, & Whiting, 2011; Mavranezouli, Megnin-Viggars, et al., 2020; Morina, Koerssen, & Pollet, 2016).

Quick Summary

Anxiety disorders and depression in children are referred to as internalizing disorders. Depression in childhood and adolescence appears to be generally similar to depression in adulthood, although there are notable differences. In childhood, depression affects boys and girls equally, but in adolescence, girls are affected almost twice as often as boys. Genetics and stressful life events play a role in depression in childhood. Research on cognitive factors in childhood depression supports the notion that attributional style also has a role; however, this work must consider the developmental stage of the child. A randomized controlled trial found that a combination of medication and cognitive behavioral therapy (CBT) was the most effective treatment for depression, but concerns about the effect of medications on suicide risk need to be addressed.

Anxiety and fear are typical in childhood. When fears interfere with functioning, such as by keeping a child from school, intervention is warranted. Theories about the causes of anxiety disorders in children are similar to theories about their causes in adulthood, though less research has been done with children on, for example, cognitive factors. Cognitive behavior therapy is an effective intervention for a number of different anxiety disorders in childhood. Other problems, such as PTSD in childhood, require additional study.

13.2 Check Your Knowledge

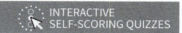
INTERACTIVE
SELF-SCORING QUIZZES

(Answers are at the end of the chapter.)
Answer the following questions.

1. What are the most common mood and anxiety disorders in children and adolescents?
2. Evidence to date indicates that time spent on smartphones _____ an increase in depression and anxiety among youth.
3. Like research with adults, studies with children find that _____ and the cognitive factor of attributional style to be associated with depression.
4. What are two broad types of depression prevention programs?
5. The symptoms for most anxiety disorders are similar for children and adults. For children age 6 and under, however, the symptoms for _____ are different.
6. What is an effective type of cognitive behavior therapy (CBT) that is used with children to treat anxiety?

Specific Learning Disorder and Intellectual Disability

Dyslexia: A Type of Specific Learning Disorder

Clinical Case

Marcus

Marcus was excited about his college major in psychology and dreamed of becoming a clinical psychologist. He eagerly signed up for as many courses as would fit into his schedule and had open seats. He sat in the front of the large lecture courses, raising his hand and contributing to the discussion whenever possible. When it came time to take the first exam, he carefully reviewed his notes and textbook. He also experienced that creeping anxiety that came whenever he took written exams. Even though he thought he studied as much if not more than the other students, he did not do well on the exams. "He didn't test well" was what he told himself. But when he thought about it, he realized that when he was reading the textbook, the words and letters sometimes got scrambled in a way that made it difficult to remember the material.

When he received his grade on the first midterm, he was worried. It contained all sorts of marks from the grader indicating that his writing was indecipherable and that he had not covered all the concepts required for the correct answers. His graduate student instructor suggested that he go for testing at the campus clinic in charge of assessments for learning disorders.

After a comprehensive assessment at the campus clinic, Marcus received a diagnosis of specific learning disorder with the dyslexia specifier. Marcus was now going to get extra time for his exams and papers—not just in his psychology classes, but in all his classes. The following semester, Marcus's grade point average went up to 3.8, and he felt confident that he was closer to achieving his goal of attending graduate school in clinical psychology.

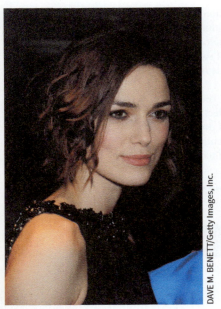

Keira Knightley, a highly successful actress, has dyslexia.

DAVE M. BENETT/Getty Images, Inc.

A **specific learning disorder** is a condition in which a person shows a problem in a specific area of academic, language, speech, or motor skills that is not due to intellectual disability or deficient educational opportunities. Children with a specific learning disorder have difficulty learning some specific skill in the affected area (e.g., math or reading), and thus their progress in school is impeded.

DSM-5-TR includes several disorders in the areas of learning, communication, and motor development. These disorders are described briefly in **Table 13.3**. They are often identified and treated within the school system rather than through mental health clinics.

Dyslexia is not named as a distinct disorder in DSM-5-TR; instead, the category *specific learning disorder* is used with one of three different specifiers: (1) impairment in reading (dyslexia), (2) impairment in written expression, or (3) impairment in math (dyscalculia). Dyscalculia involves difficulty in producing or understanding numbers, quantities, or basic arithmetic operations. An impairment in written expression refers to problems in spelling, grammar, and the clarity and organization of written work.

Dyslexia involves significant difficulty with word recognition, reading fluency, and reading comprehension. An analysis of four large epidemiological samples indicates that dyslexia is more common in boys than in girls (Rutter, Caspi, et al., 2004). In general, dyslexia affects 5–15% of school-age children (Peterson & Pennington, 2015).

VIDEO CONTENT

**Case Study: Dyslexia
Pause and Ponder**

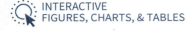

INTERACTIVE FIGURES, CHARTS, & TABLES

TABLE 13.3   Specific Learning, Communication, and Motor Disorders in DSM-5-TR

Diagnoses	Major Features
Specific learning disorder	• Reading impairment (dyslexia) • Written expression impairment • Math impairment (dyscalculia)
Communication disorders	
Speech sound disorder	• Correct comprehension and sufficient vocabulary use, but unclear speech and improper articulation. For example, *blue* comes out *bu*, and *rabbit* sounds like *wabbit*. With speech therapy, complete recovery occurs in almost all cases, and milder cases may recover spontaneously by age 8.
Childhood onset fluency disorder (stuttering)	• Difficulty with verbal fluency that is characterized by one or more of the following speech patterns: frequent repetitions or prolongations of sounds, long pauses between words, substituting easy words for those that are difficult to articulate (e.g., words beginning with certain consonants), and repeating whole words (e.g., saying "go-go-go-go" instead of just a single "go"). Up to 80% of people with stuttering recover, most of them without professional intervention, before the age of 16.
Language disorder	• Problems in developing and using language
Social (pragmatic) communication disorder	• Difficulties in using verbal and nonverbal language in social communication
Motor disorders	
Tourette's disorder	• One or more vocal and multiple motor tics (sudden, rapid movement or vocalization) that start before age 18
Developmental coordination disorder	• Difficulties in the development of motor coordination not explainable by intellectual disability or a disorder such as cerebral palsy
Stereotypic movement disorder	• Repetition of purposeless movements over and over that interferes with functioning and could even cause self-injury

Intellectual Developmental Disorder (Intellectual Disability)

Development of the DSM-5 criteria for **intellectual disability** [called intellectual developmental disorder (intellectual disability) in DSM-5-TR] was influenced by the guidelines of the American Association on Intellectual and Developmental Disabilities (AAIDD). The AAIDD's mission is to "promote progressive policies, sound research, effective practices, and universal human rights for people with intellectual and developmental disabilities" (**www.aaidd.org**). There are three components to the AAIDD definition of intellectual disability:

1. significant problems in intellectual functioning (usually assessed with an IQ test)
2. significant problems in adaptive behavior across contexts
3. problems begin before age 18

The current AAIDD guidelines are summarized in **Table 13.4**.

DSM-5-TR changed the name of this category to intellectual developmental disorder (intellectual disability) to be consistent with ICD-11, which refers to disorders of intellectual development. DSM-5-TR kept intellectual disability in parentheses to indicate its common usage. We will use the name *intellectual disability* in most of the chapter.

Assessment of Intellectual Disability

Assessment for intellectual disability will include an IQ test, but interpretation of the IQ score must be considered within the context of a more thorough assessment. In addition, adaptive functioning must be assessed in a broad range of contexts. The severity of intellectual disability is assessed in three areas: conceptual (which includes intellectual and other cognitive functioning), social, and practical.

The AAIDD approach encourages the identification of an individual's strengths and weaknesses in psychological, physical, and environmental

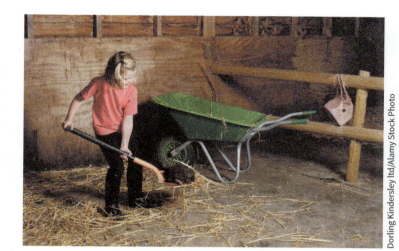

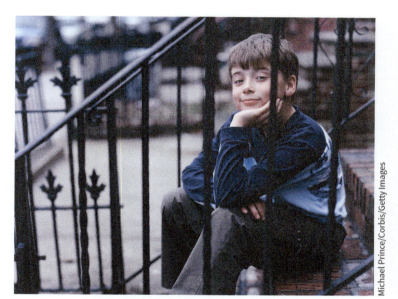

When adaptive functioning is assessed, the cultural environment must be considered. A person living in a rural community may not need the skills essential to someone living in New York City, and vice versa.

TABLE 13.4   **The AAIDD Guidelines on Intellectual Disability**

Five Assumptions Essential to the Application of the Definition

1. Limitations in present functioning must be considered within the context of community environments typical of the individual's age, peers, and culture.

2. Valid assessment considers cultural and linguistic diversity as well as differences in communication, sensory, motor, and behavioral factors.

3. Within an individual, limitations often coexist with strengths.

4. An important purpose of describing limitations is to develop a profile of needed supports.

5. With appropriate personalized supports over a sustained period, the life functioning of the person with intellectual disability generally will improve.

Source: Adapted from *Intellectual Disability: Definition, Classification, and Systems of Supports* (11th ed.), © 2002 American Association on Intellectual and Developmental Disabilities.

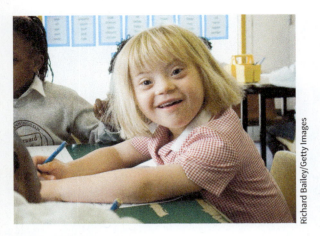

Child with Down syndrome.

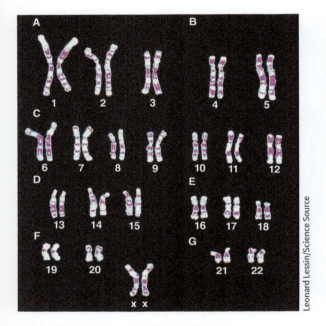

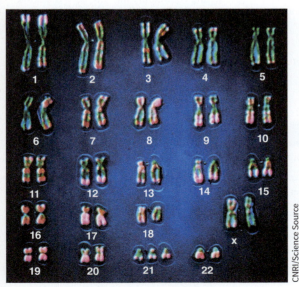

(a) The normal complement of chromosomes is 23 pairs.
(b) In Down syndrome, there are three copies (a trisomy) of chromosome 21.

dimensions, with a view toward determining the kinds and degrees of support needed to enhance the person's functioning in various contexts. Consider Roger, a 24-year-old man with an IQ of 45 who has attended a special program for people with intellectual disability since he was 6. The AAIDD approach would emphasize what is needed to maximize Roger's functioning. Thus, a clinician might discover that Roger can use the bus system if he takes a route familiar to him, and therefore he might be able to go to a movie by himself from time to time. And although Roger cannot prepare complicated meals, he might be able to learn to prepare frozen entrées in a microwave oven. The assumption is that by building on what he can do, Roger will make more progress.

In the schools, an individualized educational program (IEP) is based on the person's strengths and weaknesses and on the amount of instruction needed. Students are classified according to the classroom environment they are judged to need. This approach can lessen the stigmatizing effects of having an intellectual disability and may also encourage a focus on what can be done to improve the student's learning.

Causes of Intellectual Disability
At this time, the primary cause of intellectual disability can be identified in only 25% of the people affected. The causes that can be identified are typically neurobiological.

Genetic or Chromosomal Abnormalities One chromosomal abnormality that has been linked with intellectual disability is **Down syndrome**, also known as trisomy 21, because it refers to having an extra copy (i.e., three instead of two) of chromosome 21. It has been estimated that Down syndrome occurs in about 1 out of every 850 live births in the United States (Shin, Besser, et al., 2009).

People with Down syndrome may have intellectual disability as well as some distinctive physical signs, such as short and stocky stature; oval, upward-slanting eyes; a prolongation of the fold of the upper eyelid over the inner corner of the eye; sparse, fine, straight hair; a wide and flat nasal bridge; square-shaped ears; a large, furrowed tongue, which may protrude because the mouth is small and its roof is low; and short, broad hands.

Another chromosomal abnormality that can cause intellectual disability is **fragile X syndrome**, which involves a mutation in the *fMR1* gene on the X chromosome (see the website of the National Fragile X Foundation, **www.fragilex.org**). Physical symptoms associated with fragile X syndrome include large, underdeveloped ears and a long, thin face. Many people with fragile X syndrome have intellectual disability. Others may not have intellectual disability but may have a specific learning disorder, exhibit difficulties on neuropsychological tests, or experience mood swings. About a third of children with fragile X syndrome also exhibit autism spectrum behaviors, suggesting that the *fMR1* gene may be one of the many genes that contribute to autism spectrum disorder (Hagerman, 2006).

Recessive-Gene Diseases Several hundred recessive-gene diseases have been identified, and many of them can cause intellectual disability. Here we discuss one recessive-gene disease, phenylketonuria.

In **phenylketonuria (PKU)**, the infant, born without obvious signs of difficulty, soon begins to suffer from a deficiency of the liver enzyme phenylalanine hydroxylase. Because of this enzyme deficiency, phenylalanine and its derivative, phenylpyruvic acid, are not broken down and instead build up in the body's fluids. This buildup can damage the brain because the unmetabolized amino acid interferes with the process of myelination, the sheathing of neuron axons, which is essential for neuronal function. Myelination supports the rapid transmittal of neuronal impulses. If this condition is not properly treated, the resulting intellectual disabilities can be profound.

Although PKU is rare, with an incidence of about 1 in 15,000 live births, it is estimated that 1 person in 70 is a carrier of the recessive gene. A blood test is available for prospective parents who have reason to suspect that they might be carriers. Pregnant women who carry the recessive gene must monitor their diet closely so that the fetus will not be exposed to toxic levels of phenylalanine. State laws require testing newborns for PKU. If the test is positive, the parents are taught to provide the infant with a diet low in phenylalanine.

Infectious Diseases   While in utero, the fetus is at increased risk of intellectual disabilities resulting from maternal infectious diseases, such as rubella, cytomegalovirus, toxoplasmosis, herpes simplex, and HIV. The consequences of these diseases are most serious during the first trimester of pregnancy, when the fetus has no detectable immunological response; that is, its immune system is not developed enough to ward off infection. The mother may experience slight or no symptoms from the infection, but the effects on the developing fetus can be devastating.

Infectious diseases can also affect a child's developing brain after birth. Encephalitis and meningococcal meningitis may cause brain injury and even death if contracted in infancy or early childhood. In adulthood, these infections are usually far less serious. There are several forms of childhood meningitis, a disease in which the protective membranes of the brain are acutely inflamed and fever is very high.

Environmental Hazards   Several environmental pollutants are implicated in intellectual disability. One such pollutant is mercury, which may be ingested by eating affected fish. Another is lead, which is found in lead-based paints, smog, and even water pipes. The state of Michigan switched the water supply in the city of Flint in 2014, and because the new supply from the Flint River was not properly treated, lead from pipes carrying water to homes got into the water. It took over 2 years for the levels of lead to return to pre-2014 levels. Lead poisoning can cause kidney and brain damage as well as anemia, intellectual disabilities, seizures, and death. Lead-based paint is now prohibited in the United States, but it is still found in older homes, where children may eat pieces that flake off.

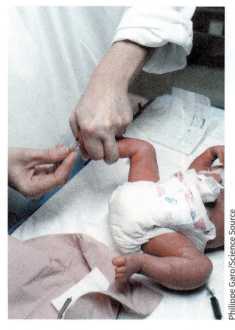

States require that newborns be tested for PKU. If excess phenylalanine is found in the blood, a special diet is recommended for the baby.

Treatment of Intellectual Disability

Residential Treatment   Although many people with intellectual disability can acquire the skills needed to function effectively in the community, some need the extra support of a residential treatment program. Ideally, adults with intellectual disability in need of such support live in small to medium-size residences that are integrated into the community. Medical care is provided, and trained, live-in supervisors and aides help with residents' special needs around the clock. Residents are encouraged to participate in household routines to the best of their abilities.

Many adults with intellectual disability have jobs and are able to live independently in their own apartments. Others live semi-independently in apartments housing three to four adults; generally, a counselor provides aid in the evening.

Behavioral Treatments   Early-intervention programs using behavioral techniques have been developed to improve the level of functioning of people with intellectual disability. Specific behavioral objectives are defined, and children are taught skills in small, sequential steps (Grey & Hastings, 2005).

To teach a child a routine, the therapist usually begins by dividing the targeted behavior, such as eating, into smaller components: pick up spoon, scoop food from plate onto spoon, bring spoon to mouth, remove food with lips, chew, and swallow food. Operant conditioning principles are then applied to teach the child these components of eating. For example, the child may be reinforced for successive approximations to picking up the spoon until he or she is able to do so. This approach to teaching new behaviors is sometimes called *applied behavior analysis*, and it is

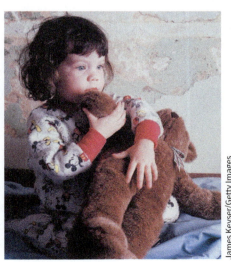

Although lead-based paint is now illegal, it can still be found in older homes. Eating these paint chips can cause lead poisoning, which can cause intellectual disability.

also used to reduce inappropriate and self-injurious behaviors (Newcomb & Hagopian, 2018). Much of the research in this area has been done with single-case experimental designs, but meta-analyses of these studies have been conducted and show support for the effectiveness of the approach (Heyvaert, Maes, et al., 2012).

A version of this treatment is called **functional communication training (FCT)** (Carr & Durand, 1985; Durand & Moskowitz, 2015). This behavioral intervention involves replacing a problem behavior (e.g., yelling) with a more socially appropriate behavior (e.g., asking or raising a hand). The approach begins with a functional analysis. What function is the problem behavior serving? For example, a child who is yelling may be thirsty and want some water. This functional analysis is used to identify a more appropriate behavior (e.g., pointing to the faucet or a glass). The new behavior results in the same desired outcome—getting a drink of water—and replaces the problematic behavior. This treatment has good empirical support (Durand & Moskowitz, 2015; Heath, Ganz, et al., 2015).

Cognitive Treatments

Many children with intellectual disability have difficulty using strategies in solving problems, and when they do use strategies, they often do not use them effectively. Thus, they can benefit from instruction in problem solving. These children may also have significant speech and language impairments and therefore benefit from interventions aimed at helping with speech and communication, broadly referred to as augmentative and alternative communication (AAC) interventions. AAC interventions include the use of sign language and other nonverbal forms of communication as well as computer-assisted techniques (Abbeduto, McDuffie, et al., 2016).

One group of researchers taught high school students with intellectual disability to make their own buttered toast and clean up after themselves (Hughes, Hugo, & Blatt, 1996). A teacher would demonstrate and verbalize the steps involved in solving a problem, such as the toaster's being upside down or unplugged. The young people learned to talk themselves through the steps using simple verbal or signed instructions. For example, when the toaster was presented upside down, the person would be taught to first state the problem ("Won't go in"), then state the response ("Turn it"), self-evaluate ("Fixed it"), and self-reinforce ("Good"). They were rewarded with praise and high fives when they verbalized and solved the problem correctly.

Another way in which communication and speech can be improved is by teaching parents how to help their children. These parent-implemented interventions have been shown to be effective (Abbeduto et al., 2016). The goal of this type of intervention is to provide parents with skills to use with their children consistently to help increase speech and communication. Because parents are with their children more than a therapist is, they have more opportunities to model and reinforce communication.

Computer-Assisted Instruction

Computer-assisted instruction is being used increasingly in educational and treatment settings. This is another type of AAC that is useful in helping people with intellectual disability (Butcher & Jameson, 2016; Luiselli & Fischer, 2016). The visual and auditory components of computers can help to maintain the attention of distractible students; the level of the material can be geared to the individual, ensuring successful experiences; and the computer can meet the need for numerous repetitions of material without becoming bored or impatient, as a human teacher might. For example, computers have been used to help people with intellectual disability learn to use an ATM (Davies, Stock, & Wehmeyer, 2003). Smartphones can be enormously helpful by providing reminders, directions, instructions, and descriptions of daily tasks.

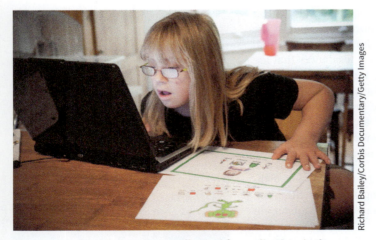

Computer-assisted instruction is well suited for applications in the treatment of intellectual disability.

Richard Bailey/Corbis Documentary/Getty Images

Quick Summary

Dyslexia is a specifier for the category *specific learning disorder* in DSM-5-TR. Other specifiers include dyscalculia (impairment in math) and impairment in written expression. Dyslexia affects 5–15% of school-age children, and it is often identified and treated in schools.

The DSM-5-TR category *intellectual developmental disorder (intellectual disability)* emphasizes the importance of assessing intellectual ability and adaptive functioning within a person's cultural group, consistent with the approach of the AAIDD. It is also important to identify an individual's strengths and weaknesses. There are a number of known causes of intellectual disability, including genetic and chromosomal abnormalities, infections, and toxins.

13.3 Check Your Knowledge

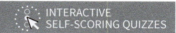 INTERACTIVE SELF-SCORING QUIZZES

(Answers are at the end of the chapter.)
Answer the following questions.

1. Which of the following is *not* one of the specific learning, communication, and motor disorders in DSM-5-TR?

    a. speech sound disorder

    b. developmental coordination disorder

    c. auditory impairment disorder

    d. language disorder

2. Which of the following is *true* about dyslexia?

    a. It affects boys more than girls.

    b. It is not a separate disorder but a type (specifier) of specific learning disorder.

    c. It affects between 5% and 15% of school-age children.

    d. All of the above are true.

3. Which of the following has *not* been established as a cause for intellectual disability?

    a. chromosomal abnormalities such as trisomy 21

    b. PKU

    c. lead poisoning

    d. All of the above have been found to cause intellectual disability.

4. Which of the following is *not* one of the components of the AAIDD definition of intellectual disability?

    a. onset in childhood

    b. deficits in language acquisition

    c. deficits in intellectual functioning

    d. deficits in adaptive functioning

Autism Spectrum Disorder

Although autism was first described over 75 years ago (see **Focus on Discovery 13.3** for the history of autism), it was not formally included in the DSM until the third edition, published in 1980. As discussed in Focus on Discovery 13.2, the rates of **autism spectrum disorder (ASD)** have been rising over the past 20 years. With this increase in prevalence has come an increase in research on the causes of this disorder.

Focus on Discovery 13.3

A Brief History of Autism Spectrum Disorder

Autism was identified in 1943 by a psychiatrist at Johns Hopkins, Leo Kanner, who, in the course of his clinical work, had noted 11 children who behaved in ways that were not common among children with another psychological disorder. He named the syndrome *early infantile autism* because he observed that "there is from the start an extreme autistic aloneness that, whenever possible, disregards, ignores, shuts out anything that comes to the child from the outside" (Kanner, 1943).

Kanner considered autistic aloneness to be the most fundamental symptom. He learned that these 11 children had been unable from the beginning of life to relate to people in the ordinary way. They were severely limited in language and had a strong, obsessive desire for everything about them to remain unchanged. Despite its early description by Kanner and others (e.g., Rimland, 1964), the disorder was not accepted into official diagnostic nomenclature until the publication of DSM-III in 1980, where it was called *autistic disorder*.

Asperger's disorder was named after Hans Asperger, who in 1944 described the syndrome as being less severe and having fewer communication deficits than autism. It was first introduced to the DSM in 1994 in DSM-IV. In this disorder, social relationships are difficult and stereotyped behavior can be intense and rigid, but language and intelligence are intact. Greater awareness about Asperger's (what we now consider a milder form of ASD) has been important for many adults who for years wondered why they were different from others. Adults with these symptoms are now more frequently recognized and treated by mental health professionals than they were 20 years ago (Gaus, 2018).

Because research suggests that Asperger's disorder does not differ qualitatively from autistic disorder, these two categories were combined in DSM-5. Researchers, clinicians, and families have referred to the "autism spectrum" for years, so, in some ways, this change fits with the language that many were using, at least in terms of the name. However, some worry that the stigma associated with the name *autism* might keep people from seeking help.

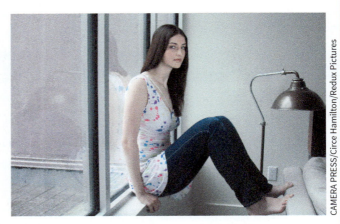

Heather Kuzmich, a finalist on the TV show *America's Next Top Model*, has what was called Asperger's disorder in DSM-IV-TR but is called autism spectrum disorder in DSM-5.

Clinical Descriptions, Prevalence, and Prognosis of Autism Spectrum Disorder

The symptoms of ASD fall into three broad domains: (1) social and emotional behavior, (2) communication, and (3) repetitive and ritualistic behaviors. These symptoms typically emerge in the first 3 years of life (Jones, Gliga, et al., 2014; Tiede & Walton, 2021). Efforts are under way to identify ASD even prior to age 3 so that intervention efforts can begin early while the brain is developing (Constantino, Charman, & Jones, 2021; Talbott & Miller, 2020). Evidence also indicates that these domains worsen from infancy to early childhood (Ozonoff & Iosif, 2019).

Social and Emotional Behavior

Children with ASD can have profound problems with the social world. They may rarely approach others and may look through or past people or turn their backs on them. For example, one study found that children with ASD rarely offered a spontaneous greeting or farewell (either verbally or by smiling, making eye contact, or gesturing) upon meeting or departing from an adult (Hobson & Lee, 1998). Children with ASD are less likely to initiate play with other children, and they are more likely to remain by themselves in social situations (Corbett, Swain, et al., 2014; Jones et al., 2014; Locke, Shih, et al., 2016).

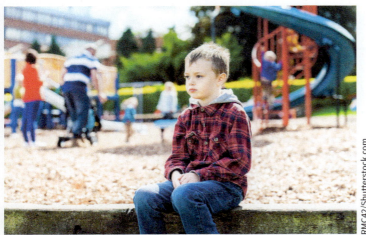

Children with ASD do not often play or socially interact with other children.

Children with ASD sometimes make eye contact, but their gaze may have an unusual quality. Typically, children gaze to gain someone's attention or to direct the other person's attention to an object; children with ASD generally do not (Dawson, Toth, et al., 2004; Tiede & Walton, 2021). This is often referred to as a problem in **joint attention**. That is, interactions that require two people to pay attention to each other, whether speaking or communicating emotion nonverbally, are impaired in children with autism.

More fine-grained analyses of gaze involve measuring eye movements and looking time. In one study, 6-month-old infants later diagnosed with ASD spent less time looking at videos of dynamic speaking faces, particularly at the eyes and mouth regions, than did typically developing children (Shic, Macari, & Chawarska, 2014). A different study measured the eye movements of infants several different times between the ages of 2 months and 24 months (Jones & Klin, 2013). At 2 months, the eye movements of infants who later were diagnosed with ASD did not differ from those of typically developing infants, suggesting that children with ASD are not born with gaze deficits. However, from 2 months to 24 months, the pattern of gaze between the two groups of infants began to diverge. Overall, the time spent looking at faces declined in the group of infants with ASD, so much so that by 2 years of age, these children were looking at the faces 50% less than children without ASD. Infants who showed a faster decline in looking time, particularly at the eyes region, were the ones who later had more social deficits. Older children with ASD are also less likely to spontaneously look at others and to respond to facial expressions (Sivaraman, Virues-Ortega, & Roeyers, 2020).

Some researchers have found that children with ASD have a deficient theory of mind that is at the core of the kinds of social dysfunctions we have described here (Gopnik, Capps, & Meltzoff, 2000; Mazza, Mariano, et al., 2017). *Theory of mind* refers to a person's understanding that other people have desires, beliefs, intentions, and emotions that may be different from one's own. This ability is crucial for understanding and successfully engaging in social interactions. Theory of mind typically develops from the ages of 2½ to 5. Children with ASD seem not to undergo this developmental milestone and thus seem unable to understand others' perspectives and emotional reactions.

Although some children with ASD can learn to understand emotional experiences, they have a good deal of difficulty with understanding others' feelings. Laboratory studies of children with ASD have found that they may recognize others' emotions without really understanding them (Capps, Rasco, et al., 1999; Capps, Yirmiya, & Sigman, 1992). For example, when asked to explain why someone was angry, a child with ASD responded "because he was yelling" (Capps, Losh, & Thurber, 2000).

Communication Difficulties

Even before they acquire language, some children with ASD show deficits in communication. By age 2, most typically developing children use words to represent objects in their surroundings and construct one- and two-word sentences to express more complex thoughts, such as "Mommy go" or "Me juice." In contrast, children with ASD lag well behind in these abilities and often show other language disturbances.

One such feature associated with ASD is *echolalia*, in which the child echoes, usually with remarkable fidelity, what they heard another person say. The teacher may ask a child with ASD, "Do you want a cookie?" The child's response may be, "Do you want a cookie?" This is immediate echolalia. In delayed echolalia, the child may be in a room with the television on and appear to be completely uninterested. Several hours later or even the next day, the child may echo a word or phrase from the television program.

Another language abnormality common in the speech of children with ASD is *pronoun reversal*, in which children refer to themselves as "he," "she," or "you" (or even by their own name). For example:

Parent:	What are you doing, Johnny?
Child:	He's here.
Parent:	Are you having a good time?
Child:	He knows it.

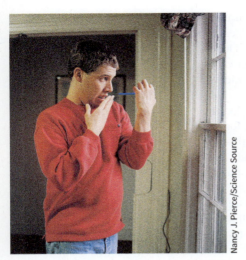

People with ASD may engage in stereotyped behavior, such as ritualistic hand movements.

Repetitive and Ritualistic Behaviors   Children with ASD can become upset over changes in their daily routines and surroundings. An offer of milk in a different drinking cup or a rearrangement of furniture may make them cry or may precipitate a temper tantrum.

Children with ASD may become focused on and preoccupied with specific things. In their play, they may continually line up toys or construct intricate patterns with household objects. As they grow older, they may become preoccupied with train schedules, subway routes, and number sequences. Children with ASD are also likely to perform a more limited number of behaviors than children without ASD and are less likely to explore new surroundings.

Children with ASD may also display stereotypical behavior, peculiar ritualistic hand movements, and other rhythmic movements, such as endless body rocking, hand flapping, and walking on tiptoe. They may spin and twirl string, crayons, sticks, and plates; twiddle their fingers in front of their eyes; and stare at fans and other spinning things. Researchers often describe these as self-stimulatory activities. The children may become preoccupied with manipulating an object and may become very upset when interrupted.

Some children with ASD become preoccupied with and form strong attachments to simple inanimate objects (e.g., keys, rocks, a wire-mesh basket, light switches, a large blanket) and to more complex mechanical objects (e.g., refrigerators and vacuum cleaners). If the object is something they can carry, they may walk around with it in their hands, and this may interfere with their learning to do more useful things.

Prevalence of Autism Spectrum Disorder   ASD begins in early childhood and can be evident in the first months of life. It affects about 1 in every 36 children. About four times more boys than girls have ASD (Maenner, Shaw, et al., 2020). It is found in all socioeconomic, ethnic, and racial groups. The diagnosis of ASD is very stable. In one study, 336 out of 400 children diagnosed with ASD early (at 14 months) retained the diagnosis at follow-up a year later; another 35 showed ASD features at follow-up but did not meet the diagnostic criteria (Pierce, Gazestani, et al., 2019).

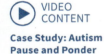

VIDEO CONTENT

Case Study: Autism Pause and Ponder

Defining Symptoms of Autism Spectrum Disorder

- Significant problems in social communication and social interactions, such as:

  1. Problems in understanding other people's emotions, reluctance to approach others, trouble with back-and-forth conversations
  2. Problems in maintaining eye contact, showing facial expressions, or using gestures to communicate with other people
  3. Problems in forming and keeping peer relationships

- Repeated and ritualistic behavior patterns, interests, or activities, such as:

  1. Repeating the same speech, movements, or use of objects over and over again in a fairly fixed and stable manner
  2. Extreme desire to maintain routines or behavior rituals; can become very upset if required to change
  3. Preoccupation with just a few interests or objects
  4. Very sensitive to sensory input or unusually interested in the sensory environment, such as being enchanted by lights or spinning objects

---

Comorbidity and ASD   Most children with ASD do not have comorbid intellectual disability (Christensen, Bilder, et al., 2016). Children who do have deficits in cognitive abilities can still be quite graceful and adept at swinging, climbing, or balancing, whereas children with intellectual disability have far more difficulty in areas of gross motor development, such as learning to walk. Sometimes children with ASD may have isolated skills that reflect great talent, such as the ability to multiply two 4-digit numbers rapidly in their heads.

As many as a third of children with ASD also have a specific learning disorder (Lichtenstein, Carlstrom, et al., 2010). In addition, ASD is also frequently comorbid with anxiety, including separation anxiety, social anxiety, ADHD, and specific phobias (Antshel, Zhang-James, et al., 2016; Johnson, Gliga, et al., 2015; Simonoff, Pickles, et al., 2008; Talbott & Miller, 2020; White, Oswald, et al., 2009).

Prognosis for Autism Spectrum Disorder   What happens to children with ASD when they reach adulthood? Generally, children with higher IQs who learn to speak before age 6 have the best outcomes. For example, one longitudinal study of children with ASD from preschool to early adulthood found that IQ scores higher than 70 predicted more strengths and fewer weaknesses in adaptive functioning as the children grew older (McGovern & Sigman, 2005), and outcomes were better for those who had interacted and engaged more with their peers. Another large prospective study followed people with ASD from age 2 to age 19. Young adults with IQ scores over 70 at age 19 were doing better socially and on adaptive functioning; 25% no longer met the criteria for ASD (Anderson, Liang, & Lord, 2014). **Focus on Discovery 13.4** describes a woman with ASD whose adult life is remarkable for professional distinction blended with the social and emotional deficits that are part of ASD.

Focus on Discovery 13.4

The Story of a Woman Living with Autism Spectrum Disorder

Temple Grandin has autism spectrum disorder. She also has a Ph.D. in animal science, runs her own business designing machinery for use with farm animals, and is on the faculty at Colorado State University. Four autobiographical books (Grandin, 1986, 1995, 2008, 2013) by her and a profile by the late neurologist Oliver Sacks (1995) provide a moving and revealing portrait of the mysteries of ASD. A highly acclaimed HBO movie based on Grandin's 1995 book, *Thinking in Pictures,* starred Clare Danes as Grandin. Grandin has also written other books about her professional work with animals.

Lacking understanding of the complexities and subtleties of human social discourse and deficient in the ability to empathize with others, Grandin sums up her relationship to the nonautistic world by saying, "Much of the time I feel like an anthropologist on Mars" (Sacks, 1995, p. 259).

Grandin was diagnosed with autism in 1950 at age 3. She had no speech at all, and doctors predicted that institutionalization would be her fate. However, with the help of a therapeutic nursery school, speech therapy, and the support of her family, she learned to speak by age 6 and began to make more contact with others. Still, as an adolescent, she was mystified by the ability of other children to understand each other's needs and wishes, to empathize, and to communicate.

In her own writings, Grandin points out that many people with ASD are great fans of *Star Trek*, especially the characters of Spock and Data. Spock is a member of the Vulcan race, purely intellectual, logical beings who eschew any consideration of the emotional side of life. Data is an android, a highly sophisticated computer housed in a human body and, like Spock, lacking in emotion. (One of the dramatic themes involving both characters was, of course, their flirtation with the experience of human emotion, portrayed with particular poignancy by Data. This is a theme in Grandin's life as well.) As Grandin (1995) wrote at age 47:

All my life I have been an observer, and I have always felt like someone who watches from the outside. I could not participate in the social interactions of high school life.

Even today, personal relationships are something I don't really understand. I've remained celibate because doing so helps me avoid the many complicated situations that are too difficult for me to handle. [M]en who want to date often don't understand how to relate to a woman. They [and I myself] remind me of Data, the android on Star Trek*. In one episode, Data's attempts at dating were a disaster. When he tried to be romantic [by effecting a change in a subroutine of his computer program], he complimented his date by using scientific terminology. Even very able adults with autism have such problems. (pp. 132–133)*

Some of the difficulties of people with ASD make them charmingly honest and trustworthy. "Lying," wrote Grandin, "is very anxiety-provoking because it requires rapid interpretations of subtle social cues [of which I am incapable] to determine whether the other person is really being deceived" (Grandin, 1995, p. 135).

Grandin's professional career is impressive. She uses her remarkable powers of visualization and her empathy for farm animals to design machines that reduce suffering, such as a chute that leads cows to slaughter via a circular route, which protects them from the fear evoked by awareness of their fate until the moment of death.

Accounts from Grandin and others with ASD can provide insight into how people adapt to their own idiosyncrasies, using the seemingly peculiar gifts they have been given and working around the difficulties they experience. Sacks took note of Grandin's own words about how she has come to think of herself. "If I could snap my fingers and be nonautistic, I would not—because then I wouldn't be me. Autism is part of who I am" (quoted in Sacks, 1995, p. 291).

This sentiment was emphasized in Grandin's most recent book (2013), where she stated that there are many things *right* with the autistic brain. In other words, some of the difficulties experienced by people with autism can also be strengths. For example, one of the reasons that social interactions are difficult for her to decipher is that they require an integration of many things happening all at once (e.g., words, facial expressions, gestures, tone of voice). However, she is quite good at concentrating on one thing at a time, and she can bring a laser focus to small details. She credits her success with animals to this ability; she is able to see a small detail that might scare an animal but that other people would ignore.

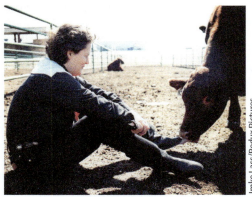

Temple Grandin, Ph.D., was diagnosed with autism in early childhood and has had a successful academic career.

Imke Lass/Redux Pictures

Causes of Autism Spectrum Disorder

The earliest theory about the cause of ASD was that psychological factors, such as bad parenting, were responsible for its development. This narrow and faulty perspective unfortunately put an undue emotional burden on parents who were told that they were at fault for their child's ASD. Evidence now shows that genetic and neurological factors are important in the cause.

Genetic Factors   Evidence suggests a strong genetic component for ASD, with heritability estimates between 0.60 and 0.90 (Bai, Yip, et al., 2019; Gaugler, Klei, et al., 2014; Tick, Bolton, et al., 2015). Twin studies have found concordance rates of 47–90% for ASD between identical twins, compared with concordance rates of 0–20% between fraternal twins (Lichtenstein et al., 2010; Tick et al., 2015). Even though genes play a big role in ASD, remember that genes do their work via the environment. Shared environmental factors (e.g., common experiences in a family; see Chapter 2) and nonshared environmental factors (e.g., peers) also account for some of the risk for ASD (Bai et al., 2019; Hallmayer, Cleveland, et al., 2011).

Studies of twins and of families with a member with ASD suggest that ASD is linked genetically to a broader spectrum of deficits in communication and social interaction. In families where more than one child had ASD or language delay, unaffected siblings also exhibited deficits in social communication and interactions (Constantino, Zhang, et al., 2010).

Molecular genetics studies try to pinpoint areas of the genome that may confer risk for ASD. Findings from GWAS have not yet provided a clear set of findings. One GWAS (Autism Spectrum Disorders Working Group of the Psychiatric Genomics Consortium, 2017) did not reveal SNPs meeting the strict statistical test thresholds required, but several genes were identified as possible markers and, importantly, these genes had been identified in other studies (Chaste, Klei, et al., 2015). Another larger GWAS with over 18,000 people with ASD (Grove, Ripke, et al., 2019) found evidence for five SNPs specific to ASD and another seven loci that were also present in schizophrenia and depression. An even larger cross-disorder GWAS analyzed data from over 750,000 people across eight different disorders and found shared SNPs between ASD and ADHD (Cross-Disorder Group of the Psychiatric Genomics Consortium, 2019). As in many of the studies of genetics we have reviewed in the book, finding genetic similarities across disorders is more common than finding specific genes or mutations for specific disorders (see Chapter 2 for more on this). Given this complexity, finding the many genes that are associated with genetic vulnerability to autism remains a challenge.

Neurobiological Factors   A number of studies examining the brain in people with ASD have been well replicated, allowing for a clearer picture of what may go wrong in the brain of a person with ASD. What remains to be figured out is why the brain goes awry early in development. It should be noted that brain imaging can be difficult with young children, and ASD can be diagnosed in toddlers. Brain-imaging studies of adolescents and adults with ASD may produce different results, not necessarily due to ASD changes but perhaps due to age changes in brain development. A key example of this is in connection with so-called brain overgrowth.

Studies using magnetic resonance imaging (MRI) found that, overall, the brains of adults and children with ASD large are larger than the brains of adults and children without ASD (Courchesne, Campbell, & Solso, 2011; Courchesne, Carnes, & Davis, 2001; Girault & Piven, 2020). What makes these findings particularly interesting and puzzling is that most children with ASD are born with brains of a relatively normal size; however, at ages 1–4, the brains of children with ASD become significantly larger (Courchesne, 2004). A longitudinal study of babies at high familial risk for ASD (i.e., someone else in the family had ASD) measured the trajectory of brain growth using MRI at 6, 12, and 24 months of age (Hazlett, Gu, et al., 2017). The researchers found that the overall growth rate of brain size was greater between 12 and 24 months and that the surface area of the brain grew faster at 12–24 months for the high-risk babies. They also found that brain size at 24 months was positively correlated with ASD symptoms. These findings suggest that the first few years of life may be a critical period of brain development for children who develop ASD.

Having a larger-than-normal brain is not necessarily a good thing, as it might indicate that neurons are not being pruned correctly. The pruning of neurons is an important part of brain maturation; older children have fewer connections between neurons than do babies. Adding further to this puzzle, brain growth in ASD appears to slow abnormally in later childhood. It is worth noting that the areas of the brain that are "overgrown" in ASD include the frontal, temporal, and cerebellar regions, which have been linked with language, social, and emotional functions.

Other areas of the brain are implicated in ASD as well. The cerebellum supports movement as well as cognition, and abnormalities in this brain area have been linked to posture, exploration, and gaze problems in ASD (Fatemi, Aldinger, et al., 2012; Hampson & Blatt, 2015; Su, Xu, et al., 2020). The cerebellum is connected to many other areas of the brain, including sensory and frontal cortices, and disruptions to these connections may help explain some of the ASD symptoms, such as theory of mind (Olson, Hoffman, et al., 2023).

Given that ASD is associated with social and emotional difficulties, it stands to reason that the areas of the brain that support these functions might be involved in ASD. That appears to be the case based on findings about brain structure, function, and connectivity. A large study by the group called Enhancing Neuroimaging Genetics Through Meta-Analysis (ENIGMA) combined data from 49 different studies that included over 3,000 people with and without ASD (van Rooij, Anagnostou, et al., 2018). The researchers found differences between those with and without ASD in the frontal cortex, amygdala, and striatum, and these differences were found in children as young as 2 years and adults as old as 64 years. Other meta-analyses have also found differences in the amygdala (Stanfield, McIntosh, et al., 2008). A meta-analysis of fMRI studies examined BOLD (blood oxygenation level dependent) responses during social and nonsocial tasks and found less activation in the striatum for both types of reward in people with ASD compared to people without ASD (Clements, Zoltowski, et al., 2018). Finally, studies show disruptions in brain connectivity of brain region networks that support social behavior (Müller & Fishman, 2018).

In sum, areas of the brain that are involved in social and emotional processes are implicated in ASD.

Treatment of Autism Spectrum Disorder

Even though genetic and neurological factors in the cause of ASD have much more empirical support than psychological factors, it is the psychological treatments that currently show the most promise, not medications.

Treatments for children with ASD are usually aimed at reducing their unusual behavior and improving their communication and social skills. In most cases, the earlier the intervention begins, the better the outcome. In a promising longitudinal study, children at high risk for developing ASD (having a parent or sibling with ASD) were studied beginning at age 14 months. Even though these children did not yet have language, the researchers were able to identify deficits in joint attention and communication that allowed for an early provisional diagnosis of ASD (Landa, Holman, & Garrett-Mayer, 2007).

Behavioral Treatment
Psychologist Ivar Lovaas developed a behavioral treatment consisting of intensive operant conditioning with young (under 4 years old) children with ASD (Lovaas, 1987). Therapy encompassed all aspects of the children's lives for more than 40 hours a week over a period of more than 2 years. Parents were also trained extensively so that treatment could continue during almost all the children's waking hours. Nineteen children receiving this intensive treatment were compared with 40 children who received a similar treatment for less than 10 hours per week. Both groups of children were rewarded for being less aggressive, more compliant, and more socially appropriate—for example, talking and playing with other children.

The results of this landmark study were dramatic and encouraging: Children in the intensive-treatment group showed a larger increase in IQ scores in 1st grade, and more children in this group were advanced to 2nd grade than were children in the other group. A follow-up of these children 4 years later indicated that the

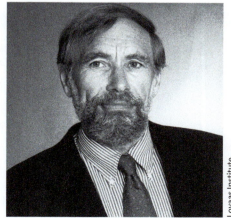

Ivar Lovaas, a behavior therapist, was noted for his operant conditioning treatment of children with autism.

intensive-treatment group maintained their gains in IQ score, adaptive behavior, and grade promotions in school (McEachin, Smith, & Lovaas, 1993). Although critics rightly pointed out weaknesses in the study's methodology and outcome measures (Schopler, Short, & Mesibov, 1989), this ambitious program demonstrated the benefits of intensive therapy with the heavy involvement of both professionals and parents in dealing with the challenges of ASD.

A meta-analysis of 22 studies using other types of intensive behavioral treatments, either in a clinic setting or with parents as the primary point of intervention, reported several noteworthy results. First, the average quality of these studies, rated on a 1 to 5 scale, with 5 being the best, was only 2.5. Few were randomized clinical trials, and many had very small sample sizes. With these limitations in mind, the overall effect sizes were large for changes in IQ score, language skills, overall communication, socialization, and daily living skills (Virués-Ortega, 2010). These results are encouraging, but it remains important to conduct more rigorous studies of these types of treatments. Unfortunately, there are still too few high-quality studies of ASD interventions to make strong conclusions about effectiveness (Sandbank, Bottema-Beutel, et al., 2020).

Another broad type of intervention is referred to as "naturalistic developmental behavioral interventions" or NDBI (Schreibman, Dawson, et al., 2015). These interventions draw from developmental psychology and behavioral principles and are delivered in a child's natural environment (e.g., home). A recent meta-analysis found that these interventions were effective, but the study quality was also a concern (Sandbank et al., 2020). One example of an NDBI is an intervention that seeks to improve children's problems in joint attention and communication. In a randomized controlled clinical trial, children ages 3 and 4 with ASD were randomly assigned to a joint attention (JA) intervention, a symbolic play (SP) intervention, or a control group (Kasari, Freeman, & Paparella, 2006). All children were already part of an early-intervention program; the JA and SP interventions were additional interventions provided to the children in 30-minute daily blocks for 6 weeks. Children in the JA and SP intervention groups showed more improvement than children in the control group, and at 6 and 12 months after the treatment, children in the JA and SP groups had greater expressive language skills than children in the control group (Kasari, Paparella, et al., 2008).

Medications   Medication treatment of ASD is less effective than behavioral treatment. The medications most commonly used for treating problem behaviors in children with ASD are antipsychotic medications, such as haloperidol (trade name Haldol), aripiprazole (trade name Abilify), and risperidone (trade name Risperdal). Some controlled studies have shown that these drugs can reduce irritability or problem behaviors like aggression or self-injury (Fung, Mahajan, et al., 2016; Hellings, Arnold, & Han, 2017; McCracken, McGough, et al., 2002). Many children do not respond positively to the medications, however, and children may develop troubling side effects, such as weight gain, fatigue, or tremors (Masi, DeMayo, et al., 2017).

13.4 Check Your Knowledge

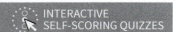
INTERACTIVE
SELF-SCORING QUIZZES

(Answers are at the end of the chapter.)
True or false?

1. All children with ASD also have intellectual disability.
2. Children with ASD have difficulty recognizing emotions in others.
3. Medication is an effective treatment for ASD.

Summary

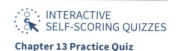
INTERACTIVE
SELF-SCORING QUIZZES
Chapter 13 Practice Quiz

Clinical Descriptions of Childhood Disorders

- Childhood disorders are often organized into two domains: externalizing disorders and internalizing disorders. Externalizing disorders are characterized by such behaviors as aggressiveness, noncompliance, overactivity, and impulsiveness; they include attention-deficit/hyperactivity disorder, conduct disorder, and oppositional defiant disorder. Internalizing disorders are characterized by such behaviors as depression, social withdrawal, and anxiety; they include childhood anxiety and mood disorders.

- Attention-deficit/hyperactivity disorder (ADHD) is a persistent pattern of inattention and/or hyperactivity and impulsivity that is more frequent and more severe than what is typically observed in children of a given age. Conduct disorder is characterized by high and widespread levels of aggression, lying, theft, vandalism, cruelty to other people and to animals, and other acts that violate laws and social norms.

- Mood and anxiety disorders in children have similarities with the adult forms of these disorders. However, differences that reflect different stages of development are also important.

- Dyslexia is a type of specific learning disorder, and it involves problems in reading.

- The AAID approach to intellectual disability specifies that deficits in intellectual functioning and adaptive behavior be considered in context. Most professionals focus more on the strengths of people with intellectual disability. This shift in emphasis is associated with increased efforts to design psychological and educational interventions that make the most of individual abilities.

- Autism spectrum disorder begins early in life. The major symptoms are difficulties in relating to other people; communication problems, consisting of either difficulties in learning language or speech irregularities such as echolalia and pronoun reversal; and deficient theory of mind.

Causes of Childhood Disorders

- There is strong evidence for genetic factors in the development of ADHD. Low birth weight and maternal smoking are also risk factors. Family factors such as parental practices can exacerbate symptoms but do not cause ADHD.

- Among the apparent etiological and risk factors for conduct disorder are genetics, inadequate learning of moral awareness and social emotions, dysfunction in brain areas including the amygdala and prefrontal cortex, and negative peer influences.

- Etiological factors for mood and anxiety disorders in children are believed to be largely the same as in adults.

- Some forms of intellectual disability have a genetic or chromosomal basis, such as the trisomy 21 that characterizes Down syndrome. Certain infectious diseases in a pregnant woman, such as toxoplasmosis and rubella, as well as illnesses that affect the child directly, such as encephalitis, can interfere with cognitive and social development. Environmental hazards, such as lead-based paint, can also cause intellectual disability.

- Compelling evidence suggests that ASD is highly heritable. Identifying ASD genes and genetic mutations has proved more difficult. Abnormalities have been found in the brains of children with ASD, including overgrowth of the brain by age 2 and abnormalities in the cerebellum, frontal cortex, amygdala, and striatum.

Treatment of Childhood Disorders

- A combined treatment including stimulant drugs, such as Adderall or Ritalin, and intensive behavioral treatment has shown effectiveness in reducing the symptoms of ADHD.

- The most promising approach to treating young people with conduct disorder involves intensive multisystemic treatment, which includes interventions focused on family, school, and peers.

- Cognitive behavior therapy is effective for mood and anxiety disorders in children and adolescents. Interpersonal therapy is effective for depression in adolescents. Medication is effective for depression among adolescents, though its use is not without controversy. Medication is also effective for anxiety when combined with a cognitive behavior therapy, such as Coping Cat.

- Behavioral treatments, such as functional communication training and computer-assisted instruction, have been used to successfully treat many of the behavioral problems of people with intellectual disability and to improve their problem-solving skills.

- The most effective treatments for ASD are psychological, involving intensive behavioral interventions and work with parents. Various drug treatments have been used but have proved less effective than behavioral interventions.

Answers to Check Your Knowledge Questions

13.1. 1. True; 2. True; 3. True; 4. False; 5. life-course-persistent; 6. ADHD, substance abuse, depression, anxiety; 7. parent management training; family checkup; multisystemic treatment.

13.2. 1. depression and specific phobia; 2. is associated with but does not cause; 3. stress; 4. Selective and universal; 5. PTSD; 6. Coping Cat.

13.3. 1. c. auditory impairment disorder; 2. d. All of the above are true; 3. d. All of the above have been found to cause intellectual disability; 4. b. deficits in language acquisition.

13.4. 1. False; 2. True; 3. False

Key Terms

attention-deficit/hyperactivity disorder (ADHD)   366
autism spectrum disorder (ASD)   395
conduct disorder   373
developmental psychopathology   366
Down syndrome (trisomy 21)   392
dyslexia   390

externalizing disorders   366
fragile X syndrome   392
functional communication training (FCT)   394
intellectual disability   391
internalizing disorders   366
joint attention   397

multisystemic treatment (MST)   378
parent management training (PMT)   377
phenylketonuria (PKU)   392
separation anxiety disorder   386
specific learning disorder   390

Late Life and Neurocognitive Disorders

LEARNING GOALS

1. Differentiate common misconceptions from established findings about age-related changes, and discuss methodological issues involved in conducting research on aging.

2. Describe the prevalence of psychological disorders in older adults and issues involved in estimating the prevalence.

3. Discuss the symptoms, causes, and treatment of differing forms of dementia.

4. Summarize the symptoms, triggers, and treatment of delirium.

Clinical Case

Henry

Henry, a 56-year-old businessman, was hospitalized for cervical disc surgery. Henry drank heavily but did not appear to have problems from his drinking. Surgery went well, and in the first couple of days, recovery seemed normal. The third night after his operation, though, Henry could not sleep and became restless. The next day he appeared severely fatigued. The next night his restlessness worsened, and he became fearful. Later that night, he thought that he saw people hiding in his room, and just before dawn, he thought that he saw strange little animals running around the room. By morning rounds, Henry was very frightened, lethargic, and incoherent. He knew who he was and where he was but did not know the date or how many days it had been since his surgery. During that day his mental status fluctuated, but by nightfall he had become grossly disoriented and agitated.

A psychiatric consultant diagnosed Henry with delirium, probably due to several factors: alcohol withdrawal, use of strong analgesics, and the stress of the operation. The treatment consisted of a reduction in pain medications, the continuous presence of a family member, and administration of 50 mg of chlorpromazine (Thorazine) three times daily and 500 mg of chloral hydrate at bedtime. Treatment reversed his confusion within 2 days, and he was able to return home in a week with no symptoms.

Adapted from Strub and Black, 1981, pp. 89–90.

In this chapter, we consider psychological disorders in late life, with a focus on dementia and delirium. We begin by reviewing some general topics relevant to understanding late life. We describe common myths about aging, and then describe some challenges and some remarkable strengths that come with growing older. Conducting research on aging is complicated by some methodological issues; we discuss evidence that the prevalence of psychological disorders such as depression, anxiety, and substance use disorder in older adults is quite low, and we critique this evidence. While rates of psychological disorders decline as people age, older adults are vulnerable to dementia and delirium (see **Figure 14.1**), and so these two conditions are a major focus of this chapter. Dementia is defined by a gradual deterioration of cognitive abilities, and delirium is an acute state of mental confusion and inability to focus attention. For dementia and delirium, we will consider the clinical description, causal factors, and treatment.

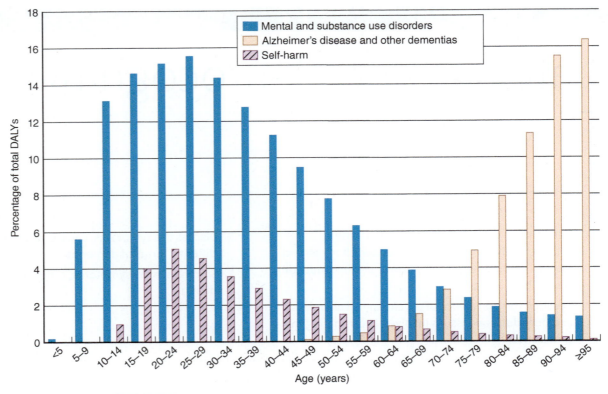

FIGURE 14.1   **The global burden of mental and substance use disorders and self-harm decreases across the life course, while the global burden of dementias increases across the life course.** (DALY = disability-adjusted life-year, which represents 1 lost year of healthy life.) Data are drawn from the Global Burden of Disease health data (2016). Reprinted from Patel, Saxena, et al., 2018.

Aging: Myths, Problems, and Methods

Older adults are usually defined as people over the age of 65, an arbitrary point set by social policies rather than any physiological process. In less than 200 years, life expectancy has almost doubled in the Western world (Oeppen & Vaupel, 2002). **Figure 14.2** shows the dramatic increase in the number of older Americans over time. As of 2016, there were 82,000

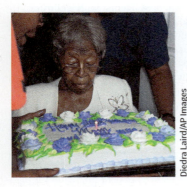

As life expectancy increases, the number of centenarians in the United States is expected to increase more than four-fold by the year 2050. Shown, Hester Ford, who died at age 115.

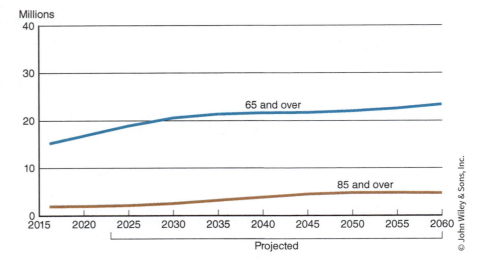

FIGURE 14.2   **The number of older adults is on the rise.**   The graph shows the number of people in the United States aged 65 and older and 85 and over, by decade of birth, for 1900–2010 and projected for 2020–2050 (U.S. Bureau of the Census, 2018).

people at least 100 years old in the United States; by 2050, that number is expected to quadruple (US Bureau of the Census, 2017). The speed of population aging is more rapid in Europe and particularly Asia than it is in the United States (Bloomberg Data, 2012). In some countries, this has raised concerns about how to address the medical and financial needs of a growing group of retired individuals. Rapid increases in the population of older adults appear to be taking a toll—countries with a sharper rise in numbers of older adults hold more negative attitudes toward older adults (North & Fiske, 2015). Worldwide, along with population aging have come rising rates of elder abuse (North & Fiske, 2015).

The social problems of aging may be especially severe for women. Although men with gray hair at the temples are seen as distinguished, wrinkles, sagging bodies, and other signs of aging in women are not valued in most cultures. The cosmetics and plastic surgery industries make billions of dollars each year exploiting the fear inculcated in women about looking their age. These attitudes toward aging, though, are not universal. Some cultures respect and revere their elders. In Abkhazia, a region of the Caucasus known for the longevity of the villagers, there is no phrase for "older people"—after age 100, individuals are called "long-living people," and each year, villagers celebrate a holiday of the long-living people (Robbins, 2007).

Myths About Late Life

Most people in the United States cling to certain assumptions about old age. Common myths include the idea that we will become doddering and befuddled. We worry that we will be unhappy, cope poorly with troubles, become focused on our poor health, and lead a lonely life.

Each of these myths has been debunked. As we will see, severe cognitive problems do not arise for most people in late life. Although a mild decline in some facets of cognitive functioning is common, different facets of cognition peak at different ages. The speed of information processing tends to peak around age 18, and short-term memory around age 25, with slow declines after that point. In contrast, people tend to accrue knowledge and vocabulary through their mid-60s, and some show increases even into their 80s (Hartshorne & Germine, 2015).

After a dip in middle age, happiness increases into late life in countries around the world (Blanchflower, 2021). Although you might suspect that these findings were artifacts of a reluctance of older individuals to describe negative feelings to researchers, laboratory studies verify that older adults are actually more skilled at regulating their emotions. For example, when shown positive and negative images, older people tend to pay more attention to the positive images (Isaacowitz, 2012) and to display less psychophysiological response to the negative images than do younger people (Kisley, Wood, & Burrows, 2007). When viewing negative images, they show more robust brain activation in regions implicated in emotion regulation than do younger people (Williams, Brown, et al., 2006). Many older people underreport somatic symptoms, perhaps because of acceptance that aches and pains are an inevitable part of aging. Even during the coronavirus disease 2019 pandemic, which threatened older more than younger age groups, older people reported more positive and fewer negative emotions (Carstensen et al., 2020).

The myth that older people are lonely has received considerable attention. The truth is that the breadth of the social activities in which older people engage is unrelated to their psychological well-being (Carstensen, 1996). As we age, our interests shift away from seeking new social interactions to cultivating a few social relationships that really matter to us, such as those with family and close friends. This phenomenon has been called **social selectivity**.

When we have less time ahead of us, we tend to place a higher value on emotional intimacy than on exploring the world. This preference applies not just to older people but also to younger people who see themselves as having limited time, such as those who are preparing to move far away from their home or who have a life-threatening illness (Frederickson & Carstensen, 1990). When we can't see a future without end, we prefer to spend our limited time with those with whom we have the closest ties rather than with casual acquaintances (Carstensen, 2021). Those unfamiliar with these age-related changes could easily misinterpret social selectivity as harmful social withdrawal.

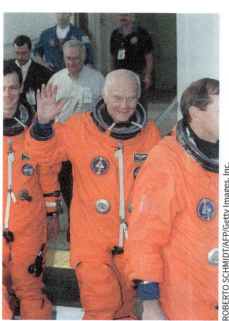

People spend billions of dollars per year on cosmetics and plastic surgery to reduce signs of aging.

As John Glenn's space flight at age 77 illustrated, advancing age need not lead to a curtailment of activities.

Many stereotypes we hold about older adults are false, but negative attitudes about older adults learned early in life persist and become negative self-perceptions as people move into their later years (Levy, 2009). These stereotypes appear to have long-term effects. Negative self-views about aging correlate with accelerated cellular aging, and they predict biomarkers of dementia (Levy, Ferrucci, et al., 2016) and earlier death (Levy, Slade, & Kasl, 2002). Not only do we need to challenge our own negative stereotypes, but we also need to help older adults challenge their views.

The Problems Experienced in Late Life

As a group, older adults have more stresses than any other age group. They have them all—physical decline and disabilities, sensory acuity deficits, loss of loved ones, the social stress of stigma toward older adults, and the cumulative effects of a lifetime of unfortunate experiences. By age 60, more than half of people have at least one medical condition that causes severe disability (Vos, Allen, et al., 2016). As people age, the quality and depth of sleep decline (Fetveit, 2009), and this decline can worsen physical, psychological, and cognitive problems unless treated (Ancoli-Israel, 2000). As one author wrote, "Late life would qualify as the Olympics of coping" (Fisher, 2011, p. 145).

Polypharmacy, the prescribing of multiple drugs to a person, is all too common. Forty percent of older adults take at least five medications (Kantor, Rehm, et al., 2015). All too often, doctors do not check to see whether the person is taking other medications or seeing other doctors. Many patients don't think to tell the doctor about over-the-counter medications, falsely assuming that those wouldn't have side effects or interactions. Once a patient is taking a medication regularly, many doctors don't consider reducing or removing that medication when symptoms dissipate (Opondo, Eslami, et al., 2012). Polypharmacy increases the risk of adverse drug reactions such as side effects and toxicity (Wastesson, Morin, et al., 2018). Often, physicians prescribe more medications to combat the side effects, thus amplifying the initial problem. Training pharmacists to monitor for polypharmacy is helpful in reducing it (Wastesson et al., 2018).

Further complicating the picture is the fact that medication side effects and toxicity are much more likely as people age. The Agency for Healthcare Research and Quality publishes a list of the many medications that are dangerous for older adults (https://www.guideline.gov/summaries/summary/49933). Across studies, it has been found that more than one-fifth of older people have been prescribed dangerous medications (Opondo et al., 2012). The STOPP/START screening tool is designed to identify dangerous medications prescribed to older patients and to suggest appropriate alternatives. Several randomized controlled trials indicate that the STOPP/START tool can reduce use of dangerous medications, as well as falls, delirium, time spent in hospitals, and medical costs (Hill-Taylor, Walsh, et al., 2016).

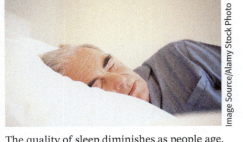

Image Source/Alamy Stock Photo

The quality of sleep diminishes as people age.

nito500/123 RF

Polypharmacy all too often creates problems for those in late life.

Research Methods in the Study of Aging

Conducting research on aging requires an understanding of several special issues. Because other factors associated with chronological age may influence findings, we must be cautious when we attribute differences between age groups solely to the effects of aging. In the field of aging, as in studies of childhood development, researchers distinguish among three kinds of effects (see **Table 14.1**):

- **Age effects** are the consequences of being a certain chronological age.
- **Cohort effects** are the consequences of growing up during a particular time period with its characteristic challenges and opportunities. For example, war and famine shape attitudes and health for decades to follow. Another example is the drastic change in the expectations for marriage over the past century, at least in Western societies, from a focus on stability to a focus on happiness and personal fulfillment.
- **Time-of-measurement effects** are confounds that arise because events at a particular point in time can have a specific effect on a variable that is being studied. For example, people tested while anticipating a major hurricane might demonstrate elevated levels of anxiety.

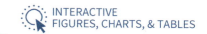
INTERACTIVE
FIGURES, CHARTS, & TABLES

TABLE 14.1   Age, Cohort, and Time-of-Measurement Effects

Age Effects	Cohort Effects	Time-of-Measurement Effects
The effects of being a certain age; e.g., being old enough to receive Social Security	The effects of having grown up during a particular time period; e.g., frugality may be increased among those who lived through the Great Depression of the 1930s	The effects of testing people at a particular time in history; e.g., people tested during the COVID-19 pandemic might express more anxiety

Researchers use two types of research designs to assess developmental change: cross-sectional and longitudinal. In cross-sectional studies, the investigator compares different age groups with regard to some variable at the same moment in time. Suppose that in 1995 we took a poll in the United States and found that many interviewees over age 80 spoke with a European accent, whereas those in their 40s and 50s did not. Could we conclude that as people grow older, they develop European accents? Hardly! Cross-sectional studies do not examine the same people over time; consequently, they do not provide clear information about how people change as they age.

In longitudinal studies, researchers periodically retest one group of people using the same measure over years or decades. For example, in the Baltimore Longitudinal Study of Aging that began in 1958, researchers have been following more than 3,000 men and women to see how their lifestyles, medical conditions, and psychological health change over time. From this study, a great deal has been learned about psychological health and aging. For example, researchers were able to combat the myth that people become unhappier over time. Rather, people who were happy at age 30 tended to be happy as they moved into late life (Costa, Metter, & McCrae, 1994). In general, longitudinal designs allow us to trace consistency or change within individuals over time. Although longitudinal studies offer fundamental advantages, results can be biased by attrition, as participants drop out of the study due to death, immobility, or lack of interest. When people are no longer available for follow-up because of death, the form of attrition is known as **selective mortality**. Selective mortality and attrition due to immobility result in a bias because findings obtained from the remaining sample are more relevant to drawing conclusions about relatively healthy people than about unhealthy people. Later in this chapter, we will discuss how these issues of cohort effects and selective mortality might influence estimates of the prevalence of psychological disorders.

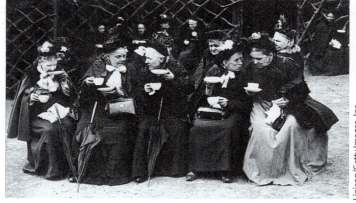

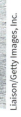
Liaison/Getty Images, Inc.

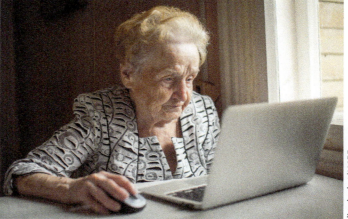
dimaberkut/123RF

Because of cohort effects, people examined over time at the same chronological age may differ considerably depending on when they were born.

Quick Summary

The number of older people in the world is burgeoning, highlighting the need for mental health professionals to understand the aging process. In contrast to stereotypes, most people as they age tend to become more effective at regulating emotions, to downplay medical symptoms, and to focus on core relationships over superficial social acquaintances and activities. Even older adults often hold negative stereotypes about aging, and the effects of such negative self-beliefs can be quite damaging. The challenges of late life do include declining health for many people. As an increasing number of chronic health problems emerge, polypharmacy becomes an issue for many. Compounding the hazards of polypharmacy is the tendency for people to become more sensitive to medication side effects and toxicity as they age.

In research on aging, it is difficult to disentangle age effects, cohort effects, and time-of-measurement effects. Cross-sectional studies do not help distinguish age and cohort effects. Longitudinal studies provide more clarity about age and cohort effects, but attrition can challenge the validity of findings. The form of attrition known as selective mortality is particularly important to consider in studies of aging.

14.1 Check Your Knowledge

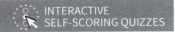
INTERACTIVE
SELF-SCORING QUIZZES

(Answers are at the end of the chapter.)
True or false?

1. The key to happiness in late life is to have many different types of social activities.

Answer the following questions.

2. How do emotions and responses to emotion-relevant stimuli change as people age?

3. How do values about social relationships tend to change as people age?

Psychological Disorders in Late Life

The DSM criteria are the same for older and younger adults. Some have criticized this approach, pointing out, for example, that the diagnostic criteria for substance use have not been adjusted to consider physiological changes in the liver and kidneys, even though a smaller quantity of alcohol or drugs may have more functional consequences as people age (Maree & Riccelli, 2018).

Because medical conditions are more common in older adults, it is particularly important to rule them out as explanations of symptoms. DSM criteria specify that a psychological disorder should not be diagnosed if the symptoms can be accounted for by a medical condition or medication side effects. Medical problems such as thyroid problems, Parkinson's disease, Alzheimer's disease, hypoglycemia, anemia, testosterone deficits, and vitamin deficiencies can produce symptoms that mimic schizophrenia, depression, or anxiety. Age-related deterioration in the vestibular system (inner-ear control of one's sense of balance) can account for panic symptoms such as severe dizziness. Depression is common after strokes or heart attacks (Carney & Freedland, 2017). Antihypertensive medication, corticosteroids, and antiparkinson medications may contribute to depression or anxiety. Cardiovascular problems can cause erectile problems. It is a complex task to disentangle medical and psychological concerns!

With this in mind, we examine the prevalence of psychological disorders in late life. We begin by discussing the best available estimates, and next we address concerns about their accuracy. We then briefly note ways that treatments can be modified to alleviate psychological disorders in older adults.

Prevalence Estimates of Psychological Disorders in Late Life

The prevalence estimates for psychological disorders defy stereotypes of unhappiness and anxiety in late life. Findings indicate that people over age 65 have the lowest prevalence of psychological disorders of all age groups. **Figure 14.3** provides 12-month estimates from the National Comorbidity Survey–Replication (NCS–R) study, which involved a representative community sample of thousands of people living in the United States who completed extensive diagnostic interviews (Gum, King-Kallimanis, & Kohn, 2009). As shown in the figure, every single disorder was less common in older adults than in younger adults. None of those aged 65 and older met the criteria for substance use disorders. Although not covered in the NCS–R study, rates of schizophrenia and personality disorders are also low among older adults (Balsis, Gleason,

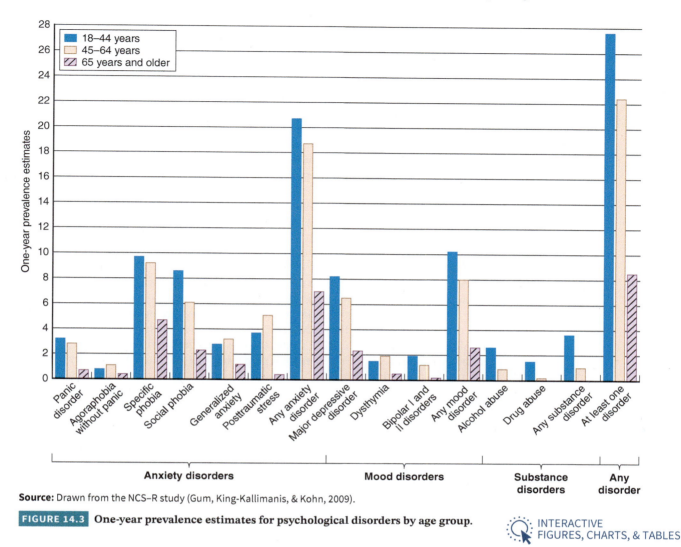

One-year prevalence estimates chart

Source: Drawn from the NCS–R study (Gum, King-Kallimanis, & Kohn, 2009).

FIGURE 14.3 **One-year prevalence estimates for psychological disorders by age group.**

INTERACTIVE FIGURES, CHARTS, & TABLES

et al., 2007; Howard, Rabins, et al., 2000). Overall, only about 8.5% of older people who took part in the NCS–R survey reported symptoms in the year before the interview that were severe enough to diagnose. Similarly low rates were observed in other countries, such as Australia (Trollor, Anderson, et al., 2007). Most people 65 years of age and older are free from serious psychological disorder.

In addition to the prevalence rates of disorders, consider the incidence rates, or how many people experience the onset of a new disorder. Most older adults who have an episode of a psychological disorder are experiencing a recurrence of a disorder that started earlier in life rather than an initial onset. For example, 97% of older adults with generalized anxiety disorder report that their symptoms began before the age of 65 (Alwahhabi, 2003), and more than 90% of older adults with major depressive disorder or agoraphobia report that their symptoms began earlier in life (Norton, Skoog, et al., 2006; Ritchie, Norton, et al., 2013). Late onset is also extremely rare for schizophrenia (Karon & VandenBos, 1998). As mentioned, then, most people with psychological disorders in late life are experiencing a continuation of symptoms that began earlier.

Why are rates of psychological disorders so low in late life? There are two completely different answers to this question. Earlier, we described some of the ways in which aging relates to more positive emotionality and more close-knit social circles. This should translate into a decrease in psychological disorders, and indeed some longitudinal studies suggest that many people who experience psychological disorders early in life grow out of those symptoms. In contrast, some have argued that methodological issues might be leading to underestimation of the prevalence of psychological disorders in late life. We turn to some of these methodological issues next.

Methodological Issues in Estimating the Prevalence of Psychological Disorders

One methodological issue is that older adults may be more uncomfortable acknowledging and discussing psychological or drug use problems than are younger people. In one study, researchers interviewed older people about depressive symptoms and then interviewed a family member about whether that older person was experiencing depressive symptoms. Among those older adults whom family members described as meeting the criteria for major depressive disorder, about one-quarter did not disclose depressive symptoms to the interviewer (Davison, McCabe, & Mellor, 2009). Discomfort discussing symptoms would certainly interfere with gathering accurate prevalence estimates.

In addition to reporting bias, there may be cohort effects. For example, many people who reached adulthood during the drug-oriented era of the 1960s continue to use drugs as they age (Zarit & Zarit, 2011). Their generation has more problems with alcohol and substance use disorders in late life than previous generations had (Substance Abuse and Mental Health Services Administration [SAMHSA], 2021).

Another factor is that people with psychological disorders are at risk for dying earlier (before age 65) for several different reasons. Heavy drinkers are at risk for premature mortality from cirrhosis. Cardiovascular disease and diabetes are more common among people with a history of anxiety disorders, depressive disorders, bipolar disorder, and alcohol use disorder (Scott, Lim, et al., 2016). Given the close ties between serious medical illness and psychological disorders, it is perhaps not surprising that the mean life expectancy of people with psychological disorders is 7 years less than that of those without psychological disorders (Plana-Ripoll, Pedersen, et al., 2019). Because people with psychological disorders may die earlier, studies on aging may suffer from selective mortality.

These three methodological issues—response biases, cohort effects, and selective mortality—could help explain the low rates of psychological disorders in late life. Most researchers, however, believe that aging is also genuinely related to better psychological health.

Treatment

Although dozens of randomized controlled trials indicate that many of the pharmacological and psychological treatments that work in earlier life are efficacious for older adults, many older adults are not offered these treatments because their psychological symptoms are not detected or diagnosed by their primary care providers. For example, in one study of older adults who met the diagnostic criteria for GAD, less than a third had received a diagnosis of an anxiety or depressive disorder from their medical provider (Calleo, Stanley, et al., 2009). Providers may falsely assume that substance use–related symptoms are signals of cognitive decline (Maree & Riccelli, 2018). The lack of treatment provision for older adults is even more pronounced among minority populations (Yarns, 2018).

When older adults do receive medication or psychological treatment, some adaptations may be important. Many psychiatric medications, including benzodiazepines, antipsychotic medications, some antidepressants, and some medications used to treat insomnia, can cause serious side effects in older adults (Mulsant & Pollock, 2015). Some psychotropic medications can be prescribed safely for older patients at lower doses. Therapists may need to adapt psychotherapies to adjust for vision or hearing loss (Brenes, Danhauer, et al., 2015; Mavandadi, Benson, et al., 2015). Telephone and internet-based delivery of therapy has been shown to be helpful, which is important for older clients with limited mobility (Xiang et al., 2020). When cognitive declines are present, including a caregiver in the therapy sessions and providing written reminders of session content can be helpful (Smoski & Areán, 2015).

Quick Summary

When older adults present with psychological symptoms, it is critically important to evaluate potential medical causes. Older adults are particularly susceptible to the negative effects of medical conditions and medications, and these effects may mimic psychological conditions.

Studies suggest lower rates of psychological disorders among older adults than among other age groups. Although methodological issues (cohort effects, selective mortality, and lack of disclosure) might help explain these low rates, it may be that people become psychologically healthier as they age.

Medications and psychological treatments have shown efficacy in addressing psychological illnesses among older adults, but providers often do not detect or diagnose psychological concerns in older adults. Treatments may need to be tailored to consider medication sensitivity, sensory deficits, limited mobility, or memory loss.

14.2 Check Your Knowledge

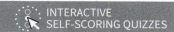 INTERACTIVE SELF-SCORING QUIZZES

(Answers are at the end of the chapter.)
True or false?

1. The DSM-5-TR provides tailored criteria to evaluate diagnoses for those in late life.

Answer the following questions.

2. Define *selective mortality*.

3. Discuss reasons older adults may not reveal psychological symptoms in interviews.

Dementia

Dementia is a descriptive term for the deterioration of cognitive abilities to the point that functioning becomes impaired. As we will discuss, there are many different causes for dementia, and the nature of symptoms depends on the type of dementia.

Dementia can lead to many different types of cognitive and other forms of impairment. Problems with memory, especially for recent events, are the most common symptom, but problems in attention, executive function, learning, language, visuospatial skill, and social cognition also occur. As dementia progresses, most people tend to develop neuropsychiatric symptoms—psychiatric symptoms that appear to be secondary to the neurological disease (Okura, Plassman, et al., 2010). The most common neuropsychiatric syndrome is depression, which affects about 50% of those with dementia, but other affective and motivational symptoms, such as apathy, anxiety, and irritability, also can develop. Sleep disturbances are common. Delusions and hallucinations can occur (American Psychiatric Association, 2013). People with dementia may lose control of their impulses; they may use coarse language, tell inappropriate jokes, shoplift, or make sexually inappropriate remarks.

Clinical Case

Ellen

"I am so glad you came," Ellen says when I greet her. She is sitting at the dining room table sipping juice, a slender, almost frail woman. But Ellen has presence. She has the posture of a dancer: shoulders back, neck elongated, head up, and the gaunt face of a once beautiful woman, with large milky hazel eyes and high patrician cheekbones. She smiles and reaches for my hand. "It is so nice of you to visit," she says. Ellen is gracious and polite, but the truth is, she doesn't remember me. She doesn't remember that we've visited a half dozen times before, that a few days ago we had tea

together, that just yesterday I sat on her bed for a half hour massaging her hands with rosemary mint lotion. Ellen, like the 43 others living at this residential care facility, has Alzheimer's disease. Her short-term memory is shot, and her long-term memory is quirky and dreamlike, with images that are sometimes bright and lucid, and other times so out of focus that she can hardly make them out. Her life is like a puzzle someone took apart when she wasn't looking. She can see some of the pieces, but she can no longer see how they fit together.

Source: Lauren Kessler, *Finding Life in the Land of Alzheimer's* (Penguin, 2007); originally published in Kessler (2004).

Defining Symptoms of Dementia

- Cognitive or behavioral symptoms that:

  1. Are reported by the patient or a knowledgeable informant or are shown on an objective cognitive assessment

  2. Interfere with the ability to function at work or at usual activities

  3. Represent a decline from previous levels of functioning and performing

4. The impairments are observed in at least two of the following domains:

   a. Ability to acquire and remember new information

   b. Reasoning, handling complex tasks, judgment

   c. Visuospatial abilities

   d. Language functions

   e. Changes in personality, behavior, or comportment

Most dementias develop very slowly over a period of years. Subtle cognitive and behavioral deficits often emerge well before a person shows the noticeable impairment of dementia. Early signs of decline, which are mild enough not to cause functional impairment, are labeled **mild cognitive impairment (MCI)**. Diagnostic criteria for dementia and MCI were developed by a panel of experts with support from the National Institute of Aging and the Alzheimer's Association (Albert, Dekosky, et al., 2011; McKhann, Knopman, et al., 2011). Acute cognitive changes due to a head injury are not diagnosed as MCI or dementia (see **Focus on Discovery 14.1** for a discussion of traumatic brain injury).

Defining Symptoms of Mild Cognitive Impairment

- Modest cognitive decline from previous levels in one or more domains, based on concerns of the patient, a close other, or a clinician.

- Cognitive domains can include memory, executive functions, language, visuospatial skills, and attentional control.

- Impairment in one or more cognitive domains compared to expectations for the patient's age and educational level or compared to baseline testing.

- Preservation of ability to function independently. The cognitive deficits do not interfere with ability to complete everyday activities (e.g., paying bills or managing medications), even though greater effort, time, or use of compensatory strategies may be required. The ability to perform complex tasks may be mildly impaired.

- The cognitive deficits are not due to vascular, traumatic, or other medical conditions.

When people experience a decline in cognitive function, all too often they assume that this is an expected part of aging. To the contrary, good clinical care involves a careful workup for problems that may be causing cognitive decline, such as infection, sleep loss, thyroid

Focus on Discovery 14.1

Traumatic Brain Injury

According to the CDC, **traumatic brain injury (TBI)** is the result of a "bump, blow, or jolt to the head that disrupts the normal function of the brain." Mild TBIs are colloquially referred to as *concussions*. Symptoms of concussion include confusion, disorientation, and lack of memory for events in the hours or day after the trauma (Carroll et al., 2004). Other symptoms include slowed speed of processing, headaches, dizziness, fatigue, and changes in mood and emotion. Concussions have been a frequent focus of media reports, as evidence has accrued on how commonly they occur in sports such as hockey, rugby, boxing, and American football (McKee, Daneshvar, et al., 2014). Most who experience a concussion recover within a matter of days or weeks, especially if they follow medical recommendations. A small percentage of people with a concussion, perhaps 10%, continue to report cognitive problems, such as deficits in attention, memory, and organizational ability, for months after the injury (Bigler, 2008). These types of long-lasting problems are more likely with repeated experiences of concussion (Goldstein, 2018).

Beyond causing symptoms in the weeks and months after the injury, there is some evidence that concussions can increase the risk of dementia late in life. There is a pressing need to understand the prevalence and severity of these long-term outcomes in order to answer important policy questions, such as whether children should play tackle football before age 12 and whether college and professional athletes should retire from their sport after a certain number of concussions.

disease, or vitamin deficiencies. About 10% of the time, cognitive declines are tied to such factors and can be reversed. Treatments to reduce any cardiovascular disease can also reduce the odds that cognitive declines will progress to dementia (Langa & Levine, 2014). Sadly, people from ethnic or racial minority groups are less likely than others to experience early detection and treatment for cognitive declines (Plassman & Potter, 2018).

Caution is warranted in diagnosing these early signs of decline. Not all people with mild cognitive symptoms develop dementia. Estimates vary, but among adults with MCI, about 10% per year will develop dementia; among adults without MCI, about 1% per year will develop dementia (Mitchell & Shiri-Feshki, 2009). It is important to provide careful psychoeducation regarding these diagnoses so that patients and family members, like Mrs. J. and her husband in the **Clinical Case**, do not assume that symptoms will necessarily progress to dementia.

Clinical Case

Mrs. J.

Mrs. J., an 81-year-old woman, contacted a neurologist for evaluation, stating, "I am forgetting things I just heard." She and her husband reported that her memory problems had started about 18 months before the appointment and had slowly worsened since then. Her husband reported that she had developed other cognitive symptoms, such as less ability to problem solve, manage time, and take initiative, along with greater distractibility. Both noticed that she had trouble remembering recent conversations, more frequently misplaced her possessions, and had difficulty remembering directions to familiar places. With

the cognitive changes, Mrs. J. became less interested in reading, she needed frequent reminders about how to use her computer and cell phone, her housekeeping declined, and she stopped cooking elaborate meals. She and her husband noted that her sleep and mood were fine, and they denied other psychological or behavioral symptoms. She was able to complete expected activities of daily living independently, and no medical cause of her cognitive symptoms was identified. After neuropsychological testing, Mrs. J. was diagnosed with mild cognitive impairment (MCI).

Source: Drawn from Langa & Levine (2014).

In 2019, the worldwide prevalence of dementia was estimated to be over 55 million (Nichols et al., 2022). Although less than 2% of people develop dementia before age 65, the prevalence increases dramatically as people age, to more than a third of people in their 90s (Prince, Bryce, et al., 2013). The prevalence of dementia among those 60 and older appears to be lower in sub-Saharan Africa (2.07%) and higher in Latin America (8.5%) than in other parts of the world (Prince et al., 2013). Although more people will be at risk for dementia as the number of older adults grows (Livingston, Sommerlad, et al., 2017), there is reason for hope. In Western countries, the percentage of older people who develop dementia has been declining over the past 25 years. Researchers speculate that this could reflect trends over time for better control of high blood pressure, higher levels of education, and more health education around issues like exercise and smoking (Alzheimer's Cohort Consortium, 2020).

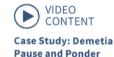

VIDEO CONTENT

Case Study: Demetia Pause and Ponder

There are many different types of dementia, and we discuss five types here: Alzheimer's disease, the most researched form; behavioral variant frontotemporal dementia, defined by the areas of the brain that are most affected; vascular dementia, caused by cerebrovascular disease; dementia with Lewy bodies, defined by the presence of Lewy bodies (a type of abnormal deposit that forms on neurons); and Huntington's disease, a genetically based form of dementia accompanied by prominent motor symptoms. See **Table 14.2** for a summary of these forms of dementia. By far the most common form of dementia is Alzheimer's disease, which accounts for more than half of the cases of dementia (Terry, 2006). We will discuss these forms of dementia separately; however, at autopsy, most people with dementia show pathology of more than one form of dementia; for example, about 75% with Alzheimer's disease also show vascular dementia (Kapasi et al., 2017).

Alzheimer's Disease

In **Alzheimer's disease**, initially described by the German neurologist Alois Alzheimer in 1906, the brain tissue irreversibly deteriorates, and death usually occurs within 12 years after the onset of cognitive symptoms. It is estimated that 4.7 to 6 million Americans are living

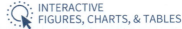

TABLE 14.2   Major Forms of Dementia

Type of Dementia	Prominent Symptoms
Alzheimer's disease	Memory loss, apathy
Behavioral variant frontotemporal dementia (FTD)	Problems with empathy, poor executive function, disinhibited behavior, compulsive or perseverative behavior, tendencies to put nonfood objects in the mouth, and apathy
Vascular dementia	Symptoms depend on the regions of the brain affected by the cardiovascular disease
Dementia with Lewy bodies (DLB)	Physical symptoms (shuffling gait, tremor, and muscle stiffness), loss of memory, visual hallucinations, fluctuating cognitive symptoms, and intense dreams
Huntington's disease	Chorea and muscle stiffness, memory and other cognitive problems

with Alzheimer's disease (Alzheimer's Association, 2023). Risk of Alzheimer's disease is 1.5 to 2-fold higher among Black and Hispanic older adults than among White older adults (Alzheimer's Association, 2023), but minority individuals often do not receive diagnosis and treatment of dementia until symptoms are more advanced (Lennon et al., 2022). In 2023, the direct and indirect costs associated with Alzheimer's disease in the United States were estimated at $345 billion (Alzheimer's Association, 2023).

The most prominent symptom of Alzheimer's disease is memory loss. The illness may begin with absentmindedness and gaps in memory for new material, as described in the **Clinical Case of Mary Ellen**. The person may leave tasks unfinished and forgotten if they are interrupted; for example, the person who had started to fill a teapot at the sink might leave the water running. It may be hard to find words. These shortcomings may be overlooked for several years but eventually interfere with daily living.

Memory loss is not the only symptom of Alzheimer's disease. Apathy is common even before the cognitive symptoms become noticeable (Balsis, Carpenter, & Storandt, 2005), and about a third of people develop full-blown depression as the illness worsens (Vinkers, Gussekloo, et al., 2004). As the disease develops, problems with language skills and word finding intensify. Visual-spatial abilities decline, which can manifest in **disorientation** (confusion with respect to time, place, or identity). The person may easily become lost, even in familiar surroundings.

As the brain deterioration progresses, the range and severity of behavioral symptoms increase. People with the disorder are typically unaware of their cognitive problems initially, and they may blame others for lost objects even to the point of developing delusions of being persecuted. As memory continues to deteriorate, the person becomes increasingly disoriented and agitated. As the dementia progresses, a parent may be unable to remember the name of a daughter or son and later may not even recall that they have children or recognize them when they come to visit. The person may forget to bathe or dress adequately. Judgment may become faulty, and the person may have difficulty comprehending situations and making plans or decisions. In the terminal phase of the illness, personality loses its sparkle and integrity. Relatives and friends say that the person is just not themselves anymore. Social involvement with others keeps narrowing. Finally, the person is oblivious to their surroundings. Among older people diagnosed with Alzheimer's, the average time to death is 4 to 8 years, but some live for 20 years or more (Alzheimer's Association, 2023).

The brains of people with Alzheimer's disease have more **plaques** (small, round deposits of beta-amyloid protein that are outside the neurons) and **neurofibrillary tangles** (twisted protein filaments composed largely of the protein tau in the axons of neurons) than would be expected for the person's age (see

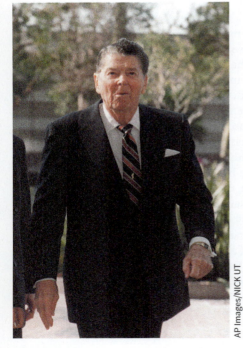
Former President Ronald Reagan died from Alzheimer's disease. His daughter wrote the following about his disease: "The past is like the rudder of a ship. It keeps you moving through the present, steers you into the future. Without it, without memory, you are unmoored, a wind-tossed boat with no anchor. You learn this by watching someone you love drift away" (Davis, 2002).

AP Images/NICK UT

Clinical Case

Mary Ellen

Mary Ellen was a 62-year-old family therapist who was enjoying her career in end-stage hospice work when she was first diagnosed with early-stage Alzheimer's disease.

> All of a sudden—but it wasn't all of a sudden, of course—I began to realize that I wasn't the gal I used to be. It was different inside my head.
>
> It was the very simple things. I would be talking with someone on the telephone, then hang up and ask myself, "Who was that? What did we talk about?" My husband John says he knew

something serious was going on when we returned from a vacation together and I told him, "I really had a great time in California. I'm so sorry you couldn't make it."

> My message to people with Alzheimer's is this: Be gentle with yourself. This disease requires that you lower your expectations of yourself. That's a hard thing for most of us to do. The fear is losing yourself, knowing that you won't bring this self to the end stage of your life. —Mary Ellen Becklenberg (Park, 2010, p. 59)

Figure 14.4). Some people produce excessive amounts of beta-amyloid, whereas others have deficiencies in the mechanisms for clearing beta-amyloid from the brain (Jack, Albert, et al., 2011). The beta-amyloid plaques are most densely present in the frontal cortex (Klunk, Engler, et al., 2004) and may be present for 20–30 years before the cognitive symptoms become noticeable (Jansen, Ossenkoppele, et al., 2015). Tangles are most densely present in the hippocampus, an area that is involved in memory. Over time, as the disease progresses, plaques and tangles spread through more of the brain (Klunk et al., 2004; Sperling, Aisen, et al., 2011). Plaques and tangles can be measured using a PET scan or in cerebrospinal fluid, and biomarkers of plaques and tangles can be measured using blood tests (Chételat et al., 2020; Ossenkoppele et al., 2022). Many scientists believe that other biological processes may be involved in the genesis of symptoms as well, including immune disturbances, brain inflammation, and problems with myelin sheaths—the insulation surrounding neurons (Blanchard et al., 2022; Neff et al., 2021).

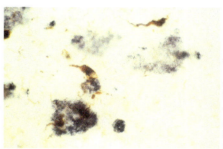

Light micrograph of a section of entorhinal cortex brain tissue affected by Alzheimer's disease, showing amyloid plaques in brown and neurofibrillary tangles in gray.

At early stages, there is a loss of synapses for acetylcholinergic (ACh) and glutamatergic neurons. Neurons also begin to die. As neurons die, the entorhinal cortex surrounding the hippocampus and then the hippocampus and other regions of the cerebral cortex

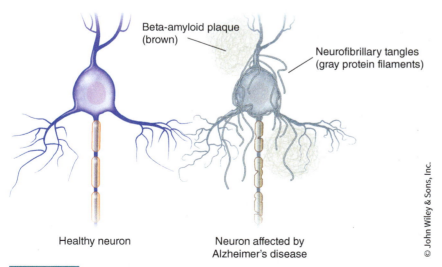

FIGURE 14.4 The brains of people with Alzheimer's disease have more plaques (small, round deposits of beta-amyloid protein that are outside the neurons) and neurofibrillary tangles (twisted protein filaments composed largely of the protein tau in the axons of neurons) than would be expected for their age.

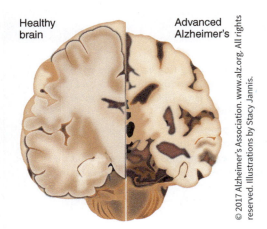

Healthy brain

Advanced Alzheimer's

FIGURE 14.5 **In Alzheimer's disease, neurons die; the entorhinal cortex, hippocampus, and other regions of the cerebral cortex shrink; and ventricles enlarge.**

shrink, and later the frontal, temporal, and parietal lobes shrink (see **Figure 14.5**). As this happens, the ventricles enlarge. The cerebellum, spinal cord, and motor and sensory areas of the cortex are less affected, which is why people with Alzheimer's do not appear to have anything physically wrong with them until late in the disease process. For some time, people with Alzheimer's are able to walk around normally, and their overlearned habits, such as making small talk, remain intact, so that in short encounters strangers may not notice anything amiss. About 25% of people with Alzheimer's disease eventually develop motor deficits.

The genetic contributions to Alzheimer's disease differ for people with the early onset form (before age 65) and those with the late onset form (65 or older). The vast majority of cases are late onset, and heritability estimates for late onset Alzheimer's disease range between 0.60 and 0.80 (Hollingworth & Williams, 2011).

The genetic polymorphism with by far the largest contribution to Alzheimer's disease is a polymorphism of a gene on chromosome 19, called the *apolipoprotein E 4 allele*, or *APOE* 4 (Lambert, Ibrahim-Verbaas et al., 2013). Whereas having one APOE 4 allele increases the risk of Alzheimer's disease to about 20%, having two APOE 4 alleles brings the risk substantially higher. The APOE 4 allele appears more related to risk of disease among White samples than among Hispanic or Black samples (Alzheimer's Association, 2023). Researchers are beginning to understand some of the ways in which the APOE 4 allele may increase risk of the disorder. People with two of this allele show overproduction of beta-amyloid plaques and less clearing of excess beta-amyloid from the brain, even before they develop symptoms of Alzheimer's disease (Bookheimer & Burggren, 2009; Wang, Najm et al., 2018). The APOE 4 allele also is related to higher levels of tau in neuronal cells (Wang et al., 2018).

In GWAS research with more than 750,000 individuals, researchers have identified 75 specific genetic loci beyond APOE 4. Many of these genetic loci appear related to the development of tangles and plaques, and some are related to microglia—cells that respond to neuronal damage in the brain (Bellenguez et al., 2022). A risk score based on the 75 loci was related to a 1.9-fold increase in AD risk among those who did not have the APOE 4 allele.

How people respond to the biological changes appears to be shaped by intellectual activity. Among people with similar levels of plaques and tangles in their brain, those who engage in more intellectual activity show fewer cognitive symptoms. That is, intellectual activity seems to protect against the expression of underlying neurobiological disease (Wilson, Scherr, et al., 2007). This type of research has led to the concept of **cognitive reserve**, or the idea that some people may be able to compensate for the disease by using alternative neuronal pathways or cognitive strategies, with the result that their cognitive symptoms are less pronounced.

Many other modifiable factors related to lifestyle appear to be related to the onset and severity of Alzheimer's disease in large-scale studies. For example, social isolation and smoking are related to a greater risk of Alzheimer's disease, while regular exercise and higher education are related to a lower risk of Alzheimer's disease (Livingston, Sommerlad et al., 2017). Exercise levels and cardiovascular fitness at mid-life are important, but it is also helpful if people improve their fitness later in life (Tari, Nauman, et al., 2019). In one study, researchers assessed lifestyle factors among thousands of older persons and then followed them for 8 years to see who showed cognitive decline. Those with at least a high school education who exercised at least once a week, remained socially active, and did not smoke sustained their cognitive functioning without decline throughout the 8 years (Yaffe, Fiocco et al., 2009). Not only do lifestyle factors predict less cognitive symptoms—lifestyle factors also have been associated with less severe biological features of the disease, such as levels of plaques in the brain (Berti, Walters, et al., 2018; Luciano, Corley, et al., 2017).

Sadly, many health-related and lifestyle risk factors are more common among minority and impoverished populations (Nianogo

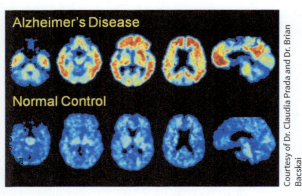

Alzheimer's Disease

Normal Control

Positron emission tomography (PET) images of the brain in a woman with Alzheimer's disease show high levels of amyloid plaque (upper series). In contrast, low levels of amyloid plaque are seen in the PET images of the brain of a woman with no Alzheimer's symptoms (lower series).

et al., 2022). As examples, rates of diabetes and cardiovascular disease are more common while access to adequate health care is more limited among Black and Hispanic individuals as compared to White non-Hispanic individuals living in the United States (Livingston et al., 2020). These health disparities, along with systemic effects of race-related stress and differences in educational opportunities, contribute to the higher rates of Alzheimer's disease among minorities (Alzheimer's Association, 2023). Despite the import of these disparities, 90% of participants in studies of dementia are White, and most samples are drawn from Europe or the United States (Mooldijk et al., 2021).

One panel of experts estimated how large the effects of modifiable factors are for dementia. Drawing from large-scale studies and meta-analyses, they concluded that 40% of dementia cases could theoretically be preventable if we were able to improve exercise and childhood education; bolster social engagement; help people not smoke or drink heavily; reduce head injuries; manage hearing loss, depression, diabetes, hypertension, and obesity; and improve air quality (Livingston et al., 2020). Despite the optimism of this statement, the conclusions were based on naturalistic studies, which cannot disentangle whether the people who engage in exercise or healthy lifestyle activities differ in some important way (on characteristics relevant to disease) from those who do not engage in these activities. We know that biological changes in the brain begin 20 years before the symptoms of Alzheimer's disease first emerge; it is plausible that those brain changes influence motivation to take part in exercise or other beneficial activities (Sabia et al., 2017). Intervention studies, described later in this chapter, that randomly assign people to take part in exercise, cognitive training, or other health-related activities help address this methodological issue.

The complexity of trying to identify the direction of effects is illustrated by the relationship of depression and Alzheimer's disease. We mentioned earlier that depression can be a consequence of dementia. Conversely, a lifetime history of depression predicts greater risk for Alzheimer's disease and other forms of dementia (Katon, Pedersen, et al., 2015). Remember, though, that biological changes begin to occur decades before the onset of Alzheimer's disease. Could those types of biological changes be causing even the depressive symptoms that precede dementia onset? To examine this question, researchers plotted cognitive and depression scores of over 10,000 people for a 28-year period (Singh-Manoux, Dugravot et al., 2017). Medical records were reviewed for diagnoses of dementia. As shown in **Figure 14.6**, among those who developed dementia, cognitive scores declined significantly 12 years before diagnosis, and cognitive decline escalated in the years before diagnosis, while depressive symptoms began to increase significantly 10 years before the dementia diagnosis—that is, *after* cognitive declines had already begun. Depressive symptoms earlier in life were unrelated to the risk of dementia. These findings indicate that the depressive symptoms observed before dementia onset may be a manifestation of the neurological decline. This may help explain why antidepressant treatment is not helpful for many people with dementia (Bingham, Flint, & Mulsant, 2019)—depression in this context may have different biological underpinnings.

Behavioral Variant Frontotemporal Dementia

As is suggested by the name, **frontotemporal dementia (FTD)** is caused by a loss of neurons in frontal and temporal regions of the brain (Pressman & Miller, 2014). FTD typically begins in the late 50s, and it progresses rapidly; death usually occurs within 5 years of the diagnosis (Kimchi & Lyketsos, 2015). FTD is rare, affecting less than 1% of the population (Pressman & Miller, 2014).

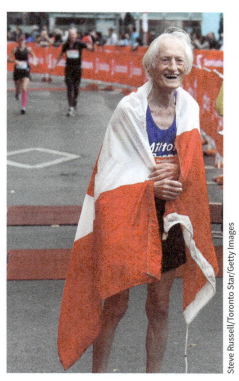

Aerobic exercise programs are of some help in improving cognitive function among older adults. Ed Whitlock is shown here completing a marathon at age 85.

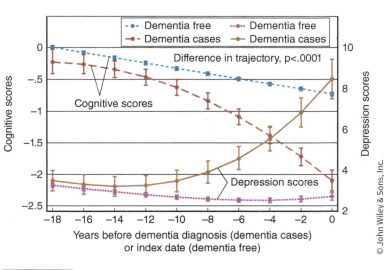

FIGURE 14.6 **Cognitive scores begin to decline 12 years before the onset of dementia.** Depression scores begin to increase a couple years later than cognitive scores, at 10 years before dementia onset (Singh-Manoux et al., 2017).

Unlike with Alzheimer's disease, memory is not severely impaired in FTD. There are multiple subtypes of FTD. The diagnostic criteria for behavioral variant FTD, the most common form, include deterioration in at least three of the following areas: empathy, executive function (cognitive capacity to plan and organize), ability to inhibit behavior, compulsive or perseverative behavior, hyperorality (tendencies to put nonfood objects in the mouth), and apathy (Rascovsky, Hodges et al., 2011), as illustrated by the **Clinical Case of Bob**. In early stages, significant others may notice changes in personality and judgment. Behavioral variant FTD affects emotions and emotion regulation more profoundly than Alzheimer's disease does (Goodkind, Gyurak et al., 2010), and in doing so, it can damage social relationships and marital satisfaction more than Alzheimer's disease does (Ascher, Sturm et al., 2010). Socially inappropriate and impulsive behaviors, such as tendencies to engage in embarrassing or sexually inappropriate comments, reckless spending, and criminal behaviors, can emerge. Apathy and reduced sexual libido are often present, and many patients show a loss of sympathy and emotional responsiveness toward their friends and family members.

Clinical Case

Bob

Bob, a 66-year-old married man, began to develop problems with understanding language. He would hear a common word, like *banana*, and be unable to think of the meaning of the word. Common objects also became confusing. He couldn't make sense of how to use a hammer or a can opener. His wife became concerned when his social and emotional responses shifted. When she turned to her husband for support about the death of a family member, he laughed instead of showing his usual tendency to comfort her. He would give $20 bills to strangers. He made embarrassing comments about obesity in grocery stores and

other public places. He became irritable and impatient, and he would express his distress without regard to the feelings of others. All of these were significant changes from his typical way of being.

Despite these changes, he seemed intellectually sharp in many other ways. He kept track of appointments, didn't repeat himself in conversation, and could remember events more clearly than his wife could. After 2 years of worsening symptoms, Bob and his wife sought help from a neurologist, who diagnosed Bob with behavioral variant frontotemporal dementia.

Drawn from Peskin, 2019.

Because a person affected by this disorder might suddenly start to overeat, chain smoke, drink alcohol, or demonstrate other behavioral symptoms, behavioral variant FTD often is misdiagnosed as a midlife crisis or as a psychological disorder such as bipolar disorder (Zhou & Seeley, 2014). The presence of apathy can result in a misdiagnosis of depression (Kimchi & Lyketsos, 2015).

FTD can be caused by many different neurobiological processes (Bang, Spina, & Miller, 2015). One of these is Pick's disease, characterized by the presence of Pick bodies (spherical inclusions) within neurons, but many other diseases or pathological processes can result in FTD. A third to a half of people with FTD show high levels of tau, the protein filaments that form the neurofibrillary tangles observed in Alzheimer's disease. About a third of FTD patients show a strong genetic component, and three specific genes appear to account for much of the risk for those cases (Moore, Nicholas, et al., 2020).

As with Alzheimer's disease, lifestyle factors appear related to how quickly FTD symptoms progress. In one study, researchers recruited 105 people who had genetic profiles related to FTD and showed no more than mild symptoms of FTD. Each year, participants underwent cognitive tests and MRI scans to assess for the early signs of disease, and they completed questionnaires regarding their cognitive and physical activity levels. Participants who were most physically and cognitively active showed much less cognitive decline over the next 1–2 years, despite evidence of atrophy on brain scans. That is, active lifestyles seemed to protect their ability to function well despite the underlying disease progression (Casaletto, Staffaroni, et al., 2020).

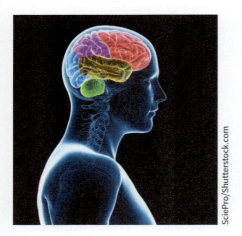

 SciePro/Shutterstock.com

In frontotemporal dementia, the frontal and temporal regions of the brain (shown in red and yellow) atrophy (shrink) as neurons in those regions die.

Vascular Dementia

Vascular dementia is caused by cerebrovascular disease. Most commonly, stroke causes a blood clot, which then impairs circulation and results in the death of neurons. About 7% of people will develop dementia in the year after a first stroke, and the risk of dementia increases with recurrent strokes (Pendlebury & Rothwell, 2009). Risk factors for vascular dementia are the same as those for cardiovascular disease in general—for example, older age, a high level of "bad" (LDL) cholesterol, cigarette smoking, and elevated blood pressure (Moroney, Tang, et al., 1999). Strokes and vascular dementias are more common in Black Americans than in White Americans (Simpkins, 2020). Because strokes and cardiovascular disease can strike different regions of the brain, the symptoms of vascular dementia vary a good deal. The onset of symptoms is usually more rapid in vascular dementia than in other forms of dementia.

Dementia with Lewy Bodies

In **dementia with Lewy bodies (DLB)**, protein deposits called *Lewy bodies* form in the brain and cause cognitive decline. As shown in **Figure 14.7**, the Lewy bodies are most often present in the olfactory bulb and the brain stem initially, and as they spread through the brain, the cognitive symptoms of DLB become noticeable. Lewy bodies are also implicated in Parkinson's disease (Goedert, Spillantini, et al., 2013). DLB is rare, affecting 1% or less of older adults and accounting for less than 10% of cases of dementia (Hogan, Fiest, et al., 2016).

The symptoms associated with this type of dementia are often hard to distinguish from the symptoms of Parkinson's (such as the shuffling gait, tremor, and muscle stiffness) and Alzheimer's disease (such as loss of memory). DLB is more likely than Alzheimer's disease to include prominent visual hallucinations and fluctuating cognitive symptoms (American Psychiatric Association, 2013). Another distinct symptom of DLB is that people often experience intense dreams accompanied by movement and vocalizing, as though they were "acting out their dreams" (McKeith, Dickson, et al., 2005).

FIGURE 14.7 In dementia with Lewy bodies (DLB), the Lewy bodies usually are initially present in the olfactory bulb and the brain stem. Cognitive symptoms become noticeable as the Lewy bodies spread through the brain. Darker areas show where denser concentrations of Lewy bodies are commonly found (Goedert et al., 2013).

Huntington's Disease

Huntington's disease is a neurocognitive disorder that involves memory problems and other cognitive symptoms like those observed with Alzheimer's disease, but it also involves distinctive symptoms of **chorea**, defined by involuntary jerky or writhing movements, and problems with voluntary movements due to muscle rigidity or contractions. The movement symptoms can interfere with a person's gait and speech.

Huntington's disease is an autosomal dominant disorder caused by a defect in a single gene, which means that a person needs only one copy of the defective gene to develop the disorder. Offspring of a parent with Huntington's disease have a 50% chance of developing the disorder. Genetic testing can be used in making the diagnosis. Although the illness can develop at any point in the life span, symptoms often first appear between ages 35 and 45, and then worsen over a period of 15–20 years after onset (Andhale & Shrivastava, 2022). Huntington's disease is extremely rare, affecting fewer than 1 in 10,000 people (Medina et al., 2022).

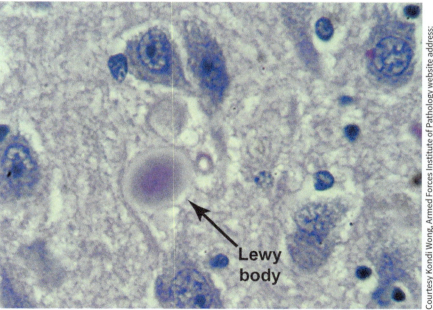

Lewy body

Courtesy Kondi Wong, Armed Forces Institute of Pathology website address: http://www.genome.gov/pressDisplay.cfm?pressDisplay.cfm?photoID=10004

Dementia with Lewy bodies (DLB) is defined by the presence of abnormal deposits called Lewy bodies. The Lewy bodies are found throughout the brain.

Treatments for Dementia

Sadly, despite hundreds of attempts to create new medications since 2000 (Park, 2016), there is no cure for dementia. Some medications are used to delay symptom progression and to address related syndromes, but no medications have been shown to restore cognitive functions (Livingston et al., 2017). There are also some psychological and lifestyle approaches to dementia, which are designed to slow cognitive decline, address related syndromes, and improve the well-being of caretakers.

Medications   Much of the treatment research has focused on Alzheimer's disease and on memory decline. Medications help slow decline, but they do not restore memory function to previous levels (Brandt & Mansour, 2016). The medications most commonly used for dementia are the cholinesterase inhibitors (drugs that interfere with the breakdown of acetylcholine), including donepezil (Aricept) and rivastigmine (Exelon). Compared to placebos, cholinesterase inhibitors have been shown to have slightly more effect in slowing memory decline for Alzheimer's disease and DLB (Livingston et al., 2017) but have not been found to be helpful for FTD or Huntington's disease. In addition to cholinesterase inhibitors, memantine (Namenda), a drug that affects glutamate receptors involved in memory, has shown small effects in placebo-controlled trials for severe Alzheimer's disease (Livingston et al., 2017). Unfortunately, many people discontinue these drugs due to aversive side effects such as nausea (Maidment, Fox, & Boustani, 2006).

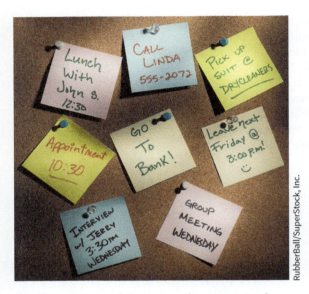

Providing memory aids is one way of compensating for memory loss.

Many studies are being conducted to test the idea that interventions that reduce plaques, tangles, or other correlates of the disorder could be helpful if applied early in the progression of the disease. The FDA recently approved two medications, Aducanumab and Leqembi, and is reviewing Donanemab, for the treatment of mild cognitive impairment or mild Alzheimer's disease, based on evidence that these medications lower levels of beta-amyloid plaques. The decision to approve Aducanumab was highly controversial as the evidence was not clear that aducanumab can slow cognitive decline (Mullard, 2021). Leqembi and Donanemab are not cures, but they both showed promise in reducing the rate of cognitive decline. Dozens of trials are ongoing to identify ways to prevent the formation of plaque buildup well before symptoms emerge in those genetically at-risk, as well as to target other proposed mechanisms early in the progression of the disease.

For those with vascular dementia, and for the many persons with Alzheimer's disease who have cardiovascular disease, one goal is to improve cardiovascular health. Blood pressure management for those with hypertension has some benefits in preventing mild cognitive impairment and slowing the onset of dementia (Hughes et al., 2020).

Although medical treatments sometimes are used to address psychological symptoms, such as the agitation and depression that commonly co-occur with dementia, there are two problems with these medication approaches. First, there is little evidence that antipsychotic medications or antidepressant medications reduce agitation or depression, and second, as noted earlier, they can have serious side effects in frail older adults (Banerjee et al., 2021; Livingston et al., 2020).

Psychological and Lifestyle Treatments   Supportive psychotherapy can help families and patients deal with the effects of the disease. The therapist provides accurate information about the illness, helps family members care for the person in the home, and encourages a realistic rather than a catastrophic attitude in dealing with the many specific challenges that this cognitive disorder presents. See **Focus on Discovery 14.2** for more detail on interventions to support caregivers.

Behavioral approaches have been shown to help compensate for memory loss and to reduce depression and disruptive behavior among people with early stages of Alzheimer's disease (Braun, 2019). For example, external memory aids such as shopping lists, calendars, phone lists, and labels can help when placed prominently as visual reminders (Buchanan, Christenson, et al., 2011). Communication strategies (asking about the reasons for distress), music, and engagement in pleasant and meaningful activities may help reduce agitation and disruptive behavior temporarily (Livingston et al., 2017).

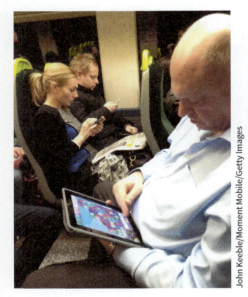

Computerized training programs have been developed with the aim of enhancing cognitive skills. Companies producing these training programs report tens of millions of users, but the effects of the programs are modest (Livingston et al., 2017).

Aerobic exercise, healthy diet, and weight loss programs may provide modest help in preventing cognitive decline before dementia has begun. Because findings are weak regarding the benefits of these programs once dementia begins, these interventions should be implemented as early as possible (Livingston et al., 2017; World Health Organization, 2019). The FINGER trial tested the effects of a

Focus on Discovery 14.2

Support for Caregivers

For every person with severe dementia who is living in an institution, there are at least two living in the community, usually supported by a family. Although many caregivers report some rewards from the role, caregiving is extremely stressful. About 40% of caregivers in the United States develop clinical depression and anxiety (Mahoney, 2005). Rates of psychological disorders are lower for caregivers living in countries such as Japan where there are more services available to assist with caretaking (Ohno et al., 2021).

Families can be helped to cope better with the daily stress of caregiving. For example, because people with Alzheimer's have difficulty placing new information into memory, they can engage in a reasonable conversation but forget the discussion within a few minutes. Family members can learn communication strategies to adapt to the memory loss. For example, families can ask questions that embed the answer. It is much easier to respond to "Was the person you just spoke to on the phone Harry or Tom?" than to "Who just called?"

Therapists can help evaluate and manage potential sources of risk due to the disease, as patients do not always recognize their limitations and may try to engage in activities beyond their abilities. Caregivers must set limits regarding dangerous activities. For example, caregivers often need to tell a relative with Alzheimer's disease that driving is off limits (and then remove the car keys, as the relative is likely to forget the new rule). As the person with Alzheimer's disease develops increasingly severe, and sometimes dangerous, limitations, family members are faced with decisions about whether their relative can continue to live at home and how to arrange legal matters. Interventions to help family members consider difficult financial and legal decisions can be helpful.

Individualized therapy programs that teach coping strategies for the caregivers (e.g., increasing pleasant activities, exercise, or social support) have been shown to relieve caregiver depression, as has a program that coupled individual psychotherapy, problem solving that targeted the challenges of specific problems caused by the dementia, and a support group (Livingston et al., 2017).

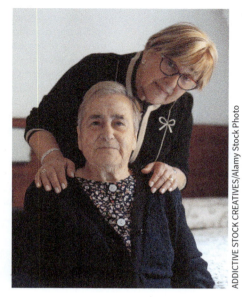

Interventions can help address some of the stress experienced by caregivers of those with dementia.

Because caregivers are so powerfully affected, respite is highly recommended. To give the caretaker a break, sometimes the person with dementia is briefly admitted to a hospital or enrolled in an adult day-care center; sometimes a healthcare worker takes over while the caregiver or the family takes a holiday. Programs offering multiple components (e.g., psychoeducation about dementia, case-management services, cognitive behavioral strategies, and respite) appear more helpful than programs that offer only education or support (Livingston et al., 2017). On the whole, though, interventions offer only modest relief from the stresses of being a caregiver (Cheng & Zhang, 2020).

multimodal intervention designed to improve diet, physical exercise, social activity, to provide cognitive training and to monitor vascular and metabolic conditions among persons at risk for but not diagnosed with dementia. Among 1,200 participants, researchers were able to show improvements in cognition, memory, and other chronic diseases as compared to those who received general health advice (Rosenberg et al., 2018).

Quick Summary

Dementia is a broad term used to describe cognitive decline, most commonly a decline in memory for recent events. As the cognitive deficits become more widespread and profound, social and occupational functioning becomes more disturbed. Dementia affects approximately 1–2% of people in their 60s but a third of people over the age of 90. The diagnosis of minor cognitive impairment refers to milder signs of cognitive decline.

There are many types of dementia, including Alzheimer's disease, frontotemporal dementia, vascular dementia, dementia with Lewy bodies (DLB), and Huntington's disease. Alzheimer's disease is characterized by plaques and neurofibrillary tangles in the brain. Memory loss is a key symptom of

Alzheimer's disease, but apathy may be present long before cognitive symptoms are observable. Risk of developing the disease is higher among those with at least one APOE 4 allele. Immune and inflammation processes, and problems with the myelin sheaths insulating neurons, may increase vulnerability to Alzheimer's disease. Lifestyle and psychological factors, such as exercise, diet, smoking, and intellectual engagement, appear to be involved as well. Frontotemporal dementia (FTD) is characterized by neuronal deterioration in the frontal and temporal lobes. Pick's disease is one form of FTD. The primary symptoms of behavioral variant FTD include marked changes in social and emotional behavior, including problems with empathy, executive function, disinhibition, compulsive behavior, hyperorality, and apathy. Vascular dementia often occurs after a stroke. The symptoms of vascular dementia depend on the brain regions that are influenced by the cerebrovascular disease. DLB is characterized by visual hallucinations, fluctuations in cognitive functioning, supersensitivity to side effects of antipsychotic medications, and intense dreams during which the person moves and talks. Huntington's disease is an autosomal dominant neurocognitive disorder that involves memory problems, other cognitive symptoms, and chorea.

The cholinesterase inhibitors and memantine are the major medical treatments for Alzheimer's disease; the cholinesterase inhibitors are also used for DLB, but these medications offer modest effects. If started before the onset of dementia, aerobic exercise, nutritional interventions, and weight loss programs may help improve cognitive functioning. Behavioral treatments can help relieve comorbid symptoms of depression. Antipsychotic and antidepressant medications can reduce agitation for those with dementia but also can have harmful side effects in this population death; behavioral treatments can safely reduce agitation. Multicomponent programs help address caregivers' needs.

14.3 Check Your Knowledge

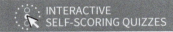
INTERACTIVE
SELF-SCORING QUIZZES

(Answers are at the end of the chapter.)
Choose the best answer.

1. A plaque is:

   a. a small, round deposit of beta-amyloid protein

   b. a filament composed of the protein tau

   c. a buildup of the myelin sheath surrounding neurons in the hippocampus

   d. a small white spot on a brain scan

2. A neurofibrillary tangle is:

   a. a small, round deposit of beta-amyloid protein

   b. a filament composed of the protein tau

   c. a buildup of the myelin sheath surrounding neurons in the hippocampus

   d. a small white spot on a brain scan

3. Behavioral variant FTD involves profound changes in:

   a. memory

   b. social and emotional behavior

   c. motor control

   d. attention

Answer the following questions.

4. Define cognitive reserve.

5. Describe the efficacy of current medical treatments for dementia.

6. What is the most prominent symptom of Alzheimer's disease?

7. Which type of dementia involves chorea?

Delirium

The term **delirium** (derived from the Latin words *de,* meaning "out of," and *lira,* meaning "track") implies a deviation from the usual state. Extreme trouble focusing attention is the hallmark symptom (Saczynski & Inouye, 2015). As illustrated in the Clinical Case of Henry at the beginning of this chapter, patients with delirium, sometimes rather suddenly, have so much trouble focusing attention that they cannot maintain a coherent stream of thought. They may have trouble answering questions because their mind wanders. As the sleep/wake cycle becomes disturbed, patients become drowsy during the day yet awake and agitated at night. Vivid dreams and nightmares are common. People with delirium may be impossible to engage in conversation because of their wandering attention and fragmented thinking. In severe delirium, speech is rambling and incoherent. Bewildered and confused, some people with delirium may become so disoriented that they are unclear about what day it is, where they are, and even who they are. Memory impairment, especially for recent events, is common.

Defining Symptoms of Delirium

- Disturbance in attention and awareness
- A change in cognition, such as disturbance in orientation, language, memory, perception, or visuospatial ability
- Symptoms not accounted for by dementia or by severely reduced arousal (e.g., a coma)

- Rapid onset (usually within hours or days) and typically fluctuation during the course of a day
- Symptoms caused by a medical condition, substance intoxication or withdrawal, or a toxin

---

Perceptual disturbances are frequent in delirium. People mistake the unfamiliar for the familiar; for example, they may state that they are at home instead of in a hospital. Although visual hallucinations are common, they are not always present. Delusions—beliefs contrary to reality—are present in about 25% of older adults with delirium (Camus, Burtin, et al., 2000). These delusions tend to be fleeting and changeable.

Swings in activity and mood accompany these disordered thoughts and perceptions. People with delirium can be erratic, ripping their clothes one moment and sitting lethargically the next. They may also shift rapidly from one emotion to another, fluctuating between depression, anxiety, fright, anger, euphoria, and irritability. They may have lucid intervals in which they become alert and coherent. Symptoms are usually worse during sleepless nights. These daily fluctuations help distinguish delirium from other syndromes, especially Alzheimer's disease.

People of any age are subject to delirium, but it is more common among children and older adults. Among older adults, it is particularly common in nursing homes and hospitals. It is the most common complication of hospitalization in older adult patients (Saczynski & Inouye, 2015).

Unfortunately, delirium is often misdiagnosed. For example, among hospitalized older adults with clear symptoms of delirium, hospital notes did not indicate delirium for 75% or more (Han, Zimmerman, et al., 2009). Physicians are particularly unlikely to detect delirium when lethargy or dementia is present (Saczynski & Inouye, 2015). Table 14.3 compares the features of dementia and delirium.

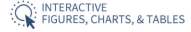

INTERACTIVE
FIGURES, CHARTS, & TABLES

TABLE 14.3   Comparative Features of Dementia and Delirium

Dementia	Delirium
Gradual deterioration of abilities	Rapid onset
Most commonly, deficits in memory for recent events	Trouble concentrating and staying with a train of thought
Caused by brain disease processes	Secondary to another medical condition
Usually progressive and nonreversible	Symptoms fluctuate over the course of a day
Treatment offers only minimal benefit	Usually reversible by treating underlying condition but potentially fatal if cause—e g., infection or malnutrition—not treated
Prevalence increases with age	Prevalence is highest in very young as well as older individuals

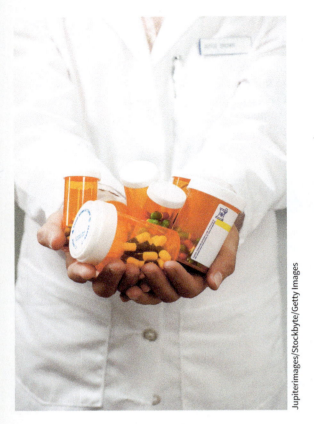

Medication misuse, whether deliberate or inadvertent, can be a serious problem among older people and can cause delirium.

Jupiterimages/Stockbyte/Getty Images

Detecting and treating delirium is of fundamental importance. The mortality rate for untreated delirium is high (Salluh, Wang, et al., 2015). Beyond the risk of death, older adults who develop delirium are at an increased risk of further cognitive decline (Goldberg et al., 2020). It is not clear why delirium predicts such bad outcomes; some believe that delirium may be an indicator of an underlying frailty that becomes apparent in the presence of medical conditions.

Triggers of Delirium

No single biological process has been identified to explain delirium (Dunne et al., 2021). As noted in the diagnostic criteria, several triggers of delirium have been identified. Drugs and drug-withdrawal reactions are the most common triggers, and dementia is related to a threefold greater risk of delirium among persons who are hospitalized (Fong & Inouye, 2022). Other common triggers include metabolic and nutritional imbalances (as in diabetes, thyroid dysfunction, kidney or liver failure, congestive heart failure, or malnutrition), dehydration, infections (such as COVID-19, pneumonia or urinary tract infections), other neurological disorders (such as head trauma, or seizures), and the stress of major surgery (Zarit & Zarit, 2011). Physical immobility and, even more, physical restraints are key risk factors (Saczynski & Inouye, 2015). As in the case of Henry at the start of this chapter, however, delirium usually has more than one cause.

Why are older adults so vulnerable to delirium? Many explanations have been offered: notably, the physical declines of late life, the increased susceptibility to chronic diseases, the many medications prescribed for older people, and the greater sensitivity to drug effects.

Treatment of Delirium

Complete recovery from delirium is possible if doctors promptly identify and treat the underlying cause. Physicians must consider all possible reversible causes of the disorder and then treat any conditions identified. Beyond treating underlying medical conditions, the most common treatment is an atypical antipsychotic medication; caution is warranted because antipsychotic medication has not been shown to reduce agitation associated with delirium and can have serious side effects among frail older adults (Finucane et al., 2020; Saczynski & Inouye, 2015). It usually takes 1 to 4 weeks for the condition to clear; it takes longer in older people than in younger people.

Because of the high rates of delirium in hospitalized older adults, preventive strategies are recommended to keep delirium from starting when an older person is hospitalized. The goal is to reduce common risk factors for delirium, such as sleep deprivation, immobility, dehydration, and visual and hearing impairment. It may help patients to stay oriented if clocks are placed within their field of vision, shades are open during the day and lights are turned off at night, and disruptions to sleep are minimized. Patients can be helped to resume walking soon after surgery, nursing staff can make sure that patients hydrate and consume enough calories, and patients' glasses and hearing aids should be returned as soon as possible after medical procedures. Family members are encouraged to be present. Implementing these preventive measures reduces the risks for delirium by more than 40% (Hshieh et al., 2015).

The high risk of delirium among people with dementia raises another set of prevention issues. Relatives of a person with dementia should learn the symptoms of delirium and know about its reversible nature so that they do not interpret the onset of delirium as a new stage of a progressive dementia. Strategies to address delirium have been found to be helpful for those with dementia (Fong & Inouye, 2022).

14.4 Check Your Knowledge

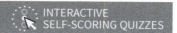
INTERACTIVE
SELF-SCORING QUIZZES

(Answers are at the end of the chapter.)
Answer the following question.

1. What is the most common symptom of delirium?

Choose the best answer.

2. Mary, a 70-year-old woman, was hospitalized for hip surgery. Although there were no immediate complications from the surgery, her son became concerned when they visited that night because she was not making any sense. Mary thanked her son for checking her into the Ritz-Carlton and laughed giddily when he told her that she was in the hospital. Half an hour later, Mary began sobbing. Although she seemed fine the next morning, symptoms of acute confusion re-emerged by lunchtime. Which diagnosis is most likely for Mary?

  a. Alzheimer's disease

  b. behavioral variant frontotemporal dementia

  c. mania

  d. delirium

Summary

INTERACTIVE
SELF-SCORING QUIZZES
Chapter 14 Practice Quiz

Aging: Issues and Methods

- As life expectancy continues to improve, it will become even more important to learn about the disorders suffered by some older people and the most effective means of treating them.

- Several stereotypes about aging are false. Generally, people in late life report low levels of negative emotion, are not inappropriately concerned with their health, and are not lonely. On the other hand, stigma, bereavement, physical disease, polypharmacy, medication sensitivity, and sleep disruption are common challenges for people as they age.

- In research studies, differences between a younger and an older group could reflect age effects, cohort effects, or time-of-measurement effects. Longitudinal studies are more helpful for untangling such effects than cross-sectional studies are, but selective attrition can bias the results of longitudinal studies.

Psychological Disorders in Late Life

- Data indicate that persons over age 65 have the lowest rates of psychological disorders of all age groups. When older people do experience a psychological disorder, the symptoms are often a recurrence of a disorder that first emerged earlier in life. It is important to rule out medical causes of psychological symptoms occurring during late life.

Neurocognitive Disorders in Late Life

- Serious cognitive disorders affect a small minority of older people. Two principal disorders have been distinguished: dementia and delirium.

- In dementia, the person's cognitive functioning declines. As the dementia progresses, the person may become oblivious to his, her or their surroundings. A variety of diseases can cause this deterioration. The most common is Alzheimer's disease. Genes play a major role in Alzheimer's disease. Lifestyle factors, such as exercise and cognitive engagement, appear to be protective.

- Other forms of dementia include frontotemporal dementia (FTD), vascular dementia, dementia with Lewy bodies (DLB), and Huntington's disease.

- Cholinesterase inhibitors and memantine can be prescribed to slow the memory decline shown in some forms of dementia, but their effects are minimal. New medications can help reduce the level of amyloid plaques and may modestly slow the rate of cognitive decline. Psychological treatments can help diminish depression. The person and the family affected by the disease can be counseled on how to make the remaining time manageable and even rewarding. Exercise and cognitive training programs can help preserve cognitive functioning if instituted early, before significant cognitive decline.

- Delirium is defined by a sudden onset of inability to sustain attention and by symptoms such as fragmented and undirected thought, incoherent speech, hallucinations, disorientation, lethargy or hyperactivity, and mood swings. Symptoms tend to vary throughout the day. Delirium is most likely to affect children and older adults. Reversing symptoms once they begin depends on addressing the underlying cause. Triggers include drug effects and withdrawal, malnutrition, metabolic disorders, dehydration, infection, neurological disorders, and surgery. Delirium is often not diagnosed. Prevention programs greatly reduce the risk of delirium.

Answers to Check Your Knowledge Questions

14.1 1. False; 2. People report more happiness, tend to attend more to positive information, and are less reactive to negative information; 3. People place more emphasis on close ties than on broader social networks.

14.2 1. False; 2. Selective mortality refers to a pattern of death among participants in longitudinal studies that is systematically related to risk factors and outcomes, such as participants with depression being more likely than those without depression to die; 3. Stigma and attitudes toward mental health problems have shifted over time, and older people may feel more embarrassed about discussing mental health symptoms.

14.3 1. a. a small, round deposit of beta-amyloid protein; 2. b. a filament composed of the protein tau; 3. b. social and emotional behavior; 4. The ability to function cognitively despite the progression of underlying biological processes involved in dementia; 5. Medications might slow decline but do not cure dementia; 6. memory loss; 7. Huntington's disease.

14.4 1. inattention; 2. d. delirium.

Key Terms

Personality Disorders

1. Explain the DSM-5-TR approach to classifying personality disorders, and identify key concerns with this approach.

2. Describe the DSM-5-TR alternative approach to personality diagnosis.

3. Discuss commonalities in causes across personality disorders.

4. Define the key features and causes of each of the personality disorders retained in the DSM-5-TR alternative approach to personality diagnosis.

5. Describe the available psychological treatments for the DSM-5-TR personality disorders.

Personality disorders are defined by enduring problems with forming a stable positive identity and with sustaining close and constructive relationships. Although all 10 of the personality disorders in DSM-5-TR are defined by extreme and inflexible traits, they cover a broad range of symptom profiles. For example, paranoid personality disorder is defined by chronic tendencies to be mistrustful and suspicious, antisocial personality disorder by patterns of irresponsibility and callous disregard for the rights of others, and dependent personality disorder by an overreliance on others. From time to time, we all behave, think, and feel in ways that are similar to symptoms of personality disorders, but an actual personality disorder is defined by the persistent, pervasive, and maladaptive ways in which these traits are expressed.

Our personalities shape almost every domain of our lives—our career choices, the quality of our relationships, the size of our social network, our favorite pastimes and preferred level of activity, our approach to tackling everyday problems, our willingness to break rules, and our typical level of well-being (Ozer & Benet-Martinez, 2006). Given how many areas of our life are shaped by personality traits, it stands to reason that the extreme and inflexible traits found in personality disorders would create problems in multiple domains. People with personality disorders experience difficulties with their identity and their relationships, and these problems are sustained for years, as illustrated in **Read More About It 15.1**. Across a review of 127 studies, personality disorders were tied to problems in friendships and family relationships (Wilson, Stroud, & Durbin, 2017). Some of the relationship problems can become quite severe. In a study of over 20,000 individuals, women with personality disorders were found to be three times as likely to experience physical assault by a partner, sexual assault, or stalking as those without a personality disorder (Walsh, Hasin, et al., 2016). Personality disorders also predict poorer physical health, even when comorbid psychological syndromes are accounted for, in both cross-sectional and longitudinal studies (Quirk, Berk, et al., 2016).

In this chapter, we begin by considering the DSM-5-TR approach to classifying personality disorders and the assessment of these disorders. We will note some concerns about the DSM-5-TR approach to personality disorders, and we will then discuss an alternative system of personality classification that has been placed after the main body of the DSM-5-TR manual, in Section III. After considering these broad issues in the classification of personality disorders, we describe factors that increase the risk of personality disorders in general. Then, we discuss specific personality disorders, including clinical descriptions and causes. We conclude with a discussion of treatment of personality disorders.

Read More About It 15.1

The Buddha and the Borderline: My Recovery from Borderline Personality Disorder Through Dialectical Behavioral Therapy, Buddhism, and Online Dating

In this book, Kiera Van Gelder shares the story of her struggles with borderline personality disorder and describes the process of growth that helped her become an international advocate for those with this syndrome. Not until she had been through numerous rounds of outpatient and inpatient treatment did she first hear the diagnosis of borderline personality disorder. In one passage, she describes the psychiatric interview that led to her diagnosis, starting with her response when asked why she was seeking therapy:

> *"At first I say it's my boyfriend, but then I tell him the whole thing. I start at the trailhead of my first suicide attempt and try to describe this overwhelming pain I've had for as long as I can remember. I show him the scars on my arms, and I name all the diagnoses I've gotten: Depression, anxiety, PTSD, and chemical dependency. I list the medications, therapies, 12-step programs, religions, and nutritional supplements I've tried. I describe my previous stay in this hospital when I was seventeen, put on a ward for the summer before I turned eighteen, and my other hospitalization in college, when I dropped out and went into AA and NA to get sober."*

> *"I've been seeing therapists for almost twenty years," I say, crying. "I've quit every substance besides caffeine and sugar. I've taken every medication psychiatrists have given me. I don't understand why I'm not getting better. Everything I touch seems to turn to shit. … I'm back at that place where I don't see the point of going on. I'm just going in circles, like circles of hell, where there's no escape."*

> … *"I'm lucky if I can hang onto a friendship longer than a year. Two years with a boyfriend is as much as I've done. And when it ends, my life falls apart."*

> … *"I admit that I've sent letters in blood when I've felt rejected, and that there have been times where I've thrown fits and kitchenware when a close friend replaces me with a boyfriend."*

> *The therapist asks, "What about anger?"*

> *"I'm terrified of it." … "The experience of having it inside me so often and having to manage it. It's like being a sword swallower, only I don't have the throat for it. Eventually the anger comes out. And it's usually scary—to others and to me."*

> *[She describes the high intensity of her emotions, their rapid shifts, and the exhaustion she feels as she experiences them].*

> *The therapist continues, "Do you cut and burn yourself regularly?"*

> *"… it depends. When I was a teenager, it was constant. Now it's periodic, mainly after breakups."*

> *The therapist then asks, "Do you have other impulsive behaviors?"*

> *I don't want to admit how many men I've slept with in the last couple of decades. Or how many credit cards I've maxed out. Or the number of times I've moved (thirty-four at the last count). "Therapists tell me I need to think more before I act. …"* (pp. 25–26)

Her initial response on hearing the diagnosis was relief—finally an explanation and a plan for treatment! The relief, though, was quickly attenuated as those in her support network began to question the diagnosis because of their worries about how deeply stigmatizing its symptoms were.

Despite the challenges of accepting the diagnosis, Van Gelder began a several year process of engaging in group and individual dialectical behavior therapy (discussed later in this chapter), along with meditative reflection. The book provides a frank glimpse into her painful process of learning coping skills to support better emotion regulation and interpersonal connection. The book illuminates the small steps she took—with support from her therapists and her support network—that contributed to change, in a way that will be helpful for those interested in becoming therapists, as well as those who want to initiate their own process of growth.

Van Gelder gives the reader insight into the many influences that weave together to contribute to her personality disorder—her emotional intensity, sensitivity to interpersonal events, early experience of abuse, and impulsive responses to emotion, as well as the difficulty others had in finding ways to acknowledge and support the intensity of her emotional experience. These vulnerabilities are well illustrated with examples drawn from her daily life. She provides poignant examples of her intense emotional responses to relationship threats and the ways in which such responses would lead others to distance and disengage—further intensifying her emotions.

The book also highlights the profound influence of the societal stigma attached to the disorder in delaying the receipt of her diagnosis and in intensifying her shame over her symptoms. As she grew stronger, she became an advocate for others with this disorder, speaking out about her own experiences. Eventually, she learned to give talks nationally and internationally, and she wrote this book, describing with candor the ups and downs she experienced during her pursuit of recovery.

Source: Van Gelder (2010).

The DSM-5-TR Approach to Classification

DSM-5-TR provides criteria for personality disorder in general as well as specific criteria for each personality disorder. The 10 different personality disorders are classified in three clusters, reflecting the idea that these disorders are characterized by odd or eccentric behavior (cluster A), dramatic or erratic behavior (cluster B), or anxious or fearful behavior (cluster C). Table 15.1 presents the key features of the DSM-5-TR personality disorders and shows their grouping in clusters.

About 7.5% of the global population meets the diagnostic criteria for a personality disorder, and the rates are higher in high-income countries than lower- or middle-income countries (Winsper, Bilgin, et al., 2019). With rates this high, it is likely that you know people who would meet the diagnostic criteria for a personality disorder.

The DSM criteria for personality disorder specify that clinicians should be sensitive to whether patterns of behavior are unusual for the person's cultural background. For example, cultures vary in the degree to which self-promotion is considered appropriate, and this is relevant to the evaluation of narcissism. Cultural attitudes toward emotion expression are relevant to evaluating the cluster C personality disorders, which involve dramatic expressions of emotion. Researchers have shown differences in the prevalence of some personality disorders between some countries (Jani, Johnson, et al., 2016) and have begun to explore how cultural values may help explain these patterns (Shou, Lay, et al., 2021).

Personality disorders tend to co-occur with psychological disorders. For example, cluster C personality disorders involve high levels of distress, and so not surprisingly, they show high comorbidity rates with mood and anxiety disorders. Cluster B personality disorders also show high rates of comorbidity with mood disorders (Friborg, Martinsen, et al., 2014; Friborg, Martinussen, et al., 2013; Grant, Chou, et al., 2008). Antisocial personality disorder is highly comorbid with substance use disorders (Krueger, Markon, et al., 2005). As a result of these

TABLE 15.1 Key Features of the DSM-5-TR Personality Disorders

INTERACTIVE FIGURES, CHARTS, & TABLES

	Key Features	Included in the Alternative DSM-5-TR Model for Personality Disorders?
Cluster A (odd/eccentric)		
Paranoid	Distrust and suspiciousness of others	No
Schizoid	Detachment from social relationships and restricted range of emotional expression	No
Schizotypal	Cognitive distortions, eccentric behavior, and lack of capacity for close relationships	Yes
Cluster B (dramatic/erratic)		
Antisocial	Disregard for and violation of the rights of others	Yes
Borderline	Instability of interpersonal relationships, self-image, and affect, as well as marked impulsivity	Yes
Histrionic	Excessive emotionality and attention seeking	No
Narcissistic	Grandiosity, need for admiration, and lack of empathy	Yes
Cluster C (anxious/fearful)		
Avoidant	Social inhibition, feelings of inadequacy, and hypersensitivity to negative evaluation	Yes
Dependent	Excessive need to be taken care of, submissive behavior, and fears of separation	No
Obsessive-compulsive	Preoccupation with order, perfection, and control	Yes

Defining Symptoms of General Personality Disorder

- An inflexible pattern of behavior and inner experience that is distinct from cultural expectations and influences at least two of the following:
  1. cognition about the self, others, and events
  2. affect
  3. interpersonal functioning
  4. impulse control

- The pattern
  1. causes significant distress or impairment
  2. is inflexible
  3. is pervasive across situations

- Onset by early adulthood
- Symptoms are stable and persistent
- Not explained by another psychological disorder, by a substance, or by a medical condition

high comorbidity levels, personality disorders are commonly encountered in treatment settings, with as many as 40% of outpatients meeting the diagnostic criteria for a personality disorder (Newton-Howes, Tyrer, et al., 2010). See **Figure 15.1** for a comparison of rates of specific personality disorders in the general community and in treatment settings. When personality disorders are comorbid with other psychological syndromes, they are associated with more severe symptoms of those psychological disorders and poorer social functioning (Ansell, Pinto, et al., 2011; Newton-Howes, Tyrer, & Johnson, 2006).

The accurate diagnosis of personality disorders requires care. When experienced clinicians use structured interviews to assess the personality disorder criteria, inter-rater reliability is adequate or good for most of the diagnoses, with one exception—experts often disagree about whether schizoid personality disorder is present. See **Table 15.2** for inter-rater reliability of personality disorder diagnoses when experts use structured diagnostic interviews. Unfortunately, most clinicians do not use structured interviews to assess personality. Unstructured clinical interviews are not reliable (Regier, Kuhl, & Kupfer, 2013), tend to miss as many as half of personality disorder diagnoses (Zimmerman & Mattia, 1999), and are less predictive than structured interviews of long-term outcomes (Samuel, Sanislow, et al., 2013).

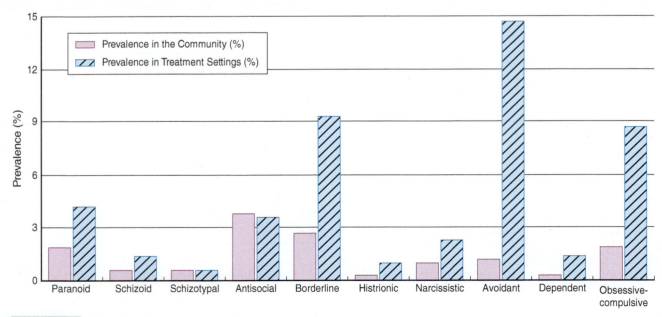

FIGURE 15.1 **Rates of DSM personality disorders in the community and in outpatient treatment settings in the United States.** Prevalence estimates for community settings are drawn from Trull, Jahng, et al. (2010) and Samuels, Eaton, et al. (2002). Prevalence estimates for treatment settings are drawn from Zimmerman, Rothschild, and Chelminski (2005).

TABLE 15.2 Inter-rater Reliability for the Personality Disorders as Assessed by Structured Interview

Diagnosis	Inter-rater Reliability (Correlation)
Paranoid	.86
Schizoid	.69
Schizotypal	.91
Antisocial	.97
Borderline	.90
Histrionic	.83
Narcissistic	.88
Avoidant	.79
Dependent	.87
Obsessive-compulsive	.85

Source: Structured interview estimates from Zanarini, Skodol, et al. (2000).

Problems with the DSM-5-TR Approach to Personality Disorders

There are some major concerns about the DSM-5-TR approach to classifying personality disorders. Here we focus on three of these concerns: These disorders are not as stable as the definition implies, the rates of comorbidity among the personality disorders are extremely high, and the thresholds for defining diagnosis are arbitrary.

Personality Disorders Are Not Stable Over Time   Although the very definition of personality disorders suggests that they should be stable over time, Figure 15.2 shows that about half of the people diagnosed with a personality disorder at one point in time did not meet the criteria for the same diagnosis when they were interviewed 2 years later. Even among patients diagnosed with a severe personality disorder, 99% did not meet the criteria for the same diagnosis when reassessed after 16 years (Zanarini, Frankenburg, et al., 2012). These results indicate that many of the personality disorders may not be as enduring as the DSM asserts. Nonetheless, even after a personality disorder remits, milder symptoms are often present, so an initial personality disorder diagnosis can predict lower functioning even 15 years later.

Personality Disorders Are Highly Comorbid   A second major problem in classifying personality disorders is that more than half of people diagnosed with a personality disorder meet the diagnostic criteria for another personality disorder (Lenzenweger, Lane, et al., 2007). Some of the personality disorders involve similar symptoms. For example, as we will describe,

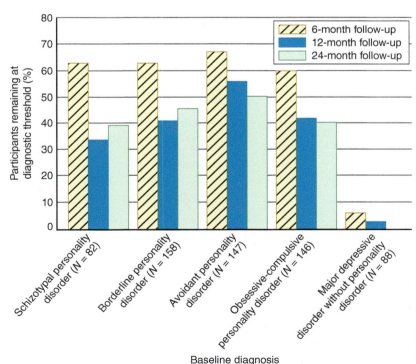

FIGURE 15.2 **Test–retest stability for personality disorders and major depressive disorder across 6-, 12-, and 24-month follow-up interviews.** Drawn from Grilo, Sanislow, et al. (2004) and Shea, Stout, et al. (2002).

the diagnostic criteria for schizotypal, avoidant, and paranoid personality disorders all emphasize social withdrawal or aloofness, and so it is not surprising that these diagnoses often co-occur.

Thresholds for Diagnosing Personality Disorders Are Arbitrary A third major problem in classifying personality disorders is that the number of symptoms required for a diagnosis is arbitrary. Many people with subsyndromal symptoms experience problems in their sense of identity and their relationships. At the same time, people who meet the diagnostic criteria for a given personality disorder are extremely varied in the severity of their functional impairment (Karukivi, Vahlberg, et al., 2017). With the exception of schizotypal personality disorder, evidence across dozens of studies suggests that personality symptoms vary along a continuum (Haslam, Holland, & Kuppens, 2012). Given this evidence, capturing the severity of symptoms and functional problems along a dimension reflecting severity may provide more helpful information than a yes/no decision about the presence of an arbitrary number of symptoms.

Quick Summary

Personality disorders are defined by longstanding and pervasive ways of being that interfere with forming and sustaining a positive self-identity and constructive relationships.

Many people with personality disorders also meet the diagnostic criteria for commonly comorbid conditions such as mood, anxiety, and substance use disorders.

In DSM-5-TR, 10 personality disorders are classified in three clusters: Cluster A personality disorders are characterized by odd or eccentric behavior, cluster B disorders by dramatic or erratic behavior, and cluster C disorders by anxious or fearful behavior.

Most personality disorders can be reliably assessed with structured clinical interviews. Unstructured clinical interviews are not reliable or sensitive and have poor predictive validity.

Most diagnoses of personality disorders remit over time, and so personality disorders are not as stable as the DSM suggests.

Personality disorders co-occur. More than half of people who meet the diagnostic criteria for one personality disorder meet the criteria for at least one other personality disorder.

Thresholds for defining personality disorders are not based on scientific evidence, and subthreshold symptoms can interfere with functioning.

15.1 Check Your Knowledge

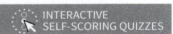
INTERACTIVE
SELF-SCORING QUIZZES

(Answers are at the end of the chapter.)
Answer the following questions.

1. Describe the inter-rater reliability levels of the DSM-5-TR personality disorder diagnoses arrived at with structured diagnostic interviews and those arrived at with unstructured diagnostic interviews.
2. List three primary concerns about the DSM-5-TR approach to classifying personality disorders.

Alternative DSM-5-TR Model for Personality Disorders

As we have discussed, the personality disorder diagnoses show poor test–retest stability and high rates of comorbidity, and the thresholds for defining a diagnosis are arbitrary. These types of concerns led the DSM-5 Committee on Personality and Personality Disorders to suggest a bold overhaul. They recommended reducing the number of personality disorders and diagnosing personality disorders based on extreme scores on personality trait measures. The American Psychological Association Board of Trustees decided to retain the personality disorder system that was in place in DSM-IV-TR but to include the alternative approach in Section III of the DSM-5 manual as an emerging approach. Although the approach to personality disorders that appears in the main text dominates clinical practice, let's consider the merits of the alternative approach.

As shown in Table 15.1, the alternative model for personality disorders includes only 6 of the 10 DSM-5-TR personality disorders. The alternative system excludes schizoid, histrionic, and dependent personality disorders because they rarely occur, and paranoid personality disorder because it usually co-occurs with other personality disorders. Much less research is available on these four personality disorders than on the others.

In the alternative DSM-5-TR model, personality disorder diagnoses are considered when a person shows persistent, stable, and pervasive impairments in personality functioning from early adulthood. If such long-term dysfunction appears to be present, the clinician considers the personality traits that explain those difficulties in functioning using two types of dimensional personality scores: five **personality trait domains** and 25 more specific **personality trait facets**, as shown in Table 15.3. These personality trait domains and facets are closely related to a very influential model of personality called the *five-factor model* (Watson, Stasik, et al., 2013). Each dimension can be evaluated using self-report items (Krueger, Derringer, et al., 2012). The profile of extreme scores on these dimensions is used to decide which personality disorder might best fit. For example, obsessive-compulsive personality disorder is defined by high scores on at least three of the following personality trait facets: rigid perfectionism, perseveration, intimacy avoidance, and restricted affectivity.

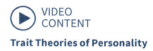

VIDEO CONTENT

Trait Theories of Personality

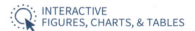

INTERACTIVE FIGURES, CHARTS, & TABLES

TABLE 15.3	The Five Personality Trait Domains and 25 Facets in the Alternative DSM-5-TR Model of Personality Disorders

Personality Trait Domain	Facet
I. Negative Affectivity (vs. Emotional Stability)	1. Anxiousness
	2. Emotional lability
	3. Hostility
	4. Perseveration
	5. Separation insecurity
	6. Submissiveness
II. Detachment (vs. Extraversion)	7. Anhedonia
	8. Depressivity
	9. Intimacy avoidance
	10. Suspiciousness
	11. Withdrawal
	12. Restricted affectivity
III. Antagonism (vs. Agreeableness)	13. Attention seeking
	14. Callousness
	15. Deceitfulness
	16. Grandiosity
	17. Manipulativeness
IV. Disinhibition (vs. Conscientiousness)	18. Distractibility
	19. Impulsivity
	20. Irresponsibility
	21. (Lack of) rigid perfectionism
	22. Risk taking
V. Psychoticism	23. Eccentricity
	24. Cognitive perceptual dysregulation
	25. Unusual beliefs and experiences

The key strengths of the focus on personality traits include the following:

- Personality trait ratings are more stable over time than are personality disorder diagnoses (Wright, Calabrese, et al., 2015).
- Twenty-five dimensional scores provide richer detail than do the categorical personality disorder diagnoses.
- Personality traits are related to many psychological disorders: Anxiety and depression are related to negative affectivity, thought disorders to psychoticism, and externalizing disorders to disinhibition and antagonism (Morey, Krueger, & Skodol, 2013).
- Personality traits robustly predict important outcomes such as happiness, relationship quality, stress, occupational outcomes, physical health, and even life expectancy (Hong, Chan, & Lim, 2020; Ingram & South, 2021; Roberts, Kuncel, et al., 2007; Wettstein, Wahl, et al., 2020).
- Clinicians rate dimensional personality approaches as more useful in communicating with clients and in planning treatment than the traditional categorical diagnostic system (Bornstein & Natoli, 2019).

Some expect that the focus on identifying personality impairment and personality trait profiles will become the major approach to personality diagnosis in the future (Sharp & Miller, 2022). Indeed, the ICD-11 has adopted the alternative approach; personality diagnosis in the ICD-11 goes one step further than the DSM-5-TR alternative approach in removing all categorical personality diagnoses with the exception of borderline personality disorder (Tyrer, Mulder, et al., 2019). In the rest of this chapter, we will focus on the approach to personality disorders that is in the main body of the DSM. But because so little is known about the four personality disorders excluded from the alternative model of DSM-5-TR, we will not discuss these disorders except to list the defining symptoms.

Quick Summary

DSM-5-TR includes an alternative model for diagnosing personality problems, which was designed to address three concerns about the traditional personality disorder approach: Personality disorders are not stable over time, they overlap substantially, and the thresholds for defining a diagnosis are arbitrary.

The alternative model includes only six personality disorders. The alternative model also provides a dimensional system for evaluating five personality trait domains and 25 more specific personality facets. These traits predict psychological syndromes and key life outcomes, and clinicians find them useful.

The alternative model is found in Section III of the DSM-5-TR.

15.2 Check Your Knowledge

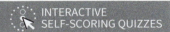
INTERACTIVE
SELF-SCORING QUIZZES

(Answers are at the end of the chapter.)
Answer the following question.

1. List two ways in which the alternative DSM-5-TR approach to personality disorders differs from the approach that appears in the main body of DSM-5-TR.

Common Risk Factors Across the Personality Disorders

Theorists over the past 100 years have tried to understand why the chronic, wide-ranging symptoms of personality disorders develop. Although psychoanalytic and behavioral theory place emphasis on parenting and early developmental influences, there is strong evidence for genetic components to these syndromes as well (Sharp, Wright, et al., 2015).

TABLE 15.4	Personality Disorders: Estimated Heritability and Effects of Child Abuse or Neglect	
Disorder	**Estimated Heritability**	**Odds Ratio of Personality Disorder After Child Abuse or Neglect**
Schizotypal	0.72	Not significantly related
Antisocial	0.69	4.97
Borderline	0.67	7.73
Narcissistic	0.71	18.21
Avoidant	0.64	Only neglect was related
Obsessive-compulsive	0.78	Too few cases to calculate

Sources: Heritability estimates from Gjerde, Czajkowski, et al. (2012); Kendler, Myers, et al. (2007); Torgersen, Lygren, et al. (2000); Torgersen, Myers, et al. (2012). Child abuse or neglect data drawn from Johnson, Cohen, et al. (1999).

Several studies have examined the heritability of personality disorders. Not only do personality disorders often co-occur, but many of the personality disorders share genetic vulnerability—people at high genetic risk for one personality disorder are also at high genetic risk for other personality disorders (Kendler, Aggen, et al., 2008). One possibility is that genetic vulnerability contributes to personality traits, such as neuroticism or impulsivity, that are related to higher risk for many different personality disorders (Sharp et al., 2015).

In contrast with the large amount of research that has focused on more severe patient samples, one genetic study is unusual in that the authors recruited a representative sample of twins through the Norwegian birth registry. To improve diagnostic reliability, the researchers combined self-ratings with interview-based ratings of personality disorder severity. Heritability estimates for all the personality disorders were at least moderately high (see **Table 15.4** for estimates for the six personality disorders we focus on).

In addition to biological factors, early adversity is present among many people who develop personality disorders. Let's consider the Children in the Community Study, one of the largest studies designed to assess the links between childhood adversity and personality disorders. In this study, researchers recruited a representative sample of 639 families with children ages 1–11. Families and children were interviewed initially in 1975, again during the period 1983–1985, and for a third time during the period 1991–1993; then the offspring were interviewed when they reached age 33. Child protective services documented childhood maltreatment for 31 of the children, and the children reported another 50 cases of abuse during their assessments. In the assessments carried out in the 1970s and 1980s, researchers conducted interviews with the parents and children to assess two aspects of parenting style: aversive parental behavior (e.g., harsh punishment, loud arguments) and lack of parental affection (e.g., little time together, poor supervision, poor communication). At the third and fourth interviews, the researchers asked questions to assess child neglect and conducted structured diagnostic interviews with the young adults to assess personality disorders. Offspring who had experienced childhood abuse or neglect were compared with a control group matched on age, parental education, and parental psychiatric disorders. In considering the role of early adversity, researchers controlled for childhood behavioral problems and parental psychiatric disorders.

Findings of this study suggest that personality disorders are strongly correlated with early adversity. As shown in **Table 15.4**, childhood abuse or neglect related to significantly higher risk of four of the six personality disorders. Children who experienced abuse or neglect were 18 times as likely as those with no history of abuse or neglect to develop narcissistic personality disorder and more than seven times as likely to develop borderline personality disorder (Johnson et al., 1999). Parenting style also predicted the onset of each of the six alternative-model DSM-5-TR personality disorders. Offspring who had experienced aversive or unaffectionate parental styles were several times more likely to develop a personality disorder than were those who had not experienced those parental styles (Johnson, Cohen, et al., 2006). Similar correlations of personality disorders with child abuse and parental conflict were shown in a study using a nationally representative samples of the Swedish and U.S. adult populations (Afifi, Mather, et al., 2011; Hengartner, Ajdacic-Gross, et al., 2013). Clearly, many people with personality disorders have had difficult experiences during their childhood.

How can we integrate the findings regarding genetic and environmental influences? The magnitude of the genetic influence on personality disorders suggests that we should be cautious as we think about parenting and early environment—many parents of those with personality disorders are likely to experience at least mild personality problems themselves as a manifestation of genetic vulnerability. Genetic studies now suggest that correlations of child abuse with personality disorder may not mean causation.

One of the first studies on this front focused on borderline personality disorder (BPD), which is a personality disorder where high rates of child abuse have been reported in dozens of studies. To determine whether genetic vulnerability and abuse are independent of each other in their effects on BPD, researchers studied 197 MZ twin pairs in which one twin, but not the other, reported childhood abuse (Bornovalova, Huibregtse, et al., 2013). If abuse, rather than genetic vulnerability, is driving BPD, twins who experienced abuse should have more BPD symptoms than their co-twins who were not abused. This was not the case. The twin pairs had similar levels of BPD symptoms. That is, childhood abuse did not predict BPD symptoms after genetic risk was controlled for. In another large twin study, childhood trauma explained less than 1% of the variance in who developed personality disorder symptoms once genetic vulnerability was considered (Berenz, Amstadter, et al., 2013).

These findings indicate that abuse may not be the driving force that sets personality disorder symptoms in motion. How can we make sense of the high rates of abuse among those with personality disorders, then? Impulsivity, emotionality, or other related traits in the parents could increase the risk that both abuse and personality disorders will occur. Findings highlight the complexity of the effect of trauma, as it often occurs within a matrix of risk factors.

Although much remains unknown, common sense still holds—child abuse and trauma have many deleterious effects, even if they are not the driving force in the development of personality disorders. The damaging effects of early adversity have been well documented, even in other studies of twins discordant for abuse (Nelson, Heath, et al., 2002). But researchers will need to conduct studies that integrate genetic vulnerability, early adversity, and child characteristics to understand how BPD personality disorder develops.

Quick Summary

The six personality disorders listed in the alternative DSM-5-TR model are all at least moderately heritable and are predicted by aversive or unaffectionate parenting. Four are tied to abuse or neglect during childhood, but some of the abuse may be tied to parental genetic vulnerability.

15.3 Check Your Knowledge

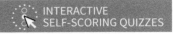 INTERACTIVE SELF-SCORING QUIZZES

(Answers are at the end of the chapter.)
Answer the following questions.

1. What is the level of heritability for personality disorders?
2. Describe the magnitude of the relationship between childhood adversity and personality disorders as observed in the Children in the Community Study.
3. What do twin studies suggest about the links between genes, trauma, and personality disorders?

Clinical Description and Causes of the Specific Personality Disorders

We now turn to the specific personality disorders. We'll consider the clinical description and the influences that shape the development of the six personality disorders listed in Table 15.4. As we consider specific risk factors, keep in mind that the genetic risk likely combines with the specific risk factors to produce symptoms.

Defining Symptoms of Paranoid Personality Disorder

Presence of four or more of the following signs of distrust and suspiciousness from early adulthood across many contexts:

- Unjustified suspiciousness of being harmed, deceived, or exploited
- Preoccupation with unwarranted doubts about the loyalty or trustworthiness of friends or associates

- Reluctance to confide in others because of suspiciousness
- Tendency to read hidden meanings into the benign actions of others
- Bearing grudges for perceived wrongs
- Angry reactions to perceived attacks on character or reputation
- Unwarranted suspiciousness of the partner's fidelity

Defining Symptoms of Schizoid Personality Disorder

Presence of four or more of the following signs of aloofness and flat affect from early adulthood across many contexts:

- Lack of desire for or enjoyment of close relationships
- Almost always prefers solitude to companionship
- Little interest in sex

- Few or no pleasurable activities
- Lack of close friends
- Indifference to praise or criticism
- Flat affect, emotional detachment, or coldness

Defining Symptoms of Histrionic Personality Disorder

Presence of five or more of the following signs of excessive emotionality and attention seeking from early adulthood across many contexts:

- Strong need to be the center of attention
- Inappropriate sexually seductive behavior
- Rapidly shifting and shallow expression of emotions

- Use of physical appearance to draw attention to self
- Speech that is excessively impressionistic and lacking in detail
- Exaggerated, theatrical emotional expression
- Being overly suggestible
- Misreading relationships as more intimate than they are

Defining Symptoms of Dependent Personality Disorder

An excessive need to be taken care of, as shown by the presence of at least five of the following from early adulthood across many contexts:

- Difficulty making decisions without excessive advice and reassurance from others
- Need for others to take responsibility for most major areas of life
- Difficulty disagreeing with others for fear of losing their support

- Difficulty doing things on own or starting projects because of lack of self-confidence
- Doing unpleasant things to obtain the approval and support of others
- Feelings of helplessness when alone because of exaggerated fears of being unable to care for self
- Urgently seeking a new relationship when one ends
- Preoccupation with fears of having to take care of self

Schizotypal Personality Disorder

The defining features of **schizotypal personality disorder** include eccentric thoughts and behavior, interpersonal detachment, and suspiciousness. Like Emily in the Clinical Case, people with this disorder may have odd beliefs or magical thinking—for instance, the belief that they can read other people's minds or see into the future. It is also common for them to have ideas of reference (the belief that events have an unusual meaning for them personally). For example, they might think that a TV program is conveying a special message designed for them. They are often suspicious of others and concerned that others might hurt them. They might also have recurrent illusions (inaccurate sensory perceptions), such as sensing the presence of a force or a person who is not actually there. In their speech, they might use words in an unusual and unclear fashion—for example, they might say "not a very talkable person" to mean a person who is not easy to talk to. Their behavior and appearance might also be eccentric—for example, they might talk to themselves or wear disheveled clothing. Their affect is flat, and they are aloof from others.

The symptoms of schizotypal personal disorder bear some similarity to the types of bizarre thinking and experiences seen in schizophrenia. In schizotypal personality disorder, though, the bizarre thinking and functional impairments are less severe than they are in schizophrenia, and neither hallucinations or full-blown delusions are present.

For many people with schizotypal personality disorder, the symptoms worsen and develop into schizophrenia over time. In a study of the medical records of the Danish population, researchers identified more than 2,500 individuals who had been diagnosed with schizotypal disorder. Across a 20-year period, about a third of the people who were initially diagnosed with schizotypal disorder were later diagnosed with schizophrenia (Hjorthøj, Albert, et al., 2018).

The genetic vulnerability for schizotypal personality disorder appears to overlap with the genetic vulnerability for schizophrenia. Family studies and adoption studies have shown that the relatives of people with schizophrenia are at increased risk for schizotypal personality disorder (Nigg & Goldsmith, 1994; Tienari, Wynne, et al., 2003). People with schizotypal personality disorder have deficits in cognitive and neuropsychological functioning that are similar to but milder than those seen with schizophrenia (Kerns, 2020). Consistent with their having deficits that are milder variants of those seen in schizophrenia, people with schizotypal personality

---

Clinical Case

Emily

Emily, a 40-year-old single woman, was referred to her employment counseling center by her boss. Her boss stated that she had always completed her clerical duties in a timely and careful manner but he was worried that her relationships with the other women who shared her office space were difficult. He said that he himself found it hard to relate to her. She was a bit eccentric and expressed herself poorly at times.

At the interview with the counselor, Emily was slightly disheveled and extremely reserved, and she had difficulty making eye contact. Emily reported that she did indeed feel very uncomfortable around others in the workplace, but that she had done her best to be polite toward her coworkers. Nonetheless, her social interactions had been a little strained from the time she started her position a couple months ago, and they had become worse after a difficult interaction in the lunchroom. Since that time, she had felt frightened around her coworkers, and she found it hard to say anything to them, even when they attended joint meetings.

When the therapist asked, Emily described the incident that seemed to intensify her problem with her coworkers. When several of her coworkers had been making fun of people who believe in extrasensory perception, Emily had explained to them that she did have a keen sixth sense of when things were about to happen. She had described knowing in advance about a car accident that happened on her block one day and occasionally being able to read minds. The more she tried to explain these experiences, the quieter the others became, and in the mornings that followed her coworkers quit making even basic greetings. As she described this incident, Emily's speech was occasionally hard to understand—her sentences became a bit disjointed, and she pronounced words in such an unusual way that the counselor had to ask her to explain what she meant a couple different times.

When the counselor asked about other areas of her life, Emily described a quiet, friendless existence. She spent most evenings and weekends alone at home. She said she was used to being alone, as she had been a lonely and teased child. She frequently thought she heard a voice saying her name, but then could find no one in the apartment who could have made the vocalization. Other times she felt as though there was a spiritual presence in her apartment, but she was not sure if that could be the case. She denied frank hallucinations. Her brother had schizophrenia, and Emily had long worried that she could develop the same disease.

disorder show difficulties on tasks involving social cognition, such as judging another person's mental state (Wastler & Lenzenweger, 2019). Furthermore, the brains of people with schizotypal personality disorder have enlarged ventricles, less temporal lobe gray matter, and neurotransmitter dysregulation similar to but less severe than what is observed in schizophrenia (Lenzenweger, 2015). Given the parallels in symptoms, the evidence that some with schizotypal personality disorder will develop schizophrenia, and the overlap in causes, the DSM-5-TR includes a reference to schizotypal personality disorder in its discussion of schizophrenia and related disorders.

Defining Symptoms of Schizotypal Personality Disorder

Presence of five or more of the following signs of unusual thinking, eccentric behavior, and interpersonal deficits from early adulthood across many contexts:

- Ideas of reference
- Odd beliefs or magical thinking (e.g., belief in extrasensory perception) not explained by subcultural norms
- Unusual perceptions

- Odd thoughts and speech
- Suspiciousness or paranoia
- Inappropriate or restricted affect
- Odd or eccentric behavior or appearance
- Lack of close friends
- Social anxiety and interpersonal fears that do not diminish with familiarity

---

Antisocial Personality Disorder and Psychopathy

Informally, laypeople often use the terms *antisocial personality disorder* and *psychopathy* interchangeably. Antisocial behavior, such as law breaking, is a core component of both, but the two syndromes differ in important ways. One difference is that antisocial personality disorder is included in DSM-5-TR, whereas psychopathy is not.

Antisocial Personality Disorder: Clinical Description   The core feature of **antisocial personality disorder (APD)** is a pervasive pattern of disregard for the rights of others (as described in the **Clinical Case of Alec**). The person with APD is distinguished by aggressive, impulsive, and callous traits. DSM-5 criteria specify the presence of conduct disorder before age 15. As adults, people with APD show irresponsible behaviors, such as working inconsistently, breaking laws, being irritable and physically aggressive, defaulting on debts, being reckless and impulsive, and neglecting to plan ahead. They show little regard for truth and little remorse for their misdeeds, even when those actions hurt family and friends.

Men are about five times more likely than are women to meet the criteria for APD (Oltmanns & Powers, 2012). About three-quarters of people with APD meet the diagnostic criteria for another disorder, with substance abuse being very common (Lenzenweger et al., 2007). More than half of prison inmates meet the diagnostic criteria for APD (Edens, Kelley, et al., 2015).

Psychopathy: Clinical Description   The concept of **psychopathy** predates the DSM diagnosis of antisocial personality disorder. In his book *The Mask of Sanity*, Hervey Cleckley (1976) drew on his clinical experience to formulate diagnostic criteria for psychopathy. The criteria for psychopathy focus on a lack of emotions, both positive and negative: Psychopathic people have no sense of shame, and their seemingly positive

---

Clinical Case

Alec

Alec, a 40-year-old man, was court-ordered to take part in a psychological assessment after being charged with manufacturing counterfeit bills. He described his history of three divorces with no remorse. His first marriage had ended in a rancorous divorce after he was discovered having two extramarital affairs simultaneously. His second marriage ended within 3 months, and he bragged about emptying her large savings account, stating, "A fool and her money are easily parted." His third wife divorced him after discovering that he had been trafficking in stolen furniture. He had a long history of petty financial and drug-related crimes, and despite his frequent drug dealing, he was deeply in debt. He was estranged from all family members, and his only friends were the regulars at his neighborhood bar.

Defining Symptoms of Antisocial Personality Disorder

- Age at least 18
- Evidence of conduct disorder before age 15
- Pervasive pattern of disregard for the rights of others since the age of 15, as shown by at least three of the following:

  1. Repeated engagement in illegal behavior(s)
  2. Deceitfulness, lying

  3. Impulsivity
  4. Irritability and aggressiveness (for example, repeated physical fights or assaults)
  5. Reckless disregard for own safety and that of others
  6. Irresponsibility, as seen in unreliable employment or financial history
  7. Lack of remorse

Focus on Discovery 15.1

Media Images of Psychopathy: Will the Real Psychopath Please Stand Up?

Media images of psychopathy vary considerably, ranging from portrayals of ruthless murderers such as Javier Bardem's character in *No Country for Old Men* to charming business tycoons to white-collar criminals. The media are quick to attach a label of psychopathy to mass murderers and other ruthless, violent offenders. At the same time, the idea that people with psychopathy use their charm, boldness, and lack of empathy to climb their way into the boardroom, where they are influencing the culture of current business practice, has become quite widespread in the media. Stories abound of remorseless capitalists who bilk their customers of money through white-collar crime, such as the one featured in the film *The Wolf of Wall Street* (Smith & Lilienfeld, 2013).

Data are available about each of these stereotypes. Some, but certainly not all, people with high levels of psychopathy engage in violence as a means of achieving their goals (Reidy, Shelley-Tremblay, & Lilienfeld, 2011). Regarding corporate success, a widely cited study did suggest that employees in a large corporate management training program obtained PCL-R scores that were somewhat higher than those of the general population, but only 3% of the employees scored above the PCL-R threshold for psychopathy (Babiak, Neumann, & Hare, 2010). Moreover, psychopathy scores were not elevated in one sample of white-collar criminals (Ragatz, Fremouw, & Baker, 2012). It is not safe to presume that someone is psychopathic just because they engage in violent or unethical behavior, have a history of white-collar crime, or are highly successful. Careful diagnosis depends on evaluating whether an entire syndrome is present.

feelings for others are merely an act. They are superficially charming and use that charm to manipulate others for personal gain. Their lack of anxiety may make it impossible for them to learn from their mistakes, and their lack of remorse leads them to behave irresponsibly and often cruelly toward others. The rule-breaking behavior of a person with psychopathy is performed impulsively, as much for thrills as for financial gain.

According to the **triarchic model of psychopathy**, three core traits underpin the symptoms of psychopathy: boldness (fearlessness), meanness (aggression and lack of remorse), and disinhibition (impulsivity) (Patrick, 2022). Meanness and disinhibition might be more core to the negative outcomes of psychopathy (Miller, Lamkin, et al., 2016; Miller & Lynam, 2012), while boldness may help explain the social poise and calm demeanor of some psychopaths (Lilienfeld, Patrick, et al., 2012). See **Focus on Discovery 15.1** for discussion of the idea that some psychopaths may be highly successful and charming.

The scale most commonly used to assess psychopathy is the Psychopathy Checklist–Revised (PCL-R; Hare, 2003). Ratings on this 20-item scale are based on an interview and a review of criminal records and mental health charts. Many self-report scales have been developed as well.

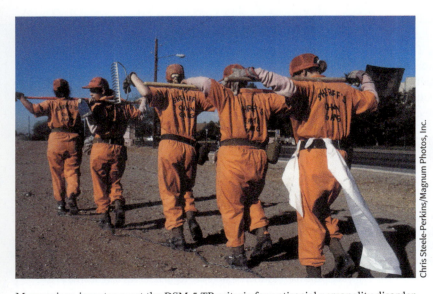

Chris Steele-Perkins/Magnum Photos, Inc.

Many prison inmates meet the DSM-5-TR criteria for antisocial personality disorder.

There are three chief differences between the criteria for APD and the definition of psychopathy as reflected on the PCL-R. First, even though the PCL-R covers many of the criteria for APD, the scale differs from the DSM-5 criteria for APD in including more affective symptoms, such as shallow affect and lack of empathy. Second, the DSM-5-TR criteria for antisocial personality disorder differ from psychopathy criteria in the requirement that a person develop symptoms before age 15. Third, APD is a categorical diagnosis, and psychopathy is rated along a dimension. When researchers conduct analyses of severity, using the number of APD symptoms as opposed to the presence or absence of the APD diagnosis, APD severity and psychopathy levels are very highly correlated (Patrick, 2022).

Causes of Antisocial Personality Disorder and Psychopathy

As we review research on the etiology of ASP and psychopathy, keep in mind an issue that makes findings a little bit hard to integrate. The research has been conducted on persons with two different diagnoses—some with APD and some with psychopathy. There may be important differences between vulnerability to APD and vulnerability to psychopathy (Baskin-Sommers, 2016; Hyde, Shaw, et al., 2016). We will discuss genetic findings based on studies of APD, and then turn toward psychological models that have been developed to explain psychopathy.

More than any other area of personality disorder research, the work on APD often considers biology conjointly with social and psychological influences. In this section, we will describe two ways in which this integrated biopsychosocial approach operates. First, in considering the social correlates of APD, we will look at how genetic and social influences work together. Second, as we discuss psychological models of psychopathy, we will note several studies that have used brain imaging to test these models. To capture these integrated models, we will deviate from our organizational approach in other sections of the text, where we have tended to separate neurobiological and psychological models.

Interactions of Genes and the Social Environment

Considerable research suggests that the genetic vulnerability for APD overlaps with the genetic vulnerability for substance use disorders, which helps explain the high rate of substance use disorders among those with APD (Krueger, Hicks, et al., 2002). Nonetheless, the social environment plays a major role in whether that genetic vulnerability is expressed in APD symptoms.

Earlier in the chapter, we described the Children in the Community study, one of the many studies showing that parenting qualities can predict antisocial behavior. Substantial prospective research also indicates that broader social factors, including poverty and exposure to violence, predict antisocial behavior (Loeber & Hay, 1997). For example, among adolescents with conduct disorder, those who are impoverished are twice as likely to develop APD as are those from higher socioeconomic backgrounds (Lahey, Loeber, et al., 2005). There is little question that childhood adversity can set the stage for the development of APD.

Adoption research has also shown that genetic, behavioral, and family influences are very hard to disentangle (Ge, Conger, et al., 1996). That is, the genetically influenced antisocial behavior of the child can provoke harsh discipline and lack of warmth, even in adoptive parents, and these parental characteristics in turn exacerbate the child's antisocial tendencies. Nonetheless, the findings of many studies indicate that social influences such as harsh discipline and poverty robustly predict APD even after genetic risk is controlled for (Jaffee, Strait, & Odgers, 2012).

Risk for Psychopathology: Insensitivity to Threat, Lack of Empathy, and Poor Executive Control

According to the triarchic model, each of the three underlying traits involved in psychopathy—boldness, meanness, and disinhibition—is correlated to specific psychological processes: threat sensitivity, lack of empathy, and poor executive control, respectively. Next, we discuss some of the evidence from self-report, laboratory, and neuro-imaging studies that these three processes are related to psychopathy.

Threat Sensitivity

A large body of work relates psychopathy, and more specifically to the trait of boldness, to deficits in the sensitivity to threat (Patrick, 2022). People with high levels of boldness show less reactivity in skin conductance and heart rate is less reactive when they are confronted with or anticipate an aversive stimulus (Patrick, Iacono, et al., 2019; Yancey, Venables, et al., 2016). Low reactivity of skin conductance to aversive stimuli (loud tones) at age 3 predicted psychopathy scores at age 28 (Glenn, Raine, et al., 2007). In addition to lower levels of skin conductance, those with psychopathy show blunted neural responsivity to aversive stimuli (Baskin-Sommers, 2016).

People with psychopathy seem unable to learn from experience; they often repeat misconduct that has been harshly punished, even if it resulted in jail time. They seem immune to the anxiety that keeps most of us from breaking the law, lying, or injuring others. Cleckley (1976) argued that people with psychopathy do not learn to avoid trouble because they are insensitive to threats. The lack of biological response to negative stimuli appears to shape this difficulty learning from aversive feedback—that is, those with high psychopathy show diminished classical conditioning when aversive stimuli such as electric shock or loud blasts of noise (the unconditioned stimulus) are repeatedly paired with a conditioned stimulus (Smith & Lilienfeld, 2015). In an interesting test of classical conditioning deficits, researchers used brain imaging to examine what happens when an unconditioned stimulus (painful pressure) is repeatedly paired with neutral pictures (the conditioned stimuli). To assess responses to the conditioned stimulus after these repeated pairings, the researchers measured the activity of the amygdala, a brain region that is implicated in emotion reactivity, and other brain regions involved in emotion (Birbaumer, Veit, et al., 2005). After conditioning, healthy control participants showed increases in amygdala activity when viewing the neutral pictures. People with high psychopathy scores, though, did not show this expected increase in amygdala activity. Weakened classical conditioning to threats could help explain why people with psychopathy are slow to learn from punishment.

Lack of Empathy   Psychopathy and particularly meanness, might be tied to a lack of empathy, defined by the capacity to share the emotional reactions of others (Blair, 2005). Several types of research provide support for this theory. When asked to identify the emotion conveyed in videos of strangers, men with psychopathy do poorly in recognizing others' fear, even though they recognize other emotions well (Brook & Kosson, 2013). Those with antisocial symptoms show less amygdala response (presumably reflecting less emotional response) when imagining others' pain than when imagining their own pain (Marsh, Finger, et al., 2013). The ventromedial prefrontal cortex, a region involved in processing social and moral information and in conditioning, is also generally less active among people with psychopathy (Baskin-Sommers, 2016). Disruptions in the connectivity of the amygdala with the ventromedial prefrontal cortex while viewing others' facial expressions of fear predicted psychopathic traits at a follow-up assessment 2 years later (Waller, Gard, et al., 2019). These behavioral and neural indicators of unresponsiveness to others' emotions appear particularly related to the meanness dimension of psychopathy (Patrick, 2022).

Borderline Personality Disorder

Borderline personality disorder (BPD) has been a major focus of research interest for several reasons: It is very common in clinical settings, very hard to treat, and associated with recurrent self-harm behavior and suicidality. As with antisocial personality disorder, BPD involves high levels of impulsivity (Mullins-Sweatt, DeShong, et al., 2019). The other core features of BPD are instability in mood and relationships.

Emotionally, people with this disorder may shift from blissful happiness to outraged explosions in the blink of an eye. Researchers have used experience sampling, in which people report on their feelings or behavior several times per day for weeks, to understand these emotional and interpersonal responses. Consistent with Kiera Van Gelder's report in **Read More About It 15.1**, findings from more than a dozen experience sampling studies show that emotions can change drastically, in a short period of time, for those with BPD (Houben, Mestdagh, et al., 2021). Most experience comorbid anxiety and depression diagnoses (Bohus, Stoffers-Winterling, et al., 2021).

BPD is also related to interpersonal hypersensitivity. Research with experience sampling and using laboratory tasks has shown that people with BPD are overly sensitive to small signs of rejection by others, and in response to those signals, they are prone to anger and aggression (Trull & Hepp, 2023). They cannot bear to be alone, have fears of abandonment, and experience chronic feelings of depression and emptiness. Of the different personality disorders, BPD is the one most closely tied to distress in romantic relationships (Wilson, Stroud, & Durbin, 2017). They may experience transient psychotic and dissociative symptoms when stressed.

People with BPD are highly impulsive, particularly in response to emotion states (Trull & Hepp, 2023). Their unpredictable, impulsive, and potentially self-damaging behavior might include gambling, reckless spending, indiscriminate sexual activity, and substance abuse. Their symptoms lead to relationship conflicts and financial crises (Powers, Gleason, & Oltmanns, 2013).

People with BPD often have not developed a clear and coherent sense of self—they experience major swings in such basic aspects of identity as their values, loyalties, and career choices. One month, they might consider a career in the business world, complete with the wardrobe and polished demeanor of a professional salesperson; the next month, they might decide to try acting, trading in their business apparel for colorful artistic garb, accompanied by a new set of interests in the arts.

Suicidal behavior is all too common with BPD. Many people with this disorder make multiple suicide attempts during their lifetime (Boisseau, Yen, et al., 2013), and some die from suicide (Soloff & Chiappetta, 2019). People with BPD are also particularly likely to engage in nonsuicidal self-injury. For example, they might slice their leg with a razor blade or burn their arm with a cigarette—behavior that is harmful but unlikely to cause death. At least two-thirds of people with BPD will engage in self-harm at some point during their lives (Stone, 1993).

Many adolescents go through periods of emotionally labile and impulsive behavior. Although some of these adolescents will be diagnosed with borderline personality disorder, it is important to note that only a small percentage of those will meet borderline personality disorder when re-interviewed as adults. Some believe that borderline personality disorder is being overdiagnosed among adolescents (Trull & Hepp, 2023).

Causes of Borderline Personality Disorder

We will begin by considering the neurobiological correlates of BPD, and then we will discuss Linehan's model of how parenting style may interact with a child's emotionality and behavior. Both types of findings highlight how important it is to consider a matrix of risk factors conjointly in trying to understand BPD.

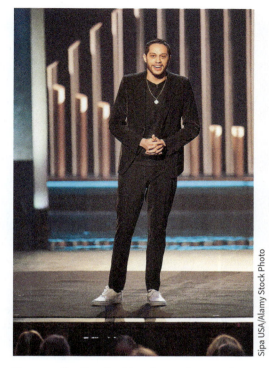

Sipa USA/Alamy Stock Photo

The comedian Pete Davidson has spoken out about his diagnosis of borderline personality disorder on *Saturday Night Live* and the *Howard Stern Show*, hoping to reduce stigma (M. Holahan, Dec. 4, 2018, *Today*, https://www.today.com/health/ borderline-personality-disorder-pete-davidson- raises-awareness-t144443).

Defining Symptoms of Borderline Personality Disorder

Presence of five or more of the following signs of instability in relationships, self-image, and impulsivity from early adulthood across many contexts:

- Frantic efforts to avoid abandonment
- Unstable interpersonal relationships in which others are either idealized or devalued
- Unstable sense of self
- Self-damaging, impulsive behaviors in at least two areas, such as spending, sex, substance abuse, reckless driving, and binge eating

- Recurrent suicidal behavior or gestures or self-injurious behavior (e.g., cutting self)
- Marked mood reactivity
- Chronic feelings of emptiness
- Recurrent bouts of intense or poorly controlled anger
- During stress, a tendency to experience transient paranoid thoughts and dissociative symptoms

---

Neurobiological Factors   Core features of BPD include heightened emotionality and impulsivity. Relatedly, neurobiological research suggests the importance of regulatory control regions (such as regions of the prefrontal cortex and anterior cingulate cortex) and regions implicated in emotion response (such as the amygdala and hippocampus) (Schulze, Schulze, et al., 2019). Several studies link BPD to diminished connectivity of brain regions involved in emotion experience and those involved in regulatory control. Consistent with this model, several studies have shown that applying repetitive transcranial magnetic stimulation (rTMS) to the dorsolateral prefrontal cortex can lead to short-term improvements in emotion regulation among persons with BPD (Chiappini, Picutti, et al., 2022). These neurobiological patterns could help explain the poor control over emotions shown by people with BPD and their impulsivity when emotions are present (Mancke, Herpertz, & Bertsch, 2015).

VIDEO
CONTENT

Case Study: Borderline Personality Disorder Pause and Ponder

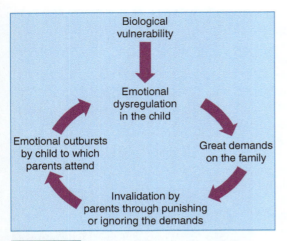

FIGURE 15.3 **Linehan's biosocial theory of borderline personality disorder.**

Interaction of Parenting with Child Vulnerability   Marsha Linehan (1987) proposes that we need to consider how parenting could amplify the vulnerabilities of some children. She argues that BPD develops when people who have difficulty controlling their emotions because of a biological vulnerability (possibly genetic) are raised in a family environment that is invalidating. In an invalidating environment, the person's efforts to communicate feelings are disregarded or even punished. Linehan argues that a vulnerability to emotional dysregulation interacts with experiences of invalidation to promote the development of BPD.

The two main hypothesized influences—emotional dysregulation and invalidation—interact with each other in a dynamic fashion (see **Figure 15.3**). For example, the emotionally dysregulated child may make enormous demands on his or her family. The exasperated parents ignore or even punish the child's outbursts, which leads the child to suppress their emotions. The suppressed emotions build up to an explosion, which then gets the attention of the parents. Thus, the parents end up reinforcing the very behaviors that they find aversive. Many other patterns are possible, of course, but what they all have in common is a chronic back-and-forth between dysregulation and invalidation.

Research on the development of BPD supports the importance of parental relationships in BPD. For example, despite some nonreplications (Stepp, Lazarus, & Byrd, 2016), longitudinal studies suggest that BPD symptoms can be predicted by difficult parental relationships, even when objective raters evaluate the quality of parenting (Belsky, Caspi, et al., 2012; Carlson, Egeland, & Sroufe, 2009; Lyons-Ruth, Bureau, et al., 2013).

Research also indicates the importance of considering the dynamic nature of the interactions between children and their parents. In one study, researchers conducted annual assessments of 2,228 girls from age 5 through 14, along with their mothers. Poor self-control (e.g., "cannot control temper outbursts") predicted an increase over time in harsh parenting, and vice versa—harsh parenting predicted worse self-control. The childhood problems with self-control predicted more BPD symptoms as the girls reached age 14 (Hallquist, Hipwell, & Stepp, 2015). These findings illustrate the importance of considering the dynamic interaction between child behavior and parenting.

Dozens of studies support the idea that emotion regulation is challenging for those with BPD. When distressed, those with BPD tend to try to suppress or avoid those experiences, rather than accepting that the emotion is present and engaging in problem-solving (Daros & Williams, 2019). The emotion regulation difficulties are correlated with many of the troubling outcomes of BPD, such as impulsivity, substance use problems, and relationship distress (Trull & Hepp, 2023).

Narcissistic Personality Disorder

People with **narcissistic personality disorder** have a grandiose view of their qualities and are preoccupied with fantasies of great success (as demonstrated by Bob in the Clinical Case). Their interpersonal relationships are disturbed by their lack of empathy, by their arrogance coupled with feelings of envy, and by their feelings of entitlement and expectations that others will do special favors for them.

People with narcissistic personality disorder view themselves as superior to others, and they overestimate their attractiveness to others and their contributions to group activities ("Others must be jealous of me; I've been responsible for the lion's share of our progress here today"). In some studies, researchers have provided participants with feedback that they were successful on a task (regardless of their actual performance) and then asked them to rate the reasons they were successful. In these types of studies, people with narcissistic personality disorder attribute successes to their abilities rather than to chance more than those without personality disorder do (Morf & Rhodewalt, 2001).

When people with narcissistic personality disorder interact with others, their primary goal is to bolster their own self-esteem (Morf & Rhodewalt, 2001). Indeed, they value being admired more than they do gaining or maintaining closeness (Campbell, Bosson, et al., 2007)—which helps explain why they are willing to do things that others find irritating. They do a lot to gain the admiration of others. They often pursue fame and wealth. In one study, independent observers were able to make snap judgments of narcissism with some accuracy from photographs, most typically by noticing the expensive clothes and overinvestment in appearance of those with narcissistic traits (Vazire, Naumann, et al., 2008). People with narcissistic personality disorder work hard in contexts in which there is a chance for recognition (Roberts, Woodman, & Sedikides, 2017). They also tend to brag a lot.

People with narcissistic personality disorder are highly likely to be vindictive and aggressive when faced with a competitive threat or a put-down (Kjærvik & Bushman, 2021). When someone else performs better than they do on a task that is relevant to self-esteem, they will denigrate the other person, even to that person's face (Roberts, Woodman, & Sedikides, 2017). Although their ability to present their strengths and project confidence is often perceived positively in brief initial interactions, their aggressive, competitive tendencies tend to wear thin over time, and others tend to rate them more negatively after just a few sessions of working together (Leckelt, Küfner, et al., 2015). That is, the antagonistic behavior associated with rivalry backfires—it paradoxically lessens confidence about having attained social status (Zeigler-Hill, Vrabel, et al., 2019).

Narcissism also tends to predict problems in romantic partnerships. People with narcissistic personality disorder are likely to seek out high-status partners whom they idealize and proudly show off, only to change partners if given an opportunity to be with a person of higher status. In a study of newlyweds, high levels of narcissistic traits among wives predicted steep declines in marital satisfaction for both the husbands and the wives over a 4-year period (Lavner, Lamkin, et al., 2016).

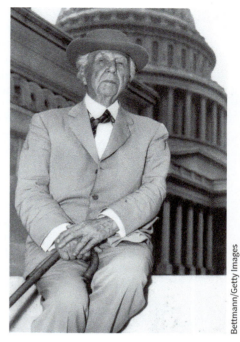

Bettmann/Getty Images

Frank Lloyd Wright, one of the most influential American architects, displayed at least some narcissistic traits. He is quoted as saying, "Early in life, I had to choose between honest arrogance and hypocritical humility. I chose honest arrogance and have seen no reason to change."

Clinical Case

Bob

Bob, a 50-year-old college professor, sought treatment only after urging from his wife. During the interview, Bob's wife noted that he seemed so focused on himself and his own advancement that he often belittled others. Bob was dismissive of these concerns, stating that he had never been the sort of person to tolerate idiots, and he could see no reason why he should begin offering such tolerance now. In rapid fire, he described his supervisor, his students, his parents, and a set of former friends as lacking the intelligence to merit his friendship. He willingly acknowledged working long hours but stated that his research had the potential to change people's lives and that other activities could not be allowed to interfere with his success. The therapist's gentle questioning of whether his expressions of superiority might provoke some interpersonal tension was met with a scathing rebuke.

Defining Symptoms of Narcissistic Personality Disorder

Presence of five or more of the following signs of grandiosity, need for admiration, and lack of empathy from early adulthood across many contexts:

- Grandiose view of one's importance
- Preoccupation with fantasies of success, power, brilliance, beauty, or ideal love
- Belief that one is special and can be understood only by other high-status people

- Extreme need for admiration
- Strong sense of entitlement
- Tendency to exploit others
- Lack of empathy
- Envious of others
- Arrogant behavior or attitudes

Given the associated tendencies toward confidence and ambition, could a small amount of narcissism be adaptive? In one study, 121 scholars with expertise in American leaders rated the degree of (subclinical) narcissism of the first 42 U.S. presidents. Presidents who were rated as relatively more narcissistic were more likely to be persuasive, won more of the popular vote, and initiated more legislation. On the other hand, they were also more likely to get in trouble for unethical behavior (Watts, Lilienfeld, et al., 2013).

Causes of Narcissistic Personality Disorder

In this section, we consider theory and research on how some people develop narcissistic personality traits. We begin by discussing parenting and then consider models of fragile self-esteem.

Parenting In one prominent account of how parenting might influence the development of narcissism, Millon (1996) hypothesized that parents who are overly indulgent promote children's beliefs that they are special (even more special than other children) and that behavioral expressions of their specialness will be tolerated by others. Several studies indicate that people with high self-rated levels of narcissism do report experiencing overindulgence from their parents (Horton, 2011). More importantly, independent ratings confirm this profile. Researchers assessed 565 children ages 7–11 and their parents twice a year for 2 years. Consistent with theory, parental tendencies to perceive their children as highly superior to others predicted an increase in their children's narcissistic traits at each time point (Brummelman, Thomaes, et al., 2015). These findings, though, are somewhat hard to reconcile with evidence, described in Table 15.4, that parental abuse or neglect is closely related to narcissistic personality disorder.

Fragile Self-Esteem Heinz Kohut (1971, 1977) developed a model of narcissism based on self-psychology, a variant of psychodynamic theory. He started from the clinical observation that the person with narcissistic personality disorder projects self-importance, self-absorption, and fantasies of limitless success on the surface. Kohut theorized that these characteristics mask a very fragile self-esteem. People with narcissistic personality disorder strive to bolster their sense of self-worth through unending quests for respect from others. Inflated self-worth and denigration of others, then, are defenses against feelings of shame. Research supports the idea that people diagnosed with narcissistic personality disorder experience shame more frequently than do those without narcissistic personality disorder (Ritter, Vater, et al., 2014).

The idea that narcissism is tied to fragile self-esteem has shaped cognitive behavioral theory and research. To assess whether people with narcissistic personality disorder have fragile self-esteem, many researchers have examined how much their self-esteem depends on external feedback (Morf & Rhodewalt, 2001). For example, when falsely told that they have done poorly on an IQ test, they show much more reactivity than others do; similarly, they show more reactivity to hearing that they have succeeded at something.

In one study, researchers used fMRI to examine vulnerability to feedback in the form of social rejection during a cyberball game. Participants were falsely led to believe that they were playing the game with two other people (Cascio, Konrath, & Falk, 2015). During one block of the game, the (sham) participants did not toss the ball to the participant. As expected, social exclusion activated neural regions associated with processing social and other forms of pain (such as the anterior insula and anterior cingulate cortex). Narcissistic traits were tied to more activation of those pain-relevant neural regions. That is, those with narcissistic tendencies were particularly sensitive to negative social interactions.

Even though some people with narcissistic personality disorder show signs of fragile self-esteem, the degree of this fragility varies across those with narcissistic personality disorder (Miller, Lynam, et al., 2017). When present, fragile self-esteem predicts poorer important outcomes, and could be why narcissistic personality disorder is related to depression and suicidality (Pincus, 2023).

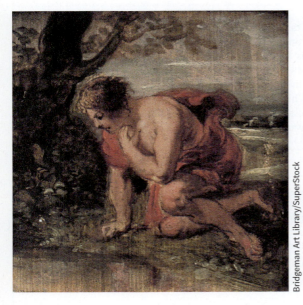

Narcissistic personality disorder draws its name from the Greek mythological figure Narcissus, who fell in love with his own reflection, was consumed by his desire, and was transformed into a flower.

Source: Peter Paul Rubens. 1577–1640 (Flemish). *Narcissus.* Museum Bojimans Van Beuningen, Rotterdam, Netherlands.

Bridgeman Art Library/SuperStock

Avoidant Personality Disorder

People with **avoidant personality disorder** are so fearful of criticism, rejection, and disapproval that they will avoid jobs or relationships to protect themselves from negative feedback. In social situations, they are restrained and timid because of an extreme fear of saying something foolish, being embarrassed, or showing signs of anxiety. They believe that they are inadequate and inferior to others, and like Leon in the Clinical Case, they are reluctant to take risks or try new activities. Even though they would like to form close relationships, their fears often make it hard for them to do so.

Clinical Case

Leon

Leon, a 45-year-old man, sought treatment for depression. During the interview, Leon described feeling depressed and socially uncomfortable for as long as he could remember. By age 5, he would experience intense anxiety when he was with other children, and his mind would "go blank" if he had to speak in front of others. He grew up dreading birthday parties, teachers' classroom questions, and meeting other children. Although he was able to play with some of the children in his neighborhood, he had never asked a woman out on a date or developed a close friendship. He took a job at the post office after graduation because it involved little social interaction.

Adapted from Spitzer, Gibbon, et al. (1994).

Avoidant personality disorder often co-occurs with social anxiety disorder (see Chapter 6), probably because the diagnostic criteria for these two disorders are so similar. The genetic vulnerabilities for avoidant personality disorder and social anxiety disorder appear to overlap (Torvik, Welander-Vatn, et al., 2016). Etiological variables related to avoidant personality disorder, then, might overlap with those of social anxiety disorder, discussed in Chapter 6.

Defining Symptoms of Avoidant Personality Disorder

A pervasive pattern of social inhibition, feelings of inadequacy, and hypersensitivity to criticism, as shown by four or more of the following from early adulthood across many contexts:

- Avoidance of occupational activities that involve significant interpersonal contact, because of fears of criticism, rejection, or disapproval
- Unwilling to get involved with people unless certain of being liked
- Restrained in intimate relationships because of the fear of being shamed or ridiculed
- Preoccupation with being criticized or rejected
- Inhibited in new interpersonal situations because of feelings of inadequacy
- Viewing self as socially inept, unappealing, or inferior
- Unusually reluctant to take risks or try new activities because they may prove embarrassing

---

Obsessive-Compulsive Personality Disorder

The person with **obsessive-compulsive personality disorder** is a perfectionist, preoccupied with details, rules, and schedules. Although order and perfectionism have their adaptive sides, particularly in fostering success in complex occupational goals, people with this disorder can pay so much attention to detail that they fail to finish projects (as illustrated in the **Clinical Case of Sarah**). They are more oriented toward work than pleasure, and social relationships often suffer as the pursuit of perfection in the workplace takes time away from family

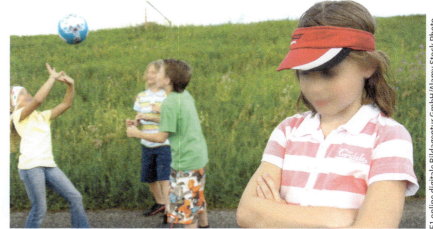

People with avoidant personality disorder often avoid interpersonal interactions, as they find them too stressful.

F1 online digitale Bildagentur GmbH/Alamy Stock Photo

and friends. Their interpersonal relationships can be impacted by their demands that everything be done the right way—their way. Even social and leisure activities can become laborious, as they excessively plan the details of upcoming events. Generally, they are serious, rigid, formal, and inflexible, especially regarding moral issues. They may be unable to discard worn-out and useless objects, even those with no sentimental value, and they are likely to be excessively frugal.

Clinical Case

Sarah

Sarah, a 22-year-old woman, was happy to attain a position as a research assistant with a highly accomplished scientist just after graduation. She was planning to pursue a career in science, and the position fit perfectly with her long-held interests. Despite Sarah's initial enthusiasm, things soon soured with her new boss. When asked to collect data using methods that she already knew well, she began by creating large spreadsheets of the planned process and then shifted gears and invested in elaborate software for project management. No matter how hard she tried, she could not move from project planning into actual data collection. When faced with writing a project description for the university ethics board review,

she wrote over 50 pages of detailed notes on potentially relevant issues but then could not find a way to describe the study in the single page allowed on the form. Although she was asked to manage eight undergraduate volunteers who worked with the team, she could not delegate tasks to them because she was so worried that they might make mistakes. Even though she worked 15-hour days, her boss asked her to resign at the end of the 3-month probationary period because she had accomplished less than her predecessor, who had worked only 20 hours a week. She was disillusioned by the experience, and she sought therapy with a sense that this was just one in a series of events in which she had gotten herself into trouble by losing sight of the forest for the trees.

Defining Symptoms of Obsessive-Compulsive Personality Disorder

Intense need for order, perfection, and control, as shown by the presence of at least four of the following from early adulthood across many contexts:

- Preoccupation with rules, details, and organization to the extent that the point of an activity is lost
- Extreme perfectionism interferes with task completion
- Excessive devotion to work to the exclusion of leisure and friendships

- Inflexibility about morals and values
- Difficulty discarding worthless items
- Reluctance to delegate unless others conform to one's standards
- Miserliness
- Rigidity and stubbornness

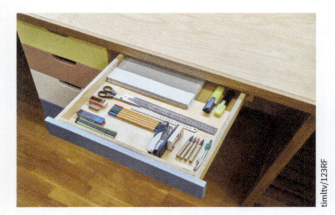

For the person with obsessive-compulsive personality disorder, the overly perfectionistic quest for order may interfere with being productive.

Those with obsessive-compulsive personality disorder have less interpersonal difficulty than do those with other personality disorders. Across studies, this personality disorder is not tied to major problems in friendships, family relationships, or romantic relationships, regardless of whether their own report or another's report is used to evaluate those relationships (Wilson, Stroud, & Durbin, 2017).

Obsessive-compulsive personality disorder is distinct from obsessive-compulsive disorder, despite the similarity in names. The personality disorder does not include the obsessions and compulsions that define the latter.

Nonetheless, there is some evidence for considering OCPD as related to OCD (Stein, Kogan, et al., 2016). People with OCD and their family members show high rates of OCPD (Bienvenu, Samuels, et al., 2012). Both conditions are related to cognitive inflexibility and to problems in tolerating uncertainty (Stein et al., 2016; Wheaton & Ward, 2020). Overall, though, relatively little is known about the risk factors for obsessive-compulsive personality disorder.

Quick Summary

People with schizotypal personality disorder are eccentric in their thoughts and behavior. Biological and cognitive studies indicate that schizotypal personality disorder and schizophrenia are related.

The key features of APD include violation of rules and a disregard for others' feeling and social norms. Psychopathy is related to antisocial personality disorder but is not defined in the DSM. Psychopathy criteria focus more on internal experiences (such as a lack of anxiety or empathy) than the antisocial personality disorder criteria do. BPD is defined by intense emotionality, impulsivity, and unstable sense of identity. Narcissistic personality disorder is characterized by highly inflated self-esteem and a focus on gaining admiration.

A harsh family environment and poverty play a role in the development of APD, and these social influences may be magnified when genetic risk for the disorder is present. Psychopathy is related to blunted responses to threat, lack of empathy, and poor executive control.

Consistent with their emotionality and impulsivity, people with BPD demonstrate diminished connectivity of the brain regions involved in emotionality and those involved in regulation. Linehan's model integrates the high rates of parental invalidation reported by people with BPD with a biologically based vulnerability to emotional dysregulation.

Across studies, those with narcissistic personality disorder report that their parents were overly indulgent; this is difficult to reconcile with the high correlation of abuse or neglect with narcissistic personality disorder. Many, but not all, of those with narcissistic personality disorder show fragile self-esteem.

People with avoidant personality disorder are timid and often feel inadequate. Avoidant personality disorder may be genetically related to social anxiety disorder.

Those with obsessive-compulsive personality disorder are intensely focused on the details of maintaining order, perfection, and control. This disorder is less related to functional impairment than are other personality disorders.

15.4 Check Your Knowledge

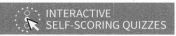
INTERACTIVE
SELF-SCORING QUIZZES

(Answers are at the end of the chapter.)
Answer the following questions.

1. Which personality disorder is most closely related to schizophrenia in family history studies?
2. Which personality disorder is most common in clinical settings?
3. Which two of the cluster B personality disorders are strongly related to impulsivity?
4. Which personality disorder is most common in prison settings?

You are the director of human resources for a large corporation. You are asked to review a set of situations in which employees had interpersonal or task-focused problems that were severe and persistent enough to raise concerns in the workplace. Name the most likely personality disorder for each of the following.

5. Mariana refuses to meet with customers. It turns out that she has called in sick the last three times her boss scheduled an appointment with her and her colleagues barely know her name. When asked, she says that meeting with any of these people makes her feel horribly nervous about potential rejection of her ideas. She asks for a position that would involve little social contact.
6. Sheila has had three subordinate employees request transfers from their department. They each stated that Sheila was too controlling, picked on small mistakes, and would not listen to new ideas for solving problems. At the interview, Sheila brought in a 15-page chart of the goals she would like to execute for the company. Despite having an inordinate number of goals, she failed to complete a single project during her first year with the company.
7. Police contact you to let you know that they have arrested Sam, one of your employees. Sam was caught at a bank trying to cash a $10,000 company check on which he had forged the signature. You learn that Sam had previously defrauded three other companies. When you meet with Sam, he does not seem the least bit sorry.

Treatment of Personality Disorders

Many people with personality disorders enter treatment for a condition other than their personality disorder. For example, a person with antisocial personality disorder might seek treatment for substance abuse, and a patient with dependent personality disorder might seek help for depression. Clinicians are encouraged to consider whether personality disorders are present because their presence predicts slower improvement in psychotherapy. Often, addressing those conditions can lead to improvements in personality function as well.

Psychotherapy is the treatment of choice for personality disorders. You might think that it would be impossible to change personality, but personality traits do change in psychotherapy. Across 207 studies, psychotherapy and other interventions led to significant changes in personality traits such as neuroticism and often did so within 6 weeks (Roberts, Luo, et al., 2017). Some treatment programs are particularly relevant to personality concerns. For example, programs designed to enhance emotion regulation skills are relevant for addressing neuroticism (Sauer-Zavala, Fournier, et al., 2021). Indeed, even with full-blown personality disorders, dozens of studies show that psychotherapy provides small but positive effects compared with treatment as usual (Budge, Moore, et al., 2013).

People with severe personality disorders might attend weekly psychotherapy sessions, or they might attend a day treatment program that offers psychotherapy in both group and individual formats for several hours per day. The length of treatment programs varies, but some day treatment programs last for months, and individual therapy sometimes lasts for a year or longer.

Psychotherapy is often supplemented with medications to treat the accompanying depression, anxiety, or cognitive symptoms that can be present (Marin, Foster, & Goodman, 2022). For example, antidepressants are used to quell some of the depressive symptoms that accompany personality disorders (Bhaduri, Thompson, & Chanen, 2019). Antipsychotic drugs (e.g., risperidone, trade name Risperdal) can help address some of the symptoms of schizotypal personality disorder (Raine, 2006). Medications, though, have not been shown to address the full spectrum of personality disorder symptoms (Marin, Foster, & Goodman, 2022).

Psychodynamic theory suggests that childhood problems are at the root of personality disorders, and so the aim of psychodynamic therapy is to help patients reconsider those early experiences, become more aware of how those experiences drive their current behaviors, and then reconsider their beliefs and responses to those early events. For example, a psychodynamic therapist might guide a man with obsessive-compulsive personality disorder to realize that his need to be perfect is based on a childhood quest to win his parents' love and that this quest does not need be carried into adulthood—that others will love him even with his imperfections.

Cognitive theory suggests that negative cognitive beliefs, such as those shown in Table 15.5, are at the heart of the personality disorders (Beck & Freeman, 1990). The aim of cognitive therapy, then, is to help a person become more aware of those beliefs and then to challenge maladaptive cognitions. For example, cognitive therapy for a perfectionistic person

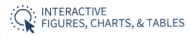
INTERACTIVE FIGURES, CHARTS, & TABLES

TABLE 15.5   **Examples of Maladaptive Cognitions Hypothesized to Be Associated with Each Personality Disorder**

Personality Disorder	Maladaptive Cognitions
Avoidant	If people get to know the real me, they will reject me.
Obsessive-compulsive	If things get disorganized, horrible mistakes will happen.
Antisocial	People ask for exploitation—they let down their guard.
Narcissistic	I am better than others, and people who can't understand that don't deserve my time.

Source: Adapted from Beck and Freeman (1990).

with obsessive-compulsive personality disorder entails first persuading the patient to accept the essence of the cognitive model—that feelings and behaviors are primarily a function of thoughts. Biases in thinking are explored, such as when the patient concludes that he or she cannot do anything right based on a trivial failure. The therapist also looks for dysfunctional assumptions or schemas that might underlie the person's thoughts and feelings—for example, the belief that it is critical for every decision to be correct.

Beyond challenging cognitions, cognitive behavioral therapy often includes other behavioral techniques. Cognitive behavioral treatment for avoidant personality disorder, for example, might involve helping a person challenge their negative beliefs about social interactions by teaching behavioral strategies for dealing with difficult social situations and by exposure treatment, in which the person gradually learns to take part in feared social situations. There is some evidence that this approach can be more helpful than psychodynamic therapy for those with avoidant personality disorder (Emmelkamp, Benner, et al., 2006).

Less is known about the treatment of specific personality disorders because treatment outcome studies often focus on a broad range of different personality disorders (c.f. Volkert, Haschild, & Taubner, 2019), with the exception of borderline personality disorder, where at least 75 randomized controlled trials have provided a strong evidence base concerning psychological treatments that work (Storebø, Stoffers-Winterling, et al., 2020). Here, then, we focus on treatments for borderline personality disorders.

People with BPD seek treatment more often than those with mood, anxiety, or substance use disorders, but the treatment process can be challenging, because they tend to show their interpersonal problems in the therapeutic relationship as much as they do in other relationships. Because these clients find it inordinately hard to trust others, therapists find it challenging to develop and maintain the therapeutic relationship. Patients alternately idealize and vilify the therapist, demanding special attention and consideration at certain times—such as therapy sessions at odd hours and countless phone calls during crisis periods—and refusing to keep appointments at other times.

Suicide is always a serious risk, but it is often difficult for the therapist to judge whether a frantic phone call at 2:00 a.m. from a BPD patient is a call for help or a manipulative gesture designed to test how special the patient is to the therapist. As in the case of Kiera Van Gelder (see Read More About It 15.1), hospitalization is sometimes needed to protect against the threat of suicide. Because of the risk of dangerous behavior and the challenges of managing the therapeutic relationship, therapists working with BPD clients often feel overwhelmed, inadequate, and at the same time overly involved (Colli, Tanzilli, et al., 2014). To combat their stress as they cope with the challenges of helping BPD clients, many therapists regularly consult with another therapist for advice and support.

Two forms of treatment have been particularly well-studied: many randomized controlled trials indicate that dialectical behavior therapy (DBT) and mentalization-based therapy are both more efficacious than control treatments such as treatment as usual Both types of treatment reduce borderline symptoms, suicidality, and the risk of self-harm, and the benefits of both types of treatment have been sustained at follow-up assessments (Bateman, Constantinou, et al., 2021; Gillespie, Murphy, & Joyce, 2022). An additional form of psychodynamic therapy, called **transference-focused therapy**, has shown positive effects in a smaller number of randomized controlled trials (Clarkin et al., 2007; Doering, Hörz, et al., 2010). Although findings clearly show that treatment can help relieve borderline personality disorder symptoms, many researchers are working to improve the treatments because effects have tended to be small to moderate, drop-out rates are high, longer-term outcomes are varied when compared to control groups, and there is some evidence of publication bias in the long-term follow-up findings—that is, it appears that positive results are more likely to have been published than negative results (Cristea, Gentili, et al., 2017; Gillespie, Murphy, & Joyce, 2022; Iliakis, Ilagan, & Choi-Kain, 2021).

Both therapies include techniques to help understand and reduce self-destructive and dangerous behaviors. Therapists examine the triggers for self-harm and other risky behaviors, and they provide the client with tools to manage and reduce those impulses.

Mentalization-based therapy integrates psychodynamic and cognitive behavioral approaches (Bateman & Fonagy, 2016). Because many people with borderline personality disorder tend to respond quickly and impulsively to emotions, **mentalization-based therapy** focuses on helping clients to be more reflective about their own feelings and those of other people, to avoid acting automatically without thinking when emotions or interpersonal stressors occur. Therapists model a reflective approach to considering mental states, and they teach skills to help the client be more contemplative about their own and other's mental states.

Dialectical behavior therapy (DBT) combines empathy and acceptance with cognitive behavioral problem solving, emotion-regulation techniques, and social skills training (Linehan, 1987). The concept of dialectics refers to the constant tension between any phenomenon (e.g., an idea or event, called the *thesis*) and its opposite (the *antithesis*), which is resolved by creating a new phenomenon (the *synthesis*). We discuss the dialectical tension between accepting clients as they are and helping them change in **Focus on Discovery 15.2.**

DBT therapists use group and individual therapy sessions to employ specific cognitive behavioral techniques in four stages. In the first stage, therapy addresses dangerously impulsive behaviors such as suicidal actions. In the second stage, the focus is on modulating the extreme emotionality and coaching the client to tolerate emotional distress. In this stage, clients are taught to mindfully notice their emotions in a nonjudgmental manner, without rushing into impulsive actions. Stage three focuses on improving relationships and self-esteem. Stage four is designed to promote connectedness and happiness. Throughout, clients learn more effective and socially acceptable ways of handling their day-to-day problems.

Focus on Discovery 15.2

Drawing From Personal Experience to Promote Acceptance and Change

Marsha Linehan developed dialectical behavior therapy to treat BPD, and it is considered the best validated approach. In a brave move, Linehan decided to speak publicly about her own experiences of BPD (Carey, 2011). Hospitalized at age 17 for her severe suicidality, she found ways to injure herself even when the staff

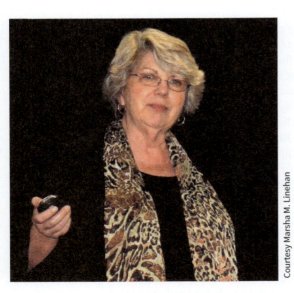

Courtesy Marsha M. Linehan

Marsha Linehan created dialectical behavior therapy, which combines cognitive behavior therapy with acceptance.

confined her to a seclusion chamber—left alone with no objects, she banged her head against the wall and floor. She remained hospitalized for 26 months. Failed treatments continued for several years, until she found a way out of the struggles on her own—through radical acceptance. She earned a Ph.D. in clinical psychology, and she drew on her own personal experiences to help others, in the process becoming one of the most productive researchers in the field of clinical psychology.

Linehan (1987) argues that a therapist must work for change, while at the same time accepting the real possibility that no changes are going to occur. Linehan's reasoning is that people with BPD are so sensitive to rejection and criticism that even gentle encouragement to behave or think differently can be misinterpreted as a serious rebuke, leading to extreme emotional reactions. When this happens, the therapist, who may have been revered a moment earlier, is suddenly vilified. Thus, while observing limits—"I would be very sad if you killed yourself, so I hope very much that you won't"—the therapist must convey to the patient that he or she is fully accepted. This is hard to do if the patient is threatening suicide, showing uncontrolled anger, or railing against imagined rebukes from the therapist. Completely accepting the patient does not mean approving of everything the patient does; rather, it means that the therapist must accept the situation for what it is.

Linehan's approach emphasizes that clients, too, must accept who they are and what they have been through. Clients are asked to accept that their childhood is now unchangeable, that their behaviors might have caused relationships to end, and that they feel emotions more intensely than others do. This approach, it is hoped, will provide a basis for understanding the self and promoting growth.

15.5 Check Your Knowledge

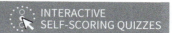
INTERACTIVE
SELF-SCORING QUIZZES

(Answers are at the end of the chapter.)
Answer the following questions.

1. What class of medication is used in the treatment of schizotypal personality disorder?
2. What types of treatments have been shown to be more helpful than treatment as usual for borderline personality disorder?
3. What are the four stages of treatment in DBT?

True or false?
4. Personality dimensions cannot be changed.

Summary

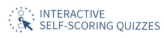
INTERACTIVE
SELF-SCORING QUIZZES

Chapter 15 Practice Quiz

- Personality disorders are defined as pervasive and persistent patterns of behavior and inner experience that disrupt functioning.
- DSM-5-TR includes 10 personality disorders, divided into three clusters.
- The odd/eccentric cluster include paranoid personality disorder, schizoid personality disorder, and schizotypal personality disorder.
- The dramatic/erratic cluster includes histrionic, antisocial, borderline, and narcissistic personality disorders.
- The anxious/fearful cluster includes avoidant personality disorder, obsessive-compulsive personality disorder, and dependent personality disorder.
- The alternative DSM-5-TR approach was designed to address several problems with the traditional diagnostic system: the lack of stability of diagnoses over time, the high levels of comorbidity, and the arbitrary thresholds for defining personality disorders. The alternative model includes six personality disorders, along with dimensional scoring of personality domain traits and facets.
- Personality disorders are usually comorbid with other disorders, such as depression and anxiety disorders, and they predict poorer outcomes for these disorders.
- Most personality disorders appear at least moderately heritable when careful research methods are used. High rates of child abuse/neglect, aversive parental behavior, and lack of parental affection are observed across many of the personality disorders, but twin studies indicate that early adversity does not predict much variance in personality disorders after genetic vulnerability is accounted for.

Clinical Description and Causes of Specific Personality Disorders

- The major symptom of schizotypal personality disorder is unusual thinking and behavior.
- Genetic, neurobiological, and cognitive research supports the idea that schizotypal personality disorder is related to schizophrenia.

- Antisocial personality disorder and psychopathy overlap a great deal but are not equivalent. The assessment of psychopathy emphasizes emotional deficits more than the criteria for antisocial personality disorder do.
- Psychopathy and antisocial behavior are related to family environment and poverty, and genes may amplify the effects of these social variables.
- Psychopathy is related to lack of response to threat, lack of responsivity to other people's pain, and poor executive control.
- The major symptom of borderline personality disorder (BPD) is unstable, highly changeable emotion and behavior.
- BPD is related to diminished connectivity of neural regions involved in emotion and those involved in regulation.
- Linehan's cognitive behavioral theory of BPD proposes an interaction between emotional dysregulation and an invalidating family environment.
- The major symptom of narcissistic personality disorder is inflated self-esteem.
- Theories about the causes of narcissism focus on overindulgent parenting and fragile self-esteem.
- The major symptom of avoidant personality disorder is fear of rejection or criticism.
- Avoidant personality disorder might be a more severe variant of social anxiety disorder.
- The major symptom of obsessive-compulsive personality disorder is a perfectionistic, detail-oriented style.

Treatment of Personality Disorders

- Psychodynamic and cognitive behavioral treatments are used for personality disorders. Pharmacological treatments can help address comorbid conditions, such as depression, and can help address the cognitive symptoms of schizotypal personality disorder.
- Cognitive behavioral treatment and psychodynamic treatment are often used to treat personality disorder. Relatively little

research has been conducted regarding the treatment of some specific personality disorders.

- Cognitive behavioral treatment for avoidant personality disorder is similar to the treatment of social anxiety disorder.

- Dialectical behavior therapy and mentalization-based therapy have been well validated as treatments for BPD.

Answers to Check Your Knowledge Questions

15.1　1. Most personality disorders can be reliably assessed when structured diagnostic interviews are used; inter-rater reliability correlations have been .79 or higher, except in the case of schizoid personality disorder, where agreement is more modest. Inter-rater reliability when clinicians use unstructured interviews to assess personality disorders is not adequate; 2. Personality disorders are not as stable as the definition in DSM-5-TR implies, they are highly comorbid with each other, and the thresholds for defining personality disorders are arbitrary.

15.2　1. six personality disorders instead of 10 and the use of personality trait domains and facets (dimensional scores).

15.3　1. Heritability estimates for the six specific personality disorders range from 0.64 to 0.78; 2. Children who experienced abuse or neglect were 18 times more likely than those with no history of abuse or neglect to develop narcissistic personality disorder, more than 7 times more likely to develop borderline personality

disorder, and about 5 times more likely to develop antisocial personality disorder. Parental neglect also increased the risk of avoidant personality disorder. All six personality disorders were related to aversive or unaffectionate parental styles; 3. Trauma explains very little of whether people will develop a personality disorder once genetic vulnerability is accounted for.

15.4　1. schizotypal personality disorder; 2. borderline personality disorder; 3. antisocial personality disorder and borderline personality disorder; 4. antisocial personality disorder; 5. avoidant personality disorder; 6. obsessive-compulsive personality disorder; 7. antisocial personality disorder.

15.5　1. antipsychotic medication; 2. dialectical behavior therapy (DBT) and mentalization-based therapy; 3. stage 1: address dangerous behaviors; stage 2: teach emotion regulation skills such as mindfulness; stage 3: improve relationships and self-esteem; stage 4: promote connectedness and happiness; 4. False.

Key Terms

antisocial personality disorder (APD)　441
avoidant personality disorder　449
borderline personality disorder (BPD)　444
dependent personality disorder　431
dialectical behavior therapy (DBT)　454
histrionic personality disorder　431
mentalization-based therapy　453

narcissistic personality disorder　446
obsessive-compulsive personality disorder　449
paranoid personality disorder　431
personality disorders　429
personality trait domains　435
personality trait facets　435

psychopathy　441
schizoid personality disorder　431
schizotypal personality disorder　440
transference-focused therapy　453
triarchic model of psychopathy　442

Legal and Ethical Issues

Amendment I Congress shall make no law respecting an establishment of religion, or prohibiting the free exercise thereof; or abridging the freedom of speech, or of the press; or the right of the people peaceably to assemble, and to petition the Government for a redress of grievances.

Amendment IV The right of the people to be secure in their persons, houses, papers, and effects, against unreasonable searches and seizures, shall not be violated... .

Amendment V No person ... shall be compelled in any criminal case to be a witness against himself, nor be deprived of life, liberty, or property, without due process of law... .

Amendment VI In all criminal prosecutions, the accused shall enjoy the right to a speedy and public trial ... to be confronted with the witnesses against him; to have compulsory process for obtaining witnesses in his favor, and to have the Assistance of Counsel for his defense.

Amendment VIII Excessive bail shall not be required, nor excessive fines imposed, nor cruel and unusual punishment inflicted.

Amendment XIII ... Neither slavery nor involuntary servitude, except as a punishment for crime whereof the party shall have been duly convicted, shall exist within the United States, or any place subject to their jurisdiction... .

Amendment XIV ... No State shall ... deprive any person of life, liberty, or property, without due process of law; nor deny to any person within its jurisdiction the equal protection of the laws.

Amendment XV ... The right of citizens of the United States to vote shall not be denied or abridged by the United States or by any State on account of race, color, or previous condition of servitude.

Jeremy

Jeremy had been hearing voices for several days. Unable to drown them out with music or talking, he became more and more troubled. The voices were telling him that he was the one chosen by God to rid the world of evil. Jeremy went to the emergency room of the local hospital seeking relief. Instead of being admitted, Jeremy was given a prescription for Haldol and sent on his way. Two days later, Jeremy took a loaded gun into a busy train station and began shooting. He killed two people and injured four others. When he was arrested, Jeremy told the police he was answering to God. His speaking was disorganized and hard to follow, and he expressed a number of paranoid beliefs.

Jeremy was found competent to stand trial because he understood that he was charged with murder and he was able to help his attorney with his defense. At trial, Jeremy entered a plea of "not guilty by reason of insanity." His defense lawyer arranged for Jeremy to be evaluated by a psychologist. The psychologist concluded that Jeremy had schizophrenia and that at the time of the crime he was unable to discern right from wrong (he thought his behavior was the right thing to do since God was directing him) and unable to conform his behavior to the requirements of the law. The prosecution did not dispute these findings, and the case was settled before going to trial. Jeremy was committed to the local forensic hospital for an indeterminate period of time. He was to remain there until he was no longer dangerous and mentally ill. Periodic evaluations would be conducted to see if Jeremy could be transferred to a less secure hospital.

After 7 years in the hospital, Jeremy had done very well. He took his prescribed medication (Zyprexa), was never in a physical altercation with other people, participated in individual and group therapy, worked in the hospital machine shop, and served as a team leader for the unit where he lived. Jeremy felt horribly remorseful for the crimes he had committed, and he recognized that he had schizophrenia that would require treatment for the rest of his life. The members of the treatment team on the unit all agreed that Jeremy was no longer dangerous and that his schizophrenia was under control with the medication. They recommended that he be transferred to a less secure psychiatric hospital. Jeremy's attorney presented the case before a judge in the courtroom that was part of the hospital. The attorneys for the state objected to Jeremy's release, arguing that Jeremy could stop taking his medications and become violent again. The judge agreed that release was premature at this time and ordered that Jeremy remain in the forensic hospital for another year before being evaluated again.

These eloquent statements describe and protect some of the rights of U.S. citizens and others residing in the United States. We open our final chapter with them because the legal and mental health systems collaborate continually, although often subtly, to deny a substantial proportion of the U.S. population their basic civil rights. With the best of intentions, judges, legislatures, legal associations, and professional mental health groups have worked over the years to balance the need to protect individual rights guaranteed in the Constitution (i.e., the rights of a person with a psychological disorder) with the need to protect society from the actions of people who have a psychological disorder and are considered dangerous to themselves or to others. This balance is not always easy to achieve, as we shall see.

In this chapter, we look in depth at the legal procedures that are involved in criminal and civil commitment. Then we turn to an examination of some important ethical issues relating to treatment and research.

Criminal Commitment

People with a psychological disorder who have broken the law or who are alleged to have done so are subject to **criminal commitment**, a procedure that confines a person in a mental or forensic hospital (see **Focus on Discovery 1.1** for a discussion of types of hospitals) either for determination of competency to stand trial or after acquittal by reason of insanity, as in the **Clinical Case of Jeremy**.

What is insanity? Insanity is a legal concept, not a psychological one. As such, it is defined by courts. In today's courts, judges and lawyers call on psychiatrists and clinical psychologists for assistance in determining whether a person meets the legal criteria for insanity. Although the insanity defense was developed to protect people's rights, in practice it often results in a greater denial of liberties than people would otherwise experience.

The Insanity Defense

The **insanity defense** is the legal argument that a defendant should not be held responsible for an illegal act if it is attributable to a psychological disorder or intellectual disability that interferes with rationality or that results from some other excusing circumstance, such as not knowing right from wrong. A staggering amount of material has been written on the insanity defense, even though it is pleaded in less than 1% of all cases that reach trial, and even when pleaded it is rarely successful (Steadman, 1979; Steadman, McGreevy, et al., 1993).

Because an insanity defense is based on the accused's mental condition at the time the crime was committed, a retrospective, often speculative, judgment is required on the part of attorneys, judges, jurors, and mental health professionals. And disagreement between defense and prosecution psychiatrists and psychologists is the rule.

It is critically important to understand that psychological disorders and crime do not go hand in hand. That is, a person can have a diagnosis of a psychological disorder and still be held fully responsible for a crime. For example, David Tarloff, a New York man with a confirmed diagnosis of schizophrenia, killed his psychologist in 2008; he was found guilty of this crime in 2014 and sentenced to life in prison without parole (his insanity defense was unsuccessful). Furthermore, someone who has no psychological disorder at all can commit the most heinous or bizarre crime, despite our tendency to think that someone must have been "crazy" to commit such an act.

Landmark Cases and Laws   Several court rulings and established principles bear on the problems of legal responsibility and psychological disorders. **Table 16.1** summarizes these rulings and principles (for more on these issues, see Frederick, Mrad, & DeMier, 2007). Even though some of these cases are over a century old, they still form the basis for insanity defenses today. We describe some of these in more detail next.

TABLE 16.1	**Landmark Cases and Laws Regarding the Insanity Defense** INTERACTIVE FIGURES, CHARTS, & TABLES
Irresistible impulse (1834)	A pathological impulse or drive that the person could not control compelled that person to commit a criminal act.
M'Naghten rule (1843)	The person did not know the nature and quality of the criminal act in which he or she engaged, or, if the person did know it, the person did not know what he or she was doing was wrong.
Durham test (1954)	The person's criminal act is the product of mental disease or defect.
American Law Institute guidelines (1962)	1. The person's criminal act is a result of "mental disease or defect" that results in the person's not appreciating the wrongfulness of the act or in the person's inability to behave according to the law (combination of M'Naghten rule and irresistible impulse).
	2. "[T]he terms 'mental disease or defect' do not include an abnormality manifested only by repeated criminal or otherwise antisocial conduct" (American Law Institute, 1962).
Insanity Defense Reform Act (1984)	1. The person's criminal act is a result of severe mental illness or defect that prevents the person from understanding the nature of his or her crime.
	2. The burden of proof is shifted from the prosecution to the defense. The defense must prove that the person is insane.
	3. The person is released from the forensic or prison hospital only after being judged to be no longer dangerous and to have recovered from mental illness. This could be longer than he or she would have been imprisoned if convicted.

Irresistible Impulse   The concept of **irresistible impulse** was formulated in 1834 in a case in Ohio. According to this concept, if a pathological impulse or uncontrollable drive compelled the person to commit the criminal act, an insanity defense is legitimate. The irresistible-impulse test was confirmed in two subsequent court cases: *Parsons v. State* and *Davis v. United States.*[1]

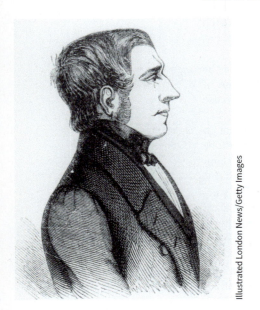

Daniel M'Naghten had a mental disorder when he tried to kill the British prime minister. His case helped to establish a legal definition for the insanity defense.

Illustrated London News/Getty Images

The M'Naghten Rule   The **M'Naghten rule** was formulated in the aftermath of a murder trial in England in 1843. The defendant, Daniel M'Naghten, had set out to kill the British prime minister, Sir Robert Peel, but had mistaken Peel's secretary for Peel. M'Naghten claimed that he had been instructed to kill Lord Peel by the "voice of God." The judges ruled that to establish a defense of insanity, it must be clearly proved that, at the time of the committing of the act, the party accused was laboring under such a defect of reason, from disease of the mind, as not to know the nature and quality of the act he was doing; or if he did know it, that he did not know what he was doing was wrong.

American Law Institute Guidelines   In 1962, the American Law Institute (ALI) proposed its own guidelines, which were intended to be more specific and informative to lay jurors than were other tests. The **American Law Institute guidelines**, sometimes referred to as the "model penal code test," state the following (American Law Institute, 1962, p. 66):

1. A person is not responsible for criminal conduct if at the time of such conduct as a result of mental disease or defect he lacks substantial capacity either to appreciate the criminality (wrongfulness) of his conduct or conform his conduct to the requirements of law.

2. As used in the article, the terms "mental disease or defect" do not include an abnormality manifested only by repeated criminal or otherwise antisocial conduct.

The first ALI guideline combines the M'Naghten rule and the concept of irresistible impulse. The phrase "substantial capacity" in the first guideline is designed to limit an insanity defense to people with the most serious psychological disorders. The second guideline concerns those who are repeatedly in trouble with the law; repetitive criminal behavior and psychopathy are not evidence for insanity.

Insanity Defense Reform Act   In a highly publicized trial in March 1981, John Hinckley Jr. was found not guilty by reason of insanity (NGRI) for his assassination attempt against President Ronald Reagan. After the verdict, the court received a flood of mail from citizens outraged that a would-be assassin of a U.S. president had not been held criminally responsible and had "only" been committed to an indefinite stay in a mental hospital. The outrage reflected the public's misperceptions about the insanity defense. People often believe that a person is "getting away" with a crime when found not guilty by reason of insanity and that he or she will be released from the hospital in short order. In reality, many people who are committed to a mental hospital stay there longer than they would have stayed in prison, had they been given a sentence (as vividly illustrated in the **Clinical Case of Michael Jones**). With respect to Hinckley, he was committed to St. Elizabeth's Hospital, a public mental hospital in Washington, D.C., for over three decades. Although he could have been released whenever his mental health was deemed adequate and he was no longer considered dangerous, this did not happen until 2016, when he was released and allowed to live with his mother with many conditions, including mandated appointments with treatment providers, restrictions on travel, and a requirement that he carry a GPS-enabled mobile phone. In 2022, at age 67, he was allowed to live independently with no restrictions.

---

[1]*Parsons v. State*, 2 So. 854, 866–67 (Ala.1887); *Davis v. United States*, 165 U.S. 373, 378 (1897).

Following the *Hinckley* verdict, the political pressure to "get tough" on criminals pushed Congress to enact the Insanity Defense Reform Act in October 1984, addressing the insanity defense for the first time at the federal level. This law, which has been adopted in all federal courts, contains several provisions designed to make it more difficult to enter an insanity plea.

- It eliminated the irresistible-impulse component of the ALI rules.

- It changed the ALI's "lacks substantial capacity ... to appreciate" to "unable to appreciate," thus making the criterion for impaired judgment more stringent.

- It stipulated that the mental disease or defect must be "severe." Mitigating circumstances such as extreme passion or "temporary insanity" do not count.

- It shifted the burden of proof from the prosecution to the defense. Instead of the prosecution's having to prove that the person was sane beyond a reasonable doubt at the time of the crime (the most stringent criterion, consistent with the constitutional requirement that people are considered innocent until proven guilty), the defense must prove that the defendant was not sane and must do so with "clear and convincing evidence" (a less stringent but still demanding standard of proof). **Table 16.2** shows the different standards of proof used in U.S. courts.

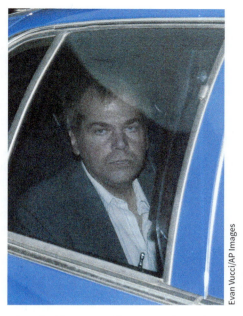

Evan Vucci/AP Images

John Hinckley Jr., President Reagan's assailant, was found not guilty by reason of insanity.

TABLE 16.2   Standards of Proof

Standard	Certainty Needed to Convict (%)
Beyond a reasonable doubt	95
Clear and convincing evidence	75
Preponderance of the evidence	51

Clinical Case

Michael Jones

To illustrate the predicament that a person can get into by raising insanity as a reason for a criminal act, we consider an infamous Supreme Court case.[1]

Michael Jones was arrested, unarmed, on September 19, 1975, for attempting to steal a jacket from a department store in Washington, DC. He was charged the next day with attempted petty larceny, a misdemeanor punishable by a maximum prison sentence of 1 year. The court ordered that he be committed to St. Elizabeth's Hospital for a determination of his competency to stand trial.

On March 2, 1976, almost 6 months after the alleged crime, a hospital psychologist reported to the court that Jones was competent to stand trial, even though he had schizophrenia. The psychologist also reported that the alleged crime resulted from his schizophrenia. This comment is noteworthy because the psychologist was not asked to offer an opinion on Jones's state of mind during the crime, only on whether Jones was competent to stand trial. Jones then pleaded not guilty by reason of insanity (NGRI). Ten days later, on March 12, the court found him NGRI and formally committed him to St. Elizabeth's Hospital for treatment of his schizophrenia.

On May 25, 1976, a customary 50-day hearing was held to determine whether Jones should remain in the hospital any longer. A psychologist from the hospital testified that Jones still suffered from schizophrenia and was a danger to himself and to others. A second hearing was held on February 22, 1977, 17 months after Jones's commitment to St. Elizabeth's, for determination of competency. The defendant demanded release since he had already been hospitalized longer than the 1-year maximum sentence he would have served had he been found guilty of the theft of the jacket. The court denied the request and returned him to St. Elizabeth's.

Ultimately, in November 1982, more than 7 years after he was first hospitalized, Jones's appeal to the Supreme Court was heard. On June 29, 1983, by a 5–4 decision, the Court affirmed the earlier decision: Jones was to remain at St. Elizabeth's. He was finally released from St. Elizabeth's in August 2004, 28 years after the crime.

---

[1] *Jones v. United States*, 463 U.S. 354 (1983).

Current Insanity Pleas

The two insanity pleas most commonly used in state and federal courts in the United States were crafted from the legal definitions and precedents we have reviewed here. In **Focus on Discovery 16.1,** we discuss two cases that illustrate how difficult it can be to mount an insanity defense. With the plea **not guilty by reason of insanity (NGRI),** there is no dispute over whether the person actually committed the crime—both sides agree that the person committed the crime. In legal terms, this is referred to as an *affirmative defense*. However, due to the person's insanity at the time of the crime, the defense attorney argues that the person should not be held responsible for and thus should be acquitted of the crime. A successful NGRI plea means the person is not held responsible for the crime due to their psychological disorder. People acquitted with the NGRI plea are committed indefinitely to a forensic hospital. That is, they will be released from a forensic hospital only if they are deemed no longer dangerous and no longer mentally ill (we discuss the difficulties in making these determinations later in the chapter).

A forensic hospital looks very much like a regular hospital except that the perimeter of the grounds is secured with gates, barbed wire, or an electric fence. Inside the hospital, doors to the different units may be locked, and there may be bars on windows on the lower floors. People do not stay in jail cells, however; they live in either individual or shared rooms. Security professionals are on hand to keep people safe. They typically do not carry weapons of any sort, and they may be dressed in regular clothing rather than uniforms.

Focus on Discovery 16.1

Insanity Versus Psychological Disorder

People charged with crimes rarely enter an insanity plea—by some estimates, less than 1% of all felony cases involve such a plea (Cirincione, Steadman, & McGreevy, 1995). And when such a plea is entered, it is rarely successful.

Here we briefly present two cases that illustrate how difficult the path to a successful insanity defense is (**Focus on Discovery 16.2,** presented later in this chapter, describes an example of an ultimately successful insanity defense). These cases show the obstacles to mounting a successful insanity defense and provide vivid examples of the critical difference between a psychological disorder and insanity. The fact that a person has a psychological disorder does not necessarily mean that the person meets the legal definition of insanity. Indeed, in these two cases the juries believed that the defendants knew right from wrong even though they had a psychological disorder and that they thus did not meet the state's legal definition of insanity.

James Holmes

In the early hours of July 20, 2012, James Holmes entered a movie theater in Aurora, Colorado, during a midnight showing of *The Dark Knight* and opened fire. He killed 12 and injured 70 others.

Three years later, his trial was held. It lasted for over 10 weeks and included hours of testimony from victims as well as from mental health professionals. The defense argued that he was mentally ill at the time of the murders. Two psychiatrists testified for the defense, arguing that he met the legal definition of insanity. The psychiatrists pointed to things he said in over 200 hours of interviews, his notebook showing incoherent and delusional thinking, and his seeking treatment from a psychiatrist prior to the killings. Two psychiatrists for the prosecution argued that he did not meet the legal definition of insanity. They noted that he was able to judge right from wrong and planned the attacks carefully ahead of time, demonstrating that he could control his behavior. In Colorado, the burden of proof rests with the prosecution: It must convince the jury that the accused person was legally sane, defined in Colorado to include both the M'Naghten rule and the irresistible-impulse standard (see Table 16.1), at the time of the crime. The jury was persuaded by the prosecution's arguments; they rejected the insanity defense and instead found him guilty. He was sentenced to prison for life without the possibility of parole.

Eddie Ray Routh

Eddie Ray Routh served in the U.S. Marine Corps during the Iraq and Afghanistan wars, and he was honorably discharged in 2011. He was diagnosed with posttraumatic stress disorder (PTSD) and prescribed antipsychotic medications, even though such medications are not typically used to treat PTSD. Review of his medical records indicated delusions and other psychotic symptoms, suggesting that he had been misdiagnosed. He continued to display psychotic symptoms, including paranoia and delusions of reference (see Chapter 9). In January 2013, he was hospitalized after exhibiting psychotic symptoms while holding his girlfriend at knifepoint. He was transferred to a VA hospital 2 days later, and the VA hospital subsequently discharged him. Less than 2 weeks later, Routh shot and killed former Marine sniper Chris Kyle (portrayed by Bradley Cooper in the film *American Sniper*) and his friend, Chad Littlefield. Kyle had taken Routh out shooting to provide support, as he had been doing for several fellow marines.

At his trial in Texas 2 years later, Routh entered a plea of not guilty by reason of insanity. In Texas, the burden of proof is on the defense to demonstrate that the defendant was legally insane at the time of the crime. The defense team argued that Routh had schizophrenia at the time of the killings, but many of the records of his prior mental health treatment were not presented at the trial. After taking less than 3 hours to deliberate, the jury rejected the insanity defense, finding Routh guilty. He was sentenced to life in prison without the possibility of parole.

The second commonly used insanity plea is **guilty but mentally ill (GBMI)**. Established in 1975, a GBMI plea allows an accused person to be found legally guilty of a crime—thus maximizing the chances of incarceration—but also allows a mental health professional to offer an opinion on how to deal with the convicted person if it is found that they had a psychological disorder when the act was committed. Thus, a person can be held morally and legally responsible for a crime but can then, in theory, be committed to a prison hospital or other facility for treatment rather than to a regular prison for punishment. In reality, however, people judged GBMI are usually put in the general prison population, where they may or may not receive treatment. If the person is still considered to be dangerous or mentally ill after serving the imposed prison sentence, they may be committed to a mental hospital under civil law proceedings.

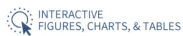

Jeffrey Dahmer was found guilty of murder; his psychological disorder did not impact the verdict.

One of the more famous cases involving something like the GBMI verdict was the 1992 conviction of Jeffrey Dahmer in Milwaukee, Wisconsin, a case which was recently revisited in a 2022 Netflix movie. He had been accused of and had admitted to butchering, cannibalizing, and having sex with the corpses of 15 boys and young men. Dahmer entered a plea of guilty, but then his attorneys argued that his psychological disorder should be considered when it came time to impose a sentence. His sanity was the sole focus of an unusual trial that had jurors listening to conflicting testimony from mental health experts about his state of mind during the killings to which he had confessed. They had to decide whether he had had a mental disease that prevented him from knowing right from wrong or from being able to control his actions. Even though there was no disagreement that he was mentally ill, with a diagnosis of a type of paraphilic disorder (see Chapter 12), Dahmer was deemed sane and therefore legally responsible for the grisly murders. The judge sentenced him to 15 consecutive life terms. Later, another inmate in prison killed him.

Critics of the GBMI verdict argue that it does not benefit criminal defendants with psychological disorders and does not result in appropriate treatment for those convicted (Woodmansee, 1996). Other critics of the GBMI verdict note that the verdict is confusing and even deceiving to jurors. Jurors believe that GBMI is not as "tough" as a guilty verdict, but in reality people receiving a GBMI verdict often spend more time incarcerated than if they had been found guilty (Melville & Naimark, 2002).

Table 16.3 compares the two insanity pleas. Only a few states allow for some or all of the GBMI provisions. Four states—Idaho, Montana, Kansas, and Utah—do not allow any insanity defense, though three of them (Idaho, Montana, and Utah) will consider mental state at the time of the crime in some form or fashion. In 2020, the U.S. Supreme Court ruled that states can determine whether or not they wish to allow any insanity defense.[2] The remaining states have some version of NGRI available. Taking a cue from the Insanity Defense Reform Act, 39 states require the burden of proof to rest with the defendant.

TABLE 16.3	**Comparing NGRI and GBMI**	INTERACTIVE FIGURES, CHARTS, & TABLES
	NGRI	**GBMI**
Responsibility for crime	Not responsible	Responsible
Where committed	Forensic hospital	Prison
Given sentence?	No	Yes
When released	When no longer dangerous and mentally ill	At end of sentence, but could then be committed civilly if dangerous and mentally ill
Treatment given?	Yes	Possibly

[2]*Kahler v. Kansas*, 589 U.S. (2020).

Quick Summary

Insanity is a legal term, not a mental health term. Meeting the legal definition is not necessarily the same thing as having a diagnosable psychological disorder. The insanity defense is the legal argument that a defendant should not be held responsible for an illegal act if it is attributable to a psychological disorder that interferes with rationality or that results from some other excusing circumstance, such as not knowing right from wrong.

The irresistible-impulse standard allowed an accused person to plead insanity if an impulse or drive that the person could not control compelled that person to commit the criminal act. The M'Naghten rule permitted an insanity plea if a person could not distinguish right from wrong at the time of the crime because of the person's psychological disorder. The Durham test specified that a person not be held responsible if the crime was the product of a mental disease or defect. The first part of the American Law Institute guidelines combines the M'Naghten rule and the concept of irresistible impulse. The second part concerns those who are repeatedly in trouble with the law; they are not to be deemed mentally ill only because they keep committing crimes. The Insanity Defense Reform Act shifted the burden of proof from the prosecution to the defense, removed the irresistible-impulse component, changed the wording regarding substantial capacity, and specified that the psychological disorder must be severe. The Jones case illustrates a number of the complexities associated with the insanity defense.

The not guilty by reason of insanity (NGRI) plea asks that an accused person not be held responsible for the crime due to his or her psychological disorder. With the guilty but mentally ill (GBMI) plea, an accused person admits to being legally guilty of a crime but can then, in theory, be committed to a prison hospital or other suitable facility for psychiatric treatment rather than to a regular prison for punishment.

16.1 Check Your Knowledge

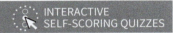 INTERACTIVE SELF-SCORING QUIZZES

(Answers are at the end of the chapter.)
Match each phrase with the correct insanity standard.

1. can't control behavior
2. found guilty
3. doesn't know right from wrong
4. affirmative defense

    a. GBMI

    b. NGRI

    c. irresistible impulse

    d. M'Naghten rule

Competency to Stand Trial

The insanity defense concerns the accused person's mental state at the time of the crime. An important issue that needs to be considered before the defense team decides what kind of defense to adopt is whether the accused person is competent to stand trial at all. In the U.S. criminal justice system, **competency to stand trial** must be decided before it can be determined whether a person is responsible for the crime of which they are accused. It is possible for a person to be judged competent to stand trial and then be judged NGRI. In **Read More About It 16.1**, we discuss a **forensic psychologist**'s efforts to assess a person's competency to stand trial in a complicated case.

The legal standard for being competent to stand trial has not changed since it was articulated by a 1960 U.S. Supreme Court decision: "The test [is] whether [the defendant] has sufficient present ability to consult with his lawyer with a reasonable degree of rational understanding, and whether he has a rational as well as a factual understanding of the proceedings against him."[3]

---

[3]*Dusky v. United States*, 362 U.S. 402 (1960).

Read More About It 16.1

Nobody's Child: A Tragedy, a Trial, and a History of the Insanity Defense

Dr. Susan Vinocour is a forensic psychologist (and former prosecutor) who was asked to evaluate a woman's competency to stand trial. The woman, Dorothy Dunn (not her real name), was charged with killing her grandson. According to the public defender assigned to her case, Dorothy appeared to have something wrong with her; thus, the attorney wanted a psychological evaluation completed for her client. The public defender wanted to know whether Dorothy was competent to stand trial as well as whether she was legally insane at the time of the alleged crime. Vinocour's evaluation of Dorothy is described unflinchingly in the book *Nobody's Child: A Tragedy, a Trial, and a History of the Insanity Defense* (Vinocour, 2020).

The case is not at all straightforward. A toddler is found dead in Dorothy's home. The toddler is Dorothy's grandson, whom she was taking care of after her oldest daughter was committed to a mental hospital. Dorothy was also caring for other children of her own in the home. Dorothy called 911, and the police officers who arrived at the home wrote in their notes that she was behaving strangely and may well have confessed to the crime (though that was an inference). The police continued to question her even after she requested an attorney. The medical examiner's autopsy indicated that the boy had died from blunt force trauma and that he had been dead for 3 days.

The book covers the interviews and psychological assessments that Vinocour conducted with Dorothy to inform her opinion about competency to stand trial. She needed to assess whether Dorothy understood the charges against her and could assist her attorney in her own defense. In the course of reading about Vinocour's evaluation, we learn a great deal about Dorothy: her life history, her cognitive ability, her psychological characteristics, and her emotional state. Vinocour uses all this information to render her opinion on competency and on whether Dorothy met the New York State definition of insanity. As the books vividly describes, this was a complex evaluation and assessment. (We won't reveal the outcomes to avoid spoilers for those who wish to read this terrific book.)

In addition to telling the story of Dorothy, the book offers an illuminating and clear history of the insanity defense. Vinocour describes the precedents across centuries and how these court cases shaped our current legal definitions and practices. In doing so, she covers the stories of several people with psychological disorders who have committed crimes. Some are considered legally insane and some are not. What accounts for the differences from cases to case? Vinocour highlights the tensions between psychological science and the law, which can unfortunately influence the judgment of psychologists, attorneys, judges, and juries. She also discusses the tension in the relationship between forensic psychologist and client. In a clinical practice outside a forensic context, a psychologist seeks to build trust, keep information confidential, and exhibit a great deal of empathy. In a forensic setting, the psychologist adopts a skeptical stance ("Is this person lying?"); records are available to all involved in the legal proceedings; and empathy may be used, but not necessarily to the benefit of the client. If showing empathy helps elicit information, it will be done.

In describing the case of Dorothy Dunn, Vinocour tells a compelling story about the law and psychology, what is like to work in her profession, and what it is like to deal with extremely difficult and tangled issues. She also shines a light on systems that often don't work as intended, whether in mental health, the law, foster care, or family support. It is a gripping tale, told honestly and directly.

The defense attorney, prosecutor, or judge may raise the question of psychological disorder whenever there is reason to believe that the accused person's mental condition might interfere with his or her upcoming trial. If, after examination, the person is deemed unable to participate meaningfully in a trial because of a psychological disorder, the trial is delayed, and the accused person is placed in a hospital with the hope that competence can be restored.

As with the insanity defense, having a psychological disorder does not necessarily mean that a person is incompetent to stand trial; a person with schizophrenia, for example, may still understand legal proceedings and be able to assist in his or her defense. In **Focus on Discovery 16.2**, we consider the case of Andrea Yates, who was found competent to stand trial despite clear agreement that she had a psychological disorder.

Being judged incompetent to stand trial can have severe consequences for a person. Bail is automatically denied, even if it would have been routinely granted had the question of incompetency not been raised. The person is usually kept in a hospital for the pretrial examination. During this period, the accused person is supposed to receive treatment to render them competent to stand trial.[4] In the meantime, the person may lose employment and undergoes the stress of being separated from family and friends and from familiar surroundings for months or even years, perhaps making their psychological state even worse and thus making it all the more difficult to show competency to stand trial.

A 1972 U.S. Supreme Court case, *Jackson v. Indiana*,[5] forced the states to make a speedier determination of incompetency. The case concerned a deaf and mute man with intellectual

---

[4]*United States v. Sherman*, 912 F.2d 907 (7th Cir. 1990).
[5]*Jackson v. Indiana*, 406 U.S. 715 (1972).

Focus on Discovery 16.2

Andrea Yates: An Example of a Successful Insanity Plea

On June 20, 2001, believing that her five children, ranging in age from 6 months to 7 years, were condemned to eternal damnation, 37-year-old Andrea Yates, who lived with her husband and children in Houston, Texas, systematically drowned each child in a bathtub. As recounted on the CNN website:

> when the police reached [the] modest brick home on Beachcomber Lane in suburban Houston, they found Andrea drenched with bathwater, her flowery blouse and brown leather sandals soaking wet. She had turned on the bathroom faucet to fill the porcelain tub and moved aside the shaggy mat to give herself traction for kneeling on the floor. It took a bit of work for her to chase down the last of the children; toward the end, she had a scuffle in the family room, sliding around on wet tile. … She dripped watery footprints from the tub to her bedroom, where she straightened the blankets around the kids in their pajamas once she was done with them. She called 911 and then her husband. "It's time. I finally did it," she said before telling him to come home and hanging up.

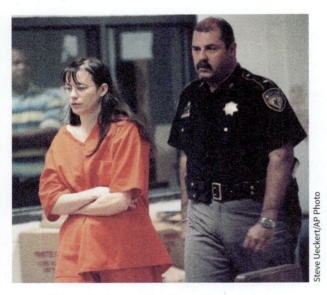

Steve Ueckert/AP Photo

Andrea Yates, who drowned her five children, pled not guilty by reason of insanity (NGRI). Although she was suffering from a psychological disorder, her initial plea was unsuccessful because she was judged capable of knowing right from wrong. After the initial verdict was thrown out, her NGRI plea was successful in the second trial.

The nation was horrified by her actions, and in the months following the murders, information came out about Yates's frequent bouts of depression, especially after giving birth, as well as her several suicide attempts and hospitalizations for severe depression.

Eight months later, her trial was held. The defense argued that she was mentally ill at the time of the murders—and for many periods of time preceding the events—and that she was unable to distinguish right from wrong when she drowned her children. The prosecution argued that she had known right from wrong and therefore should be found guilty. The defense and the prosecution agreed on two points: (1) She had murdered her children, and (2) she was mentally ill at the time of the murder. Where they disagreed was on the crucial question as to whether her psychological disorder entailed not being able to distinguish right from wrong, the M'Naghten standard for criminal responsibility.

No one disagreed that she was severely depressed, probably psychotic, when she killed her five small children. But, as we have seen, a psychological disorder is not the same as legal insanity. Employing the right–wrong principle, the jury deliberated for only 3 hours and 40 minutes on March 12, 2002, before delivering a verdict of guilty. They rejected the defense's contention that Yates could not distinguish right from wrong at the time of the crime. On March 15, the jury decided to spare her life and recommended to the presiding judge that she get life in prison and not be eligible for parole for 40 years.

The trial and the guilty verdict provoked impassioned discussion in the media and among thousands of people. How could the jury *not* have considered Yates insane? If such a person is not insane, who could be judged to be so? Should the M'Naghten rule be dropped from the laws of half the states in the United States? Didn't her phoning 911 to report what she had done prove that she knew she had done something very wrong? Didn't the careful and systematic way she killed her children reflect a mind that, despite her deep depression and delusional thinking, could formulate a complex plan and execute it successfully? Had she received proper treatment from psychiatrists, especially from the one who had recently taken her off the antidepressant medication that had been helping her and then had sent her home without adequate follow-up?

As it turns out, these questions were addressed in the Yates case after all. In January 2005, an appeals court overturned Yates's murder conviction because the jury had heard false testimony from one of the expert witnesses that may have unduly influenced their decision. A new trial was conducted, and on July 26, 2006, after 3 days of deliberation, the new jury found Yates not guilty by reason of insanity (NGRI). She was placed in a maximum-security forensic hospital in Texas. In 2007, she was transferred to a minimum-security hospital in Texas, where she remains today.

disability who was deemed not only incompetent to stand trial but also unlikely ever to become competent. The Court ruled that the length of pretrial confinement must be limited to the time it takes to determine whether treatment during this detainment is likely to render the defendant competent to stand trial. If the defendant is unlikely ever to become competent, the state must, after this period, either institute civil commitment proceedings or release the defendant. Federal and most state laws define more precisely the minimal requirements

Clinical Case

Yolanda

Yolanda, a 51-year-old African American woman, was arrested after taking a box of doughnuts from a local Quick Mart. At the time of her arrest, she claimed that she needed the doughnuts to feed the seven babies growing inside her. She said that Malcolm X was the father of her soon-to-be-born children and that she would soon assume the position of Queen of the New Cities. When asked what the New Cities were, she responded that they were a new world order that would be in place following the alignment of the clouds with the planets Jupiter, Saturn, and Venus. Yolanda's public defender immediately realized that Yolanda was not ready for trial; she asked for a competency hearing and arranged for a psychologist to conduct an evaluation. Yolanda was diagnosed with schizophrenia, and her thought disturbance was thought to be so profound that she was not able to understand that she had been charged with a crime. Furthermore, she was unable to help her attorney prepare a defense. Instead, Yolanda viewed her attorney as a threat to her unborn babies (she was not pregnant) and feared the attorney would keep her from assuming her rightful position as queen. At her competency hearing, the judge declared that Yolanda was not competent to stand trial and ordered that she be committed to the local forensic hospital for a period of 3 months, after which another competency evaluation would be held.

At the hospital, Yolanda was prescribed olanzapine (Zyprexa), and after 2 months, her thinking had become more coherent and organized. One of the unit's psychologists worked with Yolanda, teaching her about the criminal justice system. She helped Yolanda understand what the charge of theft meant and what a defense attorney, prosecuting attorney, judge, and jury were. At the end of 3 months, a different psychologist evaluated Yolanda and recommended that she now be considered competent to stand trial. Yolanda's public defender came to the hospital and met with her to discuss the case. Yolanda was able to help her attorney by telling her about her past hospitalizations and treatment history for schizophrenia. Yolanda realized that she was not pregnant but still held onto beliefs about the New Cities. Still, Yolanda understood that she had stolen the doughnuts and this was why she had to go to court. At her next competency hearing, Yolanda was deemed competent to stand trial. Two months later, she went to court again. This time, she entered a plea of not guilty by reason of insanity (NGRI). After a short trial, the judge accepted her NGRI plea, and she returned to the forensic hospital. The treatment goals were now focused on helping Yolanda recover from schizophrenia, not on restoring her competency to stand trial.

for competency to stand trial. Defendants cannot be committed for determination of competency for a period longer than the maximum possible sentence they face.[6] Most people are deemed competent to stand trial in about 6 months. As illustrated in the **Clinical Case of Yolanda**, one woman with schizophrenia became able to understand the charges against her and assist her attorney in her defense after about 5 months of treatment. People who have intellectual disabilities or a serious psychological disorder (such as schizophrenia) that requires longer hospitalization are least likely to ever be deemed competent to stand trial (Zapf & Roesch, 2011).

Medication has had an impact on the competency issue. On the one hand, if a drug such as Zyprexa temporarily produces a bit of rationality in an otherwise incompetent person, the trial may proceed. The likelihood that the defendant will again become incompetent to stand trial if the drug is withdrawn does not disqualify the person from going to court.[7] On the other hand, the individual rights of the person should protect them against forced medication, because there is no guarantee that such treatment would render the person competent to stand trial, and there is a chance that it might cause harm.

U.S. Supreme Court rulings have held that a criminal defendant generally cannot be forced to take medication in an effort to render them competent to stand trial[8] and that the defendant's civil rights must be protected, even when a drug might restore legal competency to stand trial.[9] The Court has also ruled that forced medication can be used only if alternative treatments have failed, medication is likely to be effective, medication won't interfere with a person's right to defend themselves at trial, and there is an important government interest in trying the defendant for a serious crime.[10]

---

[6]*United States v. DeBellis*, 649 F.2d 1 (1st Cir. 1981); State v. Moore, 467 N.W. 2d 201 (Wis. Ct. App. 1991).

[7]*State v. Hampton*, 218 So.2d 311 (La. 1969); *State v. Stacy*, no. 446 (Crim. App., Knoxville, Tenn., August 4, 1977); *United States v. Hayes*, 589 F.2d 811 (1979).

[8]*Riggins v. Nevada*, 504 U.S. 127 (1992).

[9]*United States v. Waddell*, 687 F. Supp. 208 (1988).

[10]*Sell v. United States*, 539 U.S. (2003).

Even if a person with a psychological disorder is found competent to stand trial, that person may not be able to serve as their own defense attorney. A 2008 U.S. Supreme Court decision[11] held that a judge may deny the right of self-representation if it is clear that the defendant would not receive a fair trial. Focus on Discovery 16.3 discusses the unusual challenge posed by dissociative identity disorder in criminal commitments.

Focus on Discovery 16.3

Dissociative Identity Disorder and the Insanity Defense

Imagine that as you are having a cup of coffee one morning, you hear pounding at the front door. There, you find two police officers. One of them asks, "Are you Jane Smith?" "Yes," you reply. "Well, ma'am, you are under arrest for grand theft and for the murder of John Doe." The officer then reads you your Miranda rights against self-incrimination, handcuffs you, and takes you to the police station, where you are permitted to call your lawyer.

This would be a scary situation for anybody. What is particularly frightening and puzzling to you and your lawyer is that you have absolutely no recollection of having committed the crime. You simply cannot account for the time period when the murder was committed—in fact, your memory is startlingly blank for that entire time. And, as if this were not bizarre enough, the detective shows you a tape in which you are clearly firing a gun at a bank teller during a holdup. "Is that you in the videotape?" asks the detective. You confer with your lawyer, saying that it certainly looks like you, including the clothes, but you are advised not to admit anything one way or the other.

Let's move forward in time now to your trial some months later. Witnesses have come forward and identified you beyond a reasonable doubt. There is no one you know who can testify that you were somewhere other than at the bank on the afternoon of the robbery and the murder. But did you murder the teller in the bank? You can assert honestly to yourself and to the jury that you did not. And yet even you have been persuaded that the person in the videotape is you—and that that person committed the robbery and the murder.

Your lawyer arranged prior to the trial to have you interviewed by a psychiatrist and a clinical psychologist, both well-known experts in forensics. Through extensive questioning, they have determined that you have dissociative identity disorder (DID, formerly called multiple personality disorder) and that the crimes were committed not by you, Jane Smith, but by your rather violent alternate personality (alter), Laura. Indeed, during one of the interviews, Laura emerged and boasted about the crime, even chuckling over the fact that you, Jane, would be imprisoned for it.

Can DID be an excusing condition for a criminal act? Should Jane Smith be held responsible for a crime committed by her alter, Laura?

Elyn Saks, a renowned legal scholar at the University of Southern California Law Center, argued that DID should be regarded as a special case in mental health law and that a new legal principle should be established. Her argument takes issue with legal practice that would hold a person with DID responsible for a crime as long as the personality acting at the time of the crime intended to commit it (Saks, 1997).

What is intriguing about Saks's argument is that she devotes a major portion of it to defining personhood. What is a person? Is a person the body we inhabit? Well, most of the time our sense of who we are as people does not conflict with the bodies we have

come to know as our own or, rather, as us. But in DID there is a discrepancy. The body that committed the crimes at the bank was Jane Smith. But it was her alter, Laura, who committed the crimes. Saks argues that, peculiar as it may sound, the law should be interested in the body only as a container for the person. It is the person who may or may not be blameworthy, not the body. Nearly all the time they are one and the same, but in the case of DID they are not. In a sense, Laura committed the murder by using Jane's body.

Then is Jane blameworthy? The person Jane did not commit the crime; she did not even know about it. For the judge to sentence Jane—or, more specifically, the body in the courtroom who usually goes by that name—would be unjust, argues Saks, for Jane is descriptively innocent. To be sure, sending Jane to prison would punish Laura, for whenever Laura would emerge, she would find herself imprisoned. But what of Jane? Saks concludes that it is unjust to imprison Jane because she is not blameworthy. Rather, we must find her not guilty by reason of dissociative identity disorder and remand her for treatment of the disorder.

DID would not, however, be a justification for a verdict of not guilty by reason of insanity (NGRI) if the alter who did not commit the crime was aware of the other alter's criminal intent and did not do anything to prevent the criminal act. Under these circumstances, argues Saks, the first alter would be complicit in the crime and would therefore be somewhat blameworthy. A comparison Saks draws is to Robert Louis Stevenson's fictional character of Dr. Jekyll and Mr. Hyde. Jekyll made the potion that caused the emergence of Mr. Hyde, his alter, with the foreknowledge that Hyde would do evil. So even though Jekyll was not present when Hyde was in charge, he would nonetheless be blameworthy because of his prior knowledge of what Hyde would do—not to mention that he, Jekyll, had concocted the potion that created his alter, Hyde.

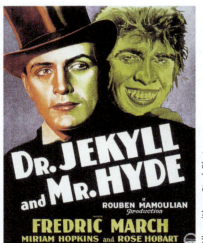

Poster for the classic film about Jekyll and Hyde.

Insanity, Intellectual Disability, and Capital Punishment

As we have just seen, an accused person's mental state may need to be taken into consideration to determine whether he or she is competent to stand trial and/or should be held legally responsible for a criminal act. On very rare occasions, the sanity or mental capacity of a person also becomes an issue after conviction. The question is, must a person who is sentenced to be put to death (i.e., capital punishment) by the state be legally sane at the time of the execution? What if the person has an intellectual disability and thus does not understand what is about to happen to him or her? The **Clinical Cases of Horace Kelly and Scott Panetti** illustrate the difficulties with capital punishment cases that involve a person with a psychological disorder.

The question of the relationship between intellectual disability and capital punishment arose in the case of Daryl Atkins, who in 1996 was convicted in Virginia for a kidnapping and murder and sentenced to death. He had an IQ score of 59, which would likely place him in the category of what is today called *intellectual disability* but was then called *moderate mental*

Clinical Cases

Horace Kelly and Scott Panetti

The question of the relationship between insanity and capital punishment arose in the case of Horace Kelly, a 39-year-old man who had been found guilty of the rape and murder of two women and the slaying of an 11-year-old boy in 1984. Although Kelly's mental state had not been an issue at the time of his trial, his lawyers argued—12 years later and just days before his scheduled execution by lethal injection—that his mental health had deteriorated during his imprisonment on death row to such an extent that one of his defense attorneys referred to him as a "walking vegetable." They made reference to a 1986 U.S. Supreme Court ruling[1] stating that it is a violation of the Eighth Amendment (which prohibits cruel and unusual punishment) for an insane individual to be executed.

Evidence of a psychological disorder during Kelly's imprisonment included psychiatrists' reports of delusions, hallucinations, and inappropriate affect. He was described by fellow inmates and by guards as hoarding his feces and smearing them on the walls of his prison cell. By 1995, after Kelly had spent 10 years on death row, one court-appointed psychiatrist had concluded that Kelly was legally insane. On the other hand, another psychiatrist reported that when Kelly was asked what being executed would mean for him, Kelly had given the rational reply that he would not be able to have a family; he was also able to name two of his victims and beat the psychiatrist in several games of tic-tac-toe. In April 1999, the U.S. Supreme Court concurred with a federal judge's June 1998 decision to stay (delay) Kelly's execution and allow his lawyers to argue, among other things, that he should not be put to death because he was insane. After these arguments, Kelly's execution was permanently stayed.

In 2007, the U.S. Supreme Court overturned another death sentence, this time in the case of Scott Panetti.[2] Panetti shot and killed his estranged wife's parents in 1992. He had been diagnosed with schizophrenia and had been hospitalized numerous times prior to the murders. At his trial, Panetti served as his own attorney (this trial took place prior to *Indiana v. Edwards*, referred to earlier), dressed up as a cowboy (he had narrowly been deemed

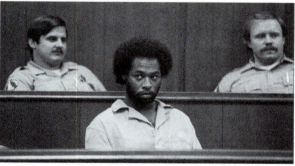

Horace Kelly was sentenced to death, but this sentence was not carried out because the courts ruled that the insane cannot be executed.

competent to stand trial). The court transcripts are filled with his incoherent ramblings. For example, he tried to subpoena Jesus Christ. In his closing arguments, he said:

> *The ability to reason correctly. Common sense, the common sense, the horse sense. This is Texas and we're not talking loopholes and if we're talking— well, let's talk a lariat. Let's talk a catch rope. ...*

A Texas court sentenced him to death, and an appeals court upheld this sentence. The U.S. Supreme Court ruled, however, that, given his mental state, Panetti could not understand why he was to be put to death and so returned the case for further evaluation of insanity by a Texas lower court. That court ruled that Panetti was competent to be executed, but just hours before his scheduled execution in 2014, an appeals court stayed the execution.

....

[1] *Ford v. Wainright*, 477 U.S. 399 (1986).

[2] *Panetti v. Quarterman*, 551 U.S. (2007).

retardation. His defense attorney argued that his intellectual limitations rendered capital punishment unconstitutional because he lacked understanding of the consequences of his actions and was therefore not as morally culpable for his acts as a person of normal intelligence.

In 2002, the U.S. Supreme Court ruled in a 6–3 decision in the case of *Atkins v. Virginia*[12] that capital punishment of people with intellectual disability constitutes cruel and unusual punishment, which is prohibited by the Eighth Amendment. The Court left open the question of what constitutes intellectual disability, however, leaving it up to the states to decide how to remain within the requirements of the Eighth Amendment.

In 2005, a Virginia jury decided that Daryl Atkins did not meet Virginia's definition of a person with intellectual disability. Thus, even though the *Atkins* case effectively abolished the practice of executing people with intellectual disabilities, Atkins himself could have been put to death in Virginia because the jury's decision paved the way for the original death sentence to be carried out. However, in 2008, a Virginia judge changed Atkins's sentence from death to life imprisonment. This change was not due to any rethinking of Atkins's mental capacity. Rather, it was due to prosecutorial misconduct (improper witness coaching) that was revealed by one of the attorneys.

In 2014, with the case of Freddie Lee Hall, the U.S. Supreme Court revised its decision to leave determination of what constitutes intellectual disability up to the states. Hall was a Florida man with an IQ score of around 70 who was convicted of murder and sentenced to death. The Court ruled that intellectual disability cannot be determined solely on the basis of an IQ score (which can vary from testing occasion to testing occasion) but must also be based on assessments of adaptive functioning over the person's lifetime.[13] In 2016, the Florida Supreme Court ruled that Hall should not be executed and should instead receive a sentence of life in prison.[14]

In 2017, the U.S. Supreme Court again revised its decision to leave things up to states. The case was that of Bobby J. Moore,[15] a Texas man with an IQ score, based on multiple tests, of between 69 and 79. Texas had argued that Moore met the criteria the state had established, but the Court ruled that those criteria were not consistent with the 2002 *Atkins* ruling.

16.2 Check Your Knowledge

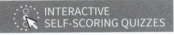 INTERACTIVE SELF-SCORING QUIZZES

(Answers are at the end of the chapter.)

True or false?

1. The *Jackson* case established that people who cannot be restored to competency should be found NGRI.

2. To be competent to stand trial, a person must be able to understand the charges and to assist their attorney.

3. The U.S. Supreme Court ruled that executing prisoners with intellectual disability constitutes cruel and unusual punishment.

Civil Commitment

Historically, governments have had a duty to protect their citizens from harm. We take for granted the right and duty of government to set limits on our freedom for the sake of protecting us. Few drivers, for example, question the legitimacy of the state's imposing limits on them by requiring seat belts or by providing traffic signals that often make them stop when they would rather go. Government has a long-established right as well as an obligation to protect us both from ourselves and from others. Civil commitment is one further way of exercising this power. **Civil commitment** is a procedure by which a person can be placed in a hospital even if they do not want to be admitted.

---

[12] *Atkins v. Virginia*, 536 U.S. 304 (2002).

[13] *Hall v. Florida*, 572 U.S. (2014).

[14] *Hall v. Florida*, SC10-1335 (2016).
[15] *Moore v. Texas*, 581 U.S. No. 15-797 (2017).

In virtually all states, a person can be committed to a hospital against their will if a judgment is made that they (1) have a psychological disorder and (2) are a danger to self—that is, the person is suicidal or unable to provide for the basic physical needs of food, clothing, and shelter—or to others. Civil commitment is supposed to last for only as long as the person remains dangerous.[16] Civil commitment affects far more people than criminal commitment.

Civil commitment procedures generally fit into one of two categories: formal and informal. Formal (or judicial) commitment is by order of a court. Any responsible citizen—usually a police officer, a relative, or a friend—can request it. If a judge believes that there is a good reason to pursue the matter, they will order a mental health examination. The person has the right to object to these attempts to "certify" them, and a court hearing can be scheduled to allow the person to present evidence against commitment.

Informal, emergency commitment of people with a psychological disorder can be accomplished without the initial involvement of the courts. The police may take any person acting in an out-of-control or dangerous manner immediately to a psychiatric hospital. Perhaps the most common informal commitment procedure is a PC, or physician's certificate. In most states, a physician, not necessarily a psychiatrist, can sign a certificate that allows a person to be hospitalized for some period of time, ranging from 24 hours to as long as 20 days. Detainment beyond this period requires formal judicial commitment.

Preventive Detention and Problems in the Prediction of Dangerousness

Based on news reports, it would seem that violence is rampant among those with psychological disorders. This is not the case (Choe, Teplin, & Abram, 2008). People with psychological disorders are more likely to be a victim of violence than a perpetrator (Choe, Teplin, & Abram, 2008; de Vries, van Busschbach, et al., 2018). Only about 3% of the violence in the United States is clearly linked to psychological disorders (Corrigan & Watson, 2005; Swanson, Holzer, et al., 1990). Moreover, about 90% of people diagnosed with psychotic disorders (primarily schizophrenia) are not violent (Swanson, et al., 1990).

Nevertheless, people with a psychological disorder are more likely to be violent than those without even though the rates are quite low (Swanson, McGinty, et al., 2015). Three factors can increase the risk of violence by people with psychological disorders: comorbid substance abuse, ineffectively treated symptoms, and prior episodes of violence. The MacArthur Violence Risk Assessment Study, a large prospective study of violent behavior among persons recently discharged from psychiatric hospitals, found that people with psychological disorders who did not also abuse substances were no more likely to engage in violence than were people without psychological disorders and substance abuse (Steadman, Mulvey, et al., 1998). This suggests that problems with substance abuse rather than psychological disorders are the main factors contributing to violence. A follow-up study with these data found that people who had delusions that others were out to get them and who felt very angry about this were more likely to be violent (Ulrich, Keers, & Coid, 2014). Meta-analyses have confirmed these findings among people with a psychotic disorder (a schizophrenia spectrum disorder, bipolar disorder, or depression with psychotic features). Paranoid symptoms are also associated with a higher risk of violence (Coid, Ullrich, et al., 2016; Douglas, Guy, & Hart, 2009; Fazel, Gulati, et al., 2009). One of the best predictors of violence in any person, whether or not that person has a psychological disorder, is whether the person has been violent in the past, a topic we discuss in the section on predicting dangerousness.

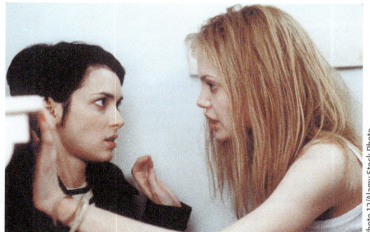

People with psychological disorders are not necessarily more likely to be violent than people without a psychological disorder, contrary to the way movies often portray someone with a disorder.

---

[16]*United States v. Debellis, 649 F.2d 1 (1st Cir. 1981).*

When people with psychological disorders do act aggressively, it is usually against family members or friends, and the incidents tend to occur at home (Desmarais, Van Dorn, et al., 2014; Steadman et al., 1998). Indeed, stranger homicide by people with psychological disorders is extremely rare (Nielssen, Bourget, et al., 2011). By and large, then, the general public is seldom affected by violence from people with psychological disorders, even though certain people with certain disorders can and will be violent. In **Focus on Discovery 16.4**, we consider the ramifications of attributing gun violence to mental illness.

The Prediction of Dangerousness   A person's likelihood of committing a dangerous act is central to civil commitment, but can mental health professionals predict dangerousness? To identify and measure risk factors for violence, mental health professionals use empirically supported methods based on clinical judgment (e.g., Historical, Clinical, and Risk Management 20, or HCR-20, now in its third version; Douglas, Hart, et al., 2014) or a combination of clinical judgment and statistical algorithms (e.g.,

---

Focus on Discovery 16.4

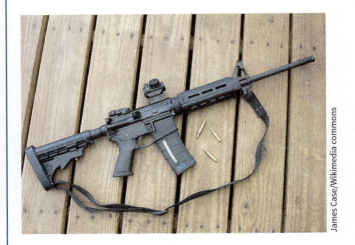

James Case/Wikimedia commons

What Is the Role of Mental Illness in Gun Violence?

Gun violence is far too common in the United States. In 2018, nearly 14,000 people were killed intentionally by a firearm (Educational Fund to Stop Gun Violence, 2020). Mass shootings, typically defined as incidents in which four or more people are killed by a gun, typically receive a good deal of attention. An example is the case of James Holmes (see **Focus on Discovery 16.1**), who entered a crowded movie theater in Aurora, Colorado, and shot and killed 12 and injured 70 others. He had schizophrenia.

Media coverage of such high-profile cases strengthens the belief that gun violence is linked to mental illness (McGinty, Kennedy-Hendricks, et al., 2016; McGinty, Webster, et al., 2014), and this belief can increase stigma (Pescosolido, 2013). Yet, not all high-profile cases of gun violence or mass shooting involve psychological disorders. In fact, most don't. For example, Brendon Tarrant, who shot and killed 51 people in a mosque in New Zealand, had no mental illness. What was revealed during this trial was that he was a white supremacist with virulent anti-immigrant

and racist views. He had carefully and methodically planned his attack over the course of 2 years.

Why then, do so many people think that gun violence and mass shootings are a result of mental illness?

One reason is a lack of understanding about the relationship between mental illness and violence. Most people are unaware that only a small percentage of gun violence incidents are carried out by people with a serious psychological disorder like schizophrenia (Smart, Morral, et al., 2020). As we have noted, research shows that people with psychological disorders are more likely to be victims of violence than perpetrators (Choe, Teplin, & Abram 2008). With respect to gun violence, one analysis suggests that less than 2% of such violence is perpetrated by people with a serious disorder, such as schizophrenia (Steadman, Monahan, et al., 2015). As we discuss in the chapter, people with psychological disorders are not necessarily more likely to be violent than people without a disorder. Factors predicting violence by people with serious psychological disorders are comorbid substance use disorders, ineffective treatments, and prior instances of violence (Choe, Teplin, & Abram 2008).

Another reason for public perceptions, though, is that some incidents, such as the mass shooting by James Holmes, do involve mental illness. Because these cases are often the ones most heavily covered by the media, people tend to link gun violence and mental illness.

Yet, people with psychological disorders are less likely to carry a gun (Swanson et al., 2015), and federal law prohibits possession of a gun by people who have been hospitalized with a psychological disorder (Rozel & Mulvey, 2017). As Rozel and Mulvey (2017, p. 461) wrote, "The amount of violence in general, and gun violence in particular, involving mentally ill individuals is so small that focusing on this aspect of the problem is largely a distraction."

Unfortunately, nearly every time a high-profile shooting receives press coverage, claims are made about mental illness being the cause even when the evidence does not support them. Blaming gun violence on mental illness does not help reduce gun violence, nor does it help people with serious mental illness (Hirschtritt & Binder, 2018).

Violence Risk Appraisal Guide [VRAG]; Quinsey, Harris, et al., 2006). These measures seem to work equally well, but even with these improved measures, accurately predicting future dangerousness remains a challenge (Skeem & Monahan, 2011).

Research suggests that violence prediction is most accurate under the following conditions (Campbell, Stefan, & Loder, 1994; Monahan, 1984; Monahan & Steadman, 1994; Steadman et al., 1998):

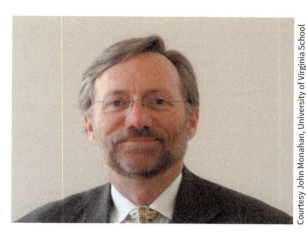

Courtesy John Monahan, University of Virginia School of Law

John Monahan is an expert on predicting dangerousness.

- If a person has been repeatedly violent in the recent past, it is reasonable to predict that they will be violent in the near future unless there have been major changes in the person's mental health or environment.

- If violence is in the person's distant past, and if it was a single but very serious act, and if that person has been incarcerated for a period of time, then violence can be expected on release if there is reason to believe that the person's mental state and physical abilities have not changed since predetention and if the person is going to return to the same environment in which they were previously violent.

- Even with no history of violence, violence can be predicted if the person is judged to be on the brink of a violent act—for example, if the person is pointing a loaded gun at an occupied building.

Violence among people with a psychological disorder is more likely when they do not receive treatment, whether as a result of lack of availability or noncompliance (Keers, Ullrich, et al., 2014; Monahan, 1992; Steadman et al., 1998). Outpatient commitment, or **assisted outpatient treatment (AOT)**, is one way of increasing medication compliance. This is an arrangement whereby a person is mandated by the court to receive treatment on an outpatient basis (i.e., not in a hospital); 47 states use some type of AOT (Berger, Dailey, et al., 2018; Torrey, 2014). To the extent that AOT increases compliance with medication regimens and other mental health treatments—and evidence indicates that it does (Munetz, Grande, et al., 1996; Torrey, 2014)—we can expect violence to be reduced. Importantly, if a person is not compliant with an AOT order, they are not sent to jail. But the person could be mandated to an inpatient setting such as a hospital (Rosenberg, 2019). One of the biggest challenges facing AOT is securing enough funding to implement these programs so that people can receive the care they need, not just during a mental health crisis, but also once they leave the program (Meldrum, Kelly, et al., 2016). For a discussion of mental health professionals' responsibilities to predict dangerousness, see **Focus on Discovery 16.5**.

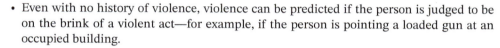

Focus on Discovery 16.5

The *Tarasoff* Case—Duty to Warn and to Protect

A person's right to privileged communication—the legal right to have the content of the therapy relationship remain confidential—is an important protection, but it is not absolute. Society has long stipulated certain conditions under which confidentiality in a relationship should not be maintained because of the harm that can befall others. A famous California court ruling in 1974[1] described circumstances in which a therapist not only may but also *must* breach the sanctity of a person's communication. First, we describe the facts of the case.

Clinical Case

In the fall of 1968, Prosenjit Poddar, a graduate student from India studying at the University of California at Berkeley, met Tatiana (Tanya) Tarasoff at a folk dancing class. They saw each other weekly during the fall, and on New Year's Eve she kissed him.

....

[1]*Tarasoff v. Regents of the University of California,* 529 P.2d 553 (Cal. 1974), vacated, reheard in bank, and affirmed, 131 Cal. Rptr. 14, 551 P.2d 334 (1976). The 1976 California Supreme Court ruling was by a 4–3 majority.

Poddar interpreted this act as a sign of formal engagement (as it might have been in India, where he was a member of the Harijan, or "untouchable," caste). But Tanya told him that she was involved with other men and indicated that she did not wish to have an intimate relationship with him.

Poddar was unhappy because of the rebuff, but he saw Tanya a few times during the spring (occasionally tape-recording their conversations to try to understand why she did not love him). Tanya left for Brazil in the summer, and Poddar, at the urging of a friend, went to the student health facility, where a psychiatrist referred him to a psychologist for therapy. When Tanya returned in October 1969, Poddar discontinued therapy. Based in part on Poddar's stated intention to purchase a gun, the psychologist notified the campus police, both orally and in writing, that Poddar was dangerous and should be taken to a community mental health center for psychiatric commitment.

The campus police interviewed Poddar, who seemed rational and promised to stay away from Tanya. They released him and notified the student health facility. No further efforts at commitment were made because the supervising psychiatrist apparently decided that there was no need and, as a matter of confidentiality, requested that the letter to the police as well as certain therapy records be destroyed.

On October 27, Poddar went to Tanya's home armed with a pellet gun and a kitchen knife. She refused to speak to him. He shot her with the pellet gun. She ran from the house; he pursued, caught, and repeatedly and fatally stabbed her. Poddar was found guilty of voluntary manslaughter rather than first- or second-degree murder.

Under the privileged communication statute of California, the counseling center psychologist properly breached the confidentiality of the professional relationship and took steps to have Poddar civilly committed, for he judged Poddar to be an imminent danger. Poddar had stated that he intended to purchase a gun, and by his other words and actions he had convinced the therapist that he was desperate enough to harm Tarasoff. What the psychologist did not do, and what the court decided he should have done, was to warn the likely victim, Tanya Tarasoff, that her former friend had bought a gun and might use it against her. As stated by the California Supreme Court in *Tarasoff v. Regents of the University of California*: "Once a therapist does in fact determine, or under applicable professional standards reasonably should have determined, that a patient poses a serious danger of violence to others, he bears a duty to exercise reasonable care to protect the foreseeable victims of that danger." The *Tarasoff* ruling requires clinicians, in deciding when to violate confidentiality, to use the very imperfect skill of predicting dangerousness.

Extending Protections from the *Tarasoff* Ruling

Since the original *Tarasoff* ruling, several other court cases have extended its protections. For example, the concept of "foreseeable victims" was extended to include close others of an identifiable victim,[2] meaning that all foreseeable victims must also be warned, even if the person had never made an explicit threat against them to the therapist,[3] as long as sufficient history of

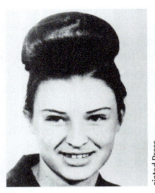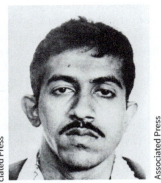

Prosenjit Poddar was convicted of manslaughter in the death of Tatiana Tarasoff. The court ruled that his therapist, who had become convinced Poddar might harm Tarasoff, should have warned her of the impending danger.

violence existed to suggest that a close other might also be harmed.

This broadening of the duty to warn and protect has placed mental health professionals in an even more difficult predicament, for the potentially violent person need not even mention the specific person they may harm. It is up to therapists to deduce the possible victims, based on what they can learn of their patient's past and present circumstances.

Other rulings have extended the duty to warn and protect to foreseeable victims of child abuse even if the possible victims are as yet unknown.[4] Further, the duty to warn was also extended to include property damage.[5] The court's conclusion about property arose in a case of arson, where injury to people could have happened. Thus, the therapist's extended duty to warn was based on the reasoning that arson is a violent act and therefore a lethal threat to people who may be in the vicinity of the fire.

Other rulings mandate that a therapist must warn a possible victim if a threat is reported by a member of the patient's family.[6] The court ruled that a close family member is, in essence, a part of the patient, and thus, a therapist does have a duty to warn potential victims if notified by a close family member of a patient.

---

[2] *Hedlund v. Superior Court,* 34 Cal.3d 695 (1983).

[3] *Jablonski by Pahls v. United States,* 712 F.2d 391 (1983).

[4] *Almonte v. New York Medical College,* 851 F. Supp. 34, 40 (D. Conn. 1994) (denying motion for summary judgment).

[5] *Peck v. Counseling Service of Addison County,* 499 A.2d 422 (Vt. 1985).

[6] *Ewing v. Goldstein,* Cal. App. 4th B163112.2d. (2004).

Protection of the Rights of People with Psychological Disorders

Several court decisions have been rendered to protect people from formal or informal civil commitment unless it is absolutely necessary. However, many rights of people with a psychological disorder are still curtailed. For example, an analysis of mental health–related bills introduced in state legislatures (Corrigan, Watson, et al., 2005) found that 75% of these bills took away liberties of people with a psychological disorder (e.g., allowing involuntary medication) and 33% took away privacy rights (e.g., sharing mental health records in the interest of public safety).

Being hospitalized against one's wishes is less likely today than in the past, in large part due to changes in health care that emphasize outpatient over inpatient care. In fact, today it is difficult to hospitalize a person who is in real need of at least a short hospital stay, and this is also problematic. People with a psychological disorder such as schizophrenia or bipolar disorder may need to spend time in a hospital when symptoms become severe. Yet, people in need of hospitalization are more likely to be sent to jails and prisons than to a hospital, a topic we return to later in this chapter.

We turn now to a discussion of several issues and trends that revolve around the protections provided to those with psychological disorders: the principle of the least restrictive alternative; the right to treatment; the right to refuse treatment; and, finally, the way in which these several themes collide in efforts to provide humane mental health treatment while respecting individual rights.

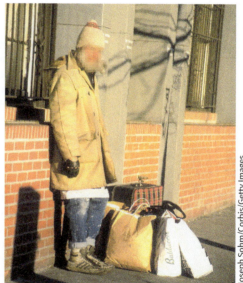

Joseph Sohm/Corbis/Getty Images

Least Restrictive Alternative   As noted earlier, civil commitment in most states rests on presumed dangerousness. The **least restrictive alternative** to freedom is to be provided when one is treating people with psychological disorders and protecting them from harming themselves and others. A number of court rulings require that only those people who cannot be adequately looked after in less restrictive settings be placed in hospitals. In general terms, mental health professionals have to provide the treatment that restricts the person's liberty to the least possible degree while remaining workable.[17] It is unconstitutional to confine a person with a psychological disorder who is nondangerous and who is capable of living on their own or with the help of willing and responsible family or friends.[18] Of course, this principle has meaning only if society provides suitable residences and treatments, which unfortunately does not happen as much as it needs to.

Right to Treatment   Another aspect of civil commitment that has come to the attention of the courts is the so-called right to treatment. If a person is deprived of liberty because they are mentally ill and is a danger to self or others, is the state not required to provide treatment to alleviate these problems?

The right to treatment was extended to all people committed under civil law in a landmark 1972 case, *Wyatt v. Stickney*.[19] In that case, an Alabama federal court ruled that treatment is the only justification for the civil commitment

Civil commitment supposedly requires that the person be dangerous. But in actual practice, the decision to commit can be based on a judgment of severe disability, as in the case of some people who are homeless.

---

[17]*In Re: Tarpley*, 556 N.E.2d, superseded by 581 N.E.2d 1251 (1991).

[18]*Project Release v. Prevost*, 722 F.2d 960 (2d Cir. 1983).

[19]*Wyatt v. Stickney*, 325 F.Supp. 781 (M.D. Ala. 1971), enforced in 334 F.Supp. 1341 (M.D. Ala. 1971), 344 F.Supp. 373, 379. (M.D. Ala.1972), *aff'd sub nom Wyatt v. Anderholt*, 503 F.2d 1305 (5th Cir. 1974).

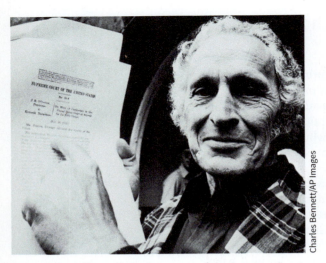

Charles Bennett/AP Images

Kenneth Donaldson, displaying a copy of the Supreme Court opinion stating that nondangerous people with psychological disorders cannot be confined against their will under civil commitment.

of people with a psychological disorder to a psychiatric hospital. This ruling, upheld on appeal, is frequently cited as ensuring the protection of people confined by civil commitment, at least to the extent that the state cannot simply "put them away" without meeting minimal standards of care. In fact, when people with intellectual disability (as opposed to those deemed to be mentally ill) are released from an institution, health officials are not relieved of their constitutional duty to provide reasonable care and safety as well as appropriate training.[20]

The *Wyatt* ruling was also significant because it set forth very specific requirements for mental hospitals—for example, they must be of a certain size and provide certain types of privacy and limit physical restraints except in emergency situations. The ruling also specified how many mental health professionals ought to be working in the hospital.

In another celebrated case, *O'Connor v. Donaldson*,[21] a civilly committed man sued two hospital doctors for his release and for monetary damages on the grounds that he had been kept against his will for 14 years without being treated and without being dangerous to himself or to others. In January 1957, at the age of 49, Kenneth Donaldson was committed to the Florida State Hospital in Chattahoochee on petition of his father, who felt that his son was delusional. At a brief court hearing, a county judge found that Donaldson had schizophrenia and committed him for "care, maintenance, and treatment."

Unfortunately, Donaldson did not receive treatment, and he was not allowed to leave the hospital despite many requests to be discharged. Finally, the U.S. Supreme Court[22] ruled that "a State cannot constitutionally confine ... a nondangerous individual who is capable of surviving safely in freedom by himself or with the help of willing and responsible family members or friends." As a result of this decision, a civilly committed person's status must be periodically reviewed, because the grounds on which the person was committed cannot be assumed to continue to be in effect forever.

Right to Refuse Treatment

Does a person committed under civil law have the right to refuse treatment or a particular kind of treatment? The answer is yes, but with qualifications.

The right of committed people to refuse medication is still debated. Some argue that because many people with a psychological disorder have no insight into their condition, they believe they do not need any treatment and thus subject themselves and their loved ones to sometimes desperate and frightening situations by refusing medication or other modes of therapy, most of which involve hospitalization. The costs of untreated psychological disorders, which are substantial, are often overlooked (Torrey, 2014).

On the other hand, there are many arguments against forcing a person to take medications. The side effects of most antipsychotic drugs are often aversive (see Chapter 9) and are sometimes harmful and irreversible in the long run. Notably, one-third or more of people who take medications do not benefit from them.

Although there is inconsistency across jurisdictions, the trend is toward granting even involuntarily committed people certain rights to refuse medication, based on the constitutional protections of freedom from physical invasion, freedom of thought, and the right to privacy. In an extension of the least-restrictive-treatment principle, the U.S. Supreme Court ruled that the government cannot force antipsychotic drugs on a person only on the supposition that at some future time they might become dangerous.[23] The threat to public safety

[20]*Thomas S. v. Flaherty*, 902 F.2d 250, cert. denied, 111 S.Ct. 373 (1990).

[21]*O'Connor v. Donaldson*, 95 S.Ct. 2486 (1975).

[22]*O'Connor v. Donaldson*, 422 U.S. 563 (1975).

[23]*United States v. Charters*, 863, F.2d 302 (1988).

has to be clear and imminent to justify the risks and restrictions that such medications pose, and it must be shown that less intrusive intervention will not likely reduce impending danger to others.

Deinstitutionalization, Civil Liberties, and Mental Health

Beginning in the 1950s, many states embarked on a policy referred to as *deinstitutionalization*, discharging as many people as possible from hospitals and discouraging admissions. Civil commitment is more difficult to achieve now than it was then, even though some people with psychological disorders very much need short stays in a hospital.

By 2010, there were approximately 14 psychiatric hospital beds for every 100,000 people in the United States; in 1955, there were 350 psychiatric hospital beds for every 100,000 people (Torrey, 2014). By some estimates, we need at least 50 hospital beds for every 100,000 people in the United States to meet the needs of people with psychological disorders—nearly four times what we currently have (Torrey, 2014). The maxim "Treat them in the community" has been in place for over 50 years, with the (incorrect) assumption being that virtually anything is preferable to institutionalization.

Unfortunately, there are woefully inadequate resources for treatment in the community. Some effective programs are described in Chapter 9, but these are very much the exception, not the rule. Rates of homelessness have soared among those with psychological disorders, and unhoused people do not have fixed addresses and need help in establishing eligibility and residency to receive benefits.

Deinstitutionalization may be a misnomer. *Transinstitutionalization* may be more apt, for declines in the number of psychiatric hospital beds have occasioned increases in the presence of people with psychological disorders in nursing homes, the mental health departments of nonpsychiatric hospitals, and, most sadly, prisons (Sisti, Segal, & Emanuel, 2015; Torrey, 2014). These settings are by and large not equipped to handle the needs of people with psychological disorders. In **Read More About It 16.2**, we highlight a recent book on the crisis involving mental illness and jails, aptly titled *Insane*.

Read More About It 16.2

Insane: America's Criminal Treatment of Mental Illness

In her 2018 book *Insane: America's Criminal Treatment of Mental Illness,* author and reporter Alisa Roth offers a blistering account of how the United States is failing to protect some of its most vulnerable citizens: those with severe mental illnesses. In a chapter called "The Asylum Fallacy," Roth traces the history of mental illness treatment in the United States, showing that people with mental illness were kept in jails *before* the development of asylums. In fact, part of the impetus for the work of Dorothea Dix and others (see Chapter 1) was to provide more humane places for people with mental illness rather than the jails and prisons of the day.

Most of the book focuses on our current predicament: Since so many hospitals in the United States have closed, people with severe mental illness have moved from hospitals to homelessness to the criminal justice system, where they often languish and do not receive the treatment they need. Many jails and prisons are doing remarkable jobs with providing treatment and support, yet they often do so without enough funding, sufficient training, and adequate facilities.

Roth's important and timely book is divided into three sections. In the first, she covers why so many people with mental illness end up in jails and prisons rather than in treatment facilities.

In the second part, she takes a close look at the lives of people inside jails and prisons, covering both people with mental illness and the corrections officers charged with keeping them and others in the facilities safe. In the third and final part of the book, she shines a light on the difficulties people with severe mental illness face when trying to get out of the criminal justice system.

She covers some of the largest jails—Cook County Jail in Chicago and L.A. County Jails in Los Angeles—describing the challenges they face in trying to manage and help people with severe mental illness. These large facilities have special mental health units, but they are always full and are not large enough to meet the demand that exists in the overall jail population. Unfortunately, being transferred from jail or prison to a state mental hospital is not always better in terms of the treatment offered. Roth also discusses competency to stand trial and the insanity defense in its various incarnations. She shows how some versions of the insanity defense, including the GBMI plea, have eroded the public's support for and faith in the insanity defense altogether.

This excellent book shows that we have a great deal of work to do when it comes to providing treatment for people with mental illness. Jails and prisons are not the answer. In some states, such as California and New York, officials are making decisions to close down mental health units or entire jails (e.g., Riker's Island) in an effort to spur state health systems to develop much-needed better alternatives.

Indeed, jails and prisons have become the new "hospitals" for people with psychological disorders in the 21st century. In the 1970s, about 5% of people in prisons had a serious psychological disorder; by 2007, between 17% and 30% of people in prisons had a serious psychological disorder (Steadman, Osher, et al., 2009; Torrey, 2014). A 2014 report by the Treatment Advocacy Center notes that 44 of the 50 states have more people with psychological disorders in prison than in the remaining psychiatric hospitals in those states (Torrey, Zdanowicz, et al., 2014). The lives of people with psychological disorders in prison are often "horrific," according to federal judge Lawrence Karlton, who ruled unconstitutional the ways in which California corrections officials were interacting with inmates with psychological disorders—for example, using pepper spray, imposing solitary confinement, and forcing them out of their cells (Steinberg, Mills, & Romano, 2015).

In a cruel twist, some states are investigating whether shuttered former mental hospitals can be reopened and repurposed to house persons who have been incarcerated and have a serious psychological disorder (Torrey, 2014). Other states are repurposing closed hospitals as tourist attractions for people interested in ghost hunting (Searles, 2013). Have we come very far from the days of the abysmal institutions that we discussed in Chapter 1? Clearly, we must do more.

Unfortunately, police officers are now called on to do the work of mental health professionals They are often the first to come into contact with a person with a psychological disorder and obliged to make decisions as to whether a person should be taken to a hospital or jail. Fortunately, many communities recognize the need for the police to receive proper training, and mental health laws passed provide funding for such training.

Another approach is to provide police departments with specialized training so that they can develop a *crisis intervention team* (*CIT*). This approach helps equip officers with the tools to engage and help people with severe mental illness. CIT International, an organization that furthers this approach, not only provides training but also facilitates partnerships among mental health services, mental health advocates, and police departments to help the mental health system work better and to keep people with mental illness out of the criminal justice system whenever possible. In 2019, HBO presented a documentary called *Ernie & Joe: Crisis Cops*, which focused on a CIT in the San Antonio, Texas, police department (see https://www.hbo.com/movies/ernie-and-joe-crisis-copshttps://www.hbo.com/documentaries/ernie-and-joe). Evidence suggests that CITs are effective in reducing the numbers of people with mental illness who end up in jail rather than in treatment and in changing police officers' attitudes and reducing stigma toward people with mental illness (Rogers, McNeil, & Binder 2019).

In addition to supporting police training, mental health laws also provide funds to set up so-called mental health courts in local communities. The idea is that people with psychological disorders who commit crimes may be better served by courts that can monitor treatment availability and adherence. A longitudinal study found that people with a psychological disorder who went through a mental health court instead of traditional court went for a longer period of time after release without reoffending or committing a violent act (McNiel & Binder, 2007).

A related program that has shown great promise is called *jail diversion*. This program, started in Miami, Florida, by Steve Leifman, a judge in the county criminal court system, was showcased in the 2020 PBS documentary *The Definition of Insanity*. Over the course of 20 years, Judge Leifman and colleagues (mental health professionals, police officers, social services personnel, and other judicial and criminal court officials) built a program that allows people with serious mental illness who have been charged with a misdemeanor or nonviolent felony to receive treatment and services (job training, group therapy, and housing assistance) to promote recovery and to keep them out of prison. Such programs have been introduced in many other states and are working to reverse recent trends that put people with mental illness in jails.

Although programs such as these are welcome insofar as they help keep people with mental illness out of jails and prisons (Kane, Evans, & Shokraneh, 2017), we still have a long way to go. Law enforcement

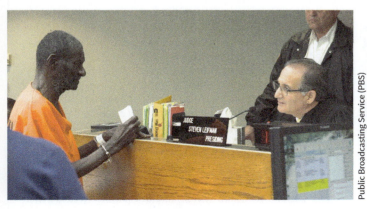

The PBS documentary, *The Definition of Insanity*, illustrates the benefits of jail diversion programs.

Public Broadcasting Service (PBS)

professionals did not ask to become the first point of contact for people with mental illness. Funding for mental health services has declined precipitously since the 1970s, and state and local governments turned to law enforcement to fill this gap.

Beginning in 2020, the tide may have begun to turn with respect to restoring much needed funding to mental health services in the United States at a level not seen in over half a century. The 2020 National Hotline Designation Act provided funding to create the 988 hotline for mental health crisis help. People in crisis can call or text this three-digit number and get in touch with someone who can provide help. In 2022, the Bipartisan Safer Communities Act provides funding for additional Certified Community Behavioral Health Clinics (CCBHCs) and telehealth services. Providing more mental health treatment in communities can hopefully reduce the need for law enforcement to step in so frequently.

Quick Summary

The legal standard for competency to stand trial requires that accused people understand the charges against them and be able to assist their attorney in the defense. Someone who is judged incompetent to stand trial receives treatment to restore competence and then returns to face charges. The *Jackson* case specified that the pretrial period could be no longer than it takes to determine whether a person will ever become competent to stand trial. The use of medication to restore competency to stand trial is permitted in limited circumstances.

The U.S. Supreme Court has ruled that it is unconstitutional (a violation of the Eighth Amendment, which prohibits cruel and unusual punishment) to execute people who are deemed legally insane or have intellectual disabilities. Individual states can determine what constitutes intellectual disability and insanity.

A person can be civilly committed to a hospital against his or her wishes if the person is mentally ill and a danger to self or others. Formal commitment requires a court order; informal commitment does not. People with psychological disorders who do not abuse substances are not necessarily more likely to engage in violence than are people who do not have psychological disorders.

Early studies on the prediction of dangerousness had several flaws. Later research has shown that violence can be more accurately predicted if any of these conditions apply: repeated acts of violence, a single serious violent act, being on the brink of violence, or medication noncompliance.

Court cases have tried to balance a person's rights with the right of society to be protected. The least restrictive alternative to freedom is to be provided when one is treating people with mental disorders and protecting them from harming themselves and others. A series of court cases have generally supported the notion that people committed to a hospital have the right to receive treatment. People with psychological disorders have the right to refuse treatment as well, except when doing so poses a danger to self or others.

Beginning in the 1950s, a large number of people were released from mental hospitals in what has been called deinstitutionalization. Unfortunately, not enough treatment options are available in the community. Jails and prisons are now the new "hospitals" for people with psychological disorders. Police officers are called on to do the work once reserved for mental health professionals. Partnerships among police, courts, and community mental health providers are a promising development for helping people with psychological disorders.

16.3 Check Your Knowledge

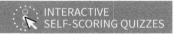

INTERACTIVE SELF-SCORING QUIZZES

(Answers are at the end of the chapter.)

True or false?

1. People with schizophrenia who have negative symptoms are more likely to be violent than those without negative symptoms.

2. Past violence is a predictor of future violence.

3. Court decisions have determined that hospitalized people do not have a right to treatment unless they are dangerous.

4. A person with schizophrenia who has many symptoms can refuse treatment if the person does not pose an imminent threat.

Ethical Dilemmas in Therapy and Research

The issues reviewed thus far place legal limits on the activities of mental health professionals. These legal constraints are important, for laws are one of society's strongest means of encouraging all of us to behave in certain ways. Mental health professionals also have ethical constraints. Ethics statements are designed to provide an ideal and to address moral issues of right and wrong that may or may not be reflected in the law. These ethics guidelines describe how mental health professionals ought to behave in their professions. Most of the time what we believe is unethical is also illegal, but sometimes existing laws are in conflict with our moral sense of right and wrong. The American Psychological Association (APA) publishes a *Code of Ethics* that covers the ethical standards that constrain research and practice in psychology (American Psychological Association, 2002; http://www.apa.org/ethics). Unfortunately, the APA itself behaved in an ethically questionable manner when it sanctioned the use of torture during the wars waged by the United States in Iraq and Afghanistan. Following an extensive independent report completed in 2015 (Hoffman, Carter, et al., 2015), the APA revised its ethics code in 2016 to explicitly state that "psychologists do not participate in, facilitate, assist or otherwise engage in torture" (American Psychological Association, 2016).

In **Focus on Discovery 16.6**, we discuss the ethical issue of whether mental health professionals should offer opinions and diagnoses of public figures.

Ethical Restraints on Research

The training of scientists equips them to pose interesting and important questions and to design meaningful research that is as free of confounds as possible. Society needs knowledge, and in a democracy a scientist has a right to seek that knowledge. However, the ordinary citizens who participate in experiments must be protected from unnecessary harm, risk, humiliation, and invasion of privacy.

Focus on Discovery 16.6

Should Mental Health Professionals Diagnose Public Figures?

In 1964, several thousand psychiatrists offered their opinions on psychological disorder diagnoses for presidential candidate Barry Goldwater in response to a request from the now-defunct *Fact* magazine. About half of the psychiatrists who responded believed Goldwater was unfit for office. Although Goldwater lost the election, he won a libel lawsuit against the magazine.

The American Psychiatric Association did not have any involvement with the article or the psychiatrists' decisions to participate, but the group nevertheless considered the issue and subsequently decided that rendering such opinions about the mental health of public figures was a breach of professional ethics. In 1973, the American Psychiatric Association adopted a new ethics rule, formally known as **Section 7.3** of the organization's ethics code but colloquially referred to as the Goldwater Rule. The rule specifies: "On occasion psychiatrists are asked for an opinion about an individual who is in the light of public attention or who has disclosed information about himself/herself through public media. In such circumstances, a psychiatrist may share with the public his or her expertise about psychiatric issues in general. However, it is unethical for a psychiatrist to offer a professional opinion unless he or she has conducted an examination and has been granted proper authorization for such a statement" (https://www.psychiatry.org/news-room/apa-blogs/apa-blog/2016/08/the-goldwater-rule).

Although the American Psychological Association does not have such a rule in its code of ethics, psychologists are strongly discouraged from offering diagnoses or other mental health opinions about public figures. One reason psychologists are discouraged from offering such opinions is that they would not be able to establish a professional relationship with the public figure and thus would be unable to do a thorough psychological assessment (see Chapter 3). However, rendering a professional opinion on the mental health of a politician is not the same thing as making a diagnosis (Lilienfeld, Miller, & Lynam, 2017).

Following the 2016 presidential election in the United States, the issue was raised again, with mental health professionals being asked for their opinions on the mental health and fitness of public figures, most notably politicians. The American Psychiatric Association reaffirmed its ethical rule in 2017, noting that the profession was tarnished by the Goldwater lawsuit and that it need not go down that road again. However, psychologists have argued that the Goldwater Rule is outdated and ought to be revised and updated to allow for discussion of the mental health of people who "hold positions of substantial power over others" (Lilienfeld, Miller, & Lynam, 2017, p. 18). Lilienfeld and colleagues were clear that this ought to be done rarely and with clear-eyed awareness of the risks (e.g., harm to the reputation of the person whose mental health is being discussed). They also argued that psychologists have a "duty to inform" when it comes to people who are of such importance.

Perhaps the most reprehensible ethical insensitivity was exhibited in the brutal experiments conducted by German physicians on concentration camp prisoners during World War II. One experiment, for example, investigated how long people lived when their heads were bashed repeatedly with a heavy stick. Clearly, such actions violate our sense of decency and morality. The Nuremberg Trials, conducted by the Allies following the war, brought these and other barbarisms to light and handed out severe punishment (including the death penalty) to some of the soldiers, physicians, and Nazi officials who had engaged in or contributed to such actions, even when they claimed that they had merely been following orders.

In response to the many instances of harm inflicted on research participants, several international codes of ethics for the conduct of scientific research were developed—the Nuremberg Code formulated in 1947 in the aftermath of

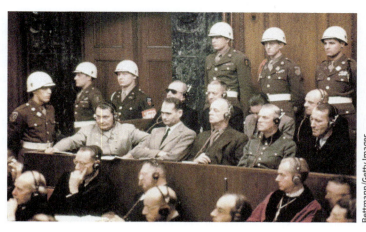

Defendants at the Nuremberg trials.

the Nazi war-crime trials, the 1964 Declaration of Helsinki, and statements from the British Medical Research Council. In 1979, the National Commission for the Protection of Human Subjects of Biomedical and Behavioral Research issued a report (the Belmont Report) that arose from hearings and inquiries into restrictions that the U.S. government might impose on research performed with prisoners, children, and people in psychiatric hospitals. The U.S. Department of Health and Human Services issued regulations as well (45 CFR part 46; https://www.hhs.gov/ohrp/regulations-and-policy/regulations/45-cfr-46/index.html), which have come to be known as "The Common Rule." These various codes and principles are continually being re-evaluated and revised as new challenges are posed to the research community. The Common Rule was revised most recently in 2017 (Menikoff, Kaneshiro, & Pritchard, 2017) and can be read online at https://www.gpo.gov/fdsys/pkg/FR-2017-01-19/pdf/2017-01058.pdf.

The proposals of behavioral researchers, many of whom conduct experiments related to psychological disorders, have been reviewed for safety and general ethical propriety by institutional review boards in medical centers, universities, and research institutes. Such committees—and this is significant—comprise not only behavioral scientists but also citizens from the community. They are able to block any research proposal, and they can require questionable aspects to be modified if, in their collective judgment, the research would put participants at too great a risk. Universities and other research institutions are required to certify researchers on the basis of special coursework and examinations concerning research ethics. Researchers who receive funds from federal agencies, such as the National Institute of Mental Health, are also required to receive specialized training in research ethics.

Informed Consent

A core component of ethical research is **informed consent**. The investigator must provide enough information to enable people to decide whether they want to be in a study. Researchers must describe the study clearly, including any risks involved. Researchers should disclose even minor risks that could occur from a study, including emotional distress from answering personal questions. There must be no coercion in obtaining informed consent. Participants must understand that they have every right not to take part in the study or to withdraw from the study at any point without penalty.

A central issue is that potential participants must be able to understand the study and associated risks. What if the prospective participant is a person with intellectual disability, unable to understand fully what is being asked? In clinical and research settings, researchers must ascertain that people are not having trouble understanding the study.

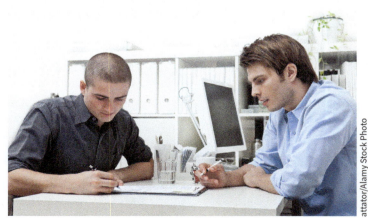

Informed consent must be obtained for research.

Still, as with the right to refuse treatment, there is recognition that people with a psychological disorder are not necessarily incapable of giving informed consent. For example, although people with schizophrenia may do more poorly than people without schizophrenia on tests designed to assess decision-making skills, people with schizophrenia can give informed consent if a more detailed procedure describing a study is included—for example, one that describes what they will be asked to do and what they will see and explains that their participation is voluntary and in no way will impact their treatment (Carpenter, Gold, et al., 2000; Wirshing, Wirshing, et al., 1998).

As with schizophrenia, having a diagnosis of Alzheimer's disease does not necessarily mean that a person cannot provide informed consent (Marson, Huthwaite, & Hebert, 2004).

These results point to the importance of examining each person individually for the ability to give informed consent, rather than assuming that a person with schizophrenia or Alzheimer's disease is unable to do so.

Confidentiality and Privileged Communication

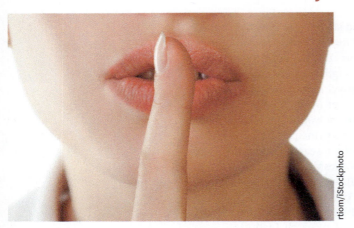

What people tell their therapist is confidential, although in certain situations confidentiality may be broken.

When people consult a psychiatrist or clinical psychologist, they are assured by professional ethics codes that what goes on in the session will remain confidential. **Confidentiality** means that nothing will be revealed to any third party except for other professionals and those intimately involved in the person's treatment.

A **privileged communication** goes even further. It is communication between parties in a confidential relationship that is protected by law. The recipient of such a communication cannot legally be compelled to disclose it as a witness. The right of privileged communication is a major exception to the courts' access to evidence in judicial proceedings. Society believes that in the long term the interests of people are best served if some communications remain off limits to the police, judges, and prosecutors. The privilege applies to such relationships as those between spouses, physician and patient, psychologist and client, religious leader and congregant, and attorney and client. The legal expression is that the patient or client "holds the privilege," which means that only they may release the other person to disclose confidential information in a legal proceeding.

There are important limits to a person's right of privileged communication, however. For example, this right is eliminated for any of the following reasons in some states:

- A person has accused a therapist of malpractice. In such a case, the therapist can divulge information about the therapy to defend themself in any legal action initiated by the person.

- The person is younger than 16, and the therapist has reason to believe that the child has been a victim of a crime such as child abuse. In fact, the psychologist is required to report to the police or to a child welfare agency within 36 hours any suspicion they have that the child has been physically or sexually abused.

- The person initiated therapy in hopes of evading the law for having committed a crime or for planning to do so.

- The therapist judges that the person is a danger to self or others and disclosure of information is necessary to ward off such danger (see **Focus on Discovery 16.5** on *Tarasoff*).

Summary

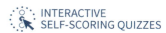
- Some civil liberties can be set aside when mental health professionals and the court judge that a psychological disorder has played a decisive role in determining a person's behavior. This may occur through criminal or civil commitment.

- There is an important difference between a psychological disorder and insanity. Insanity is a legal concept. A person can be diagnosed as mentally ill and yet be deemed sane enough both to stand trial and to be found guilty of a crime.

- Criminal commitment can send a person to a hospital either before a trial for an alleged crime, because the person is deemed incompetent to stand trial, or after an acquittal by reason of insanity.

- Several landmark cases and principles in law address the conditions under which a person who has committed a crime might be excused from legal responsibility for it—that is, not guilty by reason of insanity. These involve the presence of an irresistible impulse, the notion that some people may not be able to distinguish between right and wrong (the M'Naghten rule), or both (the ALI guidelines). The Insanity Defense Reform Act of 1984 made it harder for accused people to argue insanity as a defense.

- Two insanity pleas used today are not guilty by reason of insanity (NGRI) and guilty but mentally ill (GBMI). They differ in terms of whether a person is responsible for his or her criminal actions, where the person receives treatment, and how long the person remains committed.

- Under civil commitment, a person who is considered mentally ill and dangerous to self or to others can be committed to a hospital even if the person did not commit a crime.

- Court rulings have provided greater protection to people with psychological disorders, particularly those under civil commitment. They have the right to the least restrictive treatment setting; the right to be treated; and, in most circumstances, the right to refuse treatment, particularly any procedure that entails considerable risk.

- Ethical restraints concerning research specify what kinds of research are allowable and stipulate the duty of scientists to obtain informed consent from prospective human participants.

- In the area of therapy, ethics codes assure the right of patients to confidentiality.

Answers to Check Your Knowledge Questions

16.1   1. c; 2. a; 3. d; 4. b.

16.2   1. False; 2. True; 3. True.

16.3   1. False; 2. True; 3. False; 4. True.

Key Terms

American Law Institute guidelines   460
assisted outpatient treatment   473
civil commitment   470
competency to stand trial   464
confidentiality   482

criminal commitment   458
forensic psychologist   464
guilty but mentally ill (GBMI)   463
informed consent   481
insanity defense   459

irresistible impulse   460
least restrictive alternative   475
M'Naghten rule   460
not guilty by reason of insanity (NGRI)   462
privileged communication   482

DSM-5-TR Diagnoses

Neurodevelopmental Disorders

Intellectual Developmental Disorder

Intellectual Developmental Disorder (Intellectual Disability)

Communication Disorders

Language Disorder / Social (Pragmatic) Communication Disorder / Speech Sound Disorder / Childhood Onset Fluency Disorder (Stuttering)

Autism Spectrum Disorder

Autism Spectrum Disorder

Attention-Deficit / Hyperactivity Disorder

Attention-Deficit / Hyperactivity Disorder

Specific Learning Disorder Motor Disorders

Developmental Coordination Disorder / Stereotypic Movement Disorder / Tourette's Disorder / Persistent (Chronic) Motor or Vocal Tic Disorder / Provisional Tic Disorder

Schizophrenia Spectrum and Other Psychotic Disorders

Schizophrenia / Schizotypal Personality Disorder / Schizophreniform Disorder / Brief Psychotic Disorder / Delusional Disorder / Schizoaffective Disorder

Bipolar and Related Disorders

Bipolar I Disorder / Bipolar II Disorder / Cyclothymic Disorder

Depressive Disorders

Disruptive Mood Dysregulation Disorder / Major Depressive Disorder / Persistent Depressive Disorder / Premenstrual Dysphoric Disorder

Anxiety Disorders

Panic Disorder / Agoraphobia / Specific Phobia / Social Anxiety Disorder / Generalized Anxiety Disorder / Separation Anxiety Disorder / Selective Mutism

Obsessive-Compulsive and Related Disorders

Obsessive-Compulsive Disorder / Body Dysmorphic Disorder / Hoarding Disorder / Trichotillomania (Hair-Pulling Disorder) / Excoriation (Skin-Picking) Disorder

Trauma- and Stressor-Related Disorders

Reactive Attachment Disorder / Disinhibited Social Engagement Disorder / Acute Stress Disorder / Posttraumatic Stress Disorder / Adjustment Disorders/ Prolonged Grief Disorder

Dissociative Disorders

Depersonalization-Derealization Disorder / Dissociative Amnesia / Dissociative Identity Disorder

Somatic Symptom and Related Disorders

Somatic Symptom Disorder / Illness Anxiety Disorder / Functional Neurological Symptom Disorder (Conversion Disorder) / Psychological Factors Affecting Other Medical Conditions / Factitious Disorder

Feeding and Eating Disorders

Pica / Rumination Disorder / Avoidant Restrictive Food Intake Disorder / Anorexia Nervosa / Bulimia Nervosa / Binge Eating Disorder

Elimination Disorders

Enuresis / Encopresis

Sleep–Wake Disorders

Insomnia Disorder / Hypersomnolence Disorder / Narcolepsy / Obstructive Sleep Apnea Hypopnea / Central Sleep Apnea / Sleep-Related Hypoventilation / Circadian Rhythm Sleep–Wake Disorders / Nightmare Disorder / Rapid Eye Movement Sleep Behavior Disorder / Restless Legs Syndrome / Non-Rapid Eye Movement Sleep Arousal Disorders

Sexual Dysfunctions

Erectile Disorder / Female Orgasmic Disorder / Delayed Ejaculation / Premature (Early) Ejaculation / Female Sexual Interest / Arousal Disorder / Male Hypoactive Sexual Desire Disorder / Genito-Pelvic Pain / Penetration Disorder

Gender Dysphoria

Gender Dysphoria in Children, in Adolescents, or Adults

Disruptive, Impulse-Control, and Conduct Disorders

Oppositional Defiant Disorder / Intermittent Explosive Disorder / Conduct Disorder

Substance-Related and Addictive Disorders

Alcohol Use Disorder / Cannabis Use Disorder / Stimulant Use Disorder / Other Hallucinogen Use Disorder / Inhalant Use Disorder / Nicotine Use Disorder / Opioid Use Disorder / Phencyclidine Use Disorder / Sedative, Hypnotic, or Anxiolytic Use Disorders / Tobacco Use Disorder / Gambling Disorder

Neurocognitive Disorders

Delirium / Mild Neurocognitive Disorder / Major Neurocognitive Disorder

Personality Disorders

Antisocial Personality Disorder / Avoidant Personality Disorder / Borderline Personality Disorder / Narcissistic Personality Disorder / Obsessive-Compulsive Personality Disorder / Schizotypal Personality Disorder / Dependent Personality Disorder / Schizoid Personality Disorder / Paranoid Personality Disorder / Histrionic Personality Disorder

Paraphilic Disorders

Exhibitionistic Disorder / Fetishistic Disorder / Frotteuristic Disorder / Pedophilic Disorder / Sexual Masochism Disorder / Sexual Sadism Disorder / Transvestic Disorder / Voyeuristic Disorder

Conditions for Further Study

Attenuated Psychosis Syndrome / Depressive Episodes with Short-Duration Hypomania / Caffeine Use Disorder / Internet Gaming Disorder / Neurobehavioral Disorder Associated with Prenatal Alcohol Exposure / Suicidal Behavior Disorder / Non-Suicidal Self Injury

DSM-5-TR Classification System

Neurodevelopmental Disorders

Schizophrenia Spectrum and Other Psychotic Disorders

Bipolar and Related Disorders

Depressive Disorders

Anxiety Disorders

Obsessive-Compulsive and Related Disorders

Trauma- and Stressor-Related Disorders

Dissociative Disorders

Somatic Symptom and Related Disorders

Feeding and Eating Disorders

Elimination Disorders

Sleep–Wake Disorders

Sexual Dysfunctions

Gender Dysphoria

Disruptive, Impulse-Control, and Conduct Disorders

Substance-Related and Addictive Disorders

Neurocognitive Disorders

Personality Disorders

Paraphilic Disorders

Other Mental Disorders

Medication-Induced Movement Disorders and Other Adverse Effects of Medication

Other Conditions That May Be a Focus of Clinical Attention

ABAB design   An experimental design in which behavior is measured during a baseline period (A), during a period when a treatment is introduced (B), during the reinstatement of the conditions that prevailed in the baseline period (A), and finally during a reintroduction of the treatment (B); commonly used in operant research to isolate cause-effect relationships. Also known as a *reversal design*.

actigraphy   Devices used to record activity levels, most commonly used to study sleep and circadian rhythms.

acute stress disorder (ASD)   A short-lived reaction to a traumatic event involving symptoms such as recurrent intrusive memories or dreams, attempts to avoid reminders or thoughts about the traumatic event, changes in emotions and thoughts, and signs of hyper-arousal; if it lasts more than a month, it is diagnosed as posttraumatic stress disorder.

adoptees method   Research method that studies children who were adopted and reared completely apart from their parents, thereby eliminating the influence of being raised by disordered parents.

age effects   The consequences of being a certain chronological age. Compare *cohort effects*.

agoraphobia   Anxiety disorder in which the person fears situations from which it would be embarrassing or difficult to escape if anxiety symptoms occurred; most commonly diagnosed in some individuals with panic disorder.

allele   Any of the various forms of a particular gene.

alogia   A negative symptom in schizophrenia, marked by diminished speaking.

alternate-form reliability   The extent to which a two version of a test, measurement, or classification system produce the same scientific observation.

Alzheimer's disease   A dementia involving a progressive atrophy of cortical tissue and marked by memory impairment, intellectual deterioration, and loss of motivation. See also *neurofibrillary tangles* and *plaques*.

American Law Institute guidelines   Guidelines for an insanity defense with two articles: (1) During criminal conduct, an individual could not judge right from wrong or control his or her behavior as required by law; and (2) repetitive criminal acts are disavowed as a sole criterion. Compare *M'Naghten rule* and *irresistible impulse*.

amphetamines   A group of stimulating drugs that produce heightened levels of energy and, in large doses, nervousness, sleeplessness, and paranoid delusions.

amygdala   A subcortical structure of the temporal lobe involved in processing emotionally salient stimuli.

analogue experiment   An experimental study of a phenomenon different from but related to the actual interests of the investigator; for example, animal research used to study human disorders or research on mild symptoms used as a bridge to clinical disorders.

anhedonia   A negative symptom in schizophrenia or a symptom in depression in which the individual experiences a loss of interest and pleasure. See also *anticipatory pleasure* and *consummatory pleasure*.

anorexia nervosa   An eating disorder in which a person restricts food to the extent that extreme weight loss results, fears gaining weight, and has a distorted body image.

anterior cingulate   In the subcortical region of the brain, the anterior portion of the cingulate gyrus, stretching around the corpus callosum.

anticipatory pleasure   Expected or anticipated pleasure for events, people, or activities in the future. Compare *consummatory pleasure*.

antidepressant   Any drug that alleviates depression; also widely used to treat anxiety disorders.

antipsychotic drugs   Psychoactive drugs, such as thorazine or olanzapine, that reduce psychotic symptoms but have long-term side effects resembling symptoms of neurological diseases.

antisocial personality disorder (APD)   Personality disorder defined by the absence of concern for others' feelings or social norms and a pervasive pattern of rule breaking.

anxiety   An unpleasant feeling of distress and apprehension accompanied by increased physiological arousal. Anxiety can be assessed by self-report, by measuring physiological arousal, and by observing overt behavior.

anxiety disorders   Disorders characterized by excessive levels of fear or anxiety, including specific phobias, social anxiety disorder, panic disorder, generalized anxiety disorder, and agoraphobia.

Anxiety Sensitivity Index   A test that measures the extent to which people respond fearfully to changes in their bodily sensations and other signs of anxiety; predicts the degree to which unexplained physiological arousal leads to panic attacks.

anxiolytics   Medications, including antidepressants and benzodiazepines, used to treat anxiety disorders.

asociality   A negative symptom of schizophrenia marked by diminished interest in forming close relationships.

assisted outpatient treatment (AOT)   A form of civil commitment consistent with the principle of the least restrictive alternative, whereby the person is not hospitalized but rather is allowed to remain free in the community under legal/medical constraints that ensure, for example, that prescribed medication is taken and other treatment measures are observed.

asylums   Refuges established in Western Europe in the 15th century to confine and provide for people with mental illness; forerunners of the mental hospital.

ataque de nervios   A syndrome characterized by intense negative emotion, uncontrolled screaming or shouting, trembling, aggression, and physical sensations, usually in response to a major stressor. Most common among people from Latino cultures.

attention-deficit/hyperactivity disorder (ADHD)   A disorder in children marked by difficulties in focusing adaptively on the task at hand, inappropriate fidgeting and impulsivity, and excessive non-goal-directed behavior.

attributional style   Trait-like tendency to make a certain type of attribution for life events.

attributions   The explanations a person forms for why an event occurred.

atypical anorexia nervosa   This disorder is categorized in the DSM-5-TR as a manifestation of "Other Specified

Feeding or Eating Disorder (OSFED)." It includes all the symptoms of anorexia nervosa except for very low body weight.

autism spectrum disorder A disorder beginning in childhood that involves deficits in social communication and social interactions, repetitive and ritualistic behaviors, and in some cases severe deficits in speech. DSM-5 combined Asperger's disorder and autistic disorder into this category.

autonomic nervous system (ANS) The division of the nervous system that regulates involuntary functions; innervates endocrine glands, smooth muscle, and heart muscle; and initiates the physiological changes that are part of the expression of emotion. See also *sympathetic* and *parasympathetic nervous systems.*

avoidant personality disorder Personality disorder defined by aloofness and extreme sensitivity to potential rejection, despite desire for affiliation and affection.

avolition A negative symptom in schizophrenia in which the individual has diminished motivation or drive.

behavioral activation (BA) therapy Clinical approach to depression that seeks to increase participation in positively reinforcing activities.

behavioral inhibition The tendency to exhibit anxiety or to freeze when facing threat. In infants, it manifests as a tendency to become agitated and cry when faced with novel stimuli; may be a heritable predisposition for the development of anxiety disorders.

behavior genetics The study of individual differences in behavior that are attributable to differences in genetic makeup.

behaviorism An approach originally associated with John B. Watson, who proposed a focus on observable behavior rather than on consciousness or mental functioning.

benzodiazepines Medications that effect the neurotransmitter gamma-aminobutyric acid (GABA) that are commonly prescribed for anxiety disorders. Common examples are alprazolam (Xanax), lorazepam (Ativan), diazepam (Valium). Not recommended as the first-line approach to anxiety disorders due to side effects and risk of dependence.

Big Five Inventory-2 (BFI-2) A personality inventory that assesses five broad domains of personality: openness, conscientiousness, extraversion, agreeableness, and neuroticism.

binge eating disorder An eating disorder first included as a diagnosis in DSM-5; involves recurrent episodes of unrestrained eating.

biological arousal In the context of sexuality, increased blood flow to the genitalia.

bipolar I disorder A diagnosis defined on the basis of at least one lifetime episode of mania. Most people with this disorder also experience episodes of major depression.

bipolar II disorder A form of bipolar disorder diagnosed in those who have experienced at least one major depressive episode and at least one episode of hypomania.

blunted affect A negative symptom of schizophrenia that involves diminished outward expression of emotion.

body dysmorphic disorder (BDD) A disorder marked by preoccupation with one or more imagined or exaggerated defects in appearance—for example, facial wrinkles or excess facial or body hair.

body mass index (BMI) Measure of body fat calculated by dividing weight in kilograms by height in meters squared; considered a more valid estimate of body fat than many others.

BOLD (blood oxygenation level dependent) The signal detected by functional MRI studies of the brain; measures blood flow and thus neural activity in any given region.

borderline personality disorder (BPD) Personality disorder defined by impulsiveness and unpredictability, an uncertain self-image, intense and unstable social relationships, and extreme swings of mood.

brain networks Clusters of brain regions that are connected to one another, as indicated by correlations between activation in these regions when people perform certain types of tasks or are at rest.

brief psychotic disorder A disorder in which a person has a sudden onset of psychotic symptoms—incoherence, loose associations, delusions, hallucinations— immediately after a severely disturbing event; the symptoms last more than 1 day but no more than 1 month. Compare *schizophreniform disorder.*

bulimia nervosa An eating disorder characterized by episodic, uncontrollable eating binges followed by purging, either by vomiting or by taking laxatives.

caffeine Perhaps the world's most popular drug; a generalized stimulant of body systems, including the sympathetic nervous system. Though seldom viewed as a drug, caffeine is addictive, produces tolerance, and induces withdrawal symptoms in habitual users upon cessation of use.

case study The collection of historical or biographical information on a single individual, often including experiences in therapy.

catatonia Constellation of schizophrenia symptoms including repetitive, peculiar, complex gestures and, in some cases, an almost manic increase in overall activity level. It can also manifest itself as immobility, with a fixed posture maintained for long periods, with accompanying muscular rigidity and trancelike state of consciousness.

categorical classification An approach to assessment in which a person is or is not a member of a discrete grouping. Compare *dimensional diagnostic system.*

caudate nucleus A nucleus within the basal ganglia that is involved in learning and memory and is implicated in body dysmorphic disorder and obsessive-compulsive disorder.

chorea Involuntary movements, as shown in Huntington's disease, which usually are brief, are not rhythmic, and flow from one muscle to the next.

circadian rhythms Twenty-four-hour biological rhythms that guide activity, alertness, and body functions.

civil commitment A procedure whereby a person can be legally certified as mentally ill and dangerous and then hospitalized, even against their will. Compare *criminal commitment* and *assisted outpatient treatment.*

classical conditioning A basic form of learning, sometimes referred to as Pavlovian conditioning, in which a neutral stimulus is repeatedly paired with another stimulus (called the unconditioned stimulus, UCS) that naturally elicits a certain desired response (called the unconditioned response, UCR). After repeated trials, the neutral stimulus becomes a conditioned stimulus (CS) and evokes the same or a similar response, now called the conditioned response (CR). Compare *operant conditioning.*

clinical high-risk study A study that identifies people who show subtle or early clinical signs of a disorder, such as schizophrenia, and then follows them over time to determine who might be at risk for developing the disorder.

clinical interview   General term for conversation between a clinician and a patient that is aimed at determining diagnosis, history, causes of problems, and possible treatment options. In a structured clinical interview, the clinician uses a standardized set of questions.

clinical psychologist   An individual who has earned a Ph.D. degree or a Psy.D. degree and whose training has included an internship in a hospital or clinic.

clinical significance   The degree to which effect size is large enough to be meaningful in predicting or treating a clinical disorder. Compare *statistical significance*.

clock genes   Genetic polymorphisms that influence the strength and timing of circadian (day/night) rhythms

cocaine   A stimulating and addictive drug obtained from coca leaves that can increase attention, produce euphoria, and in large doses cause paranoia and hallucinations.

cognition   The process of knowing; the thinking, judging, reasoning, and planning activities of the human mind. Behavior is now often explained as depending on these processes.

cognitive behavior therapy (CBT)   Behavior therapy that incorporates theory and research on cognitive processes such as thoughts, perceptions, judgments, self-statements, and tacit assumptions; a blend of both the cognitive and behavioral approaches.

cognitive reserve   Intellectual capacity that allows a person to continue to think and function well despite high levels of beta-amyloid plaques or other dementia-related pathology in the brain.

cognitive restructuring   Any behavior therapy procedure that attempts to alter the manner in which a client thinks about life so that they change overt behavior and emotions.

cohort effects   The consequences of having been born in a given year and having grown up during a particular time period with characteristic challenges and opportunities. Compare *age effects*.

comorbidity   The co-occurrence of two disorders, as when a person has depression and social phobia.

competency to stand trial   A legal decision as to whether a person can participate meaningfully in their own defense by understanding the charges and assisting the attorney.

compulsion   The irresistible impulse to repeat an irrational act or thought over and over. Compare *obsession*.

concordance   As applied in behavior genetics, the similarity in psychiatric diagnosis or in other traits within a pair of twins or family members.

conditioned response (CR)   See *classical conditioning*.

conditioned stimulus (CS)   See *classical conditioning*.

conduct disorder   Pattern of extreme misconduct in childhood, such as theft, vandalism, lying, and callous behavior.

confidentiality   A principle observed by lawyers, doctors, religious leaders, psychologists, and psychiatrists which dictates that the contents of a professional and private relationship are not to be divulged to anyone else. See also *privileged communication*.

connectivity   The ways in which different brain regions are connected to one another and form networks. Structural connectivity refers to how different structures of the brain are connected via white matter. Functional connectivity refers to correlations between brain areas' blood oxygen level dependent (BOLD) signals measured with fMRI.

construct validity   The extent to which scores or ratings on an assessment instrument relate to other variables or behaviors in accordance with theory.

consummatory pleasure   Pleasure experienced in the moment or in the presence of a pleasurable stimulus. Compare *anticipatory pleasure*.

content validity   The extent to which a measure adequately samples the domain of interest.

contrast avoidance model   The theory that the chronic worry of GAD provides a functional advantage in reducing the volatility of negative emotions and psychophysiological arousal in response to severe stress.

control group   Those for whom the active condition of the independent variable is not administered, thus forming a baseline against which the effects of the active condition of the independent variable can be evaluated.

copy number variation (CNV)   Refers to variation in gene structure involving copy number changes in a defined chromosomal region; could be in the form of a deletion where a copy is deleted or an addition (duplication) where an extra copy is added.

correlation   The tendency for two variables, such as height and weight, to covary.

correlation coefficient   A statistic that provides an index of the strength and direction of a linear relationship between two variables; a correlation coefficient of .00 indicates no relationship, +1.00 indicates a perfect positive relationship, and −1.00 indicates a perfect negative relationship.

correlational method   The research strategy used to establish whether two or more variables are related without manipulating the independent variable. Relationships may be positive—as values for one variable increase, those for the other do also—or negative—as values for one variable increase, those for the other decrease. Compare *experiment*.

cortico-striatal-thalamic-cortical (CSTC) loop   Neural circuitry linking cortical regions such as the orbitofrontal cortex and anterior cingulate cortex, the caudate nucleus and other parts of the striatum, and the thalamus, implicated in obsessive-compulsive and related disorders.

cortisol   A "stress hormone" secreted by the adrenal cortices; helps the body prepare to face threats.

counseling psychologists   Mental health professionals who work with people on relationships, life goals, improving coping and resilience, and other issues impacting well-being.

crack   A rock-crystal form of cocaine that is heated, melted, and smoked.

criminal commitment   A procedure whereby a person is confined in a mental hospital either for determination of competency to stand trial or after acquittal by reason of insanity. Compare *civil commitment*.

criterion validity   The extent to which test scores are related to scores on other tests that are designed to assess the same dimension.

cross-fostering   Research method that studies offspring who were adopted and reared completely apart from their biological parents, where the adoptive parent has a particular disorder but the biological parent does not, thereby introducing the influence of being raised by disordered parents.

cross-sectional design   Studies in which different age groups are compared at the same time. Compare *longitudinal design*.

cultural competence The capacity of a therapist to understand the patient's cultural framework and its implications for therapeutic work.

cultural concepts of distress Psychological syndromes that have been observed in specific cultural groups. Nine well-studied cultural concepts of distress are described in the appendix to DSM-5.

cyclothymic disorder A form of bipolar disorder characterized by swings between elation and depression over at least a 2-year period, but with mood changes not so severe as manic or major depressive episodes.

cytokines Proteins that help initiate bodily responses to infection.

defense mechanisms In Freud's theory, reality-distorting strategies unconsciously adopted to protect the ego from anxiety.

delayed ejaculation disorder A disorder in men involving persistent delay in reaching orgasm or inability to reach orgasm.

delirium A state of intense mental confusion in which consciousness is clouded, attention cannot be sustained, and the stream of thought and speech is incoherent. Symptoms can include disorientation; dramatic emotional shifts; restlessness or lethargy; and illusions, delusions, or hallucinations.

delirium tremens (DTs) One of the withdrawal symptoms that sometimes occurs when a period of heavy alcohol consumption is terminated; marked by fever, sweating, trembling, cognitive impairment, and hallucinations.

delusional disorder A disorder in which the individual has persistent delusions but has no disorganized thinking or hallucinations.

delusions Beliefs contrary to reality, firmly held despite evidence to the contrary: delusion of control, belief that one is being manipulated by some external force, such as a cell phone tower, TV, or creature from outer space; delusion of reference, belief that one can draw strong personal meaning from seemingly trivial remarks or activities of others and completely unrelated events; grandiose, exaggerated sense of one's importance, power, knowledge, or identity; thought insertion, belief that thoughts are being inserted into one's head; thought broadcasting, belief that thoughts are broadcast out loud so others can hear them; persecutory, belief that one is being plotted against or oppressed by others.

dementia Deterioration of cognitive abilities, such as memory, judgment, abstract thought, control of impulses, and intellectual ability, that impairs functioning. See *Alzheimer's disease, dementia with Lewy bodies, frontotemporal dementia, vascular dementia,* and *Huntington's disease.*

dementia with Lewy bodies (DLB) Form of dementia that often co-occurs with Parkinson's disease; characterized by shuffling gait, memory loss, and hallucinations and delusions.

dependent variable In a psychological experiment, the behavior or outcome that is measured and is expected to change with manipulation of the independent variable.

depersonalization An alteration in perception of the self in which the individual feels estranged from the self and perhaps separated from the body; may be a temporary reaction to stress and fatigue or part of panic disorder, depersonalization/ derealization disorder, or schizophrenia.

depersonalization/derealization disorder A DSM-5-TR disorder defined by the sense that one is detached from one's self and/or experiences one's surroundings as unreal.

derealization Loss of the sense that the surroundings are real; present in several psychological disorders, such as panic disorder, depersonalization/derealization disorder, and schizophrenia.

detoxification The initial stage in weaning an addicted person from a drug; can involve medical supervision of withdrawal.

developmental psychopathology The field that studies disorders of childhood within the context of development over the life span.

diagnosis The determination that the set of symptoms or problems of a patient indicates a particular disorder.

***Diagnostic and Statistical Manual of Mental Disorders*, 5th edition, Text Revision** Currently in its fifth edition, the *Diagnostic and Statistical Manual of Mental Disorders* provides the major diagnostic guidelines for mental health syndromes in the United States. Published by the American Psychiatric Association.

dialectical behavior therapy (DBT) A therapeutic approach to borderline personality disorder that combines client-centered empathy and acceptance with behavioral problem solving, social skills training, and limit setting.

dimensional diagnostic system A diagnostic system that describes the degree of an entity that is present (e.g., a 1-to-10 scale of anxiety, where 1 represents minimal and 10, extremely severe).

directionality problem A difficulty that arises in correlational research when it is known that two variables are related but it is unclear which is causing the other.

disorganized behavior Symptom of schizophrenia that is marked by odd behaviors that do not appear organized, such as bouts of agitation, unusual dress, or childlike, silly behavior.

disorganized speech Speech that is marked by poorly organized ideas and is difficult for others to understand; also known as *formal thought disorder.*

disorganized symptoms Broad category of symptoms in schizophrenia that includes disorganized behavior and disorganized speech.

disorientation A state of mental confusion with respect to time, place, and identity of self.

dissemination The process of facilitating adoption of efficacious treatments in the community, most typically by offering clinicians guidelines about the best available treatments along with training on how to conduct those treatments.

dissociation A symptom in which some aspect of emotion, memory, or experience is inaccessible consciously.

dissociative amnesia A dissociative disorder in which the person suddenly becomes unable to recall important personal information to an extent that cannot be explained by ordinary forgetfulness.

dissociative disorders Disorders in which the normal integration of consciousness, memory, or identity is suddenly and temporarily altered; include dissociative amnesia, dissociative identity disorder (multiple personality), and depersonalization/derealization disorder.

dissociative fugue subtype Subtype of dissociative amnesia in which the person experiences total amnesia, moves, and establishes a new identity.

dissociative identity disorder (DID) A rare dissociative disorder (formerly called *multiple personality disorder*) in which two or more distinct and separate personality states are present within the same individual, each with its own memories, relationships, and behavior patterns, with only one of them dominant at any given time.

dizygotic (DZ) twins   Twins who developed from separate fertilized eggs and who are only 50% alike genetically, just like siblings born from different pregnancies involving the same father. Also called *fraternal twins*. Compare *monozygotic twins*.

dopamine   Central nervous system neurotransmitter, a catecholamine that is also a precursor of norepinephrine and apparently figures in schizophrenia and Parkinson's disease.

dorsolateral prefrontal cortex   A region of the prefrontal cortex that is involved in working memory, motor planning, organization, and regulation. Atypical activation patterns are implicated in many psychopathologies.

double-blind procedure   A method for reducing the biasing effects of the expectations of research participant and experimenter; neither is allowed to know whether the independent variable of the experiment is being applied to the participant.

Down syndrome (trisomy 21)   A form of intellectual disability caused by trisomy 21 (having a third copy of chromosome 21); also involves distinctive physical characteristics.

dyslexia   A specific learning disorder involving significant difficulty with word recognition, reading fluency, and reading comprehension.

ecological momentary assessment (EMA)   Form of self-observation involving collection of data in real time (e.g., in a diary) regarding thoughts, moods, and stressors.

Ecstasy   A hallucinogen, chemically similar to mescaline and the amphetamines. Sometimes referred to as molly.

effectiveness   How well a therapeutic treatment works in the real world with broader samples seen by nonacademic, less supervised therapists. Compare *efficacy*.

efficacy   How well a therapeutic treatment works under rarified, academic research conditions. Compare *effectiveness*.

ego   In Freud's theory, the predominantly conscious part of the personality, responsible for decision making and for dealing with reality.

electroconvulsive therapy (ECT)   A treatment that produces a convulsion by passing electric current through the brain; despite public concerns about this treatment, it can be useful in alleviating severe depression for some people.

emotions   The expressions, experiences, and physiologies that guide responses to problems and challenges in the environment.

empirically supported treatments (ESTs)   Approaches whose efficacy has been demonstrated through research that meets standards for research on psychotherapy.

epidemiology   The study of the frequency and distribution of an illness or a disorder in a population.

epigenetics   The study of changes in gene expression that are caused by something other than changes in the DNA (gene) sequence or structure, such as DNA methylation.

episodic disorder   A condition, such as major depressive disorder, whose symptoms dissipate but that tends to recur.

erectile disorder   A disorder involving recurrent and persistent inability to attain an erection or maintain it until completion of sexual activity.

exhibitionistic disorder   A disorder involving a marked preference for obtaining sexual gratification by exposing one's genitals to an unwilling observer.

exorcism   The ritualistic casting out of evil spirits.

experiment   The most powerful research technique for determining causal relationships; involves the manipulation of an independent variable, the measurement of a dependent variable, and the random assignment of participants to the several different conditions being investigated. Compare *correlational method*.

experimental effect   A statistically significant difference between two groups assigned to different conditions of the independent variable.

explicit memory   Memory involving the conscious recall of experiences; the area of deficits typically seen in dissociative amnesia. Compare *implicit memory*.

exposure and response prevention (ERP)   The most widely used and accepted treatment of obsessive-compulsive disorder and related disorders, in which the sufferer is prevented from engaging in compulsive ritual activity and instead faces the anxiety provoked by the stimulus, leading eventually to extinction of the conditioned response (anxiety).

exposure   Real-life (in vivo) or imaginal confrontation of a feared object or situation, especially as a component of systematic desensitization.

expressed emotion (EE)   Hostility, criticism, and emotional overinvolvement directed from family members toward a person with a psychological disorder.

externalizing disorders   Psychological disorders characterized by outward-directed behaviors, such as aggressiveness, noncompliance, excessive activity, and impulsiveness; the category includes alcohol and substance use disorder, attention-deficit/hyperactivity disorder, conduct disorder, oppositional defiant disorder, and antisocial personality disorder. Compare *internalizing disorders*.

external validity   The extent to which the results of a study can be considered generalizable.

extinction   The elimination of a classically conditioned response by the omission of the unconditioned stimulus. In operant conditioning, the elimination of a behavior by the omission of reinforcement.

factitious disorder   Disorder in which the individual's physical or psychological symptoms appear under voluntary control and are adopted merely to assume the role of a sick person; called *factitious disorder imposed on another*, or *Munchausen syndrome by proxy*, when a parent produces a physical illness in a child.

familial high-risk study   A study involving the offspring of people with a disorder, such as schizophrenia, who have a high probability of later developing a disorder.

family method   A research strategy in behavior genetics in which the frequency of a trait or of abnormal behavior is determined in relatives who have varying percentages of shared genes.

fear   A reaction to real or perceived immediate danger in the present; can involve arousal, or sympathetic nervous system activity.

fear circuit   Set of brain structures, including the amygdala, that tend to be activated when the individual is feeling anxious or fearful; especially active among people with anxiety disorders; this label has been criticized, as the same brain structures are involved in processing many different emotion-related experiences.

female orgasmic disorder A recurrent and persistent delay or absence of orgasm in a woman during sexual activity that is adequate in focus, intensity, and duration; in many instances, the woman may experience considerable sexual excitement.

female sexual interest/arousal disorder A DSM-5-TR disorder defined by prolonged absence of sexual desire, subjective arousal, or biological arousal.

fetal alcohol syndrome (FAS) Disrupted growth of the developing fetus and infant involving cranial, facial, and limb anomalies as well as intellectual disabilities; caused by heavy consumption of alcohol by the mother during pregnancy.

flashbacks An unpredictable recurrence of experiences from an earlier drug high.

flight of ideas A symptom of mania that involves rapidly shifting thoughts, manifested in a conversation style in which a person shifts rapidly from one topic to another with only superficial associative connections.

forensic psychologist A forensic psychologist works on issues involving psychology in legal contexts (Neal, 2018), including conducting assessments of competency to stand trial or evaluations for insanity pleas. Forensic psychologists may also provide interventions for persons in prisons or forensic hospitals; testify in child custody evaluations, or help with the selection of law enforcement applicants.

fragile X syndrome Malformation (or even breakage) of the X chromosome, associated with intellectual disability; physical symptoms include large, underdeveloped ears and a long, thin face.

frontotemporal dementia (FTD) Dementia that begins typically in the mid- to late 50s and that involves loss of neurons in the frontal and temporal lobes. The behavioral variant is characterized by deficits in executive functions such as planning, problem solving, and goal-directed behavior as well as recognition and comprehension of emotions in others. Compare *Alzheimer's disease*.

frotteuristic disorder A disorder in which the person gains sexual gratification by sexually touching an unsuspecting person, typically in public places that provide an easy means of escape.

functional communication training (FCT) A behavioral intervention for children and adults with intellectual disability where a problem behavior's function is identified and it is replaced, through shaping and reinforcement, with a more socially appropriate behavior.

functional magnetic resonance imaging (fMRI) Modification of *magnetic resonance imaging (MRI)* that allows researchers to take pictures of the brain so quickly that metabolic changes can be measured, resulting in a picture of the brain at work rather than of its structure alone.

functional neurological symptom disorder A disorder in which sensory or motor function is impaired, even though there is no detectable neurological explanation for the deficits.

gamma-aminobutyric acid (GABA) Inhibitory neurotransmitter that may be involved in the anxiety disorders.

gene expression The switching on and off of the reading (transcription and translation) of genes to form their products (usually proteins) and thus their associated phenotypes.

gene–environment interaction The influence of genetics on an individual's sensitivity or reaction to an environmental event.

generalized anxiety disorder (GAD) Disorder characterized by chronic, persistent worry.

genes The smallest portion of DNA within a chromosome that functions as a piece of functional hereditary information.

genito-pelvic pain/penetration disorder A disorder in which a woman persistently experiences pain or vaginal muscle spasms when intercourse is attempted.

genome-wide association studies (GWAS) Studies of variations in the entire human genome to identify associations of genetic variants with particular behaviors, traits, or disorders. Large sample sizes are needed for these types of studies.

genotype An individual's genetic constitution, that is, the totality of genes present in the cells of an individual; often applied to the genes contributing to a single trait. Compare *phenotype*.

ghost sickness A cultural concept of distress defined by an extreme preoccupation with death and those who have died, found among certain Native American tribes.

gray matter The neural tissue—made up largely of nerve cell bodies—that constitutes the cortex covering the cerebral hemisphere, the nuclei in lower brain areas, columns of the spinal cord, and the ganglia of the autonomic nervous system. Compare *white matter*.

guilty but mentally ill (GBMI) Insanity plea in which a mentally ill person can be held morally and legally responsible for a crime but can then, in theory, be sent to a prison hospital or other suitable facility for psychiatric treatment rather than to a regular prison for punishment. In reality, however, people judged GBMI are usually put in the general prison population, where they may or may not receive treatment. Compare *not guilty by reason of insanity (NGRI)*.

hallucinations Perceptions in any sensory modality without relevant and adequate external stimuli.

hallucinogen A drug or chemical, such as LSD, psilocybin, or mescaline, whose effects include hallucinations; often called a psychedelic.

heritability The extent to which variability in a behavior/disorder within a population can be attributed to genetic influences.

heroin An addictive narcotic drug derived from morphine.

high-risk method A research technique involving the intensive examination of people, such as the offspring of people with schizophrenia, who have a high probability of later developing a disorder.

hikikomori A syndrome involving severe withdrawal, most commonly observed among adolescent or young adult males in Japan, Taiwan, or South Korea.

hippocampus In the subcortical region of the brain, the long, tubelike structure that stretches from the septal area into the temporal lobe.

HiTOP model An approach to diagnosis that is based on research data regarding overlap in symptoms and syndromes (https://renaissance.stonybrookmedicine.edu/HITOP/AboutHiTOP).

hoarding disorder A disorder involving compulsive need to acquire objects and extreme difficulty in disposing of those objects.

hopelessness theory Cognitive theory that focuses on hopelessness as a major influence of depression—an expectation that desirable outcomes will not occur and that no available responses can change the situation.

HPA axis The neuroendocrine connections among hypothalamus, pituitary gland, and adrenal cortex, central to the body's response to stress.

Huntington's disease An autosomal dominant form of dementia characterized by symptoms of chorea, memory loss, and other cognitive symptoms.

hydrocodone   An opiate combined with other drugs such as acetaminophen to produce prescription pain medications, including the commonly abused drug Vicodin. See also *oxycodone*.

hypomania   An extremely happy or irritable mood accompanied by symptoms such as increased energy and decreased need for sleep, but without the significant functional impairment associated with mania.

hypothalamus   In the subcortical region of the brain, the structure that regulates many visceral processes, including metabolism, temperature, perspiration, blood pressure, sleeping, and appetite.

hypothesis   Specific expectation or prediction about what should occur or be found if a theory is true or valid.

iatrogenic   Inadvertently induced by treatment.

id   In Freud's theory, that part of the personality present at birth, comprising all the energy of the psyche and expressed as biological urges that strive continually for gratification.

illness anxiety disorder   A disorder defined by excessive concern and help seeking about health concerns in the absence of major physical symptoms.

imaginal exposure   Treatment for anxiety disorders and posttraumatic stress disorder that involves visualizing feared scenes for extended periods of time. Frequently used in the treatment of posttraumatic stress disorder when in vivo exposure to the initial trauma cannot be conducted.

implicit memory   Memory that underlies behavior but is based on experiences that cannot be consciously recalled; typically not compromised in cases of dissociative amnesia. Compare *explicit memory*.

incest   Sexual relations between close relatives, most often between daughter and father or between brother and sister.

incidence   In epidemiological studies of a particular disorder, the rate at which new cases occur in a given place at a given time. Compare *prevalence*.

independent variable   In a psychological experiment, the factor, experience, or treatment that is under the control of the experimenter and that is expected to have an effect on the dependent variable.

index case   The person who in a genetic investigation bears the diagnosis or trait in which the investigator is interested. Also termed proband.

information-processing biases   Tendencies to perceive events in a negative manner, for example, by attending to or remembering negative information more than positive information; hypothesized to be driven by underlying negative schemas.

informed consent   The agreement of a person to serve as a research participant or to enter therapy after being told the possible outcomes, both benefits and risks.

insanity defense   The legal argument that a defendant should not be held responsible for an illegal act if the conduct is attributable to mental illness. See also *guilty but mentally ill (GBMI)* and *not guilty by reason of insanity (NGRI)*.

intellectual disability   A disorder identified in early childhood characterized by below-average intellectual functioning associated with impairment in adaptive behavior.

intelligence test   A standardized means of assessing a person's current mental ability; for example, the Stanford-Binet test or the Wechsler Adult Intelligence Scale.

internal consistency reliability   The extent to which items on a test are related to one another.

internalizing disorders   Disorders characterized by inward-focused experiences and behaviors, such as depression, social withdrawal, and anxiety; the category includes anxiety and mood disorders. Compare *externalizing disorders*.

internal validity   The extent to which the experimental effect can be attributed confidently to the independent variable.

interoceptive conditioning   Classical conditioning of panic attacks in response to internal bodily sensations of arousal (as opposed to the external situations that trigger anxiety).

interpersonal therapy (IPT)   A short-term, here-and-now-focused psychological treatment initially developed for depression and influenced by the psychodynamic emphasis on relationships.

inter-rater reliability   The extent to which a test, measurement, or classification system produces the same scientific observation each time it is applied.

in vivo (real-life) exposure   As applied in exposure treatment, taking place in a real-life situation.

irresistible impulse   The term used in an 1834 Ohio court ruling on criminal responsibility, which determined that an insanity defense can be established by proving that the accused had an uncontrollable urge to perform the act.

joint attention   A shared focus by two people on each other when speaking or communicating emotion nonverbally. This is impaired in children with autism spectrum disorder.

khyâl cap   A syndrome characterized by symptoms similar to those of panic attacks that are triggered by a belief that a windlike substance is rising in the body. Observed in Southeast Asian groups.

law of effect   A principle of learning that holds that behavior is acquired by virtue of its consequences.

least restrictive alternative   The legal principle according to which a hospitalized person must be treated in a setting that imposes as few restrictions as possible on their freedom.

lithium   A medication useful in treating both mania and depression in bipolar disorder.

locus coeruleus   A brain region that is especially important in panic disorder; the major source in the brain of norepinephrine, which helps trigger sympathetic nervous system activity.

longitudinal design   Investigation that collects information on the same individuals repeatedly over time, perhaps over many years, in an effort to determine how phenomena change or how baseline variables predict outcomes across time. Compare *cross-sectional design*.

loose associations (derailment)   In schizophrenia, an aspect of disorganized thinking wherein the patient has difficulty sticking to one topic and drifts off on a train of associations evoked by an idea from the past.

LSD   *d*-lysergic acid diethylamide, a drug synthesized in 1938 and discovered by accident to be a hallucinogen in 1943.

magnetic resonance imaging (MRI)   A technique for measuring the structure (or, in the case of *functional magnetic resonance imaging*, the activity) of the living brain or body. The person is placed inside a large circular magnet that causes hydrogen atoms to change alignment; the return of the atoms to their original alignments when the current to the magnet is turned off is translated by a computer into pictures of brain tissue.

major depressive disorder (MDD)   An episodic disorder marked by sadness or anhedonia, along with symptoms such as feelings of worthlessness and guilt; withdrawal from others; loss of sleep, appetite, or sexual desire; and either lethargy or agitation.

male hypoactive sexual desire disorder A sexual dysfunction disorder defined by persistent absence of or deficiency in sexual fantasies and urges in men.

malingering Faking a physical or psychological incapacity to avoid a responsibility or gain an end, where the goal is readily recognized from the individual's circumstances; distinct from functional neurological symptom disorder, in which the incapacity is assumed to be beyond voluntary control.

mania Intense elation or irritability, accompanied by symptoms such as excessive talkativeness, rapid thoughts, distractibility, grandiose plans, heightened activity, and insensitivity to the negative consequences of actions.

marijuana A drug derived from the dried and ground leaves and stems of the hemp plant *Cannabis sativa*.

MDMA Methylenedioxymethamphetamine, a chemical component of Ecstasy.

means restriction An approach to suicide prevention in which access to lethal methods is reduced. Examples include keeping guns locked in cabinets, reducing the unrestricted sale of poisons, and erecting suicide barriers on bridges.

medial prefrontal cortex A region of the cortex in the anterior frontal lobes involved in executive function and emotion regulation that is implicated in mood and anxiety disorders.

mentalization-based therapy A therapeutic approach to borderline personality disorder that draws from psychodynamic and cognitive behavioral approaches to help people be more reflective about their own feelings and those of other people.

meta-analysis A quantitative method of analyzing the results of a set of studies on a topic, by standardizing the results.

methamphetamine An amphetamine derivative that is highly addictive.

mild cognitive impairment (MCI) Decline in cognitive ability that is not severe enough to cause functional impairment or to interfere with activities of daily living.

mindfulness-based cognitive therapy (MBCT) Adaptation of cognitive therapy for major depression; aims to "decenter" the person's perspective in order to break the cycle between sadness and thinking patterns.

MMPI-3 A personality inventory to assess anxiety, depression, paranoia, and other psychological dimensions, using true/false items.

M'Naghten rule An 1843 British court decision that stated that an insanity defense can be established by proving that the defendant did not know what he or she was doing or did not realize that it was wrong.

modeling Learning by observing and imitating the behavior of others or teaching by demonstrating and providing opportunities for imitation.

molecular genetics Studies that seek to determine the components of a trait that are heritable by identifying relevant genes and their functions.

monoamine oxidase inhibitors (MAOIs) A group of antidepressant drugs that prevent the enzyme monoamine oxidase from deactivating catecholamines and indolamines.

monozygotic (MZ) twins Genetically identical twins who developed from a single fertilized egg. Compare *dizygotic twins*.

mood disorders Disorders, such as depressive disorders or bipolar disorders, in which there are disabling disturbances in emotion.

moral treatment A therapeutic regimen whereby mentally ill patients were released from their restraints and were treated with compassion and dignity rather than with contempt and denigration.

Mowrer's two-factor model Mowrer's theory of conditioning according to which (1) fear is attached to a neutral stimulus by pairing it with a noxious unconditioned stimulus, and (2) a person learns to avoid the conditioned stimulus and so extinction of the conditioning is prevented.

multisystemic treatment (MST) Treatment for conduct disorder that involves delivering intensive and comprehensive therapy services in the community, targeting the adolescent, the family, the school, and, in some cases, the peer group, in ecologically valid settings and using varied techniques.

narcissistic personality disorder Personality disorder defined by extreme self-centeredness; a grandiose view of one's uniqueness, achievements, and talents; an insatiable craving for admiration and approval from others; willingness to exploit others to achieve goals; and expectation of much more from others than one is willing to give in return.

negative reinforcement The strengthening of a tendency to exhibit desired behavior by rewarding responses in that situation with the removal of an aversive stimulus.

negative symptoms Behavioral deficits in schizophrenia, which include blunted affect, anhedonia, asociality, alogia, and avolition. Compare *positive symptoms*.

negative triad In Beck's theory of depression, a person's negative views of the self, the world, and the future, in a reciprocal causal relationship with pessimistic assumptions (schemas) and cognitive biases such as selective abstraction.

NEO Personality Inventory (NEO-PI) A personality scale designed to assess the big five personality dimensions of openness to experience, neuroticism, extraversion, agreeableness, and neuroticism. In 2005, the third edition of the NEO-PI was published.

neurofibrillary tangles Abnormal protein filaments present in the axons of brain cells in patients with Alzheimer's disease.

neuron A single nerve cell.

neuropsychological tests Psychological tests, such as the Luria-Nebraska battery, that can detect impairment in different parts of the brain.

neuroticism The tendency to react to events with more frequent or greater-than-average negative affect; a strong predictor of onset of anxiety disorders and depression.

neurotransmitters Chemical substances important in transferring a nerve impulse from one neuron to another, for example, serotonin and norepinephrine.

neutral predictable unpredictable (NPU) threat task A laboratory task designed to test sensitivity to unpredictable versus predictable threats. Participants are exposed to threat conditions in which they could receive a shock. In the predictable threat condition, there is a cue warning when the shock will occur. In the unpredictable threat condition, there is no cue warning when the shock will occur.

nicotine The principal component of tobacco that is addicting.

N-methyl D-aspartate (NMDA) receptor antagonists Antidepressant medications recently approved by the FDA that have shown rapid benefits in relieving depression within days to weeks. Auvelity is an oral antidepressant; Esketamine (Spravato) is a nasal spray that was approved only for patients who did not obtain relief after trying two other antidepressants.

nonshared environment Factors distinct among family members, such as relationships with friends or specific experiences unique to a person. Compare *shared environment*.

nonsuicidal self-injury (NSSI) Behaviors that are meant to cause immediate bodily harm but are not intended to cause death.

norepinephrine A catecholamine neurotransmitter, disturbances of which have been related to mania, depression, and particularly anxiety disorders. It is also a sympathetic nervous system neurotransmitter, a hormone released in addition to epinephrine and similar in action, and a strong vasoconstrictor.

not guilty by reason of insanity (NGRI) Insanity plea that specifies an individual is not to be held legally responsible for the crime because the person had a mental illness at the time of the crime. State laws and federal law have different standards for defining *mental illness* and specifying what must be demonstrated by the defense. In most cases, the defense must show that because of the mental illness, the accused person could not conform his or her behavior to the law and did not know right from wrong when the crime was committed. Compare *guilty but mentally ill (GBMI)*.

obese Currently defined as exhibiting a body mass index (BMI) greater than 30.

obsession An intrusive and recurring thought that seems irrational and uncontrollable to the person experiencing it. Compare *compulsion*.

obsessive-compulsive disorder (OCD) A disorder involving persistent and uncontrollable thoughts and/or the performance of certain acts again and again, causing significant distress and interference with everyday functioning.

obsessive-compulsive personality disorder Personality disorder defined by inordinate difficulty with making decisions, extreme concern with details and efficiency, and poor relations with others due to demands that things be done just so, as well as the person's unduly conventional, serious, formal, and stingy emotions.

operant conditioning The acquisition or elimination of a response as a function of the environmental contingencies of reinforcement and punishment. Compare *classical conditioning*.

opioids A group of addictive sedatives that in moderate doses relieve pain and induce sleep.

orbitofrontal cortex The portion of the frontal lobe located just above the eyes; one of the brain regions that is unusually active in individuals with obsessive-compulsive disorder when symptoms are induced during functional brain imaging.

orgasm A peak of sexual pleasure, generally including ejaculation in men and contraction of the outer vaginal walls in women.

oxycodone An opiate combined with other drugs to produce prescription pain medications, including the commonly abused drug OxyContin. See also *hydrocodone*.

panic attack A sudden experience of intense apprehension, terror, and impending doom, accompanied by symptoms such as labored breathing, nausea, chest pain, feelings of choking and smothering, heart palpitations, dizziness, sweating, and trembling.

panic disorder An anxiety disorder in which the individual has sudden, inexplicable, and frequent panic attacks, and then fears the possibility of another panic attack. See also *panic attack*.

paraphilic disorders Disorders whose core feature is sexual attraction to unusual objects or unusual sexual activities that leads to social difficulties or distress.

parasympathetic nervous system The division of the autonomic nervous system that is involved with maintenance; controls many of the internal organs and is active primarily when the organism is not aroused. Compare *sympathetic nervous system*.

parent management training (PMT) Behavioral program in which parents are taught to modify their responses to their children so that prosocial rather than antisocial behavior is consistently rewarded.

PCP Phencyclidine, also known by names such as angel dust and zombie. This very powerful and hazardous drug causes profound disorientation; agitated and often violent behavior; and even seizures, coma, and death.

pedophilic disorder A paraphilic disorder defined by a sexual attraction to prepubescent children; the person has either acted on the urges or the urges create distress or dysfunction.

penile plethysmograph A device for detecting blood flow and thereby recording changes in the size of the penis.

persistent depressive disorder A DSM-5-TR disorder defined by depressive symptoms that last at least 2 years in adults or 1 year in youths.

personality disorders A group of disorders involving long-standing, inflexible, and maladaptive personality traits that impair functioning.

personality trait domains Five personality dimensions included in Section III of the DSM-5-TR manual to help supplement diagnoses of personality disorders: negative affectivity, detachment, antagonism, disinhibition, and psychoticism.

personality trait facets Narrow personality dimensions, such as anxiousness, emotional lability, hostility, perseveration, separation insecurity, and submissiveness within the broader trait of negative affectivity. See *personality trait domains*.

PET scan Computer-generated picture of the living brain, created by analysis of emissions from radioactive isotopes injected into the bloodstream.

p-hacking A problematic research practice in which researchers run multiple types of analyses in their quest to identify a significant result.

phenotype The totality of physical characteristics and behavioral traits of an individual or of a particular trait exhibited by an individual; the product of interactions between genetics and the environment over the course of development. Compare *genotype*.

phenylketonuria (PKU) A genetic deficiency in a liver enzyme, phenylalanine hydroxylase, that causes severe intellectual disability unless phenylalanine can be largely restricted from the diet.

placebo Any inactive therapy or chemical agent, or any attribute or component of such a therapy or chemical, that affects a person's behavior for reasons related to his or her expectation of change.

placebo effect The action of a drug or psychological treatment that is not attributable to any specific operations of the agent. For example, a tranquilizer can reduce anxiety both because of its special biochemical action and because the recipient expects relief. See also *placebo*.

plaques Small, round deposits of beta-amyloid protein; present in the brains of patients with Alzheimer's disease.

polygenic As applied to psychopathology or any other trait, caused by multiple genes contributing their effects, typically during multiple stages of development.

polygenic risk score A statistical method that adds up the number of SNPs a person has that are associated with a psychological disorder that also takes into account the effect size of the SNP in GWAS and the associations of the SNPs with other genetic loci.

polymorphism Any specific difference in DNA sequence that exists within a population.

positive reinforcement The strengthening of a tendency to exhibit desired behavior by rewarding responses in that situation with a desired reward.

positive symptoms Behavioral excesses in schizophrenia, such as hallucinations and delusions. Compare *negative symptoms*.

posttraumatic model (of DID) Etiological model of dissociative identity disorder that assumes the condition begins in childhood as a result of severe physical or sexual abuse. Compare *sociocognitive model (of DID)*.

posttraumatic stress disorder (PTSD) An anxiety disorder in which a particularly stressful event, such as military combat, rape, or a natural disaster, brings in its aftermath intrusive reexperiencing of the trauma, a desire to avoid reminders of the event, changes in emotions and thought patterns, and indicators of heightened arousal.

prefrontal cortex A region of the cortex in the anterior frontal lobes involved in executive function and emotion regulation that is implicated in mood and anxiety disorders, particularly in the medial (middle) regions.

premature (early) ejaculation Inability of the male to inhibit his orgasm long enough for mutually satisfying sexual relations.

prepared learning In classical conditioning theory, a biological predisposition to rapidly learn fears to evolutionarily relevant stimuli (such as dangerous animals).

prevalence In epidemiological studies of a disorder, the percentage of a population that has the disorder at a given time. Compare *incidence*.

privileged communication The communication between parties in a confidential relationship that is protected by statute, which a spouse, doctor, lawyer, religious leader, psychologist, or psychiatrist thus cannot be forced to disclose, except under unusual circumstances.

proband The person who in a genetic investigation bears the diagnosis or trait in which the investigator is interested.

pruning In neural development, the selective loss of synaptic connections, especially in the fine-tuning of brain regions devoted to sensory processing.

psilocybin A psychedelic drug that acts primarily on the serotonin system. It is the active chemical in "magic mushrooms." Although still considered a Schedule 1 (illegal) drug, there is growing evidence to suggest it may be effective for treating some people with anxiety or depression.

psychiatric nurse A nurse who receives specialized training in mental illness. An advanced practice psychiatric nurse may prescribe psychiatric medications.

psychiatrist A physician (M.D.) who completes medical training and also specialized postdoctoral training, called a *residency*, in the diagnosis, treatment, and prevention of psychological disorders.

psychoanalysis Primarily the therapy procedures pioneered by Freud, entailing free association, dream analysis, and working through transference. The term can also refer to the numerous variations on basic Freudian therapy.

psychoeducation Especially with bipolar disorder and schizophrenia, intervention to help people learn about symptoms, expected time course, triggers for symptoms, and treatment strategies.

psychological disorder The DSM-5 defines psychological disorder as a clinically significant behavioral or psychological syndrome or pattern. The definition includes a number of key features, including distress, disability or impaired functioning, violation of social norms, and dysfunction.

psychomotor agitation A symptom characterized by pacing, restlessness, or inability to sit still.

psychomotor retardation A symptom commonly observed in major depressive disorder in which the person moves their limbs and body slowly.

psychopathology The field concerned with the nature, development, and treatment of psychological disorders.

psychopathy A personality syndrome related to antisocial personality disorder but defined by unemotionality, impulsivity, manipulativeness, and irresponsibility.

psychotherapy A primarily verbal means of helping troubled individuals change their thoughts, feelings, and behavior to reduce distress and to achieve greater life satisfaction.

publication bias The tendency not to publish findings that do not support hypotheses.

questionable research practices Selective presentation of analyses that support one's hypotheses while not disclosing analyses that fail to confirm hypotheses. Believed to contribute to nonreproducibility of findings.

random assignment A method of assigning people to groups by chance (e.g., using a flip of a coin). The procedure helps to ensure that groups are comparable before the experimental manipulation begins.

randomized controlled trials (RCTs) Experiments designed to assess treatment outcomes in which clients are randomly assigned to receive either active treatment or a comparison (a placebo condition involving no treatment or an active-treatment control group that receives another treatment); the independent variable is the treatment type and the dependent variable is client outcome.

reliability The extent to which a test, measurement, or classification system produces the same scientific observation each time it is applied. Reliability types include *test–retest*, the relationship between the scores that a person achieves when he or she takes the same test twice; *inter-rater*, the relationship between the judgments that at least two raters make independently about a phenomenon; *split-half*, the relationship between two halves of an assessment instrument that have been determined to be equivalent; *alternate-form*, the relationship between scores achieved by people when they complete two versions of a test that are judged to be equivalent; and *internal consistency*, the degree to which different items of an assessment are related to one another.

replication Duplication by a research study of the findings of a previous study.

Research Domain Criteria A long-term project by the National Institute of Mental Health to develop new ways of classifying psychological disorders based on behavioral and neurobiological dimensions related to risk for psychopathology.

reuptake Cellular process by which released neurotransmitters are taken back into the presynaptic cell, terminating their present postsynaptic effect but making them available for subsequent modulation of nerve impulse transmission.

reversal design See *ABAB design*.

rumination Repetitive thought about why a person is experiencing a negative mood or sad events.

safety behaviors   Behaviors used to avoid experiencing anxiety in feared situations, such as the tendency of people with social phobia to avoid looking at other people (so as to avoid perceiving negative feedback) or the tendency of people with panic disorder to avoid exercise (so as to avoid somatic arousal that could trigger a panic attack).

schema   A mental structure for organizing information about the world.

schizoaffective disorder   Diagnosis involving either a depressive or a manic episode and symptoms of schizophrenia.

schizophrenia   A disorder characterized by disturbances in thought, emotion, and behavior; disordered thinking in which ideas are not logically related; delusional beliefs; faulty perception, such as hallucinations; disturbances in attention; disturbances in motor activity; blunted expression of emotion; reduced desire for interpersonal relations and withdrawal from people; and diminished motivation and anticipatory pleasure. See also *schizoaffective disorder, schizophreniform disorder,* and *brief psychotic disorder.*

schizophreniform disorder   Diagnosis given to people who have all the symptoms of schizophrenia for only 1 to 6 months. Compare *brief psychotic disorder.*

schizotypal personality disorder Personality disorder defined by eccentric behavior, odd beliefs and unusual perceptions (e.g., magical thinking), and interpersonal deficits.

second-generation antipsychotic drugs   Any of several drugs, such as clozapine, that are used to treat schizophrenia and produce different side effects than first-generation antipsychotics while reducing positive and disorganized symptoms at least as effectively. Side effects can be serious.

secondhand smoke   Also referred to as *environmental tobacco smoke (ETS),* the smoke from the burning end of a cigarette or other tobacco product; contains higher concentrations of ammonia, carbon monoxide, nicotine, and tar than the smoke inhaled by the smoker.

selective mortality   The tendency for less healthy individuals to die earlier than relatively healthy people, which leads to biased samples in long-term follow-up studies.

selective serotonin reuptake inhibitors (SSRIs)   A specific form of serotonin reuptake inhibitors (SRIs) with less effect on dopamine and norepinephrine levels; SSRIs inhibit the reuptake of serotonin into the presynaptic neuron so that serotonin levels in the cleft are sustained for a longer period.

separation anxiety disorder   A disorder in which the child feels intense fear and distress when away from someone on whom they are very dependent.

Serotonin 1A Partial Agonist   A new type of antidepressant approved by the FDA in 2023 that is expected to have few side effects.

serotonin   A neurotransmitter of the central nervous system whose disturbances apparently figure in depression.

serotonin–norepinephrine reuptake inhibitors (SNRIs)   Any of various drugs that inhibit the presynaptic reuptake of serotonin and norepinephrine, such that both neurotransmitters will have more prolonged effects on postsynaptic neurons.

sexual dysfunctions   DSM-5-TR disorders involving problems with sexual arousal, desire, or orgasm or pain associated with intercourse.

sexual interest   Subjective sexual desire, sometimes including sexually arousing fantasies or thoughts.

sexual masochism disorder   A paraphilic disorder defined by a sexual attraction to being subjected to pain or humiliation.

sexual sadism disorder   A paraphilic disorder defined by a sexual attraction to inflicting pain or humiliation on another person.

shared environment   Factors that family members have in common, such as income level, child-rearing practices, and parental marital status and quality. Compare *nonshared environment.*

shenjing shuairuo   A common diagnosis in China, a syndrome characterized by weakness, mental fatigue, negative emotions, and sleep problems.

sickness behavior   A syndrome triggered by illness and by pro-inflammatory cytokines, characterized by decreased motor activity, lower food consumption, social withdrawal, changes in sleep patterns, and reduced motivation to pursue rewards.

single-case experimental design   A design for an experiment conducted with a single subject. Typically, behavior is measured within a baseline condition, then during an experimental or treatment condition, and finally within the baseline condition again.

SNPs   A variation in gene sequence. Specifically, differences between people in a single nucleotide (A, T, G, or C) in the DNA sequence of a particular gene.

social anxiety disorder   A collection of fears linked to the presence of other people.

social selectivity   The late-life shift in interest away from seeking new social interactions and toward cultivating those few social relationships that matter most, such as with family and close friends.

social skills training   Behavior therapy procedures, such as modeling and behavior rehearsal, for teaching individuals how to meet others, talk to them and maintain eye contact, give and receive criticism, offer and accept compliments, make requests and express feelings, and otherwise improve their relations with other people.

social worker   A mental health professional who holds a master of social work (M.S.W.) degree.

sociocognitive model (of DID) Etiological model of dissociative identity disorder that considers the condition to be the result of learning to enact social roles, though not through conscious deception but in response to suggestion. Compare *posttraumatic model (of DID).*

somatic symptom and related disorders   DSM-5-TR disorders defined by concerns about physical symptoms. See *functional neurological symptom disorder, illness anxiety disorder, and somatic symptom disorder.*

somatic symptom disorder   A DSM-5-TR diagnosis defined by excessive concern and help seeking regarding physical symptoms.

specific learning disorders   A set of developmental disorders encompassing dyslexia and dyscalculia; characterized by failure to develop in a specific academic area to the degree expected by the child's intellectual level.

specific phobia   A consistent tendency to experience extreme fear of a specific object or circumstance, for example, fear of nonpoisonous snakes or fear of heights.

SPECT   Single photon emission computed tomography, which measures gamma rays that are produced following an injection of a radioisotope and generates images of activity in different regions of the brain.

standardization   The process of constructing a normed assessment procedure that meets the various psychometric criteria for reliability and validity.

statistical significance   A measure that indicates that a result has a low probability of having occurred by chance alone if the null hypothesis is true. Compare *clinical significance*.

stigma   The destructive beliefs and attitudes held by a society about groups considered different in some manner, such as people with mental illness.

stimulant   A drug, such as cocaine, that increases alertness and motor activity and at the same time reduces fatigue, allowing an individual to remain awake for an extended period of time.

stress   State of an organism subjected to a stressor; can take the form of increased autonomic activity and in the long term can cause breakdown of an organ or development of a psychological disorder.

striatum   A region of the brain involved in motor action and responses to reward.

structured interview   An interview in which the questions are set out in a prescribed fashion for the interviewer; assists professionals in making diagnostic decisions based on standardized criteria.

subjective arousal   In the context of sexuality, self-rated sexual excitement, which may not correlate with biological arousal for women.

substance use disorders   Disorders in which drugs such as alcohol or heroin are used to such an extent that behavior becomes maladaptive, social and occupational functioning are impaired, and control or abstinence becomes impossible. Dependence on the drug may produce tolerance and withdrawal.

suicidal ideation   Thoughts about intentionally taking one's own life.

suicide attempts   Acts intended to cause one's own death.

suicide   The intentional taking of one's own life.

superego   In Freud's theory, the part of the personality that acts as the conscience and reflects society's moral standards as learned from parents and teachers.

sympathetic nervous system   The division of the autonomic nervous system that acts on bodily systems—for example, contracting the blood vessels, reducing activity of the intestines, and increasing the heartbeat—to prepare the organism for exertion, emotional stress, or extreme cold. Compare *parasympathetic nervous system*.

synapse   Small gap between two neurons where the nerve signal passes electrically or chemically from the axon of the first to the dendrites, cell body, or axon of the second.

taijin kyofusho   A fear of offending others that has been observed in Japan and other cultures that place an emphasis on social appropriateness and hierarchy.

test–retest reliability   The extent to which a test, measurement, or classification system produces the same scientific observation each time it is applied.

theory   A formally stated and coherent set of propositions that explain and logically order a range of phenomena, generating testable predictions or hypotheses.

third-variable problem   The difficulty in the correlational method of research whereby the relationship between two variables may be attributable to a third factor.

thought–action fusion   The tendency to believe that thinking about something is as morally wrong as engaging in the action or can make the imagined event more likely to occur. Believed to contribute to the persistence of obsessions.

thought suppression   An attempt to stop a certain thought that has the paradoxical effect of inducing preoccupation with that thought; considered to intensify obsessions.

time-of-measurement effects   A possible confound in longitudinal studies that arises because the social context at a given point in time can affect a variable that is being studied.

time-out   An operant conditioning procedure in which, after bad behavior, the person is temporarily removed from a setting where reinforcers can be obtained and placed in a less desirable setting, for example, in a boring room.

tolerance   A physiological process in which greater and greater amounts of an addictive drug are required to produce the same effect.

transcranial direct current stimulation (tDCS)   A noninvasive method for stimulating brain activity by applying a continuous low current through two electrodes placed on the scalp.

transcranial magnetic stimulation (TMS)   A noninvasive method for stimulating brain activity using an electronic pulse delivered through a magnetic coil placed on the scalp. It has successfully been used to treat depression and obsessive-compulsive disorder.

transference   A person's responses to his or her analyst that seem to reflect attitudes and ways of behaving toward important people in the person's past.

transference-focused therapy   A psychodynamic therapy that has been found to be more helpful than treatment as usual for those with borderline personality disorder, in which a focus is placed on the client's responses to the therapist and how those might shed light on experiences and expectations in the client's other relationships.

transition uncertainty   A phenomenon theorized to contribute to OCD, in which people doubt the evidence for their decisions when the context changes (Fradkin et al., 2020).

traumatic brain injury (TBI)   The result of a bump, blow, or jolt to the head that disrupts brain function; in mild form, commonly referred to as a concussion.

treatment outcome research   Studies designed to assess whether medical or psychological approaches are efficacious in relieving symptoms of a disorder. See also *randomized controlled trials*.

triarchic model of psychopathy   A model suggesting that psychopathy is comprised of three core dimensions: boldness (fearlessness), meanness (aggression and lack of remorse), and disinhibition (impulsivity), and that these three dimensions relate to different psychological and neurobiological risk factors.

tricyclic antidepressants   A group of antidepressants with molecular structures characterized by three fused rings; they interfere with the reuptake of norepinephrine and serotonin.

twin method   Research strategy in behavior genetics in which concordance rates of monozygotic and dizygotic twins are compared.

unconditioned response (UCR)   See *classical conditioning*.

unconditioned stimulus (UCS)   See *classical conditioning*.

unconscious   A state of unawareness without sensation or thought; in Freud's theory, the part of the personality, in particular, the id impulses or energy, of which the ego is unaware.

vaginal plethysmograph   A device for measuring physiological signs of sexual arousal in women; the device is shaped like a tampon and is inserted into the vagina to measure increases in blood flow.

validity   In research, includes *internal validity*, the extent to which results can be confidently attributed to the manipulation of the independent variable, and *external validity*, the extent to which results can be generalized to other populations and settings. Validity as applied to psychological measures includes *content validity*, the extent to which a measure adequately samples the domain of interest, and *criterion validity*, the extent to which a measure is associated in an expected way with some other measure (the criterion). See also *construct validity*.

vascular dementia   A form of dementia caused by cerebrovascular disease, most commonly occurring after a stroke. Because the areas of the brain affected by the disease can vary, the symptoms of vascular dementia vary as well.

ventricles   Cavities deep within the brain, filled with cerebrospinal fluid, that connect to the spinal cord.

voyeuristic disorder   A disorder defined by a desire to obtain sexual gratification from watching unsuspecting others in a state of undress or having sexual relations.

white matter   Neural tissue, particularly of the brain and spinal cord, consisting of tracts or bundles of myelinated (sheathed) nerve fibers. Compare *gray matter*.

withdrawal   Negative physiological and psychological reactions evidenced when a person suddenly stops taking an addictive drug; reactions include cramps, restlessness, and even death.

Aas, M., Melle, I., Bettella, F., Djurovic, S., Le Hellard, S., et al. (2018). Psychotic patients who used cannabis frequently before illness onset have higher genetic predisposition to schizophrenia than those who did not. *Psychological Medicine, 48*, 43–49.

Abbeduto, L., McDuffie, A., Thurman, A. J., & Kover, S. T. (2016). Chapter Three: Language development in individuals with intellectual and developmental disabilities: From phenotypes to treatments. In R. M. Hodapp & D. J. Fidler (Eds.), *Fifty years of research in intellectual and developmental disabilities* (Vol. 50, pp. 71–118). Academic Press.

Abbey, A., & McAuslan, P. (2004). A longitudinal examination of male college students' perpetration of sexual assault. *Journal of Consulting and Clinical Psychology, 72*, 747–756. https://doi.org/10.1037/0022-006X.72.5.747

Abel, G. G., Becker, J. V., Mittelman, M., Cunningham-Rathner, J., Rouleau, J. L., & Murphy, W. D. (1987). Self-reported sex crimes of nonincarcerated paraphiliacs. *Journal of Interpersonal Violence, 2*, 3–25.

Abplanalp, S. J., Braff, D. L., Light, G. A., Nuechterlein, K. H., Green, M. F., & Consortium on the Genetics of Schizophrenia-2 (2022). Understanding connections and boundaries between positive symptoms, negative symptoms, and role functioning among individuals with schizophrenia: A network psychometric approach. *JAMA Psychiatry, 79*(10), 1014–1022.

Abramovitch, A., Elliott, C. M., Wilhelm, S., Steketee, G., & Wilson, A. C. (2014). Obsessive-compulsive disorder: Assessment and treatment. In P. Emmelkamp & T. Ehring (Eds.), *The Wiley handbook of anxiety disorders* (pp. 1111–1144). John Wiley & Sons, Ltd.

Abramowitz, J. S. (2018). Presidential Address: Are the obsessive-compulsive related disorders related to obsessive-compulsive disorder? A critical look at DSM-5's new category. *Behavior Therapy, 49*(1), 1–11. https://doi.org/10.1016/j.beth.2017.06.002

Abramowitz, J. S., Franklin, M. E., Schwartz, S. A., & Furr, J. M. (2003). Symptom presentation and outcome of cognitive-behavioral therapy for obsessive-compulsive disorder. *Journal of Consulting and Clinical Psychology, 71*, 1049–1057.

Abramowitz, J. S., & Jacoby, R. J. (2015). Obsessive-compulsive and related disorders: A critical review of the new diagnostic class. *Annual Review of Clinical Psychology, 11*, 165–186. https://doi.org/10.1146/annurev-clinpsy-032813-153713

Abramowitz, J. S., Nelson, C. A., Rygwall, R., & Khandker, M. (2007). The cognitive mediation of obsessive-compulsive symptoms: A longitudinal study. *Journal of Anxiety Disorders, 21*, 91–104.

Abramson, L. Y., Metalsky, G. I., & Alloy, L. B. (1989). Hopelessness depression: A theory-based subtype of depression. *Psychological Review, 96*, 358–372.

Acarturk, C., de Graaf, R., van Straten, A., Have, M. T., & Cuijpers, P. (2008). Social phobia and number of social fears, and their association with comorbidity, health-related quality of life and help seeking: A population-based study. *Social Psychiatry and Psychiatric Epidemiology, 43*, 273–279.

Acocella, J. (1999). *Creating hysteria: Women and multiple personality disorder*. Jossey-Bass.

Adam, D. (2014). *The man who couldn't stop: OCD and the true story of a life lost in thought*. Sarah Crichton Books, Farrar, Straus and Giroux.

Addington, J., Cadenhead, K. S., Cornblatt, B. A., Mathalon, D. H., McGlashan, T. H., Perkins, D. O., et al. (2012). North American Prodrome Longitudinal Study (NAPLS 2): Overview and recruitment. *Schizophrenia Research, 142*, 77–82.

Addington, J., Liu, L., Brummitt, K., Bearden, C. E., Cadenhead, K. S., Cornblatt, B. A., et al. (2020). North American Prodrome Longitudinal Study (NAPLS 3): Methods and baseline description. *Schizophrenia Research, 243*, 262–267. Advance online publication. https://doi.org/10.1016/j.schres.2020.04.010

Adler, A. (1930). *Guiding the child on the principles of individual psychology*. Greenberg.

Afifi, T. O., Mather, A., Boman, J., Fleisher, W., Enns, M. W., MacMillan, H., & Sareen, J. (2011). Childhood adversity and personality disorders: Results from a nationally representative population-based study. *Journal of Psychiatric Research, 45*(6), 814–822. https://doi.org/10.1016/j.jpsychires.2010.11.008

Agostino, H., Burstein, B., Moubayed, D., Taddeo, D., Grady, R., Vyver, E., et al. (2021). Trends in the incidence of new-onset anorexia nervosa and atypical anorexia nervosa among youth during the COVID-19 pandemic in Canada. *JAMA Network Open, 4*(12), e2137395–e2137395.

Agras, W. S., & Bohon, C. (2021). Cognitive behavioral therapy for the eating disorders. *Annual Review of Clinical Psychology, 17*, 417–438.

Agras, W. S., Crow, S. J., Halmi, K. A., Mitchell, J. E., Wilson, G. T., & Kraemer, H. C. (2000). Outcome predictors for the cognitive-behavioral treatment of bulimia nervosa: Data from a multisite study. *American Journal of Psychiatry, 157*, 1302–1308.

Agras, W. S., Lock, J., Brandt, H., Bryson, S. W., Dodge, E., Halmi, K. A., et al. (2014). Comparison of 2 family therapies for adolescent anorexia nervosa: A randomized parallel trial. *JAMA Psychiatry, 71*(11), 1279–1286.

Aguilera, A., Bruehlman-Senecal, E., Liu, N., & Bravin, J. (2018). Implementing group CBT for depression among Latinos in a primary care clinic. *Cognitive and Behavioral Practice, 25*(1), 135–144. https://doi.org/10.1016/j.cbpra.2017.03.002

Aguilera, A., Lopez, S. R., Breitborde, N. J., Kopelowicz, A., & Zarate, R. (2010). Expressed emotion and sociocultural moderation in the course of schizophrenia. *Journal of Abnormal Psychology, 119*, 875–885.

Akyüz, F., Gökalp, P. G., Erdman, S., Oflaz, S., & Karida, Ç. (2017). Conversion disorder comorbidity and childhood trauma. *Archives of Neuropsychiatry, 54*, 15–20. https://doi.org/10.5152/npa.2017.19184

Alarcon, R. D., Becker, A. E., Lewis-Fernandez, R., Like, R. C., Desai, P., Foulks, E., et al. for the Cultural Psychiatry Committee of the Group for the Advancement of Psychiatry. (2009). Issues for DSM-V: The role of culture in psychiatric diagnosis. *Journal of Nervous and Mental Disease, 197*, 559–560.

Albert, M. S., Dekosky, S. T., Dickson, D., Dubois, B., Feldman, H. H., Fox, N. C., et al. (2011). The diagnosis of mild cognitive impairment due to Alzheimer's disease: Recommendations from the National Institute on Aging–Alzheimer's Association work-groups on diagnostic guidelines for Alzheimer's disease. *Alzheimer's and Dementia: The Journal of the Alzheimer's Association, 7*, 270–279.

Alden, L. E., Buhr, K., Robichaud, M., Trew, J. L., & Plasencia, M. L. (2018). Treatment of social approach processes in adults with social anxiety disorder. *Journal of Consulting and Clinical Psychology,* *86*(6), 505–517. https://doi.org/10.1037/ccp0000306

Alegria, A. A., Radua, J., & Rubia, K. (2016). Meta-analysis of fMRI studies of disruptive behavior disorders. *American Journal of Psychiatry,* *173,* 1119–1130. https://doi.org/10.1176/appi.ajp.2016.15081089

Alegria, M., Canino, G., Shrout, P. E., Woo, M., Duan, N., & Vila, D. (2008). Prevalence of mental illness in immigrant and non-immigrant U.S. Latino groups. *American Journal of Psychiatry, 165,* 359–369.

Alegria, M., Woo, M., Cao, Z., Torres, M., Meng, X-L., & Striegel-Moore, R. (2007). Prevalence and correlates of eating disorders among Latinos in the United States. International *Journal of Eating Disorders, 40,* s15–s21.

Alexander, M. G., & Fisher, T. D. (2003). Truth and consequences: Using the bogus pipeline to examine sex differences in self-reported sexuality. *Journal of Sex Research, 40,* 27–35. https://doi.org/10.1080/00224490309552164

Allderidge, P. (1979). Hospitals, mad houses, and asylums: Cycles in the care of the insane. *British Journal of Psychiatry, 134,* 321–324.

Allen, M., D'Alessio, D., & Brezgel, K. (1995). A meta-analysis summarizing the effects of pornography: II. Aggression after exposure. *Human Communication Research, 22,* 258–283.

Alley, Z. M., Kerr, D. C. R., & Bae, H. (2020). Trends in college students' alcohol, nicotine, prescription opioid and other drug use after recreational marijuana legalization: 2008–2018. *Addictive Behaviors, 102,* 106212.

Alloy, L. B., Abramson, L. Y., Walshaw, P. D., Cogswell, A., Grandin, L. D., Hughes, M. E., et al. (2008). Behavioral approach system and behavioral inhibition system sensitivities and bipolar spectrum disorders: Prospective prediction of bipolar mood episodes. *Bipolar Disorders, 10,* 310–322.

Almerie, M. Q., Okba Al Marhi, M., Jawoosh, M., Alsabbagh, M., Matar, H. E., Maayan, N., et al. (2015). Social skills programmes for schizophrenia. *The Cochrane Database of Systematic Reviews, 2015*(6), CD009006. https://doi.org/10.1002/14651858.CD009006.pub2

Althof, S. E. (2014). Treatment of premature ejaculation: Psychotherapy, pharmacotherapy, and combined therapy. In Y. M. Binik & K. S. K. Hall (Eds.), *Principles and practice of sex therapy* (5th ed., pp. 112–137). Guilford Press.

Althof, S. E., McMahon, C. G., Waldinger, M. D., Serefoglu, E. C., Shindel, A. W., Adaikan, P. G., et al. (2014). An update of the International Society of Sexual Medicine's guidelines for the diagnosis and treatment of premature ejaculation (PE). *Sexual Medicine, 2,* 60–90. https://doi.org/10.1002/sm2.28

Altshuler, L. L., Kupka, R. W., Hellemann, G., Frye, M. A., Sugar, C. A., McElroy, S. L., et al. (2010). Gender and depressive symptoms in 711 patients with bipolar disorder evaluated prospectively in the Stanley Foundation Bipolar Treatment Outcome Network. *American Journal of Psychiatry, 167,* 708–715.

Alwahhabi, F. (2003). Anxiety symptoms and generalized anxiety disorder in the elderly: A review. *Harvard Review of Psychiatry, 11,* 180–193.

Alzheimer's Association. (2023). 2023 Alzheimer's disease facts and figures. *Alzheimer's & Dementia, 19*(4), 1598–1695. https://doi.org/10.1002/alz.13016

Alzheimer's Cohort Consortium. (2020). Twenty-seven-year time trends in dementia incidence in Europe and the United States. *Neurology, 95*(5), e519–e531. https://doi.org/10.1212/WNL.0000000000010022

American Law Institute. (1962). *Model penal code: Proposed official draft.* Author.

American Psychiatric Association. (2013). *Diagnostic and statistical manual of mental disorders* (5th ed.). https://doi.org/10.1176/appi.books.9780890425596

American Psychiatric Association (APA). (2002). *Practice guideline for the treatment of patients with bipolar disorder* (2nd ed.). American Psychiatric Association Publishing. https://psychiatryonline.org/pb/assets/raw/sitewide/practice_guidelines/guidelines/bipolar.pdf

American Psychiatric Association (APA). (2020). The American Psychiatric Association practice guideline for the treatment of patients with schizophrenia. Author. https://www.psychiatry.org/psychiatrists/practice/clinical-practice-guidelines

American Psychological Association. (2002). Criteria for evaluating treatment guidelines. *American Psychologist, 57,* 1052–1059. https://doi.org/10.1037//0003-066X.57.12.1052

American Psychological Association. (2017). Clinical practice guideline for the treatment of depression across three age cohorts. https://www.apa.org/depression-guideline/

American Psychological Association. (2019). Summary of the clinical practice guideline for the treatment of posttraumatic stress disorder (PTSD) in adults. *American Psychologist, 74*(5), 596–607. https://doi.org.libproxy.berkeley.edu/10.1037/amp0000473

Amir, N., Cashman, L., & Foa, E. B. (1997). Strategies of thought control in obsessive-compulsive disorder. *Behaviour Research and Therapy, 35,* 775–777.

Amir, N., Foa, E. B., & Coles, M. E. (1998). Negative interpretation bias in social phobia. *Behaviour Research and Therapy, 36,* 945–957.

Anand, A., Verhoeff, P., Seneca, N., Zoghbi, S. S., Seibyl, J. P., Charney, D. S., et al. (2000). Brain SPECT imaging of amphetamine-induced dopamine release in euthymic bipolar disorder patients. *American Journal of Psychiatry, 157,* 1109–1114.

Ancoli-Israel, S. (2000). Insomnia in the elderly: A review for the primary care practitioner. *Sleep, 23*(Suppl 1), S23–30; discussion S36–28.

Anderson, D. K., Liang, J. W., & Lord, C. (2014). Predicting young adult outcome among more and less cognitively able individuals with autism spectrum disorders. *Journal of Child Psychology and Psychiatry, 55,* 485–494.

Anderson, D. M., & Rees, D. I. (2021). The Public Health Effects of Legalizing Marijuana (No. 28647). https://doi.org/10.3386/w28647

Anderson, E. R., & Mayes, L. C. (2010). Race/ethnicity and internalizing disorders in youth: A review. *Clinical Psychology Review, 30*(3), 338–348.

Anderson, R. A. E., Silver, K. E., Ciampaglia, A. M., Vitale, A. M., & Delahanty, D. L. (2019). The frequency of sexual perpetration in college men: A systematic review of reported prevalence rates from 2000 to 2017. *Trauma, Violence, and Abuse.* https://doi.org/10.1177/1524838019860619

Andersson, A., Tuvblad, C., Chen, Q., Rietz, E. D., Cortese, S., Kuja-Halkola, R., et al. (2020). Research review: The strength of the genetic overlap between ADHD and other psychiatric symptoms: A systematic review and meta-analysis. *Journal of Child Psychology and Psychiatry, and Allied Disciplines, 168*(76), 406. https://doi.org/10.1111/jcpp.13233

Andersson, E., Mataix-Cols, D., & Rück, C. (2017). Computer-aided interventions for obsessive-compulsive spectrum disorders. In P. Emmelkamp & T. Ehring (Eds.), *The Wiley handbook of obsessive compulsive disorders* (pp. 663–680). John Wiley & Sons, Ltd. https://doi.org/10.1002/9781118890233.ch37

Andhale, R., & Shrivastava, D. (2022). Huntington's Disease: A Clinical Review. *Cureus, 14*(8). https://doi.org/10.7759/CUREUS.28484

Andrews, G., Basu, A., Cuijpers, P., Craske, M. G., McEvoy, P., English, C. L., & Newby, J. M. (2018). Computer therapy for the anxiety and depression disorders is effective, acceptable and practical health care: An updated meta-analysis. *Journal of Anxiety Disorders, 55*, 70–78. https://doi.org/10.1016/j.janxdis.2018.01.001

Andrilla, C. H. A., Coulthard, C., & Larson, E. H. (2017). Barriers rural physicians face prescribing buprenorphine for opioid use disorder. *Annals of Family Medicine, 15*, 359–362. https://doi.org/10.1370/afm.2099

Anglin, D. M. (2023). Racism and social determinants of psychosis. *Annual Review of Clinical Psychology, 19*(1), 277–302. https://doi.org/10.1146/annurev-clinpsy-080921-074730

Anglin, D. M., Ereshefsky, S., Klaunig, M. J., Bridgwater, M. A., Niendam, T. A., Ellman, L. M., et al. (2021). From womb to neighborhood: A racial analysis of social determinants of psychosis in the United States. *Ajp, 178*(7), 599–610. https://doi.org/10.1176/appi.ajp.2020.20071091

Anglin, D. M., Ereshefsky, S., Klaunig, M. J., Bridgwater, M. A., Niendam, T. A., Ellman, L. M., et al. (2021). From womb to neighborhood: A racial analysis of social determinants of psychosis in the United States. *AJP, 178*(7), 599–610. https://doi.org/10.1176/appi.ajp.2020.20071091

Angst, F., Stassen, H. H., Clayton, P. J., & Angst, J. (2002). Mortality of patients with mood disorders: Follow-up over 34–38 years. *Journal of Affective Disorders, 68*, 167–181.

Angst, J., Rössler, W., Ajdacic-Gross, V., Angst, F., Wittchen, H. U., Lieb, R., et al. (2019). Differences between unipolar mania and bipolar-I disorder: Evidence from nine epidemiological studies. *Bipolar Disorders, 21*(5), 437–448. https://doi.org/10.1111/bdi.12732

Ansell, E. B., Pinto, A., Edelen, M. O., Markowitz, J. C., Sanislow, C. A., Yen, S., et al. (2011). The association of personality disorders with the prospective 7-year course of anxiety disorders. *Psychological Medicine, 41*, 1019–1028.

Antshel, K. M., Zhang-James, Y., Wagner, K. E., Ledesma, A., & Faraone, S. V. (2016). An update on the comorbidity of ADHD and ASD: A focus on clinical management. *Expert Review of Neurotherapeutics, 16*(3), 279–293. https://doi.org/10.1586/14737175.2016.1146591

Anttila, V., Bulik-Sullivan, B., Finucane, H. K., Walters, R. K., Bras, J., Duncan, L., et al. (2018). Analysis of shared heritability in common disorders of the brain. *Science, 360*(6395), eaap8757.

Appignanesi, L. (2008). *Mad, bad, and sad: Women and the mind doctors.* W. W. Norton.

Arcelus, J., Mitchell, A. J., Wales, J., Nielsen, S. (2011). Mortality rates in patients with anorexia nervosa and other eating disorders. *Archives of General Psychiatry, 68*(7), 724–731. https://doi.org/10.1001/arch-genpsychiatry.2011.74

Armstrong, E. A., England, P., & Fogarty, A. C. K. (2009). Orgasm in college hookups and relationships. In B. J. Risman (Ed.), *Families as they really are* (pp. 362–377). Norton.

Armstrong, S. C., Bolling, C. F., Michalsky, M. P., Reichard, K. W.; SECTION ON OBESITY, SECTION ON SURGERY. (2019). Pediatric metabolic and bariatric surgery: Evidence, barriers, and best practices. *Pediatrics, 144*(6), e20193223.

Arnett, J. J. (2008). The neglected 95%: Why American psychology needs to become less American. *American Psychologist, 63*, 602–614.

Arnold, E. H., O'Leary, S. G., & Edwards, G. H. (1997). Father involvement and self-reported parenting of children with attention deficit hyperactivity disorder. *Journal of Consulting and Clinical Psychology, 65*, 337–342.

Arnold, L. E., Elliott, M., Sachs, L., Kraemer, H. C., Wells, K. C., Abikoff, H. B., et al. (2003). Effects of ethnicity on treatment attendance, stimulant response/dose, and 14-month outcome in ADHD. *Journal of Consulting and Clinical Psychology, 71*, 713–727.

Arnold, L. M., Keck, P. E., Jr., Collins J., Wilson, R., Fleck, D. E., Corey, K. B., et al. (2004). Ethnicity and first-rank symptoms in patients with psychosis. *Schizophrenia Research, 67*, 207–212.

Arnsten, A. F. T. (2015). Stress weakens prefrontal networks: Molecular insults to higher cognition. *Nature Neuroscience, 18*(10), 1376–1385. https://doi.org/10.1038/nn.4087

Arora, T., Alhelali, E., & Grey, I. (2020). Poor sleep efficiency and daytime napping are risk factors of depersonalization disorder in female university students. *Neurobiology of Sleep and Circadian Rhythms, 9*, 100059. https://doi.org/10.1016/J.NBSCR.2020.100059

Arseneault, L., Cannon, M., Poulton, R., Murray, R., Caspi, A., & Moffitt, T. E. (2002). Cannabis use in adolescence and risk for adult psychosis: Longitudinal prospective study. *British Medical Journal, 325*, 1212–1213.

Ascher, E. A., Sturm, V. E., Seider, B. H., Holley, S. R., Miller, B. L., & Levenson, R. W. (2010). Relationship satisfaction and emotional language in frontotemporal dementia and Alzheimer's disease patients and spousal caregivers. *Alzheimer's Disease and Associated Disorders, 24*, 49–55.

Ashbaugh, A. R., Antony, M. M., McCabe, R. E., Schmidt, L. A., & Swinson, R. P. (2005). Self-evaluative biases in social anxiety. *Cognitive Therapy and Research, 29*, 387–398.

Ashbaugh, A. R., Marinos, J., & Bujaki, B. (2017). The impact of depression and PTSD symptom severity on trauma memory. *Memory, 26*(1), 106–116. https://doi.org/10.1080/09658211.2017.1334801

Asher, M., Kauffmann, A., & Aderka, I. M. (2020). Out of sync: Nonverbal synchrony in social anxiety disorder. *Clinical Psychological Science, 8*(2), 280–294. https://doi.org/10.1177/2167702619894566

Ashok, A. H., Mizuno, Y., Volkow, N. D., & Howes, O. D. (2017). Association of stimulant use with dopaminergic alterations in users of cocaine, amphetamine, or methamphetamine: A systematic review and meta-analysis. *JAMA Psychiatry, 74*(5), 511–519.

Asmundson, G. J., Larsen, D. K., & Stein, M. B. (1998). Panic disorder and vestibular disturbance: An overview of empirical findings and clinical implications. *Journal of Psychosomatic Research, 44*, 107–120.

Attia, E., Becker, A. E., Bryant-Waugh, R., Hoek, H. W., Kreipe, R. E., Marcus, M. D., et al. (2013). Feeding and eating disorders in DSM-5. *American Journal of Psychiatry, 170*, 1237–1239.

Atwoli, L., Stein, D. J., Koenen, K. C., & McLaughlin, K. A. (2015). Epidemiology of posttraumatic stress disorder: Prevalence, correlates and consequences. *Current Opinion in Psychiatry, 28*(4), 307–311. https://doi.org/10.1097/yco.0000000000000167

Audrain-McGovern, J., Rodriguez, D., Epstein, L. H., Cuevas, J., Rodgers, K., & Wiley, E. P. (2009). Does delay discounting play an etiological role in smoking or is it a consequence of smoking? *Drug and Alcohol Dependence, 103*, 99–106.

Audrain-McGovern, J., & Tercyak, K. P. (2011). Genes, environment, and adolescent smoking: Implications for prevention. In K. S. Kendler, S. R. Jaffee, & D. Romer (Eds.), *The dynamic genome and mental health* (pp. 294–321). Oxford University Press.

Auerbach, R. P., Alonso, J., Axinn, W. G., Cuijpers, P., Ebert, D. D., Green, J. G., et al. (2016). Mental disorders among college students in the World Health Organization World Mental Health Surveys. *Psychological Medicine, 46*(14), 2955–2970. https://doi.org/10.1017/S0033291716001665

Autism Spectrum Disorders Working Group of the Psychiatric Genomics Consortium. (2017). Meta-analysis of GWAS of over 16,000 individuals with autism spectrum disorder highlights a novel locus at 10q24.32 and a significant overlap with schizophrenia. *Molecular Autism, 8*(1), 21.

Avenevoli, S., Swendsen, J., He, J.-P., Burstein, M., & Merikangas, K. R. (2015). Major depression in the national comorbidity survey adolescent supplement: Prevalence, correlates, and treatment. *Journal of the American Academy of Child & Adolescent Psychiatry, 54*(1), 37–44.e32. https://doi.org/10.1016/j.jaac.2014.10.010

Averill, L. A., Averill, C. L., Akiki, T. J., & Abdallah, C. G. (2021). Examining neurocircuitry and neuroplasticity in PTSD. In M. J. Friedman, P. P. Schnurr, & T. M. Keane (Eds.), *Handbook of PTSD: Science and practice* (3rd ed., pp. 152–167). The Guilford Press.

Aviv, R. (2018). The edge of identity. *The New Yorker*, online. https://www.newyorker.com/magazine/2018/04/02/how-a-young-woman-lost-her-identity.

Awaad, R., & Ali, S. (2015). Obsessional Disorders in al-Balkhi's 9th century treatise: Sustenance of the Body and Soul. *Journal of Affective Disorders, 180*, 185–189. https://doi.org/10.1016/j.jad.2015.03.003

Awaad, R., & Ali, S. (2016). A modern conceptualization of phobia in al-Balkhi's 9th century treatise: Sustenance of the body and soul. *Journal of Anxiety Disorders, 37*, 89–93. https://doi.org/10.1016/j.janxdis.2015.11.003

Awaad, R., & Ali, S. (2016). A modern conceptualization of phobia in al-Balkhi's 9th century treatise: Sustenance of the body and soul. *Journal of Anxiety Disorders, 37*, 89–93. https://doi.org/10.1016/j.janxdis.2015.11.003

Axelsson, E., Andersson, E., Ljótsson, B., Björkander, D., Hedman-Lagerlöf, M., & Hedman-Lagerlöf, E. (2020). Effect of internet vs face-to-face cognitive behavior therapy for health anxiety: A randomized noninferiority clinical trial. *JAMA Psychiatry, 77*(9), 915–924. https://doi.org/10.1001/jamapsychiatry.2020.0940

Aybek, S., & Vuilleumier, P. (2016). Imaging studies of functional neurologic disorders. *Handbook of Clinical Neurology, 139*, 73–84. https://doi.org/10.1016/B978-0-12-801772-2.00007-2

Azagba, S., King, J., Shan, L., & Manzione, L. (2020). Cigarette smoking behavior among menthol and nonmenthol adolescent smokers. *The Journal of Adolescent Health: Official Publication of the Society for Adolescent Medicine, 66*(5), 545–550.

Azrael, D., & Miller, M. J. (2016). Reducing suicide without affecting underlying mental health. In R. C. O'Connor & J. Pirkis (Eds.), *The international handbook of suicide prevention* (pp. 637–662). John Wiley & Sons, Ltd. https://doi.org/10.1002/9781118903223.ch36

Babchishin, K. M., Hanson, R. K., & VanZuylen, H. (2015). Online child pornography offenders are different: A meta-analysis of the characteristics of online and offline sex offenders against children. *Archives of Sexual Behavior, 44*, 45–66. https://doi.org/10.1007/s10508-014-0270-x

Babiak, P., Neumann, C. S., & Hare, R. D. (2010). Corporate psychopathy: Talking the walk. *Behavioral Sciences and the Law, 28*, 174–193.

Bae, H., & Kerr, D. C. R. (2020). Marijuana use trends among college students in states with and without legalization of recreational use: Initial and longer-term changes from 2008 to 2018. *Addiction, 115*, 1115–1124. https://doi.org/10.1111/add.14939

Bai, D., Yip, B. H. K., Windham, G. C., Sourander, A., Francis, R., Yoffe, R., et al. (2019). Association of genetic and environmental factors with autism in a 5-country cohort. *JAMA Psychiatry, 76*(10), 1035–1043.

Baik, S. Y., & Newman, M. G. (2023). The transdiagnostic use of worry and rumination to avoid negative emotional contrasts following negative events: A momentary assessment study. *Journal of Anxiety Disorders, 95*, 102679. https://doi.org/10.1016/j.janxdis.2023.102679

Bailer, J., Kerstner, T., Witthöft, M., Diener, C., Mier, D., & Rist, F. (2016). Health anxiety and hypochondriasis in the light of DSM-5. *Anxiety, Stress, & Coping, 29*, 219–239. https://doi.org/10.1080/10615806.2015.1036243

Baillargeon, J., Binswanger, I. A., Penn, J. V., Williams, B. A., & Murray, O. J. (2009). Psychiatric disorders and repeat incarcerations: The revolving prison door. *American Journal of Psychiatry, 166*(1), 103–109.

Bai, S., Guo, W., Feng, Y., Deng, H., Li, G., Nie, H., et al. (2020). Efficacy and safety of anti-inflammatory agents for the treatment of major depressive disorder: A systematic review and meta-analysis of randomised controlled trials. *Journal of Neurology, Neurosurgery and Psychiatry, 91*(1), 21–32. https://doi.org/10.1136/jnnp-2019-320912

Baker, J. H., Mitchell, K. S., Neale, M. C., & Kendler, K. S. (2010). Eating disorder symptomatology and substance use disorders: Prevalence and shared risk in a population based twin sample. *International Journal of Eating Disorders, 43*, 648–658.

Baker, T. B., & McCarthy, D. E. (2021). Smoking treatment: A report card on progress and challenges. *Annual Review of Clinical Psychology, 17*(1), 1–30. https://doi.org/10.1146/annurev-clinpsy-081219-090343

Baker, T. B., Piper, M. E., Stein, J. H., Smith, S. S., Bolt, D. M., Fraser, D. L., et al. (2016). Effects of nicotine patch vs varenicline vs combination nicotine replacement therapy on smoking cessation at 26 weeks: A randomized clinical trial. *JAMA, 315*(4), 371–379.

Bakolis, I., Hammoud, R., Stewart, R., Beevers, S., Dajnak, D., Mac-Crimmon, S., et al. (2021). Mental health consequences of urban air pollution: prospective population-based longitudinal survey. *Social Psychiatry and Psychiatric Epidemiology, 56*(9), 1587–1599.

Baldwin, D. S., Aitchison, K., Bateson, A., Curran, H. V., Davies, S., Leonard, B., et al. (2013). Benzodiazepines: Risks and benefits. A reconsideration. *Journal of Psychopharmacology, 27*(11), 967–971. https://doi.org/10.1177/0269881113503509

Ball, J. C., & Ross, A. (1991). *The effectiveness of methadone maintenance treatment*. Springer-Verlag.

Ball, T. M., Knapp, S. E., Paulus, M. P., & Stein, M. B. (2017). Brain activation during fear extinction predicts exposure success. *Depression and Anxiety, 34*(3), 257–266. https://doi.org/10.1002/da.22583

Balon, R. (2016). *Practical guide to paraphilia and paraphilic disorders*. Springer.

Balsis, S., Carpenter, B. D., & Storandt, M. (2005). Personality change precedes clinical diagnosis of dementia of the Alzheimer type. *Journal of Gerontology, 60B*, 98–101.

Balsis, S., Gleason, M. E., Woods, C. M., & Oltmanns, T. F. (2007). An item response theory analysis of DSM-IV personality disorder criteria across younger and older age groups. *Psychology and Aging, 22*, 171–185.

Bandelow, B. (2020). Current and novel psychopharmacological drugs for anxiety disorders. *Advances in Experimental Medicine and Biology, 1191*, 347–365. https://pubmed.ncbi.nlm.nih.gov/32002937/

Bandelow, B., Baldwin, D., Abelli, M., Altamura, C., Dell'Osso, B., Domschke, K., et al. (2016). Biological markers for anxiety disorders, OCD and PTSD—A consensus statement. Part I: Neuroimaging and genetics. *The World Journal of Biological Psychiatry, 17*(5), 321–365.

Bandelow, B., Baldwin, D., Abelli, M., Bolea-Alamanac, B., Bourin, M., Chamberlain, S. R., et al. (2017). Biological markers for anxiety disorders, OCD and PTSD: A consensus statement. Part II: Neurochemistry, neurophysiology and neurocognition. *The World Journal of Biological Psychiatry, 18*(3), 162–214. https://doi.org/10.1080/15622975.2016.1190867

Bandura, A., & Menlove, F. L. (1968). Factors determining vicarious extinction of avoidance behavior through symbolic modeling. *Journal of Personality and Social Psychology, 8*, 99–108.

Banerjee, S., High, J., Stirling, S., Shepstone, L., Swart, A. M., Telling, T., et al. (2021). Study of mirtazapine for agitated behaviours in dementia (SYMBAD): A randomised, double-blind, placebo-controlled trial. *The Lancet, 398*(10310), 1487–1497. https://doi.org/10.1016/S0140-6736(21)01210-1

Bang, J., Spina, S., & Miller, B. L. (2015). Frontotemporal dementia. *The Lancet, 386*, 1672–1682. https://doi.org/10.1016/S0140-6736(15)00461-4

Bantin, T., Stevens, S., Gerlach, A. L., & Hermann, C. (2016). What does the facial dot-probe task tell us about attentional processes in social anxiety? A systematic review. *Journal of Behavior Therapy and Experimental Psychiatry, 50*, 40–51.

Barbato, A., D'Avanzo, B., & Parabiaghi, A. (2018). Couple therapy for depression. *Cochrane Database Systematic. Review. 6*: CD004188.

Barber, C. (2008). *Comfortably numb*. Pantheon Books.

Barboza, G. E., Dominguez, S., & Chance, E. (2016). Physical victimization, gender identity and suicide risk among transgender men and women. *Preventive Medicine Reports, 4*, 385–390. https://doi.org/10.1016/j.pmedr.2016.08.003

Bardone-Cone, A. M., Wonderlich, S. A., Frost, R. O., Bulik, C. M., Mitchell, J., Uppala, S., et al. (2007). Perfectionism and eating disorders: Current status and future directions. *Clinical Psychology Review, 27*, 384–405.

Bar-Haim, Y., Lamy, D., Pergamin, L., Bakermans-Kranenburg, M. J., & van Ijzendoorn, M. H. (2007). Threat-related attentional bias in anxious and nonanxious individuals: A meta-analytic study. *Psychological Bulletin, 133*, 1–24.

Barkley, R. A. (1997). Behavioral inhibition, sustained attention, and executive functions: Constructing a unifying theory of ADHD. *Psychological Bulletin, 121*, 65–94.

Barkley, R. A., DuPaul, G. J., & McMurray, M. B. (1990). A comprehensive evaluation of attention deficit disorder with and without hyperactivity defined by research criteria. *Journal of Consulting and Clinical Psychology, 58*, 775–789.

Barkley, R. A., Fischer, M., Smallish, L., & Fletcher, K. (2002). The persistence of attention-deficit hyperactivity disorder into young adulthood as a function of reporting source and definition of disorder. *Journal of Abnormal Psychology, 111*, 279–289.

Barkley, R. A., Fischer, M., Smallish, L., & Fletcher, K. (2003). Does the treatment of attention-deficit/hyperactivity disorder with stimulants contribute to drug use/abuse? A 13 year prospective study. *Pediatrics, 111*, 97–109.

Barlow, D. H. (2004). *Anxiety and its disorders: The nature and treatment of anxiety and panic*. Guilford Press.

Barlow, D. H., Farchione, T. J., Bullis, J. R., Gallagher, M. W., Murray-Latin, H., Sauer-Zavala, S., et al. (2017). The unified protocol for transdiagnostic treatment of emotional disorders compared with diagnosis-specific protocols for anxiety disorders: A randomized clinical trial. *JAMA Psychiatry, 74*(9), 875–884. https://doi.org/10.1001/jamapsychiatry.2017.2164

Barrett, L. F. (2017). *How emotions are made: The secret life of the brain*. Mariner Books.

Barr, P. B., Bigdeli, T. B., & Meyers, J. L. (2022). Prevalence, comorbidity, and sociodemographic correlates of psychiatric diagnoses reported in the All of Us Research Program. *JAMA Psychiatry, 79*(6), 622–628.

Barsky, A. (2006). "Doctor, are you sure my heart is okay?" Cognitive-behavioral treatment of hypochondriasis. In R. L. Spitzer, M. B. W. First, J. B. Williams, & M. Gibbon (Eds.), *DSM-IV-TR® casebook, volume 2: Experts tell how they treated their own patients* (pp. 251–261). American Psychiatric Association.

Bart, C. P., Titone, M. K., Ng, T. H., Nusslock, R., & Alloy, L. B. (2021). Neural reward circuit dysfunction as a risk factor for bipolar spectrum disorders and substance use disorders: A review and integration. *Clinical Psychology Review, 87*, 102035. https://doi.org/10.1016/j.cpr.2021.102035

Bartlett, E. A., Zanderigo, F., Stanley, B., Choo, T.-H., Galfalvy, H. C., Pantazatos, S. P., et al. (2023). In vivo serotonin transporter and 1A receptor binding potential and ecological momentary assessment (EMA) of stress in major depression and suicidal behavior. *European Neuropsychopharmacology, 70*, 1–13. https://doi.org/10.1016/j.euroneuro.2023.01.006

Barton, J., Kyle, S. D., Varese, F., Jones, S. H., & Haddock, G. (2018). Are sleep disturbances causally linked to the presence and severity of psychotic-like, dissociative and hypomanic experiences in non-clinical populations? A systematic review. *Neuroscience and Biobehavioral Reviews, 89*, 119–131. https://doi.org/10.1016/j.neubiorev.2018.02.008

Baselmans, B. M. L., Yengo, L., van Rheenen, W., & Wray, N. R. (2021). Risk in relatives, heritability, SNP-based heritability, and genetic correlations in psychiatric disorders: A review. *Biological Psychiatry, 89*(1), 11–19.

Bas-Hoogendam, J. M., Groenewold, N. A., Aghajani, M., Freitag, G. F., Harrewijn, A., Hilbert, K., et al. (2022). ENIGMA-anxiety working group: Rationale for and organization of large-scale neuroimaging studies of anxiety disorders. *Human Brain Mapping, 43*(1), 83–112. https://doi.org/10.1002/hbm.25100

Baskin-Sommers, A. R. (2016). Dissecting antisocial behavior. *Clinical Psychological Science, 4*, 500–510. https://doi.org/10.1177/2167702615626904

Bass, J. K., Annan, J., McIvor Murray, S., Kaysen, D., Griffiths, S., Cetinoglu, T., et al. (2013). Controlled trial of psychotherapy for Congolese survivors of sexual violence. *The New England Journal of Medicine, 368*(23), 2182–2191. https://doi.org/10.1056/NEJMOA1211853

Basson, R., Althof, S. A., Davis, S., Fugl-Meyer, K., Goldstein, I., Leiblum, S., et al. (2004). Summary of the recommendations on sexual dysfunctions in women. *Journal of Sexual Medicine, 1*, 24–34.

Basson, R., Brotto, L. A., Laan, E., Redmond, G., & Utian, W. H. (2005). Assessment and management of women's sexual dysfunctions: Problematic desire and arousal. *Journal of Sexual Medicine, 2*, 291–300.

Bateman, A., Constantinou, M. P., Fonagy, P., & Holzer, S. (2021). Eight-year prospective follow-up of mentalization-based treatment versus structured clinical management for people with borderline personality disorder. *Personality Disorders: Theory, Research, and Treatment, 12*(4), 291–299. https://doi.org/10.1037/per0000422

Bateman, A., & Fonagy, P. (2016). *Mentalization-based treatment for personality disorders*. Oxford Academic. https://doi.org/10.1093/med:psych/9780199680375.001.0001

Baur, E., Forsman, M., Santtila, P., Johansson, A., Sandnabba, K., & Langstrom, N. (2016). Paraphilic sexual interests and sexually coercive behavior: A population-based twin study. *Archives of Sexual Behavior, 45*, 1163–1172. https://doi.org/10.1007/s10508-015-0674-2

Baxter, A. J., Scott, K. M., Vos, T., & Whiteford, H. A. (2013). Global prevalence of anxiety disorders: A systematic review and meta-regression. *Psychological Medicine, 43*(5), 897–910. https://doi.org/10.1017/s003329171200147x

Baxter, L. R., Ackermann, R. F., Swerdlow, N. R., Brody, A., Saxena, S., Schwartz, J. M., et al. (2000). Specific brain system mediation of obsessive-compulsive disorder responsive to either medication or behavior therapy. In W. K. Goodman, M. V. Rudorfer, & J. D. Maser (Eds.), *Obsessive-compulsive disorder: Contemporary issues in treatment* (pp. 573–610). Lawrence Erlbaum.

Beardslee, W. R., Brent, D. A., Weersing, V. R., Clarke, G. N., Porta, G., Hollon, S. D., et al. (2013). Prevention of depression in at-risk adolescents. *JAMA Psychiatry, 70*(11), 1161–1170. https://doi.org/10.1001/jamapsychiatry.2013.295

Beauchaine, T. P., Hinshaw, S. P., & Pang, K. L. (2010). Comorbidity of attention-deficit/hyperactivity disorder and early-onset conduct disorder: Biological, environmental, and developmental mechanisms. *Clinical Psychology: Science and Practice, 17*, 327–336.

Beauchaine, T. P., & McNulty, T. (2013). Comorbidities and continuities as ontogenic processes: Toward a developmental spectrum model of externalizing psychopathology. *Development and Psychopathology, 25*, 1505–1528.

Beautrais, A. L., Gibb, S. J., Fergusson, D., Horwood, L. J., & Larkin, G. L. (2009). Removing bridge barriers stimulates suicides: An unfortunate natural experiment. *Australian and New Zealand Journal of Psychiatry, 43*, 495–497.

Bechara, A. (2005). Decision making, impulse control and loss of willpower to resist drugs: A neurocognitive perspective. *Nature Neuroscience, 8*, 1458–1463.

Bechara, A., Berridge, K. C., Bickel, W. K., Morón, J. A., Williams, S. B., & Stein, J. S. (2019). A neurobehavioral approach to addiction: Implications for the opioid epidemic and the psychology of addiction. *Psychological Science in the Public Interest, 20*(2), 96–127. https://doi.org/10.1177/1529100619860513

Beck, A. T. (1967). *Depression: Clinical, experimental and theoretical aspects*. Harper & Row.

Beck, A. T. (1976). *Cognitive therapy and the emotional disorders*. International Universities Press.

Beck, A. T., & Freeman, A. (1990). *Cognitive therapy for personality disorders*. Guilford Press.

Beck, A. T., & Rector, N. A. (2005). Cognitive approaches to schizophrenia: Theory and therapy. *Annual Review of Clinical Psychology, 1*, 577–606.

Becker, B., Scheele, D., Moessner, R., Maier, W., & Hurlemann, R. (2013). Deciphering the neural signature of conversion blindness. *American Journal of Psychiatry, 170*, 121–122.

Becker, C. B., Zayfert, C., & Anderson, E. (2004). A survey of psychologists' attitudes towards and utilization of exposure therapy for PTSD. *Behaviour Research and Therapy, 42*(3), 277–292. https://doi.org/10.1016/s0005-7967(03)00138-4

Beckers, T., Hermans, D., Lange, I., Luyten, L., Scheveneels, S., & Vervliet, B. (2023). Understanding clinical fear and anxiety through the lens of human fear conditioning. *Nature Reviews Psychology, 2*(4), 233–245. https://doi.org/10.1038/s44159-023-00156-1

Beck, J. G., & Bozman, A. (1995). Gender differences in sexual desire: The effects of anger and anxiety. *Archives of Sexual Behavior, 24*, 595–612.

Beevers, C. G., Mullarkey, M. C., Dainer-Best, J., Stewart, R. A., Labrada, J., Allen, J. J. B., et al. (2019). Association between negative cognitive bias and depression: A symptom-level approach. *Journal of Abnormal Psychology, 128*(3), 212–227. https://doi.org/:10.1037/abn0000405

Beier, K. M. (2018). Preventing child sexual abuse—The Prevention Project Dunkelfeld. *The Journal of Sexual Medicine, 15*(8), 1065–1066. https://doi.org/10.1016/j.jsxm.2018.03.008

Beier, K. M., Grundmann, D., Kuhle, L. F., Scherner, G., Konrad, A., & Amelung, T. (2015). The German Dunkelfeld Project: A pilot study to prevent child sexual abuse and the use of child abusive images. *Journal of Sexual Medicine, 12*(2), 529–542. https://doi.org/10.1111/jsm.12785

Bekhbat, M., Treadway, M. T., & Felger, J. C. (2022). *Inflammation as a pathophysiologic pathway to anhedonia: Mechanisms and therapeutic implications* (pp. 397–419). https://doi.org/10.1007/7854_2021_294

Bellenguez, C., Küçükali, F., Jansen, I. E., Kleineidam, L., Moreno-Grau, S., Amin, N., et al. (2022). New insights into the genetic etiology of Alzheimer's disease and related dementias. *Nature Genetics, 54*(4), 412–436. https://doi.org/10.1038/s41588-022-01024-z

Belsky, D. W., Caspi, A., Arseneault, L., Bleidorn, W., Fonagy, P., Goodman, M., et al. (2012). Etiological features of borderline personality related characteristics in a birth cohort of 12-year-old children. *Development and Psychopathology, 24*, 251–265. https://doi.org/10.1017/s0954579411000812

Benedetti, F. (2008). Mechanisms of placebo and placebo-related effects across diseases and treatments. *Annual Review of Pharmacology and Toxicology, 48*, 33–60. https://doi.org/10.1146/ANNUREV.PHARMTOX.48.113006.094711

Benge, J. F., Wisdom, N. M., Collins, R. L., Franks, R., LeMaire, A., & Chen, D. K. (2012). Diagnostic utility of the Structured Inventory of Malingered Symptomatology for identifying psychogenic non-epileptic events. *Epilepsy & Behavior, 24*, 439–444. https://doi.org/10.1016/j.yebeh.2012.05.007

Benish, S. G., Quintana, S., & Wampold, B. E. (2011). Culturally adapted psychotherapy and the legitimacy of myth: A direct-comparison meta-analysis. *Journal of Counseling Psychology, 58*(3), 279–289. https://doi.org/10.1037/a0023626

Benjamin, C. L., Harrison, J. P., Settipani, C. A., Brodman, D. M., & Kendall, P. C. (2013). Anxiety and related outcomes in young adults 7 to 19 years after receiving treatment for child anxiety. *Journal of Consulting and Clinical Psychology, 81*(5), 865–876.

Benjet, C., Bromet, E., Karam. E. G., et al. (2016). The epidemiology of traumatic event exposure worldwide: results from the World Mental Health Survey Consortium. *Psychological Medicine, 46*, 327–343.

Bennabi, D., & Haffen, E. (2018). Transcranial direct current stimulation (tDCS): A promising treatment for major depressive disorder? *Brain Sciences, 8*(5), 81. https://doi.org/10.3390/brainsci8050081

Ben-Porath, Y. S., & Tellegen, A. (2008). *MMPI-2-RF: Manual for administration, scoring, and interpretation*. University of Minnesota Press.

Berenz, E. C., Amstadter, A. B., Aggen, S. H., Knudsen, G. P., Reichborn-Kjennerud, T., Gardner, C. O., & Kendler, K. S. (2013). Childhood trauma and personality disorder criterion counts: a co-twin control analysis. *Journal of Abnormal Psychology, 122*(4), 1070–1076. https://doi.org/10.1037/A0034238

Berger, F., Dailey, L., Johnson, B., Sinclair, E., Snook, J., & Stettin, B. (2018). *Grading the states: An analysis of involuntary psychiatric laws*. Treatment Advocacy Center. https://TreatmentAdvocacyCenter.org/Grading-the-States

Berger, F., Dailey, L. Johnson, B., Sinclair, E., Snook, J., Stettin, B. (2018). *Grading the states: An analysis of involuntary psychiatric laws*. Treatment Advocacy Center. https://www.treatmentadvocacy-center.org/grading-the-states

Berkman, E. T., Falk, E. M., & Lieberman, M. D. (2011). In the trenches of real-world self-control: Neural correlates of breaking the link between craving and smoking. *Psychological Science, 22*, 498–506.

Berk, M., Woods, R. L., Nelson, M. R., Shah, R. C., Reid, C. M., Storey, E., et al. (2020). Effect of aspirin vs placebo on the prevention of depression in older people. *JAMA Psychiatry*. https://doi.org/10.1001/jamapsychiatry.2020.1214

Berridge, K. C., Ho, C. Y., Richard, J. M., & DiFeliceantonio, A. G. (2010). The tempted brain eats: Pleasure and desire circuits in obesity and eating disorders. *Brain Research, 1350*, 43–64. https://doi.org/10.1016/j.brainres.2010.04.003

Berti, V., Walters, M., Sterling, J., Quinn, C. G., Logue, M., Andrews, R., et al. (2018). Mediterranean diet and 3-year Alzheimer brain biomarker changes in middle-aged adults. *Neurology, 90*(20), E1789–E1798. https://doi.org/10.1212/WNL.0000000000005527

Bhaduri, A., Thompson, K., & Chanen, A. (2019). Pharmacological treatment of borderline personality disorder. In *APA handbook of psychopharmacology* (pp. 451–468). American Psychological Association. https://doi.org/10.1037/0000133-020

Bhugra, D., Popelyuk, D., & McMullen, I. (2010). Paraphilias across cultures: Contexts and controversies. *Journal of Sex Research, 47,* 242–256.

Bickel, W. K., Koffarnus, M. N., Moody, L., & Wilson, A. G. (2014). The behavioral- and neuro-economic process of temporal discounting: A candidate behavioral marker of addiction. *Neuropharmacology, 76,* Part B, 518–527.

Bickel, W. K., Miller, M. L., Yi, R., Kowal, B. P., Lindquist, D. M., & Pitcock, J. A. (2007). Behavioral and neuroeconomics of drug addiction: Competing neural systems and temporal discounting processes. *Drug and Alcohol Dependence, 90,* S85–S91.

Biddinger, K. J., Emdin, C. A., Haas, M. E., Wang, M., Hindy, G., Ellinor, P. T., et al. (2022). Association of habitual alcohol intake with risk of cardiovascular disease. *JAMA Network Open, 5*(3), e223849–e223849.

Biederman, J., & Faraone, S. (2004). The Massachusetts General Hospital studies of gender influences on attention-deficit/hyperactivity disorder in youth and relatives. *Psychiatric Clinics of North America, 27,* 215–224.

Biederman, J., Monuteaux, M. C., Mick, E., Spencer, T., Wilens, T. E., Silva, J. M., et al. (2006). Young adult outcome of attention deficit hyperactivity disorder: A controlled 10-year follow-up study. *Psychological Medicine, 36,* 167–179.

Biederman, J., Petty, C. R., Monuteaux, M. C., Fried, R., Byrne, D., Mirto, T., et al. (2010). Adult psychiatric outcomes of girls with attention deficit hyperactivity disorder: 11-year follow-up in a longitudinal case-control study. *American Journal of Psychiatry, 167,* 409–417.

Bienvenu, O. J., Samuels, J. F., Wuyek, L. A., Liang, K. Y., Wang, Y., Grados, M. A., et al. (2012). Is obsessive–compulsive disorder an anxiety disorder, and what, if any, are spectrum conditions? A family study perspective. *Psychological Medicine, 42*(1), 1–13. https:// doi.org/10.1017/S0033291711000742

Bigler, E. D. (2008). Neuropsychology and clinical neuroscience of persistent post-concussive syndrome. *Journal of the International Neuropsychological Society, 14*(1), 1–22. https://doi.org/10.1017/ S135561770808017X

Bingham, K. S., Flint, A. J., & Mulsant, B. H. (2019). Management of late-life depression in the context of cognitive impairment: A review of the recent literature. *Current Psychiatry Reports, 21*(8), 1–11. https://doi.org/10.1007/s11920-019-1047-7

Binik, Y. M. (2010). The DSM diagnostic criteria for vaginismus. *Archives of Sexual Behavior, 39,* 278–291.

Binzer, M., & Kullgren, G. (1996). Conversion symptoms: What can we learn from previous studies? *Nordic Journal of Psychiatry, 50,* 143–152.

Bipolar Disorder and Schizophrenia Working Group of the Psychiatric Genomics Consortium. (2018). Genomic dissection of bipolar disorder and schizophrenia, including 28 subphenotypes. *Cell, 173,* 1705–1715.e16. https://doi.org/10.1016/j.cell.2018.05.046

Birbaumer, N., Veit, R., Lotze, M., Erb, M., Hermann, C., Grodd, W., et al. (2005). Deficient fear conditioning in psychopathy: A functional magnetic resonance imaging study. *Archives of General Psychiatry, 62,* 799–805.

Bitsko, R. H., Claussen, A. H., Lichstein, J., Black, L. I., Jones, S. E., Danielson, M. L., et al. (2022). Mental health surveillance among children—United States, 2013–2019. *MMWR Supplement, 71*(Suppl-2), 1–42. https://doi.org/10.15585/mmwr.su7102a1

Bjorkenstam, E., Burstrom, B., Vinnerljung, B., & Kosidou, K. (2016). Childhood adversity and psychiatric disorder in young adulthood: An analysis of 107,704 Swedes. *Journal of Psychiatric Research, 77,* 67–75. https://doi.org/10.1016/j.jpsychires.2016.02.018

Blachman, D. R., & Hinshaw, S. P. (2002). Patterns of friendship among girls with and without attention-deficit/hyperactivity disorder. *Journal of Abnormal Child Psychology, 30,* 625–640.

Blair, R. J. (2013). The neurobiology of psychopathic traits in youths. *Nature Reviews Neuroscience, 14*(11), 786–799.

Blair, R. J. R. (2005). Responding to the emotions of others: Dissociating forms of empathy through the study of typical and psychiatric populations. *Consciousness and Cognition, 14,* 698–718.

Blanchard, J. J., Bradshaw, K. R., Garcia, C. P., Nasrallah, H. A., Harvey, P. D., Casey, D., et al. (2017). Examining the reliability and validity of the Clinical Assessment Interview for Negative Symptoms within the Management of Schizophrenia in Clinical Practice (MOSAIC) multisite national study. *Schizophrenia Research, 185,* 137–143.

Blanchard, J. J., Squires, D., Henry, T., Horan, W. P., Bogenschutz, M., Lauriello, J., et al. (1999). Examining an affect regulation model of substance abuse in schizophrenia: The role of traits and coping. *Journal of Nervous and Mental Disease, 187,* 72–79.

Blanchard, J. W., Akay, L. A., Davila-Velderrain, J., von Maydell, D., Mathys, H., Davidson, S. M., et al. (2022). APOE4 impairs myelination via cholesterol dysregulation in oligodendrocytes. *Nature, 611*(7937), 769–779. https://doi.org/10.1038/s41586-022-05439-w

Blanchflower, D. G. (2021). Is happiness U-shaped everywhere? Age and subjective well-being in 145 countries. *Journal of Population Economics, 34*(2), 575. https://doi.org/10.1007/S00148-020-00797-Z

Blanco, C., Hoertel, N., Wall, M. M., Franco, S., Peyre, H., Neria, Y., et al. (2018). Toward understanding sex differences in the prevalence of posttraumatic stress disorder: Results from the National Epidemiologic Survey on Alcohol and Related Conditions. *The Journal of Clinical Psychiatry, 79*(2), 19420. https://doi.org/10.4088/ JCP.16M11364

Bloch, M. H., Bartley, C. A., Zipperer, L., Jakubovski, E., Landeros-Weisenberger, A., Pittenger, C., et al. (2014). Meta-analysis: Hoarding symptoms associated with poor treatment outcome in obsessive-compulsive disorder. *Molecular Psychiatry, 19*(9), 1025–1030. https://doi.org/10.1038/mp.2014.50

Bloomberg Data. (2012). Most rapidly aging countries. Data adapted from United Nations Population Division, International Labor Division. http://www.bloomberg.com/visual-data/best-and-worst/ most-rapidly-aging-countries

Boardman, J. D., Saint Onge, J. M., Haberstick, B. C., Timberlake, D. S., & Hewitt, J. K. (2008). Do schools moderate the genetic determinants of smoking? *Behavioral Genetics, 28,* 234–246.

Boegels, S. M., & Zigterman, D. (2000). Dysfunctional cognitions in children with social phobia, separation anxiety disorder, and generalized anxiety disorder. *Journal of Abnormal Child Psychology, 28,* 205–211.

Bohus, M., Stoffers-Winterling, J., Sharp, C., Krause-Utz, A., Schmahl, C., & Lieb, K. (2021). Borderline personality disorder. *The Lancet, 398*(10310), 1528–1540. https://doi.org/10.1016/ S0140-6736(21)00476-1

Boiger, M., & Mesquita, B. (2012). The construction of emotion in interactions, relationships, and cultures. *Emotion Review, 4,* 221–229.

Boisseau, C. L., Yen, S., Markowitz, J. C., Grilo, C. M., Sanislow, C. A., Shea, M. T., et al. (2013). Individuals with single versus multiple suicide attempts over 10 years of prospective follow-up. *Comprehensive Psychiatry, 54,* 238–242.

Bolívar, H. A., Klemperer, E. M., Coleman, S. R. M., DeSarno, M., Skelly, J. M., & Higgins, S. T. (2021). Contingency management for patients receiving medication for opioid use disorder: A systematic review and meta-analysis. *JAMA Psychiatry, 78*(10), 1092–1102.

Bonanno, G. A. (2004). Loss, trauma, and human resilience: Have we underestimated the human capacity to thrive after extremely aversive events? *American Psychologist, 59*, 20–28.

Bond, K., & Anderson, I. M. (2015). Psychoeducation for relapse prevention in bipolar disorder: A systematic review of efficacy in randomized controlled trials. *Bipolar Disorders, 17*, 349–362. https://doi.org/10.1111/bdi.12287

Bookheimer, S., & Burggren, A. (2009). APO 4 genotype and neurophysiological vulnerability to Alzheimer's and cognitive aging. *Annual Review of Clinical Psychology, 5*, 343–362.

Boone, L., Soenens, B., & Luyten, P. (2014). When or why does perfectionism translate into eating disorder pathology? A longitudinal examination of the moderating and mediating role of body dissatisfaction. *Journal of Abnormal Psychology, 123*, 412–418.

Boos, H. B., Aleman, A., Cahn, W., Hulshoff, H., & Kahn, R. S. (2007). Brain volumes in relatives of patients with schizophrenia: A meta-analysis. *Archives of General Psychiatry, 64*, 297–304.

Borch-Jacobsen, M. (1997, April 24). Sybil: The making of a disease? An interview with Dr. Herbert Spiegel. *New York Review of Books, 44*(7), 60.

Borkovec, T. D., Alcaine, O. M., & Behar, E. (2004). Clinical presentation and diagnostic features. In R. G. Heimberg, C. L. Turk, & D. S. Mennin (Eds.), *Generalized anxiety disorder* (pp. 77–108). Guilford Press.

Bornovalova, M. A., Huibregtse, B. M., Hicks, B. M., Keyes, M., McGue, M., & Iacono, W. (2013). Tests of a direct effect of childhood abuse on adult borderline personality disorder traits: A longitudinal discordant twin design. *Journal of Abnormal Psychology, 122*, 180–194.

Bornstein, R. F., & Natoli, A. P. (2019). Clinical utility of categorical and dimensional perspectives on personality pathology: A meta-analytic review. *Personality Disorders: Theory, Research, and Treatment, 10*(6), 479–490. https://doi.org/10.1037/per0000365

Boscarino, J. A. (2006). Posttraumatic stress disorder and mortality among U.S. Army veterans 30 years after military service. *Annals of Epidemiology, 16*, 248–256.

Boswell, R. G., & Kober, H. (2016). Food cue reactivity and craving predict eating and weight gain: A meta-analytic review. *Obesity Reviews, 17*, 159–177. https://doi.org/10.1111/obr.12354

Bourke, J. H., Langford, R. M., & White, P. D. (2015). The common link between functional somatic syndromes may be central sensitisation. *Journal of Psychosomatic Research, 78*, 228–236. https://doi.org/10.1016/j.jpsychores.2015.01.003

Bouton, M. E., Mineka, S., & Barlow, D. H. (2001). A modern learning theory perspective on the etiology of panic disorder. *Psychological Review, 108*, 4–32.

Bouton, M. E., & Waddell, J. (2007). Some biobehavioral insights into persistent effects of emotional trauma. In L. J. Kirmayer, R. Lemelson & M. Barad (Eds.), *Understanding trauma: Integrating biological, clinical, and cultural perspectives* (pp. 41–59). Cambridge University Press.

Bovin, M. J., Wells, S. Y., Rasmusson, A. M., Hayes, J. P., & Resick, P. A. (2014). Posttraumatic stress disorder. In P. Emmelkamp & T. Ehring (Eds.), *The Wiley handbook of anxiety disorders*. John Wiley & Sons, Ltd.

Bowers, W. A., & Ansher, L. S. (2008). The effectiveness of cognitive behavioral therapy on changing eating disorder symptoms and psychopathy of 32 anorexia nervosa patients at hospital discharge and one year follow-up. *Annals of Clinical Psychiatry, 20*, 79–86.

Bowyer, L., Krebs, G., Mataix-Cols, D., Veale, D., & Monzani, B. (2016). A critical review of cosmetic treatment outcomes in body dysmorphic disorder. *Body Image, 19*, 1–8. https://doi.org/10.1016/j.bodyim.2016.07.001

Boysen, G. A., & VanBergen, A. (2013). A review of published research on adult dissociative identity disorder: 2000–2010. *Journal of Nervous and Mental Disease, 201*, 5–11.

Boysen, G. A., & VanBergen, A. (2014). Simulation of multiple personalities: A review of research comparing diagnosed and simulated dissociative identity disorder. *Clinical Psychology Review, 34*, 14–28. https://doi.org/10.1016/j.cpr.2013.10.008

Bradbury, T. N. & Bodenmann, G. (2020). Interventions for couples. *Annual Review of Clinical Psychology, 16*.

Bradford, D. E., Curtin, J. J., & Piper, M. E. (2015). Anticipation of smoking sufficiently dampens stress reactivity in nicotine-deprived smokers. *Journal of Abnormal Psychology, 124*, 128–136. https://doi.org/10.1037/abn0000007

Bradford, D. E., Shapiro, B. L., & Curtin, J. J. (2013). How bad could it be? Alcohol dampens stress responses to threat of uncertain intensity. *Psychological Science, 24*, 2541–2549.

Bradford, D. E., Shireman, J. M., Sant'Ana, S. J., Fronk, G. E., Schneck, S. E., & Curtin, J. J. (2022). Alcohol's effects during uncertain and uncontrollable stressors in the laboratory. *Clinical Psychological Science: A Journal of the Association for Psychological Science, 10*(5), 885–900. https://doi.org/10.1177/21677026211061355

Brady, R. O., Jr., Gonsalvez, I., Lee, I., Öngür, D., Seidman, L. J., Schmahmann, J. D., et al. (2019). Cerebellar-prefrontal network connectivity and negative symptoms in schizophrenia. *AJP, 176*(7), 512–520. https://doi.org/10.1176/appi.ajp.2018.18040429

Brakoulias, V., Starcevic, V., Sammut, P., Berle, D., Milicevic, D., Moses, K., et al. (2011). Obsessive-compulsive spectrum disorders: A comorbidity and family history perspective. *Australasian Psychiatry, 19*, 151–155.

Brand, B. L., Myrick, A. C., Loewenstein, R. J., Classen, C. C., Lanius, R., et al. (2012). A survey of practices and recommended treatment interventions among expert therapists treating patients with dissociative identity disorder and dissociative disorder not otherwise specified. *Psychological Trauma: Theory, Research, Practice, and Policy, 4*(5), 490–500. https://doi.org/10.1037/a0026487

Brandl, F., Weise, B., Mulej Bratec, S., Jassim, N., Hoffmann Ayala, D., Bertram, T., et al. (2022). Common and specific large-scale brain changes in major depressive disorder, anxiety disorders, and chronic pain: A transdiagnostic multimodal meta-analysis of structural and functional MRI studies. *Neuropsychopharmacology, 47*(5), 1071–1080. https://doi.org/10.1038/s41386-022-01271-y

Brandon, T. H., Vidrine, J. I., & Litvin, E. B. (2007). Relapse and relapse prevention. *Annual Review of Clinical Psychology, 3*, 257–284.

Brandt, N. J., & Mansour, D. Z. (2016). Treatment of dementia: Pharmacological approaches. In M. Boltz & J. E. Galvin (Eds.), *Dementia care: An evidence-based approach* (pp. 73–95). Springer International Publishing.

Bransford, J. D., & Johnson, M. K. (1973). Considerations of some problems of comprehension. In W. G. Chase (Ed.), *Visual Information Processing*. Academic Press.

Braswell, L., & Kendall, P. C. (1988). Cognitive-behavioral methods with children. In K. S. Dobson (Ed.), *Handbook of cognitive-behavioral therapies*. Guilford Press.

Bratland-Sanda, S., & Sundgot-Borgen, J. (2013). Eating disorders in athletes: Overview of prevalence, risk factors and recommendations for prevention and treatment. *European Journal of Sport Science, 13*(5), 499–508.

Braun, K., & Champagne, F. A. (2014). Paternal influences on offspring development: Behavioral and epigenetic pathways. *Journal of Neuroendocrinology, 26*, 697–706.

Braun, M. (2019). Management of Behavioral and Psychological Symptoms in Dementia. In: Ravdin, L.D., Katzen, H.L. (eds) *Handbook on the Neuropsychology of Aging and Dementia*. Clinical Handbooks in Neuropsychology. Springer, Cham. https://doi.org/10.1007/978-3-319-93497-6_23

Breh, D. C., & Seidler, G. H. (2007). Is peritraumatic dissociation a risk factor for PTSD? *Journal of Trauma and Dissociation, 8*(1), 53–69. https://doi.org/10.1300/J229V08N01_04

Brenes, G. A., Danhauer, S. C., Lyles, M. F., Hogan, P. E., & Miller, M. E. (2015). Telephone-delivered cognitive behavioral therapy and telephone-delivered nondirective supportive therapy for rural older adults with generalized anxiety disorder: A randomized clinical trial. *JAMA Psychiatry, 72*, 1012–1020. https://doi.org/10.1001/jamapsychiatry.2015.1154

Brent, D. A., Brunwasser, S. M., Hollon, S. D., Weersing, V. R., Clarke, G. N., Dickerson, J. F., et al. (2015). Effect of a cognitive-behavioral prevention program on depression 6 years after implementation among at-risk adolescents: A randomized clinical trial. *JAMA Psychiatry, 72*(11), 1110–1118.

Breuer, J., & Freud, S. (1982). *Studies in hysteria.* (J. Strachey, Trans. and Ed., with the collaboration of A. Freud). Basic Books. (Original work published 1895).

Bridge, J. A., Iyengar, S., Salary, C. B., Barbe, R. P., Birmaher, B., Pincus, H. A., et al. (2007). Clinical response and risk for reported suicidal ideation and suicide attempts in pediatric antidepressant treatment: A meta-analysis of randomized controlled trials. *Journal of the American Medical Association, 297*, 1683–1696.

Britton, J., Grillon, C., Lissek, S., Norcross, M. A., Szuhany, K. L., Chen, G., et al. (2013). Response to learned threat: An fMRI study in adolescent and adult anxiety. *American Journal of Psychiatry, 170*, 1195–1204.

Brody, D. J., & Gu, Q. (2020). *Antidepressant use among adults: United States, 2015-2018: Key findings. Data from the National Health and Nutrition Examination Survey.* https://www.cdc.gov/nchs/products/index.htm

Bromet, E., Andrade, L. H., Hwang, I., Sampson, N. A., Alonso, J., de Girolamo, G., et al. (2011). Cross-national epidemiology of DSM-IV major depressive episode. *BMC Medicine, 9*, 90.

Brook, M., & Kosson, D. S. (2013). Impaired cognitive empathy in criminal psychopathy: Evidence from a laboratory measure of empathic accuracy. *Journal of Abnormal Psychology, 122*, 156–166.

Brooks, M. (2004). *Extreme measures: The dark visions and bright ideas of Francis Galton.* Bloomsbury.

Brooks, S., Prince, A., Stahl, D., Campbell, I. C., & Treasure, J. (2011). A systematic review and meta-analysis of cognitive bias to food stimuli in people with disordered eating behaviour. *Clinical Psychology Review, 31*, 37–51.

Brotto, L. A., & Basson, R. (2014). Group mindfulness-based therapy significantly improves sexual desire in women. *Behaviour Research and Therapy, 57*(1), 43–54. https://doi.org/10.1016/J.BRAT.2014.04.001

Brotto, L. A., & Luria, M. (2014). Sexual interest/arousal disorder in women. In Y. M. Binik & K. S. K. Hall (Eds.), *Principles and practice of sex therapy* (5th ed., pp. 17–41). Guilford Press.

Brown, A. S., & Derkits, E. J. (2010). Prenatal infections and schizophrenia: A review of epidemiologic and translational studies. *American Journal of Psychiatry, 167*, 261–280.

Brown, A. S., Schaefer, C. A., Quesenberry, C. P., Jr., Liu, L., Babulas, V. P., & Susser, E. S. (2005). Maternal exposure to toxoplasmosis and risk of schizophrenia in adult off spring. *American Journal of Psychiatry, 162*, 767–773.

Brown, G. K., Ten Have, T., Henriques, G. R., Xie, S. X., Hollander, J. E., & Beck, A. T. (2005). Cognitive therapy for the prevention of suicide attempts. *Journal of the American Medical Association, 294*, 563–570.

Brown, G. W., & Andrews, B. (1986). Social support and depression. In R. Trumbull & M. H. Appley (Eds.), *Dynamics of stress: Physiological, psychological, and social perspectives* (pp. 257–282). Plenum.

Brown, G. W., Bone, M., Dalison, B., & Wing, J. K. (1966). *Schizophrenia and social care.* Oxford University Press.

Brown, G. W., & Harris, T. O. (1978). *The Bedford College life events and difficulty schedule: Directory of contextual threat of events.* Bedford College University of London.

Brown, G. W., & Harris, T. O. (1989). Depression. In T. O. Harris & G. W. Brown (Eds.), *Life events and illness* (pp. 49–93). Guilford Press.

Brown, H. M., Waszczuk, M. A., Zavos, H. M. S., Trzaskowski, M., Gregory, A. M., & Eley, T. C. (2014). Cognitive content specificity in anxiety and depressive disorder symptoms: A twin study of cross-sectional associations with anxiety sensitivity dimensions across development. *Psychological Medicine, 44*(16), 3469–3480. https://doi.org/10.1017/S0033291714000828

Brown R. J. (2016). Dissociation and functional neurologic disorders. *Handbook of Clinical Neurology, 139*, 85–94. https://doi.org/10.1016/B978-0-12-801772-2.00008-4

Brown, R. J., Cardena, E., Nijenhuis, E., Sar, V., & Van der Hart, O. (2007). Should conversion disorder be reclassified as dissociative disorder in DSM-5? *Psychosomatics, 48*, 369–378.

Brown, R. J., Skelly, N., & Chew-Graham, C. A. (2020). Online health research and health anxiety: A systematic review and conceptual integration. *Clinical Psychology: Science and Practice, 27*(2), e12299. https://doi.org/10.1111/CPSP.12299

Brown, T. A., Forney, K. J., Klein, K. M., Grillot, C., & Keel, P. K. (2020). A 30-year longitudinal study of body weight, dieting, and eating pathology across women and men from late adolescence to later midlife. *Journal of Abnormal Psychology, 129*(4), 376–386. https://doi.org/10.1037/abn0000519

Brown, T. A., & Keel, P. K. (2023). Eating disorders in boys and men. *Annual Review of Clinical Psychology, 19*(1), 177–205. https://doi.org/10.1146/annurev-clinpsy-080921-074125

Broyd, S. J., van Hell, H. H., Beale, C., Yücel, M., & Solowij, N. (2016). Acute and chronic effects of cannabinoids on human cognition—A systematic review. *Biological Psychiatry, 79*, 557–567.

Bruce, M. L., Ten Have, T. R., Reynolds III, C. F., Katz, I. I., Schulberg, H. C., Mulsant, B. H., et al. (2004). Reducing suicidal ideation and depressive symptoms in depressed older primary care patients. *Journal of the American Medical Association, 291*, 1081–1091.

Brummelman, E., Thomaes, S., Nelemans, S. A., Orobio de Castro, B., Overbeek, G., & Bushman, B. J. (2015). Origins of narcissism in children. *Proceedings of the National Academy of Sciences, 112*, 3659–3662. https://doi.org/10.1073/pnas.1420870112

Bryant, R. A. (2021). Psychological models of PTSD. In M. J. Friedman, P. P. Schnurr, & T. M. Keane (Eds.), *Handbook of PTSD: Science and practice* (3rd ed., pp. 98–116). Guilford Press.

Buchanan, J. A., Christenson, A., Houlihan, D., & Ostrom, C. (2011). The role of behavior analysis in the rehabilitation of persons with dementia. *Behavior Therapy, 42*, 9–21.

Buchnik-Daniely, Y., Vannikov-Lugassi, M., Shalev, H., & Soffer-Dudek, N. (2021). The path to dissociative experiences: A direct comparison of different etiological models. *Clinical Psychology & Psychotherapy, 28*(5), 1091–1102. https://doi.org/10.1002/CPP.2559

Buchwald, J., Chenoweth, M. J., Palviainen, T., Zhu, G., Benner, C., Gordon, S., et al. (2021). Genome-wide association meta-analysis of nicotine metabolism and cigarette consumption measures in smokers of European descent. *Molecular Psychiatry, 26*(6), 2212–2223.

Budge, S. L., Moore, J. T., Del Re, A. C., Wampold, B. E., Baardseth, T. P., & Nienhuis, J. B. (2013). The effectiveness of evidence-based treatments for personality disorders when comparing treatment-as-usual and bona fide treatments. *Clinical Psychology Review, 33*, 1057–1066.

Buhlmann, U., Glaesmer, H., Mewes, R., Fama, J. M., Wilhelm, S., Brahler, E., & Rief, W. (2010). Updates on the prevalence of body dysmorphic disorder: A population-based survey. *Psychiatry Research, 178*(1), 171–175. https://doi.org/10.1016/j.psychres.2009.05.002

Buil, J. M., van Lier, P. A. C., Brendgen, M. R., Koot, H. M., & Vitaro, F. (2017). Developmental pathways linking childhood temperament with antisocial behavior and substance use in adolescence: Explanatory mechanisms in the peer environment. *Journal of Personality and Social Psychology, 112*(6), 948–966. https://doi.org/10.1037/pspp0000132

Bulik, C. M., & Reichborn-Kjennerud, T. (2003). Medical morbidity in binge eating disorder. https://www.interscience.wiley.com

Bulik, C. M., Wade, T. D., & Kendler, K. S. (2000). Characteristics of monozygotic twins discordant for bulimia nervosa. *International Journal of Eating Disorders, 29*, 1–10.

Bullers, S., Cooper, M. L., & Russell, M. (2001). Social network drinking and adult alcohol involvement: A longitudinal exploration of the direction of influence. *Addictive Behaviors, 26*, 181–199.

Burdick, K. E., Braga, R. J., Gopin, C. B., Malhotra, A. K. (2014). Dopaminergic influences on emotional decision making in euthymic bipolar patients. *Neuropsychopharmacology, 39*(2), 274–282. https://doi.org/10.1038/npp.2013.177.

Burke, B. L., Arkowitz, H., & Menchola, M. (2003). The efficacy of motivational interviewing: A meta-analysis of controlled clinical trials. *Journal of Consulting and Clinical Psychology, 71*, 843–861.

Burri, A., & Spector, T. (2011). Recent and lifelong sexual dysfunction in a female UK population sample: Prevalence and risk factors. *Journal of Sexual Medicine, 8*, 2420–2430.

Burstein, M., Ameli-Grillon, L., & Merikangas, K. R. (2011). Shyness versus social phobia in US youth. *Pediatrics, 128*(5), 917–925. https://doi.org/10.1542/peds.2011-1434

Burt, S. A. (2009a). Rethinking environmental contributions to child and adolescent psychopathology: A meta-analysis of shared environmental influences. *Psychological Bulletin, 135*, 608–637. https://doi.org/10.1037/a0015702

Burt, S. A. (2009b). Are there meaningful etiological differences within antisocial behavior? Results of a meta-analysis. *Clinical Psychology Review, 29*(2), 163–178.

Burt, S. A. (2009). Rethinking environmental contributions to child and adolescent psychopathology: A meta-analysis of shared environmental influences. *Psychological Bulletin, 135*, 608–637. https://doi.org/10.1037/a0015702

Burt, S. A. (2012). How do we optimally conceptualize the heterogeneity within antisocial behavior? An argument for aggressive versus non-aggressive behavioral dimensions. *Clinical Psychology Review, 32*, 263–279.

Burt, S. A. (2014). Research review: The shared environment as a key source of variability in child and adolescent psychopathology. *Journal of Child Psychology and Psychiatry, 55*(4), 304–312. https://doi.org/10.1111/jcpp.12173

Burt, S. A. (2022). The genetic, environmental, and cultural forces influencing youth antisocial behavior are tightly intertwined. *Annual Review of Clinical Psychology, 18*, 155–178.

Burt, S. A., Clark, D. A., Gershoff, E. T., Klump, K. L., & Hyde, L. W. (2021). Twin differences in harsh parenting predict youth's antisocial behavior. *Psychological Science, 32*(3), 395–409. https://doi.org/10.1177/0956797620968532

Burt, S. A., Klahr, A. M., & Klump, K. L. (2015). Do non-shared environmental influences persist over time? An examination of days and minutes. *Behavior Genetics, 45*, 24–34. https://doi.org/10.1007/s10519-014-9682-6

Burt, S. A., Klump, K. L., Gorman-Smith, D., & Neiderhiser, J. M. (2016). Neighborhood disadvantage alters the origins of children's nonaggressive conduct problems. *Clinical Psychological Science, 4*, 511–526. https://doi.org/10.1177/2167702615618164

Burt, S. A., & Neiderhiser, J. M. (2009). Aggressive versus nonaggressive antisocial behavior: Distinctive etiological moderation by age. *Developmental Psychology, 45*, 1164–1176. https://doi.org/10.1037/a0016130

Bury, B., Tiggemann, M., & Slater, A. (2017). Disclaimer labels on fashion magazine advertisements: Does timing of digital alteration information matter? *Eating Behaviors, 25*, 18–22.

Bushman, B. J., & Cooper, H. M. (1990). Effects of alcohol on human aggression: An integrative research review. *Psychological Bulletin, 107*, 341–354.

Butcher, F., Galanek, J. D., Kretschmar, J. M., & Flannery, D. J. (2015). The impact of neighborhood disorganization on neighborhood exposure to violence, trauma symptoms, and social relationships among at-risk youth. *Social Science & Medicine (1982), 146*, 300–306. https://doi.org/10.1016/J.SOCSCIMED.2015.10.013

Butcher, K. R., & Jameson, M. (2016). Computer-based instruction (CBI) within special education. In J. K. Luiselli & A. J. Fischer (Eds.), *Computer-assisted and web-based innovations in psychology, special education, and health* (pp. 211–254). Elsevier Academic Press.

Butzlaff, R. L., & Hooley, J. M. (1998). Expressed emotion and psychiatric relapse: A meta-analysis. *Archives of General Psychiatry, 55*, 547–553.

Buvat, J., Maggi, M., Gooren, L., Guay, A. T., Kaufman, J., Morgentaler, A., et al. (2010). Endocrine aspects of male sexual dysfunction. *Journal of Sexual Medicine, 7*, 1627–1656.

Cadoret, R. J., Yates, W. R., Troughton, E., Woodworth, G., & Stewart, M. A. (1995). Adoption study demonstrating two genetic pathways to drug abuse. *Archives of General Psychiatry, 52*, 42–52.

Cagle, J. (April 11, 2018). Mariah Carey: My Battle with Bipolar Disorder. *People Magazine*, https://people.com/music/mariah-carey-bipolar-disorder-diagnosis-exclusive/

Cahalan, S. (2012). *Brain on fire: My month of madness*. Free Press.

Cahill, K., Hartmann-Boyce, J., & Perera, R. (2015). Incentives for smoking cessation. *The Cochrane Database of Systematic Reviews, 5*, CD004307. https://doi.org/10.1002/14651858.CD004307.pub5

Cahill, K., Stead, L., & Lancaster, T. (2007). Nicotine receptor partial agonists for smoking cessation. *The Cochrane Database of Systematic Reviews*, CD006103.

Cahill, K., Stevens, S., Perera, R., & Lancaster, T. (2013). Pharmacological interventions for smoking cessation: an overview and network meta-analysis. *The Cochrane Database of Systematic Reviews, 5*, CD009329.

Cain, N. M., Pincus, A. L., & Holtforth, M. G. (2010). Interpersonal subtypes in social phobia: Diagnostic and treatment implications. *Journal of Personality Assessment, 92*(6), 514–527. https://doi.org/10.1080/00223891.2010.513704

Cai, N., Revez, J. A., Adams, M. J., Andlauer, T. F. M., Breen, G., Byrne, E. M., et al. (2020). Minimal phenotyping yields genome-wide association signals of low specificity for major depression. *Nature Genetics, 52*(4), 437–447. https://doi.org/10.1038/s41588-020-0594-5

Calhoun, V. D., Pekar, J. J., & Pearlson, G. D. (2004). Alcohol intoxication effects on simulated driving: Exploring alcohol-dose effects on brain activation using functional MRI. *Neuropsychopharmacology, 29*, 2197–2107.

Calleo, J., Stanley, M. A., Greisinger, A., Wehmanen, O., Johnson, M., Novy, D., et al. (2009). Generalized anxiety disorder in older medical patients: Diagnostic recognition, mental health management and service utilization. *Journal of Clinical Psychology in Medical Settings, 16*(2), 178–185. https://doi.org/10.1007/s10880-008-9144-5

Calzo, J. P., Blashill, A. J., Brown, T. A., & Argenal, R. L. (2017). Eating Disorders and Disordered Weight and Shape Control Behaviors in

Sexual Minority Populations. *Current Psychiatry Reports, 19*(8), 49. https://doi.org/10.1007/s11920-017-0801-y

Campbell, A. K., & Matthews, S. B. (2005). Darwin's illness revealed. *Postgraduate Medical Journal, 81*, 248–251. https://doi.org/10.1136/pgmj.2004.025569

Campbell, J., Stefan, S., & Loder, A. (1994). Putting violence in context. *Hospital and Community Psychiatry, 45*, 633.

Campbell, W. K., Bosson, J. K., Goheen, T. W., Lakey, C. E., & Kernis, M. H. (2007). Do narcissists dislike themselves "deep down inside"? *Psychological Science, 18*, 227–229.

Camus, V., Burtin, B., Simeone, I., Schwed, P., Gonthier, R., & Dubos, G. (2000). Factor analysis supports the evidence of existing hyperactive and hypoactive subtypes of delirium. *International Journal of Geriatric Psychiatry, 15*, 313–316.

Canli, T. (2008). Toward a neurogenetic theory of neuroticism. *Annals of the New York Academy of Sciences, 1129*(1), 153–174. https://doi.org/10.1196/annals.1417.022

Cannon, T. D. (2015). How schizophrenia develops: Cognitive and brain mechanisms underlying onset of psychosis. *Trends in Cognitive Sciences, 19*, 744–756.

Cannon, T. D., Cadenhead, K., Cornblatt, B., Woods, S. W., Addington, J., Walker, E. F., et al. (2008). Prediction of psychosis in youth at high clinical risk: A multisite longitudinal study in North America. *Archives of General Psychiatry, 65*, 28–37.

Cannon, T. D., Chung, Y., He, G., Sun, D., Jacobson, A., van Erp, T. G. M., et al. (2015). Progressive reduction in cortical thickness as psychosis develops: A multisite longitudinal neuroimaging study of youth at elevated clinical risk. *Biological Psychiatry, 77*, 147–157. https://doi.org/10.1016/j.biopsych.2014.05.023

Cannon, T. D., van Erp, T. G., Rosso, I. M., Huttunen, M., Lönqvist, J., Pirkola, T., et al. (2002). Fetal hypoxia and structural brain abnormalities in schizophrenic patients, their siblings, and controls. *Archives of General Psychiatry, 59*, 35–42.

Cannon, T. D., Yu, C., Addington, J., Bearden, C. E., Cadenhead, K. S., Cornblatt, B. A., et al. (2016). An individualized risk calculator for research in prodromal psychosis. *American Journal of Psychiatry, 173*, 980–988. https://doi.org/10.1176/appi.ajp.2016.15070890

Cano-López, J. B., García-Sancho, E., Fernández-Castilla, B., & Salguero, J. M. (2022). Empirical evidence of the metacognitive model of rumination and depression in clinical and nonclinical samples: A systematic review and meta-analysis. *Cognitive Therapy and Research, 46*(2), 367–392. https://doi.org/10.1007/s10608-021-10260-2

Cantor-Graae, E., & Selten, J.-P. (2005). Schizophrenia and migration: A meta-analysis and review. *The American Journal of Psychiatry, 162*, 12–24. https://doi.org/10.1176/appi.ajp.162.1.12

Cantor, J. M., Blanchard, R., Robichaud, L. K., & Christensen, B. K. (2005). Quantitative reanalysis of aggregate data on IQ in sexual offenders. *Psychological Bulletin, 131*, 555–568.

Cantor, J. M., & McPhail, I. V. (2015). Sensitivity and specificity of the phallometric test for hebephilia. *Journal of Sexual Medicine, 12*, 1940–1950. https://doi.org/10.1111/jsm.12970

Cappelletti, M., & Wallen, K. (2016). Increasing women's sexual desire: The comparative effectiveness of estrogens and androgens. *Hormones and Behavior, 78*, 178–193. https://doi.org/10.1016/j.yhbeh.2015.11.003

Capps, L., Losh, M., & Thurber, C. (2000). "The frog ate the bug and made his mouth sad": Narrative competence in children with autism. *Journal of Abnormal Child Psychology, 28*, 193–204.

Capps, L., Rasco, L., Losh, M., & Heerey, E. (1999). *Understanding of self-conscious emotions in high-functioning children with autism.* Paper presented at the Biennial Meeting of the Society for Research in Child Development, Albuquerque, NM.

Capps, L., Yirmiya, N., & Sigman, M. (1992). Understanding of simple and complex emotion in high-functioning children with autism. *Journal of Child Psychology and Psychiatry, 33*, 1169–1182.

Caraballo, R. S., Shafer, P. R., Patel, D., Davis, K. C., & McAfee, T. A. (2017). Quit methods used by US adult cigarette smokers, 2014–2016. *Preview of Chronic Disease, 14*, 160600. https://doi.org/10.5888/pcd14.160600

Cardinale, E. M., Breeden, A. L., Robertson, E. L., Lozier, L. M., Vanmeter, J. W., & Marsh, A. A. (2018). Externalizing behavior severity in youths with callous-unemotional traits corresponds to patterns of amygdala activity and connectivity during judgments of causing fear. *Development and psychopathology, 30*(1), 191–201. https://doi.org/10.1017/S0954579417000566

Carey, B. (2011, June 23). Expert on mental illness reveals her own fight. *The New York Times.*

Carey, B. (2017, July 24). England's mental health experiment: No-cost talk therapy. *New York Times.* https://www.nytimes.com/2017/07/24/health/england-mental-health-treatment-therapy.html?_r50 on July 28, 2017.

Carey, K. B., Carey, M. P., Maisto, S. A., & Henson, J. M. (2006). Brief motivational interventions for heavy college drinkers: A randomized controlled trial. *Journal of Consulting and Clinical Psychology, 74*, 943–954.

Carl, E., Stein, A. T., Levihn-Coon, A., Pogue, J. R., Rothbaum, B., Emmelkamp, P., et al. (2019). Virtual reality exposure therapy for anxiety and related disorders: A meta-analysis of randomized controlled trials. *Journal of Anxiety Disorders, 61*, 27–36. https://doi.org/10.1016/j.janxdis.2018.08.003

Carl, E., Witcraft, S. M., Kauffman, B. Y., Gillespie, E. M., Becker, E. S., Cuijpers, P., et al. (2020). Psychological and pharmacological treatments for generalized anxiety disorder (GAD): A meta-analysis of randomized controlled trials. *Cognitive Behaviour Therapy, 49*(1), 1–21. https://pubmed.ncbi.nlm.nih.gov/30760112/

Carlson, E. A., Egeland, B., & Sroufe, L. A. (2009). A prospective investigation of the development of borderline personality symptoms. *Development and Psychopathology, 21*, 1311–1334. https://doi.org/10.1017/S0954579409990174

Carlson, E. B., Dalenberg, C., & McDade-Montez, E. (2012). Dissociation in posttraumatic stress disorder part I: Definitions and review of research. *Psychological Trauma: Theory, Research, Practice, and Policy, 4*(5), 479–489. https://doi.org/10.1037/a0027748

Carlucci, L., Saggino, A., & Balsamo, M. (2021). On the efficacy of the unified protocol for transdiagnostic treatment of emotional disorders: A systematic review and meta-analysis. *Clinical psychology review, 87*, 101999. https://doi.org/10.1016/j.cpr.2021.1

Carmi, L., Tendler, A., Bystritsky, A., Hollander, E., Blumberger, D. M., Daskalakis, J., et al. (2019). Efficacy and safety of deep transcranial magnetic stimulation for obsessive-compulsive disorder: A prospective multicenter randomized double-blind placebo-controlled trial. *American Journal of Psychiatry, 176*(11), 931–938. https://doi.org/10.1176/appi.ajp.2019.18101180

Carney, R. M., & Freedland, K. E. (2017). Depression and coronary heart disease. *Nature Reviews Cardiology, 14*(3), 145–155. https://doi.org/10.1038/nrcardio.2016.181

Carpenter, J. K., Andrews, L. A., Witcraft, S. M., Powers, M. B., Smits, J. A. J., & Hofmann, S. G. (2018). Cognitive behavioral therapy for anxiety and related disorders: A meta-analysis of randomized placebo-controlled trials. *Wiley Online Library, 35*(6), 502–514. https://doi.org/10.1002/da.22728

Carpenter, W. T., Gold, J. M., Lahti, A. C., Queern, C. A., Conley, R. R., Bartko, J. J., et al. (2000). Decisional capacity for informed consent in schizophrenia research. *Archives of General Psychiatry, 57*, 533–538.

Carpenter, W. T., & van Os, J. (2011). Should attenuated psychosis syndrome be a DSM-5 diagnosis? *American Journal of Psychiatry, 168*, 460–463.

Carr, D. (2008). *The night of the gun: A reporter investigates the darkest story of his life. His own.* Simon & Schuster Adult Publishing Group.

Carr, E. G., & Durand, V. M. (1985). Reducing behavior problems through functional communication training. *Journal of Applied Behavior Analysis, 18*, 111–126.

Carrion, R. E., Cornblatt, B. A., Burton, C. Z., Tso, I. F., Auther, A. M., Adelsheim, S., et al. (2016). Personalized prediction of psychosis: External validation of the NAPLS-2 psychosis risk calculator with the EDIPPP project. *American Journal of Psychiatry, 173*, 989–996. https://doi.org/10.1176/appi.ajp.2016.15121565

Carroll, K. M., Kiluk, B. D., Nich, C., Gordon, M. A., Portnoy, G. A., Marino, D. R., et al. (2014). Computer-assisted delivery of cognitive-behavioral therapy: Efficacy and durability of CBT4CBT among cocaine-dependent individuals maintained on methadone. *American Journal of Psychiatry, 171*, 436–444.

Carroll, K. M., & Weiss, R. D (2017). The role of behavioral interventions in buprenorphine maintenance treatment: A review. *The American Journal of Psychiatry, 174*(8), 738–747.

Carroll, L. J., Cassidy, J. D., Holm, L., Kraus, J., Coronado, V. G., & WHO Collaborating Centre Task Force on Mild Traumatic Brain Injury (2004). Methodological issues and research recommendations for mild traumatic brain injury: the WHO Collaborating Centre Task Force on Mild Traumatic Brain Injury. *Journal of rehabilitation medicine*, (43 Suppl), 113–125. https://doi.org/10.1080/16501960410023877

Carson, A., & Lehn, A. (2016). Epidemiology. *Handbook of Clinical Neurology, 139*, 47–60. https://doi.org/10.1016/B978-0-12-801772-2.00005-9

Carstensen, L. L. (1996). Evidence for a life-span theory of socioemotional selectivity. *Current Directions in Psychological Science, 4*, 151–156.

Carstensen, L. L. (2021). Socioemotional selectivity theory: The role of perceived endings in human motivation. *The Gerontologist, 61*(8), 1188–1196. https://doi.org/10.1093/geront/gnab116

Carstensen, L. L., Shavit, Y. Z., & Barnes, J. T. (2020). Age advantages in emotional experience persist even under threat from the COVID-19 pandemic. *Psychological Science, 31*(11), 1374–1385. https://doi.org/10.1177/0956797620967

Carter, J. S., & Garber, J. (2011). Predictors of the first onset of a major depressive episode and changes in depressive symptoms across adolescence: Stress and negative cognitions. *Journal of Abnormal Psychology, 120*, 779–796.

Carvalheira, A. A., Brotto, L. A., & Leal, I. (2010). Women's motivations for sex: Exploring the Diagnostic and Statistical Manual, fourth edition, text revision criteria for hypoactive sexual desire and female sexual arousal disorders. *Journal of Sexual Medicine, 7*, 1454–1463.

Carvalho, J., & Nobre, P. (2010). Biopsychosocial determinants of men's sexual desire: Testing an integrative model. *Journal of Sexual Medicine, 8*, 754–763.

Carver, C. S., Johnson, S. L., & Joormann, J. (2008). Serotonergic function, two-mode models of self-regulation, and vulnerability to depression: What depression has in common with impulsive aggression. *Psychological Bulletin, 134*, 912–943.

Casaletto, K. B., Staffaroni, A. M., Wolf, A., Appleby, B., Brushaber, D., Coppola, G., et al. (2020). Active lifestyles moderate clinical outcomes in autosomal dominant frontotemporal degeneration. Alzheimer's & dementia: *The Journal of the Alzheimer's Association, 16*(1), 91–105. https://doi.org/10.1002/alz.12001

Cascio, C. N., Konrath, S. H., & Falk, E. B. (2015). Narcissists' social pain seen only in the brain. *Social Cognitive and Affective Neuroscience, 10*, 335–341. https://doi.org/10.1093/scan/nsu072

Caspi, A., Houts, R. M., Belsky, D. W., Goldman-Mellor, S. J., Harrington, H., Israel, S., et al. (2014). The p factor: One general psychopathology factor in the structure of psychiatric disorders? *Clinical Psychological Science, 2*, 119–137. https://doi.org/10.1177/2167702613497473

Caspi, A., & Moffitt, T. E. (2018). All for one and one for all: Mental disorders in one dimension. *American Journal of Psychiatry, 175*(9), 831–844. https://doi.org/10.1176/appi.ajp.2018.17121383

Cassin, S. E., & von Ranson, K. M. (2005). Personality and eating disorders: A decade in review. *Clinical Psychology Review, 25*(7), 895–916.

Castle, D., Beilharz, F., Phillips, K. A., Brakoulias, V., Drummond, L. M., Hollander, E., et al. (2021). Body dysmorphic disorder: A treatment synthesis and consensus on behalf of the International College of Obsessive-Compulsive Spectrum Disorders and the Obsessive Compulsive and Related Disorders network of the European College of Neuropsychopharmacology. *International Clinical Psychopharmacology, 36*(2), 61–75. https://doi.org/10.1097/YIC.0000000000000342

Catalá-López, F., Hutton, B., Núñez-Beltrán, A., Page, M. J., Ridao, M., Macías Saint-Gerons, D., et al. (2017). The pharmacological and non-pharmacological treatment of attention deficit hyperactivity disorder in children and adolescents: A systematic review with network meta-analyses of randomised trials. *PLOS ONE, 12*(7), e0180355. https://doi.org/10.1371/journal.pone.0180355

CBS. (2017). More than 12M "MeToo" Facebook posts, comments, reactions in 24 hours. https://www.cbsnews.com/news/metoo-more-than-12-million-facebook-posts-comments-reactions-24-hours/

Celebucki, C. C., Wayne, G. F., Connolly, G. N., Pankow, J. F., & Chang, E. I. (2005). Characterization of measured menthol in 48 U.S. cigarette sub-brands. *Nicotine and Tobacco Research, 7*, 523–531.

Cénat, J. M., Blais-Rochette, C., Morse, C., Vandette, M., Noorishad, P., Kogan, C., . . . Labelle, P. R. et al. (2021). Prevalence and risk factors associated with attention-deficit/hyperactivity disorder among US black individuals: A systematic review and meta-analysis. *JAMA Psychiatry, 78*(1), 21–28. https://doi.org/10.1001/jamapsychiatry.2020.2788

Center for Disease Control (CDC). (2023, May 11). *Suicide data and statistics.* https://www.cdc.gov/suicide/suicide-data-statistics.html

Centers for Disease Control (2023). Adverse Childhood Experiences. Retrieved from https://www.cdc.gov/violenceprevention/aces/index.html.

Centers for Disease Control and Prevention. (2018, August 31). 2018 Annual Surveillance Report of Drug-Related Risks and Outcomes—United States. Surveillance Special Report. Centers for Disease Control and Prevention, U.S. Department of Health and Human Services. https://www.cdc.gov/drugoverdose/pdf/pubs/2018-cdc-drug-surveillance-report.pdf

Centers for Disease Control and Prevention (CDC; 2023). *Behavioral Risk Factor Surveillance System Survey Questionnaire.* Atlanta, Georgia: U.S. Department of Health and Human Services, Centers for Disease Control and Prevention

Cerny, J. A., Barlow, D. H., Craske, M. G., & Himadi, W. G. (1987). Couples treatment of agoraphobia: A two-year follow-up. *Behavior Therapy, 18*, 401–415.

Chami, R., Reichenberger, J., Cardi, V., Lawrence, N., Treasure, J., & Blechert, J. (2021). Characterising binge eating over the course of a feasibility trial among individuals with binge eating disorder and bulimia nervosa. *Appetite, 164*, 105248.

Champagne, F. A. (2016). Epigenetic legacy of parental experiences: Dynamic and interactive pathways to inheritance. *Development and Psychopathology, 28*, 1219–1228. https://doi.org/10.1017/S0954579416000808

Chan, A. T., Sun, G. Y., Tam, W. W., Tsoi, K. K., & Wong, S. Y. (2017). The effectiveness of group-based behavioral activation in the treatment of depression: An updated meta-analysis of randomized controlled trial. *Journal of Affective Disorders, 208*, 345–354. https://doi.org/10.1016/j.jad.2016.08.026

Chan, B., Kondo, K., Freeman, M., Ayers, C., Montgomery, J., & Kansagara, D. (2019). Pharmacotherapy for cocaine use disorder—A systematic review and meta-analysis. *Journal of General Internal Medicine, 34*(12), 2858–2873.

Chan, G. C. K., Kelly, A. B., Carroll, A., & Williams, J. W. (2017). Peer drug use and adolescent polysubstance use: Do parenting and school factors moderate this association? *Addictive Behaviors, 64*, 78–81.

Chang, N. A., Jager-Hyman, S., Brown, G. K., Cunningham, A., & Stanley, B. (2016). Treating the suicidal patient. In R. C. O'Connor & J. Pirkis (Eds.), *The international handbook of suicide prevention* (pp. 416–430). John Wiley & Sons, Ltd. https://doi.org/10.1002/9781118903223.ch23

Chansatitporn, N., Charoenca, N., Sidhu, A., Lapvongwatana, P., Kungskulniti, N., & Sussman, S. (2016). Three-month effects of Project EX: A smoking intervention pilot program with Thai adolescents. *Addictive Behaviors, 61*, 20–24. https://doi.org/10.1016/j.addbeh.2016.05.003

Chard, K. M., Ricksecker, E. G., Healy, E. T., Karlin, B. E., & Resick, P. A. (2012). Dissemination and experience with cognitive processing therapy. *Journal of Rehabilitation Research and Development, 49*(5), 667–678.

Charuvastra, A., & Cloitre, M. (2008). Social bonds and posttraumatic stress disorder. *Annual Review of Psychology, 59*, 301–328.

Chassin, L., Curran, P. J., Hussong, A. M., & Colder, C. R. (1996). The relation of parent alcoholism to adolescent substance abuse: A longitudinal follow-up. *Journal of Abnormal Psychology, 105*, 70–80.

Chaste, P., Klei, L., Sanders, S. J., Hus, V., Murtha, M. T., Lowe, J. K., et al. (2015). A genome-wide association study of autism using the Simons Simplex Collection: Does reducing phenotypic heterogeneity in autism increase genetic homogeneity? *Biological Psychiatry, 77*(9), 775–784. https://doi.org/10.1016/j.biopsych.2014.09.017

Chavanne, A. V., & Robinson, O. J. (2021). The overlapping neurobiology of induced and pathological anxiety: A meta-analysis of functional neural activation. *American Journal of Psychiatry, 178*(2), 156–164. https://doi.org/10.1176/appi.ajp.2020.19111153

Chen, C., Hsu, F. C., Li, C. W., & Huang, M. C. (2019). Structural, functional, and neurochemical neuroimaging of methamphetamine-associated psychosis: A systematic review. *Psychiatry Research Neuroimaging, 292*, 23–31. https://doi.org/10.1016/j.pscychresns.2019.06.002

Cheng, P. W. C., Louie, L. L. C., Wong, Y. L., Wong, S. M. C., Leung, W. Y., Nitsche, M. A., et al. (2020 Oct). The effects of transcranial direct current stimulation (tDCS) on clinical symptoms in schizophrenia: A systematic review and meta-analysis. *Asian Journal of Psychiatry, 53*, 102392. https://doi.org/10.1016/j.ajp.2020.102392. Epub 2020 Sep 5. PMID: 32956993.

Cheng, S.-T., & Zhang, F. (2020). A comprehensive meta-review of systematic reviews and meta-analyses on nonpharmacological interventions for informal dementia caregivers. *BMC Geriatrics, 20*(1), 137. https://doi.org/10.1186/s12877-020-01547-2

Cheng, Z. H., Perko, V. L., Fuller-Marashi, L., Gau, J. M., & Stice, E. (2019). Ethnic differences in eating disorder prevalence, risk factors, and predictive effects of risk factors among young women. *Eating Behaviors, 32*, 23–30.

Chen, S., Yang, P., Chen, T., Su, H., Jiang, H., & Zhao, M. (2020). Risky decision-making in individuals with substance use disorder: A meta-analysis and meta-regression review. *Psychopharmacology, 237*(7), 1893–1908. https://doi.org/10.1007/s00213-020-05506-y

Chen, Y.-Y., Wu, K. C.-C., Wang, Y., & Yip, P. S. F. (2016). Suicide prevention through restricting access to suicide means and hotspots. In R. C. O'Connor & J. Pirkis (Eds.), *The international handbook of suicide prevention* (pp. 609–636). John Wiley & Sons, Ltd. https://doi.org/10.1002/9781118903223.ch35

Chesney, E., Goodwin, G. M., & Fazel, S. (2014). Risks of all-cause and suicide mortality in mental disorders: A meta review. *World Psychiatry, 13*, 153–160.

Chételat, G., Arbizu, J., Barthel, H., Garibotto, V., Law, I., Morbelli, S., et al. (2020). Amyloid-PET and 18F-FDG-PET in the diagnostic investigation of Alzheimer's disease and other dementias. *The Lancet Neurology, 19*(11), 951–962. https://doi.org/10.1016/S1474-4422(20)30314-8

Cheung, C. H., Rijdijk, F., McLoughlin, G., Faraone, S. V., Asherson, P., & Kuntsi, J. (2015). Childhood predictors of adolescent and young adult outcome in ADHD. *Journal of Psychiatric Research, 62*, 92–100.

Chiappini, S., Picutti, E., Chiara Alessi, M., Di Carlo, F., Miuli, A., Pettorruso, M., et al. (2022). Efficacy of noninvasive brain stimulation on borderline personality disorder core symptoms: A systematic review. *Journal of Personality Disorders, 36*(5), 505–526. https://doi.org/10.1521/pedi.2022.36.5.505

Chivers, M. L., Seto, M. C., Lalumiere, M. L., Laan, E., & Grimbos, T. (2010). Agreement of self-reported and genital measures of sexual arousal in men and women: A meta-analysis. *Archives of Sexual Behavior, 39*, 5–56.

Choe, J. Y., B.A., Teplin, L. A., & Abram, K. M. (2008). Perpetration of violence, violent victimization, and severe mental illness: Balancing public health concerns. *Psychiatric Services, 59*(2), 153–164. https://doi.org/10.1176/ps.2008.59.2.153

Chorpita, B. F., Vitali, A. E., & Barlow, D. H. (1997). Behavioral treatment of choking phobia in an adolescent: An experimental analysis. *Journal of Behavior Therapy and Experimental Psychiatry, 28*, 307–315.

Chou, Y.-H., Ton That, V., & Sundman, M. (2020). A systematic review and meta-analysis of rTMS effects on cognitive enhancement in mild cognitive impairment and Alzheimer's disease. *Neurobiology of Aging, 86*, 1–10. https://doi.org/10.1016/j.neurobiolaging.2019.08.020

Christakis, N., & Fowler, J. (2008). The collective dynamics of smoking in a large social network. *New England Journal of Medicine, 358*, 2249–2258.

Christensen, D., Bilder, D., Zahorodny, W., Pettygrove, S., Durkin, M., Fitzgerald, R., et al. (2016). Prevalence and characteristics of autism spectrum disorder among 4-year-old children in the autism and developmental disabilities monitoring network. *Journal of Developmental & Behavioral Pediatrics, 37*, 1–8. https://doi.org/10.1097/DBP.0000000000000235

Christensen, S. S., Frostholm, L., Ørnbøl, E., & Schröder, A. (2015). Changes in illness perceptions mediated the effect of cognitive behavioural therapy in severe functional somatic syndromes. *Journal of Psychosomatic Research, 78*, 363–370. https://doi.org/10.1016/j.jpsychores.2014.12.005

Chronis, A. M., Jones, H. A., & Raggi, V. L. (2006). Evidence-based psychosocial treatments for children and adolescents with attention-deficit/hyperactivity disorder. *Clinical Psychology Review, 26*, 486–502.

Chronis-Tuscano, A., Degnan, K. A., Pine, D. S., Perez-Edgar, K., Henderson, H. A., Diaz, Y., et al. (2009). Stable early maternal report of behavioral inhibition predicts lifetime social anxiety disorder in adolescence. *Journal of the American Academy of Child and Adolescent Psychiatry, 48*, 928–935.

Chu, C., Buchman-Schmitt, J. M., Stanley, I. H., Hom, M. A., Tucker, R. P., Hagan, C. R., et al. (2017). The interpersonal theory of suicide: A systematic review and meta-analysis of a decade of cross-national research. *Psychological Bulletin, 143*(12), 1313–1345. https://doi.org/10.1037/bul0000123

Cicero, T. J., Ellis, M. S., Surratt, H. L., & Kurtz, S. P. (2014). The changing face of heroin use in the United States: A retrospective analysis of the past 50 years. *Journal of the American Medical Association, Psychiatry, 71*, 821–826.

Cipriani, A., Pretty, H., Hawton, K., & Geddes, J. R. (2005). Lithium in the prevention of suicidal behavior and all-cause mortality in patients with mood disorders: A systematic review of randomized trials. *American Journal of Psychiatry, 162*, 1805–1819.

Cirincione, C., Steadman, H. J., & McGreevy, M. A. (1995). Rates of insanity acquittals and the factors associated with successful insanity pleas. *Bulletin of the American Academy of Psychiatry and Law, 23*, 399–409.

Cisler, J. M., & Koster, E. H. (2010). Mechanisms of attentional biases towards threat in anxiety disorders: An integrative review. *Clinical Psychology Review, 30*, 203–216.

Clark, D. A. (1997). Twenty years of cognitive assessment: Current status and future directions. *Journal of Consulting and Clinical Psychology, 65*, 996–1000.

Clark, D. A. (2006). *Cognitive-behavioral therapy for OCD*. Guilford Press.

Clark, D. A., & González, A. D. P. (2014). Obsessive-compulsive disorder. In P. Emmelkamp & T. Ehring (Eds.), *The Wiley handbook of anxiety disorders* (pp. 497–534). John Wiley & Sons, Ltd.

Clark, D. M. (1996). Panic disorder: From theory to therapy. In P. M. Salkovskis (Ed.), *Frontiers of cognitive therapy* (pp. 318–344). Guilford Press.

Clark, D. M., Ehlers, A., Hackmann, A., McManus, F., Fennell, M., Grey, N., et al. (2006). Cognitive therapy versus exposure and applied relaxation in social phobia: A randomized controlled trial. *Journal of Consulting and Clinical Psychology, 74*, 568–578.

Clark, D. M., Ehlers, A., McManus, F., Hackmann, A., Fennell, M., Campbell, H., et al. (2003). Cognitive therapy versus fluoxetine in generalized social phobia: A randomized control trial. *Journal of Consulting and Clinical Psychology, 71*, 1058–1067.

Clark, D. M., Salkovskis, P. M., Hackmann, A., Wells, A., Ludgate, J., & Gelder, M. (1999). Brief cognitive therapy for panic disorder: A randomized controlled trial. *Journal of Consulting and Clinical Psychology, 67*, 583–589.

Clark, D. M., & Wells, A. (1995). A cognitive model of social phobia. In R. Heimberg, M. R. Liebowitz, D. A. Hope, & F. R. Schneier (Eds.), *Social phobia: Diagnosis, assessment and treatment* (pp. 69–93). Guilford Press.

Clarkin, J. F., Levy, K. N., Lenzenweger, M. F., & Kernberg, O. F. (2007). Evaluating three treatments for borderline personality disorder: a multiwave study. *The American Journal of Psychiatry, 164*(6), 922–928. https://doi.org/10.1176/ajp.2007.164.6.922

Clauss, J. A., & Blackford, J. U. (2012). Behavioral inhibition and risk for developing social anxiety disorder: A meta-analytic study. *Journal of the American Academy of Child & Adolescent Psychiatry, 51*(10), 1066–1075.e1. https://doi.org/10.1016/j.jaac.2012.08.002

Cleckley, H. (1976). *The mask of sanity* (5th ed.). St. Louis, MO: Mosby.

Clements, C. C., Zoltowski, A. R., Yankowitz, L. D., Yerys, B. E., Schultz, R. T., & Herrington, J. D. (2018). Evaluation of the social motivation hypothesis of autism: A systematic review and meta-analysis. *JAMA Psychiatry, 75*(8), 797–808.

Cloitre, M., Courtois, C. A., Charuvastra, A., Carapezza, R., Stolbach, B. C., & Green, B. L. (2011). Treatment of complex PTSD: Results of the ISTSS expert clinician survey on best practices. *Journal of Traumatic Stress, 24*, 615–627.

Cohen, D. (2014). *A big fat crisis: The hidden forces behind the obesity epidemic and how we can end it.* Nation Books.

Cohen, J. A., Deblinger, E., Mannarino, A. P., & Steer, R. (2004). A multi-site, randomized controlled trial for children with abuse-related PTSD symptoms. *Journal of the American Academy of Child and Adolescent Psychiatry, 43*, 393–402.

Cohen, P. (2008, February 21). Midlife suicide rises, puzzling researchers. *The New York Times*, pp. 1–4.

Cohen, S., Frank, E., Doyle, W. J., Rabin, B. S., Skoner, D. P., & Gwaltney, J. M., Jr. (1998). Types of stressors that increase susceptibility to the common cold in healthy adults. *Health Psychology, 17*, 214–223.

Coid, J. W., Ullrich, S., Bebbington, P., Fazel, S., & Keers, R. (2016). Paranoid Ideation and Violence: Meta-analysis of individual subject data of 7 population Surveys. *Schizophrenia Bulletin, 42*(4), 907–915.

Coie, J. D., & Dodge, K. A. (1998). Aggression and antisocial behavior. In W. Damon & N. Eisenberg (Eds.), *Handbook of child psychology: Volume 3: Social, emotional and personality development* (pp. 779–862). John Wiley & Sons.

Cole, D. A., Ciesla, J. A., Dallaire, D. H., Jacquez, F. M., Pineda, A. Q., Lagrange, B., et al. (2008). Emergence of attributional style and its relations to depressive symptoms. *Journal of Abnormal Psychology, 117*, 16–31.

Cole, D., Zelkowitz, R., Nick, E., Lubarsky, S., & Rights, J. (2019). Simultaneously examining negative appraisals, emotion reactivity, and cognitive reactivity in relation to depressive symptoms in children. *Development and Psychopathology, 31*(4), 1527–1540. https://doi.org/10.1017/S0954579418001207

Cole, E. J., Stimpson, K. H., Bentzley, B. S., Gulser, M., Cherian, K., Tischler, C., et al. (2020). Stanford accelerated intelligent neuro-modulation therapy for treatment-resistant depression. *American Journal of Psychiatry, 177*(8), 716–726. https://doi.org/10.1176/appi.ajp.2019.19070720

Coleman, J. R. I., Gaspar, H. A., Bryois, J., Byrne, E. M., Forstner, A. J., Holmans, P. A., et al. (2020). The genetics of the mood disorder spectrum: Genome-wide association analyses of more than 185,000 cases and 439,000 controls. *Biological Psychiatry, 88*(2), 169–184. https://doi.org/10.1016/j.biopsych.2019.10.015

Colli, A., Tanzilli, A., Dimaggio, G., & Lingiardi, V. (2014). Patient personality and therapist response: An empirical investigation. *American Journal of Psychiatry, 171*, 102–108. https://doi.org/10.1176/appi.ajp.2013.13020224

Collin, G., Kahn, R. S., de Reus, M. A., Cahn, W., & van den Heuvel, M. P. (2014). Impaired rich club connectivity in unaffected siblings of schizophrenia patients. *Schizophrenia Bulletin, 40*, 438–448.

Colombo, C., Benedetti, F., Barbini, B., Campori, E., & Smeraldi, E. (1999). Rate of switch from depression into mania after therapeutic sleep deprivation in bipolar depression. *Psychiatry Research, 86*, 267–270.

Colom, F., Vieta, E., Reinares, M., Martinez-Aran, A., Torrent, C., Goikolea, J. M., & Gasto, C. (2003). Psychoeducation efficacy in bipolar disorders: Beyond compliance enhancement. *Journal of Clinical Psychiatry, 64*, 1101–1105.

Comas-Díaz, L., Hall, G. N., & Neville, H. A. (2019). Racial trauma: Theory, research, and healing: Introduction to the special issue. *American Psychologist, 74*(1), 1–5. https://doi.org/10.1037/amp0000442

Comer, S. D., Hart, C. L., Ward, A. S., Haney, M., Foltin, R. W., & Fischman, M. W. (2001). Effects of repeated oral methamphetamine administration in humans. *Psychopharmacology, 155*, 397–404.

Conduct Problems Prevention Research Group (CPPRG). (2010a). The difficulty of maintaining positive intervention effects: A look at disruptive behavior, deviant peer relations, and social skills during the middle school years. *Journal of Early Adolescence, 30*(4), 593–624.

Conduct Problems Prevention Research Group (CPPRG). (2010b). Fast track intervention effects on youth arrests and delinquency. *Journal of Experimental Criminology, 6*(2), 131–157.

Conduct Problems Prevention Research Group (CPPRG). (2011). The effects of the Fast track preventive intervention on the development of conduct disorder across childhood. *Child Development, 82*(1), 331–345.

Conduct Problems Prevention Research Group (CPPRG). (2020). *The Fast Track program for children at risk: Preventing antisocial behavior.* Guilford Press.

Constantino, J. N., Charman, T., & Jones, E. J. H. (2021). Clinical and translational implications of an emerging developmental substructure for autism. *Annual Review of Clinical Psychology, 17*(1), 365–389. https://doi.org/10.1146/annurev-clinpsy-081219-110503

Constantino, J. N., Zhang, Z., Frazier, T., Abbachi, A. M., & Law, P. (2010). Sibling recurrence and the genetic epidemiology of autism. *American Journal of Psychiatry, 167*, 1349–1356.

Cook, M., & Mineka, S. (1989). Observational conditioning of fear to fear-relevant versus fear-irrelevant stimuli in rhesus monkeys. *Journal of Abnormal Psychology, 98*, 448–459.

Cooper, A. A., Zoellner, L. A., Roy-Byrne, P., Mavissakalian, M. R., & Feeny, N. C. (2017). Do changes in trauma-related beliefs predict PTSD symptom improvement in prolonged exposure and sertraline? *Journal of Consulting and Clinical Psychology, 85*(9), 873–882. https://doi.org/10.1037/ccp0000220

Cooper, K., Martyn-St James, M., Kaltenthaler, E., Dickinson, K., Cantrell, A., Wylie, K., et al. (2015). Behavioral therapies for management of premature ejaculation: A systematic review. *Sexual Medicine, 3*, 174–188. https://doi.org10.1002/sm2.65

Cooper, M. S., & Clark, V. P. (2013). Neuroinflammation, neuroautoimmunity, and the co-morbidities of complex regional pain syndrome. *Journal of Neuroimmune Pharmacology, 8*, 452–469.

Cooper, S. E., & Dunsmoor, J. E. (2021). Fear conditioning and extinction in obsessive-compulsive disorder: A systematic review. *Neuroscience and Biobehavioral Reviews, 129*, 75–94. https://doi.org/10.1016/j.neubiorev.2021.07.026

Copeland, W. E., Angold, A., Costello, E. J., & Egger, H. (2013). Prevalence, comorbidity, and correlates of DSM-5 proposed disruptive mood dysregulation disorder. *American Journal of Psychiatry, 170*(2), 173–179.

Copeland, W. E., & McGinnis, E. W. (2021). Epidemiology of trauma and PTSD in childhood and adolescence. In M. J. Friedman, P. P. Schnurr, & T. M. Keane (Eds.), *Handbook of PTSD: Science and practice* (3rd ed., pp. 76–97). Guilford Press.

Copeland, W. E., Wolke, D., Angold, A., & Costello, E. J. (2013). Adult psychiatric outcomes of bullying and being bullied by peers in childhood and adolescence. *JAMA Psychiatry, 70*(4), 419–426. https://doi.org/10.1001/jamapsychiatry.2013.504

Copf, T. (2016). Impairments in dendrite morphogenesis as etiology for neurodevelopmental disorders and implications for therapeutic treatments. *Neuroscience & Biobehavioral Reviews, 68*, 946–978. https://doi.org/10.1016/j.neubiorev.2016.04.008

Copolov, D. L., Mackinnon, A., & Trauer, T. (2004). Correlates of the affective impact of auditory hallucinations in psychotic disorders. *Schizophrenia Bulletin, 30*, 163–171.

Corbett, B. A., Swain, D. M., Newsom, C., Wang, L., Song, Y., & Edgerton, D. (2014). Biobehavioral profiles of arousal and social motivation in autism spectrum disorders. *Journal of Child Psychology and Psychiatry, 55*, 924–934.

Correll, C. U., Cortese, S., Croatto, G., Monaco, F., Krinitski, D., Arrondo, G., et al. (2021). Efficacy and acceptability of pharmacological, psychosocial, and brain stimulation interventions in children and adolescents with mental disorders: An umbrella review. *World Psychiatry, 20*(2), 244–275. https://doi.org/10.1002/wps.20881

Correll, C. U., Solmi, M., Veronese, N., Bortolato, B., Rosson, S., Santonastaso, P., et al. (2017). Prevalence, incidence and mortality from cardiovascular disease in patients with pooled and specific severe mental illness: A large-scale meta-analysis of 3,211,768 patients and 113,383,368 controls. *World Psychiatry, 16*, 163–180. https://doi.org/10.1002/wps.20420

Corrigan, P. W. (2015). Challenging the stigma of mental illness: Different agendas, different goals. *Psychiatric Services, 66*, 1347–1349. https://doi.org/10.1176/appi.ps.201500107

Corrigan, P. W., Morris, S. B., Michaels, P. J., Rafacz, J. D., & Rüsch, N. (2012). Challenging the public stigma of mental illness: A meta-analysis of outcome studies. *Psychiatric Services, 63*, 963–973. https://doi.org/10.1176/appi.ps.201100529

Corrigan, P. W., & Nieweglowski, K. (2019). How does familiarity impact the stigma of mental illness? *Clinical Psychology Review, 70*, 40–50.

Corrigan, P. W., & Watson, A. C. (2005). Findings from the National Comorbidity Survey on the frequency of violent behavior in individuals with psychiatric disorders. *Psychiatry Research, 136*, 153–162.

Corrigan, P. W., Watson, A. C., Heyrman, J. D., Warpinski, A., Gracia, G., Slopen, N., et al. (2005). Structural stigma in state legislatures. *Psychiatric Services, 56*, 557–563.

Cortese, S., Kelly, C., Chabernaud, C., Proal, E., Di Martino, A., Milham, M. P., et al. (2012). Toward systems neuroscience of ADHD: A meta-analysis of 55 fMRI studies. *American Journal of Psychiatry, 169*(10), 1038–1055.

Costa, P. T., Metter, E. J., & McCrae, R. R. (1994). Personality stability and its contribution to successful aging. *Journal of Geriatric Psychiatry, 27*, 41–59.

Costello, J. E., Erkanli, A., & Angold, A. (2006). Is there an epidemic of child or adolescent depression? *Journal of Child Psychology and Psychiatry, 47*(12), 1263–1271.

Cougle, J. R., Timpano, K. R., Sachs-Ericsson, N., Keough, M. E., & Riccardi, C. J. (2010). Examining the unique relationships between anxiety disorders and childhood physical and sexual abuse in the national comorbidity survey-replication. *Psychiatry Research, 177*(1–2), 150–155. https://doi.org/10.1016/j.psychres.2009.03.008

Courchesne, E. (2004). Brain development in autism: Early overgrowth followed by premature arrests of growth. *Mental Retardation and Developmental Disabilities Research Reviews, 10*, 106–111.

Courchesne, E., Campbell, K., & Solso, S. (2011). Brain growth across the life span in autism: Age-specific changes in anatomical pathology. *Brain Research, 1380*, 138–145. https://doi.org/10.1016/j.brainres.2010.09.101

Courchesne, E., Carnes, B. S., & Davis, H. R. (2001). Unusual brain growth patterns in early life in patients with autistic disorder: An MRI study. *Neurology, 57*, 245–254.

Coyne, J. C. (1976). Depression and the response of others. *Journal of Abnormal Psychology, 85*, 186–193.

Coyne, J. C. (1994). Self-reported distress: Analog or ersatz depression? *Psychological Bulletin, 116*, 29–45. https://doi.org/10.1037/0033-2909.116.1.29

Crane, N. A., Burkhouse, K. L., Gorka, S. M., Klumpp, H., & Phan, K. L. (2022). Electrocortical measures of win and loss processing are associated with mesocorticolimbic functional connectivity: A combined ERP and rs-fMRI study. *Psychophysiology, 59*(12). https://doi.org/10.1111/psyp.14118

Craske, M. G., & Barlow, D. (2014). In panic disorder and agoraphobia. In D. Barlow (Ed.), *Clinical handbook of psychological disorders: A step-by-step treatment manual* (p. 768). Guilford.

Craske, M. G., Rauch, S. L., Ursano, R., Prenoveau, J., Pine, D. S., & Zinbarg, R. E. (2009). What is an anxiety disorder? *Depression and Anxiety, 26*, 1066–1085.

Craske, M. G., Sandman, C. F., & Stein, M. B. (2022). How can neurobiology of fear extinction inform treatment? *Neuroscience & Biobehavioral Reviews, 143*, 104923. https://doi.org/10.1016/j.neubiorev.2022.104923

Crean, R. D., Crane, N. A., & Mason, B. J. (2011). An evidence based review of acute and long-term effects of Cannabis use on executive cognitive functions. *Journal of Addictive Medicines, 5*, 1–8.

Crissman, H. P., Berger, M. B., Graham, L. F., & Dalton, V. K. (2017). Transgender demographics: A household probability sample of U.S. adults, 2014. *American Journal of Public Health, 107*, 213–215. https://doi.org/10.2105/ajph.2016.303571

Cristea, I. A., Gentili, C., Cotet, C. D., Palomba, D., Barbui, C., & Cuijpers, P. (2017). Efficacy of psychotherapies for borderline personality disorder: A systematic review and meta-analysis. *JAMA Psychiatry, 74*, 319–328. https://doi.org/10.1001/jamapsychiatry.2016.4287

Crits-Christoph, P., Frank, E., Chambless, D. L., Brody, C., & Karp, J. F. (1995). Training in empirically validated treatments: What are clinical psychology students learning? *Professional Psychology: Research and Practice, 26*, 514–522.

Critser, G. (2003). *Fatland: How Americans became the fattest people in the world.* Houghton Mifflin.

Cronbach, L. J., & Meehl, P. E. (1955). Construct validity in psychological tests. *Psychological Bulletin, 52*, 281–302.

Cross-Disorder Group of the Psychiatric Genomics Consortium. (2013). Identification of risk loci with shared effects on five major psychiatric disorders: A genome-wide analysis. *The Lancet, 381*, 1371–1379.

Cross-Disorder Group of the Psychiatric Genomics Consortium (2019). Genomic relationships, novel loci, and pleiotropic mechanisms across eight psychiatric disorders. *Cell, 179*(7), 1469–1482. e11. https://doi.org/10.1016/j.cell.2019.11.020

Crossley, N. A., Mechelli, A., Ginestet, C., Rubinov, M., Bullmore, E. T., & McGuire, P. (2016). Altered hub functioning and compensatory activations in the connectome: A meta-analysis of functional neuroimaging studies in schizophrenia. *Schizophrenia Bulletin, 42*, 434–442. https://doi.org/10.1093/schbul/sbv146

Crow, S. J. (2019). Pharmacologic treatment of eating disorders. *The Psychiatric Clinics of North America, 42*(2), 253–262.

Crow, S. J., Peterson, C. B., Swanson, S. A., Raymond, N. C., Specker, S., Eckert, E. D., et al. (2009). Increased mortality in bulimia nervosa and other eating disorders. *American Journal of Psychiatry, 166*, 1342–1346.

Crump, C., Sundquist, K., Winkleby, M. A., & Sundquist, J. (2013). Comorbidities and mortality in bipolar disorder: A Swedish national cohort study. *JAMA Psychiatry, 70*(9), 931–939. https://doi.org/10.1001/jamapsychiatry.2013.1394

Cuijpers, P., Berking, M., Andersson, G., Quigley, L., Kleiboer, A., & Dobson, K. S. (2013). A meta-analysis of cognitive-behavioural therapy for adult depression, alone and in comparison with other treatments. *Canadian Journal of Psychiatry, 58*(7), 376–385. https://doi.org/10.1177/070674371305800702

Cuijpers, P., Cristea, I. A., Karyotaki, E., Reijnders, M., & Huibers, M. J. H. (2016). How effective are cognitive behavior therapies for major depression and anxiety disorders? A meta-analytic update of the evidence. *World Psychiatry, 15*(3), 245–258. https://doi.org/10.1002/wps.20346

Cuijpers, P., Donker, T., Weissman, M. M., Ravitz, P., & Cristea, I. A. (2016). Interpersonal psychotherapy for mental health problems: A comprehensive meta-analysis. *American Journal of Psychiatry, 173*, 680–687. https://doi.org/10.1176/appi.ajp.2015.15091141

Cuijpers, P., Sijbrandij, M., Koole, S. L., Andersson, G., Beekman, A. T., & Reynolds, C. F. (2013). The efficacy of psychotherapy and pharmacotherapy in treating depressive and anxiety disorders: A meta-analysis of direct comparisons. *World Psychiatry, 12*, 137–148.

Culbert, K. M., Racine, S. E., & Klump, K. L. (2015). Research review: What we have learned about the causes of eating disorders—A synthesis of sociocultural, psychological, and biological research. *Journal of Child Psychology and Psychiatry, 56*(11), 1141–1164. https://doi.org/10.1111/jcpp.12441

Cummings, C. M., Caporino, N. E., & Kendall, P. C. (2014). Comorbidity of anxiety and depression in children and adolescents: 20 years after. *Psychological Bulletin, 140*(3), 816–845.

Curran, E., Adamson, G., Stringer, M., Rosato, M., & Leavey, G. (2016). Severity of mental illness as a result of multiple childhood adversities: US National Epidemiologic Survey. *Social Psychiatry and Psychiatric Epidemiology, 51*, 647–657. https://doi.org/10.1007/s00127-016-1198-3

Curry, J., Silva, S., Rohde, P., Ginsburg, G., Kratochvil, C., Simons, A., et al. (2011). Recovery and recurrence following treatment for adolescent major depression. *Archives of General Psychiatry, 68*, 263–270.

Curry, S. J., Mermelstein, R. J., & Sporer, A. K. (2009). Therapy for specific problems: Youth tobacco cessation. *Annual Review of Psychology, 60*, 229–255.

Curtis, N. M., Ronan, K. R., & Borduin, C. M. (2004). Multisystemic treatment: A meta-analysis of outcome studies. *Journal of Family Psychology, 18*(3), 411–419. https://doi.org/10.1037/0893-3200.18.3.411

Cusack, K., Jonas, D. E., Forneris, C. A., Wines, C., Sonis, J., Middleton, J. C., et al. (2016). Psychological treatments for adults with post-traumatic stress disorder: A systematic review and meta-analysis. *Clinical Psychology Review, 43*, 128–141. https://doi.org/10.1016/j.cpr.2015.10.003

Dahlenburg, S. C., Gleaves, D. H., & Hutchinson, A. D. (2019). Anorexia nervosa and perfectionism: A meta-analysis. *International Journal of Eating Disorders, 52*(3), 219–229. https://doi.org/10.1002/eat.23009

Dalenberg, C. J., Brand, B. L., Gleaves, D. H., Dorahy, M. J., Loewenstein, R. J., Cardeña, E., et al. (2012). Evaluation of the evidence for the trauma and fantasy models of dissociation. *Psychological Bulletin, 138*, 550–588. https://doi.org/10.1037/a0027447

Daley, S. E., Hammen, C., & Rao, U. (2000). Predictors of first onset and recurrence of major depression in young women during the 5 years following high school graduation. *Journal of Abnormal Psychology 109*, 525–533.

Dallman, M. F., Pecoraro, N., Akana, S. F., La Fleur, S. E., Gomez, F., Houshyar, H., et al. (2003). Chronic stress and obesity: A new view of comfort food. *Proceedings of the National Academy of Sciences, 100*, 11696–11701.

Dalmau, J., Tüzün, E., Wu, H. Y., Masjuan, J., Rossi, J. E., Voloschin, A., Baehring, J. M., Shimazaki, H., Koide, R., King, D., Mason, W., Sansing, L. H., Dichter, M. A., Rosenfeld, M. R., Lynch, D. R. (2007 Jan). Paraneoplastic anti-N-methyl-D-aspartate receptor encephalitis associated with ovarian teratoma. *Ann Neurol, 61*(1), 25–36. https://doi.org/10.1002/ana.21050. PMID: 17262855; PMCID: PMC2430743.

Daly, E. J., Trivedi, M. H., Janik, A., Li, H., Zhang, Y., Li, X., et al. (2019). Efficacy of Esketamine nasal spray plus oral antidepressant treatment for relapse prevention in patients with treatment-resistant depression. *JAMA Psychiatry, 76*(9), 893. https://doi.org/10.1001/jamapsychiatry.2019.1189

Daly, M. (2022). Prevalence of depression among adolescents in the U.S. from 2009 to 2019: Analysis of trends by sex, race/ethnicity, and income. *Journal of Adolescent Health, 70*(3), 496–499. https://doi.org/10.1016/j.jadohealth.2021.08.026

Dao, D. T., Mahon, P. B., Cai, X., Kovacsics, C. E., Blackwell, R. A., Arad, M., et al. (2010). Mood disorder susceptibility gene CACNA1C modifies mood-related behaviors in mice and interacts with sex to influence behavior in mice and diagnosis in humans. *Biological Psychiatry, 68*(9), 801–810. https://doi.org/10.1016/j.biopsych.2010.06.019

Daros, A. R., & Williams, G. E. (2019). A meta-analysis and systematic review of emotion-regulation strategies in borderline personality disorder. *Harvard Review of Psychiatry, 27*(4), 217–232. https://doi.org/10.1097/HRP.0000000000000212

Davies, A. E., Burnette, C. B., & Mazzeo, S. E. (2020). Testing a moderated mediation model of Objectification Theory among black women in the United States: The role of protective factors. *Sex Roles, 84*(4). https://doi.org/10.1007/s11199-020-01151-z

Davies, C., Segre, G., Estradé, A., Radua, J., De Micheli, A., Provenzani, U., et al. (2020). Prenatal and perinatal risk and protective factors for psychosis: A systematic review and meta-analysis. *The Lancet Psychiatry, 7*(5), 399–410.

Davies, D. K., Stock, S. E., & Wehmeyer, M. (2003). Application of computer simulation to teach ATM access to individuals with intellectual disabilities. *Education and Training in Developmental Disabilities, 38*, 451–456.

Davison, T. E., McCabe, M., & Mellor, D. (2009). An examination of the "gold standard" diagnosis of major depression in aged-care settings. *American Journal of Geriatric Psychiatry, 17*, 359–367.

Davis, P. (2002). The faces of Alzheimer's. *Time Magazine.* http://www.time.comtime/magazine/article/0,9171,1003090,00.html

Davis, S. R., Worsley, R., Miller, K. K., Parish, S. J., & Santoro, N. (2016). Androgens and female sexual function and dysfunction: Findings from the Fourth International Consultation of Sexual Medicine. *Journal of Sexual Medicine, 13*, 168–178. https://doi.org/10.1016/j.jsxm.2015.12.033

Davis, T. E., May, A., & Whiting, S. E. (2011). Evidence-based treatment of anxiety and phobia in children and adolescents: Current status and effects on the emotional response. *Clinical Psychology Review, 31*, 592–602.

Dawson, G., Toth, K., Abbott, R., Osterling, J., Munson, J., Estes, A., et al. (2004). Early social attention impairments in autism: Social orienting, joint attention, and attention to distress. *Developmental Psychology, 40*, 271–283.

Dazzi, T., Gribble, R., Wessely, S., & Fear, N. T. (2014). Does asking about suicide and related behaviours induce suicidal ideation? What is the evidence? *Psychological Medicine, 44*(16), 3361–3363. https://doi.org/10.1017/S0033291714001299

Deacon, B. J., & Abramowitz, J. S. (2004). Cognitive and behavioral treatments for anxiety disorders: A review of meta-analytic findings. *Journal of Clinical Psychology, 60*, 429–441.

Deak, J. D., & Johnson, E. C. (2021). Genetics of substance use disorders: A review. *Psychological Medicine, 51*(13), 2189–2200. https://doi.org/10.1017/S0033291721000969

Deary, I. J., & Johnson, W. (2010). Intelligence and education: Causal perceptions drive analytic processes and therefore conclusions. *International Journal of Epidemiology, 39*, 1362–1369.

De Bolle, M., De Fruyt, F., McCrae, R. R., Löckenhoff, C. E., Costa, P. T., Aguilar-Vafaie, M. E., et al. (2015). The emergence of sex differences in personality traits in early adolescence: A cross-sectional, cross-cultural study. *Journal of Personality and Social Psychology, 108*(1), 171–185. https://doi.org/10.1037/a0038497

deCharms, R. C., Maeda, F., Glover, G. H., Ludlow, D., Pauly, J. M., Soneji, D., et al. (2005). Control over brain activation and pain learned by using real-time functional MRI. *Proceedings of the National Academy of Sciences of the United States of America, 102*, 18626–18631.

De Crescenzo, F., Ciabattini, M., D'Alò, G. L., De Giorgi, R., Del Giovane, C., Cassar, C., et al. (2018). Comparative efficacy and acceptability of psychosocial interventions for individuals with cocaine and amphetamine addiction: A systematic review and network meta-analysis. *PLoS Medicine, 15*(12), e1002715. https://doi.org/10.1371/journal.pmed.1002715

Degnan, A., Berry, K., Sweet, D., Abel, K., Crossley, N., & Edge, D. (2018). Social networks and symptomatic and functional outcomes in schizophrenia: A systematic review and meta-analysis. *Social Psychiatry and Psychiatric Epidemiology, 53*, 873–888. https://doi.org/10.1007/s00127-018-1552-8

Deisenhammer, E. A., Ing, C. M., Strauss, R., Kemmler, G., Hinterhuber, H., & Weiss, E. M. (2009). The duration of the suicidal process: How much time is left for intervention between consideration and accomplishment of a suicide attempt? *Journal of Clinical Psychiatry, 70*(1), 19–24.

De Jonge, M., Bockting, C. L. H., Kikkert, M. J., Van DIjk, M. K., Van Schaik, Di. J. F., Peen, J., et al. (2019). Preventive cognitive therapy versus care as usual in cognitive behavioral therapy responders: A randomized controlled trial. *Journal of Consulting and Clinical Psychology, 87*(6), 521–529. https://doi.org/10.1037/ccp0000395

De Jongh, A., Amann, B. L., Hofmann, A., Farrell, D., & Lee, C. W. (2019). The status of EMDR therapy in the treatment of posttraumatic stress disorder 30 years after its introduction. *Journal of EMDR Practice and Research, 13*(4), 261–269. https://doi.org/10.1891/1933-3196.13.4.261

De Jong, J. T. V. M., Komproe, I. H., Van Ommeren, M., El Masri, M., Araya, M., Khaled, N., Van De Put, W., & Somasundaram, D. (2001). Lifetime events and posttraumatic stress disorder in 4 postconflict settings. *JAMA, 286*(5), 555–562. https://doi.org/10.1001/jama.286.5.555

de la Cruz, L. F., Llorens, M., Jassi, A., Krebs, G., Vidal-Ribas, P., Radua, J., et al. (2015). Ethnic inequalities in the use of secondary and tertiary mental health services among patients with obsessive-compulsive disorder. *British Journal of Psychiatry, 207*(6), 530–535. https://doi.org/10.1192/bjp.bp.114.154062

De La Cruz, L. F., Rydell, M., Runeson, B., D'Onofrio, B. M., Brander, G., Rück, C., Lichtenstein, P., Larsson, H., & Mataix-Cols, D. (2016). Suicide in obsessive–compulsive disorder: a population-based study of 36 788 Swedish patients. *Molecular Psychiatry 2016 22:11, 22*(11), 1626–1632. https://doi.org/10.1038/mp.2016.115

Delaney, K. R., Drew, B. L., & Rushton, A. (2018). Report on the APNA national psychiatric mental health advanced practice registered Nurse survey. *Journal of the American Psychiatric Nurses Association, 25*(2), 146–155. https://doi.org/10.1177/1078390318777873

Del Fabro, L., Schmidt, A., Fortea, L., Delvecchio, G., D'Agostino, A., Radua, J., Borgwardt, S., & Brambilla, P. (2021). Functional brain network dysfunctions in subjects at high-risk for psychosis: A meta-analysis of resting-state functional connectivity. *Neuroscience and biobehavioral reviews, 128*, 90–101. https://doi.org/10.1016/j.neubiorev.2021.06.020

Delis, D. C., Kramer, J. H., Kaplan, E., & Ober, B. A. (2017). *California verbal learning test-3* (3rd ed.). The Psychological Corporation.

Dell, P. F. (2006). A new model of dissociative identity disorder. *Psychiatric Clinics of North America, 29*, 1–26, vii.

DeMatteo, D., Galloway, M., Arnold, S., & Patel, U. (2015). Sexual assault on college campuses: A 50-state survey of criminal sexual assault statutes and their relevance to campus sexual assault. *Psychology, Public Policy, and Law, 21*, 227–238. https://doi.org/10.1037/law0000055

Demontis, D., Walters, R. K., Martin, J., Mattheisen, M., Als, T. D., Agerbo, E., et al. (2019). Discovery of the first genome-wide significant risk loci for attention deficit/hyperactivity disorder. *Nature Genetics, 51*(1), 63–75. https://doi.org/10.1038/s41588-018-0269-7

Demyttenaere, K., Bruffaerts, R., Posada-Villa, J., Gasquet, I., Kovess, V., Lepine, J. P., et al. (2004). Prevalence, severity, and unmet need for treatment of mental disorders in the World Health Organization World Mental Health Surveys. *JAMA: The Journal of the American Medical Association, 291*, 2581–2590. https://doi.org/10.1001/jama.291.21.2581

Dennis-Tiwary, T. A., Roy, A. K., Denefrio, S., & Myruski, S. (2019). Heterogeneity of the anxiety-related attention bias: A review and working model for future research. *Clinical Psychological Science, 7*(5), 879–899. https://doi.org/10.1177/2167702619838474

DePhilippis, D., Petry, N. M., Bonn-Miller, M. O., Rosenbach, S. B., & McKay, J. R. (2018). The national implementation of Contingency Management (CM) in the Department of Veterans Affairs: Attendance at CM sessions and substance use outcomes. *Drug and Alcohol Dependence, 185*, 367–373.

Depression Guidelines Panel. (1993). Depression in primary care: Treatment of major depression. Clinical practice guideline No. 5. (Vol. 2). U.S. Department of Health and Human Services, Public Health Service, Agency for Health Care Policy and Research.

Depue, R. A., Collins, P. F., & Luciano, M. (1996). A model of neurobiology: Environment interaction in developmental psychopathology. In M. F. Lenzenweger & J. J. Haugaard (Eds.), *Frontiers of developmental psychopathology* (pp. 44–76). Oxford University Press.

Desmarais, S. L., Van Dorn, R. A., Johnson, K. L., Grimm, K. J., Douglas, K. S., & Swartz, M. S. (2014). Community violence perpetration and victimization among adults with mental illnesses. *American Journal of Public Health, 104*(12), 2342–2349. https://doi.org/10.2105/AJPH.2013.301680

Deutsch, A. R., Chernyavskiy, P., Steinley, D., & Slutske, W. S. (2015). Measuring peer socialization for adolescent substance use: A comparison of perceived and actual friends' substance use effects. *Journal of Studies on Alcohol and Drugs, 76*, 267–277. https://doi.org/10.15288/jsad.2015.76.267

Devoe, D. J., Han, A., Anderson, A., Katzman, D. K., Patten, S. B., Soumbasis, A., et al. (2023). The impact of the COVID-19 pandemic on eating disorders: A systematic review. *International Journal of Eating Disorders, 56*(1), 5–25. https://doi.org/10.1002/eat.23704

Devoto, F., Zapparoli, L., Bonandrini, R., Berlingeri, M., Ferrulli, A., Luzi, L., et al. (2018). Hungry brains: A meta-analytical review of brain activation imaging studies on food perception and appetite in obese individuals. *Neuroscience & Biobehavioral Reviews, 94*, 271–285.

de Vries, B., van Busschbach, J. T., van der Stouwe, E. C. D., Aleman, A., van Dijk, J. J. M., Lysaker, P. H., et al. (2018). Prevalence rate and risk factors of victimization in adult patients with a psychotic disorder: A systematic review and meta-analysis. *Schizophrenia Bulletin, 45*(1), 114–126.

Devries, K. M., Mak, J. Y., Bacchus, L. J., et al. (2013) Intimate partner violence and incident depressive symptoms and suicide attempts: A systematic review of longitudinal studies. *PLoS Med, 10*: e1001439.

DeVylder, J., Anglin, D., Munson, M. R., Nishida, A., Oh, H., Marsh, J., et al. (2023). Ethnoracial variation in risk for psychotic experiences. *Schizophrenia Bulletin, 49*(2), 385–396.

de Wit, H., & Zacny, J. (2000). Abuse potential of nicotine replacement therapies. In K. J. Palmer (Ed.), *Smoking cessation* (pp. 79–92). Adis International Publications.

Dhingra, K., Boduszek, D., & O'Connor, R. C. (2015). Differentiating suicide attempters from suicide ideators using the Integrated Motivational-Volitional model of suicidal behaviour. *Journal of Affective Disorders, 186*, 211–218. https://doi.org/10.1016/j.jad.2015.07.007

Dick, D. M., Pagan, J. L., Viken, R., Purcell, S., Kaprio, J., Pulkinnen, L., et al. (2007). Changing environmental influences on substance use across development. *Twin Research and Human Genetics, 10*, 315–326.

Dickerson, S. S., & Kemeny, M. E. (2004). Acute stressors and cortisol responses: A theoretical integration and synthesis of laboratory research. *Psychological Bulletin, 130*, 355–391.

Didie, E. R., Menard, W., Stern, A. P., & Phillips, K. A. (2008). Occupational functioning and impairment in adults with body dysmorphic disorder. *Comprehensive Psychiatry, 49*, 561–569.

Dieserud, G., Roysamb, E., Braverman, M. T., Dalgard, O. S., & Ekeberg, O. (2003). Predicating repetition of suicide attempt: A prospective study of 50 suicide attempters. *Archives of Suicide Research, 7*, 1–15.

Di Forti, M., Sallis H., Allegri, F., Trotta, A., Ferraro L., Stilo, S. A., et al. (2013). Daily use, especially of high-potency Cannabis, drives the earlier onset of psychosis in Cannabis users. *Schizophrenia Bulletin, 40*, 1509–1517. https://doi.org/10.1093/schbul/sbt181

DiGangi, J. A., Gomez, D., Mendoza, L., Jason, L. A., Keys, C. B., & Koenen, K. C. (2013). Pretrauma risk factors for posttraumatic stress disorder: A systematic review of the literature. *Clinical Psychology Review, 33*(6), 728–744. https://doi.org/10.1016/j.cpr.2013.05.002

Dijk, C., van Emmerik, A. A. V. E., & Grasman, R. P. P. P. G. (2018). Social anxiety is related to dominance but not to affiliation as perceived by self and others: A real-life investigation into the psychobiological perspective on social anxiety. *Personality and Individual Differences, 124*, 66–70. https://doi.org/10.1016/j.paid.2017.11.050

DiLillo, D., Giuffre, D., Tremblay, G. C., & Peterson, L. (2001). A closer look at the nature of intimate partner violence reported by women with a history of child sexual abuse. *Journal of Interpersonal Violence, 16*, 116–132.

Dillon, B. (2010). *The hypochondriacs: Nine tormented lives.* Faber & Faber.

Dimidjian, S., Barrera, M., Martell, C., Muñoz, R. F., & Lewinsohn, P. M. (2011). The origins and current status of behavioral activation treatments for depression. *Annual Review of Clinical Psychology, 7*, 1–38.

Dimoff, J. D., & Sayette, M. A. (2017). The case for investigating social context in laboratory studies of smoking. *Addiction, 12*, 388–395. https://doi.org/10.1111/add.13503

Disabato, B., Bauer, I. E., Soares, J. C., & Sheline, Y. (2016). Neural structure and organization of mood pathology. In R. J. DeRubeis & D. R. Strunk (Eds.), *The Oxford handbook of mood disorders* (Vol. 1). Oxford University Press. https://doi.org/10.1093/oxfordhb/9780199973965.013.19

Dishion, T., Forgatch, M., Chamberlain, P., & Pelham, W. E. (2016). The Oregon model of behavior family therapy: From intervention design to promoting large-scale system change. *Special 50th Anniversary Issue: Honoring the Past and Looking to the Future: Updates on Seminal Behavior Therapy Publications on Current Therapies and Future Directions, Part II, 47*(6), 812–837.

Dishion, T. J., & Andrews, D. W. (1995). Preventing escalation in problem behaviors with high-risk young adolescents: Immediate and 1-year outcomes. *Journal of Consulting and Clinical Psychology, 63*, 538–548.

Dishion, T. J., Brennan, L. M., Shaw, D. S., McEachern, A. D., Wilson, M. N., & Jo, B. (2014). Prevention of problem behavior through annual family check-ups in early childhood: Intervention effects from home to early elementary school. *Journal of Abnormal Child Psychology, 42*, 343–354. https://doi.org/10.1007/s10802-013-9768-2

Dishion, T. J., Kim, H., & Tein, J.-Y. (2015). Friendship and adolescent problem behavior: Deviancy training and coercive joining as dynamic mediators. In T. P. Beauchaine & S. P. Hinshaw (Eds.), *The Oxford handbook of externalizing spectrum disorders* (pp. 303–311). Oxford University Press.

Dishion, T. J., Shaw, D., Connell, A., Gardner, F., Weaver, C., & Wilson, M. (2008). The family check-up with high-risk indigent families: Preventing problem behavior by increasing parents' positive behavior support in early childhood. *Child Development, 79*(5), 1395–1414. https://doi.org/10.1111/j.1467-8624.2008.01195.x

Dixon, L. B., Dickerson, F., Bellack, A. S., Bennett, M., Dickinson, D., Goldberg, R. W., et al. (2010). The 2009 schizophrenia PORT psychosocial treatment recommendations and summary statements. *Schizophrenia Bulletin, 36*, 48–70.

Dobson, K. S., Hollon, S. D., Dimidjian, S., Schmaling, K. B., Kohlenberg, R. J., Gallop, R., et al. (2008). Randomized trial of behavioral activation, cognitive therapy, and antidepressant medication in the prevention of relapse and recurrence in major depression. *Journal of Consulting and Clinical Psychology, 76*, 468–477.

Dodes, L., & Dodes, Z. (2014). *The sober truth: Debunking the bad science behind 12-step programs and the rehab industry.* Beacon Press.

Dodge, K. A. (2020). Annual Research Review: Universal and targeted strategies for assigning interventions to achieve population impact. *Journal of Child Psychology and Psychiatry, and Allied Disciplines, 61*(3), 255–267. https://doi.org/10.1111/jcpp.13141

Dodge, K. A., Bierman, K. L., Coie, J. D., Greenberg, M. T., Lochman, J. E., McMahon, R. J., et al. (2015). Impact of early intervention on psychopathology, crime, and well-being at age 25. *American Journal of Psychiatry, 172*(1), 59–70. https://doi.org/10.1176/appi.ajp.2014.13060786

Dodge, K. A., & Frame, C. L. (1982). Social cognitive biases and deficits in aggressive boys. *Child Development, 53*, 620–635.

Dodge, K. A., & Godwin, J. (2013). Social-information-processing patterns mediate the impact of preventive intervention on adolescent antisocial behavior. *Psychological Science, 24*(4), 456–465.

Doering, S., Hörz, S., Rentrop, M., Fischer-Kern, M., Schuster, P., Benecke, C., et al. (2010). Transference-focused psychotherapy v. treatment by community psychotherapists for borderline personality disorder: randomised controlled trial. *The British Journal of Psychiatry, 196*(5), 389–395. https://doi.org/10.1192/BJP.BP.109.070177

Doerr, P., Fichter, M., Pirke, K. M., & Lund, R. (1980). Relationship between weight gain and hypothalamic pituitary adrenal function in patients with anorexia nervosa. *Journal of Steroid Biochemistry, 13*, 529–537.

Dohrenwend, B. P., & Dohrenwend, B. S. (1974). Social and cultural influences on psychopathology. *Annual Review of Psychology, 25*, 417–452.

Dohrenwend, B. P., Levav, P. E., Schwartz, S., Naveh, G., Link, B. G., Skodol, A. E., et al. (1992). Socioeconomic status and psychiatric disorders: The causation–selection issue. *Science, 255*, 946–952.

Doll, H. A., & Fairburn, C. G. (1998). Heightened accuracy of self-reported weight in bulimia nervosa: A useful cognitive "distortion." *International Journal of Eating Disorders, 24*, 267–273.

Dong, D., Wang, Y., Chang, X., Luo, C., & Yao, D. (2018). Dysfunction of large-scale brain networks in schizophrenia: A meta-analysis of resting-state functional connectivity. *Schizophrenia Bulletin, 44*(1), 168–181.

Dong, D., Wang, Y., Chang, X., Luo, C., & Yao, D. (2018). Dysfunction of large-scale brain networks in schizophrenia: A meta-analysis of resting-state functional connectivity. *Schizophrenia bulletin, 44*(1), 168–181. https://doi.org/10.1093/schbul/sbx034

Donoghue, K., Elzerbi, C., Saunders, R., Whittington, C., Pilling, S., & Drummond, C. (2015). The efficacy of acamprosate and naltrexone in the treatment of alcohol dependence, Europe versus the rest of the world: A meta-analysis. *Addiction, 110*, 920–930. https://doi.org/10.1111/add.12875.

Dougall, N., Maayan, N., Soares-Weiser, K., McDermott, L. M., & McIntosh, A. (2015). *Transcranial magnetic stimulation (TMS) for schizophrenia (Review).* The Cochrane Collaboration. John Wiley & Sons, Ltd.

Dougherty, L., Smith, V., Bufferd, S., Kessel, E., Carlson, G., & Klein, D. (2016). Disruptive mood dysregulation disorder at the age of 6 years and clinical and functional outcomes 3 years later. *Psychological Medicine, 46*(5), 1103–1114. https://doi.org/10.1017/S0033291715002809

Douglas, K. S., Guy, L. S., & Hart, S. D. (2009). Psychosis as a risk factor for violence to others: A meta-analysis. *Psychological Bulletin, 135*, 679–706.

Douglas, K. S., Hart, S. D., Webster, C. D., Belfrage, H., Guy, L. S., & Wilson, C. M. (2014). Historical–clinical–risk management-20, version 3 (HCR-20V3): Development and overview. *International Journal of Forensic Mental Health, 13*(2), 93–108.

Doyle, P. M., Le Grange, D., Loeb, K., Doyle, A. C., & Crosby, R. D. (2010). Early response to family-based treatment for adolescent anorexia nervosa. *International Journal of Eating Disorders, 43*, 659–662.

Doyon, W. M., Dong, Y., Ostroumov, A., Thomas, A. M., Zhang, T. A., & Dani, J. A. (2013). Nicotine decreases ethanol-induced dopamine signaling and increases self-administration via stress hormones. *Neuron, 79*, 530–540.

Drane, D. L., Williamson, D. J., Stroup, E. S., Holmes, M. D., Jung, M., Koerner, E., et al. (2006). Cognitive impairment is not equal in patients with epileptic and psychogenic nonepileptic seizures. *Epilepsia, 47*, 1879–1886. https://doi.org/10.1111/j.1528-1167.2006.00611.x

Driessen, E., Hollon, S. D., Bockting, C. L., Cuijpers, P., & Turner, E. H. (2015). Does publication bias inflate the apparent efficacy of psychological treatment for major depressive disorder? A systematic review and meta-analysis of US National Institutes of Health-Funded trials. *PLoS One, 10*(9), e0137864. https://doi.org/10.1371/journal.pone.0137864

Drozdick, L. W., Raiford, S. E., Wahlstrom, D., & Weiss, L. G. (2018). The Wechsler Adult Intelligence Scale—Fourth Edition and the Wechsler Memory Scale—Fourth Edition. In *Contemporary intellectual assessment: Theories, tests, and issues* (4th ed., pp. 486–511). The Guilford Press.

Drury, H., Ajmi, S., Fernández de la Cruz, L., Nordsletten, A. E., & Mataix-Cols, D. (2014). Caregiver burden, family accommodation, health, and well-being in relatives of individuals with hoarding disorder. *Journal of Affective Disorders, 159*, 7–14. https://doi.org/10.1016/j.jad.2014.01.023

Dugas, M. J., Brillon, P., Savard, P., Turcotte, J., Gaudet, A., Ladouceur, R., et al. (2010). A randomized clinical trial of cognitive-behavioral therapy and applied relaxation for adults with generalized anxiety disorder. *Behavior Therapy, 41*(1), 46–58. https://doi.org/10.1016/j.beth.2008.12.004

Dugas, M. J., Marchand, A., & Ladouceur, R. (2005). Further validation of a cognitive-behavioral model of generalized anxiety disorder: Diagnostic and symptom specificity. *Journal of Anxiety Disorders, 19*, 329–343.

Dugosh, K., Abraham, A., Seymour, B., McLoyd, K., Chalk, M., & Festinger, (2016). A systematic review on the use of psychosocial interventions in conjunction with medications for the treatment of opioid addiction. *Journal of Addiction Medicine, 10*(2), 93–103.

Duits, P., Cath, D. C., Lissek, S., Hox, J. J., Hamm, A. O., Engelhard, I. M., et al. (2015). Updated meta-analysis of classical conditioning in the anxiety disorders. *Depression and Anxiety, 32*(4), 239–253. https://doi.org/10.1002/da.22353

Duncan, L., Yilmaz, Z., Gaspar, H., Walters, R., Goldstein, J., Anttila, V., et al. (2017). Significant locus and metabolic genetic correlations revealed in genome-wide association study of anorexia nervosa. *American Journal of Psychiatry, 174*, 850–858. https://doi.org/10.1176/appi.ajp.2017.16121402

Dunham, L. (2014). Difficult Girl. The New Yorker. https://www.newyorker.com/magazine/2014/09/01/difficult-girl

Dunn, E. C., Gilman, S. E., Willett, J. B., Slopen, N. B., & Molnar, B. E. (2012). The impact of exposure to interpersonal violence on gender differences in adolescent-onset major depression: Results from the National Comorbidity Survey Replication (NCS-R). *Depression and Anxiety, 29*, 392–399. https://doi.org/10.1002/da.21916

Dunner, D. L., Aaronson, S. T., Sackeim, H. A., Janicak, P. G., Carpenter, L. L., Boyadjis, T., et al. (2014). A multisite, naturalistic, observational study of transcranial magnetic stimulation for patients with pharmacoresistant major depressive disorder: Durability of benefit over a 1-year follow-up period. *Journal of Clinical Psychiatry, 75*(12), 1394–1401. https://doi.org/10.4088/JCP.13m08977

Dunne, S. S., Coffey, J. C., Konje, S., Gasior, S., Clancy, C. C., Gulati, G., et al. (2021). Biomarkers in delirium: A systematic review. *Journal of Psychosomatic Research, 147.* https://doi.org/10.1016/J.JPSYCHORES.2021.110530

DuPaul, G. J., Gormley, M. J., & Laracy, S. D. (2013). Comorbidity of LD and ADHD: Implications of DSM-5 for assessment and treatment. *Journal of Learning Disabilities, 46*(1), 43–51. https://doi.org/10.1177/0022219412464351

Durand, V. M., & Moskowitz, L. (2015). Functional communication training: Thirty years of treating challenging behavior. *Topics in Early Childhood Special Education, 35*(2), 116–126. https://doi.org/10.1177/0271121415569509

Du, X., Witthöft, M., Zhang, T., Shi, C., & Ren, Z. (2023). Interpretation bias in health anxiety: A systematic review and meta-analysis. *Psychological Medicine, 53*(1), 34–45. https://doi.org/10.1017/S0033291722003427

Dwyer-Lindgren, L., Mokdad, A. H., Srebotnjak, T., Flaxman, A. D., Hansen, G. M., & Murray, C. J. (2014). Cigarette smoking prevalence in US counties: 1996–2012. *Population Health Metrics, 12*, 5.

Dyshniku, F., Murray, M. E., Fazio, R. L., Lykins, A. D., & Cantor, J. M. (2015). Minor physical anomalies as a window into the prenatal origins of pedophilia. *Archives of Sexual Behavior, 44*, 2151–2159. https://doi.org/10.1007/s10508-015-0564-7

Eardley, I., Donatucci, C., Corbin, J., El-Meliegy, A., Hatzimouratidis, K., McVary, K., et al. (2010). Pharmacotherapy for erectile dysfunction. *Journal of Sexual Medicine, 7*, 524–540.

Eaton, W. W., Shao, H., Nestadt, G., Lee, H. B., Bienvenu, O. J., & Zandi, P. (2008). Population-based study of first onset and chronicity in major depressive disorder. *Archives of General Psychiatry, 65*(5), 513–520. https://doi.org/10.1001/archpsyc.65.5.513

Eckshtain, D., Kuppens, S., Ugueto, A., Ng, M. Y., Vaughn-Coaxum, R., Corteselli, K., et al. (2020). Meta-analysis: 13-Year follow-up of psychotherapy effects on youth depression. *Journal of the American Academy of Child and Adolescent Psychiatry, 59*(1), 45–63. https://doi.org/10.1016/j.jaac.2019.04.002

Eddy, K. T., Tabri, N., Thomas, J. J., Murray, H. B., Keshaviah, A., Hastings, E., et al. (2017). Recovery from anorexia nervosa and bulimia nervosa at 22-year follow-up. *The Journal of Clinical Psychiatry, 78*(2), 184–189. https://doi.org/10.4088/JCP.15m10393

Edenberg, H. J., Gelernter, J., & Agrawal, A. (2019). Genetics of alcoholism. *Current Psychiatry Reports, 21.* https://doi.org/10.1007/s11920-019-1008-1

Edenberg, H. J., Xuie, X., Chen, H-J., Tian, H., Weatherill, L. F., Dick, D. M., et al. (2006). Association of alcohol dehydrogenase genes with alcohol dependence: A comprehensive analysis. *Human Molecular Genetics, 15*, 1539–1549.

Edens, J. F., Kelley, S. E., Lilienfeld, S. O., Skeem, J. L., & Douglas, K. S. (2015). DSM-5 antisocial personality disorder: Predictive validity in a prison sample. *Law and Human Behavior, 39*, 123–129. https://doi.org/10.1037/lhb0000105

Edmondson, D., & von Känel, R. (2017). Post-traumatic stress disorder and cardiovascular disease. *The Lancet Psychiatry, 4*(4), 320–329. https://doi.org/10.1016/S2215-0366(16)30377-7

Educational Fund to Stop Gun Violence. (2020). Gun violence in America: 2018 data Brief. *www.efsgv.org.*

Edvardsen, J., Torgersen, S., Roysamb, E., Lygren, S., Skre, I., Onstad, S., et al. (2008). Heritability of bipolar spectrum disorders. Unity or heterogeneity? *Journal of Affective Disorders, 106*, 229–240.

Edwards, A. C., Ohlsson, H., Mocicki, E., Crump, C., Sundquist, J., Lichtenstein, P., et al. (2021). On the genetic and environmental relationship between suicide attempt and death by suicide. *American Journal of Psychiatry, 178*(11), 1060–1069. https://doi.org/10.1176/appi.ajp.2020.20121705

Egerton, A., Grace, A. A., Stone, J., Bossong, M. G., Sand, M., & McGuire, P. (2020). Glutamate in schizophrenia: Neurodevelopmental perspectives and drug development. *Schizophrenia Research, 223*, 59–70.

Egger, H. L., & Angold, A. (2006). Common emotional and behavioral disorders in preschool children: Presentation, nosology, and epidemiology. *Journal of Child Psychology and Psychiatry, 47*(3–4), 313–337.

Ehde, D. M., Dillworth, T. M., & Turner, J. A. (2014). Cognitive-behavioral therapy for individuals with chronic pain: Efficacy, innovations, and directions for research. *American Psychologist, 69*, 153–166.

Ehlers, A., & Clark, D. M. (2008). Posttraumatic stress disorder: The development of effective psychological treatments. *Nordic Journal of Psychiatry, 62*(Suppl 47), 11–18. https://doi.org/10.1080/08039480802315608

Eisen, J. L., Sibrava, N. J., Boisseau, C. L., Mancebo, M. C., Stout, R. L., Pinto, A., et al. (2013). Five-year course of obsessive-compulsive disorder: Predictors of remission and relapse. *Journal of Clinical Psychiatry, 74*, 233–239.

Elis, O., Caponigro, J. M., & Kring, A. M. (2013). Psychosocial treatments for negative symptoms in schizophrenia: Current practices and future directions. *Clinical Psychology Review, 33*, 914–928.

Elkins, I. J., King, S. M., McGue, M., & Iacono, W. G. (2006). Personality traits and the development of nicotine, alcohol, and illicit drug disorders: Prospective links from adolescence to young adulthood. *Journal of Abnormal Psychology, 115*, 26–39. https://doi.org/10.1037/0021-843X.115.1.26

Ellenberger, H. F. (1972). The story of "Anna O": A critical review with new data. *Journal of the History of the Behavioral Sciences, 8*, 267–279.

Ellickson-Larew, S., Stasik-O'Brien, S. M., Stanton, K., & Watson, D. (2020). Dissociation as a multidimensional transdiagnostic symptom. *Psychology of Consciousness: Theory Research, and Practice, 7*(2), 126–150. https://doi.org/10.1037/CNS0000218

ElSohly, M. A., Chandra, S., Radwan, M., Majumdar, C. G., & Church, J. C. (2021). A comprehensive review of cannabis potency in the United States in the last decade. *Cannabis, Cannabinoids, the Endocannabinoid System, and Psychosis, 6*(6), 603–606.

Emery, S., Kim, Y., Choi, Y. K., Szczypka, G., Wakefield, M., & Chaloupka, F. J. (2012). The effects of smoking-related television advertising on smoking and intentions to quit among adults in the United States: 1999–2007. *American Journal of Public Health, 102*, 751–757.

Emmelkamp, P. M. G., Benner, A., Kuipers, A., Feiertag, G. A., Koster, H. C., & van Apeldoorn, F. J. (2006). Comparison of brief dynamic and cognitive-behavioural therapies in avoidant personality disorder. *British Journal of Psychiatry, 189*, 60–64.

Engdahl, B., Dikel, T. N., Eberly, R., & Blank, A. (1997). Posttraumatic stress disorder in a community group of former prisoners of war: A normative response to severe trauma. *American Journal of Psychiatry, 154*, 1576–1581.

Ensink, K., Berthelot, N., Bégin, M., Maheux, J., & Normandin, L. (2017). Dissociation mediates the relationship between sexual abuse and child psychological difficulties. *Child Abuse & Neglect, 69*, 116–124. https://doi.org/10.1016/j.chiabu.2017.04.017

Erlangsen, A., Jacobsen, A. L., Ranning, A., Delamare, A. L., Nordentoft, M., & Frisch, M. (2023). Transgender identity and suicide attempts and mortality in Denmark. *JAMA, 329*(24), 2145. https://doi.org/10.1001/jama.2023.8627

Ersche, K. D., Williams, G. B., Robbins, T. W., & Bullmore, E. T. (2013). Meta-analysis of structural brain abnormalities associated with stimulant drug dependence and neuroimaging of addiction vulnerability and resilience. *Addiction, 23*, 615–624.

Espada, J. P., Gonzálvez, M. T., Orgilés, M., Guillén-Riquelme, A., Soto, D., & Sussman, S. (2015). Pilot clinic study of project EX for smoking cessation with Spanish adolescents. *Addictive Behaviors, 45*, 226. https://search.proquest.com/docview/1666836700?accountid514496

Essex, M. J., Klein, M. H., Slattey, M. J., Goldsmith, H. H., & Kalin, N. H. (2010). Early risk factors and developmental pathways to chronic high inhibition and social anxiety disorder in adolescence. *American Journal of Psychiatry, 167*, 40–46.

Etkin, A. (2019). A reckoning and research agenda for neuroimaging in psychiatry. *American Journal of Psychiatry, 176*, 507–511.

Eustis, E. H., Gallagher, M. W., Tirpak, J. W., Nauphal, M., Farchione, T. J., & Barlow, D. H. (2020). The Unified Protocol compared with diagnosis-specific protocols for anxiety disorders: 12-month follow-up from a randomized clinical trial. *General Hospital Psychiatry, 67*, 58–61. https://doi.org/10.1016/j.genhosppsych.2020.08.012

Evans-Lacko, S., Brohan, E., Mojtabai, R., & Thornicroft, G. (2011). Association between public views of mental illness and self-stigma among individuals with mental illness in 14 European countries. *Psychological Medicine, 42*, 1741–1752. https://doi.org/10.1017/S0033291711002558

Everaert, J., Vrijsen, J. N., Martin-Willett, R., van de Kraats, L., & Joormann, J. (2022). A meta-analytic review of the relationship between explicit memory bias and depression: Depression features an explicit memory bias that persists beyond a depressive episode. *Psychological Bulletin, 148*(5–6), 435–463. https://doi.org/10.1037/bul0000367

Express Scripts. (2020). America's state of mind. https://express-scripts.com/corporate

Fairbairn, C. E., & Sayette, M. A. (2013). The effect of alcohol on emotional inertia: A test of alcohol myopia. *Journal of Abnormal Psychology, 122*, 770–781. https://doi.org/10.1037/a0032980

Fairbairn, C. E., & Sayette, M. A. (2014). A social-attributional analysis of alcohol response. *Psychological Bulletin, 140*, 1361–1382.

Fairburn, C. G. (2013). *Overcoming binge eating.* Vol. 2. The Guilford Press.

Fairburn, C. G., Bailey-Straebler, S., Basden, S., Doll, H. A., Jones, R., Murphy, R., ... Cooper, Z. (2015). A transdiagnostic comparison of enhanced cognitive behaviour therapy (CBT-E) and interpersonal psychotherapy in the treatment of eating disorders. *Behaviour Research and Therapy, 70*, 64–71

Fairburn, C. G., Cooper, A., Doll, H. A., O'Connor, M. E., Bohn, K., Hawker, D. M., et al. (2009). Transdiagnostic cognitive-behavioral therapy for patients with eating disorders: A two-site trial with 60-week follow-up. *American Journal of Psychiatry, 166*, 311–319.

Fairburn, C. G., Jones, R., Peveler, R. C., Carr, S. J., Solomon, R. A., O'Connor, M. E., et al. (1991). Three psychological treatments for bulimia nervosa. *Archives of General Psychiatry, 48*, 463–469.

Fairburn, C. G., Jones, R., Peveler, R. C., Hope, R. A., & O'Connor, M. E. (1993). Psychotherapy and bulimia nervosa: The longer-term effects of interpersonal psychotherapy, behavior therapy, and cognitive therapy. *Archives of General Psychiatry, 50*, 419–428.

Fairburn, C. G., Norman, P. A., Welch, S. L., O'Connor, M. E., Doll, H. A., & Peveler, R. C. (1995). A prospective study of outcome in bulimia nervosa and the long-term effects of three psychological treatments. *Archives of General Psychiatry, 52*, 304–312.

Fairburn, C. G., Shafran, R., & Cooper, Z. (1999). A cognitive behavioural theory of anorexia nervosa. *Behaviour Research and Therapy, 37*, 1–13.

Fair, D. A., Bathula, D., Nikolas, M. A., & Nigg, J. T. (2012). Distinct neuropsychological subgroups in typically developing youth inform heterogeneity in children with ADHD. *Proceedings of the National Academy of Sciences, 109*(17), 6769–6774.

Fals-Stewart, W., O'Farrell, T. J., & Lam, W. K. K. (2009). Behavioral couple therapy for gay and lesbian couples with alcohol use disorders. *Journal of Substance Abuse Treatment, 37*, 379–387.

Faltinsen, E., Todorovac, A., Staxen Bruun, L., Hróbjartsson, A., Gluud, C., Kongerslev, M. T., et al. (2022). Control interventions in randomised trials among people with mental health disorders. *Cochrane Database of Systematic Reviews, 4*. https://doi.org/10.1002/14651858.MR000050.pub2

Fanous, A. H., Prescott, C. A., & Kendler, K. S. (2004). The prediction of thoughts of death or self-harm in a population-based sample of female twins. *Psychological Medicine, 34*, 301–312.

Faraone, S. V., Asherson, P., Banaschewski, T., Biederman, J., Buitelaar, J. K., Ramos-Quiroga, J. A., et al. (2015). Attention-deficit/hyperactivity disorder. *Nature Reviews Disease Primers, 1*(1), 15020.

Faraone, S. V., Banaschewski, T., Coghill, D., Zheng, Y., Biederman, J., Bellgrove, M. A., et al. (2021). The World Federation of ADHD International Consensus Statement: 208 evidence-based conclusions about the disorder. *Neuroscience & Biobehavioral Reviews, 128*, 789–818.

Faraone, S. V., Biederman, J., & Mick, E. (2005). The age-dependent decline of attention deficit hyperactivity disorder: A meta-analysis of follow-up studies. *Psychological Medicine, 36*, 159–165.

Faraone, S. V., & Larsson, H. (2019). Genetics of attention deficit hyperactivity disorder. *Molecular Psychiatry, 24*(4), 562–575.

Farina, A. (1976). *Abnormal psychology.* Prentice-Hall.

Farley, A. C. (2023). *Girls and their monsters: The Genain quadruplets and the making of madness in America.* Grand Central Publishing.

Fatemi, S. H., Aldinger, K. A., Ashwood, P., Bauman, M. L., Blaha, C. D., Blatt, G. J., et al. (2012). Consensus paper: Pathological role of the cerebellum in autism. *The Cerebellum, 11*(3), 777–807.

Fawcett, E. J., Power, H., & Fawcett, J. M. (2020). Women are at greater risk of OCD than men. *The Journal of Clinical Psychiatry, 81*(4), 19r13085. https://doi.org/10.4088/JCP.19r13085

Fazel, S., Gulati, G., Linsell, L., Geddes, J. R., & Grann, M. (2009). Schizophrenia and violence: systematic review and meta-analysis. *PLoS medicine, 6*(8), e1000120. https://doi.org/10.1371/journal.pmed.1000120

Feeney, A., Hock, R. S., Fava, M., Hernández Ortiz, J. M., Iovieno, N., & Papakostas, G. I. (2022). Antidepressants in children and adolescents with major depressive disorder and the influence of placebo response: A meta-analysis. *Journal of Affective Disorders, 305*, 55–64.

Feldman Barrett, L. (2017). *How emotions are made.* Houghton Mifflin Harcourt.

Felitti, V. J., Anda, R. F., Nordenberg, D., Williamson, D. F., Spitz, A. M., Edwards, V., et al. (1998). Relationship of Childhood Abuse and Household Dysfunction to Many of the Leading Causes of Death in Adults: The Adverse Childhood Experiences (ACE) Study. *American Journal of Preventive Medicine, 14*(4), 245–258.

Ferguson, S. B., Shiffman, S., & Gwaltney, C. J. (2006). Does reducing withdrawal severity mediate nicotine patch efficacy? A randomized clinical trial. *Journal of Consulting and Clinical Psychology, 74*, 1153–1161.

Fergusson, D., Doucette, S., Glass, K. C., Shapiro, S., Healy, D., Hebert, P., et al. (2005). Association between suicide attempts and selective serotonin reuptake inhibitors: Systematic review of randomised controlled trials. *British Medical Journal, 330*(7488), 396. https://doi.org/10.1136/bmj.330.7488.396

Fergusson, D. M., McLeod, G. F. H., & Horwood, L. J. (2013). Childhood sexual abuse and adult developmental outcomes: Findings from a 30-year longitudinal study in New Zealand. *Child Abuse & Neglect, 37*, 664–674. https://doi.org/10.1016/j.chiabu.2013.03.013

Fernandez de La Cruz, L., Rydell, M., Runeson, B., D'Onofrio, B. M., Brander, G., Rück, C., et al. (2016). Suicide in obsessive–compulsive disorder: A population-based study of 36788 Swedish patients. *Molecular Psychiatry, 22*(11), 1626–1632. https://doi.org/10.1038/mp.2016.115

Fernandez, E., Salem, D., Swift, J. K., & Ramtahal, N. (2015). Meta-analysis of dropout from cognitive behavioral therapy: Magnitude, timing, and moderators. *Journal of Consulting and Clinical Psychology, 83*(6), 1108–1122. https://doi.org/10.1037/CCP0000044

Ferrari, A. (2022). Global, regional, and national burden of 12 mental disorders in 204 countries and territories, 1990–2019: A systematic analysis for the Global Burden of Disease Study 2019. *The Lancet Psychiatry, 9*(2), 137–150. https://doi.org/10.1016/S2215-0366(21)00395-3

Ferrari, A., & GBD 2019 Mental Disorders Collaborators. (2022). Global, regional, and national burden of 12 mental disorders in 204 countries and territories, 1990–2019: A systematic analysis for the Global Burden of Disease Study 2019. *The Lancet Psychiatry, 9*(2), 137–150. https://doi.org/10.1016/S2215-0366(21)00395-3

Ferré, S. (2008). An update on the mechanisms of the psychostimulant effects of caffeine. *Journal of Neurochemistry, 105*, 1067–1079. https://doi.org/10.1111/j.1471-4159.2007.05196.x

Fervaha, G., Foussias, G., Agid, O., & Remington, G. (2014). Impact of primary negative symptoms on functional outcomes in schizophrenia. *European Psychiatry, 29*(7), 449–455. https://doi.org/10.1016/j.eurpsy.2014.01.007

Fetveit, A. (2009). Late-life insomnia: A review. *Geriatrics and Gerontology International, 9*, 220–234.

Feusner, J. D., Phillips, K. A., & Stein, D. J. (2010). Olfactory reference syndrome: Issues for DSM-V. *Depression and Anxiety, 27*, 592–599.

Fiellin, D. A., O'Connor, P. G., Chawarski, M., Pakes, J. P., Pantalon, M. V., & Schottenfeld, R. S. (2001). Methadone maintenance in primary care: A randomized controlled trial. *Journal of the American Medical Association, 286*, 1724–1731.

Fineberg, A. M., & Ellman, L. M. (2013). Inflammatory cytokines and neurological and neurocognitive alterations in the course of schizophrenia. *Biological Psychiatry, 73*(10), 951–966. https://doi.org/10.1016/j.biopsych.2013.01.001

Fineberg, A. M., Ellman, L. M., Schaefer, C. A., Maxwell, S. D., Shen, L., Chaudhury, N. H., et al. (2016). Fetal exposure to maternal stress and risk for schizophrenia spectrum disorders among offspring: Differential influences of fetal sex. *Psychiatry Research, 236*, 91–97.

Finkelstein, E. A., Graham, W. C., & Malhotra, R. (2014). Lifetime direct medical costs of childhood obesity. *Pediatrics, 133*, 854–862. https://doi.org/10.1542/peds.2014-0063

Finkelstein, E. A., Trogdon, J. G., Cohen, J. W., & Dietz, W. (2009). Annual medical spending attributable to obesity: Payer- and service-specific estimates. *Health Affairs, 28*, w822–w831.

Fink, H. A., Mac Donald, R., Rutks, I. R., Nelson, D. B., & Wilt, T. J. (2002). Sildenafil for male erectile dysfunction: A systematic review and meta-analysis. *Archives of Internal Medicine, 162*, 1349–1360.

Finlay-Jones, R. (1989). Anxiety. In G. W. Brown & T. O. Harris (Eds.), *Life events and illness* (pp. 95–112). Guilford Press.

Finucane, A. M., Jones, L., Leurent, B., Sampson, E. L., Stone, P., Tookman, A., & Candy, B. (2020). Drug therapy for delirium in terminally ill adults. *The Cochrane Database of Systematic Reviews, 2020*(1). https://doi.org/10.1002/14651858.CD004770.PUB3

First, M. B, Williams, J. B. W., Karg, R. S., & Spitzer R. L. (2015). *Structured Clinical Interview for DSM-5 Disorders, Clinician Version (SCID-5-CV)*. American Psychiatric Association.

Fishbain, D. A., Cutler, R., Rosomoff, H. L., & Rosomoff, R. S. (2000). Evidence-based data from animal and human experimental studies on pain relief with antidepressants: A structured review. *Pain Medicine, 1*, 310–316.

Fisher, J. E. (2011). Understanding behavioral health in late life: Why age matters. *Behavior Therapy, 42*, 143–149.

Fleming, G. E., Neo, B., Briggs, N. E., Kaouar, S., Frick, P. J., & Kimonis, E. R. (2022). Parent training adapted to the needs of children with callous–unemotional traits: A randomized controlled trial. *Special 50th Anniversary Issue: Honoring the Past and Looking to the Future: Updates on Seminal Behavior Therapy Publications on Current Therapies and Future Directions, Part II, 53*(6), 1265–1281.

Florence, C. S., Zhou, C., Luo, F., & Xu, L. (2016). The economic burden of prescription opioid overdose, abuse, and dependence in the United States, 2013. *Medical Care, 54*, 901–916.

Flygare, O., Lundström, L., Andersson, E., Mataix-Cols, D., & Rück, C. (2022). Implementing therapist-guided internet-delivered cognitive behaviour therapy for obsessive–compulsive disorder in the UK's IAPT programme: A pilot trial. *British Journal of Clinical Psychology, 61*(4), 895–910. https://doi.org/10.1111/BJC.12365

Foa, E. B., Gillihan, S. J., & Bryant, R. A. (2013). Challenges and successes in dissemination of evidence-based treatments for posttraumatic stress: Lessons learned from prolonged exposure therapy for PTSD. *Psychological Science Public Interest, 14*(2), 65–111. https://doi.org/10.1177/1529100612468841

Foa, E. B., & McLean, C. P. (2016). The efficacy of exposure therapy for anxiety-related disorders and its underlying mechanisms: The case of OCD and PTSD. *Annual Review of Clinical Psychology, 12*(1), 1–28. https://doi.org/10.1146/annurev-clinpsy-021815-093533

Foa, E. B., & Meadows, E. A. (1997). Psychosocial treatments for posttraumatic stress disorder: A critical review. *Annual Review of Psychology, 48*, 449–480.

Fobian, A. D., Long, D. M., & Szaflarski, J. P. (2020). Retraining and control therapy for pediatric psychogenic non-epileptic seizures. *Annals of Clinical and Translational Neurology, 7*(8), 1410. https://doi.org/10.1002/ACN3.51138

Foerde, K., Steinglass, J. E., Shohamy, D., & Walsh, B. T. (2015). Neural mechanisms supporting maladaptive food choices in anorexia nervosa. *Nature Neuroscience, 18*, 1571–1573. https://doi.org/10.1038/nn.4136

Fong, T. G., & Inouye, S. K. (2022). The inter-relationship between delirium and dementia: the importance of delirium prevention. *Nature Reviews Neurology, 18*(10), 579–596. https://doi.org/10.1038/s41582-022-00698-7

Fontaine, N. M. G., McCrory, E. J. P., Boivin, M., Moffitt, T. E., & Viding, E. (2011). Predictors and outcomes of joint trajectories of callous-unemotional traits and conduct problems in childhood. *Journal of Abnormal Psychology, 120*, 730–742.

Food and Drug Administration (FDA). (2019). *FDA Briefing Document Psychopharmacologic Drugs Advisory Committee (PDAC) and Drug Safety and Risk Management (DSaRM) Advisory Committee Meeting*. Food and Drug Administration. https://www.fda.gov/media/121376/

Ford, C. S., & Beach, F. A. (1951). *Patterns of sexual behavior*. Harper and Brothers.

Ford, J. M., Mathalon, D. H., Whitfield, S., Faustman, W. O., & Roth, W. T. (2002). Reduced communication between frontal and temporal lobes during talking in schizophrenia. *Biological Psychiatry, 51*, 485–492.

Forgatch, M. S., Patterson, G. R., Degarmo, D. S., & Beldavs, Z. G. (2009). Testing the Oregon delinquency model with 9-year follow-up of the Oregon Divorce Study. *Development and Psychopathology, 21*, 637–660. https://doi.org/10.1017/S0954579409000340

Forney, K. J., Holland, L. A., Joiner, T. E., & Keel, P. K. (2015). Determining empirical thresholds for "definitely large" amounts of food for defining binge-eating episodes. *Eating Disorders, 23*(1), 15–30. https://doi.org/10.1080/10640266.2014.931763

Foti, D., Carlson, J. M., Sauder, C. L., & Proudfit, G. H. (2014). Reward dysfunction in major depression: Multimodal neuroimaging evidence for refining the melancholic phenotype. *NeuroImage, 101*, 50–58. https://doi.org/10.1016/j.neuroimage.2014.06.058

Foti, D. J., Kotov, R., Guey, L. T., & Bromet, E. J. (2010). Cannabis use and the course of schizophrenia: 10-year follow-up after first hospitalization. *American Journal of Psychiatry, 167*, 987–993.

Fox, A. S., Oler, J. A., Tromp, D. P. M., Fudge, J. L., & Kalin, N. H. (2015). Extending the amygdala in theories of threat processing. *Trends in Neurosciences, 38*(5), 319–329. https://doi.org/10.1016/j.tins.2015.03.002

Fox, A. S., & Shackman, A. J. (2019). The central extended amygdala in fear and anxiety: Closing the gap between mechanistic and neuroimaging research. *Neuroscience Letters, 693*, 58–67. https://doi.org/10.1016/j.neulet.2017.11.056

Frackiewicz, E. J., Sramek, J. J., Herrera, J. M., Kurtz, N. M., & Cutler, N. R. (1997). Ethnicity and antipsychotic response. *Annals of Pharmacotherapy, 31*, 1360–1369.

Fradkin, I., Adams, R. A., Parr, T., Roiser, J. P., & Huppert, J. D. (2020). Searching for an anchor in an unpredictable world: A computational model of obsessive compulsive disorder. *Psychological Review, 127*(5), 672–699. https://doi.org/10.1037/rev0000188

Franco, A., Malhotra, N., & Simonovits, G. (2014). Publication bias in the social sciences: Unlocking the file drawer. *Science, 345*(6203), 1502–1505. https://doi.org/10.1126/science.1255484

Frank, E., Kupfer, D. J., Perel, J. M., Cornes, C., Jarrett, D. B., Mallinger, A. G., et al. (1990). Three-year outcomes for maintenance therapies in recurrent depression. *Archives of General Psychiatry, 47*(12), 1093–1099.

Frankenbach, J., Weber, M., Loschelder, D. D., Kilger, H., & Friese, M. (2022). Sex drive: Theoretical conceptualization and meta-analytic review of gender differences. *Psychological Bulletin, 148*(9–10), 621–661. https://doi.org/10.1037/BUL0000366

Franklin, J. C., Hessel, E. T., Aaron, R. V., Arthur, M. S., Heilbron, N., & Prinstein, M. J. (2010). The functions of nonsuicidal self-injury: Support for cognitive-affective regulation and opponent processes from a novel psychophysiological paradigm. *Journal of Abnormal Psychology, 119*, 850–862.

Franklin, J. C., Ribeiro, J. D., Fox, K. R., Bentley, K. H., Kleiman, E. M., Huang, X., et al. (2017). Risk factors for suicidal thoughts and behaviors: A meta-analysis of 50 years of research. *Psychological Bulletin, 143*(2), 187–232. https://doi.org/10.1037/bul0000084

Franklin, M. E., Budzyn, S., & Freeman, H. (2019). OCD spectrum disorders. In T*he Cambridge handbook of anxiety and related disorders* (pp. 805–825). Cambridge University Press. https://doi.org/10.1017/9781108140416.030

Franklin, M. E., & Foa, E. B. (2011). Treatment of obsessive compulsive disorder. *Annual Review of Clinical Psychology, 7*, 229–243.

Franklin, M. E., & Foa, E. B. (2014). Obsessive-compulsive disorder. In D. H. Barlow (Ed.), *Clinical handbook of psychological disorders* (5th ed., pp. 155–205). Guilford Press.

Franklin, M. E., Sapyta, J., Freeman, J. B., Khanna, M., Compton, S., Almirall, D., et al. (2011). Cognitive behavior therapy augmentation of pharmacotherapy in pediatric obsessive-compulsive disorder: The Pediatric OCD Treatment Study II (POTS II) randomized controlled trial. *Journal of the American Medical Association, 306*(11), 1224–1232.

Franko, D. L., & Keel, P. K. (2006). Suicidality in eating disorders: Occurrence, correlates, and clinical implications. *Clinical Psychology Review, 26*, 769–782.

Franko, D. L., Keshaviah, A., Eddy, K. T., Krishna, M., Davis, M. C., Keel, P. K., et al. (2013). A longitudinal investigation of mortality in anorexia nervosa and bulimia nervosa. *American Journal of Psychiatry, 170*(8), 917–925.

Franz, A. P., Bolat, G. U., Bolat, H., Matijasevich, A., Santos, I. S., Silveira, R. C., et al. (2018). Attention-deficit/hyperactivity disorder and very preterm/very low birth weight: A meta-analysis. *Pediatrics, 141*(1), e20171645. https://doi.org/10.1542/peds.2017-1645

Frederick, R. I., Mrad, D. F., & DeMier, R. L. (2007). *Examinations of criminal responsibility: Foundations in mental health case law*. Professional Resource Press.

Frederickson, B. L., & Carstensen, L. L. (1990). Choosing social partners: How old age and anticipated endings make people more selective. *Psychology and Aging, 5*, 335–347.

Fredrickson, B. L., & Roberts, T. A. (1997). Objectification theory: Toward understanding women's lived experience and mental health risks. *Psychology of Women Quarterly, 21*, 173–206.

Freeman, A. J., Youngstrom, E. A., Youngstrom, J. K., & Findling, R. L. (2016). Disruptive mood dysregulation disorder in a community mental health clinic: Prevalence, comorbidity and correlates. *Journal of Child and Adolescent Psychopharmacology, 26*(2), 123–130. https://doi.org/10.1089/cap.2015.0061

Freeman, C., Carpentier, L., & Weinberg, A. (2023). Effects of the COVID-19 pandemic on neural responses to reward: A quasi-experiment. *Biological Psychiatry: Cognitive Neuroscience and Neuroimaging*. https://doi.org/10.1016/j.bpsc.2023.02.009

Freeman, J., Sapyta, J., Garcia, A., Compton, S., Khanna, M., Flessner, C., et al. (2014). Family-based treatment of early childhood obsessive-compulsive disorder: The Pediatric Obsessive-Compulsive Disorder Treatment Study for Young Children (POTS Jr)—A randomized clinical trial. *JAMA Psychiatry, 71*(6), 689–698. https://doi.org/10.1001/jamapsychiatry.2014.170

Freire, R. C., Cabrera-Abreu, C., & Milev, R. (2020). Neurostimulation in anxiety disorders, post-traumatic stress disorder, and obsessive-compulsive disorder. In *Advances in Experimental Medicine and Biology, 1191*, 331–346. https://doi.org/10.1007/978-981-32-9705-0_18

Freizinger, M., Recto, M., Jhe, G., & Lin, J. (2022). Atypical anorexia in youth: Cautiously bridging the treatment gap. *Children, 9*(6).

Freud, A. (1946/1966). *The ego and mechanisms of defense*. International Universities Press.

Friborg, O., Martinsen, E. W., Martinussen, M., Kaiser, S., Øvergård, K. T., & Rosenvinge, J. H. (2014). Comorbidity of personality disorders in mood disorders: A meta-analytic review of 122 studies from 1988 to 2010. *Journal of Affective Disorders, 152*, 1–11. https://doi.org/10.1016/j.jad.2013.08.023

Friborg, O., Martinussen, M., Kaiser, S., Overgard, K. T., & Rosenvinge, J. H. (2013). Comorbidity of personality disorders in anxiety disorders: A meta-analysis of 30 years of research. *Journal of Affective Disorders, 145*, 143–155. https://doi.org/10.1016/j.jad.2012.07.004

Frick, P. J., Ray, J. V., Thornton, L. C., & Kahn, R. E. (2014). Can callous-unemotional traits enhance the understanding, diagnosis, and treatment of serious conduct problems in children and adolescents? A comprehensive review. *Psychological Bulletin, 140*, 1–57.

Fried, E. I., & Nesse, R. M. (2015). Depression sum-scores don't add up: Why analyzing specific depression symptoms is essential. *BMC Medicine, 13*(1), 72. https://doi.org/10.1186/s12916-015-0325-4

Friston, K. J. (1994). Functional and effective connectivity in neuro-imaging: A synthesis. *Human Brain Mapping, 2,* 56–78.

Fromer, M., Pocklington, A. J., Kavanagh, D. H., Williams, H. J., Dwyer, S., Gormley, P., et al. (2013). De novo mutations in schizophrenia implicate synaptic networks. *Nature, 506,* 179–184. https://doi.org/10.1038/nature12929

Fromuth, M. E., & Conn, V. E. (1997). Hidden Perpetrators: Sexual Molestation in a Nonclinical Sample of College Women. *Journal of Interpersonal Violence, 12*(3), 456–465. https://doi.org/10.1177/088626097012003009

Frost, D. O., & Cadet, J.-L. (2000). Effects of methamphetamine-induced toxicity on the development of neural circuitry: A hypothesis. *Brain Research Reviews, 34,* 103–118.

Frost, R. O., Marten, P. A., Lahart, C., & Rosenblate, R. (1990). The dimensions of perfectionism. *Cognitive Therapy and Research, 14,* 449–468.

Frost, R. O., & Steketee, G. (2010). Stuff: Compulsive hoarding and the meaning of things. Houghton Mifflin Harcourt.

Frost, R. O., Steketee, G., & Tolin, D. F. (2011). Comorbidity in hoarding disorder. *Depression and Anxiety, 28,* 876–884.

Frost, R. O., Steketee, G., & Tolin, D. F. (2012). Diagnosis and assessment of hoarding disorder. *Annual Review of Clinical Psychology, 8,* 219–242.

Frost, R. O., Tolin, D. F., Steketee, G., Fitch, K. E., & Selbo-Bruns, A. (2009). Excessive acquisition in hoarding. *Journal of Anxiety Disorders, 23*(5), 632–639. https://doi.org/10.1016/j.janxdis.2009.01.013

Frühauf, S., Gerger, H., Schmidt, H. M., Munder, T., & Barth, J. (2013). Efficacy of psychological interventions for sexual dysfunction: A systematic review and meta-analysis. *Archives of Sexual Behavior, 42,* 915–933.

Fuller, D. A., Sinclair, E., Geller, J., Quanbeck, C., & Snook, J. (2016). *Going, going, gone: Trends and consequences of eliminating state psychiatric beds, 2016.* Treatment Advocacy Center. https://www.treatmentadvocacycenter.org/storage/documents/going-going-gone.pdf

Fuller, R. K. (1988). Disulfiram treatment of alcoholism. In R. M. Rose & J. E. Barrett (Eds.), *Alcoholism: Origins and outcome* (pp. 237–250). Raven Press.

Fung, L. K., Mahajan, R., Nozzolillo, A., Bernal, P., Krasner, A., Jo, B., et al. (2016). Pharmacologic treatment of severe irritability and problem behaviors in autism: A systematic review and meta-analysis. *Pediatrics, 137*(Suppl), S124–S135. https://doi.org/10.1542/peds.2015-2851K

Furberg, H., Kim, Y., Dackor, J., Boerwinkle, E., Franceschini, N., Ardissino, D., et al. (2010). Genome-wide meta-analyses identify multiple loci associated with smoking behavior. *Nature Genetics, 42,* 441–447. https://doi.org/10.1038/ng.571

Fusar-Poli, P., Papanastasiou, E., Stahl, D., Rocchetti, M., Carpenter, W., Shergill, S., et al. (2015). Treatments of negative symptoms in schizophrenia: Meta-analysis of 168 randomized placebo-controlled trials. *Schizophrenia Bulletin, 41*(4), 892–899.

Gadalla, T., & Piran, N. (2007). Co-occurrence of eating disorders and alcohol use disorders in women: A meta analysis. *Archives of Women's Mental Health, 10,* 133–140.

Galán, C. A., Bekele, B., Boness, C., Bowdring, M., Call, C., Hails, K., et al. (2021). Editorial: A Call to Action for an Antiracist Clinical Science. *Journal of Clinical Child & Adolescent Psychology, 50*(1), 12–57. https://doi.org/10.1080/15374416.2020.1860066

Galmiche, M., Dechelotte, P., Lambert, G., & Tavolacci, M. P. (2019). Prevalence of eating disorders over the 2000–2018 period: A systematic literature review. *The American Journal of Clinical Nutrition, 109*(5), 1402–1413.

Gara, M. A., Minsky, S., Silverstein, S. M., Miskimen, T., & Strakowski, S. M. (2019). A Naturalistic Study of Racial Disparities in Diagnoses at an Outpatient Behavioral Health Clinic. *Psychiatric services (Washington, D.C.), 70*(2), 130–134. https://doi.org/10.1176/appi.ps.201800223

Garber, J. (2006). Depression in children and adolescents: Linking risk research and prevention. *American Journal of Preventative Medicine, 31,* 5104–5125.

Garber, J., Brunwasser, S. M., Zerr, A. A., Schwartz, K. T. G., Sova, K., & Weersing, V. R. (2016). Treatment and prevention of depression and anxiety in youth: Test of cross-over effects. *Depression and Anxiety, 33*(10), 939–959. https://doi.org/10.1002/da.22519

Garber, J., Clarke, G. N., Weersing, V. R., Beardslee, W. R., Brent, D. A., Gladstone, T. R., et al. (2009). Prevention of depression in at-risk adolescents: A randomized controlled trial. *Journal of the American Medical Association, 301,* 2215–2224.

Garber, J., Kelly, M. K., & Martin, N. C. (2002). Developmental trajectories of adolescents' depressive symptoms: Predictors of change. *Journal of Consulting and Clinical Psychology, 70,* 79–95.

Garb H. N. (2021). Race bias and gender bias in the diagnosis of psychological disorders. *Clinical psychology review, 90,* 102087. https://doi.org/10.1016/j.cpr.2021.102087

Gard, D. E., Kring, A. M., Germans Gard, M., Horan, W. P., & Green, M. F. (2007). Anhedonia in schizophrenia: Distinctions between anticipatory and consummatory pleasure. *Schizophrenia Research, 93,* 253–260.

Gard, D. E., Sanchez, A. H., Starr, J., Cooper, S., Fisher, M., Rowlands, A., et al. (2014). Using self-determination theory to understand motivation deficits in schizophrenia: The "why" of motivated behavior. *Schizophrenia Research, 156,* 217–222.

Gardner, M. J., Thomas, H. J., & Erskine, H. E. (2019). The association between five forms of child maltreatment and depressive and anxiety disorders: A systematic review and meta-analysis. *Child Abuse & Neglect, 96,* 104082.

Garety, P. A., Fowler, D., & Kuipers, E. (2000). Cognitive behavioral therapy for medication-resistant symptoms. *Schizophrenia Bulletin, 26,* 73–86.

Garner, D. M., Olmsted, M. P., & Polivy, J. (1983). Development and validation of a multi-dimensional eating disorder inventory for anorexia nervosa and bulimia. *International Journal of Eating Disorders, 2,* 15–34.

Garner, D. M., Vitousek, K. M., & Pike, K. M. (1997). Cognitive-behavioral therapy for anorexia nervosa. In D. M. Garner & P. E. Garfinkel (Eds.), *Handbook of treatment for eating disorders* (pp. 94–144). Guilford Press.

Garner, G. (2021). Amanda Seyfried opens up about panic attacks caused by fame: "It feels like life or death'. *People Magazine.* https://people.com/movies/amanda-seyfried-bizarre-panic-attacks-caused-by-fame/

Gartlehner, G., Gaynes, B. N., Hansen, R. A., Thieda, P., DeVeaugh-Geiss, A., Krebs, E. E., et al. (2008). Comparative benefits and harms of second-generation antidepressants: Background paper for the American College of Physicians. *Annals of Internal Medicine, 149*(10), 734–750.

Gasser, P., Holstein, D., Michel, Y., Doblin, R., Yazar-Klosinski, B., Passie, T., et al. (2014). Safety and efficacy of lysergic acid diethylamide-assisted psychotherapy for anxiety associated with life-threatening diseases. *Journal of Nervous and Mental Disease, 202,* 513–520.

Gaugler, T., Klei, L., Sanders, S. J., Bodea, C. A., Goldberg, A. P., Lee, A. B., et al. (2014). Most genetic risk for autism resides with common variation. *Nature Genetics, 46*(8), 881–885. https://doi.org/10.1038/ng.3039

Gaus, V. L. (2018). *Cognitive behavior therapy for adults with autism spectrum disorder* (2nd Ed.). Guilford Press.

Gavey, N., & Senn, C. Y. (2014). Sexuality and sexual violence. In D. L. Tolman, L. M. Diamond, J. A. Bauermeister, W. H. George, J. G. Pfaus, & L. M. Ward (Eds.), *APA handbook of sexuality and psychology, Vol. 1: Person-based approaches* (pp. 339–382). American Psychological Association.

GBD 2015 Obesity Collaborators. (2017). Health effects of overweight and obesity in 195 countries over 25 years. *New England Journal of Medicine, 377*, 13–27. https://doi.org/10.1056/NEJMoa1614362

Geddes, J. R., Burgess, S., Hawton, K., Jamison, K., & Goodwin, G. M. (2004). Long-term lithium therapy for bipolar disorder: Systematic review and meta-analysis of randomized controlled trials. *American Journal of Psychiatry, 161*, 217–222.

Gelauff, J., Stone, J., Edwards, M., & Carson, A. (2013). The prognosis of functional (psychogenic) motor symptoms: A systematic review. *Journal of Neurology, Neurosurgery and Psychiatry, 85*(2):220–226. https://doi.org/10.1136/jnnp-2013-305321

Gelernter, J., & Polimanti, R. (2021). Genetics of substance use disorders in the era of big data. *Nature reviews. Genetics, 22*(11), 712–729. https://doi.org/10.1038/s41576-021-00377-1

Geller, D. A., & March, J. (2012). Practice parameter for the assessment and treatment of children and adolescents with obsessive-compulsive disorder. *Journal of the American Academy of Child & Adolescent Psychiatry, 51*(1), 98–113.

Gentes, E. L., & Ruscio, A. M. (2011). A meta-analysis of the relation of intolerance of uncertainty to symptoms of generalized anxiety disorder, major depressive disorder, and obsessive-compulsive disorder. *Clinical Psychology Review, 31*, 923–933.

Gentzke, A. S., Wang, T. W., Cornelius, M., Park-Lee E., Ren, C., Sawdey M., et al. (2022). Tobacco product use and associated factors among middle and high school students—National Youth Tobacco Survey, United States, 2021. *Morbidity and Mortality Weekly Report Surveillance Summary, 71*(No. SS-5), 1–29. https://doi.org/10.15585/mmwr.ss7105a1

George, M. S. (2019). Whither TMS: A one-trick pony or the beginning of a neuroscientific revolution? *American Journal of Psychiatry, 176*(11), 904–910. https://doi.org/10.1176/appi.ajp.2019.19090957

Geraerts, E., Schooler, J. W., Merckelbach, H., Jelicic, M., Hauer, B. J. A., & Ambadar, Z. (2007). The reality of recovered memories: Corroborating continuous and discontinuous memories of childhood sexual abuse. *Psychological Science, 18*, 564–568.

Gerlach, A. L., Wilhelm, F. H., Gruber, K., & Roth, W. T. (2001). Blushing and physiological arousability in social phobia. *Journal of Abnormal Psychology, 110*, 247–258.

Gernsbacher, M. A., Dawson, M., & Goldsmith, H. H. (2005). Three reasons not to believe in an autism epidemic. *Current Directions in Psychological Science, 14*, 55–58.

Getahun, D., Jacobsen, S. J., Fassett, M. J., Chen, W., Demissie, K., & Rhoads, G. G. (2013). Recent trends in childhood attention-deficit/hyperactivity disorder. *JAMA Pediatrics, 167*(3), 282–288.

Ge, X., Conger, R. D., Cadoret, R. J., Neiderhiser, J. M., Yates, W., Troughton, E., et al. (1996). The developmental interface between nature and nurture: A mutual influence model of child antisocial behavior and parent behaviors. *Developmental Psychology, 32*, 574–589.

Ghaderi, A., Odeberg, J., Gustafsson, S., Råstam, M., Brolund, A., Pettersson, A., et al. (2018). Psychological, pharmacological, and combined treatments for binge eating disorder: A systematic review and meta-analysis. *PeerJ, 6*, e5113.

Giangrande, E. J., Weber, R. S., & Turkheimer, E. (2022). What do we know about the genetic architecture of psychopathology? *Annual Review of Clinical Psychology, 18*(1), 19–42. https://doi.org/10.1146/annurev-clinpsy-081219-091234

Gibson, L. E., Alloy, L. B., & Ellman, L. M. (2016). Trauma and the psychosis spectrum: A review of symptom specificity and explanatory mechanisms. *Clinical Psychology Review, 49*, 92–105.

Gignac, A., McGirr, A., Lam, R. W., & Yatham, L. N. (2015). Recovery and recurrence following a first episode of mania: A systematic review and meta-analysis of prospectively characterized cohorts. *Journal of Clinical Psychiatry, 76*(9), 1241–1248. https://doi.org/10.4088/JCP.14r09245

Gijs, L., & Brewaeys, A. (2007). Surgical treatment of gender dysphoria in adults and adolescents: Recent developments, effectiveness, and challenges. *Annual Review of Sex Research, 18*, 178–224.

Gilbert, D. T., King, G., Pettigrew, S., & Wilson, T. D. (2016). Comment on "estimating the reproducibility of psychological science." *Science, 351*(6277), 1037. https://doi.org/10.1126/science.aad7243

Gilboa-Schechtman, E., Galili, L., Sahar, Y., & Amir, O. (2014). Being "in" or "out" of the game: Subjective and acoustic reactions to exclusion and popularity in social anxiety. *Frontiers in Human Neuroscience, 8*(MAR), 147. https://doi.org/10.3389/fnhum.2014.00147

Gillan, C. M., Morein-Zamir, S., Urcelay, G. P., Sule, A., Voon, V., Apergis-Schoute, A. M., et al. (2014). Enhanced avoidance habits in obsessive-compulsive disorder. *Biological Psychiatry, 75*, 631–638.

Gillespie, C., Murphy, M., & Joyce, M. (2022). Dialectical behavior therapy for individuals with borderline personality disorder: A systematic review of outcomes after one year of follow-up. *Journal of Personality Disorders, 36*(4), 431–454.

Ginsburg, G. S., Becker-Haimes, E. M., Keeton, C., Kendall, P. C., Iyengar, S., Sakolsky, D., et al. (2018). Results from the Child/Adolescent Anxiety Multimodal Extended Long-Term Study (CAMELS): Primary anxiety outcomes. *Journal of the American Academy of Child & Adolescent Psychiatry, 57*(7), 471–480.

Girault, J. B., & Piven, J. (2020). The neurodevelopment of autism from infancy through toddlerhood. *Psychoradiology, 30*(1), 97–114.

Gjerde, L. C., Czajkowski, N., Røysamb, E., Ørstavik, R. E., Knudsen, G. P., Østby, K., et al. (2012). The heritability of avoidant and dependent personality disorder assessed by personal interview and questionnaire. *Acta Psychiatrica Scandinavica, 126*, 448–457. https://doi.org/10.1111/j.1600-0447.2012.01862.x

Glahn, D. C., Laird, A. R., Ellison-Wright, I., Thelen, S. M., Robinson, J. L., Lancaster, J. L., et al. (2008). Meta-analysis of gray matter anomalies in schizophrenia: Application of anatomic likelihood estimation and network analysis. *Biological Psychiatry, 64*, 774–781. https://doi.org/10.1016/j.biopsych.2008.03.031

Glausier, J. R., & Lewis, D. A. (2013). Dendritic spine pathology in schizophrenia. *Neuroscience, 251*, 90–107.

Gleaves, D. H. (1996). The sociocognitive model of dissociative identity disorder: A reexamination of the evidence. *Psychological Bulletin, 120*, 42–59.

Glenn, A. L., Raine, A., Venables, P. H., & Mednick, S. A. (2007). Early temperamental and psychophysiological precursors of adult psychopathic personality. *Journal of Abnormal Psychology, 116*, 508–518.

Glenn, J. J., Michel, B. D., Franklin, J. C., Hooley, J. M., & Nock, M. K. (2014). Pain analgesia among adolescent self-injurers. *Psychiatry Research, 220*(3), 921–926. https://doi.org/10.1016/j.psychres.2014.08.016

Godart, N. T., Flament, M., Perdereau, F., & Jeammet, P. (2002). Comorbidity between eating disorders and anxiety disorders: A review. *International Journal of Eating Disorders, 32*, 253–270.

Goedert, M., Spillantini, M. G., Del Tredici, K., & Braak, H. (2013). 100 years of Lewy pathology. *Nature Reviews Neurology, 9*, 13–24.

Goenjian, A. K., Walling, D., Steinberg, A. M., Karayan, I., Najarian, L. M., & Pynoos, R. (2005). A prospective study of posttraumatic stress and depressive reactions among treated and untreated adolescents 5 years after a catastrophic disaster. *American Journal of Psychiatry, 162*, 2302–2308.

Goldberg, S. B., Tucker, R. P., Greene, P. A., Davidson, R. J., Kearney, D. J., & Simpson, T. L. (2019). Mindfulness-based cognitive therapy for the treatment of current depressive symptoms: A meta-analysis. *Cognitive Behaviour Therapy, 48*(6), 445–462. https://doi.org/10.1080/16506073.2018.1556330

Goldberg, T. E., Chen, C., Wang, Y., Jung, E., Swanson, A., Ing, C., Garcia, P. S., Whittington, R. A., & Moitra, V. (2020). Association of Delirium with Long-term Cognitive Decline. *JAMA Neurology, 77*(11), 1373. https://doi.org/10.1001/jamaneurol.2020.2273

Goldfarb, D., Goodman, G. S., Larson, R. P., Eisen, M. L., & Qin, J. (2019). Long-term memory in adults exposed to childhood violence: Remembering genital contact nearly 20 years later. *Clinical Psychological Science, 7*(2), 381–396. https://doi.org/10.1177/2167702618805742

Goldin, P. R., Manber-Ball, T., Werner, K., Heimberg, R., & Gross, J. J. (2009). Neural mechanisms of cognitive reappraisal of negative self-beliefs in social anxiety disorder. *Biological Psychiatry, 66*, 1091–1099.

Goldsmith, D. R., Bekhbat, M., Mehta, N. D., & Felger, J. C. (2023). Inflammation-related functional and structural dysconnectivity as a pathway to psychopathology. *Biological Psychiatry, 93*(5), 405–418.

Goldsmith, D. R., Rapaport, M. H., & Miller, B. J. (2016). A meta-analysis of blood cytokine network alterations in psychiatric patients: Comparisons between schizophrenia, bipolar disorder and depression. *Molecular Psychiatry, 21*(12), 1696–1709. https://doi.org/10.1038/mp.2016.3

Gold, S. M., Köhler-Forsberg, O., Moss-Morris, R., Mehnert, A., Miranda, J. J., Bullinger, M., et al. (2020). Comorbid depression in medical diseases. *Nature Reviews Disease Primers, 6*(1), 69. https://doi.org/10.1038/s41572-020-0200-2

Goldstein, G. (2018). Neurocognitive disorders. In D. C. Beidel & B. C. Frueh (Eds.), *Adult psychopathology and diagnosis* (8th ed., pp. 725–755). John Wiley Inc.

Goldstein, L. H., Robinson, E. J., Chalder, T., Reuber, M., Medford, N., Stone, J., et al. (2022). Six-month outcomes of the CODES randomised controlled trial of cognitive behavioural therapy for dissociative seizures: A secondary analysis. *Seizure: European Journal of Epilepsy, 96*, 128–136. https://doi.org/10.1016/j.seizure.2022.01.016

Goldstein, R. B., Smith, S. M., Chou, S. P., Saha, T. D., Jung, J., Zhang, H., et al. (2016). The epidemiology of DSM-5 posttraumatic stress disorder in the United States: Results from the National Epidemiologic Survey on Alcohol and Related Conditions-III. *Social Psychiatry and Psychiatric Epidemiology, 51*(8), 1137–1148. https://doi.org/10.1007/S00127-016-1208-5

Goldstone, A., Javitz, H. S., Claudatos, S. A., Buysse, D. J., Hasler, B. P., de Zambotti, M., et al. (2020). Sleep disturbance predicts depression symptoms in early adolescence: Initial findings from the Adolescent Brain Cognitive Development Study. *Journal of Adolescent Health, 66*(5), 567–574. https://doi.org/10.1016/j.jadohealth.2019.12.005

Gondoli, D. M., Corning, A. F., Salafia, E., Bucchianeri, M. M., & Fitzsimmons, E. E. (2011). Heterosocial involvement, peer pressure for thinness, and body dissatisfaction among young adolescent girls. *Body Image, 8*(2), 143–148. https://doi.org/10.1016/j.bodyim.2010.12.005

Goodkind, M., Eickhoff, S. B., Oathes, D. J., Jiang, Y., Chang, A., Jones-Hagata, L. B., et al. (2015). Identification of a common neurobiological substrate for mental illness. *JAMA Psychiatry, 72*, 305–315. https://doi.org/10.1001/jamapsychiatry.2014.2206

Goodkind, M. S., Gyurak, A., McCarthy, M., Miller, B. L., & Levenson, R. W. (2010). Emotion regulation deficits in frontotemporal lobar degeneration and Alzheimer's disease. *Psychological Aging, 25*, 30–37.

Goodman, G. S., Ghetti, S., Quas, J. A., Edelstein, R. S., Alexander, K. W., Redlich, A. D., et al. (2003). A prospective study of memory for child sexual abuse: New findings relevant to the repressed-memory controversy. *Psychological Science, 14*, 113–118.

Goodman, W. K., Storch, E. A., & Sheth, S. A. (2021). Harmonizing the neurobiology and treatment of obsessive-compulsive disorder. *American Journal of Psychiatry, 178*(1), 17–29. https://doi.org/10.1176/APPI.AJP.2020.20111601/ASSET/IMAGES/LARGE/APPI.AJP.2020.20111601F1.JPEG

Goodwin, D. K. (2003). Team of Rivals: The Political Genius of Abraham Lincoln. Simon & Schuster.

Goodwin, F., & Jamison, K. (2007). *Manic-depressive illness: Bipolar disorders and recurrent depression* (2nd ed.). Oxford University Press.

Gopnik, A., Capps, L., & Meltzoff, A. N. (2000). Early theories of mind: What the theory can tell us about autism. In S. Baron-Cohen, H. Tager-Flusberg, & D. Cohen (Eds.), *Understanding other minds* (2nd ed., pp. 50–72). Oxford University Press.

Gorka, S. M., Lieberman, L., Shankman, S. A., & Phan, K. L. (2017). Startle potentiation to uncertain threat as a psychophysiological indicator of fear-based psychopathology: An examination across multiple internalizing disorders. *Journal of Abnormal Psychology, 126*(1), 8–18. https://doi.org/10.1037/abn0000233

Gottesman, I. I., Laursen, T. M., Bertelsen, A., & Mortensen, P. B. (2010). Severe mental disorders in offspring with 2 psychiatrically ill parents. *Archives of General Psychiatry, 67*, 252–257.

Gottesman, I. I., McGuffin, P., & Farmer, A. E. (1987). Clinical genetics as clues to the "real" genetics of schizophrenia. *Schizophrenia Bulletin, 13*, 23–47.

Gowing, L., Ali, R., & White, J. M. (2009). Buprenorphine for the management of opioid withdrawal. *Cochrane Database of Systematic Reviews, 3*, CD002025. https://doi.org/10.1002/14651858.CD002025.pub4

Grabe, S., & Hyde, J. S. (2006). Ethnicity and body dissatisfaction among women in the United States: A meta-analysis. *Psychological Bulletin, 132*, 622–640.

Grabe, S., Ward, L. M., & Hyde, J. S. (2008). The role of the media in body image concerns among women: A meta-analysis of experimental and correlational studies. *Psychological Bulletin, 134*, 460–476. https://doi.org/10.1037/0033-2909.134.3.460

Grace, S. A., Labuschagne, I., Kaplan, R. A., & Rossell, S. L. (2017). The neurobiology of body dysmorphic disorder: A systematic review and theoretical model. *Neuroscience and Biobehavioral Reviews, 83*, 83–96. https://doi.org/10.1016/j.neubiorev.2017.10.003

Grady, D. (July 20, 1999). A great pretender now faces the truth of illness. *The New York Times.*

Graham, C. A. (2010). The DSM diagnostic criteria for female sexual arousal disorder. *Archives of Sexual Behavior, 39*, 240–255.

Graham, C. A. (2014). Orgasm disorders in women. In Y. M. Binik & K. S. K. Hall (Eds.), *Principles and practice of sex therapy* (5th ed. ed., pp. 89–111). The Guilford Press.

Graham, C. A., Mercer, C. H., Tanton, C., Jones, K. G., Johnson, A. M., Wellings, K., et al. (2017). What factors are associated with reporting lacking interest in sex and how do these vary by gender? Findings from the third British national survey of sexual attitudes and lifestyles. *BMJ Open, 7*(9), e016942. https://doi.org/10.1136/bmjopen-2017-016942

Grandin, T. (1986). *Emergence: Labeled autistic.* Arena Press.

Grandin, T. (1995). *Thinking in pictures.* Doubleday.

Grandin, T. (2008). *The way I see it: A personal look at autism and Asperger's.* Future Horizons.

Grandin, T. (2013). *The autistic brain.* Houghton Mifflin Harcourt.

Granholm, E., Holden J. L., Link P., & McQuaid J. R. (2014). Randomized clinical trial of cognitive behavioral social skills training for schizophrenia: Improvement in functioning and experiential negative symptoms. *Journal of Consulting and Clinical Psychology, 82*, 1173–1185.

Granholm, E., McQuaid. J. R., & Holden, J. (2016). *Cognitive behavioral social skills training for schizophrenia: A practical treatment guide.* Guilford Press.

Granholm, E., McQuaid, J. R., McClure, F. S., Auslander, L. A., Perivoliotis, D., Paola Pedrelli, M. S., et al. (2005). A randomized, controlled trial for cognitive behavioral social skills training for middle-aged and older outpatients with chronic schizophrenia. *American Journal of Psychiatry, 162*, 520–529.

Grant, B. F., Chou, S. P., Goldstein, R. B., Huang, B., Stinson, F. S., Saha, T. D., et al. (2008). Prevalence, correlates, disability, and comorbidity of DSM-IV borderline personality disorder: Results from the Wave 2 National Epidemiologic Survey on Alcohol and Related Conditions. *Journal of Clinical Psychiatry, 69*, 533–545.

Grant, B. F., Goldstein, R. B., Saha, T. D., Chou, S. P., Jung, J., Zhang, H., et al. (2015). Epidemiology of DSM-5 alcohol use disorder: Results from the National Epidemiologic Survey on Alcohol and Related Conditions III. *JAMA Psychiatry, 72*, 757–766. https://doi.org/10.1001/jamapsychiatry.2015.0584

Grant, P. M., Huh, G., Perivoliotis, D., Stolar, N., & Beck, A. T. (2012). Randomized trial to evaluate the efficacy of cognitive therapy for low-functioning patients with schizophrenia. *Archives of General Psychiatry, 69*, 121–127.

Greenberg, J. L., Reuman, L., Hartmann, A. S., Kasarskis, I., & Wilhelm, S. (2014). Visual hot spots: An eye tracking study of attention bias in body dysmorphic disorder. *Journal of Psychiatric Research, 57*(1), 125–132. https://doi.org/10.1016/j.jpsychires.2014.06.015

Greenhill, L. L., Swanson, J. M., Hechtman, L., Waxmonsky, J., Arnold, L. E., Molina, B., et al., & MTA Cooperative Group (2020). Trajectories of growth associated with long-term stimulant medication in the multimodal treatment study of attention-deficit/hyperactivity disorder. *Journal of the American Academy of Child and Adolescent Psychiatry, 59*(8), 978–989. https://doi.org/10.1016/j.jaac.2019.06.019

Green, J. G., McLaughlin, K. A., Berglund, P. A., Gruber, M. J., Sampson, N. A., Zaslavsky, A. M., et al. (2010). Childhood adversities and adult psychiatric disorders in the National Comorbidity Survey Replication: Associations with first onset of DSM-IV disorders. *Archives of General Psychiatry, 67*, 113–123.

Greeven, A., van Balkom, A. J. L. M., Visser, S., Merkelbach, J. W., van Rood, Y. R., van Dyck, R., et al. (2007). Cognitive behavior therapy and paroxetine in the treatment of hypochondriasis: A randomized controlled trial. *American Journal of Psychiatry, 164*, 91–99.

Gregory, A. M., Caspi, A., Moffitt, T. E., Koenen, K., Eley, T. C., & Poulton, R. (2007). Juvenile mental health histories of adults with anxiety disorders. *American Journal of Psychiatry, 164*(2), 301–308. https://doi.org/10.1176/ajp.2007.164.2.301

Grey, I. M., & Hastings, R. P. (2005). Evidence-based practices in intellectual disability and behaviour disorders. *Current Opinion in Psychiatry, 18*, 469–475. https://doi.org/10.1097/01.yco.0000179482.54767.cf

Griffith, J. W., Zinbarg, R. E., Craske, M. G., Mineka, S., Rose, R. D., Waters, A. M., et al. (2009). Neuroticism as a common dimension in the internalizing disorders. *Psychological Medicine, 40*, 1125–1136. https://doi.org/10.1017/S0033291709991449

Griffiths, T. L. (2015). Manifesto for a new (computational) cognitive revolution. *Cognition, 135*, 21–23. https://doi.org/10.1016/j.cognition.2014.11.026

Grillon, C., Lissek, S., Rabin, S., McDowell, D., Dvir, S., & Pine, D. S. (2008). Increased anxiety during anticipation of unpredictable but not predictable aversive stimuli as a psychophysiologic marker of panic disorder. *The American Journal of Psychiatry, 165*(7), 898–904. https://doi.org/10.1176/appi.ajp.2007.07101581

Grilo, C. M., Crosby, R. D., Wilson, G. T., & Masheb, R. M. (2012). 12-month follow-up of fluoxetine and cognitive behavioral therapy for binge eating disorder. *Journal of Consulting and Clinical Psychology, 80*, 1108–1113.

Griner, D., & Smith, T. B. (2006). Culturally adapted mental health intervention: A meta-analytic review. *Psychotherapy, 43*, 531–548.

Grinker, R. R., & Spiegel, J. P. (1944). *Management of neuropsychiatric casualties in the zone of combat: Manual of military neuropsychiatry.* W.B. Saunders.

Grisham, J. R., Frost, R. O., Steketee, G., Kim, H. J., & Hood, S. (2006). Age of onset of compulsive hoarding. *Journal of Anxiety Disorders, 20*, 675–686.

Griswold, M. G., Fullman, N., Hawley, C., Arian, N., Zimsen, S. R. M., Tymeson, H. D., et al. (2018). Alcohol use and burden for 195 countries and territories, 1990–2016: A systematic analysis for the Global Burden of Disease Study 2016. *Lancet (London, England), 392*(10152), 1015–1035.

Grossman, D. (1995). *On killing: The psychological cost of learning to kill in war and society.* Little, Brown.

Grove, J., Ripke, S., Als, T. D., Mattheisen, M., Walters, R. K., Won, H., et al. (2019). Identification of common genetic risk variants for autism spectrum disorder. *Nature Genetics, 51*, 431–444. https://doi.org/10.1038/s41588-019-0344-8

Grundmann, D., Krupp, J., Scherner, G., Amelung, T., & Beier, K. M. (2016). Stability of self-reported arousal to sexual fantasies involving children in a clinical sample of pedophiles and hebephiles. *Archives of Sexual Behavior, 45*, 1153–1162. https://doi.org/10.1007/s10508-016-0729-z

Guendelman, M., Owens, E. B., Galan, C., Gard, A., & Hinshaw, S. P. (2016). Early adult correlates of maltreatment in girls with ADHD: Increased risk for internalizing problems and suicidality. *Development and Psychopathology, 28*, 1–14.

Guideline Development Panel for Treatment of Obesity, American Psychological Association. (2020). Summary of the clinical practice guideline for multicomponent behavioral treatment of obesity and overweight in children and adolescents. *American Psychologist, 75*(2), 178–188. https://doi.org/10.1037/amp0000530

Gum, A. M., King-Kallimanis, B., & Kohn, R. (2009). Prevalence of mood, anxiety, and substance-abuse disorders for older Americans in the National Comorbidity Survey-Replication. *American Journal of Psychiatry, 17*, 769–781.

Gunaratnam, S., & Alisic, E. (2017). Epidemiology of trauma and trauma-related disorders in children and adolescents. *Evidence-Based Treatments for Trauma Related Disorders in Children and Adolescents*, 29–47. https://doi.org/10.1007/978-3-319-46138-0_2

Guo, J. Y., Ragland, J. D., & Carter, C. S. (2019). Memory and cognition in schizophrenia. *Molecular Psychiatry, 24*(5), 633–642.

Gupta, C. N., Calhoun, V. D., Rachakonda, S., Chen, J., Patel, V., Liu, J., et al. (2015). Patterns of gray matter abnormalities in schizophrenia based on an international mega-analysis. *Schizophrenia Bulletin, 41*, 1133–1142. https://doi.org/10.1093/schbul/sbu177

Gustad, J., & Phillips, K. A. (2003). Axis I comorbidity in body dysmorphic disorder. *Comprehensive Psychiatry, 44*, 270–276.

Guzick, A. G., McCabe, R. E., & Storch, E. A. (2021). A review of motivational interviewing in cognitive behavioral therapy for obsessive-compulsive disorder. *Journal of Cognitive Psychotherapy, 35*(2), 116–132. https://doi.org/10.1891/JCPSY-D-20-00027

Haaga, D. A. F., Dyck, M. J., & Ernst, D. (1991). Empirical status of cognitive theory of depression. *Psychological Bulletin, 110*, 215–236.

Hacking, I. (1998). *Mad travelers: Reflections on the reality of transient mental illness.* University Press of Virginia.

Haedt-Matt, A. A., & Keel, P. K. (2011). Revisiting the affect regulation model of binge eating: A meta-analysis of studies using ecological momentary assessment. *Psychological Bulletin, 137*, 660–681.

Hagerman, R. (2006). Lessons from fragile X regarding neurobiology, autism, and neurodegeneration. *Developmental and Behavioral Pediatrics, 27,* 63–74.

Haijma, S. V., Van Haren, N., Cahn, W., Koolschijn, P. C., Hulshoff Pol, H. E., & Kahn, R. S. (2013). Brain volumes in schizophrenia: A meta-analysis in over 18 000 subjects. *Schizophrenia Bulletin, 39*(5), 1129–1138.

Halberstadt, A. L. (2015). Recent advances in the neuropsychopharmacology of serotonergic hallucinogens. *Special Issue: Serotonin, 277,* 99–120.

Hales, C. M., Carroll, M. D., Fryar, C. D., & Ogden, C. L. (2020). Prevalence of obesity and severe obesity among adults: United States, 2017–2018. NCHS Data Brief, no 360. National Center for Health Statistics.

Hales, C. M., Servais, J., Martin, C. B., Kohen, D. (2019). *Prescription drug use among adults aged 40–79 in the United States and Canada.* NCHS Data Brief, no 347. National Center for Health Statistics.

Hallett, M. (2016). Neurophysiologic studies of functional neurologic disorders. *Handbook of Clinical Neurology, 139,* 61–71. https://doi.org/10.1016/B978-0-12-801772-2.00006-0

Hallford, D. J., & Sharma, M. K. (2019). Anticipatory pleasure for future experiences in schizophrenia spectrum disorders and major depression: A systematic review and meta-analysis. *British Journal of Clinical Psychology, 58*(4), 357-383. https://doi.org/10.1111/bjc.12218

Hall, G. C., Hirschman, R., & Oliver, L. L. (1995). Sexual arousal and arousability to pedophilic stimuli in a community sample of normal men. *Behavior Therapy, 26,* 681–694.

Hall, G. C. N., Ibaraki, A. Y., Huang, E. R., Marti, C. N., & Stice, E. (2016). A meta-analysis of cultural adaptations of psychological interventions. *Behavior Therapy, 47*(6), 993–1014. https://doi.org/10.1016/j.beth.2016.09.005

Halliwell, E., Dittmar, H., & Orsborn, A. (2007). The effects of exposure to muscular male models among men: Exploring the moderating role of gym use and exercise motivation. *Body Image, 4,* 278–287.

Hall, J. T., Menton, W. H., & Ben-Porath, Y. (2022). Examining the psychometric equivalency of MMPI-3 scale scores derived from the MMPI-3 and the MMPI-2-RF-EX. *Assessment, 29*(4), 842–853. https://doi.org/10.1177/1073191121991921

Hall, K. D., Ayuketah, A., Brychta, R., Cai, H., Cassimatis, T., Chen, K. Y., et al. (2019). Ultra-processed diets cause excess calorie intake and weight gain: An inpatient randomized controlled trial of ad libitum food intake. *Cell Metabolism, 30*(1), 67–77.E3. https://doi.org/10.1016/j.cmet.2019.05.008

Hallmayer, J., Cleveland, S., Torres, A., Phillips, J., Cohen, B., Torigoe, T., et al. (2011). Genetic heritability and shared environmental factors among twin pairs with autism. *Archives of General Psychiatry, 68,* 1095–1102.

Hall, M. G., Alhassoon, O. M., Stern, M. J., Wollman, S. C., Kimmel, C. L., Perez-Figueroa, A., et al. (2015). Gray matter abnormalities in cocaine versus methamphetamine-dependent patients: A neuroimaging meta-analysis. *American Journal of Drug and Alcohol Abuse, 41,* 290–299. https://doi.org/10.3109/00952990.2015.1044607

Hallquist, M. N., Hipwell, A. E., & Stepp, S. D. (2015). Poor self-control and harsh punishment in childhood prospectively predict borderline personality symptoms in adolescent girls. *Journal of Abnormal Psychology, 124,* 549–564. https://doi.org/10.1037/abn0000058

Hall, W. D., & Lynskey, M. (2005). Is cannabis a gateway drug? Testing hypotheses about the relationship between cannabis use and the use of other illicit drugs. *Drug and Alcohol Review, 24,* 39–48.

Hamilton, J. L., Stange, J. P., Abramson, L. Y., & Alloy, L. B. (2015). Stress and the development of cognitive vulnerabilities to depression explain sex differences in depressive symptoms during adolescence. *Clinical Psychological Science, 3*(5), 702–714. https://doi.org/10.1177/2167702614545479

Hamilton, J. P., Etkin, A., Furman, D. J., Lemus, M. G., Johnson, R. F., & Gotlib, I. H. (2012). Functional neuroimaging of major depressive disorder: A meta-analysis and new integration of baseline activation and neural response data. *American Journal of Psychiatry, 169,* 693–703.

Hammen, C. (2009). Adolescent depression: Stressful interpersonal contexts and risk for recurrence. *Current Directions in Psychological Science, 18,* 200–204.

Hammen, C., & Brennan, P. (2001). Depressed adolescents of depressed and nondepressed mothers: Tests of an interpersonal impairment hypothesis. *Journal of Consulting and Clinical Psychology, 69,* 284–294.

Hammen, C., Hazel, N. A., Brennan, P. A., & Najman, J. (2012). Intergenerational transmission and continuity of stress and depression: Depressed women and their offspring in 20 years of follow-up. *Psychological Medicine, 42,* 931–942.

Hampson, D. R., & Blatt, G. J. (2015). Autism spectrum disorders and neuropathology of the cerebellum. *Frontiers in Neuroscience, 9,* 420. https://doi.org/10.3389/fnins.2015.00420

Hamshere, M. L., Langley, K., Martin, J., Agha, S. S., Stergiakouli, E., Anney, R. J., et al. (2013). High loading of polygenic risk for ADHD in children with comorbid aggression. *American Journal of Psychiatry, 170*(8), 909–916.

Hancock, J., Liu, S. X., Luo, M., & Mieczkowski, H. (March 9, 2022). Psychological well-being and social media use: A meta-analysis of associations between social media use and depression, anxiety, loneliness, eudaimonic, hedonic and social well-being. https://ssrn.com/abstract=4053961; https://doi.org/10.2139/ssrn.4053961

Hanel, P. H., & Vione, K. C. (2016). Do student samples provide an accurate estimate of the general public? *PLoS One, 11*(12), e0168354. https://doi.org/10.1371/journal.pone.0168354

Han, J. H., Zimmerman, E. E., Cutler, N., Schnelle, J., Morandi, A., Dittus, R. S., et al. (2009). Delirium in older emergency department patients: Recognition, risk factors, and psychomotor subtypes. *Academic Emergency Medicine, 16,* 193–200. https://doi.org/10.1111/j.1553-2712.2008.00339.x

Hankin, B. L., & Abramson, L. Y. (2001). Development of gender differences in depression: An elaborated cognitive vulnerability-transactional stress theory. *Psychological Bulletin, 127,* 773–796.

Hankin, B. L., Abramson, L. Y., Moffitt, T. E., Silva, P. A., McGee, R., & Angell, K. E. (1998). Development of depression from preadolescence to young adulthood: Emerging gender differences in a 10-year longitudinal study. *Journal of Abnormal Psychology, 107,* 128–140.

Hankin, B. L., Young, J. F., Abela, J. R. Z., Smolen, A., Jenness, J. L., Gulley, L. D., et al. (2015). Depression from childhood into late adolescence: Influence of gender, development, genetic susceptibility, and peer stress. *Journal of Abnormal Psychology, 124,* 803–816. https://doi.org/10.1037/abn0000089

Hansen, B., Kvale, G., Hagen, K., Havnen, A., & Öst, L. G. (2019). The Bergen 4-day treatment for OCD: Four years follow-up of concentrated ERP in a clinical mental health setting. *Cognitive Behaviour Therapy, 48*(2), 89–105. https://doi.org/10.1080/16506073.2018.1478447

Hansen, J., Hanewinkel, R., & Morgenstern, M. (2020). Electronic cigarette advertising and teen smoking initiation. *Addictive Behaviors, 103,* 106243.

Hanson, C. (1998, November 30). Dangerous therapy: The story of Patricia Burgus and multiple personality disorder. *Chicago Magazine.* http://www.chicagomag.com/Chicago-Magazine/June-1998/Dangerous-Therapy-The-Story-of-Patricia-Burgus-and-Multiple-Personality-Disorder/

Hanson, R. K., & Bussiere, M. T. (1998). Predicting relapse: A meta-analysis of sexual offender recidivism studies. *Journal of Consulting and Clinical Psychology, 66*, 348–362.

Harden, K. P., Hill, J. E., Turkheimer, E., & Emery, R. E. (2008). Gene–environment correlation and interaction in peer effects on adolescent alcohol and tobacco use. *Behavior Genetics, 38*, 339–347.

Hare, R. D. (2003). *The Hare psychopathy checklist* (Rev. ed.). Multi-Health System.

Harington, A. (2019). *Mind fixers: Psychiatry's troubled search for the biology of mental illness.* WW Norton.

Harkness, K. L., Bagby, R. M., & Kennedy, S. H. (2012). Childhood maltreatment and differential treatment response and recurrence in adult major depressive disorder. *Journal of Consulting and Clinical Psychology, 80*, 342–353.

Harkness, K. L., & Monroe, S. M. (2016). The assessment and measurement of adult life stress: Basic premises, operational principles, and design requirements. *Journal of Abnormal Psychology, 125*, 727–745. https://doi.org/10.1037/abn0000178

Harrington, A. (2008). *The cure within: A history of mind-body medicine.* W. W. Norton.

Harris, J. L., Bargh, J. A., & Brownell, K. D. (2009). Priming effects of television food advertising on eating behavior. *Health Psychology, 28*, 404–413.

Harrison, A., Fernández de la Cruz, L., Enander, J., Radua, J., & Mataix-Cols, D. (2016). Cognitive-behavioral therapy for body dysmorphic disorder: A systematic review and meta-analysis of randomized controlled trials. *Clinical Psychology Review, 48*, 43–51. https://doi.org/10.1016/j.cpr.2016.05.007

Harrop, E. N., Mensinger, J. L., Moore, M., & Lindhorst, T. (2021). Restrictive eating disorders in higher weight persons: A systematic review of atypical anorexia nervosa prevalence and consecutive admission literature. *International Journal of Eating Disorders, 54*(8), 1328–1357. https://doi.org/10.1002/eat.23519

Hartman, A. S., & Buhlmann, U. (2017). Prevalence and underrecognition of body dysmorphic disorder. In K. A. Phillips, *Body dysmorphic disorder: Advances in research and clinical practice* (pp. 49–60). Oxford University Press.

Hartmann-Boyce, J., McRobbie, H., Butler, A. R., Lindson, N., Bullen, C., Begh, R., Theodoulou, A., Notley, C., Rigotti, N. A., Turner, T., Fanshawe, T. R., & Hajek, P. (2021). Electronic cigarettes for smoking cessation. *The Cochrane Database of Systematic Reviews, 9*(9), CD010216. https://doi.org/10.1002/14651858.CD010216.pub6

Hartshorne, J. K., & Germine, L. T. (2015). When does cognitive functioning peak? The asynchronous rise and fall of different cognitive abilities across the life span. *Psychological Science, 26*, 433–443. https://doi.org/10.1177/0956797614567339

Hartz, D. T., Fredrick-Osborne, S. L., & Galloway, G. P. (2001). Craving predicts use during treatment for methamphetamine dependence: A prospective repeated measures, within-subjects analysis. *Drug and Alcohol Dependence, 63*, 269–276.

Hartz, S. M., Horton, A. C., Oehlert, M., Carey, C. E., Agrawal, A., Bogdan, R., et al. (2017). Association between substance use disorder and polygenic liability to schizophrenia. *Biological Psychiatry, 82*(10), 709–715.

Hartz, S. M., Pato, C. N., Medeiros, H., Cavazos-Rehg, P., Sobell, J. L., Knowles, J. A., et al. (2014). Comorbidity of severe psychotic disorders with measures of substance use. *JAMA Psychiatry, 71*(3), 248–254. https://doi.org/10.1001/jamapsychiatry.2013.3726

Harvey, A. G., & Bryant, R. A. (2002). Acute stress disorder: A synthesis and critique. *Psychological Bulletin, 128*, 886–902.

Harvey, A. G., Dong, L., Hein, K., Yu, S. H., Martinez, A. J., Gumport, N. B., Smith, F. L., et al. (2021). A randomized controlled trial of the Transdiagnostic Intervention for Sleep and Circadian Dysfunction (TranS-C) to improve serious mental illness [SB1] outcomes in a community setting. *Journal of Consulting and Clinical Psychology, 89*(6), 537–550. https://doi.org/10.1037/ccp0000650

Harvey, A. G., Soehner, A. M., Kaplan, K. A., Hein, K., Lee, J., Kanady, J., et al. (2015). Treating insomnia improves mood state, sleep, and functioning in bipolar disorder: A pilot randomized controlled trial. *Journal of Consulting and Clinical Psychology, 83*(3), 564–577. https://doi.org/10.1037/a0038655

Harvey, A. G., Watkins, E., Mansell, W., & Shafran, R. (2004). *Cognitive behavioural processes across psychological disorders: A transdiagnostic approach to research and treatment.* Oxford University Press.

Hasan, A., Keller, von, R., Friemel, C. M., Hall, W., Schneider, M., Koethe, D., et al. (2020). Cannabis use and psychosis: A review of reviews. *European Archives of Psychiatry and Clinical Neuroscience, 270*(4), 403–412.

Hasin, D. S., Keyes, K. M., Alderson, D., Wang, S., Aharonovich, E., & Grant, B. F. (2008). Cannabis withdrawal in the United States: Results from NESARC. *Journal of Clinical Psychiatry, 69*, 1354–1363.

Haslam, N., Holland, E., & Kuppens, P. (2012). Categories versus dimensions in personality and psychopathology: A quantitative review of taxometric research. *Psychological Medicine, 42*(5), 903–920. https://doi.org/10.1017/S0033291711001966

Hatoum, A. S., Colbert, S. M. C., Johnson, E. C., Huggett, S. B., Deak, J. D., Pathak, G. A., et al. (2023). Multivariate genome-wide association meta-analysis of over 1 million subjects identifies loci underlying multiple substance use disorders. *Nature Mental Health, 1*(3), 210–223.

Hawton, K., Witt, K. G., Taylor Salisbury, T. L., Arensman, E., Gunnell, D., Hazell, P., et al. (2016). Psychosocial interventions for self-harm in adults. *Cochrane Database of Systematic Review, (5)*, Cd012189. https://doi.org/10.1002/14651858.cd012189

Hayes, J., VanElzakker, M., & Shin, L. (2012). Emotion and cognition interactions in PTSD: A review of neurocognitive and neuroimaging studies. *Frontiers in Integrative Neuroscience, 6*(89). https://doi.org/10.3389/fnint.2012.00089

Hayes, R. D., Dennerstein, L., Bennett, C. M., Koochaki, P. E., Leiblum, S. R., & Graziottin, A. (2007). Relationship between hypoactive sexual desire disorder and aging. *Fertility and Sterility, 87*, 107–112. https://doi.org/10.1016/j.fertnstert.2006.05.071

Hayes, S. C. (2005). *Get out of your mind and into your life: The new acceptance and commitment therapy.* New Harbinger Publications.

Hazel, N. A., Hamman, C., Brennan, P. A., & Najman, J. (2008). Early childhood adversity and adolescent depression: The mediating role of continued stress. *Psychological Medicine, 38*, 581–589.

Hazlett, H. C., Gu, H., Munsell, B. C., Kim, S. H., Styner, M., Wolff, J. J., et al. (2017). Early brain development in infants at high risk for autism spectrum disorder. *Nature, 542*(7641), 348–351. https://doi.org/10.1038/nature21369

Hazlett-Stevens, H. (2020). Cultural considerations when treating anxiety disorders with mindfulness-based interventions. In *Handbook of cultural factors in behavioral health* (pp. 277–292). Springer International Publishing. https://doi.org/10.1007/978-3-030-32229-8_20

Heath, A. K., Ganz, J. B., Parker, R., Burke, M., & Ninci, J. (2015). A meta-analytic review of functional communication training across mode of communication, age, and disability. *Review Journal of Autism & Developmental Disorders, 2*, 155–166. https://doi.org/10.1007/s40489-014-0044

Hébert, M., Langevin, R., Guidi, E., Bernard-Bonnin, A. C., & Allard-Dansereau, C. (2016). Sleep problems and dissociation in preschool victims of sexual abuse. *Journal of Trauma & Dissociation*, 1–15. https://doi.org/10.1080/15299732.2016.1240739

Hechtman, L., Swanson, J. M., Sibley, M. H., Stehli, A., Owens, E. B., Mitchell, J. T., et al. (2016). Functional adult outcomes 16 years after childhood diagnosis of attention-deficit/hyperactivity disorder: MTA results. *Journal of the American Academy of Child & Adolescent Psychiatry, 55*(11), 945–952.

Hedegaard, H., Curtin, S., & Warner, M. (2020). *Increase in suicide mortality in the United States, 1999–2018. NCHS Data Brief, number 362*. National Center for Health Statistics.

Heinssen, R. K., Liberman, R. P., & Kopelowicz, A. (2000). Psychosocial skills training for schizophrenia: Lessons from the laboratory. *Schizophrenia Bulletin, 26*, 21–46.

Helfert, S., & Warschburger, P. (2011). A prospective study on the impact of peer and parental pressure on body dissatisfaction in adolescent girls and boys. *Body Image, 8*(2), 101–109. https://doi.org/10.1016/j.bodyim.2011.01.004

Hellings, J. A., Arnold, L. E., & Han, J. C. (2017). Dopamine antagonists for treatment resistance in autism spectrum disorders: Review and focus on BDNF stimulators loxapine and amitriptyline. *Expert Opinion on Pharmacotherapy, 18*(6), 581–588. https://doi.org/10.1080/14656566.2017.1308483

Helmuth, L. (2003). In sickness or in health? *Science, 302*, 808–810.

Helstrom, A. W., Blow, F. C., Slaymaker, V., Kranzler, H. R., Leong, S., & Oslin, D. (2016). Reductions in alcohol craving following naltrexone treatment for heavy drinking. *Alcohol and Alcoholism, 51*, 562–566. https://doi.org/10.1093/alcalc/agw038

Hendershot, C. S., Witkiewitz, K., George, W. H., & Marlatt, G. A. (2011). Relapse prevention for addictive behaviors. *Substance Abuse Treatment, Prevention, and Policy, 6*(1), 1–17. https://doi.org/10.1002/jeab.564

Hendrickx, L., Gijs, L., & Enzlin, P. (2015). Age-related prevalence rates of sexual difficulties, sexual dysfunctions, and sexual distress in heterosexual women: Results from an online survey in Flanders. *Journal of Sexual Medicine, 12*, 424–435. https://doi.org/10.1111/jsm.12725

Hengartner, M. P. (2018). Raising awareness for the replication crisis in clinical psychology by focusing on inconsistencies in psychotherapy research: How much can we rely on published findings from efficacy trials? *Frontiers in Psychology, 9*(FEB), 256. https://doi.org/10.3389/fpsyg.2018.00256

Hengartner, M. P., Ajdacic-Gross, V., Rodgers, S., Müller, M., & Rössler, W. (2013). Childhood adversity in association with personality disorder dimensions: New findings in an old debate. *European Psychiatry, 28*(8), 476–482. https://doi.org/10.1016/j.eurpsy.2013.04.004

Henggeler, S. W. (2011). Efficacy studies to large-scale transport: The development and validation of multisystemic therapy programs. *Annual Review of Clinical Psychology, 7*, 351–381. https://doi.org/10.1146/annurev-clinpsy-032210-104615

Henggeler, S. W., Schoenwald, S. K., Borduin, C. M., Rowland, M. D., & Cunningham, P. B. (2009). *Multisystemic therapy for antisocial behavior in children and adolescents*. Guilford Press.

Henriques, G., Wenzel, A., Brown, G. K., & Beck, A. T. (2005). Suicide attempter's reaction to survival as a risk factor for eventual suicide. *American Journal of Psychiatry, 162*, 2180–2182.

Herbenick, D., Reece, M., Schick, V., Sanders, S. A., Dodge, B., & Fortenberry, J. D. (2010a). Sexual behaviors, relationships, and perceived health status among adult women in the United States: Results from a national probability sample. *Journal of Sexual Medicine, 7*(Suppl 5), 277–290.

Herbenick, D., Reece, M., Schick, V., Sanders, S. A., Dodge, B., & Fortenberry, J. D. (2010b). Sexual behavior in the United States: Results from a national probability sample of men and women ages 14–94. *Journal of Sexual Medicine, 7*, 255–265. https://doi.org/10.1111/j.1743-6109.2010.02012.x

Herman, J. L. (1992). *Trauma and recovery*. Basic Books.

Herman, Y., Shireen, H., Bromley, S., Yiu, N., & Granholm, E. (2016). Cognitive-behavioural social skills training for first-episode psychosis: A feasibility study. *Early Intervention in Psychiatry*. https://doi.org/10.1111/eip.12379

Hershberger, A., Argyriou, E., & Cyders, M. (2020). Electronic nicotine delivery system use is related to higher odds of alcohol and marijuana use in adolescents: Meta-analytic evidence. *Addictive Behaviors, 105*, 106325.

Herzog, A., Shedden-Mora, M. C., Jordan, P., & Löwe, B. (2018). Duration of untreated illness in patients with somatoform disorders. *Journal of Psychosomatic Research, 107*, 1–6. https://doi.org/10.1016/j.jpsychores.2018.01.011

Herzog, D. B., Greenwood, D. N., Dorer, D. J., Flores, A. T., Ekeblad, E. R., Richards, A., et al. (2000). Mortality in eating disorders: A descriptive study. *International Journal of Eating Disorders, 28*, 20–26.

Hettema, J. M., Prescott, C. A., Myers, J. M., Neale, M. C., & Kendler, K. S. (2005). The structure of genetic and environmental risk factors for anxiety disorders in men and women. *Archives of General Psychiatry, 62*, 182–189.

Heyvaert, M., Maes, B., Van Den Noortgate, W., Kuppens, S., & Onghena, P. (2012). A multilevel meta-analysis of single-case and small-n research on interventions for reducing challenging behavior in persons with intellectual disabilities. *Research in Developmental Disabilities, 33*, 766–780.

Hilbert, A., Hoek, H. W., & Schmidt, R. (2017). Evidence-based clinical guidelines for eating disorders: international comparison. *Current Opinion in Psychiatry, 30*(6).

Hilbert, A., Petroff, D., Herpetz, S., Pietrowsky, R., Tuschen-Caffier, B., Vocks, S., et al. (2019). Meta-analysis of the efficacy of psychological and medical treatments for binge-eating disorder. *Journal of Consulting and Clinical Psychology, 87*, 91–105.

Hiller, W., Rief, W., & Brähler, E. (2006). Somatization in the population: From mild bodily misperceptions to disabling symptoms. *Social Psychiatry and Psychiatric Epidemiology, 41*(9), 704–712. https://doi.org/10.1007/s00127-006-0082-y

Hill-Taylor, B., Walsh, K. A., Stewart, S., Hayden, J., Byrne, S., & Sketris, I. S. (2016). Effectiveness of the STOPP/START (Screening Tool of Older Persons' potentially inappropriate Prescriptions/Screening Tool to Alert Doctors to the Right Treatment) criteria: Systematic review and meta-analysis of randomized controlled studies. *Journal of Clinical Pharmacy and Therapeutics, 41*, 158–169. https://doi.org/10.1111/jcpt.12372

Hilt, L. M., & Nolen-Hoeksema, S. (2014). Gender differences in depression. In I. H. Gotlib & C. L. Hammen (Eds.), *Handbook of depression* (3rd ed.). Guilford Press.

Hinshaw, S. P. (2002). Preadolescent girls with attention-deficit/hyperactivity disorder: I. Background characteristics, comorbidity, cognitive and social functioning, and parenting practices. *Journal of Consulting and Clinical Psychology, 70*, 1086–1098.

Hinshaw, S. P. (2007). *The mark of shame: The stigma of mental illness and an agenda for change*. Oxford University Press.

Hinshaw, S. P. (2018). Attention deficit hyperactivity disorder (ADHD): Controversy, developmental mechanisms, and multiple levels of analysis. *Annual Review of Clinical Psychology, 14*(1), 291–316. https://doi.org/10.1146/annurev-clinpsy-050817-084917

Hinshaw, S. P. (2018). Stigma, humanization, and mental health: The next frontier. *Behavior Therapist, 41*, 183–186.

Hinshaw, S. P., & Arnold, L. E. (2015). Attention-deficit hyperactivity disorder, multimodal treatment, and longitudinal outcome: Evidence, paradox, and challenge. *WIREs Cognitive Science, 6*, 39–52. https://doi.org/10.1002/wcs.1324

Hinshaw, S. P., Carte, E. T., Sami, N., Treuting, J. J., & Zupan, B. A. (2002). Preadolescent girls with attention-deficit/hyperactivity disorder: II. Neuropsychological performance in relation to subtypes and individual classification. *Journal of Consulting and Clinical Psychology, 70*, 1099–1111.

Hinshaw, S. P., & Lee, S. S. (2003). Oppositional defiant and conduct disorders. In E. J. Mash & R. A. Barkley (Eds.), *Child psychopathology* (2nd ed., pp. 144–198). Guilford Press.

Hinshaw, S. P., Owens, E. B., Sami, N., & Fargeon, S. (2006). Prospective follow-up of girls with attention-deficit/hyperactivity disorder into adolescence: Evidence for continuing cross-domain impairment. *Journal of Consulting and Clinical Psychology, 74*, 489–499.

Hinshaw, S. P., Owens, E. B., Zalecki, C., Huggins, S. P., Montenegro-Nevado, A. J., Schrodek, E., et al. (2012). Prospective follow-up of girls with attention-deficit/hyperactivity disorder into early adulthood: Continuing impairment includes elevated risk for suicide attempts and self-injury. *Journal of Consulting and Clinical Psychology, 80*(6), 1041–1051.

Hinshaw, S. P., & Scheffler, R. M. (2014). *The ADHD explosion: Myths, medication, money, and today's push for performance.* Oxford University Press.

Hinton, D. E., & Jalal, B. (2019). Dimensions of culturally sensitive CBT: Application to Southeast Asian populations. *American Journal of Orthopsychiatry, 89*(4), 493–507. https://doi.org/10.1037/ort0000392

Hinton, D. E., & Patel, A. (2017). Cultural adaptations of cognitive behavioral therapy. *Psychiatric Clinics of North America, 40*(4), 701–714. https://doi.org/10.1016/j.psc.2017.08.006

Hinton, D. E., Pich, V., Marques, L., Nickerson, A., & Pollack, M. H. (2010). Khyâl attacks: A key idiom of distress among traumatized Cambodia refugees. *Culture, Medicine, and Psychiatry, 34*, 244–278. https://doi.org/10.1007/s11013-010-9174-y

Hippocampal Threat Reactivity Interacts with Physiological Arousal to Predict PTSD Symptoms Büşra Tanriverdi, David F. Gregory, Thomas M. Olino, Timothy D. Ely, Nathaniel G. Harnett, Sanne J.H. van Rooij, Lauren A.M. Lebois, Antonia V. Seligowski, Tanja Jovanovic, Kerry J. Ressler, Stacey L. House, Francesca L. Beaudoin, Xinming An, Thomas C. Neylan, Gari D. Clifford, Sarah D. Linnstaedt, Laura T. Germine, Kenneth A. Bollen, Scott L. Rauch, John P. Haran, Alan B. Storrow, Christopher Lewandowski, Paul I. Musey, Phyllis L. Hendry, Sophia Sheikh, Christopher W. Jones, Brittany E. Punches, Michael C. Kurz, Meghan E. McGrath, Lauren A. Hudak, Jose L. Pascual, Mark J. Seamon, Elizabeth M. Datner, Claire Pearson, Robert M. Domeier, Niels K. Rathlev, Brian J. O'Neil, Leon D. Sanchez, Steven E. Bruce, Mark W. Miller, Robert H. Pietrzak, Jutta Joormann, Deanna M. Barch, Diego A. Pizzagalli, John F. Sheridan, Jordan W. Smoller, Steven E. Harte, James M. Elliott, Samuel A. McLean, Ronald C. Kessler, Karestan C. Koenen, Jennifer S. Stevens, Vishnu P. Murty. *Journal of Neuroscience,* 24 August 2022, *42*(34), 6593–6604; https://doi.org/10.1523/JNEUROSCI.0911-21.2022

Hirsch, C. R., Meeten, F., Krahe, C., & Reeder, C. (2016). Resolving ambiguity in emotional disorders: The nature and role of interpretation biases. *Annual Review of Clinical Psychology, 12*, 281–305. https://doi.org/10.1146/annurev-clinpsy-021815-093436

Hirschtritt, M. E. & Binder. R. L. (2018). A reassessment of blaming mass shootings on mental illness. *JAMA Psychiatry, 75*, 311–312.

Hjorthøj, C., Albert, N., & Nordentoft, M. (2018). Association of substance use disorders with conversion from schizotypal disorder to schizophrenia. *JAMA Psychiatry, 75*(7), 733. https://doi.org/10.1001/JAMAPSYCHIATRY.2018.0568

Hjorth, O. R., Frick, A., Gingnell, M., Hoppe, J. M., Faria, V., Hultberg, S., et al. (2021). Expression and co-expression of serotonin and dopamine transporters in social anxiety disorder: A multitracer positron emission tomography study. *Molecular Psychiatry, 26*(8), 3970–3979. https://doi.org/10.1038/s41380-019-0618-7

Ho, B.-C., Andreasen, N. C., Ziebell, S., Pierson, R., & Magnotta, V. (2011). Long-term antipsychotic treatment and brain volumes: A longitudinal study of first-episode schizophrenia. *Archives of General Psychiatry, 68*, 128–137. https://doi.org/10.1001/arch-genpsychiatry.2010.199

Hobson, R. P., & Lee, A. (1998). Hello and goodbye: A study of social engagement in autism. *Journal of Autism and Developmental Disorders, 28*, 117–127.

Hoebel, B. G., & Teitelbaum, P. (1966). Weight regulation in normal and hypothalamic hyperphagic rats. *Journal of Comparative and Physiological Psychology, 61*, 189–193.

Hoffman, D. H., Carter, D. J., Lopez, C. R.V., Benzmiller, H. L., Guo, A. X., Latifi, S. Y., & Craig, D. C. (2015, July 2). *Report to the Special Committee of the Board of Directors of the American Psychological Association: Independent review relating to APA Ethics Guidelines, national security interrogations, and torture.* Sidley Austin LLP. Retrieved from https://www.apa.org/independent-review/APA-FINAL-Report-7.2.15.pdf

Hofmann, S. G., & Gómez, A. F. (2017). Mindfulness-based interventions for anxiety and depression. *Psychiatric Clinics of North America, 40*(4), 739–749. W.B. Saunders. https://doi.org/10.1016/j.psc.2017.08.008

Hofmann, S. G., & Hinton, D. E. (2014). Cross-cultural aspects of anxiety disorders. *Current Psychiatry Reports, 16*(6), 450. https://doi.org/10.1007/s11920-014-0450-3

Hofmann, S. G., & Smits, J. A. (2008). Cognitive-behavioral therapy for adult anxiety disorders: A meta-analysis of randomized placebo-controlled trials. *The Journal of Clinical Psychiatry, 69*, 621–632.

Hogan, D. B., Fiest, K. M., Roberts, J. I., Maxwell, C. J., Dykeman, J., Pringsheim, T., et al. (2016). The prevalence and incidence of dementia with Lewy bodies: A systematic review. *Canadian Journal of Neurological Sciences, 43*(Suppl 1), S83–95. https://doi.org/10.1017/cjn.2016.2

Hogarty, G. E., Anderson, C. M., Reiss, D. J., Kornblith, S. J., Greenwald, D. P., Javna, C.D., et al. (1986). Family psychoeducation, social skills training, and maintenance chemotherapy in the aftercare treatment of schizophrenia: 1. One-year effects of a controlled study on relapse and expressed emotion. *Archives of General Psychiatry, 43*, 633–642.

Hogarty, G. E., Anderson, C. M., Reiss, D. J., Kornblith, S. J., Greenwald, D. P., Ulrich, R. F., Carter, M., et al. The Environmental-Personal Indicators in the Course of Schizophrenia (EPICS) Research Group. (1991). Family psychoeducation, social skills training, and maintenance chemotherapy in the aftercare treatment of schizophrenia. *Archives of General Psychiatry, 48*, 340–347.

Hollingshead, A. B., & Redlich, F. C. (1958). *Social class and mental illness: A community study.* John Wiley & Sons.

Hollingworth, P., & Williams, J. (2011). Genetic risk factors for dementia. *The handbook of Alzheimer's disease and other dementias* (pp. 195–234). Wiley-Blackwell.

Hollon, S. D., DeRubeis, R. J., Fawcett, J., Amsterdam, J. D., Shelton, C., Zajecka, D., et al. (2014). Effect of cognitive therapy with antidepressant medications vs. antidepressants alone on the rate of recovery in major depressive disorder: A randomized clinical trial. *JAMA Psychiatry, 71*(10), 1157–1164. https://doi.org/10.1001/jamapsychiatry.2014.1054

Hollon, S. D., Stewart, M. O., & Strunk, D. (2006). Enduring effects for cognitive behavior therapy in the treatment of depression and anxiety. *Annual Review of Psychology, 57*, 285–315.

Holmes, E. A., Brown, R. J., Mansell, W., Fearon, R. P., Hunter, E. C., Frasquilho, F., et al. (2005). Are there two qualitatively distinct forms of dissociation? A review and some clinical implications. *Clinical Psychology Review, 25*, 1–23.

Holtom-Viesel, A., & Allan, S. (2014). A systematic review of the literature on family functioning across all eating disorder diagnoses in comparison to control families. *Clinical Psychology Review, 34*, 29–43.

Holvoet, L., Huys, W., Coppens, V., Seeuws, J., Goethals, K., & Morrens, M. (2017). Fifty shades of Belgian gray: The prevalence of BDSM-related fantasies and activities in the general population. *Journal of Sexual Medicine, 14*, 1152–1159. https://doi.org/10.1016/j.jsxm.2017.07.003

Hong, R. Y., Chan, W. Y., & Lim, J. Y. R. (2020). Pathological personality traits and the experience of daily situations. *Clinical Psychological Science, 8*(2), 333–342. https://doi.org/10.1177/2167702619894902

Hong, S., Walton, E., Tamaki, E., & Sabin, J. A. (2014). Lifetime prevalence of mental disorders among Asian Americans: Nativity, gender, and sociodemographic correlates. *Asian American Journal of Psychology, 5*(4), 353–363. https://doi.org/10.1037/a0035680

Hoogman, M., Bralten, J., Hibar, D. P., Mennes, M., Zwiers, M. P., Schweren, L. S. J., et al. (2017). Subcortical brain volume differences in participants with attention deficit hyperactivity disorder in children and adults: A cross-sectional mega-analysis. *The Lancet. Psychiatry, 4*(4), 310–319.

Hooley, J. M., & St. Germain, S. A. (2013). Nonsuicidal self-injury, pain, and self-criticism. *Clinical Psychological Science, 2*(3), 297–305. https://doi.org/10.1177/2167702613509372

Horton, R. S. (2011). Parenting as a cause of narcissism: Empirical support for psychodynamic and social learning theories. In W. K. Campbell & J. D. Miller (Eds.), *The handbook of narcissism and narcissistic personality disorder: Theoretical approaches, empirical findings, and treatments* (pp. 181–190). John Wiley & Sons.

Hosang, G. M., Lichtenstein, P., Ronald, A., Lundström, S., & Taylor, M. J. (2019). Association of genetic and environmental risks for attention-deficit/hyperactivity disorder with hypomanic symptoms in youths. *JAMA Psychiatry, 76*(11), 1150–1158. https://doi.org/10.1001/jamapsychiatry.2019.1949

Houben, M., Mestdagh, M., Dejonckheere, E., Obbels, J., Sienaert, P., Van Roy, J., & Kuppens, P. (2021). The statistical specificity of emotion dynamics in borderline personality disorder. *Journal of Personality Disorders, 35*(6), 819–840.

Howard, A. L., Kennedy, T. M., Mitchell, J. T., Sibley, M. H., Hinshaw, S. P., Arnold, L. E., et al. (2020). Early substance use in the pathway from childhood attention-deficit/hyperactivity disorder (ADHD) to young adult substance use: Evidence of statistical mediation and substance specificity. *Psychology of Addictive Behaviors, 34*(2), 281–292. https://doi.org/10.1037/adb0000542

Howard, R., Rabins, P. V., Seeman, M. V., & Jeste, D. V. (2000). Late-onset schizophrenia and very-late-onset schizophrenia-like psychosis: An international consensus. The International Late-Onset Schizophrenia Group. *American Journal of Psychiatry, 157*, 172–178.

Howes, O. D., & Kapur, S. (2009). The dopamine hypothesis of schizophrenia: Version III—The final common pathway. *Schizophrenia Bulletin, 35*, 549–562. https://doi.org/10.1093/schbul/sbp006

Howes, O., McCutcheon, R., & Stone, J. (2015). Glutamate and dopamine in schizophrenia: An update for the 21st century. *Journal of Psychopharmacology, 29*, 97–115. https://doi.org/10.1177/0269881114563634

Hoza, B., Murray-Close, D., Arnold, L. E., Hinshaw, S. P., Hechtmen, L., & The MTA Cooperative Group. (2010). Time-dependent changes in positive illusory self-perceptions of children with attention-deficit/hyperactivity disorder: A developmental psychopathology perspective. *Developmental and Psychopathology, 22*, 375–390.

Hshieh, T. T., Yue, J., Oh, E., Puelle, M., Dowal, S., Travison, T., & Inouye, S. K. (2015). Effectiveness of multicomponent nonpharmacological delirium interventions: A meta-analysis. *Jamanetwork.com, 175*(4), 512–520. https://doi.org/10.1001/jamainternmed.2014.7779

Hsu, C. W., Tsai, S. Y., Tseng, P. T., Liang, C. S., Vieta, E., Carvalho, A. F., et al. (2022). Differences in the prophylactic effect of serum lithium levels on depression and mania in bipolar disorder: A dose-response meta-analysis. *European Neuropsychopharmacology, 58,* 20–29. https://doi.org/10.1016/j.euroneuro.2022.01.112

Huberman, J. S., & Chivers, M. L. (2015). Examining gender specificity of sexual response with concurrent thermography and plethysmography. *Psychophysiology, 52*(10), 1382–1395. https://doi.org/10.1111/psyp.12466

Hudson, J. I., Hiripi, E., Pope, H. G., & Kessler, R. C. (2007). The prevalence and correlates of eating disorders in the National Comorbidity Survey Replication. *Biological Psychology, 61*, 348–358.

Hudson, J. I., Lalonde, J. K., Berry, J. M., Pindyck, L. J., & Bulick, C. (2006). Binge-eating disorder as a distinct familial phenotype in obese individuals. *Archives of General Psychology, 63*, 3138–3319.

Huey, S. J., Jr., Tilley, J. L., Jones, E. O., & Smith, C. A. (2014). The contribution of cultural competence to evidence-based care for ethnically diverse populations. *Annual Review of Clinical Psychology, 10,* 305–338. https://doi.org/10.1146/annurev-clinpsy-032813-153729

Hughes, C., Hugo, K., & Blatt, J. (1996). Self-instructional intervention for teaching generalized problem-solving within a functional task sequence. *American Journal on Mental Retardation, 100*, 565–579.

Hughes, D., Judge, C., Murphy, R., Loughlin, E., Costello, M., Whiteley, W., Bosch, J., O'Donnell, M. J., & Canavan, M. (2020). Association of Blood Pressure Lowering with Incident Dementia or Cognitive Impairment. *JAMA, 323*(19), 1934. https://doi.org/10.1001/jama.2020.4249

Hughes, J. R., Higgins, S. T., Bickel, W. K., Hunt, W. K., & Fenwick, J. W. (1991). Caffeine self-administration, withdrawal, and adverse effects among coffee drinkers. *Archives of General Psychiatry, 48*, 611–617.

Huhn, M., Nikolakopoulou, A., Schneider-Thoma, J., Krause, M., Samara, M., Peter, N., et al. (2019). Comparative efficacy and tolerability of 32 oral antipsychotics for the acute treatment of adults with multi-episode schizophrenia: A systematic review and network meta-analysis. *Lancet (London, England), 394*(10202), 939–951.

Hulse, G. K., Ngo, H. T., & Tait, R. J. (2010). Risk factors for craving and relapse in heroin users treated with oral or implant naltrexone. *Biological Psychiatry, 68*, 296–302.

Human Genome Project. (2008). How many genes are in the human genome? https://www.ornl.gov/sci/techresources/Human_Genome/faq/genenumber.shtml

Hunter, E. C., Sierra, M., & David, A. S. (2004). The epidemiology of depersonalisation and derealisation. A systematic review. *Social Psychiatry and Psychiatric Epidemiology, 39*, 9–18.

Hunter, R., & MacAlpine, I. (1963). *Three hundred years of psychiatry 1535–1860.* Oxford University Press.

Huntjen, R. J. C., Postma, A., Peters, M. L., Woertman, L., & van der Hart, O. (2003). Interidentity amnesia for neutral, episodic information in dissociative identity disorder. *Journal of Abnormal Psychology, 112*, 290–297.

Hussong, A. M., Hicks, R. E., Levy, S. A., & Curran, P. J. (2001). Specifying the relations between affect and heavy alcohol use among young adults. *Journal of Abnormal Psychology, 110*, 449–461.

Hustvedt, A. (2011). *Medical muses: Hysteria in nineteenth-century Paris.* W. W. Norton.

Hyde, L. W., & Dotterer, H. L. (2022). The nature and nurture of callous-unemotional traits. *Current Directions in Psychological Science, 31*(6), 546–555. https://doi.org/10.1177/09637214221121302

Hyde, L. W., Shaw, D. S., Murray, L., Gard, A., Hariri, A. R., & Forbes, E. E. (2016). Dissecting the role of amygdala reactivity in antisocial behavior in a sample of young, low-income, urban men. *Clinical Psychological Science, 4*, 527–544. https://doi.org/10.1177/2167702615614511

Hyde, L. W., Waller, R., Trentacosta, C. J., Shaw, D. S., Neider-hiser, J. M., Ganiban, J. M., et al. (2016). Heritable and nonheritable pathways to early callous-unemotional behaviors. *American Journal of Psychiatry, 173*, 903–910. https://doi.org/10.1176/appi.ajp.2016.15111381

Hyman, S. E. (2010). The diagnosis of mental disorders: The problem of reification. *Annual Review of Clinical Psychology, 6*, 155–179.

Ibaraki, A. Y., & Nagayama Hall, G. C. (2014). The components of cultural match in psychotherapy. *Journal of Social and Clinical Psychology, 33*(10), 936–953. https://doi.org/10.1521/jscp.2014.33.10.936

Idrisov, B., Sun, P., Akhmadeeva, L., Arpawong, T. E., Kukhareva, P., & Sussman, S. (2013). Immediate and six-month effects of project EX Russia: A smoking cessation intervention pilot program. *Addictive Behaviors, 38*, 2402–2408. https://doi.org/10.1016/j.addbeh.2013.03.013

Iliakis, E. A., Ilagan, G. S., & Choi-Kain, L. W. (2021). Dropout rates from psychotherapy trials for borderline personality disorder: A meta-analysis. *Personality Disorders: Theory, Research, and Treatment, 12*(3), 193–206. https://doi.org/10.1037/per0000453

Indovina, I., Robbins, T. W., Nunez-Elizalde, A. O., Dunn, B. D., & Bishop, S. J. (2011). Fear-conditioning mechanisms associated with trait vulnerability to anxiety in humans. *Neuron, 69*, 563–571.

Ingram, S. H., & South, S. C. (2021). The longitudinal impact of *DSM–5* Section III specific personality disorders on relationship satisfaction. *Personality Disorders: Theory, Research, and Treatment, 12*(2), 140–149. https://doi.org/10.1037/per0000435

Inoue-Choi, M., Liao, L. M., Reyes-Guzman, C., Hartge, P., Caporaso, N., & Freedman, N. D. (2017). Association of long-term, low-intensity smoking with all-cause and cause-specific mortality in the National Institutes of Health–AARP Diet and Health Study. *JAMA Internal Medicine, 177*, 87–95. https://doi.org/10.1001/jamainternmed.2016.7511

Insel, T. R. (2014). The NIMH Research Domain Criteria (RDoC) Project: Precision medicine for psychiatry. *American Journal of Psychiatry, 171*, 395–397.

Insel, T. R. (2015). The NIMH experimental medicine initiative. *World Psychiatry, 14*(2), 151–153. https://doi.org/10.1002/wps.20227

Insel, T. R., Scanlan, J., Champoux, M., & Suomi, S. J. (1988). Rearing paradigm in a nonhuman primate affects response to B-CCE challenge. *Psychopharmacology, 96*, 81–86.

Institute of Medicine. (1999). *Marijuana and medicine: Assessing the science base.* National Academy Press.

Institute of Medicine. (2004). *Immunization safety review: Vaccines and autism.* Immunization Safety Review Board on Health Promotion and Disease Prevention. National Academies Press.

International Society for the Study of Dissociation. (2011). Guidelines for treating dissociative identity disorder in adults, third revision: Summary version. *Journal of Trauma and Dissociation, 12*, 188–212.

International Test Commission. (2017). *The ITC Guidelines for translating and adapting tests* (2nd ed.). www.InTestCom.org

Ioannidis, J. (2005a). Contradicted and initially stronger effects in highly cited clinical research. *JAMA: The Journal of the American Medical Association, 294*(2), 218–228. https://doi.org/10.1001/jama.294.2.218

Ioannidis, J. (2005b). Why most published research findings are false. *PLoS Medicine, 2*(8), e124. https://doi.org/10.1371/journal.pmed.0020124

Ironside, M., Kumar, P., Kang, M. S., & Pizzagalli, D. A. (2018). Brain mechanisms mediating effects of stress on reward sensitivity. *Current Opinion in Behavioral Sciences, 22*, 106–113. https://doi.org/10.1016/J.COBEHA.2018.01.016

Isaacowitz, D. M. (2012). Mood regulation in real time: Age differences in the role of looking. *Current Directions in Psychological Science, 21*, 237–242.

Ito, T., Miller, N., & Pollock, V. (1996). Alcohol and aggression: A meta-analysis on the moderating effects of inhibitory cues, triggering events, and self-focused attention. *Psychological Bulletin, 120*, 60–82.

Jack, C. R., Jr., Albert, M. S., Knopman, D. S., McKhann, G. M., Sperling, R. A., Carrillo, M. C., et al. (2011). Introduction to the recommendations from the National Institute on Aging-Alzheimer's Association workgroups on diagnostic guidelines for Alzheimer's disease. *Alzheimer's and Dementia: The Journal of the Alzheimer's Association, 7*, 257–262.

Jacobson, N. S., Roberts, L. J., Berns, S. B., & McGlinchey, J. B. (1999). Methods for defining and determining the clinical significance of treatment effects: Description, application, and alternatives. *Journal of Consulting and Clinical Psychology, 67*, 300–307.

Jaffee, S. R., Strait, L. B., & Odgers, C. L. (2012). From correlates to causes: Can quasi-experimental studies and statistical innovations bring us closer to identifying the causes of antisocial behavior? *Psychological Bulletin, 138*, 272–295.

Jagfeld, G., Lobban, F., Marshall, P., & Jones, S. H. (2021). Personal recovery in bipolar disorder: Systematic review and "best fit" framework synthesis of qualitative evidence—A POETIC adaptation of CHIME. *Journal of Affective Disorders, 292*, 375–385. https://doi.org/10.1016/j.jad.2021.05.051

Jalal, H., Buchanich, J. M., Roberts, M. S., Balmert, L. C., Zhang, K., & Burke, D. S. (2018). Changing dynamics of the drug overdose epidemic in the United States from 1979 through 2016. *Science, 361*(6408), eaau1184.

James, D. J., & Glaze, L. E. (2006). Mental health problems of prison and jail inmates. *NCJ 213600.* https://www.bjs.gov/content/pub/pdf/mhppji.pdf

Jamison, K. R. (1993). *Touched with fire: Manic-depressive illness and the artistic temperament.* Simon & Schuster.

Jamison, K. R. (1995). *The unquiet mind: A memoir of moods and madness.* Vintage Books.

Jamison, L. (2018). *The recovering: Intoxication and its aftermath.* Little Brown and Company.

Jani, S., Johnson, R. S., Banu, S., & Shah, A. (2016). Cross-cultural bias in the diagnosis of borderline personality disorder. *Bulletin of the Menninger Clinic, 80*, 146–165. https://doi.org/10.1521/bumc.2016.80.2.146

Jansen, W. J., Ossenkoppele, R., Knol, D. L., Tijms, B. M., Scheltens, P., Verhey, F. R., et al. (2015). Prevalence of cerebral amyloid pathology in persons without dementia: a meta-analysis. *JAMA, 313*(19), 1924–1938. https://doi.org/10.1001/jama.2015.4668

Jardri, R., Pouchet, A., Pins, D., & Thomas, P. (2011). Cortical activation during auditory verbal hallucinations in schizophrenia: A coordinate-based meta-analysis. *American Journal of Psychiatry, 168*, 73–81.

Jauhar, S., McKenna, P., Radua, J., Fung, E., Salvador, R., & Laws, K. R. (2014). Cognitive-behavioural therapy for the symptoms of schizophrenia: Systematic review and meta-analysis with examination of potential bias. *British Journal of Psychiatry, 204*, 20–29.

Jáuregui Renaud, K. (2015). Vestibular function and depersonalization/derealization symptoms. *Multisensory Research, 28*(5–6), 637–651. https://doi.org/10.1163/22134808-00002480

Javitt, D. C., & Kantrowitz, J. T. (2022). The glutamate/N-methyl-d-aspartate receptor (NMDAR) model of schizophrenia at 35: On the path from syndrome to disease. *Schizophrenia Research, 242*, 56–61.

Jay, M. (2016). *This way madness lies.* Thames and Hudson.

Jeans, R. F. I. (1976). An independently validated case of multiple personality. *Journal of Abnormal Psychology, 85*, 249–255.

Jennings, W. G., Perez, N. M., & Reingle Gonzalez, J. M. (2018). Conduct disorder and neighborhood effects. *Annual Review of Clinical Psychology, 14*(1), 317–341. https://doi.org/10.1146/annurev-clinpsy-050817-084911

Jensen, M., George, M. J., Russell, M. A., & Odgers, C. L. (2019). Young adolescents' digital technology use and mental health symptoms: Little evidence of longitudinal or daily linkages. *Clinical Psychological Science, 7*, 1416–1433.

Jensen, M. P., & Patterson, D. R. (2014). Hypnotic approaches for chronic pain management: Clinical implications of recent research findings. *American Psychologist, 69*, 167–177.

Jensen, P. S., Arnold, L. E., Swanson, J. M., Vitiello, B., Abikoff, H. B., Greenhill, L. L., et al. (2007). 3-year follow-up of the NIMH MTA study. *Journal of the American Academy of Child and Adolescent Psychiatry, 46*, 989–1002.

Jeong, J., Shin, S. D., Kim, H., Hong, Y. C., Hwang, S. S., & Lee, E. J. (2012). The effects of celebrity suicide on copycat suicide attempt: A multi-center observational study. *Social Psychiatry and Psychiatric Epidemiology, 47*(6), 957–965. https://doi.org/10.1007/s00127-011-0403-7

Jernigan, D., Noel, J., Landon, J., Thornton, N., & Lobstein, T. (2017). Alcohol marketing and youth alcohol consumption: A systematic review of longitudinal studies published since 2008. *Addiction, 112*, 7–20. https://doi.org/10.1111/add.13591

Jespersen, A. F., Lalumiere, M. L., & Seto, M. C. (2009). Sexual abuse history among adult sex offenders and non-sex offenders: A meta-analysis. *Child Abuse and Neglect, 33*, 179–192.

Jett, D., LaPorte, D. J., & Wanchism, J. (2010). Impact of exposure to pro-eating disorder websites on eating behaviour in college women. *European Eating Disorders Review, 18*, 410–416.

Jobes, D. A., Comtois, K. A., Brenner, L. A., Gutierrez, P. M., & O'Connor, S. S. (2016). Lessons learned from clinical trials of the Collaborative Assessment and Management of Suicidality (CAMS). In R. C. O'Connor & J. Pirkis (Eds.), *The international handbook of suicide prevention* (pp. 431–449). John Wiley & Sons, Ltd. https://doi.org/10.1002/9781118903223.ch24

Johani, F. H., Majid, M., Azme, M. H., & Nawi, A. M. (2020). Cytochrome P450 2A6 whole-gene deletion (CYP2A6*4) polymorphism reduces risk of lung cancer: A meta-analysis. *Tobacco Induced Diseases, 18*, 50. https://doi.org/10.18332/tid/122465

John, O. P., Naumann, L. P., & Soto, C. J. (2008). Paradigm shift to the integrative big-five trait taxonomy: History measurement, and conceptual issues. In O. P. John, R. W. Robins, & L. A. Pervin (Eds.), *Handbook of personality: Theory and research* (pp. 114–158). Guilford Press.

Johnson, J. G., Cohen, P., Brown, J., Smailes, E. M., & Bernstein, D. P. (1999). Childhood maltreatment increases risk for personality disorders during early adulthood. *Archives of General Psychiatry, 56*, 600–606.

Johnson, J. G., Cohen, P., Chen, H., Kasen, S., & Brook, J. S. (2006). Parenting behaviors associated with risk for offspring personality disorder during adulthood. *Archives of General Psychiatry, 63*, 579–583.

Johnson, J. G., Cohen, P., Kasen, S., & Brook, J. S. (2006). Dissociative disorders among adults in the community, impaired functioning, and axis I and II comorbidity. *Journal of Psychiatric Research, 40*(2), 131–140.

Johnson, K. R., & S. L. Johnson. (2014). Inadequate treatment of Black Americans with bipolar disorder. *Psychiatric Services, 65*(2), 255–258. https://doi.org/10.1176/appi.ps.201200590

Johnson, M. H., Gliga, T., Jones, E., & Charman, T. (2015). Annual research review: Infant development, autism, and ADHD - Early pathways to emerging disorders. *Journal of Child Psychology and Psychiatry, 56*(3), 228–247. https://doi.org/10.1111/jcpp.12328

Johnson, S. L., Cuellar, A. K., & Peckham, A. D. (2014). Risk factors for bipolar disorder. In I. H. Gotlib and C. Hammen (Eds.), *Handbook of depression* (3rd ed.). Guilford Press.

Johnson, S. L., Edge, M. D., Holmes, M. K., Carver, C. S., & Nolen-Hoeksema, S. (2012). The behavioral activation system and mania. *Annual Review of Clinical Psychology, 8*, 243–267. https://doi.org/10.1146/annurev-clinpsy-032511-143148

Johnson, S. L., Mehta, H., Ketter, T. A., Gotlib, I. H., & Knutson, B. (2019). Neural responses to monetary incentives in bipolar disorder. *NeuroImage: Clinical, 24*. https://doi.org/10.1016/j.nicl.2019.102018

Johnson, S. L. & Miklowitz, D. J. (2017). Bipolar and related disorders. In D. Beidel (Eds.), *Adult psychopathology and diagnosis* (8th ed.). Wiley and Sons.

Joiner, T. E. (2005). *Why people die by suicide*. Harvard University Press.

Jones, E. J. H., Gliga, T., Bedford, R., Charman, T., & Johnson, M. H. (2014). Developmental pathways to autism: A review of prospective studies of infants at risk. *Neuroscience & Biobehavioral Reviews, 39*, 1–33.

Jones, E., & Wessely, S. (2001). Psychiatric battle casualties: An intra- and interwar comparison. *British Journal of Psychiatry, 178*, 242–247.

Jones, J. (2022). *LGBT identification in U.S. ticks up to 7.1%*. Gallup News. https://news.gallup.com/poll/389792/lgbt-identification-ticks-up.aspx

Jones, W., & Klin, A. (2013). Attention to eyes is present but in decline in 2–6-month-old infants later diagnosed with autism. *Nature, 504*(7480), 427–431.

Joormann, J., Levens, S. M., & Gotlib, I. H. (2011). Sticky thoughts. *Psychological Science, 22*(8), 979–983. https://doi.org/10.1177/0956797611415539

Jordbru, A. A., Smedstad, L. M., Klungsoyr, O., & Martinsen, E. W. (2014). Psychogenic gait disorder: A randomized controlled trial of physical rehabilitation with one-year follow-up. *Journal of Rehabilitation Medicine, 46*, 181–187. https://doi.org/10.2340/16501977-1246

Jorm, A. F., Christensen, H., Henderson, A. S., Jacomb, P. A., Korten, A. E., & Rodgers, B. (2000). Predicting anxiety and depression from personality: Is there a synergistic effect of neuroticism and extraversion? *Journal of Abnormal Psychology, 109*, 145–149.

Josephs, A. J., Tandon, N., Yang, L. H., Duckworth, K., Torous, J., Seidman, L. J., et al. (2015). Schizophrenia: Use and misuse on twitter. *Schizophrenia Research, 165*, 111–115.

Josephs, R. A., & Steele, C. M. (1990). The two faces of alcohol myopia: Attentional mediation of psychological stress. *Journal of Abnormal Psychology, 99*, 115–126.

Joyal, C. C., & Carpentier, J. (2017). The prevalence of paraphilic interests and behaviors in the general population: A provincial survey. *Journal of Sex Research, 54*, 161–171. https://doi.org/10.1080/00224499.2016.1139034

Jungilligens, J., Paredes-Echeverri, S., Popkirov, S., Barrett, L. F., & Perez, D. L. (2022). A new science of emotion: Implications for functional neurological disorder. *Brain: A Journal of Neurology, 145*(8), 2648–2663. https://doi.org/10.1093/brain/awac204

Kafka, M. P. (2010). The DSM diagnostic criteria for fetishism. *Archives of Sexual Behavior, 39*, 357–362.

Kagan, J., & Snidman, N. (1999). Early childhood predictors of adult anxiety disorders. *Biological Psychiatry, 46*, 1536–1541.

Kamody, R. C., Grilo, C. M., & Udo, T. (2020). Disparities in DSM-5 defined eating disorders by sexual orientation among U.S. adults. *International Journal of Eating Disorders, 53*(2), 278–287. https://doi.org/10.1002/eat.23193

Kandel, D., & Kandel, E. (2015). The Gateway Hypothesis of substance abuse: Developmental, biological and societal perspectives. *Acta Paediatrica, 104*, 130–137. https://doi.org/10.1111/apa.12851

Kane, E., Evans, E., & Shokraneh, F. (2017). Effectiveness of current policing-related mental health interventions: A systematic review. *Criminal Behaviour and Mental Health, 28*(2), 108–119. https://doi.org/10.1002/cbm.2058

Kane, J. M., Durgam, S., Satlin, A., Vanover, K. E., Chen, R., Davis, R., et al. (2021). Safety and tolerability of lumateperone for the treatment of schizophrenia: A pooled analysis of late-phase placebo- and active-controlled clinical trials. *International Clinical Psychopharmacology, 36*(5).

Kane, J. M., Robinson, D. G., Schooler, N. R., Mueser, K. T., Penn, D. L., Rosenheck, R. A., et al. (2016). Comprehensive versus usual community care for first-episode psychosis: 2-year outcomes from the NIMH RAISE early treatment program. *American Journal of Psychiatry, 173*, 362–372. https://doi.org/10.1176/appi.ajp.2015.15050632

Kanner, L. (1943). Autistic disturbances of affective contact. *Nervous Child, 2*, 217–250.

Kantor, E. D., Rehm, C. D., Haas, J. S., Chan, A. T., & Giovannucci, E. L. (2015). Trends in prescription drug use among adults in the United State from 1999–2012. *Journal of the American Medical Association, 314*, 1818–1830. https://doi.org/10.1001/jama.2015.13766

Kapasi, A., DeCarli, C., & Schneider, J. A. (2017). Impact of multiple pathologies on the threshold for clinically overt dementia. *Acta Neuropathologica, 134*(2), 171. https://doi.org/10.1007/S00401-017-1717-7

Kaplan, H. S. (1974). *The new sex therapy*. Brunner/Mazel.

Kaplan, M. S., & Krueger, R. B. (2012). Cognitive-behavioral treatment of the paraphilias. *Israel Journal of Psychiatry Related Sciences, 49*, 291–296.

Kaplow, J. B., & Widom, C. S. (2007). Age of onset of child maltreatment predicts long-term mental health outcomes. *Journal of Abnormal Psychology, 116*, 176–187.

Kaptchuk, T. J., Kelley, J. M., Conboy, L. A., Davis, R. B., Kerr, C. E., Jacobson, E. E., et al. (2008). Components of placebo effect: Randomised controlled trial in patients with irritable bowel syndrome. *British Medical Journal, 336*, 999–1003.

Karam, E. G., Friedman, M. J., Hill, E. D., Kessler, R. C., McLaughlin, K. A., Petukhova, M., et al. (2014). Cumulative traumas and risk thresholds: 12-month PTSD in the World Mental Health (WMH) surveys. *Depression and Anxiety, 31*(2), 130. https://doi.org/10.1002/da.22169

Karcher, N. R., Klaunig, M. J., Elsayed, N. M., Taylor, R. L., Jay, S. Y., & Schiffman, J. (2022). Understanding associations between race/ethnicity, experiences of discrimination, and psychotic-like experiences in middle childhood. *Journal of the American Academy of Child and Adolescent Psychiatry, 61*, 1262–1272.

Karlin, B. E., Brown, G. K., Trockel, M., Cunning, D., Zeiss, A. M., & Barr Taylor, C. (2012). National dissemination of cognitive behavioral therapy for depression in the department of veterans affairs health care system: Therapist and patient-level outcomes. *Journal of Consulting and Clinical Psychology, 80*(5), 707–718. https://doi.org/10.1037/a0029328

Karlin, B. E., & Cross, G. (2014). From the laboratory to the therapy room: National dissemination and implementation of evidence-based psychotherapies in the U.S. Department of Veterans Affairs health care system. *American Psychologist, 69*(1), 19–33. https://doi.org/10.1037/a0033888

Karlin, B. E., & Cross, G. (2014). From the laboratory to the therapy room: National dissemination and implementation of evidence-based psychotherapies in the U.S. Department of Veterans Affairs health care system. *American Psychologist, 69*(1), 19–33. https://doi.org/10.1037/a0033888

Karlin, B. E., Ruzek, J. I., Chard, K. M., Eftekhari, A., Monson, C. M., Hembree, E. A., et al. (2010). Dissemination of evidence-based psychological treatments for posttraumatic stress disorder in the Veterans Health Administration. *Journal of Traumatic Stress, 23*(6), 663–673. https://doi.org/10.1002/jts.20588

Karney, B. R. & Bradbury, T. N. (2020). Research on marital satisfaction and stability in the 2010's: Challenging conventional wisdom. *Journal of Marriage and Family, 82*, 1100-116.

Karon, B. P., & VandenBos, G. R. (1998). Schizophrenia and psychosis in elderly populations. In I. H. Nordhus, G. R. VandenBos, S. Berg, & P. Fromholt (Eds.), *Clinical geropsychology* (pp. 219–227). American Psychological Association.

Karukivi, M., Vahlberg, T., Horjamo, K., Nevalainen, M., & Korkeila, J. (2017). Clinical importance of personality difficulties: Diagnostically sub-threshold personality disorders. *BMC Psychiatry, 17*(1). https://doi.org/10.1186/s12888-017-1200-y

Kasari, C., Freeman, S., & Paparella, T. (2006). Joint attention and symbolic play in young children with autism: A randomized controlled intervention study. *Journal of Child Psychology and Psychiatry, 47*, 611–620.

Kasari, C., Paparella, T., Freeman, S., & Jahromi, L. B. (2008). Language outcome in autism: Randomized comparison of joint attention and play interventions. *Journal of Consulting and Clinical Psychology, 76*, 125–137.

Kassel, J. D., & Shiffman, S. (1997). Attentional mediation of cigarette smoking's effect on anxiety. *Health Psychology, 16*, 359–368.

Kassel, J. D., & Unrod, M. (2000). Smoking, anxiety, and attention: Support for the role of nicotine in attentionally mediated anxiolysis. *Journal of Abnormal Psychology, 109*, 161–166.

Kato, M., Hori, H., Inoue, T., Iga, J., Iwata, M., Inagaki, T., et al. (2021). Discontinuation of antidepressants after remission with antidepressant medication in major depressive disorder: A systematic review and meta-analysis. *Molecular Psychiatry, 26*(1), 118–133. https://doi.org/10.1038/s41380-020-0843-0

Katon, W., Pedersen, H. S., Ribe, A. R., Fenger-Gron, M., Davydow, D., Waldorff, F. B., et al. (2015). Effect of depression and diabetes mellitus on the risk for dementia: A national population-based cohort study. *JAMA Psychiatry, 72*, 612–619. https://doi.org/10.1001/jamapsychiatry.2015.0082

Kaya, C., Gunes, M., Gokce, A. M., & Kalkan, S. (2015). Is sexual function in female partners of men with premature ejaculation compromised? *Journal of Sex & Marital Therapy, 41*, 379–383. https://doi.org/10.1080/0092623X.2014.915905

Kaye, J. T., Bradford, D. E., Magruder, K. P., & Curtin, J. J. (2017). Probing for neuroadaptations to unpredictable stressors in addiction: Translational methods and emerging evidence. *Journal of Studies on Alcohol and Drugs, 78*, 353–371. https://doi.org/10.15288/jsad.2017.78.353

Kaye, W. H., Wierenga, C. E., Bailer, U. F., Simmons, A. N., & Bischoff-Grethe, A. (2013). Nothing tastes as good as skinny feels: The neurobiology of anorexia nervosa. *Trends in Neuroscience, 36*, 110–120, https://doi.org/10.1016/j.tins.2013.01.003

Kazdin, A. (2011). *Single-case research designs: Methods for clinical and applied settings* (2nd ed.). Oxford University Press.

Kazdin, A. E. (2005). *Parent management training: Treatment for oppositional, aggressive, and antisocial behavior in children and adolescents*. Oxford University Press.

Keane, T. M., Zimering, R. T., & Caddell, J. (1985). A behavioral formulation of posttraumatic stress disorder in Vietnam veterans. *The Behavior Therapist, 8*, 9–12.

Keel, P. K. (2018). Eating disorders. In J. N. Butcher & J. M. Hooley (Eds.), *APA Handbook of psychopathology: Understanding, assessing, and treating adult mental disorders*. American Psychological Association.

Keel, P. K., Baxter, M. G., Heatherton, T. F., & Joiner, T. E. (2007). A 20-year longitudinal study of body weight, dieting, and eating disorder symptoms. *Journal of Abnormal Psychology, 116*, 422–432.

Keel, P. K., & Brown, T. A. (2010). Update on course and outcome in eating disorders. *International Journal of Eating Disorders, 43*, 195–204.

Keel, P. K., Gravener, J. A., Joiner, T. E., Jr., & Haedt, A. A. (2010). Twenty-year follow-up of bulimia nervosa and related eating disorders not otherwise specified. *International Journal of Eating Disorders, 43*, 492–497.

Keel, P. K., & Klump, K. L. (2003). Are eating disorders culture-bound syndromes? Implications for conceptualizing their etiology. *Psychological Bulletin, 129*, 747–769.

Keel, P. K., Mitchell, J. E., Davis, T. L., & Crow, S. J. (2002). Long-term impact of treatment in women diagnosed with bulimia nervosa. *International Journal of Eating Disorders, 31*, 151–158.

Keers, R., Ullrich, S., DeStavola, B. L., & Coid, J. W. (2014). Association of violence with emergence of persecutory delusions in untreated schizophrenia. *American Journal of Psychiatry, 171*, 332–339.

Kelley, M. E., Wan, C. R., Broussard, B., Crisafio, A., Cristofaro, S., Johnson, S., et al. (2016). Marijuana use in the immediate 5-year pre-morbid period is associated with increased risk of onset of schizophrenia and related psychotic disorders. *Schizophrenia Research, 171*, 62–67.

Kellner, C. H., Fink, M., Knapp, R., Petrides, G., Husain, M., Rummans, T., et al. (2005). Relief of expressed suicidal intent by ECT: A consortium for research in ECT study. *American Journal of Psychiatry, 162*, 977–982.

Kelly, A. B., Chan, G. C. K., Toumbourou, J. W., O'Flaherty, M., Homel, R., Patton, G. C., et al. (2012). Very young adolescents and alcohol: Evidence of a unique susceptibility to peer alcohol use. *Addictive Behaviors, 37*, 414–419.

Kelly, J. F., Humphreys, K., & Ferri, M. (2020). Alcoholics Anonymous and other 12-step programs for alcohol use disorder. *Cochrane Database of Systematic Reviews, 3*(3), CD012880.

Kendall, P. C., Aschenbrand, S. G., & Hudson, J. L. (2003). Child-focused treatment of anxiety. In A. E. Kazdin & J. R. Weisz (Eds.), *Evidence-based psychotherapies for children and adolescents* (pp. 81–100). Guilford Press.

Kendall, P. C., & Beidas, R. S. (2007). Trial for dissemination of evidence-based practices for youth: Flexibility within fidelity. *Professional Psychology: Research and Practice, 38*, 13–20.

Kendall, P. C., Cummings, C. M., Villabø, M. A., Narayanan, M. K., Treadwell, K., Birmaher, B., et al. (2016). Mediators of change in the Child/Adolescent Anxiety Multimodal Treatment Study. *Journal of Consulting and Clinical Psychology, 84*(1), 1–14. https://doi.org/10.1037/a0039773

Kendall, P. C., Flannery-Schroeder, E. C., Panichelli-Mindel, S., Southam-Gerow, M., Henin, A., & Warman, M. (1997). Therapy for youths with anxiety disorders: A second randomized clinical trial. *Journal of Consulting and Clinical Psychology, 65*, 366–380.

Kendall, P. C., Hudson, J. L. Gosch, E., Flannery-Schroeder, E., & Suveg, C. (2008). Cognitive–behavioral therapy for anxiety disordered youth: A randomized clinical trial evaluating child and family modalities. *Journal of Consulting and Clinical Psychology, 76*, 282–297.

Kendall, P. C., Safford, S., Flannery-Schroeder, E., & Webb, A. (2004). Child anxiety treatment: Outcomes in adolescence and impact on substance use and depression at 7.4-year follow-up. *Journal of Consulting and Clinical Psychology, 72*, 276–287.

Kendler, K. S., Aggen, S. H., Czajkowski, N., et al. (2008). The structure of genetic and environmental risk factors for DSM-IV personality disorders: A multivariate twin study. *Archives of General Psychiatry, 65*, 1438–1446. https://doi.org/10.1001/archpsyc.65.12.1438

Kendler, K. S., Aggen, S. H., Knudsen, G. P., Roysamb, E., Neale, M. C., & Reichborn-Kjennerud, T. (2011). The structure of genetic and environmental risk factors for syndromal and subsyndromal common DSM-IV Axis I and all Axis II disorders. *The American Journal of Psychiatry, 168*(1), 29–39. https://doi.org/10.1176/appi.ajp.2010.10030340

Kendler, K. S., Aggen, S. H., Knudsen, G. P., Røysamb, E., Neale, M. C., & Reichborn-Kjennerud, T. (2011). The structure of genetic and environmental risk factors for syndromal and subsyndromal common DSM-IV Axis I and all Axis II disorders. *The American Journal of Psychiatry, 168*(1), 29–39. https://doi.org/10.1176/appi.ajp.2010.10030340

Kendler, K. S., Chen, X., Dick, D., Maes, H., Gillespie, N., Neale, M. C., et al. (2012). Recent advances in the genetic epidemiology and molecular genetics of substance use disorders. *Nature Neuroscience, 15*, 181–189.

Kendler, K. S., & Gardner, C. O. (2014). Sex differences in the pathways to major depression: A study of opposite-sex twin pairs. *American Journal of Psychiatry, 171*(4), 426–435. https://doi.org/10.1176/appi.ajp.2013.13101375

Kendler, K. S., Gardner, C. O., Gatz, M., & Pedersen, N. L. (2007). The sources of co-morbidity between major depression and generalized anxiety disorder in a Swedish national twin sample. *Psychological Medicine, 37*(3), 453–462. https://doi.org/10.1017/S0033291706009135

Kendler, K. S., Jacobson, K. C., Prescott, C. A., & Neale, M. C. (2003). Specificity of genetic and environmental risk factors for use and abuse/dependence of cannabis, cocaine, hallucinogens, sedatives, stimulants, and opiates in male twins. *American Journal of Psychiatry, 160*, 687–695.

Kendler, K. S., Jacobson, K., Myers, J. M., & Eaves L. J. (2008). A genetically informative developmental study of the relationship between conduct disorder and peer deviance in males. *Psychological Medicine, 38*, 1001–1011.

Kendler, K. S., Lönn, S. L., Salvatore, J., Sundquist, J., & Sundquist, K. (2016). Effect of marriage on risk for onset of alcohol use disorder: A longitudinal and co-relative analysis in a Swedish national sample. *American Journal of Psychiatry, 173*, 911–918. https://doi.org/10.1176/appi.ajp.2016.15111373

Kendler, K. S., Myers, J., & Prescott, C. A. (2002). The etiology of phobias: An evaluation of the stress-diathesis model. *Archives of General Psychiatry, 59*, 242–249.

Kendler, K. S., Myers, J., Torgersen, S., Neale, M. C., & Reichborn-Kjennerud, T. (2007). The heritability of cluster A personality disorders assessed by both personal interview and questionnaire. *Psychological Medicine, 37*, 655–665. https://doi.org/10.1017/s0033291706009755

Kendler, K. S., Ohlsson, H., Sundquist, J., & Sundquist, K. (2019). A contagion model for within-family transmission of drug abuse. *American Journal of Psychiatry, 176*(3), 239–248. https://doi.org/10.1176/appi.ajp.2018.18060637

Kendler, K. S., & Prescott, C. A. (1998). Cannabis use, abuse, and dependence in a population-based sample of female twins. *American Journal of Psychiatry, 155*, 1016–1022.

Kendler, K. S., Prescott, C. A., Myers, J., & Neale, M. C. (2003). The structure of genetic and environmental risk factors for common psychiatric and substance use disorders in men and women. *Archives of General Psychiatry, 60*, 929–937.

Kendrick, T., Pilling, S., Mavranezouli, I., Megnin-Viggars, O., Ruane, C., Eadon, H., et al. (2022). Management of depression in adults: Summary of updated NICE guidance. *BMJ (Clinical Research Ed.), 378*. https://doi.org/10.1136/BMJ.O1557

Kenwood, M. M., Kalin, N. H., & Barbas, H. (2022). The prefrontal cortex, pathological anxiety, and anxiety disorders. *Neuropsychopharmacology, 47*(1), 260–275. https://doi.org/10.1038/s41386-021-01109-z

Kerns, J. G. (2020). Cluster a personality disorders. In C. LeJeuz & K. L. Graff (Eds.), *The Cambridge handbook of personality disorders* (pp. 195–211). Cambridge University Press. https://doi.org/10.1017/9781108333931.037

Kessler, D. A. (2009). *The end of overeating.* Rodale.

Kessler, L. (2004, August 22). Dancing with Rose: A strangely beautiful encounter with Alzheimer's patients provides insights that challenge the way we view the disease. *Los Angeles Times Magazine.*

Kessler, R. C. (2003). Epidemiology of women and depression. *Journal of Affective Disorders, 74*, 5–13.

Kessler, R. C., Aguilar-Gaxiola, S., Alonso, J., Chatterji, S., Lee, S., Ormel, J., et al. (2009). The global burden of mental disorders: An update from the WHO World Mental Health (WMH) Surveys. *Epidemiologia e Psichiatria Sociale, 18*, 23–33.

Kessler, R. C., Aguilar-Gaxiola, S., Alonso, J., Chatterji, S., Lee, S., & Üstün, T. B. (2009). The WHO World Mental Health (WMH) Surveys. *Psychiatrie (Stuttgart, Germany), 6*(1), 5–9.

Kessler, R. C., Angermeyer, M., Anthony, J. C., de Graaf, R., Demyttenaere, K., Gasquet, I., et al. (2007). Lifetime prevalence and age-of-onset distributions of mental disorders in the World Health Organization's World Mental Health Survey Initiative. *World Psychiatry, 6*, 168–176.

Kessler, R. C., Avenevoli, S., Costello, E. J., Georgiades, K., Green, J. G., Gruber, M. J., et al. (2012). Prevalence, persistence, and sociodemographic correlates of DSM-IV disorders in the National Comorbidity Survey Replication Adolescent Supplement. *Archives of General Psychiatry, 69*(4), 372–380. https://doi.org/10.1001/archgenpsychiatry.2011.160

Kessler, R. C., Berglund, P. A., Chiu, W. T., Deitz, A. C., Hudson, J. I., Shahly, V., et al. (2013). The prevalence and correlates of binge eating disorder in the World Health Organization World Mental Health Surveys. *Biological Psychiatry, 73*(9), 904–914.

Kessler, R. C., Berglund, P., Demler, O., Jin, R., Koretz, D., Merikangas, K. R., et al. (2003). The epidemiology of major depressive disorder: Results from the National Comorbidity Survey Replication (NCS-R). *Journal of the American Medical Association, 289*, 3095–3105.

Kessler, R. C., Berglund, P., Demler, O., Jin, R., Merikangas, K. R., & Walters, E. E. (2005). Lifetime prevalence and age-of-onset distributions of DSM-IV disorders in the National Comorbidity Survey Replication. *Archives of General Psychiatry, 62*(6), 593–602.

Kessler, R. C., Berglund, P., Demler, O., Jin, R., Merikangas, K. R., & Walters, E. E. (2005). Lifetime prevalence and age-of-onset distributions of DSM-IV disorders in the national comorbidity survey replication. *Archives of General Psychiatry, 62*, 593–602.

Kessler, R. C., Birnbaum, H. G., Shahly, V., Bromet, E., Hwang, I., McLaughlin, K. A., et al. (2010). Age differences in the prevalence and co-morbidity of DSM-IV major depressive episodes: Results from the WHO World Mental Health Survey Initiative. *Depression and Anxiety, 27*, 351–364.

Kessler R. C., Chiu, W. T., Demler, O., & Walters, E. E. (2005). Prevalence, severity, and comorbidity of 12-month DSM-IV disorders in the National Comorbidity Survey replication. *Archives of General Psychiatry, 62*, 617–627.

Kessler, R. C., Chiu, W. T., Jin, R., Ruscio, A. M., Shear, K., & Walters, E. E. (2006). The epidemiology of panic attacks, panic disorder, and agoraphobia in the National Comorbidity Survey replication. *Archives of General Psychiatry, 63*, 415–424.

Kessler, R. C., Hwang, I., LaBrie, R., Petukhova, M., Sampson, N. A., Winters, K. C., et al. (2008). The prevalence and correlates of DSM-IV pathological gambling in the National Comorbidity Survey Replication. *Psychological Medicine, 38*, 1351–1360.

Kessler, R. C., McLaughlin, K. A., Green, J. G., Gruber, M. J., Sampson, N. A., Zaslavsky, A. M., et al. (2010). Childhood adversities and adult psychopathology in the WHO World Mental Health Surveys. *British Journal of Psychiatry, 197*, 378–385.

Kessler, R. C., Petukhova, M., Sampson, N. A., Zaslavsky, A. M., & Wittchen, H. U. (2012). Twelve-month and lifetime prevalence and lifetime morbid risk of anxiety and mood disorders in the United States. *International Journal of Methods in Psychiatric Research, 21*, 169–184.

Kessler, R. C., Sampson, N. A., Berglund, P., Gruber, M. J., Al-Hamzawi, A., Andrade, L., et al. (2015). Anxious and non-anxious major depressive disorder in the World Health Organization World Mental Health Surveys. *Epidemiology and Psychiatric Sciences, 24*(3), 210–226. https://doi.org/10.1017/S2045796015000189

Keyes, K. M., Maslowsky, J., Hamilton, A., & Schulenberg, J. (2015). The great sleep recession: Changes in sleep duration among US adolescents, 1991–2012. *Pediatrics, 135*(3), 460–468. https://doi.org/10.1542/peds.2014-2707

Keyes, K. M., Rutherford, C., Hamilton, A., Barocas, J. A., Gelberg, K. H., Mueller, P. P., et al. (2022). What is the prevalence of and trend in opioid use disorder in the United States from 2010 to 2019? Using multiplier approaches to estimate prevalence for an unknown population size. *Drug and Alcohol Dependence Reports, 3*, 100052.

Keys, A., Brozek, J., Hsu, L. K. G., McConoha, C. E., & Bolton, B. (1950). *The biology of human starvation.* University of Minnesota Press.

Khan, O., Ferriter, M., Huband, N., Powney, M. J., Dennis, J. A., & Duggan, C. (2015). Pharmacological interventions for those who have sexually offended or are at risk of offending. In *Cochrane database of systematic reviews* (Vol. 2015, Issue 2). John Wiley and Sons Ltd. https://doi.org/10.1002/14651858.CD007989.pub2

Kiang, M. V., Basu, S., Chen, J., & Alexander, M. J. (2019). Assessment of changes in the geographical distribution of opioid-related mortality across the United States by opioid type, 1999–2016. *JAMA Network Open, 2*(2), e190040–e190040.

Kiecolt-Glaser, J. K., & Glaser, R. (2002). Depression and immune function: Central pathways to morbidity and mortality. *Journal of Psychosomatic Research, 53*, 873–876.

Kieseppa, T., Partonen, T., Haukka, J., Kaprio, J., & Lonnqvist, J. (2004). High concordance of bipolar I disorder in a nationwide sample of twins. *American Journal of Psychiatry, 161*, 1814–1821.

Kiesler, C. A. (1991). Changes in general hospital psychiatric care. *American Psychologist, 46*, 416–421.

Kiluk, B. D., Nich, C., Buck, M. B., Devore, K. A., Frankforter, T. L., LaPaglia, D. M., et al. (2018). Randomized clinical trial of computerized and clinician-delivered CBT in comparison with standard outpatient treatment for substance use disorders: Primary within-treatment and follow-up outcomes. *American Journal of Psychiatry, 175*(9), 853–863. https://doi.org/10.1176/appi.ajp.2018.17090978

Kiluk, B. D., Ray, L. A., Walthers, J., Bernstein, M., Tonigan, J. S., & Magill, M. (2019). Technology-delivered cognitive-behavioral interventions for alcohol use: A meta-analysis. Alcoholism, *Clinical and Experimental Research, 43*(11), 2285–2295. https://doi.org/10.1111/acer.14189

Kimchi, E. Z., & Lyketsos, C. G. (2015). Dementia and mild neurocognitive disorders. In D. C. Steffens, D. G. Blazer, & M. E. Thakur (Eds.), *The American Psychiatric Publishing textbook of geriatric psychiatry.* APA.

Kim, D. D., & Basu, A. (2016). Estimating the medical care costs of obesity in the United States: Systematic review, meta-analysis, and empirical analysis. *Value in Health, 19*, 602–613.

Kim, E. (2005). The effect of the decreased safety behaviors on anxiety and negative thoughts in social phobics. *Journal of Anxiety Disorders, 19*, 69–86.

Kimerling, R., Weitlauf, J. C., & Street, A. E. (2021). Gender issues in PTSD. In M. J. Friedman, P. P. Schnurr & T. M. Keane (Eds.), Handbook of PTSD: Science and practice (3rd ed., pp. 229–245, 670 Pages). The Guilford Press.

Kim, H., & Newman, M. G. (2022). Avoidance of negative emotional contrast from worry and rumination: An application of the Contrast Avoidance Model. *Journal of Behavioral and Cognitive Therapy, 32*(1), 33–43. https://doi.org/10.1016/j.jbct.2021.12.007

Kim, M. J., Loucks, R. A., Palmer, A. L., Brown, A. C., Solomon, K. M., Marchante, A. N., et al. (2011). The structural and functional connectivity of the amygdala: From normal emotion to pathological anxiety. *Behavioural Brain Research, 223*, 403–410.

King, A. C., McNamara, P. J., Hasin, D. S., & Cao, D. (2014). Alcohol challenge responses predict future alcohol use disorder symptoms: A 6-year prospective study. *Biological Psychiatry, 75*, 798–806.

King, D. L., Delfabbro, P. H., Perales, J. C., Deleuze, J., Király, O., Krossbakken, E., et al. (2019). Maladaptive player-game relationships in problematic gaming and gaming disorder: A systematic review. *Clinical Psychology Review, 73*, 101777.

Kirkbride, J. B., Barker, D., Cowden, F., Stamps, R., Yang, M., Jones, P. B., et al. (2008). Psychoses, ethnicity and socioeconomic status. *The British Journal of Psychiatry, 193*, 18–24. https://doi.org/10.1192/bjp.bp.107.041566

Kirkpatrick, B., Fenton, W., Carpenter, W. T., & Marder, S. R. (2006). The NIMH-MATRICS consensus statement on negative symptoms. *Schizophrenia Bulletin, 32*, 296–303.

Kirmayer, L. J. (2001). Cultural variations in the clinical presentation of depression and anxiety: Implications for diagnosis and treatment. *Journal of Clinical Psychiatry, 62*(Suppl. 13), 22–28.

Kirmayer, L. J. (2001). Cultural variations in the clinical presentation of depression and anxiety: Implications for diagnosis and treatment. *Journal of Clinical Psychiatry, 62*(Suppl. 23), 22–28.

Kisley, M. A., Wood, S., & Burrows, C. L. (2007). Looking at the sunny side of life: Age-related change in an event-related potential measure of the negativity bias. *Psychological Science, 18*, 838.

Kjærvik, S. L., & Bushman, B. J. (2021). The link between narcissism and aggression: A meta-analytic review. *Psychological Bulletin, 147*(5), 477–503. https://doi.org/10.1037/bul0000323

Klein, D. N., & Kotov, R. (2016). Course of depression in a 10-year prospective study: Evidence for qualitatively distinct subgroups. *Journal of Abnormal Psychology, 125*(3), 337–348. https://doi.org/10.1037/abn0000147

Klein, D. N., Schwartz, J. E., Rose, S., & Leader, J. B. (2000). Five-year course and outcome of dysthymic disorder: A prospective, naturalistic follow-up study. *American Journal of Psychiatry, 157*, 931–939.

Klein, D. N., Shankman, S. A. M. A., & Rose, S. M. A. (2006). Ten-year prospective follow-up study of the naturalistic course of dysthymic disorder and double depression. *American Journal of Psychiatry, 163*, 872–880.

Kleinman, A. (1986). *Social origins of distress and disease: Depression, neurasthenia, and pain in modern China.* Yale University Press.

Kleinplatz, P. J. (2014). The paraphilias: An experiential approach to "dangerous" desires. In Y. M. Binik & K. S. K. Hall (Eds.), *Principles and practice of sex therapy* (5th ed.). Guilford Press.

Kleinplatz, P. J. (2018). History of the treatment of female sexual dysfunction(s). Annual *Review of Clinical Psychology, 14*(1), 29–54. https://doi.org/10.1146/annurev-clinpsy-050817-084802

Klerman, G. L., Weissman, M. M., Rounsaville, B. J., & Chevron, E. S. (1984). *Interpersonal psychotherapy of depression.* Basic Books.

Klimentidis, Y. C., Beasley, T. M., Lin, H. Y., Murati, G., Glass, G. E., Guyton, M., et al. (2011). Canaries in the coal mine: A cross-species analysis of the plurality of obesity epidemics. *Proceedings of the Royal Society B: Biological Sciences, 278*, 1626–1632.

Klonsky, E. D., May, A. M., & Saffer, B. Y. (2016). Suicide, suicide attempts, and suicidal ideation. *Annual Review of Clinical Psychology, 12*, 307–330. https://doi.org/10.1146/annurev-clinpsy-021815-093204

Klump, K. L., Culbert, K. M., & Sisk, C. L. (2017). Sex differences in binge eating: Gonadal hormone effects across development. *Annual Review of Clinical Psychology, 13*, 183–207. https://doi.org/10.1146/annurev-clinpsy-032816-045309

Klump, K. L., McGue, M., & Iacono, W. G. (2002). Genetic relationships between personality and eating attitudes and behaviors. *Journal of Abnormal Psychology, 111*, 380–389.

Klunk, W. E., Engler, H., Nordberg, A., Wang, Y., Blomqvist, G., & Holt, D. P. (2004). Imaging brain amyloid in Alzheimer's disease with Pittsburgh Compound-B. *Annals of Neurology, 55*, 306–319.

Knight, R. A., & King, M. (2012). Typologies for child molesters: The generation of a new structural model. In B. K. Schwartz (Ed.), *The sexual offender.* Civic Research Institute.

Knight, R. A., & Sims-Knight, J. (2011). Risk factors for sexual violence. In J. White, M. Koss, & A. E. Kazdin (Eds.), *Violence against women and children, Volume 1: Mapping the terrain.* American Psychological Association.

Knox, K. L., Pflanz, S., Talcott, G. W., Campise, R. L., Lavigne, J. E., Bajorska, A., et al. (2010). The US Air Force suicide prevention program: Implications for public health policy. *American Journal of Public Health, 100*, 2457–2463.

Kober, H., & Boswell, R. G. (2018). Potential psychological & neural mechanisms in binge eating disorder: Implications for treatment. *Clinical Psychology Review, 60*, 32–44.

Kochanek, K. D., Murphy, S. L., Xu, J., & Tejada-Vera, B. (2016). *Deaths: Final data for 2014.* National Vital Statistics Reports. https://www.cdc.gov/nchs/data/nvsr/nvsr65/nvsr65_04.pdf

Koenen, K. C., Moffitt, T. E., Poulton, R., Martin, J., & Caspi, A. (2007). Early childhood factors associated with the development of post-traumatic stress disorder: Results from a longitudinal birth cohort. *Psychological Medicine, 37*, 181–192.

Koenen, K. C., Ratanatharathorn, A., Ng, L., McLaughlin, K. A., Bromet, E. J., Stein, D. J., et al. (2017). Posttraumatic stress disorder in the World Mental Health Surveys. *Psychological Medicine, 47*(13), 2260–2274. https://doi.org/10.1017/S0033291717000708

Köhler, C. A., Freitas, T. H., Maes, M., de Andrade, N. Q., Liu, C. S., Fernandes, B. S., et al. (2017). Peripheral cytokine and chemokine alterations in depression: A meta-analysis of 82 studies. *Acta Psychiatrica Scandinavica, 135*(5), 373–387. https://doi.org/10.1111/acps.12698

Kohn, M. L. (1968). Social class and schizophrenia: A critical review. In D. Rosenthal & S. S. Kety (Eds.), *The transmission of schizophrenia.* Pergamon Press.

Kohut, H. (1971). *The analysis of the self.* International Universities Press.

Kohut, H. (1977). *The restoration of the self.* International Universities Press.

Kolar, D. R., Rodriguez, D. L., Chams, M. M., & Hoek, H. W. (2016). Epidemiology of eating disorders in Latin America: A systematic review and meta-analysis. *Current Opinion in Psychiatry, 29*, 363–371.

Kolker R. (2020). *Hidden Valley Road: Inside the mind of an American family.* Doubleday.

Konnopka, A., Schaefert, R., Heinrich, S., Kaufmann, C., Luppa, M., Herzog, W., et al. (2012). Economics of medically unexplained symptoms: A systematic review of the literature. *Psychotherapy and Psychosomatics, 81*, 265–275.

Konova, A. B., Lopez-Guzman, S., Urmanche, A., Ross, S., Louie, K., Rotrosen, J., et al. (2020). Computational markers of risky decision-making for identification of temporal windows of vulnerability to opioid use in a real-world clinical setting. *JAMA Psychiatry, 77*(4), 368–377.

Konrad, A., Kuhle, L. F., Amelung, T., & Beier, K. M. (2018). Is emotional congruence with children associated with sexual offending in pedophiles and hebephiles from the community? *Sexual Abuse: A Journal of Research and Treatment, 30*(1), 3–22. https://doi.org/10.1177/1079063215620397

Koob, G. F., & Le Moal. (2008). Addiction and the brain antireward system. *Annual Review of Psychology, 59*, 29–53

Kopala-Sibley, D., & Klein, D. N. (2017). Depressive disorders: Presentation, classification, developmental trajectories, and course. In N. L. Cohen (Ed.), *Public health perspectives on depressive disorders* (pp. 13–39, Chapter XI). Johns Hopkins University Press. https://search.proquest.com/docview/1981171433?accountid=14496

Kopelowicz, A., Liberman, R. P., & Zarate, R. (2006). Recent advances in social skills training for schizophrenia. *Schizophrenia Bulletin, 32*(suppl_1), S12–S23.

Koshiyama, D., Fukunaga, M., Okada, N., Morita, K., Nemoto, K., Usui, K., et al. (2020). White matter microstructural alterations across four major psychiatric disorders: Mega-analysis study in 2937 individuals. *Molecular Psychiatry, 25*(4), 883–895. https://doi.org/10.1038/s41380-019-0553-7

Kotov, R., Gamez, W., Schmidt, F., & Watson, D. (2010). Linking "big" personality traits to anxiety, depressive, and substance use disorders: A meta-analysis. *Psychological Bulletin, 136*, 768–821.

Kotov, R., Krueger, R. F., Watson, D., Achenbach, T. M., Althoff, R. R., Bagby, R. M., et al. (2017, in press). The hierarchical taxonomy of psychopathology (HiTOP): A dimensional alternative to traditional nosologies. *Journal of Abnormal Psychology.* https://doi.org/10.1037/abn0000258

Kotov, R., Krueger, R. F., Watson, D., Achenbach, T. M., Althoff, R. R., Bagby, R. M., et al. (2017). The hierarchical taxonomy of psychopathology (HITOP): A dimensional alternative to traditional nosologies. *Journal of Abnormal Psychology, 126*(4), 454–477. https://doi.org/10.1037/abn0000258

Koyama, A., Miyake, Y., Kawakami, N., Tsuchiya, M., Tachimori, H., & Takeshima, T. (2010). Lifetime prevalence, psychiatric comorbidity and demographic correlates of "hikikomori" in a community population in Japan. *Psychiatry Research, 176*(1), 69–74. https://doi.org/10.1016/j.psychres.2008.10.019

Kraemer, H. C. (2014). The reliability of clinical diagnoses: State of the art. *Annual Review of Clinical Psychology, 10*, 111–130. https://doi.org/10.1146/annurev-clinpsy-032813-153739

Krain, A. L., Wilson, A. M., Arbuckle, R., Castellanos, F. X., & Milham, M. P. (2006). Distinct neural mechanisms of risk and ambiguity: A meta-analysis of decision-making. *Special Issue: Educational Neuroscience, 32*(1), 477–484.

Kranzler, H. R., & van Kirk, J. (2001). Efficacy of naltrexone and acamprosate for alcoholism treatment: A meta analysis. *Alcoholism: Clinical and Experimental Research, 25*, 1335–1341.

Krebs, G., de la Cruz, L. F., Rijsdijk, F. V., Rautio, D., Enander, J., Rück, C., et al. (2022). The association between body dysmorphic symptoms and suicidality among adolescents and young adults: A genetically informative study. *Psychological Medicine, 52*(7), 1268–1276. https://doi.org/10.1017/S0033291720002998

Kreslake, J. M., Wayne, G. F., Alpert, H. R., Koh, H. K., & Connolly, G. N. (2008). Tobacco industry control of menthol in cigarettes and targeting of adolescents and young adults. *American Journal of Public Health, 98*, 1685–1692.

Kreslake, J., Wayne, G. F., & Connolly, G. (2008). The menthol smoker: Tobacco industry research on consumer sensory perception of menthol cigarettes and its role in smoking behavior. *Nicotine & Tobacco Research, 10*, 705–715. https://doi.org/10.1080/14622200801979134

Kreyenbuhl, J., Buchanan, R. W., Dickerson, F. B., & Dixon, L. B. (2010). The Schizophrenia Patient Outcomes Research Team (PORT): Updated treatment recommendations 2009. *Schizophrenia Bulletin, 36*, 94–103.

Kreyenbuhl, J., Zito, J. M., Buchanan, R. W., Soeken, K. L., & Lehman, A. F. (2003). Racial disparity in the pharmacological management of schizophrenia. *Schizophrenia Bulletin, 29*, 183–193.

Krieger, T., Bur, O. T., Weber, L., Wolf, M., Berger, T., Watzke, B., & Munder, T. (2023). Human contact in internet-based interventions for depression: A pre-registered replication and meta-analysis of randomized trials. *Internet Interventions, 32*, 100617. https://doi.org/10.1016/j.invent.2023.100617

Kring, A. M., & Barch, D. M. (2014). The motivation and pleasure dimension of negative symptoms: Neural substrates and behavioral outputs. *European Neuropsychopharmacology, 24*, 725–736.

Kring, A. M., & Elis O. (2013). Emotion deficits in people with schizophrenia. *Annual Review of Clinical Psychology, 9*, 409–433.

Krinsley, K. E., Gallagher, J., Weathers, F. W., Kutter, C. J., & Kaloupek, D. G. (2003). Consistency of retrospective reporting about exposure to traumatic events. *Journal of Traumatic Stress, 16*, 399–409.

Kronstein, P. D., Ishida, E., Khin, N. A., Chang, E., Hung, H. M., Temple, R. J., et al. (2015). Summary of findings from the FDA regulatory science forum on measuring sexual dysfunction in depression trials. *Journal of Clinical Psychiatry, 76*, 1050–1059. https://doi.org/10.4088/JCP.14r09699

Krstic, S., Neumann, C. S., Roy, S., Robertson, C. A., Knight, R. A., & Hare, R. D. (2017). Using latent variable- and person-centered approaches to examine the role of psychopathic traits in sex offenders. *Personal Disorders.* https://doi.org/10.1037/per0000249

Krueger (1999). The structure of common mental disorders. *Archives of General Psychiatry, 56*, 921–926.

Krueger, R. B. (2010a). The DSM diagnostic criteria for sexual masochism. *Archives of Sexual Behavior, 39*, 346–356.

Krueger, R. B. (2010b). The DSM diagnostic criteria for sexual sadism. *Archives of Sexual Behavior, 39*, 325–345.

Krueger, R. F., Derringer, J., Markon, K. E., Watson, D., & Skodol, A. E. (2012). Initial construction of a maladaptive personality trait model and inventory for DSM-5. *Psychological Medicine, 42*, 1879–1890.

Krueger, R. F., Hicks, B. M., Patrick, C. J., Carlson, S. R., Iacono, W. G., & McGue, M. (2002). Etiologic connections among substance dependence, antisocial behavior, and personality: Modeling the externalizing spectrum. *Journal of Abnormal Psychology, 111*(3), 411–424. https://doi.org/10.1037/0021-843X.111.3.411

Krueger, R. F., Markon, K. E., Patrick, C. J., & Iacono, W. G. (2005). Externalizing psychopathology in adulthood: A dimensional-spectrum conceptualization and its implications for DSM-V. *Journal of Abnormal Psychology, 114*, 537–550.

Krueger, R. F., Markon, K. E., Patrick, C. J., & Iacono, W. G. (2005). Externalizing psychopathology in adulthood: A dimensional-spectrum conceptualization and its implications for DSM-V. *Journal of Abnormal Psychology, 114*, 537–550. https://doi.org/10.1037/0021-843X.114.4.537

Krystal, J. H., Cramer, J. A., Krol, W. F., Kirk, G. F., Rosenheck R. A. (2001). Naltrexone in the treatment of alcohol dependence. *New England Journal of Medicine, 345*, 1734–1739.

Kulkarni, M., Barrad, A., & Cloitre, M. (2014). In P. Emmelkamp & T. Ehring (Eds.), *The Wiley handbook of anxiety disorders*. John Wiley & Sons, Ltd.

Kunst-Wilson, W. R., & Zajonc, R. B. (1980). Affective discrimination of stimuli that cannot be recognized. *Science, 207*, 557–558.

Kurian, B. T., Ray, W. A., Arbogast, P. G., Fuchs, D. C., Dudley, J. A., & Cooper, W. O. (2007). Effect of regulatory warnings on antidepressant prescribing for children and adolescents. *Archives of General Psychiatry, 161*, 690–696.

Kurtz, M. M., & Mueser, K. T. (2008). A meta-analysis of controlled research on social skills training for schizophrenia. *Journal of Consulting and Clinical Psychology, 76*, 491–504. https://doi.org/10.1037/0022-006X.76.3.491

Kuyken, W., Hayes, R., Barrett, B., Byng, R., Dalgleish, T., Kessler, D., et al. (2015). Effectiveness and cost-effectiveness of mindfulness-based cognitive therapy compared with maintenance antidepressant treatment in the prevention of depressive relapse or recurrence (prevent): A randomised controlled trial. *The Lancet, 386*(9988), 63–73. https://doi.org/10.1016/S0140-6736(14)62222-4

Kvaale, E. P., Haslam, N., & Gottdiener, W. H. (2013). The "side effects" of medicalization: A meta-analytic review of how biogenetic explanations affect stigma. *Clinical Psychology Review, 33*, 782–794.

Kwok, W. (2014). Is there evidence that social class at birth increases risk of psychosis? A systematic review. *International Journal of Social Psychiatry, 60*, 801–808.

Kyaga, S., Landen, M., Boman, M., Hultman, C. M., Langstrom, N., & Lichtenstein, P. (2013). Mental illness, suicide and creativity: 40-year prospective total population study. *Journal of Psychiatric Research, 47*(1), 83–90. https://doi.org/10.1016/j.jpsychires.2012.09.010

LaFrance, W. C., Baird, G. L., Barry, J. J., Blum, A. S., Frank Webb, A., Keitner, G. I., et al. (2014). Multicenter pilot treatment trial for psychogenic nonepileptic seizures: A randomized clinical trial. *JAMA Psychiatry, 71*(9), 997–1005. https://doi.org/10.1001/jamapsychiatry.2014.817

Lagisetty, P. A., Ross, R., Bohnert, A., Clay, M., & Maust, D. T. (2019). Buprenorphine treatment divide by race/ethnicity and payment. *JAMA Psychiatry, 76*(9), 979–981.

Lahey, B. B., Lee, S. S., Sibley, M. H., Applegate, B., Molina, B. S. G., & Pelham, W. E. (2016). Predictors of adolescent outcomes among 4–6-year-old children with attention-deficit/hyperactivity disorder. *Journal of Abnormal Psychology, 125*(2), 168–181. https://doi.org/10.1037/abn0000086

Lahey, B. B., Loeber, R., Burke, J. D., & Applegate, B. (2005). Predicting future antisocial personality disorder in males from a clinical assessment in childhood. *Journal of Consulting and Clinical Psychology, 73*, 389–399.

Lahey, B. B., Van Hulle, C. A., Singh, A. L., Waldman, I. D., & Rathouz, P. J. (2011). Higher-order genetic and environmental structure of prevalent forms of child and adolescent psychopathology. *Archives of General Psychiatry, 68*(2), 181–189.

Lahey, B. B., & Waldman, I. D. (2012). Phenotypic and causal structure of conduct disorder in the broader context of prevalent forms of psychopathology. *Journal of Child Psychology and Psychiatry, 53*, 536–557.

Lambert, J. C., Ibrahim-Verbaas, C. A., Harold, D., Naj, A. C., Sims, R., Bellenguez, C., et al. (2013). Meta-analysis of 74,046 individuals identifies 11 new susceptibility loci for Alzheimer's disease. *Nature Genetics, 45*, 1452–1458. https://doi.org/10.1038/ng.2802

Lambert, M. J. (2004). Psychotherapeutically speaking—updates from the Division of Psychotherapy (29). https://www.divisionofpsychotherapy.org/updates.php

Lambert, M. J., & Ogles, B. M. (2004). The efficacy and effectiveness of psychotherapy. In M. J. Lambert (Ed.), *Bergin and Garfield's handbook of psychotherapy and behavior change* (5th ed., pp. 139–193). John Wiley & Sons.

Lamb, H. R., Weinberger, L. E., & DeCuir, W. J. (2002). The police and mental health. *Psychiatry Services, 53*, 1266–1271.

Lambrou, C., Veale, D., & Wilson, G. (2011). The role of aesthetic sensitivity in body dysmorphic disorder. *Journal of Abnormal Psychology, 120*, 443–453.

Lam, D. H., Jones, S. H., & Hayward, P. (2010). *Cognitive therapy for bipolar disorder: A therapist's guide to concepts, methods and practice* (2nd ed.). Wiley Press.

Lam, M., Chen, C.-Y., Li, Z., Martin, A. R., Bryois, J., Ma, X., et al. (2019). Comparative genetic architectures of schizophrenia in East Asian and European populations. *Nature Genetics, 51*(12), 1670–1678.

Landa, R. J., Holman, K. C., & Garrett-Mayer, E. (2007). Social and communication development in toddlers with early and later diagnosis of autism spectrum disorders. *Archives of General Psychiatry, 64*, 853–864.

Landgrebe, M., Barta, W., Rosengarth, K., Frick, U., Hauser, S., Langguth, B., et al. (2008). Neuronal correlates of symptom formation in functional somatic syndromes: A fMRI study. *NeuroImage, 41*, 1336–1344.

Langa, K. M., & Levine, D. A. (2014). The diagnosis and management of mild cognitive impairment: A clinical review. *Journal of the American Medical Association, 312*, 2551–2561. https://doi.org/10.1001/jama.2014.13806

Lang, A. R., Goeckner, D. J., Adessor, V. J., & Marlatt, G. A. (1975). Effects of alcohol on aggression in male social drinkers. *Journal of Abnormal Psychology, 84*, 508–518.

Lange, S., Probst, C., Gmel, G., Rehm, J., Burd, L., & Popova, S. (2017). Global prevalence of fetal alcohol spectrum disorder among children and youth: A systematic review and meta-analysis. *JAMA Pediatrics, 171*(10), 948–956. https://doi.org/10.1001/jamapediatrics.2017.1919

Lang, K., Kerr-Gaffney, J., Hodsoll, J., Jassi, A., Tchanturia, K., & Krebs, G. (2021). Is poor global processing a transdiagnostic feature of body dysmorphic disorder and anorexia nervosa? A meta-analysis. *Body Image, 37*, 94–105. https://doi.org/10.1016/j.bodyim.2021.01.012

Långström, N., & Seto, M. C. (2006). Exhibitionistic and voyeuristic behavior in a Swedish national population survey. *Archives of Sexual Behavior, 35*, 427–435. https://doi.org/10.1007/s10508-006-9042-6

Larson, R. P., Cartwright, A. E., & Goodman, G. S. (Eds.). (2016). Understanding and evaluating the testimony of child victims and witnesses in the legal system. *Behavioral Sciences & the Law, 34*, 1–245.

Larsson, H., Chang, Z., D'Onofrio, B. M., & Lichtenstein, P. (2014). The heritability of clinically diagnosed attention deficit hyperactivity disorder across the lifespan. *Psychological Medicine, 44*(10), 2223–2229. https://doi.org/10.1017/S0033291713002493

Latthe, P., Mignini, L., Gray, R., Hills, R., & Khan, K. (2006). Factors predisposing women to chronic pelvic pain: Systematic review. *British Medical Journal, 332*, 749–755. https://doi.org/10.1136/bmj.38748.697465.55

Lau, J. Y. F., Gregory, A. M., Goldwin, M. A., Pine, D. S., & Eley, T. C. (2007). Assessing gene–environment interactions on anxiety symptom subtypes across childhood and adolescence. *Development and Psychopathology, 19*, 1129–1146.

Laumann, E. O., Paik, A., & Rosen, R. C. (1999). Sexual dysfunction in the United States: Prevalence and predictors. *Journal of the American Medical Association, 281*, 537–544.

Laursen, T. M., Nordentoft, M., & Mortensen, P. B. (2014). Excess early mortality in schizophrenia. *Annual Review of Clinical Psychology, 10*, 425–448. https://doi.org/10.1146/annurev-clinpsy-032813-153657

Lavender, J. M., Utzinger, L. M., Cao, L., Wonderlich, S. A., Engel, S. G., Mitchell, J. E., et al. (2016). Reciprocal associations between negative affect, binge eating, and purging in the natural environment in women with bulimia nervosa. *Journal of Abnormal Psychology, 125*(3), 381–386. https://doi.org/10.1037/abn0000135

Lavner, J. A., Lamkin, J., Miller, J. D., Campbell, W. K., & Karney, B. R. (2016). Narcissism and newlywed marriage: Partner characteristics and marital trajectories. *Personality Disorders, 7*, 169–179. https://doi.org/10.1037/per0000137

Leahy, R. L. (2003). *Cognitive therapy techniques: A practitioner's guide* (2nd ed.). Guilford Press.

LeBeau, R. T., Glenn, D., Liao, B., Wittchen, H. U., Beesdo-Baum, K., Ollendick, T., & Craske, M. G. (2010). Specific phobia: a review of DSM-IV specific phobia and preliminary recommendations for DSM-V. *Depression and anxiety, 27*(2), 148–167. https://doi.org/10.1002/da.20655

Lebowitz, E. R., Marin, C., Martino, A., Shimshoni, Y., & Silverman, W. K. (2020). Parent-based treatment as efficacious as cognitive-behavioral therapy for childhood anxiety: A randomized noninferiority study of supportive parenting for anxious childhood emotions. *Journal of the American Academy of Child & Adolescent Psychiatry, 59*(3), 362–372. https://doi.org/10.1016/j.jaac.2019.02.014

Leckelt, M., Küfner, A. C. P., Nestler, S., & Back, M. D. (2015). Behavioral processes underlying the decline of narcissists' popularity over time. *Journal of Personality and Social Psychology: Personality Processes and Individual Differences, 109*, 856–871. https://doi.org/10.1037/pspp0000057

LeDoux, J. E., & Pine, D. S. (2016). Using neuroscience to help understand fear and anxiety: A two-system framework. *American Journal of Psychiatry, 173*(11), 1083–1093. https://doi.org/10.1176/appi.ajp.2016.16030353

Leeners, B., Hengartner, M. P., Rössler, W., Ajdacic-Gross, V., & Angst, J. (2014). The role of psychopathological and personality covariates in orgasmic difficulties: A prospective longitudinal evaluation in a cohort of women from age 30 to 50. *Journal of Sexual Medicine, 11*, 2928–2937. https://doi.org/10.1111/jsm.12709

Lee, S., Ng, K. L., Kwok, K., & Fung, C. (2010). The changing profile of eating disorders at a tertiary psychiatric clinic in Hong Kong (1987–2007). *International Journal of Eating Disorders, 43*, 307–314.

Lee, S. S., Humphreys, K. L., Flory, K., Liu, R., & Glass, K. (2011). Prospective association of childhood attention-deficit/hyperactivity disorder (ADHD) and substance use and abuse/dependence: A meta-analytic review. *Clinical Psychology Review, 31*(3), 328–341.

Lee, S. S., Lahey, B., Owens, E. B., & Hinshaw, S. P. (2008). Few preschool boys and girls with ADHD are well-adjusted during adolescence. *Journal of Abnormal Child Psychology, 36*, 373–383.

Lefaucheur, J.-P., André-Obadia, N., Antal, A., Ayache, S. S., Baeken, C., Benninger, D. H., et al. (2014). Evidence-based guidelines on the therapeutic use of repetitive transcranial magnetic stimulation (rTMS). *Clinical Neurophysiology, 125*(11), 2150–2206.

Legault, E., & Laurence, J. P. (2007). Recovered memories of childhood sexual abuse: Social worker, psychologist, and psychiatrist reports of beliefs, practices, and cases. *Australian Journal of Clinical and Experimental Hypnosis, 35*, 111–133.

Le Grange, D., Crosby, R. D., Rathouz, P. J., & Leventhal, B. L. (2007). A randomized controlled comparison of family-based treatment and supportive psychotherapy for adolescent bulimia nervosa. *Archives of General Psychiatry, 64*, 1049–1056.

Le Grange, D., Fitzsimmons-Craft, E. E., Crosby, R. D., Hay, P., Lacey, H., Bamford, B., et al. (2014). Predictors and moderators of outcome for severe and enduring anorexia nervosa. *Behaviour Research and Therapy, 56*, 91–98.

Le Grange, D., Hughes, E. K., Court, A., Yeo, M., Crosby, R. D., & Sawyer, S. M. (2016). Randomized clinical trial of parent-focused treatment and family-based treatment for adolescent anorexia nervosa. *Journal of the American Academy of Child & Adolescent Psychiatry, 55*(8), 683–692.

Le Grange, D., & Rienecke, R. (2018). Family therapy. In W. S. Agras & A. Robinson (Eds.), *The Oxford handbook of eating disorders* (2nd ed.). Oxford University Press. https://www.oxfordhandbooks.com/view/10.1093/oxfordhb/9780190620998.001.0001/oxfordhb-9780190620998

Lehn, A., Gelauff, J., Hoeritzauer, I., Ludwig, L., McWhirter, L., Williams, S., et al. (2016). Functional neurological disorders: Mechanisms and treatment. *Journal of Neurology, 263*, 611–620. https://doi.org/10.1007/s00415-015-7893-2

LeMoult, J., & Gotlib, I. H. (2019). Depression: A cognitive perspective. *Clinical Psychology Review, 69*, 51–66. https://doi.org/10.1016/j.cpr.2018.06.008

Lennon, J. C., Aita, S. L., Bene, V. A. D., Rhoads, T., Resch, Z. J., Eloi, J. M., & Walker, K. A. (2022). Black and White individuals differ in dementia prevalence, risk factors, and symptomatic presentation. *Alzheimer's & Dementia, 18*(8), 1461–1471. https://doi.org/10.1002/ALZ.12509

Lenzenweger, M. (2015). Schizotypic psychopathology: Theory evidence, and future directions. In P. Blaney, R. B. Krueger, & T. Millon (Eds.), *Oxford textbook of psychopathology* (pp. 729–767). Oxford University Press.

Lenzenweger, M. F., Lane, M. C., Loranger, A. W., & Kessler, R. C. (2007). DSM-IV personality disorders in the National Comorbidity Survey Replication. *Biological Psychiatry, 62*, 553–564.

Leon, G. R., Fulkerson, J. A., Perry, C. L., & Early-Zald, M. B. (1995). Prospective analysis of personality and behavioral vulnerabilities and gender influences in the later development of disordered eating. *Journal of Abnormal Psychology, 104*, 140–149.

Leon, G. R., Fulkerson, J. A., Perry, C. L., Peel, P. K., & Klump, K. L. (1999). Three to four year prospective evaluation of personality and behavioral risk factors for later disordered eating in adolescent girls and boys. *Journal of Youth and Adolescence, 28*, 181–196.

Lesh, T., Niendam, T. A., Minznberg, M., J., & Carter, C. S. (2012). Cognitive control deficits in schizophrenia: Mechanisms and meaning. *Neuropsychopharmacology Reviews, 36*, 316–338.

Leslie, D. L., & Rosenheck, R. A. (2004). Incidence of newly diagnosed diabetes attributable to atypical antipsychotic medications. *American Journal of Psychiatry, 161*, 1709–1711.

Leucht, S., Leucht, C., Huhn, M., Chaimani, A., Mavridis, D., Helfer, B., et al. (2017). Sixty years of placebo-controlled antipsychotic drug trials in acute schizophrenia: Systematic review, Bayesian meta-analysis, and meta-regression of efficacy predictors. *The American Journal of Psychiatry*, appiajp201716121358. https://doi.org/10.1176/appi.ajp.2017.16121358

Levenson, J. S., & Grady, M. D. (2016). The influence of childhood trauma on sexual violence and sexual deviance in adulthood. *Traumatology, 22*, 94–103. https://doi.org/10.1037/trm0000067

Levy, B. (2009). Stereotype embodiment: A psychosocial approach to aging. *Current Directions in Psychological Science, 18*(6), 332–336. https://doi.org/10.1111/j.1467-8721.2009.01662.x

Levy, B. R., Ferrucci, L., Zonderman, A. B., Slade, M. D., Troncoso, J., & Resnick, S. M. (2016). A culture–brain link: Negative age stereotypes predict Alzheimer's disease biomarkers. *Psychology and Aging, 31*, 82–88. https://doi.org/10.1037/pag0000062

Levy, B. R., Slade, M. D., & Kasl, S. V. (2002). Longitudinal benefit of positive self-perceptions of aging on functional health. *Journal of Gerontology: Psychological Sciences, 57B*, 409–417.

Lewinsohn, P. M. (Ed.). (1974). *A behavioral approach to depression.* Springer Publishing.

Lewinsohn, P. M., Rohde, P., Seeley, J. R., Klein, D. N., & Gotlib, I. H. (2000). Natural course of adolescent major depressive disorder in a community sample: Predictors of recurrence in young adults. *American Journal of Psychiatry, 157*, 1584–1591.

Lewis-Fernandez, R., & Aggarwal, N. K. (2013). Culture and psychiatric diagnosis. *Advances in Psychosomatic Medicine, 33*, 15–30. https://doi.org/10.1159/000348725

Liao, W.-W., Asri, M., Ebler, J., Doerr, D., Haukness, M., Hickey, G., et al. (2023). A draft human pangenome reference, *Nature, 617*(7960), 312–324.

Liberman, R. P., Eckman, T. A., Kopelowicz, A., & Stolar, D. (2000). *Friendship and intimacy module.* Available from Psychiatric Rehabilitation Consultants, PO Box 2867, Camarillo, CA 93011.

Liberzon, I. (2018). Searching for intermediate phenotypes in posttraumatic stress disorder. *Biological Psychiatry, 83*(10), 797–799. https://doi.org/10.1016/j.biopsych.2017.06.005

Lichtenstein, P., Carlstrom, E., Ramstam, M., Gillberg, C., & Anckarsater, H. (2010). The genetics of autism spectrum disorders and related neuropsychiatric disorders in childhood. *American Journal of Psychiatry, 167*, 1357–1363.

Lickel, J., Nelson, E., Lickel, A. H., & Deacon, B. (2008). Interoceptive exposure exercises for evoking depersonalization and derealization: A pilot study. *Journal of Cognitive Psychotherapy, 22*(4), 321–330. https://doi.org/10.1891/0889-8391.22.4.321

Lieberman, J. A., Stroup, T. S., McEvoy, J. P., Swartz, M. S., Rosenheck, R. A., Perkins, D. O., et al. (2005). Effectiveness of antipsychotic drugs in patients with chronic schizophrenia. *New England Journal of Medicine, 353*, 1209–1223.

Liechti, M. E., Baumann, C., Gamma, A., & Vollenweider, F. X. (2000). Acute psychological effects of 3, 4 methylenedioxymethamphetamine (MDMA, "Ecstasy") are attenuated by the serotonin uptake inhibitor citalopram. *Neuropsychopharmacology, 22*, 513–521.

Lilienfeld, S. O. (2007). Psychological treatments that cause harm. *Perspectives on Psychological Science, 2*, 53–70.

Lilienfeld, S. O., Lynn, S. J., Kirsch, I., Chaves, J. F., Sarbin, T. R., & Ganaway, G. K. (1999). Dissociative identity disorder and the sociogenic model: Recalling lessons from the past. *Psychological Bulletin, 125*, 507–523.

Lilienfeld, S. O., Lynn, S. J., Ruscio, J., & Beyerstein, B. L. (2010). Sad, mad, and bad: Myths about mental illness. In S. O. Lilienfeld, S. J. Lynn, J. Ruscio, & B. L. Beyerstein (Eds.), *50 great myths of popular psychology: Shattering widespread misconceptions about human behavior* (pp. 181–208). John Wiley & Sons.

Lilienfeld, S. O., Miller, J. D., & Lynam, D. R. (2017). The Goldwater rule: Perspectives from, and implications for, psychological science. *Perspectives in Psychological Science, 13*(1), 3–27. https://doi.org/10.1177/1745691617727864

Lilienfeld, S. O., Patrick, C. J., Benning, S. D., Berg, J., Sellbom, M., & Edens, J. F. (2012). The role of fearless dominance in psychopathy: Confusions, controversies, and clarifications. *Personality Disorders: Theory, Research, and Treatment, 3*, 327–340. https://doi.org/10.1037/a0026987

Lilienfeld, S. O., Wood, J. M., & Garb, H. N. (2000). The scientific status of projective techniques. *Psychological Science in the Public Interest, 1*, 27–66.

Lilly, R., Quirk, A., Rhodes, T., & Stimson, G. V. (2000). Sociality in methadone treatment: Understanding methadone treatment and service delivery as a social process. *Drugs: Education, Prevention and Policy, 7*, 163–178.

Li, L., Wu, C., Gan, Y., Qu, X., & Lu, Z. (2016). Insomnia and the risk of depression: A meta-analysis of prospective cohort studies. *BMC Psychiatry, 16*(1), 375. https://doi.org/10.1186/s12888-016-1075-3

Li, M. D., Cheng, R., Ma, J. Z., & Swan, G. E. (2003). A meta-analysis of estimated genetic and environmental effects on smoking behavior in male and female adult twins. *Addiction, 98*, 23–31.

Lim, R. F. (2015). *Clinical manual of cultural psychiatry* (2nd ed.). American Psychiatric Association.

Linardon, J., Wade, T. D., de la Piedad Garcia, X., & Brennan, L. (2017). The efficacy of cognitive-behavioral therapy for eating disorders: A systematic review and meta-analysis. *Journal of Consulting and Clinical psychology, 85*(11), 1080–1094. https://doi.org/10.1037/ccp0000245

Lindemann, E., & Finesinger, I. E. (1938). The effect of adrenalin and mecholyl in states of anxiety in psychoneurotic patients. *American Journal of Psychiatry, 95*, 353–370.

Lindson-Hawley, N., Aveyard, P., & Hughes, J. R. (2012). Reduction versus abrupt cessation in smokers who want to quit. *Cochrane Database of Systematic Reviews, 11*, CD008033. https://doi.org/10.1002/14651858.CD008033.pub3

Linehan, M. M. (1987). Dialectical behavior therapy for borderline personality disorder. *Bulletin of the Menninger Clinic, 51*, 261–276.

Linehan, M. M. (1993). *Cognitive-behavioral treatment of borderline personality disorder.* Guilford Press.

Linehan, M. M., Comtois, K., Murray, A. M., Brown, M. A., Gallop, R. J., Heard, H. L., et al. (2006). Two-year randomized controlled trial and follow-up of dialectical behavior therapy vs. therapy by experts for suicidal behaviors and borderline personality disorder. *Archives of General Psychiatry, 63*(7), 757–766. https://doi.org/10.1001/archpsyc.63.7.757

Lin, N., Bacala, L., Martin, S., Bratiotis, C., & Muroff, J. (2023). Hoarding disorder: The current evidence in conceptualization, intervention, and evaluation. *Psychiatric Clinics of North America, 46*(1), 181–196. https://doi.org/10.1016/j.psc.2022.10.007

Linnet, K. M., Dalsgaard, S., Obel, C., Wisborg, K., Henriksen, T. B., Rodriguez, A., et al. (2003). Maternal life-style factors in pregnancy risk of attention deficit hyperactivity disorder and associated behaviors: Review of the current evidence. *American Journal of Psychiatry, 160*, 1028–1040.

Littlewood, D. L., Kyle, S. D., Carter, L.-A., Peters, S., Pratt, D., & Gooding, P. (2019). Short sleep duration and poor sleep quality predict next-day suicidal ideation: An ecological momentary assessment study. *Psychological Medicine, 49*(3), 403–411. https://doi.org/10.1017/S0033291718001009

Liu, H., Petukhova, M. V., Sampson, N. A., Aguilar-Gaxiola, S., Alonso, J., Andrade, L. H., et al. (2017). Association of DSM-IV posttraumatic stress disorder with traumatic experience type and history in the World Health Organization World Mental Health Surveys. *JAMA Psychiatry, 74*, 270–281. https://doi.org/10.1001/jamapsychiatry.2016.3783

Livingstone-Banks, J., Norris, E., Hartmann-Boyce, J., West, R., Jarvis, M., & Hajek, P. (2019). Relapse prevention interventions for smoking cessation. *Cochrane Database of Systematic Reviews, 2*(2), CD003999.

Livingston, G., Huntley, J., Sommerlad, A., Ames, D., Ballard, C., Banerjee, S., et al. (2020). Dementia prevention, intervention, and care: 2020 report of the Lancet Commission. *The Lancet, 396*(10248), 413–446. https://doi.org/10.1016/S0140-6736(20)30367-6

Livingston, G., Sommerlad, A., Orgeta, V., Costafreda, S. G., Huntley, J., Ames, D., et al. (2017). Dementia prevention, intervention, and care. *The Lancet, 390*(10113), 2673–2734. https://doi.org/10.1016/S0140-6736(17)31363-6

Lobmaier, P. P., Kunøe, N., Gossop, M., & Waal, H. (2011), Naltrexone depot formulations for opioid and alcohol dependence: A systematic review. *CNS Neuroscience & Therapeutics, 17*, 629–636. https://doi.org/10.1111/j.1755-5949.2010.00194.x

Locke, J., Shih, W., Kretzmann, M., & Kasari, C. (2016). Examining playground engagement between elementary school children with and without autism spectrum disorder. *Autism, 20*(6), 653–662. https://doi.org/10.1177/1362361315599468

Lock, J., Le Grange, D., Agras, S., Moye, A., Bryson, S. W., & Jo, B. (2010). Randomized clinical trial comparing family-based treatment with adolescent-focused individual therapy for adolescents with anorexia nervosa. *Archives of General Psychiatry, 67*, 1025–1032.

Lock, J., Le Grange, D., Agras, W. S., & Dare, C. (2001). *Treatment manual for anorexia nervosa: A family-based approach.* Guilford Press.

Loeber, R., Burke, J. D., Lahey, B. B., Winters, A., & Zera, M. (2000). Oppositional defiant and conduct disorder: A review of the past 10 years, Part I. *Journal of the American Academy of Child and Adolescent Psychiatry, 39*, 1468–1484.

Loeber, R., & Hay, D. (1997). Key issues in the development of aggression and violence from childhood to early adulthood. *Annual Review of Psychology, 48*, 371–410.

Loeber, R., & Keenan, K. (1994). Interaction between conduct disorder and its comorbid conditions: Effects of age and gender. *Clinical Psychology Review, 14*, 497–523.

Loeb, K. L., Walsh, B. T., Lock, J., le Grange, D., Jones, J., Marcus, S., et al. (2007). Open trial of family-based treatment for full and partial anorexia nervosa in adolescence: Evidence of successful dissemination. *Journal of the American Academy of Child and Adolescent Psychiatry, 46*, 792–800.

Logue, M. W., van Rooij, S. J. H., Dennis, E. L., Davis, S. L., Hayes, J. P., Stevens. J. S., et al. (2018). Smaller hippocampal volume in posttraumatic stress disorder: A multisite ENIGMA-PGC study: Subcortical volumetry results from Posttraumatic Stress Disorder Consortia. *Biological Psychiatry, 83*(3), 244–253. https://doi.org/10.1016/j.biopsych.2017.09.006

Longshore, D., Hawken, A., Urada, D., & Anglin, M. (2006). Evaluation of the Substance Abuse and Crime Prevention Act: SACPA cost-analysis report (first and second years). https://www.uclaisap.org/prop36/html/reports.html

Longshore, D., Urada, D., Evans, E., Hser, Y. I., Prendergast, M., & Hawken, A. (2005). Evaluation of the Substance Abuse and Crime Prevention Act: 2004 report. Department of Alcohol and Drug Programs, California Health and Human Services Agency.

Longshore, D., Urada, D., Evans, E., Hser, Y. I., Prendergast, M., Hawken, A., et al. (2003). Evaluation of the Substance Abuse and Crime Prevention Act. https://www.uclaisap.org/prop36/html/reports.html

Looper, K. J., & Kirmayer, L. J. (2002). Behavioral medicine approaches to somatoform disorders. *Journal of Consulting and Clinical Psychology, 70*, 810–827.

Loos, R. J. F., & Yeo, G. S. H. (2022). The genetics of obesity: From discovery to biology. *Nature Reviews Genetics, 23*(2), 120–133.

Lopez-Ibor, J. J., Jr. (2003). Cultural adaptations of current psychiatric classifications: Are they the solution? *Psychopathology, 36*, 114–119.

Lopez, S. (2008). *The soloist: A lost dream, an unlikely friendship, and the redemptive power of music.* Putnam.

López, S. R. (1989). Patient variable biases in clinical judgment: Conceptual overview and methodological considerations. *Psychological Bulletin, 106*, 184–203.

López, S. R. (1994). Latinos and the expression of psychopathology: A call for direct assessment of cultural influences. In C. Telles & M. Karno (Eds.), *Latino mental health: Current research and policy perspectives.* UCLA.

López, S. R. (1996). Testing ethnic minority children. In B. B. Wolman (Ed.), *The encyclopedia of psychology, psychiatry, and psychoanalysis.* Holt.

López, S. R. (2002). Teaching culturally informed psychological assessment: Conceptual issues and demonstrations. *Journal of Personality Assessment, 79*, 226–234.

Lopez, S. R., Barrio, C., Kopelowicz, A., & Vega, W. A. (2012). From documenting to eliminating disparities in mental health care for Latinos. *American Psychologist, 67*, 511–523.

Lopez, S. R., Garcia, J. I. R., Ullman, J. B., Kopelowicz, A., Jenkins, J., Breitborde, N. J. K., et al. (2009). Cultural variability in the manifestation of expressed emotion. *Family Process, 48*, 179–194.

López, S. R., & Guarnaccia, P. J. (2016). Cultural dimensions of psychopathology: The social world's impact on mental disorders. In J. E. Maddux, & B. A. Winstead (Eds.), *Psychopathology: Foundations for a contemporary understanding* (4th ed., pp. 59–75). Routledge/Taylor & Francis Group.

Lopez, S. R., Lopez, A. A., & Fong, K. T. (1991). Mexican Americans' initial preferences for counselors: The role of ethnic factors. *Journal of Counseling Psychology, 38*, 487–496.

LoPiccolo, J., & Lobitz, W. C. (1972). The role of masturbation in the treatment of orgasmic dysfunction. *Archives of Sexual Behavior, 2*, 163–171.

Loughman, A., & Haslam, N. (2018). Neuroscientific explanations and the stigma of mental disorder: A meta-analytic study. *Cognitive Research: Principles and Implications, 3*(1), 43.

Lovaas, O. I. (1987). Behavioral treatment and normal educational and intellectual functioning in young autistic children. *Journal of Consulting and Clinical Psychology, 55*, 3–9.

Lowe, M. R., Arigo, D., Butryn, M. L., Gilbert, J. R., Sarwer, D., & Stice, E. (2016). Hedonic hunger prospectively predicts onset and maintenance of loss of control eating among college women. *Health Psychology, 35*, 238–244. https://doi.org/10.1037/hea0000291

Loyer Carbonneau, M., Demers, M., Bigras, M., & Guay, M.-C. (2021). Meta-analysis of sex differences in ADHD symptoms and associated cognitive deficits. *Journal of Attention Disorders, 25*(12), 1640–1656. https://doi.org/10.1177/1087054720923736

Lubin, G., Werbeloff, N., Halperin, D., Shmushkevitch, M., Weiser, M., & Knobler, H. Y. (2010). Decrease in suicide rates after a change of policy reducing access to firearms in adolescents: A naturalistic epidemiological study. *Suicide and Life-Threatening Behavior, 40*(5), 421–424. https://doi.org/10.1521/suli.2010.40.5.421

Luciano, M., Corley, J., Cox, S. R., Hernández, M. C. V., Craig, L. C. A., Dickie, D. A., et al. (2017). Mediterranean-type diet and brain structural change from 73 to 76 years in a Scottish cohort. *Neurology, 88*(5), 449–455. https://doi.org/10.1212/WNL.0000000000003559

Ludwig, L., Pasman, J. A., Nicholson, T., Aybek, S., David, A., Tuck, S., et al. (2018). Stressful life events and maltreatment in conversion (functional neurological) disorder: systematic review and meta-analysis of case-control studies. *The Lancet Psychiatry, 5*(4), 307–320. https://doi.org/10.1016/S2215-0366(18)30051-8

Luhrmann, T. M., Padmavati, R., Tharoor, H., & Osei, A. (2015). Differences in voice-hearing experiences of people with psychosis in the USA, India and Ghana: Interview-based study. *The British Journal of Psychiatry, 206*, 41–44. https://doi.org/10.1192/bjp.bp.113.139048

Luiselli, J. K., & Fischer, A. J. (2016). *Computer-assisted and web-based innovations in psychology, special education, and health.* Elsevier, Academic Press. https://doi.org/10.1016/C2014-0-01763-7

Lumley, M. N., & Harkness, K. L. (2007). Specificity in the relations among childhood adversity, early maladaptive schemas, and symptom profiles in adolescent depression. *Cognitive Therapy and Research, 31*, 639–657.

Luo, F., Florence, C. S., Quispe-Agnoli, M., Ouyang, L., & Crosby, A. E. (2011). Impact of business cycles on US suicide rates, 1928–2007. *American Journal of Public Health, 101*, 1139–1146.

Lydecker, J. A., & Grilo, C. M. (2022). Psychiatric comorbidity as predictor and moderator of binge-eating disorder treatment outcomes: An analysis of aggregated randomized controlled trials. *Psychological Medicine, 52*(16), 4085–4093. https://doi.org/10.1017/S0033291721001045

Lynn, S. J., Berg, J. M., Lilienfeld, S. O., Merckelbach, H., Giesbrecht, T., Van-Heugten-van der Kloet, D., et al. (2018). Dissociative disorders. In D. C. Beidel & B. C. Frueh (Eds.), *Adult psychopathology and diagnosis* (pp. 451–495). John Wiley & Sons.

Lynn, S. J., Lock, T., Loftus, E. F., Krackow, E., & Lilienfeld, S. O. (2003). The remembrance of things past: Problematic memory recovery techniques in psychotherapy. In S. J. Lynn & S. O. Lilienfeld (Eds.), *Science and pseudoscience in clinical psychology* (pp. 205–239). Guilford Press.

Lynn, S. J., Polizzi, C., Merckelbach, H., Chiu, C.-D., Maxwell, R., van Heugten, D., et al. (2022). Dissociation and dissociative disorders reconsidered: Beyond sociocognitive and trauma models toward a transtheoretical framework. *Annual Review of Clinical Psychology, 18*(1), 259–289. https://doi.org/10.1146/annurev-clinpsy-081219-102424

Lyons-Ruth, K., Bureau, J.-F., Easterbrooks, M. A., Obsuth, I., & Hennighausen, K. (2013). Parsing the construct of maternal insensitivity: Distinct longitudinal pathways associated with early maternal withdrawal. *Attachment and Human Development, 15.* https://doi.org/10.10 80/14616734.2013.841051

MacDonald, A. W., III, & Chafee, D. (2006). Translational and developmental perspective on N-methyl-D-aspartate synaptic deficits in schizophrenia. *Development and Psychopathology, 18,* 853–876.

Mac Giollabhui, N., Hamilton, J. L., Nielsen, J., Connolly, S. L., Stange, J. P., Varga, S., et al. (2018). Negative cognitive style interacts with negative life events to predict first onset of a major depressive episode in adolescence via hopelessness. *Journal of Abnormal Psychology, 127*(1), 1–11. https://doi.org/10.1037/abn0000301

Mac Giollabhui, N., Ng, T. H., Ellman, L. M., & Alloy, L. B. (2021). The longitudinal associations of inflammatory biomarkers and depression revisited: Systematic review, meta-analysis, and meta-regression. *Molecular Psychiatry, 26*(7), 3302–3314. https://doi.org/10.1038/s41380-020-00867-4

MacGregor, M. W. (1996). Multiple personality disorder: Etiology, treatment, and techniques from a psychodynamic perspective. *Psychoanalytic Psychology, 13,* 389–402.

Mackey, S., & Paulus, M. (2013). Are there volumetric brain differences associated with the use of cocaine and amphetamine-type stimulants? *Neuroscience & Biobehavioral Reviews, 37,* 300–316.

Macy, B. (2018). *Dopesick: Dealers, doctors, and the drug company that addicted America.* Little Brown & Company.

Macy, B. (2022). *Raising Lazarus: Hope, justice, and the future of America's overdose crisis.* Little Brown & Company.

Maenner, M. J., Graves, S. J., Peacock, G., Honein, M. A., Boyle, C. A., & Dietz, P. M. (2021). Comparison of 2 case definitions for ascertaining the prevalence of autism spectrum disorder among 8-year-old children. *American Journal of Epidemiology, 190*(10), 2198–2207.

Maenner, M. J., Shaw, K. A., Baio, J., Washington, A., Patrick, M., DiRienzo, M., et al. (2020). Prevalence of autism spectrum disorder among children aged 8 years—Autism and Developmental Disabilities Monitoring Network, 11 Sites, United States, 2016. *MMWR Surveillance Summary, 69*(No. SS-4), 1–12. https://doi.org/10.15585/mmwr.ss6904a1

Maenner, M. J., Warren, Z., Williams, A. R., Amoakohene, E., Bakian, A. V., Bilder, D. A., et al. (2023). Prevalence and characteristics of autism spectrum disorder among children aged 8 years—Autism and Developmental Disabilities Monitoring Network, 11 Sites, United States, 2020. *Morbidity and Mortality Weekly Report. Surveillance Summaries 72*(2), 1–14. https://doi.org/10.15585/mmwr.ss7202a1

Magill, M., & Ray, L. A. (2009). Cognitive-behavioral treatment with adult alcohol and illicit drug users: a meta-analysis of randomized controlled trials. *Journal of Studies on Alcohol and Drugs, 70*(4), 516–527. https://doi.org/10.15288/jsad.2009.70.516

Magill, M., Ray, L., Kiluk, B., Hoadley, A., Bernstein, M., Tonigan, J. S., et al. (2019). A meta-analysis of cognitive-behavioral therapy for alcohol or other drug use disorders: Treatment efficacy by contrast condition. *Journal of Consulting and Clinical Psychology, 87*(12), 1093–1105. https://doi.org/10.1037

Mahmood, Z., Keller, A. V., Burton, C. Z., Vella, L., Matt, G. E., McGurk, S. R., et al. (2019). Modifiable predictors of supported employment outcomes among people with severe mental illness. *Psychiatric Services, 70*(9), 782–792. https://doi.org/10.1176/appi.ps.201800562

Mahoney, R. (2005). Anxiety and depression in family caregivers of people with Alzheimer disease: The LASER-AD Study. *American Journal of Geriatric Psychiatry, 13*(9), 795–801. https://doi.org/10.1176/appi.ajgp.13.9.795

Maidment, I., Fox, C., & Boustani, M. (2006). Cholinesterase inhibitors for Parkinson's disease dementia. *Cochrane Database of Systematic Reviews, 1,* CD004747.

Maietta, J. E., Paul, N. B., & Allen, D. N. (2020). Cultural considerations for schizophrenia spectrum disorders Part I: Symptoms, diagnosis, and prevalence. In L. T. Benuto, F. R. Gonzalez, & J Singer (Eds.), *Handbook of cultural factors in behavioral health.* Springer. https://doi.org/10.1007/978-3-030-32229-8_26

Mallory, A. B., Stanton, A. M., & Handy, A. B. (2019). Couples' sexual communication and dimensions of sexual function: A meta-analysis. *Journal of Sex Research, 56*(7), 882–898. https://doi.org/10.1080/00224499.2019.1568375

Mancebo, M. C., Eisen, J. L., Sibrava, N. J., Dyck, I. R., & Rasmussen, S. A. (2011). Patient utilization of cognitive-behavioral therapy for OCD. *Behavior Therapy, 42,* 399–412.

Mancke, F., Herpertz, S. C., & Bertsch, K. (2015). Aggression in borderline personality disorder: A multidimensional model. *Personality Disorders: Theory, Research, and Treatment, 6,* 278–291. https://doi.org/10.1037/per0000098

Mandelli, L., Draghetti, S., Albert, U., De Ronchi, D., & Atti, A. (2020). Rates of comorbid obsessive-compulsive disorder in eating disorders: A meta-analysis of the literature. *Journal of Affective Disorders, 277,* 927–939. https://doi.org/10.1016/j.jad.2020.09.003

Mann, R. E., Hanson, R. K., & Thornton, D. (2010). Assessing risk for sexual recidivism: Some proposals on the nature of psychologically meaningful risk factors. *Sexual Abuse: A Journal of Research and Treatment, 22,* 191–217.

March, D., Hatch, S. L., Morgan, C., Kirkbride, J. B., Bresnahan, M., Fearon, P., et al. (2008). Psychosis and place. *Epidemiologic Reviews, 30,* 84–100. https://doi.org/10.1093/epirev/mxn006

March, J., Silva, S., Petrycki, S., Curry, J., Wells, K., Fairbank, J., et al. (2004). Fluoxetine, cognitive-behavioral therapy, and their combination for adolescents with depression: Treatment for Adolescents with Depression Study (TADS) randomized controlled trial. *Journal of the American Medical Association, 292,* 807–820.

Marconi, A., Di Forti, M., Lewis, C. M., Murray, R. M., & Vassos, E. (2016). Meta-analysis of the association between the level of cannabis use and risk of psychosis. *Schizophrenia Bulletin, 42*(5), 1262–1269.

Marcus, D. K., Gurley, J. R., Marchi, M. M., & Bauer, C. (2007). Cognitive and perceptual variables in hypochondriasis and health anxiety: A systematic review. *Clinical Psychology Review, 27,* 127–139.

Maree, R. D., & Riccelli, C. A. (2018). Substance-related and addictive disorders. In *Psychiatric disorders late in life* (pp. 217–227). Springer International Publishing. https://doi.org/10.1007/978-3-319-73078-3_20

Margraf, J., Ehlers, A., & Roth, W. T. (1986). Sodium lactate infusions and panic attacks: A review and critique. *Psychosomatic Medicine, 48,* 23–51.

Margulies, D. M., Weintraub, S., Basile, J., Grover, P. J., & Carlson, G. A. (2012). Will disruptive mood dysregulation disorder reduce false diagnosis of bipolar disorder in children? *Bipolar Disorders, 14*(5), 488–496. https://doi.org/10.1111/j.1399-5618.2012.01029.x

Marin, L. K., Foster, C., & Goodman, M. (2022). Pharmacotherapy for personality disorders. In *Personality disorders and pathology: Integrating clinical assessment and practice in the DSM-5 and ICD-11 era* (pp. 305–321). American Psychological Association. https://doi.org/10.1037/0000310-014

Marin, M. F., Zsido, R. G., Song, H., Lasko, N. B., Killgore, W. D. S., Rauch, S. L., et al. (2017). Skin conductance responses and neural activations during fear conditioning and extinction recall across anxiety disorders. *JAMA Psychiatry, 74*(6), 622–631. https://doi.org/10.1001/jamapsychiatry.2017.0329

Marks, I. M., & Cavanagh, K. (2009). Computer-aided psychological treatments: Evolving issues. *Annual Review of Clinical Psychology, 5*, 121–141.

Marlatt, G. A., & Gordon, J. R. (Eds.). (1985). *Relapse prevention: Maintenance strategies in the treatment of addictive behaviors.* Guilford Press.

Marmar, C. R., Schlenger, W., Henn-Haase, C., Qian, M., Purchia, E., Li, M., et al. (2015). Course of posttraumatic stress disorder 40 years after the Vietnam War: Findings from the National Vietnam Veterans Longitudinal Study. *JAMA Psychiatry, 72*(9), 875–881. https://doi.org/10.1001/jamapsychiatry.2015.0803

Marques, J. K., Wiederanders, M., Day, D. M., Nelson, C., & van Ommeren, A. (2005). Effects of a relapse prevention program on sexual recidivism: Final results from California's Sex Offender Treatment and Evaluation Project (SOTEP). *Sexual Abuse: A Journal of Research and Treatment, 17*, 79–107.

Marsh, A. A., & Blair, R. J. (2008). Deficits in facial affect recognition among antisocial populations: A meta-analysis. *Neuroscience and Biobehavioral Reviews, 32*(3), 454–465.

Marsh, A. A., Finger, E. C., Fowler, K. A., Adalio, C. J., Jurkowitz, I. T. N., Schechter, J. C., et al. (2013). Empathic responsiveness in amygdala and anterior cingulate cortex in youths with psychopathic traits. *Journal of Child Psychology and Psychiatry, 54*, 900–910. https://doi.org/10.1111/jcpp.12063

Marsh, R. J., Dorahy, M. J., Verschuere, B., Butler, C., Middleton, W., & Huntjens, R. J. C. (2018). Transfer of episodic self-referential memory across amnesic identities in dissociative identity disorder using the Autobiographical Implicit Association Test. *Journal of Abnormal Psychology, 127*(8), 751–757. https://doi.org/10.1037/abn0000377

Marsman, A., van den Heuvel, M. P., Klomp, D. W. J., Kahn, R. S., Luijten, P. R., & Hulshoff Pol, H. E. (2013). Glutamate in schizophrenia: A focused review and meta-analysis of (1)H-MRS studies. *Schizophrenia Bulletin, 39*, 120–129. https://doi.org/10.1093/schbul/sbr069

Marson, D. C., Huthwaite, J. S., & Hebert, K. (2004). Testamentary capacity and undue influence in the elderly: A jurisprudent therapy perspective. *Law and Psychology Review, 28*, 71–96.

Martell, C. R., Addis, M. E., & Jacobson, N. S. (2001). *Ending depression one step at a time: The new behavioral activation approach to getting your life back.* Oxford University Press.

Martin, A., & Jacobi, F. (2006). Features of hypochondriasis and illness worry in the general population in Germany. *Psychosomatic Medicine, 68*, 770–777.

Martinasek, M. P., McGrogan, J. B., & Maysonet, A. (2016). A systematic review of the respiratory effects of inhalational marijuana. *Respiratory Care, 61*, 1543–1551. https://doi.org/10.4187/respcare.04846

Marx, R. F., & Didziulis, V. (2009, February 27). A life, interrupted. *The New York Times.* http://www.nytimes.com/2009/03/01/nyregion/thecity/01miss.html?mcubz=0

Marx, R. F. (September 29, 2017). A teacher vanishes again. This time, in the Virgin Islands. *The New York Times.* https://www.nytimes.com/2017/09/29/nyregion/missing-teacher-virgin-islands.html

Masi, A., DeMayo, M. M., Glozier, N., & Guastella, A. J. (2017). An overview of autism spectrum disorder, heterogeneity and treatment options. *Neuroscience Bulletin, 33*(2), 183–193.

Masters, W. H., & Johnson, V. E. (1970). *Human sexual inadequacy.* Little, Brown.

Mathew, I., Gardin, T. M., Tandon, N., Eack, S., Francis, A. N., Seidman, L. J., et al. (2014). Medial temporal lobe structures and hippocampal subfields in psychotic disorders: Findings from the Bipolar-Schizophrenia Network on Intermediate Phenotypes (B-SNIP) study. *Journal of the American Medical Association, Psychiatry, 71*, 769–777.

Mathews, A., & MacLeod, C. (2002). Induced processing biases have causal effects on anxiety. *Cognition and Emotion, 16*, 331–354.

Mathews, C. A., Mackin, R. S., Chou, C.-Y., Uhm, S. Y., David Bain, L., Stark, S. J., et al. (2018). Randomised clinical trial of community-based peer-led and psychologist-led group treatment for hoarding disorder. Cambridge.Org. https://doi.org/10.1192/bjo.2018.30

Matsuda, L. A., Lolait, S. J., Brownstein, M. J., Young, A. C., & Bonner, T. I. (1990). Structure of a cannabinoid receptor and functional expression of the cloned cDNA. *Nature, 346*, 561–564.

Matthews, M., Nigg, J. T., & Fair, D. A. (2014). Attention deficit hyperactivity disorder. *Current Topics in Behavioral Neurosciences, 16*, 235–266.

Mattick, R. P., Breen, C., Kimber, J., & Davoli, M. (2014). Buprenorphine maintenance versus placebo or methadone maintenance for opioid dependence. *Cochrane Database of Systematic Reviews, 2014*(2), CD002207.

Maunder, R. D., & White, F. A. (2019). Intergroup contact and mental health stigma: A comparative effectiveness meta-analysis. *Clinical Psychology Review, 72*, 101749.

Mavandadi, S., Benson, A., DiFilippo, S., Streim, J. E., & Oslin, D. (2015). A telephone-based program to provide symptom monitoring alone vs. symptom monitoring plus care management for late-life depression and anxiety: A randomized clinical trial. *JAMA Psychiatry, 72*, 1211–1218. https://doi.org/10.1001/jamapsychiatry.2015.2157

Mavranezouli, I., Mayo-Wilson, E., Dias, S., Kew, K., Clark, D. M., Ades, A. E., et al. (2015). The cost effectiveness of psychological and pharmacological interventions for social anxiety disorder: A model-based economic analysis. *PLoS One, 10*(10), e0140704. https://doi.org/10.1371/journal.pone.0140704

Mavranezouli, I., Megnin-Viggars, O., Daly, C., Dias, S., Stockton, S., Meiser-Stedman, R., et al. (2020). Research review: Psychological and psychosocial treatments for children and young people with post-traumatic stress disorder: A network meta-analysis. *Journal of Child Psychology and Psychiatry, 61*(1), 18–29. https://doi.org/10.1111/jcpp.13094

May, A. M., & Klonsky, E. D. (2016). What distinguishes suicide attempters from suicide ideators? A meta-analysis of potential factors. *Clinical Psychology: Science and Practice, 23*(1), 5–20. https://doi.org/10.1111/cpsp.12136

Mayer, E. A., Berman, S., Suyenobu, B., Labus, J., Mandelkern, M. A., Naliboff, B. D., et al. (2005). Differences in brain responses to visceral pain between patients with irritable bowel syndrome and ulcerative colitis. *Pain, 115*, 398–409.

Mayes, S. D., Mathiowetz, C., Kokotovich, C., Waxmonsky, J., Baweja, R., Calhoun, S. L., et al. (2015). Stability of disruptive mood dysregulation disorder symptoms (irritable-angry mood and temper outbursts) throughout childhood and adolescence in a general population sample. *Journal of Abnormal Child Psychology, 43*(8), 1543–1549.

Mayes, S. D., Waxmonsky, J. D., Calhoun, S. L., & Bixler, E. O. (2016). Disruptive mood dysregulation disorder symptoms and association with oppositional defiant and other disorders in a general population child sample. *Journal of Child and Adolescent Psychopharmacology, 26*(2), 101–106. https://doi.org/10.1089/cap.2015.0074

Mayo-Wilson, E., Dias, S., Mavranezouli, I., Kew, K., Clark, D. M., Ades, A. E., et al. (2014). Psychological and pharmacological interventions for social anxiety disorder in adults: A systematic review and network meta-analysis. *The Lancet Psychiatry, 1*(5), 368–376. https://doi.org/10.1016/S2215-0366(14)70329-3

May, P. A., Chambers, C. D., Kalberg, W. O., Zellner, J., Feldman, H., Buckley, D., et al. (2018). Prevalence of fetal alcohol spectrum disorders in 4 US communities. *JAMA, 319*(5), 474–482. https://doi.org/10.1001/jama.2017.21896

Mazza, M., Mariano, M., Peretti, S., Masedu, F., Pino, M. C., & Valenti, M. (2017). The role of theory of mind on social information processing in children with autism spectrum disorders: A mediation analysis. *Journal of Autism and Developmental Disorders, 47*, 1369–1379.

Mazziotta, J. (2018). Emma Stone on the Anxiety and Panic Attacks that 'Still Haunt Me to This Day'. *People Magazine.* https://people.com/health/emma-stone-anxiety-panic-attacks-mental-health/

McCabe, R. E., McFarlane, T., Polivy, J., & Olmsted, M. (2001). Eating disorders, dieting, and the accuracy of self-reported weight. *International Journal of Eating Disorders, 29*, 59–64.

McCabe, S. E., Schulenberg, J. E., Wilens, T. E., Schepis, T. S., McCabe, V. V., & Veliz, P. T. (2023). Prescription stimulant medical and nonmedical use among US secondary school students, 2005 to 2020. *JAMA Network Open, 6*(4), e238707–e238707.

McCracken, J. T., McGough, J., Shah, B., Cronin, P., Hong, D., Aman, M. G., et al. (2002). Risperidone in children with autism and serious behavioral problems. *New England Journal of Medicine, 347*(5), 314–321.

McCracken, L. M., & Vowles, K. E. (2014). Acceptance and commitment therapy and mindfulness for chronic pain: Model, process, and progress. *American Psychologist, 69*, 178–187.

McCrady, B. S., Epstein, E. E., Cook, S., Jensen, N., & Hildebrandt, T. (2009). A randomized trial of individual and couple behavioral alcohol treatment for women. *Journal of Consulting and Clinical Psychology, 77*(2), 243–256. https://doi.org/10.1037/a0014686

McCrady, B. S., Wilson, A. D., Muñoz, R. E., Fink, B. C., Fokas, K., & Borders, A. (2016). Alcohol-focused behavioral couple therapy. *Family Process, 55*(3), 443–459. https://doi.org/10.1111/famp.12231

McCrae, R. R., Costa, P. T., & Martin, T. A. (2005). The NEO-PI-3: A more readable Revised NEO Personality Inventory. *Journal of Personality Assessment, 84*(3), 261–270. https://doi.org/10.1207/s15327752jpa8403_05

McCullough, J. P., Klein, D. N., Keller, M. B., Holzer, C. E., Davis, S. M., Korenstein, S. G., et al. (2000). Comparison of DSM-III major depression and major depression superimposed on dysthymia (double depression): Validity of the distinction. *Journal of Abnormal Psychology, 109*, 419–427.

McDonagh, M. S., Dana, T., Kopelovich, S. L., Monroe-DeVita, M., Blazina, I., Bougatsos, C., et al. (2022). Psychosocial interventions for adults with schizophrenia: An overview and update of systematic reviews. *Psychiatric Services, 73*(3), 299–312. https://doi.org/10.1176/appi.ps.202000649

McEachin, J. J., Smith, T., & Lovaas, O. I. (1993). Long-term outcome for children with autism who received early intensive behavioral treatment. *American Journal on Mental Retardation, 97*, 359–372.

McElroy, S. L., Guerdjikova, A. I., Mori, N., & Romo-Nava, F. (2019). Progress in developing pharmacologic agents to treat bulimia nervosa. *CNS Drugs, 33*(1), 31–46. https://doi.org/10.1007/s40263-018-0594-5

McEvoy, P. M., & Mahoney, A. E. J. (2012). To be sure, to be sure: Intolerance of uncertainty mediates symptoms of various anxiety disorders and depression. *Behavior Therapy, 43*(3), 533–545. https://doi.org/10.1016/j.beth.2011.02.007

McEwan, K., Gilbert, P., & Duarte, J. (2012). An exploration of competitiveness and caring in relation to psychopathology. *British Journal of Clinical Psychology, 51*(1), 19–36. https://doi.org/10.1111/j.2044-8260.2011.02010.x

McFarlane, W. R. (2016). Family interventions for schizophrenia and the psychoses: A review. *Family Process, 55*, 460–482. https://doi.org/10.1111/famp.12235

McGinty, E. E., Kennedy-Hendricks, A., Choksy, S. & Barry, C. L. (2016). Trends in news media coverage of mental illness in the United States: 1995–2014. *Health Affairs, 35*, 1121–1129.

McGinty, E. E., Webster, D. W., Jarlenski, M., & Barry, C. L. (2014). News media framing of serious mental illness and gun violence in the United State. *American Journal of Public Health, 104*, 406–413.

McGlashan, T. H., & Hoffman, R. E. (2000). Schizophrenia as a disorder of developmentally reduced synaptic connectivity. *Archives of General Psychiatry, 57*, 637–648.

McGovern, C. W., & Sigman, M. (2005). Continuity and change from early childhood to adolescence in autism. *Journal of Child Psychology and Psychiatry, 46*, 401–408.

McGue, M., Pickens, R. W., & Svikis, D. S. (1992). Sex and age effects on the inheritance of alcohol problems: A twin study. *Journal of Abnormal Psychology, 101*, 3–17.

McHugh, R. K., Hearon, B. A., & Otto, M. W. (2010). Cognitive-behavioral therapy for substance use disorders. *Psychiatric Clinics of North America, 33*(3), 511–525.

McHugh, R. K., Votaw, V. R., Sugarman, D. E., & Greenfield, S. F. (2018). Sex and gender differences in substance use disorders. *Clinical Psychology Review, 66*, 12–23.

McIntyre, R. S., Berk, M., Brietzke, E., Goldstein, B. I., López-Jaramillo, C., Kessing, L. V., et al. (2020). Bipolar disorders. *The Lancet, 396*(10265), 1841–1856. https://doi.org/10.1016/S0140-6736(20)31544-0

McKee, A. C., Daneshvar, D. H., Alvarez, V. E., & Stein, T. D. (2014). The neuropathology of sport. *Acta Neuropathologica, 127*(1), 29–51. https://doi.org/10.1007/s00401-013-1230-6

McKeith, I. G., Dickson, D. W., Lowe, J., Emre, M., O'Brien, J. T., Feldman, H., et al. (2005). Diagnosis and management of dementia with Lewy bodies: Third report of the DLB consortium. *Neurology, 65*, 1863–1872.

McKhann, G. M., Knopman, D. S., Chertkow, H., Hyman, B. T., Jack, C. R., Jr., Kawas, C. H., et al. (2011). The diagnosis of dementia due to Alzheimer's disease: Recommendations from the National Institute on Aging–Alzheimer's Association workgroups on diagnostic guidelines for Alzheimer's disease. *Alzheimer's & Dementia: The Journal of the Alzheimer's Association, 7*, 263–269.

McKinley, N. M., & Hyde, J. S. (1996). The objectified body consciousness scale: Development and validation. *Psychology of Women Quarterly, 20*, 181–216.

McKinnon, M. C., Palombo, D. J., Nazarov, A., Kumar, N., Khuu, W., & Levine, B. (2015). Threat of death and autobiographical memory. *Clinical Psychological Science, 3*, 487–502. doi:10.1177/2167702614542280

McKown, C., & Weinstein, R. S. (2003). The development and consequences of stereotype consciousness in middle childhood. *Child Development, 74*, 498–515.

McLaughlin K. A., Koenen K. C., Bromet E. J., Karam E. G., Liu H., Petukhova M., Ruscio A. M., et al. (2017). Childhood adversities and post-traumatic stress disorder: Evidence for stress sensitisation in the World Mental Health Surveys. *British Journal of Psychiatry, 211*(5), 280–288. https://doi.org/10.1192/bjp.bp.116.197640

McLean, C. P., Asnaani, A., Litz, B. T., & Hofmann, S. G. (2011). Gender differences in anxiety disorders: Prevalence, course of illness, comorbidity and burden of illness. *Journal of Psychiatric Research, 45*(8), 1027–1035. https://doi.org/10.1016/j.jpsychires.2011.03.006

McLeod, B. D., Weisz, J. R., & Wood, J. J. (2007). Examining the association between parenting and childhood anxiety: A meta-analysis. *Clinical Psychology Review, 27*, 155–172.

McManus, F., Surawy, C., Muse, K., Vazquez-Montes, M., & Williams, J. M. (2012). A randomized clinical trial of mindfulness-based cognitive therapy versus unrestricted services for health anxiety (hypochondriasis). *Journal of Consulting and Clinical Psychology, 80*, 817–828.

McMaster, K., & Johnson, S. (2014). Inadequate treatment of Black Americans with bipolar disorder. *Psychiatric Services (Washington, D.C.), 65*, 255–258.

McMillan, K. A., & Asmundson, G. J. G. (2016). PTSD, social anxiety disorder, and trauma: An examination of the influence of trauma type on comorbidity using a nationally representative sample. *Psychiatry Research, 246*, 561–567. https://doi.org/10.1016/j.psychres.2016.10.036

McNally, R. J. (2003). *Remembering trauma*. Belknap Press of Harvard University Press.

McNally, R. J., Lasko, N. B., Clancy, S. A., Macklin, M. L., Pitman, R. K., & Orr, S. P. (2004). Psychophysiological responding during script-driven imagery in people reporting abduction by space aliens. *Psychological Science, 15*, 493–497.

McNiel, D. E., & Binder, R. L. (2007). Effectiveness of a mental health court in reducing criminal recidivism and violence. *American Journal of Psychiatry, 164*, 1395–1403.

McPhail, I. V, Hermann, C. A., Fernane, S., Fernandez, Y. M., Nunes, K. L., & Cantor, J. M. (2019). Validity in phallometric testing for sexual interests in children: A meta-analytic review. *Assessment, 26*(3), 535–551. https://doi.org/10.1177/1073191117706139

McTeague, L. M., & Lang, P. J. (2012). The anxiety spectrum and the reflex physiology of defense: From circumscribed fear to broad distress. *Depression and Anxiety, 29*, 264–281.

McTeague, L. M., Rosenberg, B. M., Lopez, J. W., Carreon, D. M., Huemer, J., Jiang, Y., et al. (2020). Identification of common neural circuit disruptions in emotional processing across psychiatric disorders. *American Journal of Psychiatry, 177*(5), 411–421. https://doi.org/10.1176/appi.ajp.2019.18111271

Meana, M., Binik, I., Khalife, S., & Cohen, D. (1998). Affect and marital adjustment in women's ratings of dyspareunic pain. *Canadian Journal of Psychiatry, 43*, 381–385.

Medford, N. (2012). Emotion and the unreal self: Depersonalization disorder and de-affectualization. *Emotion Review, 4*(2), 139–144. https://doi.org/10.1177/1754073911430135

Medina, A., Mahjoub, Y., Shaver, L., & Pringsheim, T. (2022). Prevalence and incidence of Huntington's disease: An updated systematic review and meta-analysis. *Movement Disorders, 37*(12), 2327–2335. https://doi.org/10.1002/MDS.29228

Mednick, S. A., & Schulsinger, F. (1968). Some premorbid characteristics related to breakdown in children with schizophrenic mothers. In D. Rosenthal & S. S. Kety (Eds.), *The transmission of schizophrenia*. Pergamon Press.

Mehler, P. S. (2011). Medical complications of bulimia nervosa and their treatments. *International Journal of Eating Disorders, 44*, 95–104.

Meier, M. H., Caspi, A., Ambler, A., Harrington, H., Houts, R., Keefe, R. S. E., et al. (2012). Persistent cannabis users show neuropsychological decline from childhood to midlife. *Proceedings of the National Academy of Sciences, 109*, E2657–E2664.

Meier, M. H., Caspi, A., Knodt, R. A., Hall, W., Ambler, A., Harrington, H., et al. (2022). Long-term cannabis use and cognitive reserves and hippocampal volume in midlife. *AJP, 179*(5), 362–374. https://doi.org/10.1176/appi.ajp.2021.21060664

Meier, M. H., Caspi, A., Reichenberg, A., Keefe, R. S., Fisher, H. L., Harrington, H., et al. (2014). Neuropsychological decline in schizophrenia from the premorbid to the postonset period: Evidence from a population-representative longitudinal study. *American Journal of Psychiatry, 171*, 91–101.

Meier, S. M., Mattheisen, M., Mors, O., Schendel, D. E., Mortensen, P. B., & Plessen, K. J. (2016). Mortality among persons with obsessive-compulsive disorder in Denmark. *JAMA Psychiatry, 73*(3), 268–274. https://doi.org/10.1001/jamapsychiatry.2015.3105

Meijer, A., Conradi, H. J., Bos, E. H., Thombs, B. D., van Melle, J. P., & de Jonge, P. (2011). Prognostic association of depression following myocardial infarction with mortality and cardiovascular events:

A meta-analysis of 25 years of research. *General Hospital Psychiatry, 33*(3), 203–216. https://doi.org/10.1016/j.genhosppsych.2011.02.007

Meldrum, M. L., Kelly, E. L., Calderon, R., Brekke, J. S., & Braslow, J. T. (2016). Implementation status of assisted outpatient treatment Programs: A national survey. *Psychiatric Services, 67*(6), 630–635. https://doi.org/10.1176/appi.ps.201500073

Melisse, B., de Beurs, E., & van Furth, E. F. (2020). Eating disorders in the Arab world: A literature review. *Journal of Eating Disorders, 8*(1), 59.

Melnik, T., Soares, B. G. O., & Nasello, A. G. (2008). The effectiveness of psychological interventions for the treatment of erectile dysfunction: Systematic review and meta-analysis, including comparisons to sildenafil treatment, intracavernosal injection, and vacuum devices. *Journal of Sexual Medicine, 5*, 2562–2574.

Meltzer, H. Y. (2003). Suicide in schizophrenia. *Journal of Clinical Psychiatry, 64*, 1122–1125.

Melville, J. D., & Naimark, D. (2002). Punishing the insane: The verdict of guilty but mentally ill. *Journal of the American Academy of Psychiatry and the Law, 30*, 553–555.

Mendrek, A., & Mancini-Marïe, A. (2016). Sex/gender differences in the brain and cognition in schizophrenia. *Neuroscience & Biobehavioral Reviews, 67*, 57–78.

Menikoff, J., Kaneshiro, J., & Pritchard, I. (2017). The common rule, updated. *New England Journal of Medicine, 376*, 613–615.

Mennin, D. S., Heimberg, R. G., & Turk, C. L. (2004). Clinical presentation and diagnostic features. In R. G. Heimberg, C. L. Turk, & D. S. Mennin (Eds.), *Generalized anxiety disorder* (pp. 3–28). Guilford Press.

Menzies, L., Chamberlain, S. R., Laird, A. R., Thelen, S. M., Sahakian, B. J., & Bullmore, E. T. (2008). Integrating evidence from neuroimaging and neuropsychological studies of obsessive-compulsive disorder: The orbitofronto-striatal model revisited. *Neuroscience and Biobehavioral Reviews, 32*, 525–549.

Merckelbach, H., Boskovic, I., Pesy, D., Dalsklev, M., & Lynn, S. J. (2017). Symptom overreporting and dissociative experiences: A qualitative review. *Consciousness and Cognition, 49*, 132–144. https://doi.org/10.1016/j.concog.2017.01.007

Merckelbach, H., Dekkers, T., Wessel, I., & Roefs, A. (2003). Dissociative symptoms and amnesia in Dutch concentration camp survivors. *Comprehensive Psychiatry, 44*, 65–69.

Merikangas, K. R., He, J.-P., Burstein, M., Swanson, S. A., Avenevoli, S., Cui, L., et al. (2010). Lifetime prevalence of mental disorders in U.S. adolescents: Results from the National Comorbidity Survey Replication–Adolescent Supplement (NCS-A). *Journal of the American Academy of Child & Adolescent Psychiatry, 49*(10), 980–989.

Merikangas, K. R., Jin, R., He, J., Kessler, R. C., Lee, S., Sampson, N. A., et al. (2011). Prevalence and correlates of bipolar spectrum disorder in the World Mental Health Survey Initiative. *Archives of General Psychiatry, 68*, 241–251.

Merlo, L. J., Lehmkuhl, H. D., Geffken, G. R., & Storch, E. A. (2009). Decreased family accommodation associated with improved therapy outcome in pediatric obsessive-compulsive disorder. *Journal of Consulting and Clinical Psychology, 77*(2), 355–360. https://doi.org/10.1037/A0012652

Meston, C. M., & Buss, D. (2009). *Why women have sex: Women reveal the truth about their sex lives, from adventure to revenge (and everything in between)*. St. Martin's Press.

Meston, C. M., & Gorzalka, B. B. (1995). The effects of sympathetic activation on physiological and subjective sexual arousal in women. *Behaviour Research and Therapy, 33*, 651–664.

Meyer, B., Johnson, S. L., & Winters, R. (2001). Responsiveness to threat and incentive in bipolar disorder: Relations of the BIS/BAS scales with symptoms. *Journal of Psychopathology and Behavioral Assessment, 23*, 133–143.

Meyer, V. (1966). Modification of expectations in cases with obsessional rituals. *Behaviour Research and Therapy, 4,* 273–280.

Micale, V., Kucerova, J., & Sulcova, A. (2013). Leading compounds for the validation of animal models of psychopathology. *Cell and Tissue Research, 354*(1), 309–330. https://doi.org/10.1007/s00441-013-1692-9

Michael, T., Blechert, J., Vriends, N., Margraf, J., & Wilhelm, F. H. (2007). Fear conditioning in panic disorder: Enhanced resistance to extinction. *Journal of Abnormal Psychology, 116,* 612–617.

Michal, M., Adler, J., Wiltink, J., Reiner, I., Tschan, R., Wölfling, K., et al. (2016). A case series of 223 patients with depersonalization-derealization syndrome. *BMC Psychiatry, 16,* 11.

Miech, R. A., Johnston, L. D., O'Malley, P. M., Bachman, J. G., Schulenberg, J. E., & Patrick, M. E. (2020). *Monitoring the future national survey results on drug use, 1975–2019: Volume I, Secondary school students.* Institute for Social Research, The University of Michigan.

Miech, R. A., Johnston, L. D., Patrick, M. E., O'Malley, P. M., Bachman, J. G., & Schulenberg, J. E. (2023). *Monitoring the future national survey results on drug use, 1975–2022: Secondary school students.* Monitoring the Future Monograph Series. Institute for Social Research, University of Michigan. https://monitoringthefuture.org/results/publications/monographs/

Miech, R. A., Johnston, L. D., Patrick, M. E., O'Malley, P. M., Bachman, J. G., & Schulenberg, J. E. (2023). Monitoring the future national survey results on drug use, 1975–2022: Secondary school students. University of Michigan Institute for Social Research. https://monitoringthefuture.org/wp-content/uploads/2022/12/mtf2022.pdf

Miech, R., Johnston, L., O'Malley, P. M., Bachman, J. G., & Patrick, M. E. (2019). Trends in adolescent vaping, 2017–2019. *New England Journal of Medicine, 381*(15), 1490–1491. https://doi.org/10.1056/NEJMc1910739

Miech, R., Patrick, M. E., O'Malley, P. M., & Johnston, L. D. (2017). E-cigarette use as a predictor of cigarette smoking: Results from a 1-year follow-up of a national sample of 12th grade students. *Tobacco Control, 26*(e2), e106–e111. https://doi.org/10.1136/tobaccocontrol-2016-053291

Miers, A. C., Blöte, A. W., Bokhorst, C. L., & Westenberg, M. (2009). Negative self-evaluations and the relation to performance level in socially anxious children and adolescents. *Behaviour Research and Therapy, 47,* 1043–1049.

Miers, A. C., Blöte, A. W., Heyne, D. A., & Westenberg, P. M. (2014). Developmental pathways of social avoidance across adolescence: The role of social anxiety and negative cognition. *Journal of Anxiety Disorders, 28*(8), 787–794. https://doi.org/10.1016/j.janxdis.2014.09.008

Mikami, A. Y., Huang-Pollack, C. L., Pfiffner, L. J., McBurnett, K., & Hangai, D. (2007). Social skills differences among attention-deficit/hyperactivity disorder types in a chat room assessment task. *Journal of Abnormal Child Psychology, 35,* 509–521.

Mikami, A. Y., Miller, M., & Lerner, M. D. (2019). Social functioning in youth with attention-deficit/hyperactivity disorder and autism spectrum disorder: Transdiagnostic commonalities and differences. *Clinical Psychology Review, 68,* 54–70.

Mikami, A. Y., Szwedo, D. E., Ahmad, S. I., Samuels, A. S., & Hinshaw, S. P. (2015). Online social communication patterns among emerging adult women with histories of childhood attention-deficit/hyperactivity disorder. *Journal of Abnormal Psychology, 124*(3), 576–588. https://doi.org/10.1037/abn0000053

Mikhail, M. E., Keel, P. K., Burt, S. A., Neale, M., Boker, S., & Klump, K. L. (2020). Low emotion differentiation: An affective correlate of binge eating? *International Journal of Eating Disorders, 53*(3), 412–421. https://doi.org/10.1002/eat.23207

Miklowitz, D. J., Efthimiou, O., Furukawa, T. A., Scott, J., McLaren, R., Geddes, J. R., & Cipriani, A. (2021). Adjunctive psychotherapy for bipolar disorder: A systematic review and component network meta-analysis. *JAMA Psychiatry, 78*(2), 141–150. https://doi.org/10.1001/jamapsychiatry.2020.2993

Miklowitz, D. J., George, E. L., Richards, J. A., Simoneau, T. L., & Suddath, R. L. (2003). A randomized study of family-focused psychoeducation and pharmacotherapy in the outpatient management of bipolar disorder. *Archives of General Psychiatry, 60,* 904–912.

Miklowitz, D. J., & Goldstein, M. J. (1997). *Bipolar disorder: A family-focused treatment approach* (2nd ed.). Guilford Press.

Miklowitz, D. J., Otto, M. W., Frank, E., Reilly-Harrington, N. A., Wisniewski, S. R., Kogan, J. N., et al. (2007). Psychosocial treatments for bipolar depression: A 1-year randomized trial from the systematic treatment enhancement program. *Archives of General Psychiatry, 64,* 419–427.

Miklowitz, D. J., & Taylor, D.O. (2005). Family-focused treatment of the suicidal bipolar patient. Unpublished manuscript.

Miller, J. D., Lamkin, J., Maples-Keller, J. L., & Lynam, D. R. (2016). Viewing the triarchic model of psychopathy through general personality and expert-based lenses. *Personality Disorders: Theory, Research, and Treatment, 7,* 247–258. https://doi.org/10.1037/per0000155

Miller, J. D., & Lynam, D. R. (2012). An examination of the Psychopathic Personality Inventory's nomological network: A meta-analytic review. *Personality Disorders: Theory, Research, and Treatment, 3,* 305–326. https://doi.org/10.1037/a0024567

Miller, J. D., Lynam, D. R., Hyatt, C. S., & Campbell, W. K. (2017). Controversies in narcissism. *Annual Review of Clinical Psychology, 13,* 291–315. https://doi.org/10.1146/annurev-clinpsy-032816-045244

Miller-Johnson, S., Coie, J. D., Maumary-Gremaud, A., & Bierman, K. (2002). Peer rejection and aggression and early starter models of conduct disorder. *Journal of Abnormal Child Psychology, 30*(3), 217–230.

Miller, T. J., McGlashan, T. H., Rosen, J. L., Somjee, L., Markovich, P. J., Stein, K., et al. (2002). Prospective diagnosis of the initial prodrome for schizophrenia based on the structured interview for prodromal syndromes: Preliminary evidence of interrater reliability and predictive validity. *American Journal of Psychiatry, 159,* 863–865.

Miller, T. Q., & Volk, R. J. (1996). Weekly marijuana use as a risk factor for initial cocaine use: Results from a six wave national survey. *Journal of Child and Adolescent Substance Abuse, 5,* 55–78.

Miller, W. R., & Rollnick, S. (Eds.). (1991). *Motivational interviewing: Preparing people to change addictive behavior.* Guilford Press.

Millon, T. (1996). *Disorders of personality: DSM-IV and beyond* (2nd ed.). John Wiley & Sons.

Mineka, S., & Öhman, A. (2002a). Born to fear: Nonassociative vs. associative factors in the etiology of phobias. *Behaviour Research and Therapy, 40,* 173–184.

Mineka, S., & Öhman, A. (2002b). Phobias and preparedness: The selective, automatic, and encapsulated nature of fear. In *Biological Psychiatry* (Vol. 52, Issue 10, pp. 927–937). Elsevier. https://doi.org/10.1016/S0006-3223(02)01669-4

Mineka, S., & Sutton, J. (2006). Contemporary learning theory perspectives on the etiology of fear and phobias. In M. G. Craske, D. Hermans, & D. Vansteenwegen (Eds.), *Fear and learning: From basic processes to clinical implications* (pp. 75–97). American Psychological Association.

Mineka, S., Williams, A. L., Wolitzky-Taylor, K., Vrshek-Schallhorn, S., Craske, M. G., Hammen, C., et al. (2020). Five-year prospective neuroticism–stress effects on major depressive episodes: Primarily additive effects of the general neuroticism factor and stress. *Journal of Abnormal Psychology.* https://doi.org/10.1037/abn0000530

Mineka, S., Williams, A. L., Wolitzky-Taylor, K., Vrshek-Schallhorn, S., Craske, M. G., Hammen, C., et al. (2020). Five-year prospective neuroticism–stress effects on major depressive episodes: Primarily additive effects of the general neuroticism factor and stress. *Journal of Abnormal Psychology.* https://doi.org/10.1037/abn0000530

Mineka, S., & Zinbarg, R. (1998). Experimental approaches to the anxiety and mood disorders. In J. G. Adair, D. Belanger, & K. L. Dion (Eds.), *Advances in psychological science, Volume 1: Social personal and cultural aspects* (pp. 429–454). Psychology Press.

Mineka, S., & Zinbarg, R. (2006). A contemporary learning theory perspective on the etiology of anxiety disorders: It's not what you thought it was. *The American Psychologist, 61,* 10–26.

Mirsky, A. F., Bieliauskas, L. A., Duncan, C. C., & French, L. M. (2013). Letter to the editor. *Schizophrenia Research, 148*(1–3), 186–187.

Mitchell, A. J., & Shiri-Feshki, M. (2009). Rate of progression of mild cognitive impairment to dementia—Meta-analysis of 41 robust inception cohort studies. *Acta Psychiatrica Scandinavica, 119,* 252–265. https://doi.org/10.1111/j.1600-0447.2008.01326.x

Mitchell, J. M., Bogenschutz, M., Lilienstein, A., Harrison, C., Kleiman, S., Parker-Guilbert, K., et al. (2021). MDMA-assisted therapy for severe PTSD: A randomized, double-blind, placebo-controlled phase 3 study. *Nature Medicine, 27*(6), 1025–1033.

Mitchell, K. R., Jones, K. G., Wellings, K., Johnson, A. M., Graham, C. A., Datta, J., et al. (2016). Estimating the prevalence of sexual function problems: The impact of morbidity criteria. *Journal of Sex Research, 53*(8), 955–967. https://doi.org/10.1080/00224499.2015.1089214

Mittal, V. A., Ellman, L. M., & Cannon, T.D. (2008). Gene-environment interaction and covariation in schizophrenia: The role of obstetric complications. *Schizophrenia Bulletin, 34,* 1083–1094.

Moberg, C. A., Bradford, D. E., Kaye, J. T., & Curtin, J. J. (2017). Increased startle potentiation to unpredictable stressors in alcohol dependence: Possible stress neuroadaptation in humans. *Journal of Abnormal Psychology, 126,* 441–453. https://doi.org/10.1037/abn0000265

Moffitt, T. E. (1993). Adolescence-limited and life-course-persistent antisocial behavior: A developmental taxonomy. *Psychological Review, 100,* 674–701.

Moffitt, T. E. (2007). A review of research on the taxonomy of life-course persistent versus adolescence-limited antisocial behavior. In D. J. Flannery, A. T. Vazsonyi, & I. D. Waldman (Eds.), *The Cambridge handbook of violent behavior and aggression* (pp. 49–74). Cambridge University Press.

Moffitt, T. E., Caspi, A., Harrington, H., & Milne, B. J. (2002). Males on the life-course persistent and adolescence-limited antisocial pathways: Follow-up at age 26. *Development and Psychopathology, 14,* 179–207.

Moffitt, T. E., Caspi, A., Harrington, H., Milne, B. J., Melchior, M., Goldberg, D., et al. (2007). Generalized anxiety disorder and depression: Childhood risk factors in a birth cohort followed to age 32. *Psychological Medicine, 37,* 441–452.

Moffitt, T. E., Caspi, A., Taylor, A., Kokaua, J., Milne, B. J., Polanczyk, G., et al. (2010). How common are common mental disorders? Evidence that lifetime prevalence rates are doubled by prospective versus retrospective ascertainment. *Psychological Medicine, 40*(6), 899–909. https://doi.org/10.1017/S0033291709991036

Moffitt, T. E., Caspi, A., Taylor, A., Kokaua, J., Milne, B. J., Polanczyk, G., et al. (2010). How common are common mental disorders? Evidence that lifetime prevalence rates are doubled by prospective versus retrospective ascertainment. *Psychological Medicine, 40*(6), 899–909. https://doi.org/10.1017/S0033291709991036

Moffitt, T. E., Caspi, A., Taylor, A., Kokaua, J., Milne, B. J., Polanczyk, G., et al. (2010). How common are common mental disorders? Evidence that lifetime prevalence rates are doubled by prospective versus retrospective ascertainment. *Psychological Medicine, 40*(6), 899–909. https://doi.org/10.1017/S0033291709991036

Mogensen, H., Möller, J., Hultin, H., & Mittendorfer-Rutz, E. (2016). Death of a close relative and the risk of suicide in Sweden—A large scale register-based case-crossover study. *PloS One, 11*(10), e0164274. https://doi.org/10.1371/journal.pone.0164274

Mohajerin, B., Lynn, S. J., Bakhtiyari, M., & Dolatshah, B. (2020). Evaluating the Unified Protocol in the Treatment of Dissociative Identify Disorder. *Cognitive and Behavioral Practice, 27*(3), 270–289. https://doi.org/10.1016/J.CBPRA.2019.07.012

Mojtabai, R., Stuart, E. A., Hwang, I., Susukida, R., Eaton, W. W., Sampson, N., et al. (2015). Long-term effects of mental disorders on employment in the National Comorbidity Survey ten-year follow-up. *Social Psychiatry and Psychiatric Epidemiology, 50*(11), 1657–1668. https://doi.org/10.1007/s00127-015-1097-z

Mokros, A., & Banse, R. (2019). The "Dunkelfeld" project for self-identified pedophiles: A reappraisal of its effectiveness. *The Journal of Sexual Medicine, 16*(5), 609–613. https://doi.org/10.1016/J.JSXM.2019.02.009

Molina, B. S. G., Hinshaw, S. P., Swanson, J. M., Arnold, L. E., Vitiello, B., Jensen, P. S., et al. (2009). The MTA at 8 years: Prospective follow-up of children treated for combined-type ADHD in a multisite study. *Journal of the American Academy of Child and Adolescent Psychiatry, 48,* 484–500.

Molina, B. S., Hinshaw, S. P., Eugene Arnold, L., Swanson, J. M., Pelham, W. E., Hechtman, L., et al. (2013). Adolescent substance use in the multimodal treatment study of attention-deficit/hyper-activity disorder (ADHD) (MTA) as a function of childhood ADHD, random assignment to childhood treatments, and subsequent medication. *Journal of the American Academy of Child and Adolescent Psychiatry, 52*(3), 250–263.

Monahan, J. (1984). The prediction of violent behavior: Toward a second generation of theory and policy. *American Journal of Psychiatry, 141,* 10–15.

Monahan, J. (1992). Mental disorder and violent behavior: Perceptions and evidence. *American Psychologist, 47,* 511–521.

Monahan, J., & Steadman, H. (1994). Toward a rejuvenation of risk assessment research. In J. Monahan & H. Steadman (Eds.), *Violence and mental disorder: Developments in risk assessment.* University of Chicago Press.

Moniz, E. (1936). *Tentatives operatoires dans le traitement de certaines psychoses.* Mason.

Monroe, S. M., & Harkness, K. L. (2022). Major depression and its recurrences: Life course matters. *Annual Review of Clinical Psychology, 18*(1), 329–357. https://doi.org/10.1146/annurev-clinpsy-072220-021440

Monstrey, S., Vercruysse, H., & De Cuypere, G. (2009). Is gender reassignment surgery evidence based? Recommendation for the seventh version of the WPATH Standards of Care. *International Journal of Transgenderism, 11,* 206–214. https://doi.org/10.1080/15532730903383799

Monteleone, A. M., Pellegrino, F., Croatto, G., Carfagno, M., Hilbert, A., Treasure, J., et al. (2022). Treatment of eating disorders: A systematic meta-review of meta-analyses and network meta-analyses. *Neuroscience & Biobehavioral Reviews, 142,* 104857.

Montgomery, S. C. (2018). *American Foundation for Suicide Prevention resources for journalists.* https://afsp.org/for-journalists#resources-for-reporting-on-suicide

Monzani, B., Rijsdijk, F., Harris, J., & Mataix-Cols, D. (2014). The structure of genetic and environmental risk factors for dimensional representations of DSM-5 obsessive-compulsive spectrum disorders. *JAMA Psychiatry, 71*(2), 182–189. https://doi.org/10.1001/jamapsychiatry.2013.3524

Mooldijk, S. S., Licher, S., & Wolters, F. J. (2021). Characterizing demographic, racial, and geographic diversity in dementia research: A systematic review. *JAMA Neurology, 78*(10), 1255–1261. https://doi.org/10.1001/jamaneurol.2021.2943

Moore, A. A., Blair, R. J., Hettema, J. M., & Roberson-Nay, R. (2019). The genetic underpinnings of callous-unemotional traits: A systematic research review. *Neuroscience and Biobehavioral Reviews, 100*, 85–97. https://doi.org/10.1016/j.neubiorev.2019.02.018

Moore, A. A., Silberg, J. L., Roberson-Nay, R., & Mezuk, B. (2017). Life course persistent and adolescence limited conduct disorder in a nationally representative US sample: Prevalence, predictors, and outcomes. *Social Psychiatry and Psychiatric Epidemiology, 52*(4), 435–443. https://doi.org/10.1007/s00127-017-1337-5

Moore, K. M., Nicholas, J., Grossman, M., McMillan, C. T., Irwin, D. J., Massimo, L., et al. (2020). Age at symptom onset and death and disease duration in genetic frontotemporal dementia: An international retrospective cohort study. *The Lancet Neurology, 19*(2), 145–156. https://doi.org/10.1016/S1474-4422(19)30394-1

Moore, T. H. M., Zammit, S., Lingford-Hughes, A., Barnes, T. R. E., Jones, P. B., Burke, M., et al. (2007). Cannabis use and risk of psychotic or affective mental health outcomes: A systematic review. *The Lancet, 370*, 319–328.

Morales, I., & Berridge, K. C. (2020). "Liking" and "wanting" in eating and food reward: Brain mechanisms and clinical implications. *Physiology & Behavior, 227*, 113152.

Moran, E. K., Prevost, C., Culbreth, A. J., & Barch, D. M. (2023). Effort-cost decision-making in psychotic and mood disorders. *Journal of Psychopathology and Clinical Science, 132*(4), 490–498. https://doi.org/10.1037/abn0000822

Moreland, K., Wing, S., Diez Roux, A., & Poole, C. (2002). Neighborhood characteristics associated with the location of food stores and food services places. *American Journal of Preventive Medicine, 22*, 23–29.

Moreland-Russell, S., Harris, J., Snider, D., Walsh, H., Cyr, J., & Barnoya, J. (2013). Disparities and menthol marketing: Additional evidence in support of point of sale policies. *International Journal of Environmental Research and Public Health, 10*, 4571–4583. https://doi.org/10.3390/ijerph10104571

Morey, L. C., Krueger, R. F., & Skodol, A. E. (2013). The hierarchical structure of clinician ratings of proposed DSM–5 pathological personality traits. *Journal of Abnormal Psychology, 122*, 836–841. https://doi.org/10.1037/a0034003

Morf, C. C., & Rhodewalt, F. (2001). Unraveling the paradoxes of narcissism: A dynamic self-regulatory processing model. *Psychological Inquiry, 12*, 177–196.

Morgan, C. A. I., Hazlett, G., Wang, S., Richardson, E. G. J., Schnurr, P., & Southwick, S. M. (2001). Symptoms of dissociation in humans experiencing acute, uncontrollable stress: A prospective investigation. *American Journal of Psychiatry, 158*, 1239–1247.

Morgan, M. J. (2000). Ecstasy (MDMA): A review of its possible persistent psychological effects. *Psychopharmacology, 152*, 230–248.

Morgan, V. A., Mitchell, P. B., & Jablensky, A. V. (2005). The epidemiology of bipolar disorder: Sociodemographic, disability and service utilization data from the Australian National Study of low prevalence (psychotic) disorders. *Bipolar Disorders, 7*(4), 326–337. https://doi.org/10.1111/j.1399-5618.2005.00229.x

Morina, N., Koerssen, R., & Pollet, T. V. (2016). Interventions for children and adolescents with posttraumatic stress disorder: A meta-analysis of comparative outcome studies. *Clinical Psychology Review, 47*, 41–54. https://doi.org/10.1016/j.cpr.2016.05.006

Morina, N., Wicherts, J. M., Lobbrecht, J., & Priebe, S. (2014). Remission from post-traumatic stress disorder in adults: a systematic review and meta-analysis of long term outcome studies. *Clinical Psychology Review, 34*(3), 249–255. https://doi.org/10.1016/J.CPR.2014.03.002

Morland, L. A., Glassman, L. H., Greene, C. J., Hoffman, J. E., & Rosen, C. (2021). Treating PTSD using telemental health technology. In M. J. Friedman, P. P. Schnurr, & T. M. Keane (Eds.), *Handbook of PTSD: Science and practice* (3rd ed., pp. 535–550). Guilford Press.

Moroney, J. T., Tang, M. X., Berglund, L., Small, S., Merchant, C., Bell, K., et al. (1999). Low-density lipoprotein cholesterol and the risk of dementia with stroke. *Journal of American Medical Association, 282*, 254–260.

Mortberg, E., Clark, D. M., & Bejerot, S. (2011). Intensive group cognitive therapy and individual cognitive therapy for social phobia: Sustained improvement at 5-year follow-up. *Journal of Anxiety Disorders, 25*, 994–1000.

Moser, C., & Kleinplatz, P. J. (2020). Conceptualization, history, and future of the paraphilias. *Annual Review of Clinical Psychology, 16*(1). https://doi.org/10.1146/annurev-clinpsy-050718-095548

Mowrer, O. H. (1947). On the dual nature of learning: A reinterpretation of "conditioning" and "problem-solving." *Harvard Educational Review, 17*, 102–148.

Moyer, C. E., Shelton, M. A., & Sweet, R. A. (2015). Dendritic spine alterations in schizophrenia. *Dendritic Spine Dysgenesis in Neuropsychiatric Disease, 601*, 46–53.

MTA Cooperative Group. (1999a). A 14-month randomized clinical trial of treatment strategies for attention-deficit/hyperactivity disorder. *Archives of General Psychiatry, 56*, 1073–1086.

MTA Cooperative Group. (1999b). Moderators and mediators of treatment response for children with attention-deficit/hyperactivity disorder. *Archives of General Psychiatry, 56*, 1088–1096.

Muehlenhard, C. L., & Shippee, S. K. (2010). Men's and women's reports of pretending orgasm. *Journal of Sex Research, 47*, 552–567.

Muehlenkamp, J. J., Claes, L., Havertape, L., & Plener, P. L. (2012). International prevalence of adolescent non-suicidal self-injury and deliberate self-harm. *Child and Adolescent Psychiatry and Mental Health, 6*, 10–10. https://doi.org/10.1186/1753-2000-6-10

Mueller, A., Hong, D. S., Shepard, S., & Moore, T. (2017). Linking ADHD to the neural circuitry of attention. *Trends in Cognitive Sciences, 21*(6), 474–488.

Mueller-Pfeiffer, C., Rufibach, K., Perron, N., Wyss, D., Kuenzler, C., Prezewowsky, C., et al. (2012). Global functioning and disability in dissociative disorders. *Psychiatry Research, 200*, 475–481.

Mueser, K. T., Deavers, F., Penn, D. L., & Cassisi, J. E. (2013). Psychosocial treatments for schizophrenia. *Annual Review of Clinical Psychology, 9*, 465–497.

Mueser, K. T., Penn, D. L., Addington, J., Brunette, M. F., Gingerich, S., Glynn, S. M., et al. (2015). The NAVIGATE program for first-episode psychosis: Rationale, overview, and description of psychosocial components. *Psychiatric Services, 66*, 680–690. https://doi.org/10.1176/appi.ps.201400413

Mukherjee, S. (2016). *The gene: An intimate history.* Scribner.

Mullard, A. (2021). Landmark Alzheimer's drug approval confounds research community. *Nature, 594*(7863), 309–310. https://doi.org/10.1038/D41586-021-01546-2

Müller, R.-A., & Fishman, I. (2018). Brain connectivity and neuroimaging of social networks in autism. *Trends in Cognitive Sciences, 22*(12), 1103–1116.

Mullins-Sweatt, S. N., DeShong, H. L., Lengel, G. J., Helle, A. C., & Krueger, R. F. (2019). Disinhibition as a unifying construct in understanding how personality dispositions undergird psychopathology. *Journal of Research in Personality, 80*, 55–61. https://doi.org/10.1016/j.jrp.2019.04.006

Mulsant, B. H., & Pollock, B. G. (2015). Psychopharmacology. In D. C. Steffens, D. G. Blazer, & M. E. Thakur (Eds.), *The American Psychiatric Publishing textbook of geriatric psychiatry.* American Psychiatric Publishing.

Munetz, M. R., Grande, T., Kleist, J., & Peterson, G. A. (1996). The effectiveness of outpatient civil commitment. *Psychiatric Services, 47*, 1251–1253.

Munro, S., Thomas, K. L., & Abu-Shaar, M. (1993). Molecular characterization of a peripheral receptor for cannabinoids. *Nature, 365*, 61–65.

Murphy, J. (1976). Psychiatric labeling in cross-cultural perspective. *Science, 191*, 1019–1028.

Murphy, J. A., & Byrne, G. J. (2012). Prevalence and correlates of the proposed DSM-5 diagnosis of chronic depressive disorder. *Journal of Affective Disorders, 139*(2), 172–180. https://doi.org/10.1016/j.jad.2012.01.033

Murphy, S. E. (2017). Nicotine metabolism and smoking: Ethnic differences in the role of P450 2A6. *Chemical Research in Toxicology, 30*, 410–419. https://doi.org/10.1021/acs.chemrestox.6b00387

Murray-Close, D., Hoza, B., Hinshaw, S. P., Arnold, L. E., Swanson, J., Jensen, P. S., et al. (2010). Developmental processes in peer problems of children with attention-deficit/hyperactivity disorder in the Multimodal Treatment Study of Children with ADHD: Developmental cascades and vicious cycles. *Developmental and Psychopathology, 22*, 785–802.

Murray, G. K., Lin, T., Austin, J., McGrath, J. J., Hickie, I. B., & Wray, N. R. (2021). Could polygenic risk scores be useful in psychiatry?: A review. *JAMA Psychiatry, 78*(2), 210–219. https://doi.org/10.1001/jamapsychiatry.2020.3042

Murray, R. M., Bhavsar, V., Tripoli, G., & Howes, O. (2017). 30 years on: How the neurodevelopmental hypothesis of schizophrenia morphed into the developmental risk factor model of psychosis. *Schizophrenia Bulletin, 43*(6), 1190–1196.

Murray, S. B., Nagata, J. M., Griffiths, S., Calzo, J. P., Brown, T. A., Mitchison, D., et al. (2017). The enigma of male eating disorders: A critical review and synthesis. *Clinical Psychology Review, 57*, 1–11.

Muse, K., McManus, F., Hackmann, A., & Williams, M. (2010). Intrusive imagery in severe health anxiety: Prevalence, nature and links with memories and maintenance cycles. *Behaviour Research and Therapy, 48*, 792–798.

Mustonen, T. K., Spencer, S. M., Hoskinson, R. A., Sachs, D. P. L., & Garvey, A. J. (2005). The influence of gender, race, and menthol content on tobacco exposure measures. *Nicotine and Tobacco Research, 7*, 581–590.

Myin-Germeys, I., van Os, J., Schwartz, J. E., Stone, A. A., & Delespaul, P. A. (2001). Emotional reactivity to daily life stress in schizophrenia. *Archives of General Psychiatry, 58*, 1137–1144.

Nagayama Hall, G. C., & Huang, E. R. (2020). Behavioral health service delivery with Asian Americans. In L. T. Benuto, F. R. Gonzalez, & J. Singer (Eds.), *Handbook of cultural factors in behavioral health* (pp. 131–142). Springer International Publishing. https://doi.org/10.1007/978-3-030-32229-8_10

Nagendra, A., Weiss, D. M., Merritt, C., Cather, C., Sosoo, E. E., Mueser, K. T., et al. (2023). Clinical and psychosocial outcomes of Black Americans in the Recovery After an Initial Schizophrenia Episode Early Treatment Program (RAISE-ETP) study. *Social Psychiatry and Psychiatric Epidemiology, 58*(1), 77–89.

Nakai, Y., Nin, K., Noma, S., Teramukai, S., Fujikawa, K., & Wonderlich, S. A. (2018). Changing profile of eating disorders between 1963 and 2004 in a Japanese sample. *International Journal of Eating Disorders, 51*(8), 953–958. https://doi.org/10.1002/eat.22935

Naragon-Gainey, K. (2010). Meta-analysis of the relations of anxiety sensitivity to the depressive and anxiety disorders. *Psychological Bulletin, 136*(1), 128–150. https://doi.org/10.1037/a0018055

Natale, M., Entin, E., & Jaffe, J. (1979). Vocal interruptions in dyadic communication as a function of speech and social anxiety. *Journal of Personality and Social Psychology, 37*(6), 865–878. https://doi.org/10.1037/0022-3514.37.6.865

Nathan, D. (2011). *Sybil exposed: The extraordinary story behind the famous multiple personality case.* Free Press.

Nathan, P. E., & Gorman, J. M. (2015). Challenges to implementing evidence-based treatments. In P. E. Nathan & J. M. Gorman (Eds.), *A guide to treatments that work* (4th ed.). Oxford University Press

National Academies of Sciences, Engineering, and Math. (2019). Reproducibility and replicability in science. In *Reproducibility and Replicability in Science*. Washington, DC: National Academies Press. https://doi.org/10.17226/25303

National Academies of Sciences, Engineering, and Medicine. (2017). *The health effects of cannabis and cannabinoids: The current state of evidence and recommendations for research.* The National Academies Press. https://doi.org/10.17226/24625

National Academies of Sciences, Engineering, and Medicine. (2018). *Public health consequences of e-cigarettes.* The National Academies Press. https://doi.org/10.17226/24952

National Academies of Sciences, Engineering, and Medicine. (2019). *Medications for opioid use disorder save lives.* Washington, DC: The National Academies Press. https://doi.org/10.17226/25310

National Center for Health Statistics (NCHS). (2023). https://www.cdc.gov/nchs/nvss/vsrr/drug-overdose-data.htm#source

National Collaborating Centre for Mental Health. (2017). Eating disorders: Recognition and treatment. https://www.nice.org.uk/guidance/ng69

NCD Risk Factor Collaboration (NCD-RisC). (2017). Worldwide trends in body-mass index, underweight, overweight, and obesity from 1975 to 2016: A pooled analysis of 2416 population-based measurement studies in 128•9 million children, adolescents, and adults. *Lancet (London, England), 390*(10113), 2627–2642. https://doi.org/10.1016/S0140-6736(17)32129-3

Neale, J. M., & Oltmanns, T. (1980). *Schizophrenia.* John Wiley & Sons.

Neal, T. M. S. (2018). Forensic psychology and correctional psychology: Distinct but related subfields of psychological science and practice. *American Psychologist, 73*, 651–662. https://doi.org/10.1037/amp0000227.

Neff, R. A., Wang, M., Vatansever, S., Guo, L., Ming, C., Wang, Q., et al. (2021). Molecular subtyping of Alzheimer's disease using RNA sequencing data reveals novel mechanisms and targets. *Science Advances, 7*(2). https://doi.org/10.1126/sciadv.abb5398

Neisser, U. (1976). *Cognition and reality.* Freeman.

Nelson, E. C., Heath, A. C., Madden, P. A. F., Cooper, M. L., Dinwiddie, S. H., Bucholz, K. K., et al. (2002). Association between self-reported childhood sexual abuse and adverse psychosocial outcomes: Results from a twin study. *Archives of General Psychiatry, 59*, 139–145.

Nelson, E. C., Heath, A. C., Madden, P. A. F., Cooper, M. L., Dinwiddie, S. H., Bucholz, K. K., et al. (2002). Association between self-reported childhood sexual abuse and adverse psychosocial outcomes: Results from a twin study. *Archives of General Psychiatry, 59*, 139–145.

Nelson, J. C. (2006). The STAR*D study: A four-course meal that leaves us wanting more. *American Journal of Psychiatry, 163*, 1864–1866.

Nelson, L. D., Simmons, J., & Simonsohn, U. (2018). Psychology's renaissance. *Annual Review of Psychology, 69*, 511–534. https://doi.org/10.1146/ANNUREV-PSYCH-122216-011836

Neugebauer, R. (1979). Mediaeval and early modern theories of mental illness. *Archives of General Psychiatry, 36*, 477–484.

Neumeister, A., Daher, R. J., & Charney, D. S. (2005). Anxiety disorders: Noradrenergic neurotransmission. *Handbook of Experimental Pharmacology, 169*, 205–223.

Newby, J. M., Smith, J., Uppal, S., Mason, E., Mahoney, A. E. J., & Andrews, G. (2018). Internet-based cognitive behavioral therapy versus psychoeducation control for illness anxiety disorder and somatic symptom disorder: A randomized controlled trial. *Journal of Consulting and Clinical Psychology, 86*(1), 89–98. https://doi.org/10.1037/ccp0000248

Newcomb, E. T., & Hagopian, L. P. (2018). Treatment of severe problem behaviour in children with autism spectrum disorder and intellectual disabilities. *International Review of Psychiatry, 30*(1), 96–109. https://doi.org/10.1080/09540261.2018.1435513

Newlands, R. T., Brito, J., & Denning, D. M. (2020). Cultural considerations in the treatment of sexual dysfunction. *Handbook of Cultural Factors in Behavioral Health*, 345–361. https://doi.org/10.1007/978-3-030-32229-8_25

Newman, M. G., & Llera, S. J. (2011). A novel theory of experiential avoidance in generalized anxiety disorder: A review and synthesis of research supporting a contrast avoidance model of worry. *Clinical Psychology Review, 31*(3), 371–382. https://doi.org/10.1016/j.cpr.2011.01.008

Newman, M. G., Rackoff, G. N., Zhu, Y., & Kim, H. (2023). A transdiagnostic evaluation of contrast avoidance across generalized anxiety disorder, major depressive disorder, and social anxiety disorder. *Journal of Anxiety Disorders, 93*, 102662.

Newton-Howes, G., Tyrer, P., Anagnostakis, K., Cooper, S., Bowden-Jones, O., & Weaver, T. (2010). The prevalence of personality disorder, its comorbidity with mental state disorders, and its clinical significance in community mental health teams. *Social Psychiatry and Psychiatric Epidemiology, 45*, 453–460.

Newton-Howes, G., Tyrer, P., & Johnson, T. (2006). Personality disorder and the outcome of depression: Meta-analysis of published studies. *British Journal of Psychiatry, 188*, 13–20.

Ng, M., Fleming, T., Robinson, M., Thomson, B., Graetz, N., Margono, C., et al. (2014). Global, regional, and national prevalence of overweight and obesity in children and adults during 1980–2013: A systematic analysis for the Global Burden of Disease Study 2013. *The Lancet.* https://doi.org/10.1016/S0140-6736(14)60460-8

Ng, T. H., Alloy, L. B., & Smith, D. V. (2019). Meta-analysis of reward processing in major depressive disorder reveals distinct abnormalities within the reward circuit. *Translational Psychiatry, 9*(1), 293. https://doi.org/10.1038/s41398-019-0644-x

Ng, T. H., Chung, K.-F., Ho, F. Y.-Y., Yeung, W.-F., Yung, K.-P., & Lam, T.-H. (2015). Sleep–wake disturbance in interepisode bipolar disorder and high-risk individuals: A systematic review and meta-analysis. *Sleep Medicine Reviews, 20*, 46–58. https://doi.org/10.1016/j.smrv.2014.06.006

Nianogo, R. A., Rosenwohl-Mack, A., Yaffe, K., Carrasco, A., Hoffmann, C. M., & Barnes, D. E. (2022). Risk factors associated with Alzheimer disease and related dementias by sex and race and ethnicity in the US. *JAMA Neurology, 79*(6), 584–591. https://doi.org/10.1001/jamaneurol.2022.0976

Nicholls, L. (2008). Putting the new view classification scheme to an empirical test. *Feminism and Psychology, 18*, 515–526.

Nichols, E., Steinmetz, J. D., Vollset, S. E., Fukutaki, K., Chalek, J., Abd-Allah, F., et al. (2022). Estimation of the global prevalence of dementia in 2019 and forecasted prevalence in 2050: An analysis for the Global Burden of Disease Study 2019. *The Lancet Public Health, 7*(2), e105–e125. https://doi.org/10.1016/S2468-2667(21)00249-8

Nicolini, H., Salin-Pascual, R., Cabrera, B., & Lanzagorta, N. (2017). Influence of culture in obsessive-compulsive disorder and its treatment. *Current Psychiatry Reviews, 13*(4), 285. https://doi.org/10.2174/2211556007666180115105935

Niederkrotenthaler, T., Fu, K.-W., Yip, P. S. F., Fong, D. Y. T., Stack, S., Cheng, Q., et al. (2012). Changes in suicide rates following media reports on celebrity suicide: A meta-analysis. *Journal of Epidemiology and Community Health, 66*(11), 1037–1042. https://doi.org/10.1136/jech-2011-200707

Nielsen, G., Stone, J., Matthews, A., Brown, M., Sparkes, C., Farmer, R., et al. (2015). Physiotherapy for functional motor disorders: A consensus recommendation. *Journal of Neurology, Neurosurgery and Psychiatry, 86*(10), 1113–1119. https://doi.org/10.1136/JNNP-2014-309255/-/DC1

Nielssen, O., Bourget, D., Laajasalo, T., Liem, M., Labelle, A., Hakkanen-Nyholm, H., et al. (2011). Homicide of strangers by people with a psychotic illness. *Schizophrenia Bulletin, 37*, 572–579.

Nigg, J. T., & Casey, B. J. (2005). An integrative theory of attention-deficit/hyperactivity disorder based on the cognitive and affective neurosciences. *Development and Psychopathology, 17*, 785–806.

Nigg, J. T., Elmore, A. L., Natarajan, N., Friderici, K. H., & Nikolas, M. A. (2016). Variation in an iron metabolism gene moderates the association between blood lead levels and attention-deficit/hyperactivity disorder in children. *Psychological Science, 27*(2), 257–269. https://doi.org/10.1177/0956797615618365

Nigg, J. T., & Goldsmith, H. H. (1994). Genetics of personality disorders: Perspectives from personality and psychopathology research. *Psychological Bulletin, 115*, 346–380.

Nigg, J. T., Lewis, K., Edinger, T., & Falk, M. (2012). Meta-analysis of attention-deficit/hyperactivity disorder or attention-deficit/hyperactivity disorder symptoms, restriction diet, and synthetic food color additives. *Journal of the American Academy of Child & Adolescent Psychiatry, 51*(1), 86–97.e8. https://doi.org/10.1016/j.jaac.2011.10.015

Nilsen, F. M., & Tulve, N. S. (2020). A systematic review and meta-analysis examining the interrelationships between chemical and non-chemical stressors and inherent characteristics in children with ADHD. *Environmental Research, 180*, 108884.

Nobre, P. J., & Pinto-Gouveia, J. (2008). Cognitions, emotions, and sexual response: Analysis of the relationship among automatic thoughts, emotional responses, and sexual arousal. *Archives of Sexual Behavior, 37*, 652–661.

Nock, M. K. (2009). Why do people hurt themselves? New insights into the nature and function of self-injury. *Current Directions in Psychological Science, 18*, 78–83.

Nock, M. K. (2010). Self-injury. *Annual Review of Clinical Psychology, 6*, 339–363.

Nock, M. K., Hwang, I., Sampson, N. A., & Kessler, R. C. (2010). Mental disorders, comorbidity and suicidal behavior: Results from the National Comorbidity Survey Replication. *Molecular Psychiatry, 15*(8), 868–876.

Nock, M. K., Hwang, I., Sampson, N., Kessler, R. C., Angermeyer, M., Beautrais, A., et al. (2009). Cross-national analysis of the associations among mental disorders and suicidal behavior: Findings from the WHO world mental health surveys. *PLOS Medicine, 6*(8), e1000123–e1000123. https://doi.org/10.1371/journal.pmed.1000123

Nock, M. K., Hwang, I., Sampson, N., Kessler, R. C., Angermeyer, M., Beautrais, A., et al. (2009). Cross-national analysis of the associations among mental disorders and suicidal behavior: findings from the WHO World Mental Health Surveys. *PLoS medicine, 6*(8), e1000123. https://doi.org/10.1371/journal.pmed.1000123

Nock, M. K., Kazdin, A. E., Hiripi, E., & Kessler, R. C. (2006). Prevalence, subtypes, and correlates of DSM-IV conduct disorder in the National Comorbidity Survey Replication. *Psychological Medicine, 36*, 699–710.

Nock, M. K., & Kessler, R. C. (2006). Prevalence of and risk factors for suicide attempts versus suicide gestures: Analysis of the National Comorbidity Survey. *Journal of Abnormal Psychology, 115*(3), 616–623. https://doi.org/10.1037/0021-843X.115.3.616

Nock, M. K., & Mendes, W. B. (2008). Physiological arousal, distress tolerance, and social problem-solving deficits among adolescent self-injurers. *Journal of Consulting and Clinical Psychology, 76*, 28–38.

Nock, M. K., Prinstein, M. J., & Sterba, S. K. (2009). Revealing the form and functions of self-injurious thoughts and behaviors: A real-time ecological assessment study among adolescents and young adults. *Journal of Abnormal Psychology, 118*, 816–827.

Nolen-Hoeksema, S. (1991). Responses to depression and their effects on the duration of depressive episodes. *Journal of Abnormal Psychology, 100*, 569–582.

Nolen-Hoeksema, S. (2000). The role of rumination in depressive disorders and mixed anxiety/depressive symptoms. *Journal of Abnormal Psychology, 109*, 504–511.

Noll, S. M., & Fredrickson, B. L. (1998). A mediational model linking self-objectification, body shame, and disordered eating. *Psychology of Women Quarterly, 22*, 623–636.

Nonnemaker, J., Hersey, J., Homsi, G., Busey, A., Allen, J., & Vallone, D. (2013). Initiation with menthol cigarettes and youth smoking uptake. *Addiction, 108*, 171–178.

Noordermeer, S., & Oosterlaan, J. (2023). Attention deficit-hyperactivity disorder. In R. F. Krueger & P. H. Blaney (Eds.), *Oxford textbook of psychopathology (4th Ed.,* pp. 474–491). Oxford Academic Press.

Nordentoft, M., Mortensen, P., & Pedersen, C. (2011). Absolute risk of suicide after first hospital contact in mental disorder. *Archives of General Psychiatry, 68*(10), 1058–1064. https://doi.org/10.1001/archgenpsychiatry.2011.113

Nordsletten, A. E., Reichenberg, A., Hatch, S. L., de la Cruz, L. F., Pertusa, A., Hotopf, M., et al. (2013). Epidemiology of hoarding disorder. *British Journal of Psychiatry, 203*, 445–452.

North, M. S., & Fiske, S. T. (2015). Modern attitudes toward older adults in the aging world: A cross-cultural meta-analysis. *Psychological Bulletin, 141*, 993–1021. https://doi.org/10.1037/a0039469

Norton, M. C., Skoog, I., Toone, L., Corcoran, C., Tschanz, J. T., Lisota, R. D., et al. (2006). Three-year incidence of first-onset depressive syndrome in a population sample of older adults: The Cache County Study. *American Journal of Geriatric Psychiatry, 14*, 237–245.

Nuss, P. (2015). Anxiety disorders and GABA neurotransmission: A disturbance of modulation. *Neuropsychiatric Disorders and Treatment, 11*, 165–175. https://doi.org/10.2147/ndt.s58841

Nutt, D., Erritzoe, D., & Carhart-Harris, R. (2020). Psychedelic psychiatry's brave new world. *Cell, 181*(1), 24–28.

Obbels, J., Vansteelandt, K., Verwijk, E., Dols, A., Bouckaert, F., Oudega, M. L., et al. (2019). MMSE changes during and after ECT in late-life depression: A prospective study. *American Journal of Geriatric Psychiatry, 27*(9), 934–944. https://doi.org/10.1016/j.jagp.2019.04.006

O'Callaghan, P., McMullen, J., Shannon, C., Rafferty, H., & Black, A. (2013). A randomized controlled trial of trauma-focused cognitive behavioral therapy for sexually exploited, war-affected Congolese girls. *Journal of the American Academy of Child and Adolescent Psychiatry, 52*(4), 359–369. https://doi.org/10.1016/j.jaac.2013.01.013

Odgers, C. (2018). Smartphones are bad for some teens, not all. *Nature, 554*(7693), 432–434. https://doi.org/10.1038/d41586-018-02109-8

Odgers, C. L., & Jensen, M. R. (2020). Annual research review: Adolescent mental health in the digital age: Facts, fears, and future directions. *Journal of Child Psychology and Psychiatry, and Allied Disciplines, 61*(3), 336–348. https://doi.org/10.1111/jcpp.13190

Odgers, C. L., Moffitt, T. E., Broadbent, J. M., Dickson, N., Hancox, R. J., Harrington, H., et al. (2008). Female and male antisocial trajectories: From childhood origins to adult outcomes. *Development and Psychopathology, 20*, 673–716.

Oei, T. P. S., & Dingle, G. (2008). The effectiveness of group cognitive behavior therapy for unipolar depressive disorders. *Journal of Affective Disorders, 107*, 5–21.

Oeppen, J., & Vaupel, J. W. (2002). Broken limits to life expectancy. *Science, 296*, 1029–1031. https://doi.org/10.1126/science.1069675

O'Farrell, T. J., & Clements, K. (2012). Review of outcome research on marital and family therapy in treatment for alcoholism. *Journal of Marital and Family Therapy, 38*, 122–144. https://doi.org/10.1111/j.1752-0606.2011.00242.x

Ogloff, J. R. P., Cutajar, M. C., Mann, E., & Mullen, P. (2012). Child sexual abuse and subsequent offending and victimisation: A 45-year follow-up study. *Trends and Issues in Crime and Criminal Justice, 440*, 1–6.

O'Hara, C. B., Campbell, I. C., & Schmidt, U. (2015). A reward-centred model of anorexia nervosa: A focused narrative review of the neurological and psychophysiological literature. *Neuroscience & Biobehavioral Reviews, 52*, 131–152.

Öhman, A., Flykt, A., & Esteves, F. (2001). Emotion drives attention: Detecting the snake in the grass. *Journal of Experimental Psychology: General, 137*, 466–478.

Öhman, A., & Mineka, S. (2003). The malicious serpent: Snakes as a prototypical stimulus for an evolved module of fear. *Current Directions in Psychological Science, 12*, 5–9.

Ohno, S., Chen, Y., Sakamaki, H., Matsumaru, N., Yoshino, M., & Tsukamoto, K. (2021). Burden of caring for Alzheimer's disease or dementia patients in Japan, the US, and EU: Results from the National Health and Wellness Survey: A cross-sectional survey. *Journal of Medical Economics, 24*(1), 266–278. https://doi.org/10.1080/13696998.2021.1880801

Ohtani, T., Levitt, J. J., Nestor, P. G., Kawashima, T., Asami, T., Shenton, M. E., et al. (2014). Prefrontal cortex volume deficit in schizophrenia: A new look using 3T MRI with manual parcellation. *Schizophrenia Research, 152*(1), 184–190.

Okura, T., Plassman, B. L., Steffens, D. C., Llewellyn, D. J., Potter, G. G., & Langa, K. M. (2010). Prevalence of neuropsychiatric symptoms and their association with functional limitations in older adults in the United States: The aging, demographics, and memory study. *Journal of the American Geriatrics Society, 58*, 330–337. https://doi.org/10.1111/j.1532-5415.2009.02680.x

Olatunji, B. O., Etzel, E. N., Tomarken, A. J., Ciesielski, B. G., & Deacon, B. (2011). The effects of safety behaviors on health anxiety: An experimental investigation. *Behavior Research and Therapy, 49*, 719–728. https://doi.org/10.1016/j.brat.2011.07.008

Olatunji, B. O., Kauffman, B. Y., Meltzer, S., Davis, M. L., Smits, J. A. J., & Powers, M. B. (2014). Cognitive-behavioral therapy for hypochondriasis/health anxiety: A meta-analysis of treatment outcome and moderators. *Behavior Research and Therapy, 58*, 65–74. https://doi.org/10.1016/j.brat.2014.05.002

olde Hartman, T. C., Borghuis, M. S., Lucassen, P. L., van de Laar, F. A., Speckens, A. E., & van Weel, C. (2009). Medically unexplained symptoms, somatisation disorder and hypochondriasis: Course and prognosis. A systematic review. *Journal of Psychosomatic Research, 66*, 363–377. https://doi.org/10.1016/j.jpsychores.2008.09.018

Oldham-Cooper, R., & Loades, M. (2017). Disorder-specific versus generic cognitive-behavioral treatment of anxiety disorders in children and young people: A systematic narrative review of evidence for the effectiveness of disorder-specific CBT compared with the disorder-generic treatment, Coping Cat. *Journal of Child and Adolescent Psychiatric Nursing, 30*(1), 6–17. https://doi.org/10.1111/jcap.12165

Olff, M., Langeland, W. L., Draijer, N., & Gersons, B. P. R. (2007). Gender differences in posttraumatic stress disorder. *Psychological Bulletin, 133*, 183–204.

Olfson, M., Gerhard, T., Huang, C., Crystal, S., & Stroup, T. S. (2015). Premature mortality among adults with schizophrenia in the United States. *JAMA Psychiatry, 72*, 1172–1181. https://doi.org/10.1001/jamapsychiatry.2015.1737

Olson, I. R., Hoffman, L. J., Jobson, K. R., Popal, H. S., & Wang, Y. (2023). Little brain, little minds: The big role of the cerebellum in social development. *Developmental Cognitive Neuroscience, 60*, 101238.

Oltmanns, T. F., & Powers, A. D. (2012). Gender and personality disorder. In T. A. Widiger (Ed.), *The Oxford handbook of personality disorders* (1st ed.). Oxford University Press.

O'Neal, J. M. (1984). First person account: Finding myself and loving it. *Schizophrenia Bulletin, 10*, 109–110.

Open Science Collaboration. (2015). Estimating the reproducibility of psychological science. *Science, 349*(6251). https://doi.org/10.1126/science.aac4716

Opondo, D., Eslami, S., Visscher, S., de Rooij, S. E., Verheij, R., Korevaar, J. C., et al. (2012). Inappropriateness of medication prescriptions to elderly patients in the primary care setting: A systematic review. *PLOS ONE, 7*, e43617. https://doi.org/10.1371/journal.pone.0043617

O'Rahilly, S., & Farooqi, I. S. (2008). Human obesity as a heritable disorder of the central control of energy balance. *International Journal of Obesity, 32*(Suppl 7) S55–S61. https://doi.org/10.1038/ijo.2008.239

Oram, S., Khalifeh, H., & Howard, L. M. (2017). Violence against women and mental health. *The Lancet: Psychiatry, 4*, 159–170.

Ormel, J., Jeronimus, B. F., Kotov, R., Riese, H., Bos, E. H., Hankin, B., et al. (2013). Neuroticism and common mental disorders: Meaning and utility of a complex relationship. *Clinical Psychology Review, 33*(5), 686–697. https://doi.org/10.1016/j.cpr.2013.04.003

Ormel, J., Jeronimus, B. F., Kotov, R., Riese, H., Bos, E. H., Hankin, B., et al. (2013). Neuroticism and common mental disorders: Meaning and utility of a complex relationship. *Clinical Psychology Review, 33*(5), 686–697. https://doi.org/10.1016/j.cpr.2013.04.003

Osborne, K. J., & Mittal, V. A. (2019). External validation and extension of the NAPLS-2 and SIPS-RC personalized risk calculators in an independent clinical high-risk sample. *Psychiatry Research, 279*, 9–14. https://doi.org/10.1016/j.psychres.2019.06.034

Osman, S., Cooper, M. J., Hackman, A., & Veale, D. (2004). Spontaneously occurring images and early memories in people with body dysmorphic disorder. *Memory, 12*(4), 428–436. https://doi.org/10.1080/09658210444000043

Ossenkoppele, R., van der Kant, R., & Hansson, O. (2022). Tau biomarkers in Alzheimer's disease: Towards implementation in clinical practice and trials. *The Lancet Neurology, 21*(8), 726–734. https://doi.org/10.1016/S1474-4422(22)00168-5

Otgaar, H., Howe, M. L., Patihis, L., Merckelbach, H., Lynn, S. J., Lilienfeld, S. O., et al. (2019). The return of the repressed: The persistent and problematic claims of long-forgotten trauma. *Perspectives on Psychological Science, 14*(6), 1072–1095. https://doi.org/10.1177/1745691619862306

Owens, E. B., & Hinshaw, S. P. (2019). Adolescent mediators of unplanned pregnancy among women with and without childhood ADHD. *Journal of Clinical Child & Adolescent Psychology, 49*(2), 229–238. https://doi.org/10.1080/15374416.2018.1547970

Owens, E. B., Zalecki, C., Gillette, P., & Hinshaw, S. P. (2017). Girls with childhood ADHD as adults: Cross-domain outcomes by diagnostic persistence. *Journal of Consulting and Clinical Psychology.* https://doi.org/10.1037/ccp0000217

Ozer, D. J., & Benet-Martinez, V. (2006). Personality and the prediction of consequential outcomes. *Annual Review of Psychology, 57*, 401–421.

Ozonoff, S., & Iosif, A.-M. (2019). Changing conceptualizations of regression: What prospective studies reveal about the onset of autism spectrum disorder. *Neuroscience & Biobehavioral Reviews, 100*, 296–304.

Pacchiarotti, I., Bond, D. J., Baldessarini, R. J., Nolen, W. A., Grunze, H., Licht, R. W., et al. (2013). The International Society for Bipolar Disorders (ISBD) task force report on antidepressant use in bipolar disorders. *American Journal of Psychiatry, 170*, 1249–1262.

Pagliaccio, D., Pizzagalli, D., Auerbach, R., & Kirshenbaum, J. (2023). Neural sensitivity following stress predicts anhedonia symptoms: A 2-year multi-wave, longitudinal study. *Research Square.* https://doi.org/10.21203/rs.3.rs-3060116/v1

Papageorgiou, C., & Wells, A. (2003). An empirical test of a clinical metacognitive model of rumination and depression. *Cognitive Therapy and Research, 27*(3), 261–273. https://doi.org/10.1023/A:1023962332399

Paquin, V., Lapierre, M., Veru, F., & King, S. (2021). Early environmental upheaval and the risk for schizophrenia. *Annual Review of Clinical Psychology, 17*(1), 285–311. https://doi.org/10.1146/annurev-clinpsy-081219-103805

Parees, I., Saifee, T. A., Kassavetis, P., Kojovic, M., Rubio-Agusti, I., Rothwell, J. C., et al. (2012). Believing is perceiving: Mismatch between self-report and actigraphy in psychogenic tremor. *Brain, 135*, 117–123. https://doi.org/10.1093/brain/awr292

Paris, J. (2019). Suicidality in borderline personality disorder. *Medicina (Lithuania), 55*(6). https://doi.org/10.3390/medicina55060223

Park, A. (2010, October 31). New research on understanding Alzheimer's. *Time.*

Park, A. (2016, Feb 16, 2016). Alzheimer's from a new angle. *Time.*

Park, E., Livingston, J. A., Wang, W., Kwon, M., Eiden, R. D., & Chang, Y.-P. (2020). Adolescent E-cigarette use trajectories and subsequent alcohol and marijuana use. *Addictive Behaviors, 103*, 106213.

Park, S. L., Murphy, S. E., Wilkens, L. R., Stram, D. O., Hecht, S. S., & Le Marchand, L. (2017). Association of CYP2A6 activity with lung cancer incidence in smokers: The multiethnic cohort study. *PLOS ONE, 12*, e0178435. https://doi.org/10.1371/journal.pone.0178435

Patel, R., Spreng, R. N., Shin, L. M., & Girard, T. A. (2012). Neurocircuitry models of posttraumatic stress disorder and beyond: A meta-analysis of functional neuroimaging studies. *Neuroscience & Biobehavioral Reviews, 36*(9), 2130–2142. https://doi.org/10.1016/j.neubiorev.2012.06.003

Patel, V., Chisholm, D., Parikh, R., Charlson, F. J., Degenhardt, L., Dua, T., et al. (2016). Addressing the burden of mental, neurological, and substance use disorders: Key messages from Disease Control Priorities. *The Lancet, 387*(10028), 1672–1685.

Patel, V., Saxena, S., Lund, C., Thornicroft, G., Baingana, F., Bolton, P., et al. (2018). The Lancet Commission on global mental health and sustainable development. *The Lancet, 392*(10157), 1553–1598. https://doi.org/10.1016/S0140-6736(18)31612-X

Patihis, L., Ho, L. Y., Loftus, E. F., & Herrera, M. E. (2021). Memory experts' beliefs about repressed memory. *Memory, 29*(6), 823–828. https://doi.org/10.1080/09658211.2018.1532521

Patihis, L., Ho, L. Y., Tingen, I. W., Lilienfeld, S. O., & Loftus, E. F. (2014). Are the "memory wars" over? A scientist-practitioner gap in beliefs about repressed memory. *Psychological Science, 25*(2), 519–530. https://doi.org/10.1177/0956797613510718

Patihis, L., & Pendergrast, M. H. (2019). Reports of recovered memories of abuse in therapy in a large age-representative U.S. national sample: Therapy type and decade comparisons. *Clinical Psychological Science, 7*(1), 3–21. https://doi.org/10.1177/2167702618773315

Patrick, C. J. (2022). Psychopathy: Current knowledge and future directions. *Annual Review of Clinical Psychology, 18*(1), 387–415. https://doi.org/10.1146/annurev-clinpsy-072720-012851

Patrick, C. J., Iacono, W. G., & Venables, N. C. (2019). Incorporating neurophysiological measures into clinical assessments: Fundamental challenges and a strategy for addressing them. *Psychological Assessment, 31*(12), 1512–1529. https://doi.org/10.1037/pas0000713

Patronek, G. J., & Nathanson, J. N. (2009). A theoretical perspective to inform assessment and treatment strategies for animal hoarders. *Clinical Psychology Review, 29*, 274–281.

Patterson, G. R. (1982). *Coercive family process*. Castilia.

Paul, N. B., Maietta, J. E., & Allen, D. N. (2020). Cultural considerations for schizophrenia spectrum disorders II: Assessment and treatment. In L. T. Benuto, F. R., Gonzalez, & J., Singer (Eds.), *Handbook of cultural factors in behavioral health*. Springer. https://doi.org/10.1007/978-3-030-32229-8_27

Paulus, M. P., Tapert, S. F. & Schuckit, M. A. (2005). Neural activation patterns of methamphetamine-dependent subjects during decision making predict relapse. *Archives of General Psychiatry, 62*, 761–768.

Paxton, S. J., Schutz, H. K., Wertheim, E. H., & Muir, S. L. (1999). Friendship clique and peer influences on body image concerns, dietary restraint, extreme weight-loss behaviors, and binge eating in adolescent girls. *Journal of Abnormal Psychology, 108*, 255–264.

Payne, A., & Blanchard, E. B. (1995). A controlled comparison of cognitive therapy and self-help support groups in the treatment of irritable bowel syndrome. *Journal of Consulting and Clinical Psychology, 63*, 779–786.

Peat, C. M., Berkman, N. D., Lohr, K. N., Brownley, K. A., Bann, C. M., Cullen, K., et al. (2017). Comparative effectiveness of treatments for binge-eating disorder: Systematic review and meta-analysis. *European Eating Disorders Review, 25*, 317–328.

Peck, C. P., Schroeder, R. W., Heinrichs, R. J., Vondran, E. J., Brockman, C. J., Webster, B. K., et al. (2013). Differences in MMPI-2 FBS and RBS scores in brain injury, probable malingering, and conversion disorder groups: A preliminary study. *Clinical Neuropsychologist, 27*, 693–707. doi:10.1080/13854046.2013.779032

Pedersen, M. G., Stevens, H., Pedersen, C. B., Nørgaard-Pedersen, B., & Mortensen, P. B. (2011). Toxoplasma infection and later development of schizophrenia in mothers. *American Journal of Psychiatry, 168*, 814–821. https://doi.org/10.1176/appi.ajp.2011.10091351

Pediatric OCD Treatment Study (POTS) Team. (2004). Cognitive-behavior therapy, sertraline, and their combination for children and adolescents with obsessive-compulsive disorder: The pediatric OCD treatment study (POTS) randomized controlled trial. *Journal of the American Medical Association, 292*, 1969–1976.

Pelham, W. E., Gnagy, E. M., Greiner, A. R., Hoza, B., Hinshaw, S. P., Swanson, J. M., et al. (2000). Behavioral versus behavioral plus pharmacological treatment for ADHD children attending a summer treatment program. *Journal of Abnormal Child Psychology, 28*, 507–525.

Pelham, W. E., III, Page, T. F., Altszuler, A. R., Gnagy, E. M., Molina, B. S. G., & Pelham, W. E., Jr. (2020). The long-term financial outcome of children diagnosed with ADHD. *Journal of Consulting and Clinical Psychology, 88*(2), 160–171. https://doi.org/10.1037/ccp0000461

Pendlebury, S. T., & Rothwell, P. M. (2009). Risk of recurrent stroke, other vascular events and dementia after transient ischaemic attack and stroke. *Cerebrovascular Diseases, 27*(Suppl 3), 1–11.

Penn, D. L., & Mueser, K. T. (1996). Research update on the psychosocial treatment of schizophrenia. *American Journal of Psychiatry, 153*, 607–617.

Pentz, M. A., Shin, H., Riggs, N., Unger, J. B., Collison, K. L., & Chou, C. (2015). Parent, peer, and executive function relationships to early adolescent e-cigarette use: A substance use pathway? *Addictive Behaviors, 42*, 73–78. https://doi.org/10.1016/j.addbeh.2014.10.040

Penzes, P., Cahill, M. E., Jones, K. A., VanLeeuwen, J. E., & Woolfrey, K. M. (2011). Dendritic spine pathology in neuropsychiatric disorders. *Nature Neuroscience, 14*, 285–293.

Pérez-Fuentes, G., Olfson, M., Villegas, L., Morcillo, C., Wang, S., & Blanco, C. (2013). Prevalence and correlates of child sexual abuse: A national study. *Comprehensive Psychiatry, 54*, 16–27. https://doi.org/10.1016/j.comppsych.2012.05.010

Perkonigg, A., Pfister, H., Stein, M. B., Hofler, M., Lieb, R., Maercker, A., et al. (2005). Longitudinal course of posttraumatic stress disorder and posttraumatic stress. *American Journal of Psychiatry, 162*, 1320–1327.

Persing, J. S., Stuart, S. P., Noyes, R., & Happel, R. L. (2000). Hypochondriasis: The patient's perspective. *International Journal of Psychiatry in Medicine, 30*, 329–342.

Perugi, G., Akiskal, H. S., Giannotti, D., Frare, F., Di Vaio, S., & Cassano, G. B. (1997). Gender-related differences in body dysmorphic disorder. *Journal of Nervous and Mental Disease, 185*, 578–582.

Pescosolido B. A. (2013). The public stigma of mental illness: What do we think; what do we know; what can we prove?. *Journal of Health and Social Behavior, 54*(1), 1–21. https://doi.org/10.1177/0022146512471197

Pescosolido, B. A., Halpern-Manners, A., Luo, L., & Perry, B. (2021). Trends in public stigma of mental illness in the US, 1996–2018. *JAMA Network Open, 4*(12), e2140202–e2140202.

Pescosolido, B. A., Martin, J. K., Long, J. S., Medina, T. R., Phelan, J. C., & Link, B. G. (2010). "A disease like any other?" A decade of change in public relations to schizophrenia, depression and alcohol dependence. *American Journal of Psychiatry, 167*, 1321–1330.

Pescosolido, B. A., Medina, T. R., Martin, J. K., & Long, J. S. (2013). The "backbone" of stigma: identifying the global core of public prejudice associated with mental illness. *American Journal of Public Health, 103*, 853–860.

Peskin, S. M. (2019, November 7). The loneliness of frontotemporal dementia. *New York Times*.

Pessoa, L. (2023). How many brain regions are needed to elucidate the neural bases of fear and anxiety? *Neuroscience & Biobehavioral Reviews, 146*, 105039. https://doi.org/10.1016/j.neubiorev.2023.105039

Petersen, J. L., & Hyde, J. S. (2010). A meta-analytic review of research on gender differences in sexuality, 1993–2007. *Psychological Bulletin, 136*, 21–38. https://doi.org/10.1037/a0017504

Peterson, A. L., Foa, E. B., & Riggs, D. S. (2019). Prolonged Exposure. In B. A. Moore & W. E. Penk (Eds.), *Treating PTSD in military personnel: A clinical handbook* (pp. 46–62). Guilford Press.

Peterson, C. B., Mitchell, J. E., Crow, S. J., Crosby, R. D., & Wonderlich, S. A. (2009). The efficacy of self-help group treatment and therapist-led group treatment for binge eating disorder. *American Journal of Psychiatry, 166*, 1347–1354.

Peterson, R. L., & Pennington, B. F. (2015). Developmental dyslexia. *Annual Review of Clinical Psychology, 11*, 283–307. https://doi.org/10.1146/annurev-clinpsy-032814-112842

Petry, N. M., Alessi, S. M., & Hanson, T. (2007). Contingency management improves abstinence and quality of life in cocaine abusers. *Journal of Consulting and Clinical Psychology, 75*, 307–315.

Petry, N. M., Alessi, S. M., Olmstead, T. A., Rash, C. J., & Zajac, K. (2017). Contingency management treatment for substance use disorders: How far has it come, and where does it need to go? *Psychology of Addictive Behaviors, 31*(8), 897–906.

Pettinati, H. M., Oslin, D. W., Kampman, K. M., Dundon, W. D., Xie, H., Gallis, T. L., et al. (2010). A double-blind, placebo-controlled trial combining sertraline and naltrexone for treating co-occuring depression and alcohol dependence. *American Journal of Psychiatry, 167*, 668–675.

Pharoah, F., Mari, J. J., Rathbone, J., & Wong, W. (2010). Family intervention for schizophrenia. *Cochrane Database of Systematic Reviews*, (12).

Phillips, D. P. (1974). The influence of suggestion on suicide: Substantive and theoretical implications of the Werther effect. *American Sociological Review, 39*, 340–354.

Phillips, D. P. (1985). The Werther effect. *The Sciences, 25*, 33–39.

Phillips, K. A. (2005). *The broken mirror: Understanding and treating body dysmorphic disorder*. Oxford University Press.

Phillips, K. A. (2006). "I look like a monster": Pharmacotherapy and cognitive-behavioral therapy for body dysmorphic disorder. In R. L. Spitzer, M. B. First, J. B. W. Williams, & M. Gibbon (Eds.), *DSM-IV-TR Case Book (Vol. 2) Experts tell how they treated their own patients* (pp. 263–276). American Psychiatric Publishing.

Phillips, K. A., Menard, W., Quinn, E., Didie, E. R., & Stout, R. L. (2013). A 4-year prospective observational follow-up study of course and predictors of course in body dysmorphic disorder. *Psychological Medicine, 43*, 1109–1117.

Phillips, K. A., Pinto, A., Hart, A. S., Coles, M. E., Eisen, J. L., Menard, W., et al. (2012). A comparison of insight in body dysmorphic disorder and obsessive-compulsive disorder. *Journal of Psychiatric Research, 46*, 1293–1299.

Phillips, K. A., Wilhelm, S., Koran, L. M., Didie, E. R., Fallon, B. A., Feusner, J., et al. (2010). Body dysmorphic disorder: Some key issues for DSM-V. *Depression and Anxiety, 27*, 573–591.

Phillips, L. J., Francey, S. M., Edwards, J., & McMurray, N. (2007). Stress and psychosis: Towards the development of new models of investigation. *Clinical Psychology Review, 27*, 307–317.

Piacentini, J., Bennett, S., Compton, S. N., Kendall, P. C., Birmaher, B., Albano, A. M., et al. (2014). 24- and 36-week outcomes for the Child/Adolescent Anxiety Multimodal Study (CAMS). *Journal of the American Academy of Child and Adolescent Psychiatry, 53*(3), 297–310.

Pickett, K. E., & Wilkinson, R. G. (2010). Inequality: An underacknowledged source of mental illness and distress. *The British Journal of Psychiatry, 197*(6), 426–428. https://doi.org/10.1192/bjp.bp.109.072066

Pierce, J. M., Petry, N. M., Stitzer, M. L., Blaine, J., Kellog, S., Satterfield, F., et al. (2006). Effects of lower-cost incentives on stimulant abstinence in methadone maintenance treatment. *Archives of General Psychiatry, 63*, 201–208.

Pierce, J. P., Choi, W. S., Gilpin, E. A., Farkas, A. J., & Berry, C. C. (1998). Tobacco ads, promotional items linked with teen smoking. *Journal of the American Medical Association, 279*, 511–515.

Pierce, K., & Courchesne, E. (2001). Evidence for a cerebellar role in reduced exploration and stereotyped behavior in autism. *Biological Psychiatry, 49*, 655–664.

Pierce, K., Gazestani, V. H., Bacon, E., Barnes, C. C., Cha, D., Nalabolu, S., et al. (2019). Evaluation of the diagnostic stability of the early autism spectrum disorder phenotype in the general population starting at 12 months. *JAMA Pediatrics, 173*(6), 578–587.

Pietrzak, R. H., Goldstein, R. B., Southwick, S. M., & Grant, B. F. (2011). Personality disorders associated with full and partial posttraumatic stress disorder in the U.S. population: Results from wave 2 of the National Epidemiologic Survey on Alcohol and Related Conditions. *Journal of Psychiatric Research, 45*(5), 678–686. https://doi.org/10.1016/j.jpsychires.2010.09.013

Pike, K. M., & Dunne, P. E. (2015). The rise of eating disorders in Asia: A review. *Journal of Eating Disorders, 3*, 33. https://doi.org/10.1186/s40337-015-0070-2

Pike, K. M., Walsh, B. T., Vitousek, K., Wilson, G. T., & Bauer, J. (2003). Cognitive behavior therapy in the posthospitalization treatment of anorexia nervosa. *American Journal of Psychiatry, 160*, 2046–2049.

Pila, E., Murray, S. B., Le Grange, D., Sawyer, S. M., & Hughes, E. K. (2019). Reciprocal relations between dietary restraint and negative affect in adolescents receiving treatment for anorexia nervosa. *Journal of Abnormal Psychology, 128*(2), 129–139. https://doi.org/10.1037/abn0000402

Pilhatsch, M., Vetter, N. C., Hubner, T., Ripke, S., Muller, K. U., Marxen, M., et al. (2014). Amygdala-function perturbations in healthy mid-adolescents with familial liability for depression. *Journal of the American Academy of Child & Adolescent Psychiatry, 53*, 559–558.

Pillinger, T., McCutcheon, R. A., Vano, L., Mizuno, Y., Arumuham, A., Hindley, G., et al. (2020). Comparative effects of 18 antipsychotics on metabolic function in patients with schizophrenia, predictors of metabolic dysregulation, and association with psychopathology: A systematic review and network meta-analysis. *The Lancet. Psychiatry, 7*(1), 64–77.

Pilowsky, L. S., Bressan, R. A., Stone, J. M., Erlandsson, K., Mulligan, R. S., Krystal, J. H., et al. (2006). First in vivo evidence of an NMDA receptor deficit in medication-free schizophrenic patients. *Molecular Psychiatry, 11*, 118–119. https://doi.org/10.1038/sj.mp.4001751

Pincus, A. L. (2023). Narcissistic personality disorder and pathological narcissism. In R. F. Krueger & P. H. Blaney (Eds.), *Oxford textbook of psychopathology* (pp. 628–649). Oxford University Press. https://doi.org/10.1093/med-psych/9780197542521.003.0027

Pineles, S. L., & Mineka, S. (2005). Attentional biases to internal and external sources of potential threat in social anxiety. *Journal of Abnormal Psychology, 114*, 314–318.

Piper, A., Jr., Pope, H. G., Jr., & Borowiecki, J. J. I. (2000). Custer's last stand: Brown, Scheflin, and Whitfiled's latest attempt to salvage "dissociative amnesia." *Journal of Psychiatry and the Law, 28*, 149–213.

Pistorello, J., Jobes, D. A., Gallop, R., Compton, S. N., Locey, N. S., Au, J. S., et al. (2020). A randomized controlled trial of the Collaborative Assessment and Management of Suicidality (CAMS) versus treatment as usual (TAU) for suicidal college students. *Archives of Suicide Research*. https://doi.org/10.1080/13811118.2020.1749742

Pitcher, D., Parkin, B., & Walsh, V. (2021). Transcranial magnetic stimulation and the understanding of behavior. *Annual Review of Psychology, 72*, 97–121. https://doi.org/10.1146/annurev-psych-081120-013144

Pittenger, C. (2023). The pharmacological treatment of obsessive-compulsive disorder. *Psychiatric Clinics of North America, 46*(1), 107–119. https://doi.org/10.1016/j.psc.2022.11.005

Pittig, A., Treanor, M., LeBeau, R. T., & Craske, M. G. (2018). The role of associative fear and avoidance learning in anxiety disorders: Gaps and directions for future research. *Neuroscience and Biobehavioral Reviews, 88*, 117–140. https://doi.org/10.1016/j.neubiorev.2018.03.015

Plana-Ripoll, O., Pedersen, C. B., Agerbo, E., Holtz, Y., Erlangsen, A., Canudas-Romo, V., et al. (2019). A comprehensive analysis of mortality-related health metrics associated with mental disorders: a nationwide, register-based cohort study. *The Lancet, 394*(10211), 1827–1835. https://doi.org/10.1016/S0140-6736(19)32316-5

Plassman, B. L., & Potter, G. G. (2018). Epidemiology of dementia and mild cognitive impairment. In *APA handbook of dementia* (pp. 15–39). American Psychological Association. https://doi.org/10.1037/0000076-002

Plomin, R. (1999). Genetics and general cognitive ability. *Nature, 402*, C25–C29.

Plomin, R., DeFries, J. C., Craig, I. W., & McGuffin, P. (2003). *Behavioral genetics in the postgenomic era*. APA Books.

Polivy, J., Herman, C. P., & Howard, K. (1988). The restraint scale: Assessment of dieting. In M. Hersen & A. S. Bellack (Eds.), *Dictionary of behavioral assessment techniques* (pp. 377–380). Pergamon Press.

Pollan, M. (2018). *How to change your mind: What the new science of psychedelics teaches us about consciousness, dying, addiction, depression, and transcendence*. Penguin Press.

Ponniah, K., Magiati, I., & Hollon, S. D. (2013). An update on the efficacy of psychological treatments for obsessive-compulsive disorder in adults. *Journal of Obsessive-Compulsive and Related Disorders, 2*(2), 207–218. https://doi.org/10.1016/j.jocrd.2013.02.005

Pope, H. G. J., Oliva, P. S., Hudson, J. I., Bodkin, J. A., & Gruber, A. J. (1999). Attitudes toward DSM-IV dissociative disorders diagnoses among board-certified American psychiatrists. *American Journal of Psychiatry, 156*, 321–323.

Pope, H. G. J., Poliakoff, M. B., Parker, M. P., Boynes, M., & Hudson, J. J. (2006). Is dissociative amnesia a culture-bound syndrome? Findings from a survey of historical literature. *Psychological Medicine, 37,* 1067–1068.

Pope, K. S. (1998). Pseudoscience, cross-examination, and scientific evidence in the recovered memory controversy. *Psychology, Public Policy, and Law, 4,* 1160–1181.

Postlethwaite, A., Kellett, S., & Mataix-Cols, D. (2019). Prevalence of Hoarding Disorder: A systematic review and meta-analysis. *Journal of Affective Disorders, 256,* 309–316. https://doi.org/10.1016/J.JAD.2019.06.004

Poulsen, S., Lunn, S., Daniel, S. I., Folke, S., Mathiesen, B. B., Katznelson, H., et al. (2014). A randomized controlled trial of psychoanalytic psychotherapy or cognitive-behavioral therapy for bulimia nervosa. *American Journal of Psychiatry, 171*(1), 109–116.

Powell, R. A., & Gee, T. L. (2000). "The effects of hypnosis on dissociative identity disorder: A reexamination of the evidence": Reply. *Canadian Journal of Psychiatry, 45,* 848–849.

Powers, A. D., Gleason, M. E., & Oltmanns, T. F. (2013). Symptoms of borderline personality disorder predict interpersonal (but not independent) stressful life events in a community sample of older adults. *Journal of Abnormal Psychology, 122,* 469–474. https://doi.org/10.1037/a0032363

Powers, A. R., Addington, J., Perkins, D. O., Bearden, C. E., Cadenhead, K. S., Cannon, T. D., et al. (2020). Duration of the psychosis prodrome. *Schizophrenia Research, 216,* 443–449. https://doi.org/10.1016/j.schres.2019.10.051

Powers, M. B., Vedel, E., & Emmelkamp, P. M. G. (2008). Behavioral couples therapy (BCT) for alcohol and drug use disorders: A meta-analysis. *Clinical Psychology Review, 28,* 952–962.

Powers, R. (2017). *No one cares about crazy people: The chaos and heartbreak of mental health in America.* Hachette Books.

Pressman, P. S., & Miller, B. L. (2014). Diagnosis and management of behavioral variant frontotemporal dementia. *Biological Psychiatry, 75,* 574–581.

Price, D. D., Craggs, J. G., Zhou, Q., Verne, G. N., Perlstein, W. M., & Robinson, M. E. (2009). Widespread hyperalgesia in irritable bowel syndrome is dynamically maintained by tonic visceral impulse input and placebo/nocebo factors: Evidence from human psychophysics, animal models, and neuroimaging. *NeuroImage, 47,* 995–1001.

Prien, R. F., & Potter, W. Z. (1993). Maintenance treatment for mood disorders. In D. L. Dunner (Ed.), *Current psychiatric therapy.* Saunders.

Primack, B. A., Bost, J. E., Land, S. R., & Fine, M. J. (2007). Volume of tobacco advertising in African American markets: Systematic review and meta-analysis. *Public Health Reports, 122,* 607–615.

Prince, M., Bryce, R., Albanese, E., Wimo, A., Ribeiro, W., & Ferri, C. P. (2013). The global prevalence of dementia: A systematic review and metaanalysis. *Alzheimer's and Dementia: The Journal of the Alzheimer's Association, 9,* 63–75.e62. https://doi.org/10.1016/j.jalz.2012.11.007

Prinstein, M. J., Heilbron, N., Guerry, J. D., Franklin, J. C., Rancourt, D., Simon, V., et al. (2010). Peer influence and nonsuicidal self injury: Longitudinal results in community and clinically-referred adolescent samples. *Journal of Abnormal Child Psychology, 38*(5), 669–682. https://doi.org/10.1007/s10802-010-9423-0

Prinstein, M. J., Nesi, J., & Telzer, E. H. (2020). Commentary: An updated agenda for the study of digital media use and adolescent development—Future directions following Odgers & Jensen (2020). *Journal of Child Psychology and Psychiatry, and Allied Disciplines, 61*(3), 349–352. https://doi.org/10.1111/jcpp.13219

Proudfit, G. H. (2015). The reward positivity: From basic research on reward to a biomarker for depression. *Psychophysiology, 52*(4), 449–459. https://doi.org/10.1111/psyp.12370

Pruessner, M., Cullen, A. E., Aas, M., & Walker, E. F. (2017). The neural diathesis-stress model of schizophrenia revisited: An update on recent findings considering illness stage and neurobiological and methodological complexities. *Neuroscience & Biobehavioral Reviews, 73,* 191–218.

Przeworski, A., & Newman, M. G. (2006). Efficacy and utility of computer-assisted cognitive behavioural therapy for anxiety disorders. *The Clinical Psychologist, 10,* 43–53.

Puhl, R. M., Himmelstein, M. S., & Pearl, R. L. (2020). Weight stigma as a psychosocial contributor to obesity. *American Psychologist, 75*(2), 274–289. https://doi.org/10.1037/amp0000538

Puhl, R. M., Latner, J. D., O'Brien, K., Luedicke, J., Forhan, M., & Danielsdottir, S. (2016). Cross-national perspectives about weight-based bullying in youth: Nature, extent and remedies. *Pediatric Obesity, 11*(4), 241–250. https://doi.org/10.1111/ijpo.12051

Pujols, Y., Seal, B. N., & Meston, C. M. (2010). The association between sexual satisfaction and body image in women. *Journal of Sexual Medicine, 7,* 905–916.

Purves, K. L., Coleman, J. R. I., Meier, S. M., Rayner, C., Davis, K. A. S., Cheesman, R., et al. (2020). A major role for common genetic variation in anxiety disorders. *Molecular Psychiatry, 25*(12), 3292–3303. https://doi.org/10.1038/s41380-019-0559-1

Putnam, F. W. (1996). A brief history of multiple personality disorder. *Child and Adolescent Psychiatric Clinics of North America, 5,* 263–271.

Quigley, L., Thiruchselvam, T., & Quilty, L. C. (2022). Cognitive control biases in depression: A systematic review and meta-analysis. *Psychological Bulletin, 148*(9–10), 662–709. https://doi.org/10.1037/bul0000372

Quiles Marcos, Y., Quiles Sebastián, M. J., Pamies Aubalat, L., Botella Ausina, J., & Treasure, J. (2013). Peer and family influence in eating disorders: A meta-analysis. *European Psychiatry, 28*(4), 199–206.

Quinones, S. (2015). *Dreamland: The true tale of America's opiate epidemic.* Bloomsbury Press.

Quinsey, V. L., Harris, G. T., Rice, M. E., & Cormier, C. A. (2006). *Violent offenders: Appraising and managing risk* (2nd ed.). American Psychological Association.

Quirk, S. E., Berk, M., Chanen, A. M., Koivumaa-Honkanen, H., Brennan-Olsen, S. L., Pasco, J. A., & Williams, L. J. (2016). Population prevalence of personality disorder and associations with physical health comorbidities and health care service utilization: A review. *Personality Disorders: Theory, Research, and Treatment, 7,* 136–146. https://doi.org/10.1037/per0000148

Rachman, S. (2012). Health anxiety disorders: A cognitive construal. *Behaviour Research and Therapy, 50,* 502–512.

Rachman, S. J. (1977). The conditioning theory of fear acquisition: A critical examination. *Behaviour Research and Therapy, 15,* 375–387.

Rachman, S. J., & DeSilva, P. (1978). Abnormal and normal obsessions. *Behaviour Research and Therapy, 16,* 233–248.

Rachman, S. J., & Wilson, G. T. (1980). *The effects of psychological therapy* (2nd ed.). Pergamon Press.

Ragatz, L. L., Fremouw, W., & Baker, E. (2012). The psychological profile of white-collar offenders: Demographics, criminal thinking, psychopathic traits, and psychopathology. *Criminal Justice and Behavior, 39,* 978–997.

Ragland, J. D., Laird, A. R., Ranganath, C., Blumenfeld, R. S., Gonzales, S. M., & Glahn, D. C. (2009). Prefrontal activation deficits during episodic memory in schizophrenia. *AJP, 166*(8), 863–874. https://doi.org/10.1176/appi.ajp.2009.08091307

Raine, A. (2006). Schizotypal personality: Neurodevelopmental and psychosocial trajectories. *Annual Review of Clinical Psychology, 2,* 291–326.

Raison, C. L., Capuron, L., & Miller, A. H. (2006). Cytokines sing the blues: Inflammation and the pathogenesis of depression. *Trends in Immunology, 27,* 24–31.

Ranganathan, M., & D'Souza, D. C. (2006). The acute effects of cannabinoids on memory in humans: A review. *Psychopharmacology, 188*, 425–444. https://doi.org/10.1007/s00213-006-0508-y

Rapee, R., Mattick, R., & Murrell, E. (1986). Cognitive mediation in the affective component of spontaneous panic attacks. *Journal of Behavior Therapy and Experimental Psychiatry, 17*, 245–253.

Rapee, R. M., Schniering, C. A., & Hudson, J. L. (2009). Anxiety disorders during childhood adolescence: Origins and treatment. *Annual Review of Clinical Psychology, 5*, 311–341.

Rapoport, M. J., Lanctot, K. L., Streiner, D. L., Bedard, M., Vingilis, E., Murray, B., et al. (2009). Benzodiazepine use and driving: A meta-analysis. *Journal of Clinical Psychiatry, 70*, 663–673.

Rascovsky, K., Hodges, J. R., Knopman, D., Mendez, M. F., Kramer, J. H., Neuhaus, J., et al. (2011). Sensitivity of revised diagnostic criteria for the behavioural variant of frontotemporal dementia. *Brain: A Journal of Neurology, 134*, 2456–2477.

Rasic, D., Hajek, T., Alda, M., & Uher, R. (2014). Risk of mental illness in offspring of parents with schizophrenia, bipolar disorder, and major depressive disorder: A meta-analysis of family high-risk studies. *Schizophrenia Bulletin, 40*, 28–38.

Rastrelli, G., Corona, G., Mannucci, E., & Maggi, M. (2015). Vascular and chronological age in subjects with erectile dysfunction: A cross-sectional study. *Journal of Sexual Medicine, 12*, 2303–2312. https://doi.org/10.1111/jsm.13044

Rawson, R. A., Martinelli-Casey, P., Anglin, M. D., Dickow, A., Frazier, Y., Gallagher, C., et al. (2004). A multi-site comparison of psychosocial approaches for the treatment of methamphetamine dependence. *Addiction, 99*, 708–717.

Ray, L. A., & Grodin, E. N. (2021). Clinical neuroscience of addiction: What clinical psychologists need to know and why. *Annual Review of Clinical Psychology, 17*(1), 465–493. https://doi.org/10.1146/annurev-clinpsy-081219-114309

Reardon, K. W., Smack, A. J., Herzhoff, K., & Tackett, J. L. (2019). An N-pact factor for clinical psychological research. *Journal of Abnormal Psychology, 128*, 493–499. https://doi.org/10.1037/abn0000435

Reas, D. L., & Grilo, C. M. (2015). Pharmacological treatment of binge eating disorder: Update review and synthesis. *Expert Opinion on Pharmacotherapy, 16*(10), 1463–1478. https://doi.org/10.1517/14656566.2015.1053465

Reas, D. L., Williamson, D. A., Martin, C. K., & Zucker, N. L. (2000). Duration of illness predicts outcome for bulimia nervosa: A long-term follow-up study. *International Journal of Eating Disorders, 27*, 428–434.

Reba-Harrelson, L., Von Holle, A., Hamer, R. M., Swann, R., Reyes, M. L., & Bulik, C. M. (2009). Patterns and prevalence of disordered eating and weight control behaviors in women ages 25–45. *Eating and Weight Disorders, 14*(4), e190–198.

Redding, N. (2009). *Methland: The death and life of an American small town.* Bloomsbury USA.

Reed, B. D., Harlow, S. D., Plegue, M. A., & Sen, A. (2016). Remission, relapse, and persistence of vulvodynia: A longitudinal population-based study. *Journal of Women's Health, 25*, 276–283. https://doi.org/10.1089/jwh.2015.5397

Rees, E., Walters, J., Georgieva, L., Isles, A., Chambert, K., Richards, A., et al. (2014). Analysis of copy number variations at 15 schizophrenia-associated loci. *The British Journal of Psychiatry, 204*(2), 108–114. https://doi.org/10.1192/bjp.bp.113.131052

Regeer, E. J., Ten Have, M., Rosso, M. L., van Roijen, L. H., Vollebergh, W., & Nolen, W. A. (2004). Prevalence of bipolar disorder in the general population: A reappraisal study of the Netherlands Mental Health Survey and Incidence Study. *Acta Psychiatrica Scandinavica, 110*, 374–382.

Regier, D. A., Kuhl, E. A., & Kupfer, D. J. (2013). The DSM-5: Classification and criteria changes. *World Psychiatry, 12*, 92–98.

Regier, D. A., Narrow, W. E., Clarke, D. E., Kraemer, H. C., Kuramoto, S. J., Kuhl, E. A., et al. (2013). DSM-5 field trials in the United States and Canada, Part II: Test-retest reliability of selected categorical diagnoses. *American Journal of Psychiatry, 170*, 59–70.

Reichenberg, A., Avshalom, C., Harrington, H, Houts, R., Keefe, R. S. E., Murray, R. M., et al. (2010). Static and dynamic cognitive deficits in childhood preceding adult schizophrenia: A 30-year study. *American Journal of Psychiatry, 167*, 160–169.

Reid, J. E., Laws, K. R., Drummond, L., Vismara, M., Grancini, B., Mpavaenda, D., et al. (2021). Cognitive behavioural therapy with exposure and response prevention in the treatment of obsessive-compulsive disorder: A systematic review and meta-analysis of randomised controlled trials. *Comprehensive Psychiatry, 106*. https://doi.org/10.1016/J.COMPPSYCH.2021.152223

Reidy, D. E., Shelley-Tremblay, J. F., & Lilienfeld, S. O. (2011). Psychopathy, reactive aggression, and precarious proclamations: A review of behavioral, cognitive, and biological research. *Aggression and Violent Behavior, 16*, 512–524.

Reisner, S. L., Katz-Wise, S. L., Gordon, A. R., Corliss, H. L., & Austin, S. B. (2016 Aug). Social Epidemiology of Depression and Anxiety by Gender Identity. *Journal of Adolescent Health, 59*(2), 203–208. https://doi.org/10.1016/j.jadohealth.2016.04.006.

Reitsma, M. B., Fullman, N., Ng, M., Salama, J. S., Abajobir, A., Abate, K. H., et al. (2017). Smoking prevalence and attributable disease burden in 195 countries and territories, 1990–2015: A systematic analysis from the Global Burden of Disease Study 2015. *Lancet, 389*, 1885–1906.

Ren, W., Qiu, H., Yang, Y., Zhu, X., Zhu, C., Mao, G., et al. (2019). Randomized controlled trial of cognitive behavioural therapy for depressive and anxiety symptoms in Chinese women with breast cancer. *Psychiatry Research, 271*, 52–59. https://doi.org/10.1016/j.psychres.2018.11.026

Rescorla, L. A., Achenbach, T. M., Ivanova, M. Y., Harder, V. S., Otten, L., Bilenberg, N., et al. (2011). International comparisons of behavioral and emotional problems in preschool children: Parents' reports from 24 societies. *Journal of Clinical Child & Adolescent Psychology, 40*(3), 456–467. https://doi.org/10.1080/15374416.2011.563472

Resick, P. A., Bovin, M. J., Calloway, A. L., Dick, A. M., King, M. W., Mitchell, K. S., et al. (2012). A critical evaluation of the complex PTSD literature: Implications for DSM-5. *Journal of Traumatic Stress, 25*, 241–251.

Resick, P. A., Nishith, P., & Griffin, M. G. (2003). How well does cognitive-behavioral therapy treat symptoms of complex PTSD? An examination of child sexual abuse survivors within a clinical trial. *CNS Spectrums, 8*, 351–355.

Resick, P. A., Suvak, M. K., Johnides, B. D., Mitchell, K. S., & Iverson, K. M. (2012). The impact of dissociation on PTSD treatment with cognitive processing therapy. *Depression and Anxiety, 29*, 718–730.

Reynolds, S., Wilson, C., Austin, J., & Hooper, L. (2012). Effects of psychotherapy for anxiety in children and adolescents: A meta-analytic review. *Clinical Psychology Review, 32*(4), 251–262.

Rhee, S. H., & Waldman, I. D. (2002). Genetic and environmental influences on antisocial behavior: A meta-analysis of twin and adoption studies. *Psychological Bulletin, 128*, 490–529.

Rhode, P., Seeley, J. R., Kaufman, N. K, Clarke, G. N., & Stice, E. (2006). Predicting time to recovery among depressed adolescents treated in two psychosocial group interventions. *Journal of Consulting and Clinical Psychology, 74*, 80–88.

Ribeiro, J. D., Franklin, J. C., Fox, K. R., Bentley, K. H., Kleiman, E. M., Chang, B. P., et al. (2016). Self-injurious thoughts and behaviors as risk factors for future suicide ideation, attempts, and death: A meta-analysis of longitudinal studies. *Psychological Medicine, 46*(2), 225–236. https://doi.org/10.1017/S0033291715001804

Ribeiro, W. S., Bauer, A., Andrade, M. C. R., York-Smith, M., Pan, P. M., Pingani, L., et al. (2017). Income inequality and mental illness-related morbidity and resilience: A systematic review and meta-analysis. *The Lancet. Psychiatry, 4*(7), 554–562.

Richards, D. A., Ekers, D., McMillan, D., Taylor, R. S., Byford, S., Warren, F. C., et al. (2016). Cost and outcome of behavioural activation versus cognitive behavioural therapy for depression (COBRA): A randomised, controlled, non-inferiority trial. *The Lancet, 388*(10047), 871–880. https://doi.org/10.1016/S0140-6736(16)31140-0

Richards, R. L., Kinney, D. K., Lunde, I., Benet, M., & Merzel, A. (1988). Creativity in manic-depressives, cyclothymes, their normal relatives, and control subjects. *Journal of Abnormal Psychology, 97*, 281–288.

Richters, J., De Visser, R. O., Rissel, C. E., Grulich, A. E., & Smith, A. M. A. (2008). Demographic and psychosocial features of participants in bondage and discipline, "sadomasochism" or dominance and submission (BDSM): Data from a national survey. *Journal of Sexual Medicine, 5*, 1660–1668. https://doi.org/10.1111/j.1743-6109.2008.00795.x

Ridley, M. (2003). *Nature via nurture: Genes, experience, and what makes us human.* HarperCollins.

Rief, W., & Broadbent, E. (2007). Explaining medically unexplained symptoms—models and mechanisms. *Clinical Psychology Review, 27*, 821–841.

Rief, W., Buhlmann, U., Wilhelm, S., Borkenhagen, A., & Brähler, E. (2006). The prevalence of body dysmorphic disorder: A population-based survey. *Psychological Medicine, 36*, 877–885.

Rief, W., & Martin, A. (2014). How to use the new DSM-5 somatic symptom disorder diagnosis in research and practice: A critical evaluation and a proposal for modifications. *Annual Review of Clinical Psychology, 10*, 339–367. https://doi.org/10.1146/annurev-clinpsy-032813-153745

Riggs, D. S., Rothbaum, B. O., & Foa, E. B. (1995). A prospective examination of symptoms of posttraumatic stress disorder in victims of nonsexual assault. *Journal of Interpersonal Violence, 10*(2), 201–214. https://doi.org/10.1177/0886260595010002005

Rimland, B. (1964). *Infantile autism.* Appleton-Century-Crofts.

Rios, J. A. & Sireci, S. G. (2014). Guidelines versus practices in cross-lingual assessment: A disconcerting disconnect. *International Journal of Testing, 14*, 289–312. https://doi.org/10.1080/15305058.2014.924006

Ripke, S., Neale, B. M., Corvin, A., Walters, J. T. R., Farh, K.-H., Holmans, P. A., et al. (2014). Biological insights from 108 schizophrenia-associated genetic loci. *Nature, 511*, 421–427. https://doi.org/10.1038/nature13595

Ripke, S., Sanders, A. R., Kendler, K. S., Levinson, D. F., Sklar, P., Holmans, P. A., et al. (2011). Genome-wide association study identifies five new schizophrenia loci. *Nature Genetics, 43*, 969–976. https://doi.org/10.1038/ng.940

Ritchie, K., Norton, J., Mann, A., Carriere, I., & Ancelin, M. L. (2013). Late-onset agoraphobia: General population incidence and evidence for a clinical subtype. *American Journal of Psychiatry, 170*, 790–798.

Ritter, K., Vater, A., Rusch, N., Schroder-Abe, M., Schutz, A., Fydrich, T., et al. (2014). Shame in patients with narcissistic personality disorder. *Psychiatry Research, 215*, 429–437.

Ritter, P. S., Höfler, M., Wittchen, H.-U., Lieb, R., Bauer, M., Pfennig, A., et al. (2015). Disturbed sleep as risk factor for the subsequent onset of bipolar disorder—Data from a 10-year prospective-longitudinal study among adolescents and young adults. *Journal of Psychiatric Research, 68*, 76–82. https://doi.org/10.1016/j.jpsychires.2015.06.005

Robbins, J. (2007). *Healthy at 100.* Ballantine Books.

Robbins, S. J., Ehrman, R. N., Childress, A. R., Cornish, J. W., & O'Brien, C. P. (2000). Mood state and recent cocaine use are not associated with levels of cocaine cue reactivity. *Drug and Alcohol Dependence, 59*, 33–42.

Roberto, C. A. (2020). How psychological insights can inform food policies to address unhealthy eating habits. *American Psychologist, 75*(2), 265–273. https://doi.org/10.1037/amp0000554

Roberts, A. L., Austin, S. B., Corliss, H. L., Vandermorris, A. K., & Koenen, K. C. (2010). Pervasive trauma exposure among US sexual orientation minority adults and risk of posttraumatic stress disorder. *Ajph.Aphapublications.Org, 100*(12), 2433–2441. https://doi.org/10.2105/AJPH.2009.168971

Roberts, A. L., Gilman, S. E., Breslau, J., Breslau, N., & Koenen, K. C. (2011). Race/ethnic differences in exposure to traumatic events, development of post-traumatic stress disorder, and treatment-seeking for post-traumatic stress disorder in the United States. *Psychological Medicine, 41*, 71–83. https://doi.org/10.1017/S0033291710000401

Roberts, B. W., Kuncel, N. R., Shiner, R., Caspi, A., & Goldberg, L. R. (2007). The power of personality: The comparative validity of personality traits, socioeconomic status, and cognitive ability for predicting important life outcomes. *Perspectives on Psychological Science, 2*, 313–345.

Roberts, B. W., Luo, J., Briley, D. A., Chow, P. I., Su, R., & Hill, P. L. (2017). A systematic review of personality trait change through intervention. *Psychological Bulletin, 143*, 117–141. https://doi.org/10.1037/bul0000088

Roberts, N. A., & Reuber, M. (2014). Alterations of consciousness in psychogenic nonepileptic seizures: Emotion, emotion regulation and dissociation. *Epilepsy & Behavior, 30*, 43–49. https://doi.org/10.1016/j.yebeh.2013.09.035

Roberts, N. P., Kitchiner, N. J., Kenardy, J., Lewis, C. E., & Bisson, J. I. (2019). Early psychological intervention following recent trauma: A systematic review and meta-analysis. *European Journal of Psychotraumatology, 10*(1). https://doi.org/10.1080/20008198.2019.1695486

Roberts, R., Woodman, T., & Sedikides, C. (2017). Pass me the ball: Narcissism in performance settings. *International Review of Sport and Exercise Psychology*, 1–24. https://doi.org/10.1080/1750984X.2017.1290815

Robinson, D. G., Schooler, N. R., John, M., Correll, C. U., Marcy, P., Addington, J., et al. (2014). Prescription practices in the treatment of first-episode schizophrenia spectrum disorders: Data from the National RAISE-ETP Study. *American Journal of Psychiatry, 172*(3), 237–248. https://doi.org/10.1176/appi.ajp.2014.13101355

Robinson, J., Pirkis, J., & O'Connor, R. C. (2016). Suicide clusters. In R. C. O'Connor & J. Pirkis (Eds.), *The international handbook of suicide prevention* (pp. 758–774). John Wiley & Sons, Ltd. https://doi.org/10.1002/9781118903223.ch43

Robinson, T. E., & Berridge, K. C. (1993). The neural basis of drug craving: An incentive sensitization theory of addiction. *Brain Research Reviews, 18*, 247–191.

Robinson, T. E., & Berridge, K. C. (2003). Addiction. *Annual Review of Psychology, 54*, 25–53.

Robison, A. J., Thakkar, K. N., & Diwadkar, V. A. (2020). Cognition and reward circuits in schizophrenia: Synergistic, not separate. *Biological Psychiatry, 87*(3), 204–214.

Rodgers, N., McDonald, S., & Wootton, B. M. (2021). Cognitive behavioral therapy for hoarding disorder: An updated meta-analysis. *Journal of Affective Disorders, 290*, 128–135. https://doi.org/10.1016/j.jad.2021.04.067

Rodolico, A., Bighelli, I., Avanzato, C., Concerto, C., Cutrufelli, P., Mineo, L., et al. (2022). Family interventions for relapse prevention in schizophrenia: a systematic review and network meta-analysis. *The Lancet. Psychiatry, 9*(3), 211–221.

Rodriguez, C. I., Herman, D., Alcon, J., Chen, S., Tannen, A., Essock, S., et al. (2012). Prevalence of hoarding disorder in individuals at potential risk of eviction in New York City: A pilot study. *The Journal of Nervous and Mental Disease, 200*(1), 91–94. https://doi.org/10.1097/NMD.0B013E31823F678B

Rodriguez-Seijas, C., Eaton, N. R., & Krueger, R. F. (2015). How transdiagnostic factors of personality and psychopathology can inform clinical assessment and intervention. *Journal of Personality Assessment, 97*, 425–435. https://doi.org/10.1080/00223891.2015.1055752

Rodriguez-Seijas, C., Eaton, N. R., & Pachankis, J. E. (2019). Prevalence of psychiatric disorders at the intersection of race and sexual orientation: Results from the national epidemiologic survey of alcohol and related conditions-III. *Journal of Consulting and Clinical Psychology, 87*(4), 321–331. https://doi.org/10.1037/ccp0000377

Rodriguez-Seijas, C., McClendon, J., Wendt, D. C., Novacek, D. M., Ebalu, T., Hallion, L., Hassan, N. Y., Huson, K., Spielmans, G. I., Folk, J. B., Khazem, L. R., Neblett, E. W., Cunningham, T. J., Hampton-Anderson, J., Steinman, S. A., Hamilton, J. L., & Mekawi, Y (2024). The next generation of clinical science: Moving toward antiracism. *Clinical Psychological Science*

Roehrig, J. P., & McLean, C. P. (2010). A comparison of stigma toward eating disorders versus depression. *International Journal of Eating Disorders, 43*, 671–674.

Roemer, L., Williston, S. K., Eustis, E. H., & Orsillo, S. M. (2013). Mindfulness and acceptance-based behavioral therapies for anxiety disorders. *Current Psychiatry Reports, 15*(11), 410. https://doi.org/10.1007/s11920-013-0410-3

Rogeberg, O., & Elvik, R. (2016). The effects of cannabis intoxication on motor vehicle collision revisited and revised. *Addiction, 111*, 1348–1359.

Rogers, M. S., McNiel, D. E., & Binder, R. L. (2019). Effectiveness of Police Crisis Intervention Training Programs. *The journal of the American Academy of Psychiatry and the Law, 47*(4), 414–421. https://doi.org/10.29158/JAAPL.003863-19

Rohde, P., Arigo, D., Shaw, H., & Stice, E. (2018). Relation of self-weighing to future weight gain and onset of disordered eating symptoms. *Journal of Consulting and Clinical Psychology, 86*(8), 677–687. https://doi.org/10.1037/ccp0000325

Roll, J. M., Petry, N. M. D., Stitzer, M. L., Brecht, M. L., Peirce, J. M., McCann, M. J., et al. (2006). Contingency management for the treatment of methamphetamine use disorders. *American Journal of Psychiatry, 163*(11), 1993–1999. https://doi.org/10.1176/ajp.2006.163.11.1993

Rolon-Arroyo, B., Arnold, D. H., & Harvey, E. A. (2013). The predictive utility of conduct disorder symptoms in preschool children: A 3-year follow-up study. *Child Psychiatry and Human Development, 45*, 329–337.

Romanelli, R. J., Wu, F. M., Gamba, R., Mojtabai, R., & Segal, J. B. (2014). Behavioral therapy and serotonin reuptake inhibitor pharmacotherapy in the treatment of obsessive-compulsive disorder: A systematic review and meta-analysis of head-to-head randomized controlled trials. *Depression and Anxiety, 31*(8), 641–652. https://doi.org/10.1002/da.22232

Root, T. L., Pinheiro, A. P., Thornton, L., Strober, M., Fernandez-Aranda, F., Brandt, H., et al. (2010). Substance use disorders in women with anorexia nervosa. *International Journal of Eating Disorders, 43*, 14–21.

Rose, J. E., & Behm, F. M. (2014). Combination treatment with varenicline and bupropion in an adaptive smoking cessation paradigm. *American Journal of Psychiatry, 171*, 1199–1205.

Rose, J., E., Brauer, L. H., Behm, F. M., Cramblett, M. Calkins, K., & Lawhon, D. (2004). Psychopharmacological interactions between nicotine and ethanol. *Nicotine & Tobacco Research, 6*, 133–144.

Rose, J. E., Herskovic, J. E., Behm, F. M., & Westman, E. C. (2009). Precessation treatment with nicotine patch significantly increases abstinence rates relative to conventional treatment. *Nicotine and Tobacco Research, 11*, 1067–1075.

Rosenberg, A., Ngandu, T., Rusanen, M., Antikainen, R., Bäckman, L., Havulinna, S., et al. (2018). Multidomain lifestyle intervention benefits a large elderly population at risk for cognitive decline and dementia regardless of baseline characteristics: The FINGER trial. *Alzheimer's & Dementia, 14*(3), 263–270. https://doi.org/10.1016/J.JALZ.2017.09.006

Rosenberg, K. P. (2019). *Bedlam: An intimate journey into America's mental health crisis.* Avery/Penguin Random House.

Rosen, N. O., Brotto, L. A., & Zucker, K. J. (2018). Sexual dysfunctions and paraphilic disorders. In *Adult psychopathology and diagnosis* (8th ed., pp. 571–632). John Wiley & Sons Inc.

Rosen, R. C., Miner, M. M., & Wincze, J. P. (2014). Erectile dysfunction: Integration of medical and psychological approaches. In Y. M. Binik & K. S. K. Hall (Eds.), *Principles and practice of sex therapy* (5th ed., pp. 61–88). Guilford Press.

Rösner, S., Hackl-Herrweth, A., Leucht, S., Lehert, P., Vecchi, S., & Soyka, M. (2010). Acamprosate for alcohol dependence. *Cochrane Database of Systematic Reviews, 9*, CD004332. https://doi.org/10.1002/14651858.CD004332.pub2

Rossello, J., Bernal, G., & Rivera-Medina, C. (2008). Individual and group CBT and IPT for Puerto Rican adolescents with depressive symptoms. *Cultural Diversity and Ethnic Minority Psychology, 14*, 234–245.

Roth, A. (2018). *Insane: America's criminal treatment of mental illness.* Basic Books.

Rothbaum, B. O., Foa, E. B., Murdock, T., Riggs, D. S., & Walsh, W. (1992). A prospective examination of posttraumatic stress disorder in rape victims. *Journal of Traumatic Stress, 5*, 455–475.

Rothenberg, W. A., Lansford, J. E., Godwin, J. W., Dodge, K. A., Copeland, W. E., Odgers, C. L., et al. (2023). Intergenerational effects of the Fast Track intervention on the home environment: A randomized control trial. *Journal of Child Psychology and Psychiatry, and Allied Disciplines, 64*(5), 820–830. https://doi.org/10.1111/jcpp.13648

Roughgarden, J. (2004). *Evolution's rainbow: Diversity, gender and sexuality in nature and people.* University of California Press.

Rouleau, C. R., & von Ranson, K. M. (2011). Potential risks of pro-eating disorder websites. *Clinical Psychology Review, 31*, 525–531.

Rowland, D. L., Adamski, B. A., Neal, C. J., Myers, A. L., & Burnett, A. L. (2015). Self-efficacy as a relevant construct in understanding sexual response and dysfunction. *Journal of Sex & Marital Therapy, 41*, 60–71. https://doi.org/10.1080/0092623X.2013.811453

Rozel, J. S., & Mulvey, E. P. (2017). The link between mental illness and firearm violence: Implications for social policy and clinical practice. *Annual Review of Clinical Psychology, 13*(1), 445–469. https://doi.org/10.1146/annurev-clinpsy-021815-093459

Rubin, D. C., Berntsen, D., & Bohni, M. K. (2008). A memory-based model of posttraumatic stress disorder: Evaluating basic assumptions underlying the PTSD diagnosis. *Psychological Review, 115*, 985–1011.

Rubinstein, T. B., McGinn, A. P., Wildman, R. P., & Wylie-Rosett, J. (2010). Disordered eating in adulthood is associated with reported weight loss attempts in childhood. *International Journal of Eating Disorders, 43*, 663–666.

Rucker, J. J. H., Iliff, J., & Nutt, D. J. (2018). Psychiatry & the psychedelic drugs. Past, present & future. *Psychedelics: New Doors, Altered Perceptions, 142*, 200–218.

Ruglass, L. M., Smith, K. Z., Killeen, T. K., & Hien, D. A. (2019). Pharmacological treatment of trauma and stressor-related disorders. In *APA handbook of psychopharmacology* (pp. 281–307). American Psychological Association. https://doi.org/10.1037/0000133-013

Ruscio, A. M. (2019). Normal versus pathological mood: Implications for diagnosis. *Annual Review of Clinical Psychology, 15*(1), 179–205. https://doi.org/10.1146/annurev-clinpsy-050718-095644

Ruscio, A. M., Brown, T. A., Chiu, W. T., Sareen, J., Stein, M. B., & Kessler, R. C. (2008). Social fears and social phobia in the USA: Results from the National Comorbidity Survey Replication. *Psychological Medicine, 38*, 15–28.

Ruscio, A. M., Stein, D. J., Chiu, W. T., & Kessler, R. C. (2010). The epidemiology of obsessive-compulsive disorder in the national comorbidity survey replication. *Molecular Psychiatry, 15*(1), 53–63.

Rush, A. J., Trivedi, M., Wisniewski, S. R., Nierenberg, A. A., Stewart, J. W., Warden, D., et al. (2006). Acute and longer-term outcomes in depressed outpatients requiring one or several treatment steps: A STAR-D report. *American Journal of Psychiatry, 163*, 1905–1917.

Rush, A. J., Trivedi, M., Wisniewski, S. R., Nierenberg, A. A., Stewart, J. W., Warden, D., et al. (2006). Acute and longer-term outcomes in depressed outpatients requiring one or several treatment steps: A STAR*D report. *American Journal of Psychiatry, 163*, 1905–1917.

Rutter, M., Caspi, A., Fergusson, D., Horwood, L. J., Goodman, R., Maughan, B., et al. (2004). Sex differences in developmental reading disability: New findings from 4 epidemiological studies. *Journal of the American Medical Association, 291*, 2007–2012.

Rutter, M., & Silberg, J. (2002). Gene-environment interplay in relation to emotional and behavioral disturbance. *Annual Review of Psychology, 53*, 463–490.

Ruzek, J. I. (2021). Technology based interventions for PTSD. In M. J. Friedman, P. P. Schnurr, & T. M. Keane (Eds.), *Handbook of PTSD: Science and practice* (3rd ed., pp. 518–534). Guilford Press.

Ryberg, W., Zahl, P. H., Diep, L. M., Landrø, N. I., & Fosse, R. (2019). Managing suicidality within specialized care: A randomized controlled trial. *Journal of Affective Disorders, 249*, 112–120. https://doi.org/10.1016/j.jad.2019.02.022

Saad, L. (2015, July 29). Americans' coffee consumption is steady, few want to cut back. https://www.gallup.com/poll/184388/americans-coffee-consumption-steady-few-cut-back.aspx

Sabia, S., Dugravot, A., Dartigues, J.-F., Abell, J., Elbaz, A., Kivimäki, M., & Singh-Manoux, A. (2017). Physical activity, cognitive decline, and risk of dementia: 28 year follow-up of Whitehall II cohort study. *BMJ, 357*, j2709. https://doi.org/10.1136/bmj.j2709

Sacks, O. (1995). *An anthropologist on Mars*. Knopf.

Saczynski, J. S. D., & Inouye, S. K. (2015). Delirium. In D. C. Steffens, D. G. Blazer, & M. E. Thakur (Eds.), *The American Psychiatric Publishing textbook of geriatric psychiatry*. APA.

Sakel, M. (1938). The pharmacological shock treatment of schizophrenia. *Nervous and Mental Disease Monograph, 62*.

Saks, E. R. (1997). *Jekyll on trial: Multiple personality disorder and criminal law*. New York University Press.

Saks, E. R. (2007). *The center cannot hold: My journey through madness*. Hyperion.

Salamone, J. D. (2000). A critique of recent studies on placebo effects of antidepressants: Importance of research on active placebos. *Psychopharmacology, 152*, 1–6.

Salamone, J. D., & Correa, M. (2012). The mysterious motivational functions of mesolimbic dopamine. *Neuron, 76*, 470–485.

Salkovskis, P. M. (1996). Cognitive-behavioral approaches to understanding obsessional problems. In R. M. Rapee (Ed.), *Current controversies in anxiety disorders*. Guilford Press.

Salk, R. H., Hyde, J. S., & Abramson, L. Y. (2017). Gender differences in depression in representative national samples: Meta-analyses of diagnoses and symptoms. *Psychological Bulletin, 143*(8), 783–822. https://doi.org/10.1037/bul0000102

Salluh, J. I. F., Wang, H., Schneider, E. B., Nagaraja, N., Yenokyan, G., Damluji, A., et al. (2015). Outcome of delirium in critically ill patients: Systematic review and meta-analysis. *BMJ (Online), 350*, 1–10. https://doi.org/10.1136/bmj.h2538

Salter, D., McMillan, D., Richards, M., Talbot, T., Hodges, J., Bentovim, A., et al. (2003). Development of sexually abusive behaviour in sexually victimised males: A longitudinal study. *Lancet, 361*, 471–476.

SAMHSA. (2020). Key substance use and mental health indicators in the United States: Results from the 2019 National Survey on Drug Use and Health. *HHS Publication No. PEP19-5068, NSDUH Series H-54*, 170, 51–58. https://www.samhsa.gov/data/

SAMHSA. (2022). Mental Health Annual Report 2015-2020: Use of Mental Health Services: National Client Level Data. https://www.samhsa.gov/data/data-we-collect/mh-cld-mental-health-client-level-data

SAMSHA. (2020). Key substance use and mental health indicators in the United States: Results from the 2019 National Survey on Drug Use and Health. HHS Publication No. PEP19-5068, NSDUH Series H-54, 170, 51–58. https://www.samhsa.gov/data/

Samuel, D. B., Sanislow, C. A., Hopwood, C. J., Shea, M. T., Skodol, A. E., Morey, L. C., et al. (2013). Convergent and incremental predictive validity of clinician, self-report, and structured interview diagnoses for personality disorders over 5 years. *Journal of Consulting and Clinical Psychology, 81*, 650–659.

Samuels, J., Eaton, W. W., Bienvenu, O. J., 3rd, Brown, C. H., Costa, P. T., Jr, & Nestadt, G. (2002). Prevalence and correlates of personality disorders in a community sample. *The British journal of psychiatry, 180*, 536–542. https://doi.org/10.1192/bjp.180.6.536

Samuels, J. F., Bienvenu, O. J., 3rd, Pinto, A., Fyer, A. J., McCracken, J. T., Rauch, S. L., et al. (2007). Hoarding in obsessive-compulsive disorder: Results from the OCD Collaborative Genetics Study. *Behaviour Research and Therapy, 45*, 673–686.

Sandbank, M., Bottema-Beutel, K., Crowley, S., Cassidy, M., Dunham, K., Feldman, J. I., et al. (2020). Project AIM: Autism intervention meta-analysis for studies of young children. *Psychological Bulletin, 146*(1), 1–29. https://doi.org/10.1037/bul0000215

Santomauro, D. F., Mantilla Herrera, A. M., Shadid, J., Zheng, P., Ashbaugh, C., Pigott, D. M., et al. (2021). Global prevalence and burden of depressive and anxiety disorders in 204 countries and territories in 2020 due to the COVID-19 pandemic. *The Lancet, 398*(10312), 1700–1712. https://doi.org/10.1016/S0140-6736(21)02143-7

Santtila, P., Antfolk, J., Räfså, A., Hartwig, M., Sariola, H., Sandnabba, N. K., et al. (2015). Men's sexual interest in children: One-year incidence and correlates in a population-based sample of Finnish male twins. *Journal of Child Sexual Abuse, 24*, 115–134. https://doi.org/10.1080/10538712.2015.997410

Sara, S. J. (2009). The locus coeruleus and noradrenergic modulation of cognition. *Nature Reviews Neuroscience, 10*, 211–223.

Sareen, J., Cox, B. J., Stein, M. B., Afifi, T. O., Fleet, C., & Asmundson, G. J. G. (2007). Physical and mental comorbidity, disability, and suicidal behavior associated with posttraumatic stress disorder in a large community sample. *Psychosomatic Medicine, 69*(3), 242–248. https://doi.org/10.1097/PSY.0B013E31803146D8

Sarginson, J., Webb, R. T., Stocks, S. J., Esmail, A., Garg, S., & Ashcroft, D. M. (2017). Temporal trends in antidepressant prescribing to children in UK primary care, 2000–2015. *Journal of Affective Disorders, 210*, 312–318.

Sarpal, D. K., Argyelan, M., Robinson, D. G., Szeszko, P. R., Karlsgodt, K. H., John, M., et al. (2016). Baseline striatal functional connectivity as a predictor of response to antipsychotic drug treatment. *American Journal of Psychiatry, 173*, 69–77. https://doi.org/10.1176/appi.ajp.2015.14121571

Sartorius, N., Jablensky, A., Korten, A., Ernberg, G., Anker, M., Cooper, J. E., et al. (1986). Early manifestations and first-contact incidence of schizophrenia in different cultures: A preliminary report on the initial evaluation phase of the WHO Collaborative Study on Determinants of Outcome of Severe Mental Disorders. *Psychological Medicine, 16*, 909–928.

Sarwer, D. B., & Heinberg, L. J. (2020). A review of the psychosocial aspects of clinically severe obesity and bariatric surgery. *American Psychologist, 75*(2), 252–264. https://doi.org/10.1037/amp0000550

Sauer-Zavala, S., Fournier, J. C., Jarvi Steele, S., Woods, B. K., Wang, M., Farchione, T. J., & Barlow, D. H. (2021). Does the unified protocol really change neuroticism? Results from a randomized trial. *Psychological Medicine, 51*(14), 2378–2387. https://doi.org/10.1017/S0033291720000975

Saveanu, R., Etkin, A., Duchemin, A. M., Goldstein-Piekarski, A., Gyurak, A., Debattista, C., et al. (2015). The international study to predict optimized treatment in depression (iSPOT-D). Outcomes from the acute phase of antidepressant treatment. *Journal of Psychiatric Research, 61*, 1–12. https://doi.org/10.1016/j.jpsychires.2014.12.018

Saxena, A., & Dodell-Feder, D. (2022). Explaining the association between urbanicity and psychotic-like experiences in pre-adolescence: The indirect effect of urban exposures. *Frontiers in Psychiatry, 13*.

Saxena, S. (2015). Pharmacotherapy of compulsive hoarding. In R. O. Frost & G. Steketee (Eds.), *The Oxford handbook of hoarding and acquiring*. Oxford University Press.

Sayette, M. A. (2017). The effects of alcohol on emotion in social drinkers. *Behaviour Research and Therapy, 88*, 76–89.

Sayette, M. A., Creswell, K. G., Dimoff, J. D., Fairbairn, C. E., Cohn, J. F., Heckman, B. W., et al. (2012). Alcohol and group formation. *Psychological Science, 23*, 869–878. https://doi.org/10.1177/0956797611435134

Sayette, M. A., Marchetti, M. A., Herz, R. S., Martin, L. M., & Bowdring, M. A. (2019). Pleasant olfactory cues can reduce cigarette craving. *Journal of Abnormal Psychology, 128*(4), 327–340. https://doi.org/10.1037/abn0000431

Schaefer, J. D., Caspi, A., Belsky, D. W., Harrington, H., Houts, R., Horwood, L. J., et al. (2017). Enduring mental health: Prevalence and prediction. *Journal of Abnormal Psychology, 126*(2), 212–224. https://doi.org/10.1037/abn0000232

Schaefer, L. M., Smith, K. E., Anderson, L. M., Cao, L., Crosby, R. D., Engel, S. G., et al. (2020). The role of affect in the maintenance of binge-eating disorder: Evidence from an ecological momentary assessment study. *Journal of Abnormal Psychology, 129*(4), 387–396. https://doi.org/10.1037/abn0000517

Scharfenort, R., Menz, M., & Lonsdorf, T. B. (2016). Adversity-induced relapse of fear: Neural mechanisms and implications for relapse prevention from a study on experimentally induced return-of-fear following fear conditioning and extinction. *Translational Psychiatry, 6*(7), e858–e858. https://doi.org/10.1038/tp.2016.126

Schecter, R., & Grether, J. K. (2008). Continuing increases in autism reported to California's Developmental Services System. *Archives of General Psychiatry, 65*, 19–24.

Scherk, H., Pajonk, F. G., & Leucht, S. (2007). Second-generation antipsychotic agents in the treatment of acute mania: A systematic review and meta-analysis of randomized controlled trials. *Archives of General Psychiatry, 64*, 442–455.

Schieber, K., Kollei, I., de Zwaan, M., & Martin, A. (2015). Classification of body dysmorphic disorder - What is the advantage of the new DSM-5 criteria? *Journal of Psychosomatic Research, 78*(3), 223–227. https://doi.org/10.1016/j.jpsychores.2015.01.002

Schieber, K., Kollei, I., de Zwaan, M., Müller, A., & Martin, A. (2013). Personality traits as vulnerability factors in body dysmorphic disorder. *Psychiatry Research, 210*(1), 242–246. https://doi.org/10.1016/J.PSYCHRES.2013.06.009

Schilder, P. (1953). *Medical psychology*. International Universities Press.

Schlam, T. R., Cook, J. W., Baker, T. B., Hayes-Birchler, T., Bolt, D. M., Smith, S. S., et al. (2018). Can we increase smokers' adherence to nicotine replacement therapy and does this help them quit? *Psychopharmacology, 235*(7), 2065–2075. https://doi.org/10.1007/s00213-018-4903-y

Schmidt, N. B., Zvolensky, M. J., & Maner, J. K. (2006). Anxiety sensitivity: Prospective prediction of panic attacks and Axis I pathology. *Journal of Psychiatric Research, 40*(8), 691–699. https://doi.org/10.1016/j.jpsychires.2006.07.009

Schmid, Y., Enzler, F., Gasser, P., Grouzmann, E., Preller, K. H., Vollenweider, F. X., et al. (2015). Acute effects of lysergic acid diethylamide in healthy subjects. *Biological Psychiatry, 78*, 544–553.

Schmitz, A., & Grillon, C. (2012). Assessing fear and anxiety in humans using the threat of predictable and unpredictable aversive events (the NPU-threat test). *NatureProtocols, 7*(3), 527–532. https://www.nature.com/nprot/journal/v7/n3/abs/nprot.2012.001.html#supplementary-information

Schmucker, M., Lösel, F. The effects of sexual offender treatment on recidivism: an international meta-analysis of sound quality evaluations. J Exp Criminol 11, 597–630 (2015). https://doi-org.libproxy.berkeley.edu/10.1007/s11292-015-9241-z

Schnab, D. W., & Trinh, N. G. (2004). Do artificial food colors promote hyperactivity in children with hyperactive syndromes? A meta-analysis of double-blind placebo-controlled trials. *Journal of Developmental and Behavioral Pediatrics, 25*, 425–434.

Schoenbaum, M., Kessler, R. C., Gilman, S. E., Colpe, L. J., Heeringa, S. G., Stein, M. B., et al. (2014). Predictors of suicide and accident death in the Army Study to Assess Risk and Resilience in Servicemembers (Army STARRS) results from the Army Study to Assess Risk and Resilience in Servicemembers (Army STARRS). *JAMA Psychiatry, 71*(5), 493–503. https://doi.org/10.1001/jamapsychiatry.2013.4417

Schopler, E., Short, A., & Mesibov, G. (1989). Relation of behavioral treatment to "normal functioning": Comment on Lovaas. *Journal of Consulting and Clinical Psychology, 57*, 162–164.

Schramm, E., Kriston, L., Zobel, I., et al. (2017). Effect of disorder-specific vs nonspecific psychotherapy for chronic depression: A randomized clinical trial. *JAMA Psychiatry, 74*(3), 233–242. https://doi.org/10.1001/jamapsychiatry.2016.3880

Schreiber, F. L. (1973). *Sybil*. Regnery.

Schreibman, L., Dawson, G., Stahmer, A. C., Landa, R., Rogers, S. J., McGee, G. G., et al. (2015). Naturalistic developmental behavioral interventions: Empirically validated treatments for autism spectrum disorder. *Journal of Autism and Developmental Disorders, 45*, 2411–2428. https://doi.org/10.1007/s10803-015-2407-8

Schuler, M., Mohnke, S., Amelung, T., Dziobek, I., Lemme, B., Borchardt, V., et al. (2019). Empathy in pedophilia and sexual offending against children: A multifaceted approach. *Journal of Abnormal Psychology, 128*(5), 453–464. https://doi.org/10.1037/abn0000412

Schulze, L., Schulze, A., Renneberg, B., Schmahl, C., & Niedtfeld, I. (2019). Neural correlates of affective disturbances: A comparative meta-analysis of negative affect processing in borderline personality disorder, major depressive disorder, and posttraumatic stress disorder. *Biological Psychiatry: Cognitive Neuroscience and Neuroimaging, 4*(3), 220–232. https://doi.org/10.1016/j.bpsc.2018.11.004

Schumer, M. C., Chase, H. W., Rozovsky, R., Eickhoff, S. B., & Phillips, M. L. (2023). Prefrontal, parietal, and limbic condition-dependent differences in bipolar disorder: A large-scale meta-analysis of functional neuroimaging studies. *Molecular Psychiatry*. https://doi.org/10.1038/s41380-023-01974-8

Schwab, S. G., & Wildenauer, D. B. (2013). Genetics of psychiatric disorders in the GWAS era: An update on schizophrenia. *European Archives of Psychiatry and Clinical Neuroscience, 263*, 147–154. https://doi.org/10.1007/s00406-013-0450-z

Schwartz, C. (2022). The age of distracti-pression. *New York Times*. https://www.nytimes.com/2022/07/09/style/medication-depression-anxiety-adhd.html?referringSource=articleShare

Schwartz, E. K., Docherty, N. M., Najolia, G. M., & Cohen, A. S. (2019). Exploring the racial diagnostic bias of schizophrenia using behavioral and clinical-based measures. *Journal of Abnormal Psychology, 128*, 263–271.

Schwartz, M. B., Chambliss, O. H., Brownell, K. D., Blair, S., & Billington, C. (2003). Weight bias among health professionals specializing in obesity. *Obesity Research, 11*, 1033–1039.

Schwartz, M. W., Seeley, R. J., Zeltser, L. M., Drewnowski, A., Ravussin, E., Redman, L. M., et al. (2017). Obesity pathogenesis: An Endocrine Society scientific statement. *Endocrine Reviews, 38*(4), 267–296. https://doi.org/10.1210/er.2017-00111

Schwartz, R. C., & Blankenship, D. M. (2014). Racial disparities in psychotic disorder diagnosis: A review of empirical literature. *World Journal of Psychiatry, 4*(4), 133–140. https://doi.org/10.5498/wjp.v4.i4.133

Scott, J., Graham, A., Yung, A., Morgan, C., Bellivier, F., & Etain, B. (2022). A systematic review and meta-analysis of delayed help-seeking, delayed diagnosis and duration of untreated illness in bipolar disorders. *Acta Psychiatrica Scandinavia, 146*(5): 389-405. https://doi.org/10.1111/acps.13490

Scott, K., Koenen, K. C., Aguilar-Gaxiola, S., Alonso, J., Angermeyer, M. C., et al., (2013). Associations between lifetime traumatic events and subsequent chronic physical conditions: a cross-national, cross-sectional study. *PLOS ONE 8*, 11.

Scott, K. M., Lim, C., Al-Hamzawi, A., Alonso, J., Bruffaerts, R., Caldas-de-Almeida, J. M., et al. (2016). Association of mental disorders with subsequent chronic physical conditions: World Mental Health Surveys from 17 countries. *JAMA Psychiatry, 73*(2), 150–158. https://doi.org/10.1001/jamapsychiatry.2015.2688

Scull, A. (2022). *Desperate remedies: Psychiatry's turbulent quest to cure mental illness*. Belknap Press.

Searles, J. (2013, October 10). Getting into the spirit. *The New York Times*, p. TR10.

Seedat, S., Scott, K. M., Angermeyer, M., Berglund, P., Bromet, E., Brugha, T., et al. (2009). Cross-national associations between gender and mental disorders in the World Health Organization World Mental Health Surveys. *Archives of General Psychiatry, 66*, 785–795.

Seeman, P. (2013). Schizophrenia and dopamine receptors. *European Neuropsychopharmacology, 23*, 999–1009.

Segal, J. Z. (2015). The rhetoric of female sexual dysfunction: Faux feminism and the FDA. *Canadian Medical Association Journal, 187*, 915–916. https://doi.org/10.1503/cmaj.150363

Segal, Z. V., Kennedy, S., Gemar, M., Hood, K., Pedersen, R., & Buis, T. (2006). Cognitive reactivity to sad mood provocation and the prediction of depressive relapse. *Archives of General Psychiatry, 63*, 749–755.

Segal, Z. V., Williams, J. M. G., & Teasdale, J. D. (2003). Mindfulness-based cognitive therapy for depression: A new approach to preventing relapse. *Psychotherapy Research, 13*, 123–125.

Segal, Z. V., Williams, J. M., & Teasdale, J. D. (2001). *Mindfulness-based cognitive therapy for depression*. Guilford Press.

Segerstrom, S. C., & Miller, G. E. (2004). Psychological stress and the immune system: A meta-analytic study of 30 years of inquiry. *Psychological Bulletin, 130*, 601–630.

Sehatzadeh, S., Daskalakis, Z. J., Yap, B., Tu, H.-A., Palimaka, S., Bowen, J. M., & O'Reilly, D. J. (2019). Unilateral and bilateral repetitive transcranial magnetic stimulation for treatment-resistant depression: A meta-analysis of randomized controlled trials over 2 decades. *Journal of Psychiatry and Neuroscience, 44*(3), 151–163. https://doi.org/10.1503/jpn.180056

Seidman, L. J., Shapiro, D. I., Stone, W. S., Woodberry, K. A., Ronzio, A., Cornblatt, B. A., et al. (2016). Association of neuro-cognition with transition to psychosis: Baseline functioning in the second phase of the North American Prodrome Longitudinal Study. *JAMA Psychiatry, 73*, 1239–1248. https://doi.org/10.1001/jamapsychiatry.2016.2479

Sekar, A., Bialas, A. R., de Rivera, H., Davis, A., Hammond, T. R., Kamitaki, N., et al. (2016). Schizophrenia risk from complex variation of complement component 4. *Nature, 530*, 177–183. https://doi.org/10.1038/nature16549

Selby, E. A., Wonderlich, S. A., Crosby, R. D., Engel, S. G., Panza, E., Mitchell, J. E., et al. (2013). Nothing tastes as good as thin feels: Low positive emotion differentiation and weight-loss activities in anorexia nervosa. *Clinical Psychological Science, 2*, 514–531. https://doi.org/10.1177/2167702613512794.

Seligman, M. E., Maier, S. F., & Geer, J. H. (1968). Alleviation of learned helplessness in the dog. *Journal of Abnormal Psychology, 73*, 256–262.

Seligman, M. E. P. (1971). Phobias and preparedness. *Behavior Therapy, 2*, 307–320.

Seligman, R., & Kirmayer, L. J. (2008). Dissociative experience and cultural neuroscience: Narrative, metaphor and mechanism. *Culture, Medicine and Psychiatry, 32*, 31–64. https://doi.org/10.1007/s11013-007-9077-8

Sellbom, M., Kremyar, A. J., & Wygant, D. B. (2021). Mapping MMPI-3 scales onto the hierarchical taxonomy of psychopathology. *Psychological Assessment, 33*(12), 1153–1168. https://doi.org/10.1037/pas0001049

Sellers, R., Harold, G. T., Smith, A. F., Neiderhiser, J. M., Reiss, D., Shaw, D., et al. (2019). Disentangling nature from nurture in examining the interplay between parent–child relationships, ADHD, and early academic attainment. *Psychological Medicine*, 1–8.

Selye, H. (1950). *The physiology and pathology of exposure to stress*. Acta.

Semkovska, M., & McLoughlin, D. M. (2010). Objective cognitive performance associated with electroconvulsive therapy for depression: A systematic review and meta-analysis. *Biological Psychiatry, 68*(6), 568–577. https://doi.org/10.1016/j.biopsych.2010.06.009

Sensky, T., Turkington, D., Kingdon, D., Scott, J. L., Scott, J., Siddle, R., et al. (2000). A randomized controlled trial of cognitive-behavioural therapy for persistent symptoms in schizophrenia resistant to medication. *Archives of General Psychiatry, 57*, 165–172.

Seto, M. C., & Eke, A. W. (2017). Correlates of admitted sexual interest in children among individuals convicted of child pornography offenses. *Law and Human Behavior, 41*, 305–313. https://doi.org/10.1037/lhb0000240

Shackman, A. J., Salomons, T. V., Slagter, H. A., Fox, A. S., Winter, J. J., & Davidson, R. J. (2011). The integration of negative affect, pain and cognitive control in the cingulate cortex. *Nature Reviews Neuroscience, 12*, 154–167.

Shackman, A. J., Tromp, D. P. M., Stockbridge, M. D., Kaplan, C. M., Tillman, R. M., & Fox, A. S. (2016). Dispositional negativity: An integrative psychological and neurobiological perspective. *Psychological Bulletin, 142*(12), 1275–1314. American Psychological Association. https://doi.org/10.1037/bul0000073

Shapiro, F. (1999). Eye movement desensitization and reprocessing (EMDR) and the anxiety disorders: Clinical and research implications of an integrated psychotherapy treatment. *Journal of Anxiety Disorders, 13*, 35–67.

Sharp, C., & Miller, J. D. (2022). Ten-year retrospective on the *DSM–5* alternative model of personality disorder: Seeing the forest for the trees. *Personality Disorders: Theory, Research, and Treatment, 13*(4), 301–304. https://doi.org/10.1037/per0000595

Sharp, C., Wright, A. G. C., Fowler, J. C., Frueh, B. C., Allen, J. G., Oldham, J., & Clark, L. A. (2015). The structure of personality pathology: Both general ("g") and specific ("s") factors? *Journal of Abnormal Psychology, 124*, 387–398. https://doi.org/10.1037/abn0000033

Shaw, D. S., Dishion, T. J., Supplee, L., Gardner, F., & Arnds, K. (2006). Randomized trial of a family-centered approach to the prevention of early conduct problems: 2-year effects of the family check-up in early childhood. *Journal of Consulting and Clinical Psychology, 74*, 1–9.

Shaw, J., & Porter, S. (2015). Constructing rich false memories of committing crime. *Psychological Science, 26*(3), 291–301. https://doi.org/10.1177/0956797614562862

Sheffield, J. M., Huang, A. S., Rogers, B. P., Blackford, J. U., Heckers, S., & Woodward, N. D. (2021). Insula sub-regions across the psychosis spectrum: Morphology and clinical correlates. *Translational Psychiatry, 11*(1).

Shenk, D. (2010). *The genius is in all of us: Why everything you've been told about genetics, talent, and IQ is wrong.* Doubleday.

Shepherd, B. F., Brochu, P. M., & Rodriguez Seijas, C. (2022). A critical examination of disparities in eating disorder symptoms by sexual orientation among US adults in the NESARC-III. *International Journal of Eating Disorders, 55*(6), 790–800.

Sher, K. J., Grekin, E. R., & Williams, N. A. (2005). The development of alcohol use disorders. *Annual Review of Clinical Psychology, 1*, 493–523.

Sher, K. J., Walitzer, K. S., Wood, P. K., & Brent, E. F. (1991). Characteristics of children of alcoholics: Putative risk factors, substance use and abuse, and psychopathology. *Journal of Abnormal Psychology, 100*, 427–448.

Sher, K. J., Wood, M. D., Wood, P. K., & Raskin, G. (1996). Alcohol outcome expectancies and alcohol use: A latent variable cross-lagged panel study. *Journal of Abnormal Psychology, 105*, 561–574.

Shic, F., Macari, S., & Chawarska, K. (2014). Speech disturbs face scanning in 6-month-old infants who develop autism spectrum disorder. *Biological Psychiatry, 75*(3), 231–237.

Shi, C., Taylor, S., Witthöft, M., Du, X., Zhang, T., Lu, S., et al. (2022). Attentional bias toward health-threat in health anxiety: A systematic review and three-level meta-analysis. *Psychological Medicine, 52*(4), 604–613. https://doi.org/10.1017/S0033291721005432

Shields, G. S., Bonner, J. C., & Moons, W. G. (2015). Does cortisol influence core executive functions? A meta-analysis of acute cortisol administration effects on working memory, inhibition, and set-shifting. *Psychoneuroendocrinology, 58*, 91–103. https://doi.org/10.1016/j.psyneuen.2015.04.017

Shields, G. S., Hunter, C. L., & Yonelinas, A. P. (2022). Stress and memory encoding: What are the roles of the stress-encoding delay and stress relevance? *Learning & Memory, 29*(2), 48–54. https://doi.org/10.1101/LM.053469.121

Shields, G. S., Sazma, M. A., McCullough, A. M., & Yonelinas, A. P. (2017). The effects of acute stress on episodic memory: A meta-analysis and integrative review. *Psychological Bulletin, 143*, 636–675. https://doi.org/10.1037/bul0000100

Shiner, B., D'Avolio, L. W., Nguyen, T. M., Zayed, M. H., Young-Xu, Y., Desai, R. A., et al. (2013). Measuring use of evidence-based psychotherapy for posttraumatic stress disorder. *Administration and Policy in Mental Health, 40*(4), 311–318. https://doi.org/10.1007/s10488-012-0421-0

Shin, M., Besser, L. M., Kucik, J. E., Lu, C., Siffel, C., & Correa, A. (2009). Prevalence of Down syndrome among children and adolescents in 10 regions of the United States. *Pediatrics, 124*, 1565–1571.

Shou, Y., Lay, S. E., De Silva, H. S., Xyrakis, N., & Sellbom, M. (2021). Sociocultural influences on psychopathy traits: A cross-national investigation. *Journal of Personality Disorders, 35*(2), 194–216. https://doi.org/10.1521/PEDI_2019_33_428

Siegel, J. S., Daily, J. E., Perry, D. A., & Nicol, G. E. (2023). Psychedelic drug legislative reform and legalization in the US. *JAMA Psychiatry, 80*(1), 77–83. https://doi.org/10.1001/jamapsychiatry.2022.4101

Silove, D., Alonso, J., Bromet, E., Gruber, M., Sampson, N., Scott, K., et al. (2015). Pediatric-onset and adult-onset separation anxiety disorder across countries in the World Mental Health Survey. *American Journal of Psychiatry, 172*(7), 647–656. https://doi.org/10.1176/appi.ajp.2015.14091185

Silove, D., & Klein, L. (2021). Culture, trauma, and traumatic stress among refugees, asylum seekers, and postconflict populations. In M. J. Friedman, P. P. Schnurr, & T. M. Keane (Eds.), *Handbook of PTSD: Science and practice* (3rd ed., pp. 483–500). Guilford Press.

Simeon, D. (2009). Depersonalization disorder. In P. F. Dell & J. A. O'Neil (Eds.), *Dissociation and dissociative disorders: DSM-5 and beyond* (pp. 441–442). Routledge.

Simeon, D., Gross, S., Guralnik, O., Stein, D. J., Schmeidler, J., & Hollander, E. (1997). Feeling unreal: 30 cases of DSM-III-R depersonalization disorder. *American Journal of Psychiatry, 154*, 1107–1112.

Simeon, D., Guralnik, O., Hazlett, E. A., Spiegel-Cohen, J., Hollander, E., & Buchsbaum, M. S. (2000). Feeling unreal: A PET study of depersonalization disorder. *American Journal of Psychiatry, 157*(11), 1782–1788. https://doi.org/10.1176/appi.ajp.157.11.1782

Simeon, D., Knutelska, M., Nelson, D., & Guralnik, O. (2003). Feeling unreal: Depersonalization disorder update of 117 cases. *Journal of Clinical Psychiatry, 64*, 990–997.

Simmons, J. P., Nelson, L. D., & Simonsohn, U. (2011). False-positive psychology. *Psychological Science, 22*(11), 1359–1366. https://doi.org/10.1177/0956797611417632

Simon, J. A., Kingsberg, S. A., Portman, D., Williams, L. A., Krop, J., Jordan, R., et al. (2019). Long-term safety and efficacy of bremelanotide for hypoactive sexual desire disorder. *Obstetrics and Gynecology, 134*(5), 909. https://doi.org/10.1097/AOG.0000000000003514

Simonoff, E., Pickles, A., Charman, T., Chandler, S., Loucas, T., & Baird, G. (2008). Psychiatric disorders in children with autism spectrum disorders: Prevalence, comorbidity, and associated factors in a population-derived sample. *Journal of the American Academy of Child & Adolescent Psychiatry, 47*(8), 921–929.

Simpkins, A. N. (2020). Impact of race-ethnic and economic disparities on rates of vascular dementia in the national inpatient sample database from 2006-2014. *Journal of Stroke and Cerebrovascular Diseases, 29*(5), 104731. https://doi.org/10.1016/J.JSTROKECEREBROVASDIS.2020.104731

Singh-Manoux, A., Dugravot, A., Fournier, A., et al. (2017). Trajectories of depressive symptoms before diagnosis of dementia: A 28-year follow-up study. *JAMA Psychiatry, 74*, 712–718. https://doi.org/10.1001/jamapsychiatry.2017.0660

Singh, S. P., Harley, K., & Suhail, K. (2013). Cultural specificity of emotional overinvolvement: A systematic review. *Schizophrenia Bulletin, 39*, 449–463.

Sisti, D. A., Segal, A. G., & Emanuel, E. J. (2015). Improving long-term psychiatric care: Bring back the asylum. *JAMA, 313*, 243–244.

Sivaraman, M., Virues-Ortega, J., & Roeyers, H. (2020). Social referencing skills in children with autism spectrum disorder: A systematic review. *Research in Autism Spectrum Disorders, 72*, 101528.

Sjögren, M., Nielsen A. S. M., Hasselbalch, K. C., Wøllo, M., & Hansen, J. S. (2019). A systematic review of blood-based serotonergic biomarkers in bulimia nervosa. *Psychiatry Research, 279*, 155–171. https://doi.org/10.1016/j.psychres.2018.12.167

Skeem, J. L., & Monahan, J. (2011). Current directions in violence risk assessment. *Current Directions in Psychological Science, 20*, 38–42.

Slade, T., Chapman, C., Swift, W., Keyes, K., Tonks, Z., & Teesson, M. (2016). Birth cohort trends in the global epidemiology of alcohol use and alcohol-related harms in men and women: Systematic review and metaregression. *BMJ Open, 6*, e011827. https://doi.org/10.1136/bmjopen-2016-011827

Slevec, J. H., & Tiggemann, M. (2011). Predictors of body dissatisfaction and disordered eating in middle-aged women. *Clinical Psychology Review, 31*, 515–524.

Smart, R. G., & Ogburne, A. C. (2000). Drug use and drinking among students in 36 countries. *Addictive Behaviors, 25*, 455–460.

Smart, R., Morral, A. R., Smucker, S., Cherney, S., Schell, T. L., Peterson, S., Ahluwalia, S. C., Cefalu, M., Xenakis, L., Ramchand, R., & Gresenz, C. R. (2020). *The science of gun policy: A critical synthesis of research evidence on the effects of gun Policies in the United States* (2nd ed.). RAND Corporation. https://www.rand.org/pubs/research_reports/RR2088-1.html

Smeland, O. B., Bahrami, S., Frei, O., Shadrin, A., O'Connell, K., Savage, J., et al. (2020). Genome-wide analysis reveals extensive genetic overlap between schizophrenia, bipolar disorder, and intelligence. *Molecular Psychiatry, 25*(4), 844–853.

Smith, D. (2012). *Monkey mind.* Simon & Schuster.

Smith, D. G., & Robbins, T. W. (2013). The neurobiological underpinnings of obesity and binge eating: A rationale for adopting the Food Addiction Model. *Biological Psychiatry, 73*, 804–810.

Smith, G. T., Goldman, M. S., Greenbaum, P. E., & Christiansen, B. A. (1995). Expectancy for social facilitation from drinking: The divergent paths of high expectancy and low expectancy adolescents. *Journal of Abnormal Psychology, 104*, 32–40.

Smith, K. E., Ellison, J. M., Crosby, R. D., Engel, S. G., Mitchell, J. E., Crow, S. J., et al. (2017). The validity of DSM-5 severity specifiers for anorexia nervosa, bulimia nervosa, and binge-eating disorder. *International Journal of Eating Disorders, 50*(9), 1109–1113.

Smith, M. L., Glass, G. V., & Miller, T. I. (1980). *The benefits of psychotherapy.* Johns Hopkins University Press.

Smith, P. H., Kasza, K. A., Hyland, A., Fong, G. T., Borland, R., Brady, K., et al. (2015). Gender differences in medication use and cigarette smoking cessation: Results from the International Tobacco Control Four Country Survey. *Nicotine & Tobacco Research, 17*(4), 463–472.

Smith, S. F., & Lilienfeld, S. O. (2013). Psychopathy in the workplace: The knowns and unknowns. *Aggression and Violent Behavior, 18*, 204–218.

Smith, S. F., & Lilienfeld, S. O. (2015). The response modulation hypothesis of psychopathy: A meta-analytic and narrative analysis. *Psychological Bulletin 141*, 1145–1177. https://doi.org/10.1037/bul0000024

Smit, K., Voogt, C., Hiemstra, M., Kleinjan, M., Otten, R., & Kuntsche, E. (2018). Development of alcohol expectancies and early alcohol use in children and adolescents: A systematic review. *Clinical Psychology Review, 60*, 136–146.

Smoller, J. W. (2016). The genetics of stress-related disorders: PTSD, depression, and anxiety disorders. *Neuropsychopharmacology: Official Publication of the American College of Neuropsychopharmacology, 41*(1), 297–319. https://doi.org/10.1038/NPP.2015.266

Smoller, J. W., Andreassen, O. A., Edenberg, H. J., Faraone, S. V., Glatt, S. J., & Kendler, K. S. (2019). Psychiatric genetics and the structure of psychopathology. *Molecular Psychiatry, 24*(3), 409–420.

Smoski, M. J., & Areán, P. A. (2015). Individual and group psychotherapy. In D. C. Steffens, D. G. Blazer, & M. E. Thakur (Eds.), *The American Psychiatric Publishing textbook of geriatric psychiatry.* American Psychiatric Publishing.

Smyth, J., Wonderlich, S. A., Heron, K. E., Sliwinski, M. J., Crosby, R. D., Mitchell, J. E., et al. (2007). Daily and momentary mood and stress are associated with binge eating and vomiting in bulimia nervosa patients in the natural environment. *Journal of Consulting and Clinical Psychology, 75*, 629–638.

Sniekers, S., Stringer, S., Watanabe, K., Jansen, P. R., Coleman, J. R. I., Krapohl, E., et al. (2017). Genome-wide association meta-analysis of 78,308 individuals identifies new loci and genes influencing human intelligence. *Nature Genetics, 11*, 201. https://doi.org/10.1038/ng.3869

Snowden, L. R. (2012). Health and mental health policies' role in better understanding and closing African American–White American disparities in treatment access and quality of care. *American Psychologist, 67*(7), 524–531. https://doi.org/10.1037/a0030054

Sobell, L. C., Sobell, M. B., & Agrawal, S. (2009). Randomized controlled trial of a cognitive-behavioral motivational intervention in a group versus individual format for substance use disorders. *Psychology of Addictive Behaviors: Journal of the Society of Psychologists in Addictive Behaviors, 23*, 672–683.

Sobell, M. B., & Sobell, L. C. (1993). *Problem drinkers: Guided self-change treatment.* Guilford Press.

Sobell, M. B., & Sobell, L. C. (2005). Guided self-change model of treatment for substance use disorders. *Journal of Cognitive Psychotherapy*, (3), 199–210.

Södersten, P., Bergh, C., Leon, M., & Zandian, M. (2016). Dopamine and anorexia nervosa. *Neuroscience & Biobehavioral Reviews, 60*, 26–30.

Solis, E. C., van Hemert, A. M., Carlier, I. V. E., Wardenaar, K. J., Schoevers, R. A., Beekman, A. T. F., et al. (2021). The 9-year clinical course of depressive and anxiety disorders: New NESDA findings. *Journal of Affective Disorders, 295*, 1269–1279. https://doi.org/10.1016/j.jad.2021.08.108

Soloff, P. H., & Chiappetta, L. (2019). 10-year outcome of suicidal behavior in borderline personality disorder. *Journal of Personality Disorders, 33*(1), 82–100. https://doi.org/10.1521/PEDI_2018_32_332

Solway, A., Lin, Z., & Vinaik, E. (2020). Transfer of information across repeated decisions in general and in obsessive-compulsive disorder. *Proceedings of the National Academy of Sciences, 118*(1). https://doi.org/10.1073/pnas.2014271118.

Sordo, L., Barrio, G., Bravo, M. J., Indave, B. I., Degenhardt, L., Wiessing, L., et al. (2017). Mortality risk during and after opioid substitution treatment: Systematic review and meta-analysis of cohort studies. *BMJ, 357*, j1550. https://doi.org/10.1136/bmj.j1550

Soto, C. J., & John, O. P. (2016). The Next Big Five Inventory (BFI-2): Developing and Assessing a Hierarchical Model With 15 Facets to Enhance Bandwidth, Fidelity, and Predictive Power. *Journal of Personality and Social Psychology.* https://doi.org/10.1037/pspp0000096

South, S. C. (2021). Pathology in relationships. *Annual Review of Clinical Psychology, 17*(1), 577–601. https://doi.org/10.1146/annurev-clinpsy-081219-115420

Spencer, M. R., Warner, M., & Chisewski, J. A. (2023). Estimates of drug overdose deaths involving fentanyl, methamphetamine, cocaine, heroin, and oxycodone: United States, 2021. *NVSS, 27.* https://stacks.cdc.gov/view/cdc/125504

Spence, S. H., & Rapee, R. M. (2016). The etiology of social anxiety disorder: An evidence-based model. *Expanding the Impact of Cognitive Behaviour Therapy: A Special Edition in Honor of G. Terence Wilson, 86*, 50–67.

Sperling, R. A., Aisen, P. S., Beckett, L. A., Bennett, D. A., Craft, S., Fagan, A. M., et al. (2011). Toward defining the preclinical stages of Alzheimer's disease: Recommendations from the National Institute on Aging-Alzheimer's Association workgroups on diagnostic guidelines for Alzheimer's disease. *Alzheimer's and Dementia: The Journal of the Alzheimer's Association, 7*, 280–292.

Spitzer, R. L., Gibbon, M., Skodol, A. E., Williams, J. B. W., & First, M. B. (Eds.). (1994). *DSM-IV casebook: A learning companion to the Diagnostic and Statistical Manual of Mental Disorders* (4th ed.). American Psychiatric Press.

Sprich, S., Biederman, J., Crawford, M. H., Mundy, E., & Faraone, S. V. (2000). Adoptive and biological families of children and adolescents with ADHD. *Journal of the American Academy of Child and Adolescent Psychiatry, 39*, 1432–1437.

Springer, K. S., Levy, H. C., & Tolin, D. F. (2018). Remission in CBT for adult anxiety disorders: A meta-analysis. *Clinical Psychology Review, 61*, 1–8. https://doi.org/10.1016/j.cpr.2018.03.002

Sprooten, E., Rasgon, A., Goodman, M., Carlin, A., Leibu, E., Lee, W. H., et al. (2017). Addressing reverse inference in psychiatric neuroimaging: Meta-analyses of task-related brain activation in common mental disorders. *Human Brain Mapping, 38*, 1846–1864.

Stack, S. (2000). Media impacts on suicide: A quantitative review of 293 findings. *Social Science Quarterly, 81*, 957–971.

Stacy, A. W., Newcomb, M. D., & Bentler, P. M. (1991). Cognitive motivation and drug use: A 9-year longitudinal study. *Journal of Abnormal Psychology, 100*, 502–515.

Stanfield, A. C., McIntosh, A. M., Spencer, M. D., Philip, R., Gaur, S., & Lawrie, S. M. (2008). Towards a neuroanatomy of autism: A systematic review and meta-analysis of structural magnetic resonance imaging studies. *European Psychiatry, 23*(4), 289–299.

Stanley, B., Brown, G. K., Brenner, L. A., Galfalvy, H. C., Currier, G. W., Knox, K. L., Chaudhury, S. R., et al. (2018). Comparison of the safety planning intervention with follow-up vs usual care of suicidal patients treated in the emergency department. *JAMA Psychiatry, 75*(9), 894–900. https://doi.org/10.1001/jamapsychiatry.2018.1776

Stapinski, L. A., Abbott, M. J., & Rapee, R. M. (2010). Evaluating the cognitive avoidance model of generalised anxiety disorder: Impact of worry on threat appraisal, perceived control and anxious arousal. *Behaviour Research and Therapy, 48*(10), 1032–1040. https://doi.org/10.1016/j.brat.2010.07.005

Stapinski, L. A., Bowes, L., Wolke, D., Pearson, R. M., Mahedy, L., Button, K. S., et al. (2014). Peer victimization during adolescence and risk for anxiety disorders in adulthood: A prospective cohort study. *Depression and Anxiety, 31*(7), 574–582. https://doi.org/10.1002/da.22270

Staugaard, S. R. (2010). Threatening faces and social anxiety: A literature review. *Clinical Psychology Review, 30*, 669–690.

Stead, L. F., Perera, R., Bullen, C., Mant, D., Hartmann-Boyce, J., Cahill, K., et al. (2012). Nicotine replacement therapy for smoking cessation. *Cochrane Database of Systematic Reviews, 11*. https://doi.org/10.1002/14651858.CD000146.pub4

Steadman, H. J. (1979). *Beating a rap: Defendants found incompetent to stand trial*. University of Chicago Press.

Steadman, H. J., McGreevy, M. A., Morrissey, J. P., Callahan, L. A., Robbins, P. C., & Cirincione, C. (1993). *Before and after Hinckley: Evaluating insanity defense reform*. Guilford Press.

Steadman, H. J., Monahan, J., Pinals, D. A., Vesselinov, R., & Robbins, P. C. (2015). Gun violence and victimization of strangers by persons with a mental illness: Data from the MacArthur Violence Risk Assessment Study. *Psychiatric Services, 66*(11), 1238–1241. https://doi.org/10.1176/appi.ps.201400512

Steadman, H. J., Mulvey, E. P., Monahan, J., Robbins, P. C., Appelbaum, P. S., Grisso, T., Roth, L. H., & Silver, E. (1998). Violence by people discharged from acute psychiatric inpatient facilities and by others in the same neighborhoods. *Archives of General Psychiatry, 55*, 393–401.

Steadman, H. J., Osher, F. C., Robbins, P. C., Case, B., & Samuels, S. (2009). Prevalence of serious mental illness among jail inmates. *Psychiatric Services, 60*, 761–765.

Steele, C. M., & Josephs, R. A. (1988). Drinking your troubles away: 2. An attention-allocation model of alcohol's effects on psychological stress. *Journal of Abnormal Psychology, 97*, 196–205.

Steele, C. M., & Josephs, R. A. (1990). Alcohol myopia: Its prized and dangerous effects. *American Psychologist, 45*, 921–933.

Steel, Z., Silove, D., Giao, N. M., Phan, T. T., Chey, T., Whelan, A., et al. (2009). International and indigenous diagnoses of mental disorder among Vietnamese living in Vietnam and Australia. *British Journal of Psychiatry, 194*, 326–333. https://doi.org/10.1192/bjp.bp.108.050906

Steel, Z., Silove, D., Giao, N. M., Phan, T. T., Chey, T., Whelan, A., et al. (2009). International and indigenous diagnoses of mental disorder among Vietnamese living in Vietnam and Australia. *The British Journal of Psychiatry: The Journal of Mental Science, 194*(4), 326–333. https://doi.org/10.1192/bjp.bp.108.050906

Steenkamp, M. M., Litz, B. T., & Marmar, C. R. (2020). First-line psychotherapies for military-related PTSD. *JAMA, 323*(7), 656–657. https://doi.org/10.1001/JAMA.2019.20825

Steiger, H., Gauvin, L., Jabalpurwala, S., & Séguin, J. R. (1999). Hypersenstivity to social interactions in bulimic syndromes: Relationship to binge eating. *Journal of Consulting and Clinical Psychology, 67*, 765–775.

Steinberg, D., Mills, D., & Romano, M. (2015). *When did prisons become acceptable mental healthcare facilities?* Stanford Law School Three Strikes Project, February 19, 2015. https://law.stanford.edu/publications/when-did-prisons-become-acceptable-mental-health-care-facilities-2/

Steinberg, D., Mills, D., & Romano, M. (2015). *When did prisons become acceptable mental healthcare facilities?* Stanford Law School Three Strikes Project. https://law.stanford.edu/publications/when-did-prisons-become-acceptable-mental-healthcare-facilities-2/

Steinberg, M. (1994). *Structured clinical interview for DSM-IV dissociative disorders (SCID-D)*. American Psychiatric Press.

Steinbrecher, N., Koerber, S., Frieser, D., & Hiller, W. (2011). The prevalence of medically unexplained symptoms in primary care. *Psychosomatics, 52*(3), 263–271. https://doi.org/10.1016/j.psym.2011.01.007

Stein, D. J., Aguilar-Gaxiola, S., Alonso, J., Bruffaerts, R., De Jonge, P., Liu, Z., et al. (2014). Associations between mental disorders and subsequent onset of hypertension. *General Hospital Psychiatry, 36*, 142–149.

Stein, D. J., Koenen, K. C., Friedman, M. J., Hill, E., McLaughlin, K. A., Petukhova, M., et al. (2013). Dissociation in posttraumatic stress disorder: Evidence from the World Mental Health surveys. *Biological Psychiatry, 73*, 302–312.

Stein, D. J., Kogan, C. S., Atmaca, M., Fineberg, N. A., Fontenelle, L. F., Grant, J. E., et al. (2016). The classification of Obsessive–Compulsive and Related Disorders in the ICD-11. *Journal of Affective Disorders, 190*, 663–674. https://doi.org/10.1016/j.jad.2015.10.061

Stein, D. J., Phillips, K. A., Bolton, D., Fulford, K. W., Sadler, J. Z., & Kendler, K. S. (2010). What is a mental/psychiatric disorder? From DSM-IV to DSM-V. *Psychological Medicine, 40*, 1759–1765.

Stein, E. A., Pankiewicz, J., Harsch, H. H., Cho, J. K., Fuller, S. A., Hawkins M., et al. (1998). Nicotine-induced limbic cortical activation in the human brain: A functional MRI study. *American Journal of Psychiatry, 155*, 1009–1015.

Steinglass, J. E., & Foerde, K. (2018). Reward system abnormalities in anorexia nervosa: Navigating a path forward. *JAMA Psychiatry, 75*(10), 993–994.

Steinglass, J. E., & Walsh, B. T. (2016). Neurobiological model of the persistence of anorexia nervosa. *Journal of Eating Disorders, 4*(19), 1–7. https://doi.org/10.1186/s40337-016-0106-2

Steinhausen, H.-C. (2002). The outcome of anorexia nervosa in the 20th century. *American Journal of Psychiatry, 159*, 1284–1293. https://doi.org/10.1176/appi.ajp.159.8.1284

Steinhausen, H., & Weber, S. (2009). The outcome of bulimia nervosa: Findings from one-quarter century of research. *American Journal of Psychiatry, 166*, 1331–1341.

Steketee, G., & Frost, R. O. (2003). Compulsive hoarding: Current status of the research. *Clinical Psychology Review, 23*, 905–927.

Steketee, G., & Frost, R. O. (2015). Phenomenology of hoarding. In R. O. Frost & G. Steketee (Eds.), *The Oxford handbook of hoarding and acquiring*. Oxford University Press.

Stephens, S., Elchuk, D., Davidson, M., & Williams, S. (2022). A review of childhood sexual abuse perpetration prevention programs. *Current Psychiatry Reports, 24*(11), 679–685. https://doi.org/10.1007/S11920-022-01375-8/METRICS

Stepp, S. D., Lazarus, S. A., & Byrd, A. L. (2016). A systematic review of risk factors prospectively associated with borderline personality disorder: Taking stock and moving forward. *Personality Disorders: Theory, Research, and Treatment, 7*, 316–323. https://doi.org/10.1037/per0000186

Stern, A. M. (2015). *Eugenic nation: Faults and frontiers of better breeding in modern America*. University of California Press.

Stern, A. M., Novak, N. L., Lira, N., O'Connor, K., Harlow, S., & Kardia, S. (2017). California's sterilization survivors: An estimate and call for redress. *American Journal of Public Health, 107*, 50–54.

Stewart, M. O., Raffa, S. D., Steele, J. L., Miller, S. A., Clougherty, K. F., Hinrichsen, G. A., et al. (2014). National dissemination of interpersonal psychotherapy for depression in veterans: Therapist and patient-level outcomes. *Journal of Consulting and Clinical Psychology, 82*(6), 1201–1206. https://doi.org/10.1037/a0037410

Stice, E. (2001). A prospective test of the dual-pathway model of bulimic pathology: Mediating effects of dieting and negative affect. *Journal of Abnormal Psychology, 110*, 124–135.

Stice, E. (2002). Risk and maintenance factors for eating pathology: A meta-analytic review. *Psychological Bulletin, 128*(5), 825–848. https://doi.org/10.1037/0033-2909.128.5.825

Stice, E. (2016). Interactive and mediational etiologic models of eating disorder onset: Evidence from prospective studies. *Annual Review of Clinical Psychology, 12*, 359–381. https://doi.org/10.1146/annurev-clinpsy-021815-093317

Stice, E., Becker, C. B., & Yokum, S. (2013). Eating disorder prevention: Current evidence-base and future directions. *International Journal of Eating Disorders, 46*(5), 478–485.

Stice, E., & Burger, K. (2019). Neural vulnerability factors for obesity. *Clinical Psychology Review, 68*, 38–53.

Stice, E., Burton, E. M., & Shaw, H. (2004). Prospective relations between bulimic pathology, depression, and substance abuse: Unpacking comorbidity in adolescent girls. *Journal of Consulting and Clinical Psychology, 72*, 62–71.

Stice, E., & Desjardins, C. D. (2018). Interactions between risk factors in the prediction of onset of eating disorders: Exploratory hypothesis generating analyses. *Expanding the Impact of Cognitive Behaviour Therapy: a Special Edition in Honor of G. Terence Wilson, 105*, 52–62.

Stice, E., Durant, S., Rohde, P., & Shaw, H. (2014). Effects of a prototype internet dissonance-based eating disorder prevention program at 1- and 2-year follow-up. *Health Psychology, 33*, 1558–1567. https://doi.org/10.1037/hea0000090

Stice, E., Marti, C. N., & Rohde, P. (2013). Prevalence, incidence, impairment, and course of the proposed eating disorder diagnoses in an 8-year prospective community study of young women. *Journal of Abnormal Psychology, 122*, 445–457.

Stice, E., Marti, C. N., Shaw, H., & Rohde, P. (2019). Meta-analytic review of dissonance-based eating disorder prevention programs: Intervention, participant, and facilitator features that predict larger effects. *Clinical Psychology Review, 70*, 91–107.

Stice, E., Marti, C. N., Spoor, S., Presnell, K., & Shaw, H. (2008). Dissonance and healthy weight eating disorder prevention programs: Long-term effects from a randomized efficacy trial. *Journal of Consulting and Clinical Psychology, 76*, 329–240.

Stice, E., Rohde, P., Shaw, H., & Gau, J. M. (2017). Clinician-led, peer-led, and Internet-delivered dissonance-based eating disorder prevention programs: Acute effectiveness of these delivery modalities. *Journal of Consulting and Clinical Psychology, 85*, 883–895. https://doi.org/10.1037/ccp0000211.

Stice, E., Rohde, P., Shaw, H., & Gau, J. M. (2020). Clinician-led, peer-led, and internet-delivered dissonance-based eating disorder prevention programs: Effectiveness of these delivery modalities through 4-year follow-up. *Journal of Consulting and Clinical Psychology, 88*(5), 481–494. https://doi.org/10.1037/ccp0000493

Stice, E., Rohde, P., Shaw, H., & Marti, C. N. (2013). Efficacy trial of a selective prevention program targeting both eating disorders and obesity among female college students: 1- and 2-year follow-up effects. *Journal of Consulting and Clinical Psychology, 81*(1), 183–189.

Stice, E., & Van Ryzin, M. J. (2018). A prospective test of the temporal sequencing of risk factor emergence in the dual pathway model of eating disorders. *Journal of Abnormal Psychology, 128*, 119–128.

Stice, E., & Yokum, S. (2016). Neural vulnerability factors that increase risk for future weight gain. *Psychological Bulletin, 142*, 447–471.

Stone, A. A., Schneider, S., & Smyth, J. M. (2023). Evaluation of Pressing Issues in Ecological Momentary Assessment. *Annual Review of Clinical Psychology, 19*, 107–131. https://doi.org/10.1146/annurev-clinpsy-080921-083128

Stone, J., LaFrance, W. C., Jr., Levenson, J. L., & Sharpe, M. (2010). Issues for DSM-5: Conversion disorder. *American Journal of Psychiatry, 167*, 626–627.

Stone, J., Smyth, R., Carson, A., Lewis, S., Prescott, R., Warlow, C., et al. (2005). Systematic review of misdiagnosis of conversion symptoms and "hysteria." *British Medical Journal, 331*, 989.

Stone, M. B., Yaseen, Z. S., Miller, B. J., Richardville, K., Kalaria, S. N., & Kirsch, I. (2022). Response to acute monotherapy for major depressive disorder in randomized, placebo controlled trials submitted to the US Food and Drug Administration: Individual participant data analysis. *BMJ*, e067606. https://doi.org/10.1136/bmj-2021-067606

Stone, M. H. (1993). *Abnormalities of personality. Within and beyond the realm of treatment*. W. W. Norton.

Storebø, O. J., Stoffers-Winterling, J. M., Völlm, B. A., Kongerslev, M. T., Mattivi, J. T., Jørgensen, M. S., et al. (2020). Psychological therapies for people with borderline personality disorder. *Cochrane Database of Systematic Reviews, 2020*(11). https://doi.org/10.1002/14651858.CD012955.pub2

Stossel, S. (2014, January/February). Surviving anxiety. *Atlantic Monthly*, 1–6.

Stotzer, R. L. (2009). Violence against transgender people: A review of United States data. *Aggression and Violent Behavior, 14*(3), 170–179.

Stoving, R. K., Hangaard, J., Hansen-Nord, M., & Hagen, C. (1999). A review of endocrine changes in anorexia nervosa. *Journal of Psychiatric Research, 33*, 139–152.

Strain, E. C., Bigelow, G. E., Liebson, I. A., & Stitzer, M. L. (1999). Moderate- vs low-dose methadone in the treatment of opioid dependence. *Journal of the American Medical Association, 281*, 1000–1005.

Strauss, A. Y., Fradkin, I., McNally, R. J., Linkovski, O., Anholt, G. E., & Huppert, J. D. (2020). Why check? A meta-analysis of checking in obsessive-compulsive disorder: Threat vs. distrust of senses. *Clinical Psychology Review, 75*. https://doi.org/10.1016/j.cpr.2019.101807

Streeton, C., & Whelan, G. (2001). Naltrexone, a relapse prevention maintenance treatment of alcohol dependence: A meta-analysis of randomized controlled trials. *Alcohol and Alcoholism, 36*, 544–552.

Streltzer, J., & Johansen, L. G. (2006). Prescription drug dependence and evolving beliefs about chronic pain management. *American Journal of Psychiatry, 163*, 594–598.

Striegel-Moore, R. H., & Franco, D. L. (2008). Should binge eating disorder be included in the DSM-V? A critical review of the state of the evidence. *Annual Review of Clinical Psychology, 4*, 305–324.

Stringer, S., Minica, C. C., Verweij, K. J. H., Mbarek, H., Bernard, M., Derringer, J., et al. (2016). Genome-wide association study of lifetime cannabis use based on a large meta-analytic sample of 32,330 subjects from the International Cannabis Consortium. *Translational Psychiatry, 6*, e769. https://doi.org/10.1038/tp.2016.36

Strober, M., Freeman, R., Lampert, C., Diamond, J., & Kaye, W. (2000). Controlled family study of anorexia nervosa and bulimia nervosa: Evidence of shared liability and transmission of partial syndromes. *American Journal of Psychiatry, 157*, 393–401.

Strother, E., Lemberg, R., Stanford, S. C., & Turberville, D. (2012). Eating disorders in men: Underdiagnosed, undertreated, and misunderstood. *Eating Disorders, 20*(5), 346–355. https://doi.org/10.1080/10640266.2012.715512

Strub, R. L., & Black, F. W. (1981). *Organic brain syndromes: An introduction to neurobehavioral disorders.* F. A. Davis.

Stumpf, B. P., de Souza, L. C., Mourão, M. S. F., Rocha, F. L., Fontenelle, L. F., & Barbosa, I. G. (2022). Cognitive impairment in hoarding disorder: A systematic review. *CNS Spectrums*, 1–13. https://doi.org/10.1017/S1092852922000153

Sturm, R. A., Duffy, D. L., Zhao, Z. Z., et al. (2008). A single SNP in an evolutionary conserved region within intron 86 of the HERC2 gene determines human blue-brown eye color. *American Journal of Human Genetics, 82*, 424–431.

Styron, W. (1992). *Darkness visible: A memoir of madness.* Vintage.

Substance Abuse and Mental Health Services Administration. (2022). Results from the 2021 National Survey on Drug Use and Health: Detailed tables. https://www.samhsa.gov/data/release/2021-national-survey-drug-use-and-health-nsduh-releases#detailed-tables

Substance Abuse and Mental Health Services Administration (SAMHSA). (2021). Results from the 2021 National Survey on Drug Use and Health: Summary of National Findings. NSDUH Series H-44, HHS Publication No. (SMA) 12-4713. SAMHSA, Center for Behavioral Health Statistics and Quality.

Substance Abuse and Mental Health Services Administration (SAMHSA). (2022). Key substance use and mental health indicators in the United States: Results from the 2021 National Survey on Drug Use and Health (HHS Publication No. PEP22-07-01-005, NSDUH Series H-57). Center for Behavioral Health Statistics and Quality, Substance Abuse and Mental Health Services Administration. https://www.samhsa.gov/data/report/2021-nsduh-annual-national-report

Substance Abuse and Mental Health Services Administration (SAMHSA). (2022). *Key substance use and mental health indicators in the United States: Results from the 2021 National Survey on Drug Use and Health* (HHS Publication No. PEP22-07-01-005, NSDUH Series H-57). Rockville, MD: Center for Behavioral Health Statistics and Quality, Substance Abuse and Mental Health Services Administration. Retrieved from https://www.samhsa.gov/data/report/2021-nsduh-annual-national-report

Substance Abuse and Mental Health Services Administration (SAMHSA). (2022). Mental Health Annual Report 2015-2020: Use of Mental Health Services: National Client Level Data *(https://www.samhsa.gov/data/data-we-collect/mh-cld-mental-health-client-level-data).*

Suchy, Y., Eastvold, A. D., Strassberg, D. S., & Franchow, E. I. (2014). Understanding processing speed weaknesses among pedophilic child molesters: Response style vs. neuropathology. *Journal of Abnormal Psychology, 123*, 273–285.

Sue, S., Zane, N., Nagayama Hall, G. C., & Berger, L. K. (2009). The case for cultural competency in psychotherapeutic interventions. *Annual Review of Psychology, 60*, 525–548. https://doi.org/10.1146/annurev.psych.60.110707.163651

Su, L.-D., Xu, F.-X., Wang, X.-T., Cai, X.-Y., & Shen, Y. (2020). Cerebellar dysfunction, cerebro-cerebellar connectivity and autism spectrum disorders. *Neuroscience, 462*, 320–327.

Sullivan, P. F., Agrawal, A., Bulik, C. M., Andreassen, O. A., Børglum, A. D., Breen, G., et al. (2018). Psychiatric genomics: An update and an agenda. *American Journal of Psychiatry, 175*, 15–27. https://doi.org/10.1176/appi.ajp.2017.17030283

Sullivan, P. F., Daly, M. J., & O'Donovan, M. (2012). Genetic architectures of psychiatric disorders: The emerging picture and its implications. *Nature Reviews Genetics, 13*, 537–551.

Sullivan, P. F., & Geschwind, D. H. (2019). Defining the genetic, genomic, cellular, and diagnostic architectures of psychiatric disorders. *Cell, 177*(1), 162–183. https://doi.org/10.1016/j.cell.2019.01.015

Sullivan, P. F., Kendler, K. S., & Neale, M. C. (2003). Schizophrenia as a complex trait: Evidence from a meta-analysis of twin studies. *Archives of General Psychiatry, 60*(12), 1187–1192.

Sullivan, P. F., Neale, M. C., & Kendler, K. S. (2000). Genetic epidemiology of major depression: Review and meta-analysis. *American Journal of Psychiatry, 157*, 1552–1562.

Summers, A., & Swan, R. (2006). Sinatra: The Life Corgi Books.

Sun, D., Phillips, L., Velakoulis, D., Yung, A., McGorry, P. D., Wood, S. J., et al. (2009). Progressive brain structural changes mapped as psychosis develops in "at risk" individuals. *Schizophrenia Research, 108*, 85–92.

Sussman, S., Dent, C. W., McAdams, L., Stacy, A. W., Burton, D., & Flay, B. R. (1994). Group self-identification and adolescent cigarette smoking: A 1-year prospective study. *Journal of Abnormal Psychology, 103*, 576–580.

Sussman, S., Miyano, J., Rohrbach, L. A., Dent, C. W., & Sun, P. (2007). Six-month and one-year effects of project EX-4: A classroom-based smoking prevention and cessation intervention program. *Addictive Behaviors, 32*, 3005–3014. https://doi.org/10.1016/j.addbeh.2007.06.016

Sutker, P. B., Uddo, M., Brailey, K., Vasterling, J. J., & Errera, P. (1994). Psychopathology in war-zone deployed and nondeployed Operation Desert Storm troops assigned grave registration duties. *Journal of Abnormal Psychology, 103*, 383–390.

Suzuki, K., Takei, N., Kawai, M., Minabe, Y., & Mori, N. (2003). Is taijin kyofusho a culture-bound syndrome? *American Journal of Psychiatry, 160*(7), 1358.

Swain, J., Koszycki, D., Shlik, J., & Bradwein, J. (2003). Pharmacological challenge agents in anxiety. In D. Nutt & J. C. Ballenger (Eds.), *Anxiety disorders* (pp. 269–295). Blackwell.

Swanson, J., Hinshaw, S. P., Arnold, L. E., Gibbons, R., Marcus, S., Hur, K., et al. (2007). Secondary evaluations of MTA 36-month outcomes: Propensity score and growth mixture model analyses. *Journal of the American Academy of Child and Adolescent Psychiatry, 46*, 1002–1013.

Swanson, J. W., Holzer, C. E., Ganju, V. K., & Jono, R. T. (1990). Violence and psychiatric disorder in the community: Evidence from the Epidemiological Catchment Area surveys. *Hospital and Community Psychiatry, 41*, 761–770.

Swanson, J. W., McGinty, E. E., Fazel, S., & Mays, V. M. (2015). Mental illness and reduction of gun violence and suicide: Bringing epidemiologic research to policy. *Annals of Epidemiology, 25*(5), 366–376.

Swartz, J. R., Williamson, D. E., & Hariri, A. R. (2015). Developmental change in amygdala reactivity during adolescence: Effects of family history of depression and stressful life events. *American Journal of Psychiatry, 172*(3), 276–283. https://doi.org/10.1176/appi.ajp.2014.14020195

Szechtman, H., & Woody, E. Z. (2004). Obsessive-compulsive disorder as a disturbance of security motivation. *Psychological Review, 111,* 111–127.

Tackett, J. L., Brandes, C. M., King, K. M., & Markon, K. E. (2019). Psychology's replication crisis and clinical psychological science. *Annual Review of Clinical Psychology, 15,* 579–604. https://doi.org/10.1146/annurev-clinpsy-050718-095710

TADS team. (2007). The Treatment for Adolescents with Depression Study (TADS): Long Term Effectiveness and Safety Outcomes. *Archives of General Psychiatry, 64,* 1132–1144.

Tajika, A., Ogawa, Y., Takeshima, N., Hayasaka, Y., & Furukawa, T. A. (2015). Replication and contradiction of highly cited research papers in psychiatry: 10-year follow-up. *British Journal of Psychiatry, 207,* 357–362. https://doi.org/10.1192/bjp.bp.113.143701

Talbott, M. R., & Miller, M. R. (2020). Future directions for infant identification and intervention for autism spectrum disorder from a transdiagnostic perspective. *Journal of Clinical Child & Adolescent Psychology, 49*(5), 688–700. https://doi.org/10.1080/15374416.2020.1790382

Talih, S., Balhas, Z., Eissenberg, T., Salman, R., Karaoghlanian, N., El Hellani, A., et al. (2015). Effects of user puff topography, device voltage, and liquid nicotine concentration on electronic cigarette nicotine yield: Measurements and model predictions. *Nicotine & Tobacco Research, 17,* 150–157.

Tambs, K., Czajkowsky, N., Røysamb, E., Neale, M. C., Reichborn-Kjennerud, T., Aggen, S. H., et al. (2009). Structure of genetic and environmental risk factors for dimensional representations of DSM-IV anxiety disorders. *The British Journal of Psychiatry: The Journal of Mental Science, 195*(4), 301–307. https://doi.org/10.1192/bjp.bp.108.059485

Tamir, M. Schwartz, S. H., Oishi, S., & Kim, M. Y. (2017). The secret to happiness: Feeling good or feeling right? *Journal of Experimental Psychology. General, 146*(10), 1448–1459. https://doi.org/10.1037/xge0000303

Tang, S. X., & Gur, R. E. (2017). Longitudinal perspectives on the psychosis spectrum in 22q11.2 deletion syndrome. *American Journal of Medical Genetics Part A, 176*(10), 2192–2202. https://doi.org/10.1002/ajmg.a.38500

Tao, K. W., Owen, J., Pace, B. T., & Imel, Z. E. (2015). A meta-analysis of multicultural competencies and psychotherapy process and outcome. *Journal of Counseling Psychology, 62*(3), 337–350. https://doi.org/10.1037/cou0000086

Tarbox, S. I., Addington, J., Cadenhead, K., Cannon, T., Cornblatt, B., Perkins, D., et al. (2013). Premorbid functional development and conversion to psychosis in clinical high-risk youths. *Development and Psychopathology, 25,* 1171–1186.

Tari, A. R., Nauman, J., Zisko, N., Skjellegrind, H. K., Bosnes, I., Bergh, S., et al. (2019). Temporal changes in cardiorespiratory fitness and risk of dementia incidence and mortality: A population-based prospective cohort study. *The Lancet Public Health, 4*(11), e565–e574. https://doi.org/10.1016/S2468-2667(19)30183-5

Tarrier, N., Taylor, K., & Gooding, P. (2008). Cognitive-behavioral interventions to reduce suicide behavior. *Behavior Modification, 32,* 77–108.

Task Force on Promotion and Dissemination of Psychological Procedures. (1995). Training in and dissemination of empirically-validated psychological treatments: Report and recommendations. *The Clinical Psychologist, 48,* 3–23.

Taylor, A., & Kim-Cohen, J. (2007). Meta-analysis of gene-environment interactions in developmental psychopathology. *Development and Psychopathology, 19,* 1029–1037.

Taylor, C. T., & Alden, L. E. (2011). To see ourselves as others see us: An experimental integration of the intra- and interpersonal consequences of self-protection in social anxiety disorder. *Journal of Abnormal Psychology, 120,* 129–141.

Taylor, J., Iacono, W. G., & McGue, M. (2000). Evidence for a genetic etiology of early-onset delinquency. *Journal of Abnormal Psychology, 109,* 634–643.

Taylor, L. E., Swerdfeger, A. L., & Eslick, G. D. (2014). Vaccines are not associated with autism: An evidence-based meta-analysis of case-control and cohort studies. *Vaccine, 32*(29), 3623–3629.

Taylor, S. (2011). Early versus late onset obsessive-compulsive disorder: Evidence for distinct subtypes. *Clinical Psychology Review, 31*(7), 1083–1100. https://doi.org/10.1016/j.cpr.2011.06.007

Taylor, S. (2020). Anxiety sensitivity. In *Clinical handbook of fear and anxiety: Maintenance processes and treatment mechanisms.* (pp. 65–80). American Psychological Association. https://doi.org/10.1037/0000150-004

Taylor, S., & Asmundson, G. J. (2012). Etiology of hypochondriasis: A preliminary behavioral-genetic investigation. *International Journal of Genetics and Gene Therapy Journal, 2,* 1. https://doi.org/10.5348/ijggt-2011-1-sr-1

Teachman, B. A., & Allen, J. P. (2007). Development of social anxiety: Social interaction predictors of implicit and explicit fear of negative evaluation. *Journal of Abnormal Child Psychology, 35,* 63–78.

Teasdale, J. D., Segal, Z. V., Williams, J. M., Ridgeway, V. A., Soulsby, J. M., & Lau, M. A. (2000). Prevention of relapse/recurrence in major depression by mindfulness-based cognitive therapy. *Journal of Consulting and Clinical Psychology,* 68, 615–623. https://doi.org/10.1037/0022-006X.68.4.615

Telch, M. J., & Harrington, P. J. (2011). Anxiety sensitivity and unexpectedness of arousal in mediating affective response to 35% carbon dioxide inhalation. Unpublished Manuscript.

Telch, M. J., Shermis, M. D., & Lucas, J. A. (1989). Anxiety sensitivity: Unitary personality trait or domain-specific appraisals? *Journal of Anxiety Disorders, 3,* 25–32.

ter Kuile, M. M., Both, S., & van Lankveld, J. J. (2012). Sexual dysfunctions in women. In P. Sturmey & M. Hersen (Eds.), *Handbook of evidence-based practice in clinical psychology, adult disorders* (Vol. 2, pp. 413–436). John Wiley & Sons.

ter Kuile, M. M., & Reissing, E. D. (2014). Lifelong vaginismus. In Y. M. Binik & K. S. K. Hall (Eds.), *Principles and practice of sex therapy* (5th ed., pp. 177–194). Guilford Press.

Terlizzi, E. P., & Norris, T. (2021). Mental health treatment among adults: United States, 2020. *NCHS Data Brief, 419,* 1–8.

Terlizzi, E. P., & Zablotsky, B. (2020). *Mental health treatment among adults: United States, 2019.* NCHS Data Brief, no 380. National Center for Health Statistics.

Terry, R. D. (2006). Alzheimer's disease and the aging brain. *Journal of Geriatric Psychiatry and Neurology, 19,* 125–128.

Thapar, A. (2018). Discoveries on the genetics of ADHD in the 21st century: New findings and their implications. *American Journal of Psychiatry, 175*(10), 943–950. https://doi.org/10.1176/appi.ajp.2018.18040383

Thapar, A., Rice, F., Hay, D., Boivin, J., Langley, K., van den Bree, M., et al. (2009). Prenatal smoking might not cause attention-deficit/hyperactivity disorder: Evidence from a novel design. *Biological Psychiatry, 66*(8), 722–727.

Theodoulou, A., Chepkin, S. C., Ye, W., Fanshawe, T. R., Bullen, C., Hartmann-Boyce, J., et al. (2023). Different doses, durations and modes of delivery of nicotine replacement therapy for smoking cessation. *Cochrane Database of Systematic Reviews, 6*(6), CD013008.

Thibaut, F., Cosyns, P., Fedoroff, J. P., Briken, P., Goethals, K., & Bradford, J. M. W. (2020). The World Federation of Societies of Biological Psychiatry (WFSBP) 2020 guidelines for the pharmacological treatment of paraphilic disorders. *The World Journal of Biological Psychiatry: The Official Journal of the World Federation of Societies of Biological Psychiatry, 21*(6), 412–490. https://doi.org/10.1080/15622975.2020.1744723

Thibaut, F., De La Barra, F., Gordon, H., Cosyns, P., & Bradford, J. M. (2010). The World Federation of Societies of Biological Psychiatry (WFSBP) guidelines for the biological treatment of paraphilias. *World Journal of Biological Psychiatry, 11*, 604–655.

Thoits, P. A. (1985). Self-labeling processes in mental illness: The role of emotional deviance. *American Journal of Sociology, 92*, 221–249.

Thompson, A., Petrie, T., & Anderson, C. (2017). Eating disorders and weight control behaviors change over a collegiate sport season. *Journal of Science and Medicine in Sport, 20*(9), 808–813. https://doi.org/10.1016/j.jsams.2017.03.005

Thompson, P. M., Hayashi, K. M., Simon, S. L., Geaga, J. A., Hong, S. A., Sui, Y., et al. (2004). Structural abnormalities in the brains of human subjects who use methamphetamine. *Journal of Neuroscience, 24*, 6028–6036.

Tick, B., Bolton, P., Happé, F., Rutter, M., & Rijsdijk, F. (2015). Heritability of autism spectrum disorders: A meta-analysis of twin studies. *Journal of Child Psychology and Psychiatry, 57*(5), 585–595. https://doi.org/10.1111/jcpp.12499

Tiede, G., & Walton, K. (2021). Social endophenotypes in autism spectrum disorder: A scoping review. *Development and Psychopathology, 33*(4), 1381–1409. https://doi.org/10.1017/S0954579420000577

Tiefer, L., Hall, M., & Tavris, C. (2002). Beyond dysfunction: A new view of women's sexual problems. *Journal of Sex and Marital Therapy, 28*, 225–232.

Tienari, P., Wynne, L. C., Laksy, K., Moring, J., Nieminen, P., Sorri, A., et al. (2003). Genetic boundaries of the schizophrenia spectrum: Evidence from the Finnish adoptive family study of schizophrenia. *American Journal of Psychiatry, 160*, 1587–1594.

Tienari, P., Wynne, L. C., Moring, J., Läksy, K., Nieminen, P., Sorri, A., et al. (2000). Finnish adoptive family study: Sample selection and adoptee DSM-III diagnoses. *Acta Psychiatrica Scandinavica, 101*, 433–443.

Tiggemann, M., & Williams, E. (2012). The role of self-objectification in disordered eating, depressed mood, and sexual functioning among women: A comprehensive test of Objectification Theory. *Psychology of Women Quarterly, 36*(1), 66–75. https://doi.org/10.1177/0361684311420250

Timpano, K. R., Bainter, S. A., Goodman, Z. T., Tolin, D. F., Steketee, G., & Frost, R. O. (2020). A network analysis of hoarding symptoms, saving and acquiring motives, and comorbidity. *Journal of Obsessive-Compulsive and Related Disorders, 25*, 10. https://doi.org/10.1016/j.jocrd.2020.100520

Timpano, K. R., Broman-Fulks, J. J., Glaesmer, H., Exner, C., Rief, W., Olatunji, B. O., et al. (2013). A taxometric exploration of the latent structure of hoarding. *Psychological Assessment, 25*, 194–203.

Timpano, K. R., Muroff, J., & Steketee, G. (2016). A review of the diagnosis and management of hoarding disorder. *Current Treatment Options in Psychiatry, 3*(4), 394–410. https://doi.org/10.1007/s40501-016-0098-1

Tinghög, P., Malm, A., Arwidson, C., Sigvardsdotter, E., Lundin, A., &Saboonchi, F. (2017). Prevalence of mental ill health, traumas and postmigration stress among refugees from Syria resettled in Sweden after 2011: a population-based survey. *BMJ Open, 7*(12). https://doi.org/10.1136/BMJOPEN-2017-018899

Tjaden, P., & Thoennes, N. (2006). *Extent, nature, and consequences of rape victimization: Findings from the National Violence Against Women Survey.* National Institute of Justice.

Tolin, D. F., & Foa, E. B. (2006). Sex differences in trauma and posttraumatic stress disorder: A quantitative review of 25 years of research. *Psychological Bulletin, 132*, 959–992.

Tolin, D. F., Frost, R. O., Steketee, G., Gray, K., & Fitch, K. (2008). The economic and social burden of compulsive hoarding. *Psychiatry Research, 160*, 200–211.

Tolin, D. F., Frost, R. O., Steketee, G., & Muroff, J. (2015). Cognitive behavioral therapy for hoarding disorder: A meta-analysis. *Depression and Anxiety, 32*(3), 158–166. https://doi.org/10.1002/da.22327

Tolin, D. F., Frost, R. O., Steketee, G., & Muroff, J. (2021). Cognitive behavioral therapy for hoarding disorder: A meta-analysis. *FOCUS, 19*(4), 468–476. https://doi.org/10.1176/APPI.FOCUS.19403

Tolin, D. F., Kiehl, K. A., Worhunsky, P., Book, G. A., & Maltby, N. (2009). An exploratory study of the neural mechanisms of decision making in compulsive hoarding. *Psychological Medicine, 39*, 325–336.

Tolin, D. F., Stevens, M. C., Villavicencio, A. L., Norberg, M. M., Calhoun, V. D., Frost, R. O., et al. (2012). Neural mechanisms of decision making in hoarding disorder. *Archives of General Psychiatry, 69*, 832–841.

Tolin, D. F., Worhunsky, P., & Maltby, N. (2004). Sympathetic magic in contamination-related OCD. *Journal of Behavior Therapy and Experimental Psychiatry, 35*, 193–205.

Tomiyama, A. J. (2019). Stress and Obesity. *Annual Review of Psychology, 70*(1), 703–718. https://doi.org/10.1146/annurev-psych-010418-102936

Tomlinson R. C., Hyde L. W., Dotterer H. L., Klump K. L., & Burt S. A. (2022). Parenting moderates the etiology of callous-unemotional traits in middle childhood. *Journal of Child Psychology and Psychiatry, 63*(8), 912–920. https://doi.org/10.1111/jcpp.13542

Tompkins, M. A., & Hartl, T. L. (2013). Family interventions for hoarding. In R. O. Frost & G. Steketee (Eds.), *The Oxford handbook of hoarding and acquiring* (pp. 303–315). Oxford University Press.

Tonstad, S., Tonnesen, P., Hajek, P., Williams, K. E., Billing, C. B., & Reeves, K. R. (2006). Varenicline Phase 3 Study Group. Effect of maintenance therapy with varenicline on smoking cessation: A randomized controlled trial. *JAMA, 296*, 64–71.

Topiwala, A., Allan, C. L., Valkanova, V., Zsoldos, E., Filippini, N., Sexton, C., et al. (2017). Moderate alcohol consumption as risk factor for adverse brain outcomes and cognitive decline: Longitudinal cohort study. *British Medical Journal, 357*, j2353. https://doi.org/10.1136/bmj.j2353

Torgersen, S., Lygren, S., Oien, P. A., Skre, I., Onstad, S., Edvardsen, J., et al. (2000). A twin study of personality disorders. *Comprehensive Psychiatry, 41*, 416–425. https://doi.org/10.1053/comp.2000.16560

Torgersen, S., Myers, J., Reichborn-Kjennerud, T., Røysamb, E., Kubarych, T. S., & Kendler, K. S. (2012). The heritability of cluster B personality disorders assessed both by personal interview and questionnaire. *Journal of Personality Disorders, 26*, 848–866. https://doi.org/10.1521/pedi.2012.26.6.848

Torres, U. S., Portela-Oliveira, E., Borgwardt, S., & Busatto, G. F. (2013). Structural brain changes associated with antipsychotic treatment in schizophrenia as revealed by voxel-based morphometric MRI: An activation likelihood estimation meta-analysis. *BMC Psychiatry, 13*, 139. https://doi.org/10.1186/1471-244X-13-342

Torrey, E. F. (2014). *American psychosis: How the federal government destroyed the mental illness treatment system.* Oxford University Press.

Torrey, E. F., Kennard, A. D., Eslinger, D., Lamb, R., & Pavle, J. (2010). *More mentally ill persons are in jails and prisons than hospitals: A survey of the state.* Treatment Advocacy Center and the National Sheriffs' Association.

Torrey, E. F., Zdanowicz, M. T., Kennard, A. D., Lamb, H. R., Eslinger, D., Biasotti, M. C., & Fuller, D. A. (2014). *The treatment of persons with mental illness in prisons and jails: A state survey.* Treatment Advocacy Center.

Torvik, F. A., Welander-Vatn, A., Ystrom, E., Knudsen, G. P., Czajkowski, N., Kendler, K. S., et al. (2016). Longitudinal associations between social anxiety disorder and avoidant personality disorder: A twin study. *Journal of Abnormal Psychology, 125*(1), 114–124. https://doi.org/10.1037/abn0000124

Torvik, F. A., Welander-Vatn, A., Ystrom, E., Knudsen, G. P., Czajkowski, N., Kendler, K. S., & Reichborn-Kjennerud, T. (2016). Longitudinal associations between social anxiety disorder and avoidant personality disorder: A twin study. *Journal of Abnormal Psychology, 125,* 114–124. https://doi.org/10.1037/abn0000124

Tost, H., Champagne, F. A., & Meyer-Lindenberg, A. (2015). Environmental influence in the brain, human welfare and mental health. *Nature Neuroscience, 18,* 1421–1431. https://doi.org/10.1038/nn.4108

Toufexis, A., Blackman, A., & Drummond, T. (1996, April 29). Why Jennifer got sick. *Time.*

Touyz, S., Le Grange, D., Lacey, H., Hay, P., Smith, R., Maguire, S., et al. (2013). Treating severe and enduring anorexia nervosa: A randomized controlled trial. *Psychological Medicine, 43,* 2501–2511.

Tran, G. Q., Haaga, D. A. F., & Chambless, D. L. (1997). Expecting that alcohol will reduce social anxiety moderates the relation between social anxiety and alcohol consumption. *Cognitive Therapy and Research, 21,* 535–553.

Traviss-Turner, G. D., West, R. M., & Hill, A. J. (2017). Guided self-help for eating disorders: A systematic review and metaregression. *European Eating Disorders Review, 25*(3), 148–164. https://doi.org/10.1002/erv.2507

Treadway, M. T., Bossaller, N. A., Shelton, R. C., & Zald, D. H. (2012). Effort-based decision-making in major depressive disorder: A translational model of motivational anhedonia. *Journal of Abnormal Psychology, 121*(3), 553–558. https://doi.org/10.1037/a0028813

Treadway, M. T., & Pizzagalli, D. A. (2014). Imaging the pathophysiology of major depressive disorder—from localist models to circuit-based analysis. *Biology of Mood & Anxiety Disorders, 4*(1), 5. https://doi.org/10.1186/2045-5380-4-5

Treatment Advocacy Center. (2019). Delayed and deteriorating: Serious mental illness and psychiatric boarding in emergency departments. https://www.treatmentadvocacycenter.org/storage/documents/backgrounders/delayed_and_deteriorating.pdf

Treat, T. A., & Viken, R. J. (2010). Cognitive processing of weight and emotional information in disordered eating. *Current Directions in Psychological Science, 19,* 81–85.

Trent, M., Dooley, D. G., & Dougé, J. (2019). The impact of racism on child and adolescent health. *Pediatrics, 144*(2), 14. https://doi.org/10.1542/peds.2019-1765

Trevillion, K., Oram, S., Feder, G., & Howard, L. M. (2012). Experiences of domestic violence and mental disorders: A systematic review and meta-analysis. *PLoS One, 7:* e51740.

Treynor, W., Gonzalez, R., & Nolen-Hoeksema, S. (2003). Rumination reconsidered: A psychometric analysis. *Cognitive Therapy and Research, 27,* 247–259.

Trickey, D., Siddaway, A. P., Meiser-Stedman, R., Serpell, L., & Field, A. P. (2012). A meta-analysis of risk factors for post-traumatic stress disorder in children and adolescents. *Clinical Psychology Review, 32*(2), 122–138.

Trierweiler, S. J., Neighbors, H. W., Munday, C., Thompson, E. E., Binion, V. J., & Gomez, J. P. (2000). Clinician attributions associated with the diagnosis of schizophrenia in African American and non–African American patients. *Journal of Consulting and Clinical Psychology, 68,* 171–175.

Trinder, H., & Salkovaskis, P. M. (1994). Personally relevant intrusions outside the laboratory: Long-term suppression increases intrusion. *Behaviour Research and Therapy, 32,* 833–842.

Trivedi, M. H., Rush, A. J., Wisniewski, S. R., Nierenberg, A. A., Warden, D., Ritz, L., et al. (2006). Evaluation of outcomes with citalopram for depression using measurement-based care in STAR*D: Implications for clinical practice. *American Journal of Psychiatry, 163,* 28–40.

Trollor, J. N., Anderson, T. M., Sachdev, P. S., Brodaty, H., & Andrews, G. (2007). Prevalence of mental disorders in the elderly: The Australian national mental health and well-being survey. *American Journal of Geriatric Psychiatry, 15*(6), 455–466. https://doi.org/10.1097/JGP.0b013e3180590ba9

Trottier, D., Benbouriche, M., & Bonneville, V. (2019). A meta-analysis on the association between rape myth acceptance and sexual coercion perpetration. *The Journal of Sex Research,* 1–8. https://doi.org/10.1080/00224499.2019.1704677

Trower, P., & Gilbert, P. (1989). New theoretical conceptions of social anxiety and social phobia. *Clinical Psychology Review, 9*(1), 19–35. https://doi.org/10.1016/0272-7358(89)90044-5

Trubetskoy, V., Pardiñas, A. F., Qi, T., Panagiotaropoulou, G., Awasthi, S., Bigdeli, T. B., et al. (2022). Mapping genomic loci implicates genes and synaptic biology in schizophrenia, *Nature, c604*(7906), 502–508.

Trujillo, M., Brown, A., Watson, D., Croft-Caderao, K., & Chmielewski, M. (2022). The Dissociative Experiences Scale: An empirical evaluation of long-standing concerns. *Psychology of Consciousness: Theory, Research, and Practice.* https://doi.org/10.1037/cns0000334

Trull, T. J., & Hepp, J. (2023). Borderline personality disorder: contemporary approaches to conceptualization and etiology. In R. F. Krueger & P. H. Blaney (Eds.), *Oxford textbook of psychopathology* (pp. 650–677). Oxford University Press. https://doi.org/10.1093/med-psych/9780197542521.003.0028

Trull, T. J., Jahng, S., Tomko, R. L., Wood, P. K., & Sher, K. J. (2010). Revised NESARC personality disorder diagnoses: gender, prevalence, and comorbidity with substance dependence disorders. *Journal of personality disorders, 24*(4), 412–426. https://doi.org/10.1521/pedi.2010.24.4.412.

Trzaskowski, M., Zavos, H. M. S., Haworth, C. M. A., Plomin, R., & Eley, T. C. (2012). Stable genetic influence on anxiety-related behaviours across middle childhood. *Journal of Abnormal Child Psychology, 40*(1), 85–94. https://doi.org/10.1007/s10802-011-9545-z

Tsai, J. L. (2017). Ideal affect in daily life: implications for affective experience, health, and social behavior. *Current Opinion in Psychology, 17,* 118-128.

Tsai, J. L. (2017). Ideal affect in daily life: Implications for affective experience, health, and social behavior. *Current Opinion in Psychology, 17,* 118–128.

Tsai, J. L., Knutson, B. K., & Fung, H. H. (2006). Cultural variation in affect valuation. *Journal of Personality and Social Psychology, 90,* 288–307.

Tsuang, M. T., Lyons, M. J., Meyer, J. M., Doyle, T., Eisen, S. A., Goldberg, J., et al. (1998). Co-occurrence of abuse of different drugs in men: The role of drug-specific and shared vulnerabilities. *Archives of General Psychiatry, 55,* 967–972.

Turkheimer, E. (2000). Three laws of behavior genetics and what they mean. *Current Directions in Psychological Science, 9,* 160–164.

Turkheimer, E., Haley, A., Waldron, M., D'Onofrio, B., & Gottesman, I. I. (2003). Socioeconomic status modifies the heritability of IQ in young children. *Psychological Science, 6*, 623–628.

Turkington, D., Kingdom, D., & Turner, T. (2002). Effectiveness of a brief cognitive-behavioural intervention in the treatment of schizophrenia. *British Journal of Psychiatry, 180*, 523–527.

Turkington, D., Kingdon, D., & Weiden, P.J. (2006). Cognitive behavior therapy for schizophrenia. *American Journal of Psychiatry, 163*, 365–373.

Turner, C. M. (2006). Cognitive-behavioral theory and therapy for obsessive-compulsive disorder in children and adolescents: Current status and future directions. *Clinical Psychology Review*, 26, 912–948.

Turner, E. H., Matthews, A. M., Linardatos, E., Tell, R. A., & Rosenthal, R. (2008). Selective publication of antidepressant trials and its influence on apparent efficacy. *New England Journal of Medicine, 358*, 252–260.

Twenge, J. M. (2020). Why increases in adolescent depression may be linked to the technological environment. *Genetics, 32*, 89–94.

Twenge, J. M., Cooper, A. B., Joiner, T. E., Duffy, M. E., & Binau, S. G. (2019). Age, period, and cohort trends in mood disorder indicators and suicide-related outcomes in a nationally representative dataset, 2005–2017. *Journal of Abnormal Psychology, 128*(3), 185–199. https://doi.org/10.1037/abn0000410

Tyrer, P., Mulder, R., Kim, Y.-R., & Crawford, M. J. (2019). The development of the ICD-11 classification of personality disorders: An amalgam of science, pragmatism, and politics. *Annual Review of Clinical Psychology, 15*(1), 481–502. https://doi.org/10.1146/annurev-clinpsy-050718-095736

Tyrer, P., Wang, D., Crawford, M., Dupont, S., Cooper, S., Nourmand, S., et al. (2021). Sustained benefit of cognitive behaviour therapy for health anxiety in medical patients (CHAMP) over 8 years: A randomised-controlled trial. *Psychological Medicine, 51*(10), 1714–1722. https://doi.org/10.1017/S003329172000046X

Uchinuma, Y., & Sekine, Y. (2000). Dissociative identity disorder (DID) in Japan: A forensic case report and the recent increase in reports of DID. *International Journal of Psychiatry in Clinical Practice, 4*, 155–160.

Udo, T., & Grilo, C. M. (2018). Prevalence and correlates of DSM-5-defined eating disorders in a nationally representative sample of U.S. adults. *Biological Psychiatry, 84*(5), 345–354. https://doi.org/10.1016/j.biopsych.2018.03.014

UK ECT Review Group. (2003). Efficacy and safety of electro-convulsive therapy in depressive disorders: A systematic review and meta-analysis. *The Lancet, 361*, 799–808.

Ulrich, S., Keers, R., & Coid, J. W. (2014). Delusions, anger and serious violence: New findings from the MacArthur violence risk assessment study. *Schizophrenia Bulletin, 40*, 1174–1181.

Unschuld, P. G., Buchholz, A. S., Varvaris, M., van Zijl, P. C., Ross, C. A., Pekar, J. J., et al. (2014). Prefrontal brain network connectivity indicates degree of both schizophrenia risk and cognitive dysfunction. *Schizophrenia Bulletin, 40*, 653–664.

Urada, D., Evans, E., Yang, J., Conner, B. T., Campos, M., Brecht, L., et al. (2009). Evaluation of proposition 36: The substance abuse and crime prevention act of 2000: 2009 report. https://www.uclaisap.org/prop36/html/reports.html

US Bureau of the Census. (2017). *National Population Projections Tables: Main Series*. Retrieved May 27, 2023, from https://www.census.gov/data/tables/2017/demo/popproj/2017-summary-tables.html

U.S. Bureau of the Census. (2018). *Population estimates*. U.S. Census Bureau, Population Division.

U.S. Department of Health and Human Services. (2001). Mental health: Culture, race, and ethnicity—A supplement to mental health: A report of the Surgeon General. U.S. Department of Health and Human Services, Substance Abuse and Mental Health Services Administration, Center for Mental Health Services.

U.S. Department of Health and Human Services. (2014). The health consequences of smoking—50 years of progress: A report of the Surgeon General. U.S. Department of Health and Human Services, Centers for Disease Control and Prevention, National Center for Chronic Disease Prevention and Health Promotion, Office on Smoking and Health.

U.S. Department of Health and Human Services. (2016b). *Facing addiction in America: The Surgeon General's report on alcohol, drugs, and health*. HHS, Office of the Surgeon General.

U.S. Department of Health and Human Services (USDHHS). (2014). 2014 National healthcare disparities report. https://www.ahrq.gov/research/findings/nhqrdr/2014chartbooks/effectivetx/eff-slidesm-hsa.html

US Preventive Services Task Force (USPSTF) (2022a). Screening for anxiety in children and adolescents: US Preventive Services Task Force recommendation statement. *JAMA, 328*(14), 1438–1444.

US Preventive Services Task Force (USPSTF) (2022b). Screening for depression and suicide risk in children and adolescents: US Preventive Services Task Force recommendation statement. *JAMA, 328*(15), 1534–1542.

Vafale, N., & Kober, H. (2022). Association of drug cues and craving with drug use and relapse: A systematic review and meta-analysis. *JAMA Psychiatry, 79*, 641–650.

Valadez, E. A., Pine, D. S., Fox, N. A., & Bar-Haim, Y. (2022). Attentional biases in human anxiety. *Neuroscience & Biobehavioral Reviews*, 142, 104917. https://doi.org/10.1016/j.neubiorev.2022.104917

Valencia, M., Racon, M. L., Juarez, F., & Murow, E. (2007). A psychosocial skills training approach in Mexican outpatients with schizophrenia. *Psychological Medicine, 37*, 1393–1402.

Valenti, A. M., Narendran, R., & Pristach, C. A. (2003). Who are patients on conventional antipsychotics? *Schizophrenia Bulletin, 29*, 195–200.

Vallati, M., Cunningham, S., Mazurka, R., Stewart, J. G., Larocque, C., Milev, R. V., et al. (2020). Childhood maltreatment and the clinical characteristics of major depressive disorder in adolescence and adulthood. *Journal of Abnormal Psychology, 129*(5), 469–479. https://doi.org/10.1037/abn0000521

Vancampfort, D., Stubbs, B., Mitchell, A. J., De Hert, M., Wampers, M., Ward, P. B., et al. (2015), Risk of metabolic syndrome and its components in people with schizophrenia and related psychotic disorders, bipolar disorder and major depressive disorder: a systematic review and meta-analysis. *World Psychiatry, 14*, 339-347. https://doi.org/10.1002/wps.20252

Vance, S., Cohen-Kettenis, P., Drescher, J., Meyer-Bahlburg, H., Pfafflin, F., & Zucker, K. (2010). Opinions about the DSM gender identity disorder diagnosis: Results from an international survey administered to organizations concerned with the welfare of transgender people. *International Journal of Transgenderism, 12*, 1–14.

Vandeleur, C. L., Fassassi, S., Castelao, E., Glaus, J., Strippoli, M.-P. F., Lasserre, A. M., et al. (2017). Prevalence and correlates of DSM-5 major depressive and related disorders in the community. *Psychiatry Research, 250*, 50–58. https://doi.org/10.1016/j.psychres.2017.01.060

van der Leeuw, G., Gerrits, M. J., Terluin, B., Numans, M. E., van der Feltz-Cornelis, C. M., van der Horst, H. E., et al. (2015). The association between somatization and disability in primary care patients. *Journal of Psychosomatic Research, 79*, 117–122. https://doi.org/10.1016/j.jpsychores.2015.03.001

van Dessel, N., den Boeft, M., van der Wouden, J. C., Kleinstäuber, M., Leone, S. S., Terluin, B., et al. (2014). Non-pharmacological interventions for somatoform disorders and medically unexplained physical symptoms (MUPS) in adults. *Cochrane Database of Systematic Reviews*, Issue 11. Art. No.: CD011142. https://doi.org/10.1002/14651858.CD011142.pub2. Accessed 22 February 2024.

Van Diermen, L., Van Den Ameele, S., Kamperman, A. M., Sabbe, B. C. G., Vermeulen, T., Schrijvers, D., et al. (2018). Prediction of electroconvulsive therapy response and remission in major depression: Meta-analysis. *British Journal of Psychiatry, 212*(2), 71–80. https://doi.org/10.1192/bjp.2017.28

Van Diest, I. (2019). Interoception, conditioning, and fear: The panic threesome. *Psychophysiology, 56*(8), e13421. https://doi.org/10.1111/psyp.13421

van Erp, T. G. M., Hibar, D. P., Rasmussen, J. M., Glahn, D. C., Pearlson, G. D., Andreassen, O. A., et al. (2016). Subcortical brain volume abnormalities in 2028 individuals with schizophrenia and 2540 healthy controls via the ENIGMA consortium. *Molecular Psychiatry, 21*(4), 547–553.

van Erp, T. G. M., Walton, E., Hibar, D. P., Schmaal, L., Jiang, W., Glahn, D. C., et al. (2018). Cortical brain abnormalities in 4474 individuals with schizophrenia and 5098 control subjects via the Enhancing Neuro Imaging Genetics Through Meta Analysis (ENIGMA) Consortium. *Biological Psychiatry, 84*(9), 644–654.

Van Gelder, K. (2010). *The Buddha and the borderline: My recovery from borderline personality disorder through dialectical behavioral therapy, Buddhism, and online dating.* New Harbinger Publications, Inc.

van Hees, M. L. J. M., Rotter, T., Ellermann, T., & Evers, S. M. A. A. (2013). The effectiveness of individual interpersonal psychotherapy as a treatment for major depressive disorder in adult outpatients: A systematic review. *BMC Psychiatry, 13*(1), 22. https://doi.org/10.1186/1471-244x-13-22

van Hoeken, D., Burns, J. K., & Hoek, H. W. (2016). Epidemiology of eating disorders in Africa. *Current Opinion in Psychiatry, 29*, 372–377.

van Lankveld, J. J., Granot, M., Weijmar Schultz, W. C., Binik, Y. M., Wesselmann, U., Pukall, C. F., et al. (2010). Women's sexual pain disorders. *Journal of Sexual Medicine, 7*, 615–631.

Vannikov-Lugassi, M., & Soffer-Dudek, N. (2018). No time like the present: Thinking about the past and the future is related to state dissociation among individuals with high levels of psychopathological symptoms. *Frontiers in Psychology, 9*(DEC). https://doi.org/10.3389/FPSYG.2018.02465

Van Ommeren, M., De Jong, J. T. V. M., Sharma, B., Komproe, I., Thapa, S. B., & Cardeña, E. (2001). Psychiatric disorders among tortured Bhutanese refugees in Nepal. *Archives of General Psychiatry, 58*(5), 475–482. https://doi.org/10.1001/archpsyc.58.5.475

van Os, J., Kenis, G., & Rutten, B. P. (2010). The environment and schizophrenia. *Nature, 468*, 203–212.

van Rooij, D., Anagnostou, E., Arango, C., Auzias, G., Behrmann, M., Busatto, G. F., et al. (2018). Cortical and subcortical brain morphometry differences between patients with autism spectrum disorder and healthy individuals across the lifespan: Results from the ENIGMA ASD Working Group. *American Journal of Psychiatry, 175*(4), 359–369. https://doi.org/10.1176/appi.ajp.2017.17010100

van Rooij, S. J. H., Stevens, J. S., Ely, T. D., Hinrichs, R., Michopoulos, V., Winters, S. J., et al. (2018). The role of the hippocampus in predicting future posttraumatic stress disorder symptoms in recently traumatized civilians. *Biological Psychiatry, 84*(2), 106–115. https://doi.org/10.1016/j.biopsych.2017.09.005

Vanwesenbeeck, I., Have, M. T., & de Graaf, R. (2014). Associations between common mental disorders and sexual dissatisfaction in the general population. *British Journal of Psychiatry, 205*, 151–157. https://doi.org/10.1192/bjp.bp.113.135335

Varlet, V., Farsalinos, K., Augsburger, M., Thomas, A., & Etter, J. F. (2015). Toxicity assessment of refill liquids for electronic cigarettes. *International Journal of Environmental Research and Public Health, 12*, 4796–4815.

Vassos, E., Pedersen, C. B., Murray, R. M., Collier, D. A., & Lewis, C. M. (2012). Meta-analysis of the association of urbanicity with schizophrenia. *Schizophrenia Bulletin, 38*(6), 1118–1123.

Vaughan, E. P., Frick, P. J., Robertson, E. L., Ray, J. V., Thornton, L. C., Wall Myers, T. D., et al. (2022). Interpersonal relationships and callous-unemotional traits during adolescence and young adulthood: An investigation of bidirectional effects in parent, peer, and romantic relationships. *Clinical Psychological Science, 11*(3), 391–408. https://doi.org/10.1177/21677026221101070

Vaughn-Coaxum, R. A., Mair, P., & Weisz, J. R. (2016). Racial/ethnic differences in youth depression indicators: An item response theory analysis of symptoms reported by White, Black, Asian, and Latino youths. *Clinical Psychological Science: A Journal of the Association for Psychological Science, 4*(2), 239–253. https://doi.org/10.1177/2167702615591768

Vazire, S., Naumann, L. P., Rentfrow, P. J., & Gosling, S. D. (2008). Portrait of a narcissist: Manifestations of narcissism in physical appearance. *Journal of Research in Personality, 42*, 1439–1447.

Veale, D. (2004). Advances in a cognitive behavioural model of body dysmorphic disorder. *Body Image, 1*, 113–125.

Veehof, M. M., Oskam, M. J., Schreurs, K. M., & Bohlmeijer, E. T. (2011). Acceptance-based interventions for the treatment of chronic pain: A systematic review and meta-analysis. *Pain, 152*, 533–542.

Vervliet, B., Craske, M. G., & Hermans, D. (2013). Fear extinction and relapse: State of the art. *Annual Review of Clinical Psychology, 9*(1), 215–248. https://doi.org/10.1146/annurev-clinpsy-050212-185542

Vila-Rodriguez, F., Panenka, W. J., Lang, D. J., Thornton, A. E., Vertinsky, T., Wong, H., et al. (2013). The hotel study: multimorbidity in a community sample living in marginal housing. *American Journal of Psychiatry, 170*, 1413–1422.

Villarosa, L. (2022). Under the skin: The hidden toll of racism on American lives. Doubleday

Villemure, C., & Bushnell, M. C. (2009). Mood influences supraspinal pain processing separately from attention. *Journal of Neuroscience, 29*, 705–715.

Vinkers, D. J., Gussekloo, J., Stek, M. L., Westendorp, R. G. J., & van der Mast, R. C. (2004). Temporal relation between depression and cognitive impairment in old age: Prospective population based study. *British Medical Journal, 329*, 881.

Vinocour, S. (2020). *Nobody's child: A tragedy, a trial, and a history of the insanity defense.* W. W. Norton & Company.

Virués-Ortega, J. (2010). Applied behavior analytic intervention for autism in early childhood: Meta-analysis, meta-regression and dose–response meta-analysis of multiple outcomes. *Clinical Psychology Review, 30*, 387–399.

Visscher, P. M., Wray, N. R., Zhang, Q., Sklar, P., McCarthy, M. I., Brown, M. A., & Yang, J. (2017). 10 years of GWAS discovery: Biology, function, and translation. *American Journal of Human Genetics, 101*(1), 5–22.

Visser, S. N., Danielson, M. L., Bitsko, R. H., Holbrook, J. R., Kogan, M. D., Ghandour, R. M., et al. (2014). Trends in the parent-report of health care provider-diagnosed and medicated attention-deficit/hyperactivity disorder: United States, 2003–2011. *Journal of the American Academy of Child and Adolescent Psychiatry, 53*(1), 34–46.e32. https://doi.org/10.1016/j.jaac.2013.09.001

Vitaliani, R., Mason, W., Ances, B., Zwerdling, T., Jiang, Z., & Dalmau, J. (2005). Paraneoplastic encephalitis, psychiatric symptoms, and hypoventilation in ovarian teratoma. *Annals of Neurology, 58*(4), 594–604. https://doi.org/10.1002/ana.20614

Vittengl, J. R., Clark, L. A., Dunn, T. W., & Jarrett, R. B. (2007). Reducing relapse and recurrence in unipolar depression: A comparative meta-analysis of cognitive-behavior therapy's effects. *Journal of Consulting and Clinical Psychology, 75*, 475–488.

Vogt, D., Smith, B., Elwy, R., Martin, J., Schultz, M., Drainoni, M. L., et al. (2011). Predeployment, deployment, and postdeployment risk factors for posttraumatic stress symptomatology in female and male OEF/OIF veterans. *Journal of Abnormal Psychology, 120*, 819–831.

Volkert, J., Hauschild, S., & Taubner, S. (2019). Mentalization-Based Treatment for Personality Disorders: Efficacy, Effectiveness, and New Developments. *Current Psychiatry Reports, 21*(4), 25. https://doi.org/10.1007/s11920-019-1012-5

Volkow, N. D. (2020). Personalizing the treatment of substance use disorders. American *Journal of Psychiatry, 177*(2), 113–116. https://doi.org/10.1176/appi.ajp.2019.19121284

Volkow, N. D., & Boyle, M. (2018). Neuroscience of addiction: Relevance to prevention and treatment. *American Journal of Psychiatry, 175*(8), 729–740. https://doi.org/10.1176/appi.ajp.2018.17101174

Volkow, N. D., Jones, E. B., Einstein, E. B., & Wargo, E. M. (2019). Prevention and treatment of opioid misuse and addiction: A review. *JAMA Psychiatry, 76*(2), 208–216.

Volkow, N. D., Wang, G. J., Fischman, M. W., & Foltin, R. W. (1997). Relationship between subjective effects of cocaine and dopamine transporter occupancy. *Nature, 386*, 827–830.

von Krafft-Ebing, R. (1902). *Psychopathia sexualis*. Physicians and Surgeons Books.

Voogt, C., Beusink, M., Kleinjan, M., Otten, R., Engels, R., Smit, K., et al. (2017). Alcohol-related cognitions in children (aged 2–10) and how they are shaped by parental alcohol use: A systematic review. *Drug and Alcohol Dependence, 177*, 277–290.

Vos, T., Allen, C., Arora, M., Barber, R. M., Bhutta, Z. A., Brown, A., et al. (2016). Global, regional, and national incidence, prevalence, and years lived with disability for 310 diseases and injuries: A systematic analysis for the Global Burden of Disease Study 2015. *The Lancet, 388*, 1545–1602. https://doi.org/10.1016/S0140-6736(16)31678-6

Vrshek-Schallhorn, S., Doane, L. D., Mineka, S., Zinbarg, R. E., Craske, M. G., & Adam, E. K. (2013). The cortisol awakening response predicts major depression: Predictive stability over a 4-year follow-up and effect of depression history. *Psychological Medicine, 43*(3), 483–493.

Wadden, T. A., Tronieri, J. S., & Butryn, M. L. (2020). Lifestyle modification approaches for the treatment of obesity in adults. *American Psychologist, 75*(2), 235–251. https://doi.org/10.1037/amp0000517

Wade, C. L., Kallupi, M., Hernandez, D. O., Breysse, E., de Guglielmo, G., Crawford, E., et al. (2017). High-frequency stimulation of the subthalamic nucleus blocks compulsive-like re-escalation of heroin taking in rats. *42*, 1850–1859. https://doi.org/10.1038/npp.2016.270

Wade, K. A., Garry, M., & Pezdek, K. (2018). Deconstructing rich false memories of committing crime: Commentary on Shaw and Porter (2015). *Psychological Science, 29*(3), 471–476. https://doi.org/10.1177/0956797617703667

Wade, T. D., & Bulik, C. (2018). Genetic influences on eating disorders. In W. S. Agras & A. Robinson (Eds.), *The Oxford handbook of eating disorders* (2nd ed.). Oxford University Press. https://www.oxford-handbooks.com/view/10.1093/oxfordhb/9780190620998.001.0001/oxfordhb-9780190620998

Wagner, E. F., Hospital, M. M., Graziano, J. N., Morris, S. L., & Gil, A. G. (2014). A randomized controlled trial of guided self-change with minority adolescents. *Journal of Consulting and Clinical Psychology, 82*(6), 1128–1139. https://doi.org/10.1037/a0036939

Wahl, O. F. (1999). Mental health consumers' experience of stigma. *Schizophrenia Bulletin, 25*, 467–478.

Wakefield, J. C. (2011). DSM-5 proposed diagnostic criteria for sexual paraphilias: Tensions between diagnostic validity and forensic utility. *International Journal of Law and Psychiatry, 34*, 195–209. https://pornpen.ai/make?tags=OYUwdiBOCGAuD2kC8B3eBbcB9ADgC3gWBn-wE8AyWaYAZyTAFd0AjKLY+BnAGmehpBZmASxbxuVWljwN-QQ+PGY1uAM2gBjQdDwhg0cZJq5hwKsIA2RvNGGR1DWNxqx-S5wWrBUapbuABu7JDwmpA+GrDC8GBY9ug0BI7q5oQ6RszwA-CakODae3EkpIEYqDJBAA10.1016/j.ijlp.2011.04.012

Wakefield, J. C. (2013). The DSM-5 debate over the bereavement exclusion: Psychiatric diagnosis and the future of empirically supported treatment. *Clinical Psychology Review, 33*, 825–845. https://doi.org/10.1016/j.cpr.2013.03.007

Wakefield, J. C. (2015). DSM-5, psychiatric epidemiology and the false positives problem. *Epidemiology and Psychiatric Sciences, 24*, 188–196. https://doi.org/10.1017/s2045796015000116

Waldinger, M. D., Quinn, P., Dilleen, M., Mundayat, R., Schweitzer, D. H., & Boolell, M. (2005). A multinational population survey of intravaginal ejaculation latency time. *Journal of Sexual Medicine, 2*, 492–497.

Walker, E. F., Davis, D. M., & Savoie, T. D. (1994). Neuromotor precursors of schizophrenia. *Schizophrenia Bulletin, 20*, 441–451.

Walker, E. F., Grimes, K. E., Davis, D. M., & Adina, J. (1993). Childhood precursors of schizophrenia: Facial expressions of emotion. *American Journal of Psychiatry, 150*, 1654–1660.

Walker, E. F., Kestler, L., Bollini, A., & Hochman, K. (2004). Schizophrenia: Etiology and course. *Annual Review of Psychology, 55*, 401–430.

Walker, E. F., Mittal, V., & Tessner, K. (2008). Stress and the hypothalamic pituitary adrenal axis in the developmental course of schizophrenia. *Annual Review of Clinical Psychology, 4*, 189–216.

Walker, E. F., Trotman, H. D., Pearce, B. D., Addington, J., Cadenhead, K. S., Cornblatt, B. A., et al. (2013). Cortisol levels and risk for psychosis: Initial findings from the North American prodrome longitudinal study. *Biological Psychiatry, 74*, 410–417.

Walker, R. D., & Bigelow, D. A. (2015). Evidence-informed, culture-based interventions and best practices in American Indian and Alaska Native communities. In P. E. Nathan & J. M. Gorman (Eds.), *A guide to treatments that work* (4th ed., pp. 23–54). Oxford University Press.

Walkup, J. T., Albano, A. M., Piacentini, J., Birmaher, B., Comptom, S. N., Sherrill, J. T., et al. (2008). Cognitive behavioral therapy, sertraline, or a combination in childhood anxiety. *New England Journal of Medicine, 359*, 2753–2766.

Waller, R., Gard, A. M., Shaw, D. S., Forbes, E. E., Neumann, C. S., & Hyde, L. W. (2019). Weakened functional connectivity between the amygdala and the ventromedial prefrontal cortex Is longitudinally related to psychopathic traits in low-income males during early adulthood. *Clinical Psychological Science, 7*(3), 628–635. https://doi.org/10.1177/2167702618810231

Waller, R., & Hyde, L. W. (2018). Callous-unemotional behaviors in early childhood: The development of empathy and prosociality gone awry. *Current Opinion in Psychology, 20*, 11–16. https://doi.org/10.1016/j.copsyc.2017.07.037

Waller, R., Hyde, L. W., Klump, K. L., & Burt, S. A. (2018). Parenting is an environmental predictor of callous-unemotional traits and aggression: A monozygotic twin differences study. *Journal of the American Academy of Child and Adolescent Psychiatry, 57*(12), 955–963. https://doi.org/10.1016/j.jaac.2018.07.882

Waller, R., Wagner, N. J., Barstead, M. G., Subar, A., Petersen, J. L., Hyde, J. S., et al. (2020). A meta-analysis of the associations between callous-unemotional traits and empathy, prosociality, and guilt. *Clinical Psychology Review, 75*, 101809.

Walsh, B. T. (2013). The enigmatic persistence of anorexia nervosa. *American Journal of Psychiatry, 170*, 477–484. https://doi.org/10.1176/appi.ajp.2012.12081074

Walsh, B. T., Hagan, K. E., & Lockwood, C. (2023). A systematic review comparing atypical anorexia nervosa and anorexia nervosa. *International Journal of Eating Disorders, 56*(4), 798–820. https://doi.org/10.1002/eat.23856

Walsh, K., Hasin, D., Keyes, K. M., & Koenen, K. C. (2016). Associations between gender-based violence and personality disorders in U.S. women. *Personality Disorders: Theory, Research, and Treatment, 7,* 205–210. https://doi.org/10.1037/per0000158

Walsh, T., McClellan, J. M., McCarthy, S. E., Addington, A. M., Pierce, S. B., Cooper, G. M., et al. (2008). Rare structural variants disrupt genes in neurodevelopmental pathways in schizophrenia. *Science, 320,* 539–543.

Walters, K. S., & Hope, D. A. (1998). Analysis of social behavior in individuals with social phobia and nonanxious participants using a psychobiological model. *Behavior Therapy, 29*(3), 387–407. https://doi.org/10.1016/S0005-7894(98)80039-7

Wang, C., Najm, R., Xu, Q., Jeong, D. E., Walker, D., Balestra, M. E., et al. (2018). Gain of toxic apolipoprotein E4 effects in human iPSC-derived neurons is ameliorated by a small-molecule structure corrector article. *Nature Medicine, 24*(5), 647–657. https://doi.org/10.1038/s41591-018-0004-z

Wang, D. A., Hagger, M. S., & Chatzisarantis, N. L. D. (2020). Ironic effects of thought suppression: A meta-analysis. *Perspectives on Psychological Science.* https://doi.org/10.1177/1745691619898795. Online in advance of print.

Wang, P. S., Aguilar-Gaxiola, S., Alonso, J., Angermeyer, M. C., Borges, G., Bromet, E. J., et al. (2007). Use of mental health services for anxiety, mood, and substance disorders in 17 countries in the WHO World Mental Health Surveys. *The Lancet, 370,* 841–850.

Wang, P. S., Lane, M. C., Olfson, M., Pincus, H. A., Wells, K. B., & Kessler, R. C. (2005). Twelve-month use of mental health services in the United States: Results from the National Comorbidity Survey Replication. *Archives of General Psychiatry, 62,* 629–640.

Wang Weijun, E. (2019). *The collected schizophrenias: Essays.* Graywolf Press.

Wardle, J., Chida, Y., Gibson, E. L., Whitaker, K. L., & Steptoe, A. (2011). Stress and adiposity: A meta-analysis of longitudinal studies. *Obesity, 19*(4), 771–778.

Ward, T. B., & Beech, A. (2006). An integrated theory of sexual offending. *Aggression and Violent Behavior, 11,* 44–63.

Ware, J., McIvor, L., & Fernandez, Y. M. (2021). Behavioral control models in managing sexual deviance. *Sexual Deviance,* 311–323. https://doi.org/10.1002/9781119771401.CH20

Warwick, H. M. C., & Salkovskis, P. M. (2001). Cognitive-behavioral treatment of hypochondriasis. In D. R. Lipsitt & V. Starcevic (Eds.), *Hypochondriasis: Modern perspectives on an ancient malady* (pp. 314–328). Oxford University Press.

Washington, A. (2017, March, 3). Demi Lovato to be honored for mental health advocacy. Billboard. Retrieved from http://www.billboard.com/articles/news/7710060/demi-lovato-honored-mentalhealth-advocacy

Wastesson, J. W., Morin, L., Tan, E. C. K., & Johnell, K. (2018). An update on the clinical consequences of polypharmacy in older adults: a narrative review. *Expert Opinion on Drug Safety, 17*(12), 1185–1196. https://doi.org/10.1080/14740338.2018.1546841

Wastler, H. M., & Lenzenweger, M. F. (2019). Self-referential hypermentalization in schizotypy. *Personality Disorders: Theory, Research, and Treatment.* https://doi.org/10.1037/per0000344

Waszczuk, M. A., Zavos, H. M., Gregory, A. M., & Eley, T. C. (2014). The phenotypic and genetic structure of depression and anxiety disorder symptoms in childhood, adolescence, and young adulthood. *JAMA Psychiatry, 71,* 905–916.

Waters, A., Hill, A., & Waller, G. (2001). Internal and external antecedents of binge eating episodes in a group of women with bulimia nervosa. *International Journal of Eating Disorders, 29,* 17–22.

Waters, A. M., Peters, R. M., Forrest, K. E., & Zimmer-Gembeck, M. (2014). Fear acquisition and extinction in offspring of mothers with anxiety and depressive disorders. *Developmental Cognitive Neuroscience, 7,* 30–42. https://doi.org/10.1016/j.dcn.2013.10.007

Watkins, E. R. (2008). Constructive and unconstructive repetitive thought. *Psychological Bulletin, 134,* 163–206.

Watkins, P. C. (2002). Implicit memory bias in depression. *Cognition and Emotion, 16,* 381–402.

Watson, D., Stasik, S. M., Ro, E., & Clark, L. A. (2013). Integrating normal and pathological personality: Relating the DSM-5 trait-dimensional model to general traits of personality. *Assessment, 20,* 312–326. https://doi.org/10.1177/1073191113485810

Watson, H. J., & Rees, C. S. (2008). Meta-analysis of randomized, controlled treatment trials for pediatric obsessive-compulsive disorder. *Journal of Child Psychology and Psychiatry, and Allied Disciplines, 49*(5), 489–498. https://doi.org/10.1111/j.1469-7610.2007.01875.x

Watson, H. J., Yilmaz, Z., Thornton, L. M., Hübel, C., Coleman, J. R. I., Gaspar, H. A., et al. (2019). Genome-wide association study identifies eight risk loci and implicates metabo-psychiatric origins for anorexia nervosa. *Nature Genetics, 51*(8), 1207–1214.

Watson, J. B., & Rayner, R. (1920). Conditioned emotional reactions. *Journal of Experimental Psychology, 3*(1), 1–14.

Watson, J. B., & Rayner, R. (1920). Conditioned emotional reactions. *Journal of Experimental Psychology, 3,* 1–14.

Watts, A. L., Lilienfeld, S. O., Smith, S. F., Miller, J. D., Campbell, W. K., Waldman, I. D., et al. (2013). The double-edged sword of grandiose narcissism: Implications for successful and unsuccessful leadership among U.S. presidents. *Psychological Science, 24,* 2379–2389.

Weaton, M. G., & Van Meter, A. (2015). Comorbidity in hoarding disorder. In R. O. Frost & G. Steketee (Eds.), *The Oxford handbook of hoarding and acquiring.* Oxford University Press.

Webster, C., Douglas, K., Eaves, D., & Hart, S. (1997). *HCR-20: Assessing risk for violence (Version 2).* Simon Fraser University.

Weeks, J. W., Heimberg, R. G., & Heuer, R. (2011). Exploring the role of behavioral submissiveness in social anxiety. *Journal of Social and Clinical Psychology, 30*(3), 217–249. https://doi.org/10.1521/jscp.2011.30.3.217

Weeks, J. W., Srivastav, A., Howell, A. N., & Menatti, A. R. (2016). "Speaking more than words": Classifying men with social anxiety disorder via vocal acoustic analyses of diagnostic interviews. *Journal of Psychopathology and Behavioral Assessment, 38*(1), 30–41. https://doi.org/10.1007/s10862-015-9495-9

Wegner, D. M., Schneider, D. J., Carter, S. R., & White, T. L. (1987). Paradoxical effects of thought suppression. *Journal of Personality and Social Psychology, 53,* 5–13.

Weickert, C. S., Fung, S. J., Catts, V. S., Schofield, P. R., Allen, K. M., Moore, L. T., et al. (2013). Molecular evidence of N-methyl-D-aspartate receptor hypofunction in schizophrenia. *Molecular Psychiatry, 18,* 1185–1192. https://doi.org/10.1038/mp.2012.137

Weierich, M. R., & Nock, M. K. (2008). Posttraumatic stress symptoms mediate the relation between childhood sexual abuse and nonsuicidal self-injury. *Journal of consulting and clinical psychology, 76*(1), 39–44. https://doi.org/10.1037/0022-006X.76.1.39

Weierich, M. R., & Nock, M. K. (2008). Posttraumatic stress symptoms mediate the relation between childhood sexual abuse and nonsuicidal self-injury. *Journal of Consulting and Clinical Psychology, 76,* 39–44.

Weiler, M., Stieger, K. C., Long, J. M., & Rapp, P. R. (2020). Transcranial magnetic stimulation in Alzheimer's disease: Are we ready? *eNeuro, 7*(1), ENEURO.0235–19.2019.

Weinberg, A., Kujawa, A., & Riesel, A. (2022). Understanding trajectories to anxiety and depression: Neural responses to errors and rewards as indices of susceptibility to stressful life events. *Current Directions in Psychological Science, 31*(2), 115–123. https://doi.org/10.1177/09637214211049228

Weinberger, D. R. (1987). Implications of normal brain development for the pathogenesis of schizophrenia. *Archives of General Psychiatry, 44*, 660–669.

Weinberger, J. M., Houman, J., Caron, A. T., & Anger, J. (2019). Female sexual dysfunction: A systematic review of outcomes across various treatment modalities. *Sexual Medicine Reviews, 7*(2), 223–250. https://doi.org/10.1016/j.sxmr.2017.12.004

Weiner, B., Frieze, I., Kukla, A., Reed, L. Rest, S., & Rosenbaum, R. M. (1971). Perceiving the causes of success and failure. In E. E. Jones, et al. (Eds.), *Attribution: Perceiving the causes of behavior*. General Learning Press.

Weiner, D. B. (1994). Le geste de Pinel: The history of psychiatric myth. In M. S. Micale & R. Porter (Eds.), *Discovering the history of psychiatry*. Oxford University Press.

Weingarden, H., Curley, E. E., Renshaw, K. D., & Wilhelm, S. (2017). Patient-identified events implicated in the development of body dysmorphic disorder. *Body Image, 21*, 19–25. https://doi.org/10.1016/j.bodyim.2017.02.003

Weingarden, H., Hoeppner, S. S., Snorrason, I., Greenberg, J. L., Phillips, K. A., & Wilhelm, S. (2021). Rates of remission, sustained remission, and recurrence in a randomized controlled trial of cognitive behavioral therapy versus supportive psychotherapy for body dysmorphic disorder. *Depression Anxiety, 38*, 700–707. https://doi.org/10.1002/da.23148

Weinstock, J., Massura, C. E., & Petry, N. M. (2013). Professional and pathological gamblers: Similarities and differences. *Journal of Gambling Studies, 29*, 205–216.

Weisberg, R. B., Brown, T. A., Wincze, J. P., & Barlow, D. H. (2001). Causal attributions and male sexual arousal: The impact of attributions for a bogus erectile difficulty on sexual arousal, cognitions, and affect. *Journal of Abnormal Psychology, 110*, 324–334.

Weisberg, R. W. (1994). Genius and madness? A quasi-experimental test of the hypothesis that manic-depression increases creativity. *Psychological Science, 5*, 361–367.

Weisholz, D. (September 17, 2020). Lady Gaga reveals how her 'catatonic state' depression influenced new album. *Today*, https://www.today.com/popculture/lady-gaga-reveals-how-depression-influenced-new-album-t191884

Weiss, R. D., Potter, J. S., Fiellin, D. A., Byrne, M., Connery, H. S., Dickinson, W., et al. (2011). Adjunctive counseling during brief and extended buprenorphine-naloxone treatment for prescription opioid dependence: A 2-phase randomized controlled trial. *Archives of General Psychiatry, 68*, 1238–1246. https://doi.org/10.1001/archgenpsychiatry.2011.121

Weisz, J. R., Kuppens, S., Ng, M. Y., Eckshtain, D., Ugueto, A. M., Vaughn-Coaxum, R., et al. (2017). What five decades of research tells us about the effects of youth psychological therapy: A multilevel meta-analysis and implications for science and practice. *American Psychologist, 72*(2), 79–117. https://doi.org/10.1037/a0040360

Weisz, J. R., Suwanlert, S. C., Wanchai, W., & Bernadette, R. (1987). Over- and under-controlled referral problems among children and adolescents from Thailand and the United States: The wat and wai of cultural differences. *Journal of Consulting and Clinical Psychology, 55*, 719–726.

Weisz, J. R., Weiss, B., Suwanlert, S., & Chaiyasit, W. (2003). Syndromal structure of psychopathology in children of Thailand and the United States. *Journal of Consulting and Clinical Psychology, 71*, 375–385.

Weisz, J. R., Weiss, B., Suwanlert, S., & Chaiyasit, W. (2006). Culture and youth psychopathology: Testing the syndromal sensitivity model in Thai and American adolescents. *Journal of Consulting and Clinical Psychology, 74*(6), 1098–1107. https://doi.org/10.1037/0022-006X.74.6.1098

Wellcome Trust. (2022). *Sleep, circadian rhythms and mental health: Advances, gaps, challenges and opportunities.*

Wells, K. C., Epstein, J. N., Hinshaw, S. P., Conners, C. K., Klaric, J. Abikoff, H. B., et al. (2000). Parenting and family stress treatment outcomes in attention deficit hyperactivity disorder (ADHD): An empirical analysis in the MTA study. *Journal of Abnormal Child Psychology, 28*, 543–553.

Wender, P. H., Kety, S. S., Rosenthal, D., Schulsinger, F., Ortmann, J., & Lunde, I. (1986). Psychiatric disorders in the biological and adoptive families of adopted individuals with affective disorders. *Archives of General Psychiatry, 43*, 923–929.

Wenzel, A., & Spokas, M. (2014). Cognitive and information processing approaches to understanding suicidal behaviors. In M. K. Nock (Ed.), *The Oxford handbook of suicide and self-injury*. Oxford University Press.

Werner-Seidler, A., Spanos, S., Calear, A. L., Perry, Y., Torok, M., O'Dea, B., et al. (2021). School-based depression and anxiety prevention programs: An updated systematic review and meta-analysis. *Clinical Psychology Review, 89*, 102079.

Wessel, L. (2017). False: Vaccination can cause autism. *Science, 356*, 368.

Westen, D. (1998). The scientific legacy of Sigmund Freud: Toward a psychodynamically informed psychological science. *Psychological Bulletin, 124*, 333–371.

Westman, J., Hällgren, J., Wahlbeck, K., Erlinge, D., Alfredsson, L., & Ösby, U. (2013). Cardiovascular mortality in bipolar disorder: A population-based cohort study in Sweden. *BMJ Open, 3*(4), e002373. https://doi.org/10.1136/bmjopen-2012-002373

Wettstein, M., Wahl, H.-W., & Siebert, J. S. (2020). 20-year trajectories of health in midlife and old age: Contrasting the impact of personality and attitudes toward own aging. *Psychology and Aging, 35*(6), 910–924. https://doi.org/10.1037/pag0000464

Wheaton, M. G., & Ward, H. E. (2020). Intolerance of uncertainty and obsessive-compulsive personality disorder. *Personality Disorders: Theory, Research, and Treatment, 11*(5), 357–364. https://doi.org/10.1037/per0000396

Whisman, M. (2007). Marital distress and DSM-IV psychiatric disorders in a population-based national survey. *Journal of Abnormal Psychology, 116*, 638–643. https://doi.org/10.1037/0021-843X.116.3.638

Whisman, M. A., & Bruce, M. L. (1999). Marital dissatisfaction and incidence of major depressive episode in a community sample. *Journal of Abnormal Psychology, 108*, 674–678.

Whisman, M. A., Sheldon, C. T., & Goering, P. (2000). Psychiatric disorders and dissatisfaction with social relationships: Does type of relationship matter? *Journal of Abnormal Psychology, 109*, 803–808.

Whisman, M. A., & Uebelacker, L. A. (2006). Impairment and distress associated with relationship discord in a national sample of married or cohabiting adults. *Journal of Family Psychology, 20*, 369–377.

Whitaker, R. (2002). *Mad in America*. Perseus.

White, J., Moore, L., Cannings-John, R., Hawkins, J., Bonell, C., Hickman, M., Zammit, S., & Adara, L. (2023 May). Association Between Gender Minority Status and Mental Health in High School Students. *Journal of Adolescent Health, 72*(5), 811–814. https://doi.org/10.1016/j.jadohealth.2022.12.028.

White, S. W., Oswald, D., Ollendick, T., & Scahill, L. (2009). Anxiety in children and adolescents with autism spectrum disorders. *Clinical Psychology Review, 29*, 216–229.

WHO. (2013). *Global and regional estimates of violence against women: Prevalence and health effects of intimate partner violence and non-partner sexual violence*. World Health Organization.

Widom, C. S. (2014). Longterm consequences of child maltreatment. In J. Korbin & R. Krugman (Eds.), *Handbook of child maltreatment*. Child Maltreatment (Contemporary Issues in Research and Policy), vol. 2 (pp. 225–247). Springer.

Wiech, K., & Tracey, I. (2009). The influence of negative emotions on pain: Behavioral effects and neural mechanisms. *NeuroImage, 47,* 987–994.

Wieder, L., Brown, R. J., Thompson, T., & Terhune, D. B. (2022). Hypnotic suggestibility in dissociative and related disorders: A meta-analysis. *Neuroscience and biobehavioral reviews, 139,* 104751. https://doi.org/10.1016/j.neubiorev.2022.104751

Wilcox, C. E., Pommy, J. M., & Adinoff, B. (2016). Neural circuitry of impaired emotion regulation in substance use disorders. *American Journal of Psychiatry, 173,* 344–361. https://doi.org/10.1176/appi.ajp.2015.15060710

Wildes, J. E., Emery, R. E., & Simons, A. D. (2001). The roles of ethnicity and culture in the development of eating disturbance and body dissatisfaction: A meta-analytic review. *Clinical Psychology Review, 21,* 521–551.

Wilding, J. P. H., Batterham, R. L., Davies, M., Van Gaal, L. F., Kandler, K., Konakli, K., et al., & STEP 1 Study Group (2022). Weight regain and cardiometabolic effects after withdrawal of semaglutide: The STEP 1 trial extension. *Diabetes, Obesity & Metabolism, 24*(8), 1553–1564. https://doi.org/10.1111/dom.14725

Wilfley, D. E., Welch, R. R, Stein, R. I., Spurrell, E. B., Cohen, L. R., Saelens, B. E., et al. (2002). A randomized comparison of group cognitive-behavioral therapy and group interpersonal psychotherapy for the treatment of overweight individuals with binge eating disorder. *Archives of General Psychiatry, 59,* 713–721.

Wilhelm, S., Buhlmann, U., Hayward, L. C., Greenberg, J. L., & Dimaite, R. (2010). A cognitive-behavioral treatment approach for body dysmorphic disorder. *Cognitive and Behavioral Practice, 17,* 241–247.

Wilkinson, R. G., & Pickett, K. (2018). *The inner level: How more equal societies reduce stress, restore sanity and improve everyone's wellbeing.* Penguin Random House.

Wilkinson, S. T., Ballard, E. D., Bloch, M. H., Mathew, S. J., Murrough, J. W., Feder, A., et al. (2018). The effect of a single dose of intravenous ketamine on suicidal ideation: A systematic review and individual participant data meta-analysis. *American Journal of Psychiatry, 175*(2), 150–158. https://doi.org/10.1176/appi.ajp.2017.17040472

Wilkop, M., Wade, T. D., Keegan, E., & Cohen-Woods, S. (2023). Impairments among DSM-5 eating disorders: A systematic review and multilevel meta-analysis. *Clinical Psychology Review, 101,* 102267.

Williams, A. M., Galovski, T. E., & Resick P.A. (2019). Cognitive processing therapy. In B. A. Moore & W. E. Penk (Eds.), *Treating PTSD in military personnel: A clinical handbook* (pp. 63–77). The Guilford Press.

Williams, L. M. (2017). Defining biotypes for depression and anxiety based on large-scale circuit dysfunction: A theoretical review of the evidence and future directions for clinical translation. *Depression and Anxiety, 34*(1), 9–24. https://doi.org/10.1002/da.22556

Williams, L. M., Brown, K. J., Palmer, D., Liddell, B. J., Kemp, A. H., Olivieri, G., et al. (2006). The mellow years? Neural basis of improving emotional stability over age. *The Journal of Neuroscience, 26,* 6422–6430. https://doi.org/10.1523/jneurosci.0022-06.2006

Williamson, V., Creswell, C., Fearon, P., Hiller, R. M., Walker, J., & Halligan, S. L. (2017). The role of parenting behaviors in childhood post-traumatic stress disorder: A meta-analytic review. *Clinical Psychology Review, 53,* 1–13.

Wilson, A. J., & Stein, D. J. (2019). Pharmacological treatment of anxiety disorders. In S. M. Evans & K. M. Carpenter (Eds.), *APA handbooks in psychology® series. APA handbook of psychopharmacology* (pp. 195–215). American Psychological Association. https://doi.org/10.1037/0000133-009

Wilson, D. (2011, April 13). As generics near, makers tweak erectile drugs. *New York Times,* p. B11.

Wilson, G. T. (1995). Psychological treatment of binge eating and bulimia nervosa. *Journal of Mental Health (UK), 4,* 451–457.

Wilson, G. T. (2018). Cognitive-behavioral therapy for eating disorders. In W. S. Agras & A. Robinson (Eds.), *The Oxford handbook of eating disorders* (2nd ed.). Oxford University Press.

Wilson, G. T., Wilfley, D. E., Agras, W. S., & Bryson, S. W. (2010). Psychological treatments of binge eating disorder. *Archives of General Psychiatry, 67,* 94–101.

Wilson, G. T., & Zandberg, L. J. (2012). Cognitive -behavioral guided self-help for eating disorders: Effectiveness and scalability. *Clinical Psychology Review, 32,* 343–357.

Wilson, R. S., Scherr, P. A., Schneider, J. A., Tang, Y., & Bennett, D. A. (2007). Relation of cognitive activity to risk of developing Alzheimer's disease. *Neurology, 69,* 1191–1920.

Wilson, S., Stroud, C. B., & Durbin, C. E. (2017). Interpersonal dysfunction in personality disorders: A meta-analytic review. *Psychological Bulletin, 143,* 677–734. https://doi.org/10.1037/bul0000101

Wincze, J. P., Steketee, G., & Frost, R. O. (2007). Categorization in compulsive hoarding. *Behaviour Research and Therapy, 45,* 63–72.

Wincze, J. P., & Weisberg, R. B. (2015). *Sexual dysfunction, third edition: A guide for assessment and treatment.* Guilford Publications.

Wingfield, N., Kelly, N., Serdar, K., Shivy, V. A., & Mazzeo, S. E. (2011). College students' perceptions of individuals with anorexia and bulimia nervosa. *International Journal of Eating Disorders, 44,* 369–375.

Winsper, C., Bilgin, A., Thompson, A., Marwaha, S., Chanen, A. M., Singh, S. P., Wang, A., & Furtado, V. (2019). The prevalence of personality disorders in the community: A global systematic review and meta-analysis. *Cambridge.Org.* https://doi.org/10.1192/bjp.2019.166

Wirshing, D. W., Wirshing, W. C., Marder, S. R., Liberman, R. P., & Mintz, J. (1998). Informed consent: Assessment of comprehension. *American Journal of Psychiatry, 155,* 1508–1511.

Wismeijer, A. A. J., & van Assen, M. A. L. M. (2013). Psychological characteristics of BDSM practitioners. *Journal of Sexual Medicine, 10*(8), 1943–1952. https://doi.org/10.1111/jsm.12192

Witkiewitz, K., & Marlatt, G. A. (2004). Relapse prevention for alcohol and drug problems: That was Zen, this is Tao. *American Psychologist, 59,* 224–235.

Wittchen, H. U., Gloster, A. T., Beesdo-Baum, K., Fava, G. A., & Craske, M. G. (2010). Agoraphobia: A review of the diagnostic classificatory position and criteria. *Depression and Anxiety, 27,* 113–133.

Wittchen, H. U., & Jacobi, F. (2005). Size and burden of mental disorders in Europe—A critical review and appraisal of 27 studies. *European Neuropsychopharmacology, 15,* 357–376.

Witthöft, M., Gropalis, M., & Weck, F. (2018). Somatic symptom and related disorders. In J. H. Butcher & J. M. Hooley (Eds.), *APA handbook of psychopathology: Understanding, assessing, and treating adult mental disorders* (Vol. 1, pp. 531–556). American Psychological Association. https://doi.org/10.1037/0000064-022

Witthoft, M., & Rubin, G. J. (2013). Are media warnings about the adverse health effects of modern life self-fulfilling? An experimental study on idiopathic environmental intolerance attributed to electromagnetic fields (IEI-EMF). *Journal of Psychosomatic Research, 74,* 206–212. https://doi.org/10.1016/j.jpsychores.2012.12.002

Wodarczyk, A., Cubaa, W. J., Gauszko-Węgielnik, M., & Szarmach, J. (2021). Dissociative symptoms with intravenous ketamine in treatment-resistant depression exploratory observational study. *Medicine, 100*(29), E26769. https://doi.org/10.1097/MD.0000000000026769

Wolitzky, D. (1995). Traditional psychoanalytic psychotherapy. In A. S. Gurman & S. B. Messer (Eds.), *Essential psychotherapies: Theory and practice.* Guilford Press.

Wolitzky-Taylor, K. B., Horowitz, J. D., Powers, M. B., & Telch, M. J. (2008). Psychological approaches in the treatment of specific phobias: A meta-analysis. *Clinical Psychology Review, 28,* 1021–1037.

Wonderlich, S. A., Gordon, K. H., Mitchell, J. E., Crosby, R. D., Engel, S. G., & Walsh, B. T. (2009). The validity and clinical utility of binge eating disorder. *International Journal of Eating Disorders, 42,* 687–705.

Wong, Q. J. J., & Rapee, R. M. (2016). The aetiology and maintenance of social anxiety disorder: A synthesis of complimentary theoretical models and formulation of a new integrated model. *Journal of Affective Disorders, 203,* 84–100.

Woodberry, K. A., Giuliano, A. J., & Seidman, L. J. (2008). Premorbid IQ in schizophrenia: A meta-analytic review. *American Journal of Psychiatry, 165,* 579–587.

Woodmansee, M. A. (1996). The guilty but mentally ill verdict: Political expediency at the expense of moral principle. *Notre Dame Journal of Law, Ethics and Public Policy,* 10, 341–387.

Woods, S. W., Addington, J., Cadenhead, K. S., Cannon, T. D., Cornblatt, B. A., Heinssen, R., et al. (2009). Validity of the prodromal risk syndrome for first psychosis: Findings from the North American Prodrome Longitudinal Study. *Schizophrenia Bulletin, 35,* 894–908. https://doi.org/10.1093/schbul/sbp027

Woody, S. R., Lenkic, P., Bratiotis, C., Kysow, K., Luu, M., Edsell-Vetter, J., et al. (2020). How well do hoarding research samples represent cases that rise to community attention? *Behaviour Research and Therapy, 126.* https://doi.org/10.1016/j.brat.2020.103555

Woo, J. S., Brotto, L. A., & Gorzalka, B. B. (2011). The role of sex guilt in the relationship between culture and women's sexual desire. *Archives of Sexual Behavior, 40,* 385–394.

World Health Organization. (2015). Global health observatory data repository: Human resources data by country. https://apps.who.int/gho/data/view.main.MHHR

World Health Organization (2018). Adverse Childhood Experiences International Questionnaire. In Adverse Childhood Experiences International Questionnaire (ACE-IQ). [website]: Geneva: WHO.

World Health Organization. (2018). *International classification of diseases for mortality and morbidity statistics* (11th revision). https://icd.who.int/browse11/l-m/en

World Health Organization. (2019). *WHO guidelines on risk reduction for cognitive decline and dementia.* World Health Organization.

World Health Organization. (2020). Obesity and overweight fact sheet. https://www.who.int/news-room/fact-sheets/detail/obesity-and-overweight

World Health Organization (WHO). (2021). Suicide worldwide in 2019: Global health estimates. *World Health Organization, Geneva,* Licence: CC BY-NC-SA 3.0 IGO. https://apps.who.int/iris/rest/bitstreams/1350975/retrieve

Worthington, M. A., Miklowitz, D. J., O'Brien, M., Addington, J., Bearden, C. E., Cadenhead, K. S., et al. (2020). Selection for psychosocial treatment for youth at clinical high risk for psychosis based on the North American Prodrome Longitudinal Study individualized risk calculator. *Early Intervention in Psychiatry, 15*(1), 96–103. Advance online publication. https://doi.org/10.1111/eip.12914

Wouda, J. C., Hartman, P. M., Bakker, R. M., Bakker, J. O., van de Wiel, H. B. M., & Schultz, W. C. (1998). Vaginal plethysmography in women with dyspareunia. *Journal of Sex Research, 35,* 141–147.

Wright, A. G., Calabrese, W. R., Rudick, M. M., Yam, W. H., Zelazny, K., Williams, T. F., Rotterman, J. H., & Simms, L. J. (2015). Stability of the DSM-5 Section III pathological personality traits and their longitudinal associations with psychosocial functioning in personality disordered individuals. *Journal of abnormal psychology, 124*(1), 199–207.

Wright, A. G. C., Krueger, R. F., Hobbs, M. J., Markon, K. E., Eaton, N. R., & Slade, T. (2013). The structure of psychopathology: Toward an expanded quantitative empirical model. *Journal of Abnormal Psychology, 122*(1), 281–294. https://doi.org/10.1037/a0030133

Wright, A. G. C., Krueger, R. F., Hobbs, M. J., Markon, K. E., Eaton, N. R., & Slade, T. (2013). The structure of psychopathology: Toward an expanded quantitative empirical model. *Journal of Abnormal Psychology, 122*(1), 281–294. https://doi.org/10.1037/a0030133

Wu, H., Siafis, S., Hamza, T., Schneider-Thoma, J., Davis, J. M., Salanti, G., et al. (2022). Antipsychotic-induced weight gain: Dose-response meta-analysis of randomized controlled trials. *Schizophrenia Bulletin, 48*(3), 643–654.

Wykes, T., Steel, C., Everitt, T., & Tarrier, N. (2008). Cognitive behavior therapy for schizophrenia: Effect sizes, clinical models, and methodological rigor. *Schizophrenia Bulletin, 34,* 523–537.

Xia, J., Merinder, L. B., & Belgamwar, M. R. (2011). Psychoeducation for schizophrenia. *Schizophrenia Bulletin, 37,* 21–22.

Xiang, X., Wu, S., Zuverink, A., Tomasino, K. N., An, R., & Himle, J. A. (2020). Internet-delivered cognitive behavioral therapies for late-life depressive symptoms: a systematic review and meta-analysis. *Aging & Mental Health, 24*(8), 1196–1206. https://doi.org/10.1080/13607863.2019.1590309

Yaffe, K., Fiocco, A. J., Lindquist, K., Vittinghoff, E., Simonsick, E. M., Newman, A. B., et al. (2009). Predictors of maintaining cognitive function in older adults. *Neurology, 72,* 2029–2035.

Yancey, J. R., Venables, N. C., & Patrick, C. J. (2016). Psychoneurometric operationalization of threat sensitivity: Relations with clinical symptom and physiological response criteria. *Psychophysiology, 53*(3), 393–405. https://doi.org/10.1111/psyp.12512

Yang, F., Fang, X., Tang, W., Hui, L., Chen, Y., Zhang, C., et al. (2019). Effects and potential mechanisms of transcranial direct current stimulation (tDCS) on auditory hallucinations: A meta-analysis. *Psychiatry Research, 273,* 343–349.

Yang, X., Huang, J., Zhu, C., Wang, Y., Cheung, E. F. C., Chan, R. C. K., et al. (2014). Motivational deficits in effort-based decision making in individuals with subsyndromal depression, first-episode and remitted depression patients. *Psychiatry Research, 220*(3), 874–882. https://doi.org/10.1016/j.psychres.2014.08.056

Yap, M. B. H., & Jorm, A. F. (2015). Parental factors associated with childhood anxiety, depression, and internalizing problems: A systematic review and meta-analysis. *Journal of Affective Disorders, 175,* 424–440.

Yarns, B. C. (2018). Psychotherapy. In *Psychiatric disorders late in life* (pp. 297–306). Springer International Publishing. https://doi.org/10.1007/978-3-319-73078-3_27

Yerkes, R. M., & Dodson, J. D. (1908). The relation of strength of stimulus to rapidity of habit formation. *Journal of Comparative and Neurological Psychology, 18,* 459–482.

Yilmaz, Z., Hardaway, J. A., & Bulik, C. M. (2015). Genetics and epigenetics of eating disorders. *Advances in Genomics and Genetics, 5,* 131–150. https://doi.org/10.2147/AGG.S55776

Yilmaz, Z., Zai, C. C., Hwang, R., Mann, S., Arenovich, T., Remington, G., et al. (2012). Antipsychotics, dopamine D2 receptor occupancy and clinical improvement in schizophrenia: A meta-analysis. *Schizophrenia Research, 140,* 214–220.

Yoon, S., Kim, T. D., Kim, J., & Lyoo, I. K. (2021). Altered functional activity in bipolar disorder: A comprehensive review from a large-scale network perspective. *Brain and Behavior, 11*(1). https://doi.org/10.1002/brb3.1953

Young, E. S., Farrell, A. K., Carlson, E. A., Englund, M. M., Miller, G. E., Gunnar, M. R., et al. (2019). The dual impact of early and concurrent life stress on adults' diurnal cortisol patterns: A prospective study. *Psychological Science, 30*(5), 739–747. https://doi.org/10.1177/0956797619833664

Younglove, J. A., & Vitello, C. J. (2003). Community notification provisions of "Megan's Law" from a therapeutic jurisprudence perspective: A case study. *American Journal of Forensic Psychology, 21,* 25–38.

Yu, J., Zhou, P., Yuan, S., Wu, Y., Wang, C., Zhang, N., et al. (2022). Symptom provocation in obsessive–compulsive disorder: A voxel-based meta-analysis and meta-analytic connectivity modeling. *Journal of Psychiatric Research, 146*, 125–134. https://doi.org/10.1016/j.jpsychires.2021.12.029

Yung, A. R., McGorry, P. D., McFarlane, C. A., & Patton, G. (1995). The PACE Clinic: Development of a clinical service for young people at high risk of psychosis. *Australian Psychiatry, 3*, 345–349.

Yung, A. R., Phillips, L. J., Hok, P. Y., & McGorry, P. D. (2004). Risk factors for psychosis in an ultra high-risk group: Psychopathology and clinical features. *Schizophrenia Research, 67*, 131–142.

Yung, A. R., Woods, S. W., Ruhrmann, S., Addington, J., Schultze-Lutter, F., Cornblatt, B. A., et al. (2012). Whither the attenuated psychosis syndrome? *Schizophrenia Bulletin, 38*, 1130–1134.

Yu, S., Galimov, A., Sussman, S., Jeong, G. C., & Shin, S. R. (2019). Three-month effects of Project EX: A smoking intervention pilot program with Korean adolescents. *Addictive Behaviors Reports, 9*, 100152.

Zanarini, M. C., Frankenburg, F. R., Reich, D. B., & Fitzmaurice, G. M. (2012). Attainment and stability of sustained symptomatic remission and recovery among patients with borderline personality disorder and axis II comparison subjects: A 16-year prospective follow-up study. *American Journal of Psychiatry, 169*(5), 476–483. https://doi.org/10.1176/appi.ajp.2011.11101550

Zanarini, M. C., Skodol, A. E., Bender, D., Dolan, R., Sanislow, C., Schaefer, E., et al. (2000). The Collaborative Longitudinal Personality Disorders Study: Reliability of axis I and II diagnoses. *Journal of Personality Disorders, 14*, 291–299.

Zanelli, J., Mollon, J., Sandin, S., Morgan, C., Dazzan, P., et al. (2019). Cognitive change in schizophrenia and other psychoses in the decade following the first episode. *American Journal of Psychiatry, 176*, 811–819.

Zane, M. D. (1984). Psychoanalysis and contextual analysis of phobias. *Journal of the American Academy of Psychoanalysis, 12*, 553–568.

Zanov, M. V., & Davison, G. C. (2010). A conceptual and empirical review of 25 years of cognitive assessment using the Articulated Thoughts in Simulated Situations (ATSS) think-aloud paradigm. *Cognitive Therapy and Research, 34*, 282–291.

Zapf, P. A., & Roesch, R. (2011). Future directions in the restoration of competency to stand trial. *Current Directions in Psychological Science, 20*(1), 43–47.

Zareian, B., & Klonsky, E. D. (2020). Connectedness and suicide. In A. C. Page & W. G. K. Stritzke (Eds.), *Alternatives to suicide: Beyond risk and toward a life worth living* (Chapter 7, pp. 135–158). Academic Press. https://doi.org/10.1016/B978-0-12-814297-4.00007-8

Zarit, S. H., & Zarit, J. M. (2011). *Mental disorders in older adults: Fundamentals of assessment and treatment* (2nd ed.). Guilford Press.

Zeigler-Hill, V., Vrabel, J. K., McCabe, G. A., Cosby, C. A., Traeder, C. K., Hobbs, K. A., & Southard, A. C. (2019). Narcissism and the pursuit of status. *Journal of Personality, 87*(2), 310–327. https://doi.org/10.1111/jopy.12392

Zellers, S., Ross, J., Saunders, G., Ellingson, J., Walvig, T., Anderson, J., et al. (2023). Recreational cannabis legalization has had limited effects on a wide range of adult psychiatric and psychosocial outcomes. *Psychological Medicine*, 1–10. https://doi.org/10.1017/S0033291722003762

Zhang, T. Y., & Meaney, M. J. (2010). Epigenetics and the environmental regulation of the genome and its function. *Annual Review of Psychology, 61*, 439–466.

Zhao, J., Stockwell, T., Naimi, T., Churchill, S., Clay, J., & Sherk, A. (2023). Association between daily alcohol intake and risk of all-cause mortality: A systematic review and meta-analyses. *JAMA Network Open, 6*(3), e236185–e236185.

Zhao, J., Stockwell, T., Roemer, A., Naimi, T., & Chikritzhs, T. (2017). Alcohol consumption and mortality from coronary heart disease: An updated meta-analysis of cohort studies. *Journal of Studies on Alcohol and Drugs, 78*(3), 375–386. https://doi.org/10.15288/jsad.2017.78.375

Zheng, H., Sussman, S., Chen, X., Wang, Y. Xia, J., Gong, J., et al. (2004). Project EX—A teen smoking cessation initial study in Wuhan, China. *Addictive Behaviors, 29*, 1725–1733.

Zhou, J., & Seeley, W. W. (2014). Network dysfunction in Alzheimer's disease and frontotemporal dementia: Implications for psychiatry. *Biological Psychiatry, 75*, 565–573.

Zhukovsky, P., Wainberg, M., Milic, M., Tripathy, S. J., Mulsant, B. H., Felsky, D., et al. (2022). Multiscale neural signatures of major depressive, anxiety, and stress-related disorders. *Proceedings of the National Academy of Sciences, 119*(23). https://doi.org/10.1073/pnas.2204433119

Zimmerman, M., & Mattia, J. I. (1999). Differences between clinical and research practices in diagnosing borderline personality disorder. *American Journal of Psychiatry, 156*, 1570–1574.

Zimmerman, M., Rothschild, L., & Chelminski, I. (2005). The prevalence of DSM-IV personality disorders in psychiatric outpatients. *The American journal of psychiatry, 162*(10), 1911–1918. https://doi.org/10.1176/appi.ajp.162.10.1911

Zimmermann, K., Walz, C., Derckx, R. T., Kendrick, K. M., Weber, B., Dore, B., et al. (2017). Emotion regulation deficits in regular marijuana users. *Human Brain Mapping, 38*, 4270–4279. https://doi.org/10.1002/hbm.23671

Zinbarg, R. E., Mineka, S., Bobova, L., Craske, M. G., Vrshek-Schallhorn, S., Griffith, J. W., et al. (2016). Testing a hierarchical model of neuroticism and its cognitive facets: Latent structure and prospective prediction of first onsets of anxiety and unipolar mood disorders during 3 years in late adolescence. *Clinical Psychological Science, 4*(5), 805–824. https://doi.org/10.1177/2167702615618162

Zinbarg, R. E., Mineka, S., Bobova, L., Craske, M. G., Vrshek-Schallhorn, S., Griffith, J. W., et al. (2016). Testing a hierarchical model of neuroticism and its cognitive facets: Latent structure and prospective prediction of first onsets of anxiety and unipolar mood disorders during 3 years in late adolescence. *Clinical Psychological Science, 4*(5), 805–824. https://doi.org/10.1177/2167702615618162

Zinzow, H. M., & Thompson, M. (2015). Factors associated with use of verbally coercive, incapacitated, and forcible sexual assault tactics in a longitudinal study of college men. *Aggressive Behavior, 41*, 34–43. https://doi.org/10.1002/ab.21567

Zmigrod, L., Garrison, J. R., Carr, J., & Simons, J. S. (2016). The neural mechanisms of hallucinations: A quantitative meta-analysis of neuroimaging studies. *Neuroscience & Biobehavioral Reviews, 69*, 113–123.

Zohar, A. H., & Felz, L. (2001). Ritualistic behavior in young children. *Journal of Abnormal Child Psychology, 29*, 121–128.

Zuckerbrot, R. A., Cheung, A., Jensen, P. S., Stein, R. E. K., Laraque, D.; GLAD-PC Steering Group (2018). Guidelines for Adolescent Depression in Primary Care (GLAD-PC): Part I: Practice preparation, identification, assessment, and initial management. *Pediatrics, 141*(3), e20174081.

Zucker, K. J. (2005). Gender identity disorder in children and adolescents. *Annual Review of Clinical Psychology, 1*, 467–492. https://doi.org/10.1146/annurev.clinpsy.1.102803.144050

Subject Index